SEVENTH EDITION

Fitness Professional's Handbook

Edward T. Howley, PhD
Dixie L. Thompson, PhD
University of Tennessee, Knoxville
Editors

HUMAN KINETICS

Library of Congress Cataloging-in-Publication Data

Names: Howley, Edward T., 1943- , author. | Thompson, Dixie L., 1960- , author.
Title: Fitness professional's handbook / Edward T. Howley, Dixie L. Thompson.
Description: Seventh edition. | Champaign, IL : Human Kinetics, [2017] | Includes bibliographical references and index.
Identifiers: LCCN 2016000215 | ISBN 9781492523376 (print)
Subjects: | MESH: Exercise--physiology | Physical Fitness--physiology | Health Behavior | Exercise Therapy | Nutritional Physiological Phenomena
Classification: LCC GV481 | NLM QT 256 | DDC 613.7--dc23 LC record available at http://lccn.loc.gov/2016000215

ISBN: 978-1-4925-2337-6 (print)

The web addresses cited in this text were current as of May 2016, unless otherwise noted.

Senior Acquisitions Editor: Amy N. Tocco; **Developmental Editor:** Judy Park; **Senior Managing Editor:** Carly S. O'Connor; **Copyeditor:** Alisha Jeddeloh; **Indexer:** Susan Danzi Hernandez; **Permissions Manager:** Dalene Reeder; **Senior Graphic Designer:** Keri Evans; **Cover Designer:** Keith Blomberg; **Photograph (cover):** LuckyBusiness/Getty Images; **Photographer (interior):** Neil Bernstein, unless otherwise noted; **Photographs (interior):** © Human Kinetics, unless otherwise noted; **Photo Asset Manager:** Laura Fitch; **Visual Production Assistant:** Joyce Brumfield; **Photo Production Manager:** Jason Allen; **Senior Art Manager:** Kelly Hendren; **Illustrations:** © Human Kinetics, unless otherwise noted; **Printer:** Walsworth

We thank the University of Tennessee, Knoxville, for assistance in providing the location for the photo shoot for this book.

Printed in the United States of America 10 9 8 7 6 5 4 3 2 1

The paper in this book was manufactured using responsible forestry methods.

Human Kinetics
Website: www.HumanKinetics.com

United States: Human Kinetics
P.O. Box 5076
Champaign, IL 61825-5076
800-747-4457
e-mail: info@hkusa.com

Canada: Human Kinetics
475 Devonshire Road Unit 100
Windsor, ON N8Y 2L5
800-465-7301 (in Canada only)
e-mail: info@hkcanada.com

Europe: Human Kinetics
107 Bradford Road
Stanningley
Leeds LS28 6AT, United Kingdom
+44 (0) 113 255 5665
e-mail: hk@hkeurope.com

Australia: Human Kinetics
57A Price Avenue
Lower Mitcham, South Australia 5062
08 8372 0999
e-mail: info@hkaustralia.com

New Zealand: Human Kinetics
P.O. Box 80
Mitcham Shopping Centre, South Australia 5062
0800 222 062
e-mail: info@hknewzealand.com

E6716

To Ann, for her love and support, and to my children and grandchildren who show us that the future is bright.

—Ed Howley

To my parents, Jean and Felton Thompson, for their unwavering love and support.

—Dixie Thompson

CONTENTS

PREFACE

You are in the right place at the right time. Now more than ever, there is a pressing need for most people to increase their physical activity level. In every community, both private (e.g., fund-raising groups for cancer prevention) and government agencies (e.g., health departments, public schools) promote the integration of regular physical activity into our day-to-day routines. There is no question that regular physical activity and structured exercise are good for us—the evidence is overwhelming. The fitness professional is well suited to help individuals, as well as whole communities, make activity-related choices that will improve health and wellness. This text will help you learn the basics that fitness professionals need. You will learn how to screen participants for exercise programs, evaluate the various fitness components, and prescribe exercise to improve each fitness component. In addition, you will learn how to help people with chronic disease (e.g., hypertension) and specific conditions (e.g., pregnancy). Recent advances in how to approach these issues demanded a revision of the text, and we hope you enjoy the result.

Updates to the Seventh Edition

At regular intervals, both professional societies, such as the American College of Sports Medicine (ACSM), and government agencies, such as the Centers for Disease Control and Prevention (CDC), update physical activity recommendations for the general public and for special segments of the population such as older adults and people with chronic diseases. We have used the latest and best information throughout this text to bring you up-to-date information that will help you help others. While the new edition of *ACSM's Guidelines for Exercise Testing and Prescription* is due to be published in 2017, we have been graciously granted an advance copy in order to provide you with the most current recommendations. Throughout this book we've made updates as needed per 10th edition ACSM updates, but where recommendations stand you'll see us reference the 9th edition as well.

Given the aging of the population and the chronic diseases that accompany it, the development of the Exercise is Medicine program by ACSM will be of interest to many readers, whether they are pursuing a career in fitness, allied health, or medicine. If you are an undergraduate student, you have many career options. Regardless of whether you pursue a career in the fitness industry or in an allied health field, you will find the information in this textbook valuable as you build your professional skill set. The Exercise is Medicine program emphasizes the importance of communication between professionals in medicine and allied health with those in the fitness arena when patients are discharged. This textbook will help that conversation along by giving you a sound foundation on which to prescribe exercise and deliver physical activity and fitness programs for various populations.

In this edition of the text, every chapter has been updated based on the latest standards, guidelines, and research, be they related to special populations or low-back pain (LBP) and injury prevention. Here is a snapshot of the major changes made for each chapter:

- Chapter 1, Health, Fitness, and Performance, provides an introduction to the FITT (frequency, intensity, time, and type of exercise) principle for exercise prescription. It updates the leading causes of death, introduces the debate about whether we should focus more on changing sedentary behavior or on changing physical activity, and expands the section on sport performance as a lead-in to a new chapter dealing with that topic.
- Chapter 2, Health Risk Appraisal, includes the revised Physical Activity Readiness Questionnaire for Everyone (PAR-Q+) that provides a more streamlined screening process. Also, the new American College of Sports Medicine's preparticipation health screening process is described in detail.
- Chapter 3, Functional Anatomy and Biomechanics, includes a reorganization of the information on bones and joints, muscle groups, and exercise tips by region of the body to simplify the review of this material. In addition, muscle involvement in selected activities has been combined with common mechanical errors to emphasize interrelationships between them.
- Chapter 4, Exercise Physiology, presents new information on the consequences of exercise-induced muscle damage (rhabdomyolysis), the stroke volume (SV) response of elite endurance athletes to exercise, and the criteria for achieving maximal oxygen uptake.

- Chapter 5, Nutrition, provides updated information on the 2015-2020 Dietary Guidelines for Americans.
- Chapter 6, Energy Costs of Physical Activity, adds new focus on how to generate realistic estimates of the calories a client expends during exercise. Information on devices used to track physical activity and estimate energy expenditure (e.g., accelerometers) has been updated, and the role of body weight in energy expenditure during exercise has been expanded.
- Chapter 7, Assessment of Cardiorespiratory Fitness, provides updates on the Canadian Aerobic Fitness Test (CAFT) and the Progressive Aerobic Cardiovascular Endurance Run (PACER).
- Chapter 8, Assessment of Body Composition, includes more graphics to help the reader visualize skinfold measurement sites.
- Chapter 9, Assessment of Muscular Fitness, includes expanded information on testing protocols (e.g., familiarization, RM testing), new research insights, and updated ACSM recommendations for healthy people and clients with cardiovascular disease (CVD).
- Chapter 10, Assessment of Flexibility and Low-Back Function, introduces a variety of new concepts, including relative flexibility and the role of lumbopelvic rhythm in back function. New testing tools used to assess range of motion (ROM) and muscle length in both a clinical and fitness setting have been added. An expanded discussion on how to interpret the results of spine and hip flexion (hamstring) tests has been included.
- Chapter 11, Exercise Prescription for Cardiorespiratory Fitness, weaves the FITT principle into the discussion of the exercise dose associated with health outcomes. The importance of progression in an exercise prescription has been expanded, and examples of walk and run programs using a progression-based approach have been added.
- Chapter 12, Exercise Prescription for Weight Management, provides updated obesity statistics.
- Chapter 13, Exercise Prescription for Muscular Fitness, includes an expanded section on the health-related benefits of resistance training. Research updates have been added, along with new ACSM recommendations on resistance training.
- Chapter 14, Exercise Prescription for Flexibility and Low-Back Function, expands the discussion of spinal stability, including the roles of the active, passive, and neural systems and the contrast between local and global stabilizing systems. The most recent research on the importance of the neutral spine position for safe exercise and the optimal ways to activate the deep abdominal layers for core strengthening has been added. Current recommendations for stretching exercises for the spine and extremities are described, including pictures of typical exercises. Finally, new research on the role of Pilates, yoga, tai chi, and aquatic exercise for flexibility is presented.
- Chapter 15, Training for Performance, is a new chapter that discusses the application of training principles to improve athletic performance. Topics include training to improve performance during aerobic, sprint, and explosive power events. In addition, concurrent strength and endurance training and high-intensity interval training (HIIT) are discussed. Tips and examples for designing workouts and training programs are also included.
- Chapter 16, Exercise for Children and Youth, provides an update to the Fitnessgram and summarizes the midcourse report for the Physical Activity Guidelines for Americans as they relate to children and youth.
- Chapter 17, Exercise and Older Adults, expands the discussion on the influence of exercise on changes in cardiorespiratory fitness (CRF) and muscle mass with age. Additional detail on balance exercises has been added.
- Chapter 18, Exercise and Women's Health, incorporates the most recent recommendations for exercise during pregnancy.
- Chapter 19, Exercise and Heart Disease, updates statistics on CVD and CHD with the latest information from the American Heart Association. The discussion of how atherosclerosis develops and progresses has been extensively revised, and the discussion of peripheral artery disease (PAD) has been expanded. Finally, common medications for CVD have been added.
- Chapter 20, Exercise and Obesity, includes updated statistics on adult and childhood obesity and includes information on the latest FDA-approved drugs for weight loss.
- Chapter 21, Exercise and Diabetes, provides the latest information on how exercise can be helpful in the management of this common metabolic disease.
- Chapter 22, Exercise and Pulmonary Disease, updates the statistics on the prevalence of chronic obstructive pulmonary disease (COPD), asthma, bronchitis, and emphysema, as well as the list of medications used to treat pulmonary disease. Finally, the section dealing with the classification

of the severity of COPD has been updated with current guidelines.

- Chapter 23, Behavior Change, expands the emphasis on both the transtheoretical model of behavior change and self-determination theory (SDT). Examples and strategies for using SDT to facilitate behavior change and enhance motivation for physical activity have been added. New information on time management as a strategy for behavior change and on the role of weight bias and its effects on practitioners and clients has been included.
- Chapter 24, ECG and Exercise Performance, adds new illustrations to simplify the discussion of how electrical activity moves across and through the heart. The distinction between cardiac arrest and heart attack has been clarified, and additional detail on the risks associated with atrial fibrillation has been added.
- Chapter 25, Injury Prevention and Treatment, provides detailed information on the development of emergency action plans (EAP). New information on delayed-onset muscle soreness (DOMS), exertional rhabdomyolysis, community-associated methicillin-resistant *Staphylococcus aureus* (CA-MRSA), sickle cell trait (SCT), and traumatic brain injury (TBI) has been included.
- Chapter 26, Legal Considerations, provides updates on injury data and a more detailed description of the professional standard of care. New sections on scope of practice and the professional standard of care associated with HIIT programs have been added. Finally, new case law examples on risk management have been included.

Although many updates have been made, former users of the text will be comfortable with this new edition. The text continues to use *ACSM's Guidelines for Exercise Testing and Prescription* as a primary source of standards and expectations for fitness professionals. This has been and remains the standard-setting reference for professionals delivering fitness programs in any setting, whether in health clubs or hospitals. Consequently, the text is helpful to those interested in taking ACSM certification exams as well as exams offered by other organizations.

In addition, we have included study questions at the end of each chapter to help students review for regular examinations. This edition also includes many reproducible forms, interesting sidebars, useful key points, case study questions and answers, key terms and a glossary, and extensive references, making it a useful textbook for students as well as a valuable reference for practitioners.

Intended Audience

This text continues to be written for the upper-level undergraduate or beginning graduate student with a general background in anatomy and physiology. The purpose of the text is to enable people with limited knowledge of fitness testing and prescription to screen participants, carry out standardized fitness tests to evaluate the major components of fitness, and write appropriate exercise prescriptions. Many academic programs incorporate laboratory experiences to drive the mastery of skills needed to accomplish these tasks. In that way, the class is not simply an academic experience but one that allows a person to move into practicum or internship experiences with the requisite skills and abilities. This text will work seamlessly with most laboratory experiences associated with fitness assessment because of its attention to detail regarding the most common fitness tests, from pretest concerns to posttest evaluation of results.

Text Organization

Part I, Physical Activity: Links to Health, Fitness, and Performance, contains two chapters that provide an overview of the connections among health, fitness, and performance; general information to set up the remainder of the text; and a step-by-step approach to screening participants for fitness programs.

Part II, Scientific Foundations, covers basic anatomy, biomechanics, and exercise physiology, useful for a quick review. In addition, chapters are provided on nutrition assessment and how to evaluate the caloric cost of activity, both of which are central to energy balance.

Part III, Fitness Assessment, provides extensive detail on how to assess CRF, body composition, flexibility, and muscular strength and endurance.

Part IV, Exercise Prescription for Health, Fitness, and Performance, provides a separate chapter on how to deal with the test results for each of the fitness components assessed in part III, and it describes how to formulate an exercise prescription consistent with a client's goals and abilities. A new chapter, Training for Performance, has been added to this section to address the needs of people with performance-related goals.

Part V, Special Populations, provides chapters on exercise testing and prescription for the following: children and youth, older adults, women, and people with heart disease, obesity, diabetes, or pulmonary disease.

Part VI, Comprehensive Exercise Program Considerations, leads off with a chapter on scientific approaches to changing behavior, exercise electrocardiograms (ECGs), injury prevention and treatment, and legal considerations.

Special Features in the Seventh Edition

There are many items in the textbook that will help you identify and retain key information.

- **Objectives** quickly outline the main points of the chapter and highlight the learning goals for the topics covered.
- **Key Points** summarize important facts.
- **Glossary terms** are highlighted throughout the text, giving students a quick reference to terms as they are introduced. Full definitions are provided in the glossary at the end of the book.
- **Research Insight** boxes cover important research topics for each chapter. Additional highlight boxes on special topics and tips can be found in each chapter as well.
- **Procedures** for common fitness tests are highlighted so that they are easy to find and use.
- **Review Questions** covering important material are included at the end of every chapter.
- **Case Studies** let readers to practice the concepts covered in the chapter.
- **Answers to Case Studies** are provided so that readers can quickly check their work.
- **Video** icons let readers know when a demonstration is available on a topic. Here is what the video icon looks like:

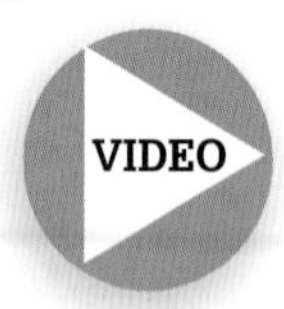

- **References** are numbered and organized by chapter at the end of the book. These resources will help the reader discover additional sources of information.

Web Resource

A valuable feature of this text for students is the web resource, which includes 24 video clips that correspond to key techniques covered in the book. (Note: You must have an Internet connection in order to view this streaming video content.) The web resource also includes fillable and printable versions of many forms found in the text, as well as periodically updated references from the authors. For more information, see Accessing the Web Resource.

Instructor Resources

In addition to the thoroughly updated content, this edition also offers several instructor resources to aid in teaching a class with this textbook:

- The updated **instructor guide** includes a syllabus; course outlines that detail lecture topics and lab and classroom activities; initial and final practical exams, including checklists for easy grading; and a laboratory notebook that students can use to track their completion of 12 fitness assessment and programming activities.
- The **test package** includes more than 650 questions, including true-or-false, fill-in-the-blank, multiple-choice, short-answer, and essay questions. The questions have been updated to reflect the new content added to the text.
- The Microsoft PowerPoint **presentation package** contains over 700 slides that present the textbook material in a lecture-friendly format, including art, photos, and tables pulled from the text.
- The **image bank** contains most of the art, tables, content photos, and reproducible forms from the text. Instructors may print the reproducible forms and use the art, tables, and photos to create class presentations.
- New to the seventh edition are **chapter quizzes**. These ready-made quizzes are learning management system (LMS) compatible and can be used to measure student learning of the most important concepts for each chapter. They include over 350 unique questions in multiple-choice, fill-in-the-blank, essay, short-answer, and true-or-false formats.

We hope that this book is helpful to you, whether you are using it as a textbook or as a resource to help you stay up to date.

ACCESSING THE WEB RESOURCE

Throughout *Fitness Professional's Handbook, Seventh Edition,* you will notice references to a web resource and online video. The web resource offers fillable and printable forms from the book along with video clips demonstrating concepts and fitness tests presented in the chapters.

The web resource can be accessed by visiting www.HumanKinetics.com/FitnessProfessionalsHandbook. If you purchased a new print book, follow the directions included on the orange-framed page at the front of your book. That page includes access steps and the unique key code that you'll need the first time you visit the *Fitness Professional's Handbook* website. If you purchased an e-book from HumanKinetics.com, follow the access instructions that were e-mailed to you following your purchase.

When a demonstration is available on a topic, you will see a video icon that looks like this:

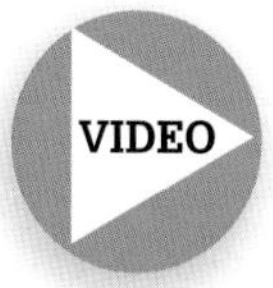

To view the videos, go to www.HumanKinetics.com/FitnessProfessionalsHandbook and select Web Resource in the ancillary items box in the upper left corner of the screen. You'll then see a page with options for accessing either the forms or the videos. Click the videos button and then select the link for the chapter's videos you want to watch. The video numbers along the right side of the player correspond with video number cross-references in the book, and the title under the player corresponds with the exercise or procedure title in the book. Scroll through the list of clips until you find the video you want to watch. Select that clip and the full video will play.

To access the forms, click on the forms button. Here is a list of the forms available in the web resource:

Form 2.2 Exercise Preparticipation Health Status Questionnaire (HSQ)

Form 2.3 Sample Medical Clearance Form

Form 5.1 Sample Food Log

Form 7.1 Pretest Instructions for a Fitness Test

Appendix 7.1 Consent Form

Form 13.1 Weekly Resistance Training Log

Form 23.1 Behavioral Contract

Form 25.1 Sample Emergency Action Plan

ACKNOWLEDGMENTS

We have been blessed with wonderful authors over the many editions of this textbook. It was a pleasure to work with them to organize and present, in a user-friendly way, crucial information to help fitness professionals move forward in their careers. We would like to recognize and thank the following for their contributions to previous editions:

Sue Carver, ATC, MPT, CMT
Ralph La Forge, MS
Jean Lewis, EdD (deceased)
Wendell Liemohn, PhD
Kyle McInnis, ScD

Physical Activity: Links to Health, Fitness, and Performance

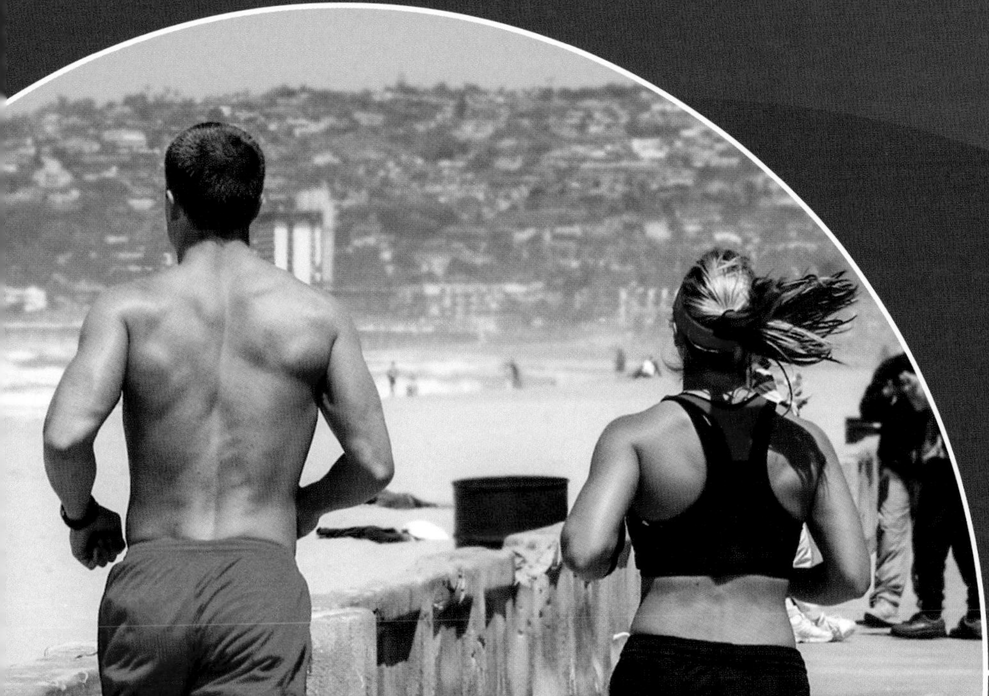

Galina Barskaya/fotolia.com

PART I

Physical activity is an essential element in health and well-being. With that in mind, we wrote this book for current and future fitness professionals who help individuals, communities, and groups gain the benefits of regular physical activity in a positive and safe environment.

The chapters of part I provide the background underlying the study of physical activity and its relevance to fitness. In chapter 1, we summarize the current evidence regarding physical activity and health, and we provide insights into the connections among health, fitness, and performance. In chapter 2 we provide a process for screening potential fitness participants and recommend criteria for medical referrals and the development of supervised and unsupervised programs.

1

Health, Fitness, and Performance

Edward T. Howley

OBJECTIVES

The reader will be able to do the following:

1. Contrast the physical activity requirements for achieving health benefits, fitness, and performance.
2. Contrast the top three leading causes of death with the top three behavioral factors that lead to early death.
3. Describe the difference between absolute and relative intensity for physical activity.
4. Explain the difference between moderate-intensity and vigorous-intensity physical activity, and how volume of physical activity is calculated.
5. List the health-related benefits gained through regular participation in physical activity and exercise.
6. Contrast the changes in physical activity guidelines over the past 40 years in terms of exercise volume, intensity, and outcomes.
7. Describe the *2008 Physical Activity Guidelines for Americans* recommendations for moderate-intensity and vigorous-intensity physical activity for realizing substantial health benefits.
8. Describe the physical activity guidelines for increasing or maintaining strength.
9. Define *adverse events* and explain how the potential for such events affects the intensity of physical activity recommended for those who have been sedentary.
10. Explain why lack of physical activity and low levels of fitness are more important to address than being overweight as far as the risk of chronic disease is concerned.
11. Describe the difference between health-related fitness and performance-related fitness.
12. Describe the continuum of physical activity recommendations for realizing health, fitness, and performance goals.

1

One of the main questions we address throughout this text is "How much exercise is enough?" In order to answer that question, we must first address another: "Enough for what?" In other words, what is your client's goal? Is it fitness, **performance**, or avoidance of disease? Exercise recommendations usually describe the frequency (number of days per week), **intensity** (strenuousness of the activity), and duration (time) you should be active in each session. As figure 1.1 shows, the frequency (F), intensity (I), time (T), and type (T) of activity vary depending on the goal. On the left side of the figure, we see that avoidance of disease (e.g., lowering the risk of heart disease, type 2 diabetes, and so on) can be achieved with moderate-intensity activity done 30 min per day, 5 days per wk. To achieve **cardiorespiratory fitness (CRF)**, as well as the health benefits associated with moderate-intensity physical activity, vigorous (hard) exercise is done 3 to 4 days per wk, 30 to 45 min per day, which is equivalent to jogging or running about 3 mi (5 km) 3 to 4 days per wk. What about those who want to be elite marathon runners? In contrast to the previous two examples, elite marathon runners work at the extreme end of the intensity scale (very hard) for hours every day. Few elite marathoners run less than 100 mi (161 km) per week (12), which is about 10 times what is needed to achieve a reasonable level of CRF.

We begin with this example because this text focuses on the amount of physical activity and exercise needed for health and fitness rather than on the performance of elite athletes. That said, the information on nutrition, CRF, body composition, strength, and flexibility forms the foundation for those who want to achieve performance-related goals, and chapter 15 focuses on the topic of training for performance. In this chapter we discuss how physical activity is connected to health, fitness, and performance. Later chapters provide more extensive detail about how to help sedentary people become active, active people become fit, and fit people realize performance-related goals.

Health and Avoidance of Disease

What does being healthy mean? For some it is the simple avoidance of disease, but it is also more than that. **Health** has long been defined as a "state of complete physical, mental, and social well-being and not merely the absence of disease or infirmity" (42). **Positive health** is associated with our capacity to enjoy life and withstand challenges. **Negative health** is associated with morbidity (incidence of disease) and premature mortality (38). The highest quality of life includes mental alertness and curiosity, positive emotional feelings, meaningful relationships with others, awareness and involvement in societal strivings, recognition of the broader forces of life, and the physical capacity to accomplish personal goals with vigor. Although physical activity plays a major role in the physical dimension, it also contributes to learning, relationships, and a sense of our limitations when confronting environmental challenges. An optimal quality of life requires us to strive, grow, and develop, though we may never achieve the highest level of positive health. So, what are the risks or challenges to our health and well-being?

Factors Affecting Health and Disease

The leading causes of death describe the specific diseases linked to dying. In 2011, the top five leading causes of death were heart disease (23.7%), malignant neoplasms (cancers) (22.9%), chronic lower respiratory diseases (5.7%), cerebrovascular diseases (stroke) (5.1%), and accidents (unintentional injuries) (4.8%) (21). Although infectious diseases are not in the top five, we are advised each year to make sure that our flu shots and other vaccinations are up to date in order to prevent a problem from occurring or to reduce the impact of the disease when it

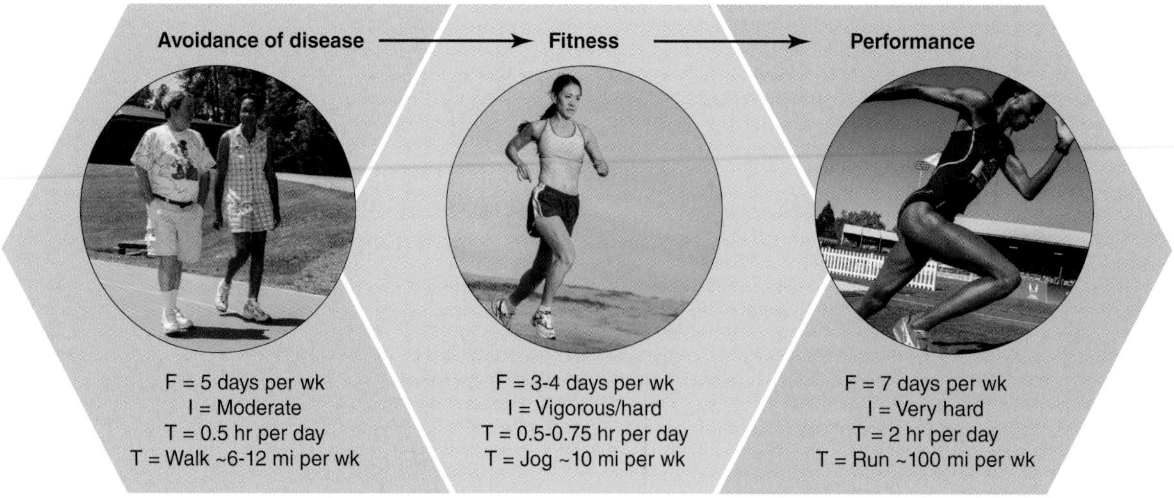
Avoidance of disease
Fitness
Performance
F = 5 days per wk
I = Moderate
T = 0.5 hr per day
T = Walk ~6-12 mi per wk
F = 3-4 days per wk
I = Vigorous/hard
T = 0.5-0.75 hr per day
T = Jog ~10 mi per wk
F = 7 days per wk
I = Very hard
T = 2 hr per day
T = Run ~100 mi per wk

FIGURE 1.1 How much physical activity is enough?

occurs. Most of the top five leading causes of death are chronic degenerative diseases whose onset can be delayed or prevented. Risk factors associated with chronic diseases can be divided into three categories (see figure 1.2) (41).

Inherited or Biological Factors

These factors include the following:

- Age—older adults have more chronic diseases than younger people.
- Sex—men develop cardiovascular disease (CVD) at an earlier age than women, but women experience more strokes than men (6).
- Race—African Americans develop about 30% more heart disease than non-Hispanic white Americans (39).
- Susceptibility to disease—several diseases have a genetic component that increases the potential for having them.

People can achieve health and fitness goals up to their genetic potential, but it is not possible to establish the relative portion of a person's health that is determined by heredity. Although heredity influences physical activity, fitness, and health (31), most people can lead healthy or unhealthy lives regardless of their genetic makeup. Thus, genetic background neither dooms a person to poor health nor guarantees good health.

Environment

We are born not only with fixed genetic potentials but also into environments that affect our development. An environment includes physical factors (e.g., climate, water, altitude, pollution), socioeconomic factors (e.g., income, housing, education, workplace), and family (e.g., parental values, divorce, extended family, friends) that affect our opportunities to be active, our levels of fitness, and our health statuses. Some elements, such as our nutrition or the air we breathe and water we drink, affect us directly. Other elements, such as the values and behaviors of people we admire, influence us indirectly. When working with clients, it is important to understand many aspects of their past and current circumstances in order to help them make lifestyle changes.

Behaviors

Whereas the leading causes of death describe the diseases that are killing us, the *actual causes* of death describe behaviors that are linked to those diseases (see the right side of figure 1.2). That smoking is at the top of the list should be no surprise given its connection to both lung cancer and CVD. In fact, it is the number one actual cause of death, accounting for 18% of all deaths (26, 27). The existence of smoking-cessation programs and laws restricting areas where people can smoke speak to the seriousness with which our society takes that risk to health. The number two actual cause of death is poor diet and physical inactivity (15.2%), with alcohol consumption coming in at number three (3.5%). The emphasis on healthy eating at work and school and the creation of new parks and bike trails to enhance opportunities to be physically active are examples of responses to these actual causes of death. Figure 1.3 shows that healthy eating and physical activity affect a large number of factors that influence health and disease. Clearly, your ability to help your clients establish and reinforce the behaviors of healthy eating and physical activity will do much to improve their health and well-being. (See chapter 5 for information on nutrition and chapter 23 for steps to help clients change their behaviors.) This chapter introduces the role that physical activity and fitness play in a healthy lifestyle. However, before we begin, we need to review a few terms that will be important in the following sections of this chapter.

Important Definitions

We will introduce you to key terms as we move through the chapters of the text; however, we need to begin here in order to facilitate your understanding of the various parts of an exercise prescription or physical activity recommendation (10, 37, 38).

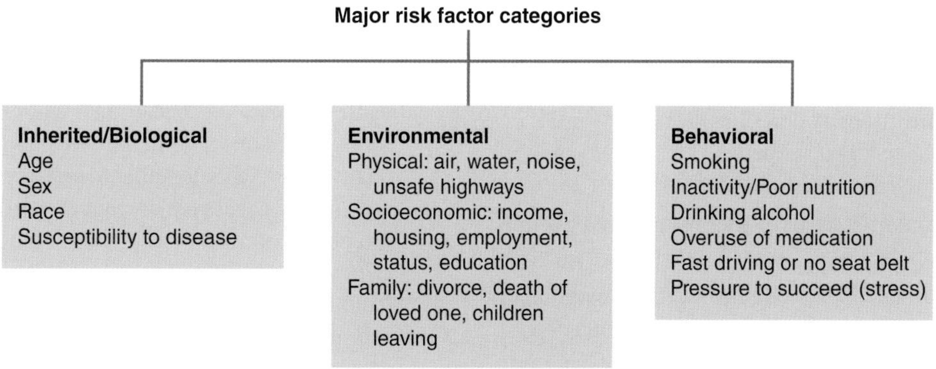

FIGURE 1.2 Major categories of risk factors with examples of each.
Adapted from Healthy People, 1979, *The Surgeon General's report on health promotion and disease prevention.*

HE	Health benefits	PA
✓	Lowers risk for heart disease	✓
✓	Reduces risk for certain cancers	✓
✓	Lowers blood pressure	✓
✓	Improves lipid profile	✓
✓	Prevents obesity	✓
✓	Prevents diabetes	✓
✓	Builds healthy bones	✓
✓	Enhances immune function	✓
?	Relieves stress, improves mood, promotes self-esteem	✓
X	Increases functional health	✓

FIGURE 1.3 Effect of healthy eating (HE) and physical activity (PA) on health benefits.

Reprinted, by permission, from R.A. Carpenter.

- **Physical activity** is defined as any bodily movement produced by skeletal muscle that results in energy expenditure. It is associated with occupation, leisure time, household chores, and sport.
- **Exercise** is a subset of physical activity that is planned, structured, and repetitive and has the objective of improving or maintaining physical fitness.
- **Physical fitness** refers to a set of health- or skill-related attributes that can be measured by specific tests.
- **Health-related fitness** refers to muscular strength and endurance, CRF, flexibility, and body composition (relative leanness).
- **Skill-related (performance-related) fitness** refers to agility, balance, coordination, speed, power, and reaction time that are linked to games, sport, dance, and so on.
- **Absolute intensity** describes the rate of work (i.e., how much energy is expended per minute) and can be expressed in a number of ways:
  - Kilocalories (kcal) of energy produced per min ($kcal \cdot min^{-1}$)
  - Milliliters of oxygen consumed per kilogram of body weight per minute ($ml \cdot kg^{-1} \cdot min^{-1}$)
  - Metabolic equivalents (METs), where 1 MET is taken as resting metabolic rate (RMR) and is equal to 3.5 $ml \cdot kg^{-1} \cdot min^{-1}$; exercise intensity is given as a multiple of the MET (e.g., 3 METs, 6 METs)
- **Relative intensity** describes the degree of effort required to expend energy and is influenced by CRF or maximal aerobic power ($\dot{V}O_2max$). A person with a CRF of 10 METs who is working at 6 METs is at a relative intensity of 60% $\dot{V}O_2max$ (6 METs ÷ 10 METs × 100%). You will see more on this in chapter 11.
- **Moderate intensity** refers to an absolute intensity of 3 to 5.9 METs and a relative intensity of 40% to 59% $\dot{V}O_2max$.
- **Vigorous intensity** refers to an absolute intensity of 6 or more METs and a relative intensity of 60% to 84% $\dot{V}O_2max$.
- **Frequency** refers to the number of days per week physical activity is done.
- **Duration** refers to the amount of time a physical activity is done.
- **Volume** refers to the total amount of energy expended or work accomplished in an activity, and it is equal to the product of the absolute intensity, frequency, and time. For example, a person expending 5 $kcal \cdot min^{-1}$ for 20 min on 3 days per wk will have an exercise volume of 300 $kcal \cdot wk^{-1}$ (5 $kcal \cdot min^{-1}$ × 20 min per day × 3 days per wk). The volume can also be expressed using the MET scale: A 10 MET activity done 3 days per wk for 20 min per day generates a volume of 600 $MET\text{-}min \cdot wk^{-1}$ (10 METs × 3 days per wk × 20 min per day).

Physical Activity and Health

From the beginning of recorded history, philosophers and health professionals have observed that regular physical activity is an essential part of a healthy life. Hippocrates wrote the following in *On Regimen in Acute Diseases,* about 400 BC:

> Eating alone will not keep a man [woman] well; he [she] must also take exercise. For food and exercise, while possessing opposite qualities, yet work together to produce health. . . . And it is necessary, as it appears, to discern the power of various exercises, both natural exercises and artificial, to know which of them tends to increase flesh and which to lessen it; and not only this, but also to proportion exercise to bulk of food, to the constitution of the patient, to the age of the individual . . . (23)

Over the past four decades, thousands of studies have examined the relationship between physical activity and the risk of various diseases and death. The overwhelming conclusion is that regular participation in physical activity results in a reduced risk of numerous diseases and of death from all causes. As shown in figure 1.4, regular participation in physical activity reduces the risk of death from all causes by about 40% (relative risk decreased from 1.0 to 0.6). Doing physical activity on a regular basis also has been shown to have a similar impact on the following (37):

- Cardiorespiratory health: Physical activity reduces the risk of heart disease and stroke, lowers blood pressure (BP), improves the blood lipid profile, and increases CRF.
- Metabolic health: Physical activity reduces the risk of developing type 2 diabetes and helps to control blood glucose in those who already have type 2 diabetes.
- Musculoskeletal health: Physical activity slows the loss of bone density that occurs with aging, and it lowers the risk of hip fractures. In addition, it improves pain management in people with arthritis. Finally, progressive muscle-strengthening activities increase or preserve muscle mass, strength, and power.
- Cancer: Physically active people have a significantly lower risk of colon cancer and breast cancer. In addition, there is some evidence that physical activity reduces the risk of endometrial cancer and lung cancer.
- Mental health: Physical activity lowers the risk of depression and age-related cognitive decline, and it improves the quality of sleep.

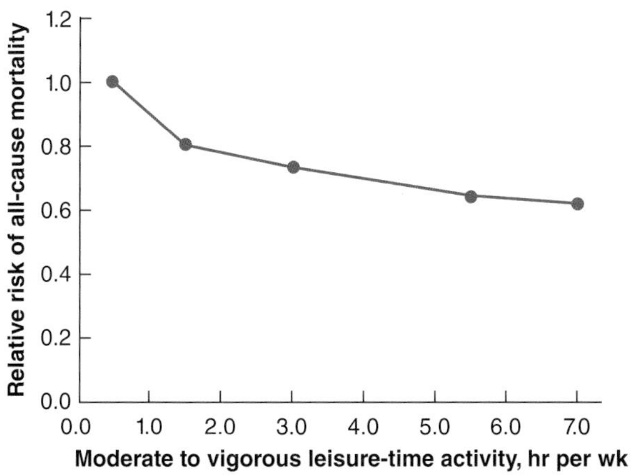

FIGURE 1.4 Dose–response of physical activity related to all-cause mortality.

Reprinted from U.S. Department of Health and Human Services, 2008, *Physical activity guidelines advisory report.*

- Functional ability and fall prevention: Physical activity reduces the risk of functional limitations (e.g., ability to do activities of daily living), and for those older adults at risk of falling, physical activity is safe and reduces this risk.

Physical Activity Guidelines

Given the large number of benefits derived from participation in physical activity, it should be no surprise that professional societies such as the American College of Sports Medicine (ACSM), the American Heart Association (AHA), and various governmental agencies (e.g., Centers for Disease Control and Prevention [CDC]) have developed physical activity guidelines for the general public. The following paragraphs provide a brief overview showing how the focus of these guidelines shifted from fitness to public health outcomes and finally to obesity over the past 40 years.

Focus on Intensity

In the early and mid-1970s, three major organizations published guidelines or recommendations for improving fitness and health:

1. In 1972, the AHA published *Exercise Testing and Training of Apparently Healthy Individuals: A Handbook for Physicians* (5). The exercise prescription was to begin at a relative intensity of 60% $\dot{V}O_2$max for 15 to 20 min, 3 days per wk.
2. In 1973, the YMCA published it first edition of *The Y's Way to Physical Fitness* (16). The exercise prescription was to exercise at 80% $\dot{V}O_2$max for 40 to 45 min, 3 days per wk.
3. In 1975, ACSM published the first edition of *ACSM's Guidelines for Exercise Testing and Prescription* (1). The exercise prescription was to exercise at ~70% to 90% $\dot{V}O_2$max for 20 to 45 min, 3 to 5 days per wk.

In each case the focus was on higher-intensity exercise, with both CRF and health outcomes being important.

Focus on Volume

In 1978, ACSM published its first position stand (2): "The Recommended Quantity and Quality of Exercise for Developing and Maintaining Fitness in Healthy Adults." The focus was on improving CRF as well as achieving health outcomes. The emphasis was again on higher-intensity exercise to achieve these goals. However, in that same year, a now classic study on Harvard alumni by Paffenbarger, Wing, and Hyde (29) showed a 36% lower risk of developing a heart attack in those who accumulated

2,000 kilocalories or more of leisure-time physical activity per week (that did not have to be done at a high intensity). This study and many that followed shifted the focus to three variables associated with physical activity guidelines:

- Activity volume (e.g., kilocalories expended) rather than intensity
- Health outcomes (e.g., reduced risk of heart attack) rather than CRF
- Leisure-time activity rather than structured exercise programs

Throughout the 1980s there was a growing body of research showing a strong relationship between regular participation in physical activity and a lower risk of chronic disease. It became clear that we needed to rethink our understanding of how physical activity and exercise were linked to a reduced risk of chronic disease (8-10). Dr. William Haskell took a leadership role in helping us to understand the potential links among physical activity, fitness, and health (18, 19). Figure 1.5 shows the following:

- In our earliest understanding, we thought that physical activity improved fitness, which, in turn, was linked to improved health outcomes (figure 1.5*a*).
- However, it was just as likely that physical activity could improve health and fitness separately and by different mechanisms (figure 1.5*b*).
- Lastly, some physical activity programs could improve fitness and not health outcomes, and vice versa (figure 1.5*c*).

These distinctions helped shape our understanding of how physical activity is connected to fitness and health outcomes—that is, physical activity could achieve health outcomes independent of fitness.

One of the most important decisions that accelerated the drive to promote physical activity in a public health context occurred in 1992, when the AHA made physical inactivity a major risk factor for CVD, the same as smoking, high BP, and high serum cholesterol (15). Following up on that important decision, in 1995 the ACSM and CDC published their public health physical activity recommendation to reduce the risk of chronic disease (30): "Every U.S. adult should accumulate 30 min or more of moderate-intensity physical activity on most, preferably all, days of the week." The shift in focus was clearly spelled out, with exercise volume (total kilocalories expended) being crucial and somewhat independent of intensity (as long as it was equal to or higher than moderate intensity). It is important to remember that this was a minimum recommendation (*at least* 30 min, 5 times per wk) for realizing health benefits. In the following year, the U.S. Surgeon General's report on physical activity and health was published (36). This document supported the 1995 ACSM and CDC statement and brought even more attention to the need for Americans to become physically active. The emphasis on physical activity from a public health perspective also was incorporated into subsequent editions of *ACSM's Guidelines for Exercise Testing and Prescription.*

Focus on Weight

The United States and many other industrialized countries have seen an incredible increase in the prevalence of overweight and obesity over the last 20 years. In the United States, 34.9% of adults are obese, and the combined overweight and obesity prevalence is 68.5% (28). The increase in obesity during the 1990s prompted the Institute of Medicine (IOM) to evaluate the research on how much physical activity was needed to prevent weight

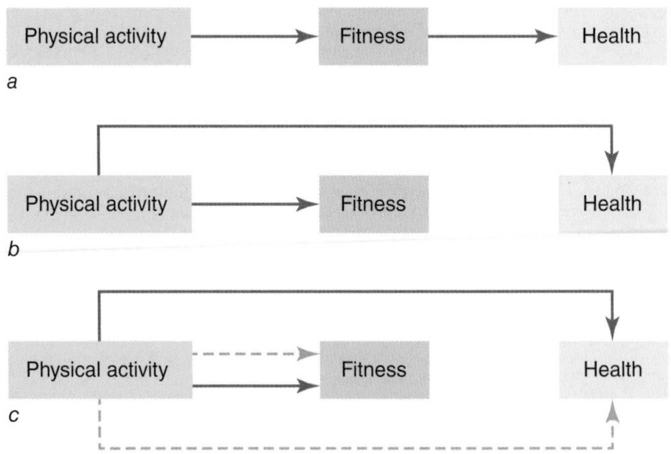

FIGURE 1.5 Possible causal relations among physical activity, physical fitness, and health. Original models *(a)* assumed that health gains due to physical activity were dependent on improved fitness, but a later model *(b)* proposed that physical activity can improve both health and fitness separately, and probably by different mechanisms. Consistent with *(b)*, the last model *(c)* suggests that some physical activity programs can improve one and not the other.

gain (22). The IOM recommended 60 min of moderate-intensity activity to prevent weight gain and achieve the full health benefits of physical activity, twice the amount that ACSM and the CDC recommended for reducing the risk of chronic diseases. This was supported by recommendations from the International Association for the Study of Obesity (IASO) to do 45 to 60 min of physical activity to prevent weight gain (33) and the International Obesity Task Force (IOTF) recommendation of 60 to 90 min of activity to prevent weight regain in those who have lost a great deal of weight (13). In 2005, the *Dietary Guidelines for Americans* endorsed the ACSM and CDC recommendation of 30 min of physical activity to reduce the risk of chronic diseases, the IOM recommendation of 60 min to prevent weight gain, and the IOTF recommendation of 60 to 90 min to sustain weight loss (40).

Current Physical Activity Guidelines

As you can imagine, there was confusion among both fitness professionals and the general public about how much activity was enough. Which was it—30, 60, or 90 min? Was moderate-intensity activity the only way to achieve these various goals? In 2007, ACSM and the AHA published an updated position stand on physical activity and health that addressed some of these questions (20):

- Moderate or vigorous: The position stand supported the 1995 minimum recommendation of 30 min of moderate-intensity activity 5 days per wk for reducing the risk of chronic disease. However, one could do 20 min of vigorous-intensity activity 3 days per wk to achieve the same goal or do some combination of both.
- More is better: Doing more than the minimum (e.g., doing 60 min of moderate-intensity activity 5 days per wk) increases health benefits.

This brief historical tour through physical activity recommendations shows how guidelines change as we learn more about the effects of physical activity. The review also provides a jumping-off point for a comprehensive series of recommendations that affects much of what is presented in this text. In 2008, the U.S. Department of Health and Human Services (HHS) published Physical Activity Guidelines for Americans—the first set of national physical activity recommendations related to health and fitness (37). This document was based on an extensive review of the literature that was carried out by an advisory committee (38). These guidelines provide physical activity recommendations for children and adolescents, adults, older adults (65 yr and older), women during and following pregnancy, people with disabilities, and people with chronic medical conditions. You will read more about the specific guidelines for each of these populations as you

RESEARCH INSIGHT

Should We Focus on Physical Activity or Sedentary Behavior?

There is no question that we spend a great deal of time sitting, be it at work, in a car, or in front of the TV or computer. Over the past decade, investigators have pointed to a link between sedentary behavior and increased risk of chronic diseases—even in people who meet the physical activity guidelines! These investigators examined the relationship between hours of sedentary behavior and chronic disease while controlling for the amount of moderate and vigorous physical activity done by the participants. This relationship has been puzzling because it suggests that there is some biological mechanism associated with being sedentary (other than not being active) that is linked to a higher risk of these diseases.

A recent study has provided new insights into this issue. Maher et al. (25) examined the relationship between 11 biomarkers for chronic disease (e.g., BP, fasting blood glucose, HDL [high-density lipoprotein] cholesterol) and time spent in sedentary behavior. When the investigators controlled for the amount of moderate-intensity and vigorous-intensity physical activity (as had been done in previous studies), they found (as in previous studies) that sedentary behavior was linked to 8 out of the 11 the biomarkers. However, when they controlled for the total physical activity done by the participants (light + moderate + vigorous), almost all of the biomarker links to sedentary behavior disappeared. This strongly suggests that because previous investigations did not consider light activity in their analyses, they drew erroneous conclusions. Further, it indicates that light physical activity has health benefits, which is important given that a large fraction of total physical activity done by many segments of the population, such as older adults, is classified as light. Lastly, while we certainly want to encourage people to reduce time spent in sedentary behaviors, our focus should be on promoting physical activity, be it of a light, moderate, or vigorous intensity.

move through the textbook; however, the following findings from the advisory committee's report are provided to help prepare you for what is ahead (38):

- Substantial health-related benefits occur at a volume of activity in the range of 500 to 1,000 MET-min · wk^{-1}. If you did a brisk walk at a moderate intensity of 3.5 METs for 150 min, you would meet the low end of that range (3.5 METs · 150 min · wk^{-1} = 525 MET-min · wk^{-1}). Another person could do vigorous activity at 7 METs for half that time and accomplish the same volume of activity. One min of vigorous-intensity physical activity is equal to 2 min at a moderate intensity. This is important because moderate-intensity activity accommodates the fitness levels of most individuals, and a fit person who can do vigorous-intensity activity can accomplish the recommended volume in a shorter time.
- Many health outcomes follow a dose–response relationship with physical activity, meaning that, in general, more is better (see the later section on adverse events).
- For those who cannot meet the lower end of the guideline, it is recommended that they be as active as they can; some activity is better than none.
- The health-related benefits of physical activity are independent of body weight, so overweight and obese adults should engage in a program of regular physical activity regardless of whether weight is being lost.

Strength Training

In the previous discussion, little was said about muscle-strengthening activities because the vast majority of studies examining the relationship between physical activity and chronic disease measured only aerobic activity. That said, ACSM has recommended exercises to enhance muscular strength and endurance since their 1990 position stand (3), and that has remained the case since then. As you might expect, the *2008 Physical Activity Guidelines for Americans* also provides guidelines for improving muscular strength and endurance. Recommendations include the following (20, 37):

- Do 8 to 10 exercises for the major muscle groups: legs, hips, back, chest, shoulders, and arms.
- To maximize strength development, use a resistance that allows 8 to 12 repetitions (number of times each lift is done in 1 set) of each exercise, at which point fatigue is experienced.
- One set of each exercise is sufficient, although more can be gained with 2 or 3 sets.
- Do resistance training on 2 or more nonconsecutive days each week.

There is no question that muscular strength and endurance activities provide benefits, including improvements in muscle mass, strength, and bone health (37). But there is also evidence that resistance training is associated with a lower risk of all-cause mortality, potentially linked to the role that increased muscle mass plays in glucose metabolism (20), as well as a lower risk of cancer mortality (32). Chapter 13 provides more details about the importance of resistance training in an exercise program to improve health and reduce the risk of chronic diseases (7).

Individuals need adequate muscular strength and endurance to be able to carry out activities of daily living (ADLs), do leisure activities (e.g., gardening, mowing, sport), and realize performance goals. An increase in muscle mass has implications beyond sport performance, because muscle mass determines to a large extent the number of calories expended per day (see chapter 12). This is tied to energy balance and the ability to maintain body weight as we age. In addition, adequate endurance of the muscles in the trunk (core) is important to reduce the risk of low-back pain (see chapter 14). As strength declines with aging, the ability of older adults to maintain an independent lifestyle is compromised (see chapter 17). The evaluation of muscular strength and endurance is discussed in chapter 9, and the design of programs to improve muscular strength and endurance is presented in chapter 13.

In spite of what we know about the effects of aerobic and resistance training on health and fitness, participation rates by adults over the age of 18 are not what they should be. However, results are more encouraging for aerobic activity than for resistance training. In 2011, 51.6% of American adults met the 2008 physical activity guidelines described earlier. In contrast, only 29.3% met the resistance training guidelines, and only 20.6% met both guidelines (17). We have our work cut out for us.

Adverse Events

In contrast to the many benefits of participating in physical activity, there is also the potential for an adverse outcome: an injury or medical complication (e.g., heart attack). Figure 1.6 captures factors that can increase the risk of injury associated with participation in physical activity. The risk is greater for older, less fit individuals who have little experience doing physical activity. The risk of musculoskeletal injuries increases with the amount of activity done (i.e., more risk for someone jogging 30 mi [48 km] a week compared with 10 mi [16 km] a week), as well as the amount of increase in physical activity, be it intensity or volume, when changing workouts. Participation in collision sports has a higher injury risk than participation in noncollision sports, and lastly, both equipment and environmental factors can contribute to injury risk. Cardiac events such as a heart attack or sudden death are rare, but the risk is higher when someone becomes more active

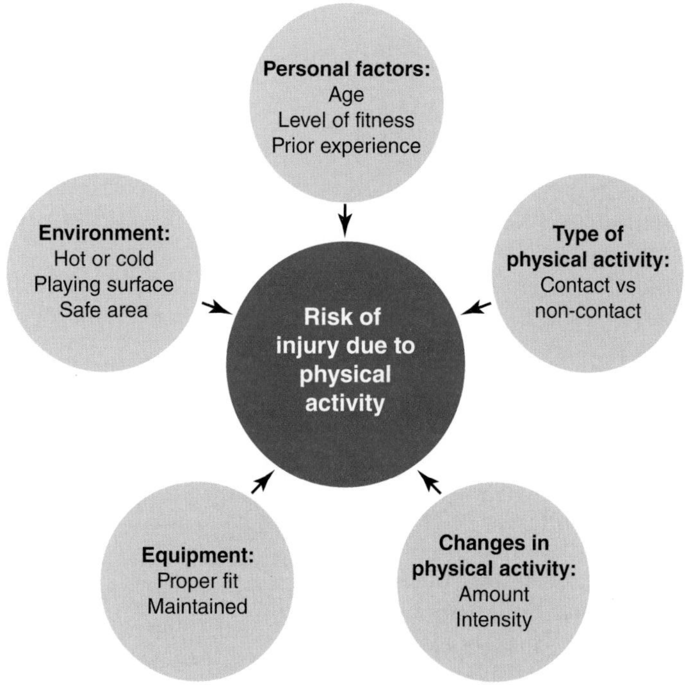
Personal factors:
Age
Level of fitness
Prior experience
Environment:
Hot or cold
Playing surface
Safe area
Type of physical activity:
Contact vs non-contact
Risk of injury due to physical activity
Equipment:
Proper fit
Maintained
Changes in physical activity:
Amount
Intensity

FIGURE 1.6 Factors affecting the risk of injury due to participation in physical activity.

than usual, emphasizing the need for a progressive introduction to physical activity (4). Figure 1.7 illustrates that although the risk of a cardiac event increases for an active person during exercise, the overall risk of cardiac arrest is considerably lower for the rest of the day compared with a sedentary person. The good news is that healthy people have a low risk of adverse events when participating in moderate-intensity physical activity such as brisk walking (38). To reduce the risks associated with exercise testing and participation in physical activity programs, you will learn how to

- screen individuals using health-risk questionnaires (chapter 2),
- measure important physiological variables at rest before taking exercise tests (chapters 7, 8, 9, 10), and
- gradually progress a sedentary person through a physical activity program (chapters 11, 13, 14).

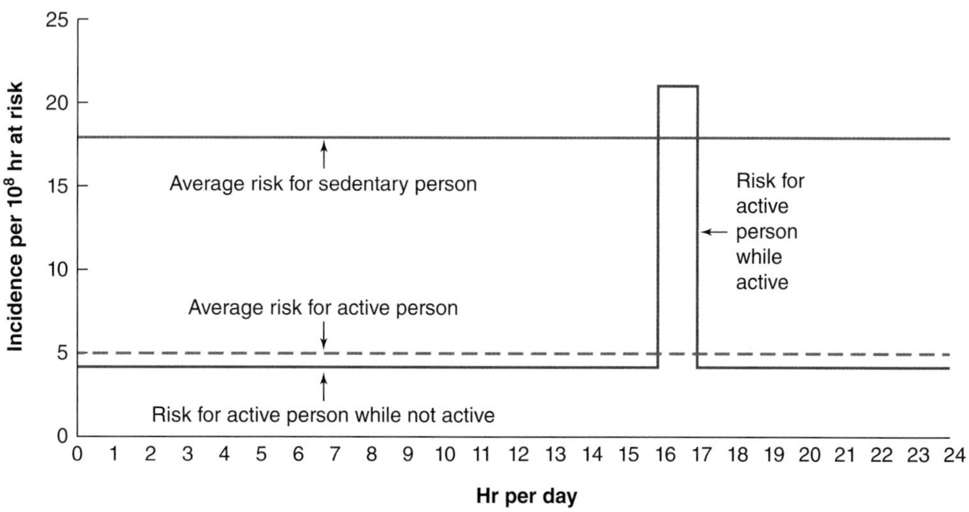

FIGURE 1.7 Activity-related cardiac risk. Strenuous activity is not recommended for a sedentary person and is not shown on this graph.

Reprinted from Office of Disease Prevention and Health Promotion, 2016, *Physical activity guidelines advisory committee report part G. Section 10: Adverse events.* Available: http://health.gov/paguidelines/report/G10_adverse.aspx#_Toc199768228

KEY POINT

Current physical activity guidelines recommend moderate-intensity or vigorous-intensity aerobic physical activity to realize substantial health benefits along with strengthening exercises to help maintain muscle mass and bone health. These recommendations have evolved as a result of a growing research base that shows beyond any doubt the substantial health benefits that can be realized through regular physical activity.

Fitness

Figure 1.1 presented health (avoidance of disease), fitness, and performance as three distinct goals, with a physical activity recommendation tied to each. It should be clear at this point, however, that health and fitness goals are not so much distinct as connected. They are two sides of the same coin—a coin that represents an investment in achieving health outcomes through regular participation in physical activity. As previously stated, health outcomes are realized by doing a minimum of

- 150 min per wk of moderate-intensity physical activity, or
- 75 min per wk of vigorous-intensity physical activity.

The vigorous-intensity recommendation is the traditional exercise prescription for increasing or maintaining CRF.

Intensity: Moderate Versus Vigorous

Are there any benefits to doing vigorous versus moderate physical activity? Swain and Franklin (35) addressed this question in a systematic review of the literature examining the relationship of physical activity to the incidence of **coronary heart disease (CHD)** and risk factors for CHD. In their review, it was important to control for the total energy expenditure associated with the physical activity in order to accurately compare the difference between moderate-intensity and vigorous-intensity activity (because for any duration of vigorous activity, more energy would be expended compared with moderate activity). Their findings follow.

- The vast majority of epidemiological studies found a greater reduction in the risk of CVD with vigorous-intensity (≥6 METs) than with moderate-intensity (3-5.9 METs) physical activity. In addition, more favorable risk-factor profiles were observed for people engaged in vigorous as opposed to moderate activity.
- Clinical intervention studies generally showed greater improvement in diastolic blood pressure (DBP), glucose control, and CRF after vigorous-intensity physical activity versus moderate-intensity activity. However, there was no intensity effect on improvements in systolic blood pressure (SBP), blood lipid profile, or body-fat loss.

Thus, although moderate-intensity physical activity was good, vigorous-intensity activity was better. In addition, one can obtain faster and larger gains in CRF with vigorous-intensity exercise programs (see chapter 11). However, as mentioned, fitness professionals must use good judgment when working with individual clients, recognizing that vigorous-intensity exercise is associated with more adverse events and that some clients may simply wish to stay with a successful moderate-intensity program that meets their needs rather than progress to a vigorous-intensity exercise program.

Fitness or Fatness: Which Is More Important?

Some investigators, notably Dr. Steven Blair and associates with the Aerobics Research Institute in Dallas, have used CRF as an index of physical activity, reasoning that more-active people would have higher levels of CRF. Many of the classic studies linking physical activity to various health outcomes have used this approach and have both confirmed and expanded on what we know from research that uses questionnaires or objective measures of physical activity (e.g., pedometers or accelerometers) to obtain information on the activity levels of individuals. The advantage of using CRF as a measure of physical activity is that it can be objectively determined using treadmill or cycle ergometer tests (see chapter 7), and it is easily tracked over time. Having information on CRF as a measure of physical activity also allows us to ask another question: Which is more important in terms of health status, having a higher level of physical activity or having a lower body fatness?

This is no small question given our attention to the obesity epidemic. As we will see in chapters 8, 12, and 20, obesity is linked to a variety of chronic diseases. However, from a health-promotion perspective, should we focus more on getting people to be physically active or on achieving a healthy body weight? Figure 1.8 is an example of the kind of data that allow one to separate the impact of fitness from fatness (11). In this study, investigators measured the CRF and body fatness of individuals with diabetes and then followed them over time to determine how many died from CVD. Those who had a high fitness score and were at a normal body weight were used as the reference group to compare with the others; this group was assigned a risk value of 1.0. As you can see, for the normal-weight group, those who had low fitness levels had about a fourfold greater risk of dying from CVD compared with those who had high fitness levels, indicating the importance of being fit. This was also true for the other weight classes. In contrast, as you look across the figure, moving from normal weight to overweight and then to obese had little impact on the risk of dying from CVD in this group of subjects. Similar observations have been made for a wide variety of health outcomes (14, 24, 34). In addition, recent work shows that a change in fitness, not fatness, is the best predictor of future health outcomes.

The message is clear: Being physically active provides substantial health benefits independent of body weight. This is consistent with a central theme of the Physical Activity Guidelines for Americans: Health-related benefits of physical activity occur in people of all body weights and whether one is gaining or losing weight. The primary focus, then, should be on getting people physically active so they can realize the health benefits and then deal with body weight as the physical activity program is being established. This is a powerful message to current and future fitness professionals.

Performance

The term *performance* means different things to different people. At its most basic level, it means being able to complete daily tasks efficiently; at a higher level, it speaks to an ability to engage successfully in sport-related performance.

Completing Daily Tasks

To get through the day efficiently, we must have fundamental motor skills that allow us to accomplish various tasks.

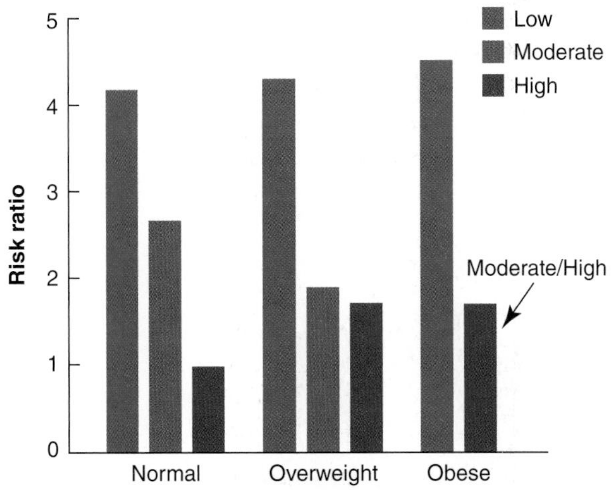

FIGURE 1.8 Effect of fitness (low, moderate, high) and fatness on the risk of death from CVD in men with diabetes.

Based on Church et al. 2005.

We must be able to move from place to place and push, pull, pick up, carry, and perform other tasks requiring the hands and arms. Moderate levels of **muscular strength** and **endurance**, **flexibility**, **body composition** or **relative leanness**, and CRF are essential for these routine tasks. Although successful daily living is important at all ages, it is a top priority for the elderly because it allows them to live independently. In addition, a person's lifestyle adds other needs. Contrast, for example, a computer programmer, a firefighter, and a parent staying at home with an infant. The computer programmer needs stretching and relaxation activities to prevent low-back and postural problems and can benefit from short activity breaks. The firefighter is sedentary for most of the time but must be able to respond quickly with near-maximal levels of anaerobic energy and muscular strength and endurance, all within an adverse environment with heavy equipment. Thus, this person must engage in regular vigorous aerobic, anaerobic, and resistance exercise to maintain the conditioning necessary to respond to emergencies. The parent needs flexibility, strength, and endurance to lift and carry the infant and other items through an obstacle course of toys, clothes, and so on (in addition to learning to perform these tasks under sleep deprivation). The term *functional fitness* has entered our vocabulary to describe fitness programming that uses a variety of exercises to simulate routine tasks rather than using traditional aerobic or resistance training exercises.

Achieving Desired Sport Performance

Some clients may want to engage in selected sports such as tennis, basketball, and golf or in high-performance endurance competitions such as triathlons, 100K bike races, or 10K runs. In addition to requiring good physical fitness, most of these activities require specific motor abilities—**agility**, **balance**, **coordination**, **power**, and **speed**—as well as the particular skills of the sport.

Clearly, high fitness levels are desirable as an athletic base, but individuals also have specific needs depending on their sport. Compare, for example, 10K runners, basketball

KEY POINT

Being physically fit (achieving appropriate levels of CRF, body composition, strength, and flexibility) is linked to a low risk of health problems and an improved ability to engage in daily tasks with adequate energy. A higher level of these fitness components is associated with sport performance, along with attention to the unique skills related to each sport or game.

players, and golfers. The runners rely on aerobic power that comes from distance running, with careful stretching before and after. Basketball players depend on aerobic and anaerobic energy, coordination, and specific passing, shooting, and defensive skills. Golfers require a moderate cardiorespiratory base, muscular power, and coordination of a complex skill used in a variety of settings (e.g., fairway, sand traps, woods). Although it is beyond the scope of this textbook to discuss performance across all sports and competitions, chapter 15 addresses the topic of training for performance to provide a connection between our focus on fitness and what is needed for performance. We direct the interested reader to the Human Kinetics website (www.humankinetics.com) for information on publications dealing with performance of a wide variety of sports.

Pulling It All Together

We end this chapter where we began, with the question of how much exercise is enough. At this point you know that the goals of health, fitness, and performance represent a continuum of outcomes that result from regular participation in physical activity and exercise (see figure 1.9). It is clear that participation in both moderate- and vigorous-intensity physical activity is associated with numerous substantial health benefits and improvement in the various fitness components of CRF, body fatness, flexibility, and strength. Achieving a level of fitness is a first step in the quest to realizing performance-related goals. The progression from moderate physical activity to structured vigorous exercise programs and then sports and games reflects a logical pathway that minimizes risk and maximizes the chance of success along the way (see chapter 11 for more on progression).

One of the most frustrating yet exciting aspects of dealing with health problems is that people can modify their health status and control major health risks. The frustrating side is that many people find it difficult to change an unhealthy lifestyle. The exciting element is that, with help, they can gain control of their health. Fitness professionals are at the cutting edge of health in much the same way scientists discovering vaccines for major diseases were at the turn of the 20th century. The opportunity to help people alter their unhealthy lifestyles carries the responsibility of making recommendations based on the best scientific evidence available. This text will lead you through the steps to evaluate health-related risk factors and behaviors, test the various fitness components, and prescribe exercise to improve each.

KEY POINT

Fitness professionals live in an exciting time because of the increasing evidence and recognition that regular physical activity is essential to a good life. It is a worthwhile challenge to motivate people to begin and continue an active lifestyle, especially when there is so much competition for everyone's time.

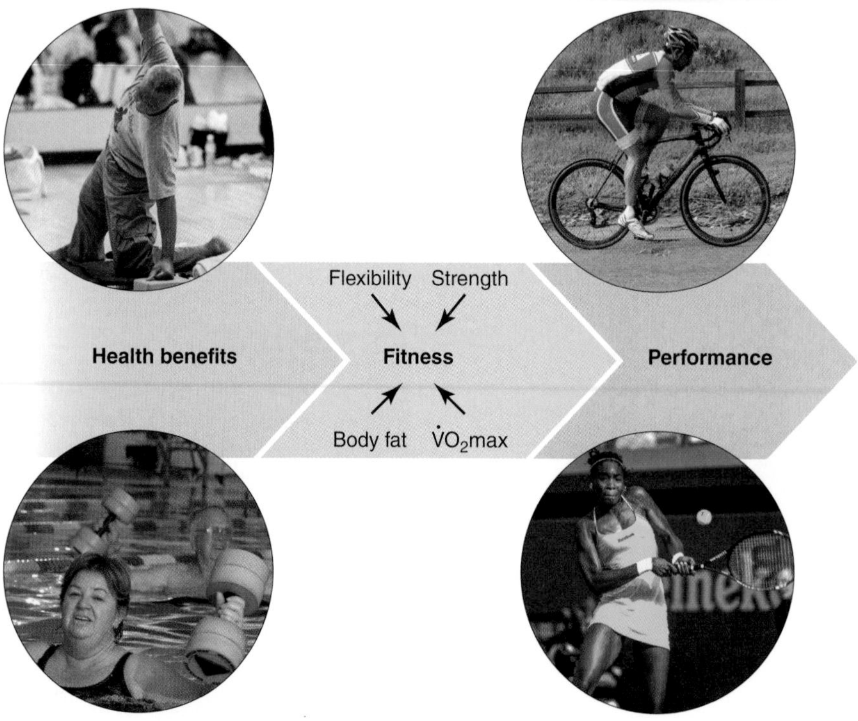

FIGURE 1.9 The continuum of health, fitness, and performance outcomes linked to physical activity.

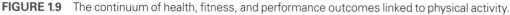

LEARNING AIDS

REVIEW QUESTIONS

1. What is the difference in the physical activity requirements for achieving health benefits, fitness, and performance?
2. List the top three leading causes of death and compare them with the behaviors linked to the top three actual causes of death.
3. What is the difference between absolute and relative intensity?
4. What is moderate-intensity and vigorous-intensity physical activity in terms of METs?
5. Calculate the volume of physical activity done per week for someone exercising at 5 METs for 40 min per day, 3 days per wk.
6. How does regular participation in physical activity affect the top two leading causes of death?
7. What do the *2008 Physical Activity Guidelines for Americans* recommend for moderate-intensity and vigorous-intensity physical activity in order to realize substantial health benefits?
8. Describe the physical activity guidelines for increasing or maintaining strength.
9. What are adverse events, and how can they be minimized?
10. What impact does fitness versus fatness have on the risk of chronic disease?
11. What performance-related fitness components are linked to sport?
12. Describe the continuum of physical activity recommendations for realizing health, fitness, and performance goals.

CASE STUDIES

1. A client complains that she has been deceived by all the physical activity recommendations you have given her over the past several years. She just read a government report indicating that a person only has to do moderate-intensity physical activity (walking) to achieve health benefits. She wants to know if she should continue her vigorous exercise program in which she exercises at her target heart rate (THR) for 30 min 3 to 4 days per wk or whether she should switch to a walking program. How do you respond?
2. You have just presented a speech on physical fitness to a local service club. One of the members says that he knows of two men who died in incidents related to exercise during the past few years and that he has read of other exercise-related deaths. He has decided that it is safer to lead a quiet life and not take the risk of exercising. How do you respond?
3. You are working with an obese client who has been sedentary for several years. He indicates that he would like to lose weight before beginning a physical activity program. What information might you provide to encourage him to begin a moderate-intensity physical activity program as plans are developed to accomplish weight-loss goals?

Answers to Case Studies

1. You might state that the physical activity recommendations in the government report were aimed at people who are currently sedentary and not those who are habitually active and involved in strenuous exercise. In addition, you might indicate that participation in more strenuous exercise is associated with other health-related benefits (increases in CRF, or $\dot{V}O_2max$) that are more difficult to achieve with moderate-intensity exercise.

2. You might respond by admitting that there are risks related to exercise, but the risk of death is very low for someone making the transition from a sedentary lifestyle to one involving moderate-intensity physical activity. Moreover, people die while sleeping or after eating and yet few people advocate the cessation of those activities. In addition, deterioration of the cardiovascular system through sedentary living causes a much higher risk of major health problems compared with being active. Finally, exercise-related risks can be minimized by starting slowly and gradually increasing the amount and intensity of exercise.
3. You might begin by telling him that the health-related benefits of physical activity occur in all people, independent of body weight or body fatness. Further, it is important to establish a pattern of physical activity as one of the new behaviors needed to help maintain the weight loss once the goal is achieved.

2

Health Risk Appraisal

Michael Shipe

OBJECTIVES

The reader will be able to do the following:

1. Understand the purpose of evaluating the health status of potential participants in fitness programs and identify appropriate instruments for the preparticipation health screening process.
2. Identify the presence of cardiovascular, metabolic, or renal disease, including signs and symptoms.
3. Describe the categories of participants who should receive medical clearance before undergoing exercise testing or participation.
4. Identify primary risk factors for cardiovascular disease and understand how they are used in providing educational counseling regarding disease prevention and management.
5. Understand how to classify fitness test results relative to the participant's age and sex.
6. Recommend an appropriate fitness program for participants based on their preparticipation health screening and fitness test results.

Fitness professionals in both clinical and commercial settings will encounter people with low CRF and an array of health and medical conditions. The fitness professional is responsible for properly screening prospective exercise participants to determine whether medical clearance is warranted before they begin a regular physical activity program. To screen an exercise participant, the fitness professional should begin with a preparticipation screening questionnaire, such as the Physical Activity Readiness Questionnaire for Everyone (PAR-Q+) or the preparticipation health status questionnaire (HSQ) (1, 2, 23). (These two questionnaires are discussed in detail later in this chapter.) The choice of questionnaire should be based on the characteristics (e.g., age, disease state) of the participant.

In some instances, medical clearance or referral of the participant to a clinic-based supervised exercise program may be necessary before starting an unsupervised exercise program. Unfortunately, there are no universal guidelines for determining when medical clearance is necessary before exercise participation or when supervised exercise in a clinical setting is warranted. To help the fitness professional make these decisions, this chapter provides the recommendations of the AHA and ACSM. When in doubt, the fitness professional should rely on the participant's primary care physician and the fitness director (or medical director) of the facility to make the final decision regarding approval for exercise participation.

Initially, the participant's preparticipation HSQ should be evaluated to ascertain if medical clearance is necessary prior to beginning an exercise program based upon the following: (1) the individual's current physical activity level (PAL), (2) known cardiovascular (CV), metabolic, or renal disease or signs and symptoms of these diseases, and (3) desired exercise intensity. Addressing these three factors will help the fitness professional identify those individuals who should not pursue unaccustomed vigorous intensity exercise that may expose them to an unnecessary increased risk for sudden cardiac death or acute myocardial infarction (1, 2, 24). Participants who do not require medical clearance may undergo a fitness test and the results should be evaluated relative to age and sex norms. The fitness professional now has the necessary information to develop an appropriate exercise prescription for improving the participant's health and fitness in relation to present health status and physical activity level. To maintain up-to-date records of the participant's health status, readminister the preparticipation HSQ annually and fitness tests semiannually (3).

Preactivity Screening

The AHA and ACSM recommend that exercise facilities provide their adult members with a preparticipation HSQ that is consistent with the exercise programs they plan to pursue. Although an exercise facility may not have a legal responsibility to conduct a preparticipation HSQ, this screening is in the best interest of exercise participants. Further, the results of the preparticipation HSQ should be interpreted and documented by qualified staff (1-5).

Regarding apparently healthy people, the risk of cardiovascular events during physical activity is remarkably low (adjusted risk of 1 to 3 per 1,000,000 participant hr), although increased age, greater physical activity level, and the presence of CVD risk factors are associated with greater risk (10, 11, 17). A well-designed and properly evaluated preparticipation HSQ serves several purposes, including identifying symptoms of chronic diseases that increase the risk of cardiovascular events during exercise participation, recognizing people with clinically significant diseases or conditions that warrant participation in medically supervised programs, and determining if people should seek medical clearance prior to fitness testing or exercise participation (5). Preparticipation screening is the first step in the fitness professional's health risk appraisal of exercise participants, and it includes the following categories:

- **M**ake a classification as to whether or not the individual currently exercises regularly
- **R**eview medical history for established CV, metabolic, or renal disease
- **P**ertinent signs and symptoms of CV, metabolic, or renal disease identified
- **L**evel of desired aerobic exercise intensity
- **E**stablish if medical clearance is necessary
- **A**dministration of fitness tests and evaluation of results
- **S**etup of exercise prescription
- **E**valuation of progress with follow-up tests

It may help the fitness professional to remember the recommended health risk appraisal categories and the order in which they are performed by using the acronym *MR. PLEASE*, which could represent the participant asking, "Mister, may I please exercise?" This protocol expands on previous recommendations for working with new clients in fitness settings (12).

Two standard preparticipation screening questionnaires commonly used in the fitness industry are the PAR-Q+ and the preparticipation HSQ (1, 3, 28). Each level of MR. PLEASE is discussed in detail following the descriptions of the PAR-Q+ and the preparticipation HSQ, and additional categories of the health risk appraisal are discussed afterwards.

Physical Activity Readiness Questionnaire for Everyone

The Physical Activity Readiness Questionnaire for Everyone (PAR-Q+; see form 2.1 on page 20 for the first page of the form or www.eparmedx.com for the complete form) was designed by the Canadian government to replace the Physical Activity Readiness Questionnaire (PAR-Q). It is an updated preparticipation screening questionnaire for people who want to pursue moderate (i.e., 40%-59% $\dot{V}O_2R$) to vigorous (i.e., ≥60% $\dot{V}O_2R$) physical activity. The PAR-Q+ is designed (and has been validated) to reduce the barriers to physical activity participation for people with and without established chronic disease. The original PAR-Q produced an inordinate number of false positives with older adults (60 yr and older), especially among those with orthopedic problems. This resulted in almost 20% of participants being referred to medical personnel before being cleared for physical activity versus only 1% for the present version (29). If participants answer *no* to all seven questions in the self-administered questionnaire (form 2.1), they are cleared for physical activity participation (28, 29).

If participants answer *yes* to any of the seven questions on the PAR-Q+, they are directed to complete 10 additional questions about whether they have signs or symptoms of chronic disease or established chronic disease (i.e., orthopedic, cancer, cardiovascular, metabolic, or pulmonary disease). If each response is *no* to the additional questions, then the person is cleared for physical activity participation. If participants answer *yes* to any of the additional questions, they are directed to contact a qualified exercise professional (CSEP-CEP) or complete an online questionnaire, the ePARmed-X+ (http://eparmedx.com), to further clarify the risk associated with exercise participation (7, 28, 29).

The ePARmed-X+ is an interactive online tool that provides a more extensive questionnaire about the presence of specific medical conditions (e.g., diabetes, low-back pain, arrhythmias), whether a physician is actively managing the conditions, and how severe the conditions are. Based on their answers, participants are recommended to either visit their physician or a qualified exercise professional with advanced university training for further information regarding appropriate exercise participation (7, 28, 29).

Most facilities offer unsupervised vigorous-intensity exercise to a clientele with varying medical histories, fitness levels, and physical activity goals, Thus, the remainder of this chapter addresses how to identify people who can safely pursue vigorous-intensity exercise independently, as well as those who need medical clearance before doing so.

Exercise Preparticipation Health Status Questionnaire

The preparticipation HSQ (see form 2.2 on page 21) is a preparticipation screening that classifies a client's current physical activity level; provides the fitness professional with enough information to quickly and accurately identify the presence of cardiovascular, metabolic, or renal disease by recognizing their major signs and symptoms; and identifies pertinent medical conditions that may affect the client's ability to begin exercising safely. The preparticipation HSQ provided in this text is based upon new recommendations for preparticipation screening proposed by the ACSM. As in the PAR-Q+, the preparticipation HSQ has been redesigned, as past pre-screening protocols were likely to result in excessive referrals to physicians for medical clearance, which could possibly discourage the client's pursuit and maintenance of a regular exercise program. The goals of the new screening process are to identify individuals: (1) who warrant medical clearance before beginning an exercise program or increasing the frequency, intensity, or volume of their current program, (2) who have clinically significant disease(s) that could benefit from participating in a medically supervised program, and (3) who have medical conditions that preclude them from exercise participation until these conditions subside or are more effectively controlled (1, 2, 24).

Assessing the presence of a client's primary risk factors for CVD (e.g., hypertension) to determine their CVD risk classification (i.e., low, moderate, or high) as part of the decision making process for medical clearance prior to exercise participation is no longer recommended. Yet fitness professional are encouraged to evaluate the CVD risk factor assessment as part of the health risk appraisal (1, 2). The information from this questionnaire should be evaluated *before* conducting any fitness testing or recommending exercise prescriptions.

A completed preparticipation HSQ will contain a significant amount of personal health information, which is protected under the Health Insurance Portability and Accountability Act of 1996 (HIPAA) (20). Thus, a completed preparticipation HSQ should be kept in a secure location and be accessible only by designated staff. A participant's medical history and fitness test results constitute personal health information. This information should be shared only with other health care professionals who will be working with the participant and should only be discussed in a private setting in which fellow staff or participants cannot overhear. For instance, a violation of HIPAA regulations would occur if a participant's medical conditions or body composition results were discussed with another participant or staff member when other people could listen in on the conversation. Additional legal concerns that may be involved in the exercise testing and prescription process are addressed in chapter 26.

Fitness professionals should note the patient information release form at the end of the preparticipation HSQ. Participants must provide their signature in this section so that their health care professional may release their pertinent medical information to the fitness professional, if warranted, in accordance with HIPAA regulations (20).

Aside from legal rights that protect personal health information, the fitness professional should consider that many participants may feel uncomfortable sharing their medical history. Using a professional yet conversational style to ask questions about medical diagnoses may help to alleviate the discomfort that clients may feel.

FORM 2.1 The PAR-Q+

PAR-Q+

The Physical Activity Readiness Questionnaire for Everyone

Regular physical activity is fun and healthy, and more people should become more physically active every day of the week. Being more physically active is very safe for MOST people. This questionnaire will tell you whether it is necessary for you to seek further advice from your doctor OR a qualified exercise professional before becoming more physically active.

GENERAL HEALTH QUESTIONS

Please read the 7 questions below carefully and answer each one honestly: check YES or NO.	YES	NO
1) Has your doctor ever said that you have a heart condition **OR** high blood pressure?	☐	☐
2) Do you feel pain in your chest at rest, during your daily activities of living, **OR** when you do physical activity?	☐	☐
3) Do you lose balance because of dizziness **OR** have you lost consciousness in the last 12 months? Please answer **NO** if your dizziness was associated with over-breathing (including during vigorous exercise).	☐	☐
4) Have you ever been diagnosed with another chronic medical condition (other than heart disease or high blood pressure)?	☐	☐
5) Are you currently taking prescribed medications for a chronic medical condition?	☐	☐
6) Do you have a bone or joint problem that could be made worse by becoming more physically active? Please answer **NO** if you had a joint problem in the past, but it does not limit your current ability to be physically active. For example, knee, ankle, shoulder or other.	☐	☐
7) Has your doctor ever said that you should only do medically supervised physical activity?	☐	☐

If you answered NO to all of the questions above, you are cleared for physical activity.
Go to Page 4 to sign the PARTICIPANT DECLARATION. You do not need to complete Pages 2 and 3.

- Start becoming much more physically active – start slowly and build up gradually.
- Follow Canada's Physical Activity Guidelines for your age (www.csep.ca/guidelines).
- You may take part in a health and fitness appraisal.
- If you have any further questions, contact a qualified exercise professional such as a Canadian Society for Exercise Physiology - Certified Exercise Physiologist® (CSEP-CEP) or a CSEP Certified Personal Trainer® (CSEP-CPT).
- If you are over the age of 45 yr and **NOT** accustomed to regular vigorous to maximal effort exercise, consult a qualified exercise professional (CSEP-CEP) before engaging in this intensity of activity.

If you answered YES to one or more of the questions above, COMPLETE PAGES 2 AND 3.

Delay becoming more active if:

- You are not feeling well because of a temporary illness such as a cold or fever - wait until you feel better
- You are pregnant - talk to your health care practitioner, your physician, a qualified exercise professional, and/or complete the **ePARmed-X+ at www.eparmedx.com** before becoming more physically active
- Your health changes - answer the questions on Pages 2 and 3 of this document and/or talk to your doctor or qualified exercise professional (CSEP-CEP or CSEP-CPT) before continuing with any physical activity program.

OSHF

FORM 2.2 Exercise Preparticipation Health Status Questionnaire (HSQ)

This questionnaire identifies adults for whom vigorous physical activity might be inappropriate or adults who should receive medical clearance before beginning a regular physical activity program.

SECTION 1: PERSONAL AND EMERGENCY CONTACT INFORMATION

Name: ____

Date of birth: ____

Address: ____

Phone: ____

Physician's name: ____

Height: ____

Weight: ____

Person to contact in case of emergency: _______________________________

Phone: ____

SECTION 2: CURRENT AND PLANNED PHYSICAL ACTIVITY LEVEL

Have you been performing planned, structured physical activity for at least 30 minutes a day at a moderate intensity on at least 3 days per week for at least the last 3 months?

❍Yes ❍No

Please note the frequency, intensity, time, and type of exercise you plan to perform

____

Please check all true statements for Sections 3-4

SECTION 3: MEDICAL CONDITIONS

Have you had or do you currently have:

______ A heart attack

______ Heart surgery, cardiac catheterization, or coronary angioplasty

______ Pacemaker, implantable cardiac defibrillator/rhythm disturbance

______ Heart valve disease

______ Heart failure

______ Heart transplantation

______ Congenital heart disease

______ Diabetes

______ Renal disease

If any of the statements were marked for this section, STOP—you should consult with a health care provider before engaging in or resuming exercise. You may need to use a facility with a medically qualified staff.

If no symptoms were marked, continue to section 4.

SECTION 4: SYMPTOMS

Do you currently experience

______ Chest discomfort with exertion

______ Unreasonable breathlessness

(continued)

Form 2.2 *(continued)*

______ Dizziness, fainting, or blackouts
______ Ankle swelling
______ Unpleasant awareness of a forceful, rapid, or irregular heart rate
______ Burning or cramping sensations in your lower legs when walking a short distance

The fitness professional should be informed immediately of any changes that occur in your health status.

SECTION 5: PRESCRIBED MEDICATIONS

Are you currently taking any medication? ❍Yes ❍No

If yes, please list all of your prescribed medications and how often you take them, whether daily (D) or as needed (PRN).

____

Of the medications you have listed, are there any you do not take as prescribed?

____

To be completed by fitness professional:

Medical clearance required: ❍Yes ❍No

If *yes*, note date when it was received: _______________________________________

PATIENT INFORMATION RELEASE FORM

If it is recommended that you receive medical clearance prior to exercise participation, you agree that it is permissible to seek this approval from your physician in compliance with the Health Insurance Portability and Accountability Act of 1996 (HIPAA).

Participant signature: ____

Date: _______________________________________

Fitness staff signature: ____

Date: _______________________________________

From E.T. Howley and D.L. Thompson, 2017, *Fitness professional's handbook,* 7th ed. (Champaign, IL: Human Kinetics). Based on American College of Sports Medicine 2014, *ACSM's guidelines for exercise testing and prescription*, 9th ed. (Philadelphia: PA: Lippincott, Williams, & Wilkins).

For instance, when participants have checked the box for having a heart attack, relevant questions providing further insight into their medical history would include the following: "Are your heart symptoms present? If so, are they stable?" "Has your heart attack affected your activities of daily life?" "Have you been able to return to the activities you were doing before the event?" "Did you participate in cardiac rehabilitation?" "Were you given any restrictions?" The participant's responses should be documented on the preparticipation HSQ. Reviewing the form conversationally allows the fitness professional to learn more about the participant's health status and to convey **empathy**, making participants more likely to perceive the fitness professional as being genuinely concerned with helping them improve their health.

No questionnaire can address all possible medical conditions that might warrant physician consent. Thus, the fitness professional should ask additional questions relevant to the participant's medical history while reviewing the preparticipation HSQ. The line of questioning should be directed by any condition that is checked as being present. In doing so, medical diagnoses or symptoms that may place the participant at additional cardiovascular risk during exercise are more likely to be addressed. A fitness facility may want to make minor alterations to the preparticipation HSQ so that it is more applicable to its participant population.

If prospective exercise participants refuse to complete a preparticipation screening form, then they cannot be properly screened according to the standards of care for fitness facilities advocated by the AHA and ACSM. When participants object to preparticipation screening procedures, the fitness professional should inform them of the benefits of screening and the potential risks of not completing the screening, as well as reassure them that all information is kept private, confidential, and secure. If prospective participants still refuse, ACSM recommends that they be permitted to sign a release or waiver before exercising. An example of a preparticipation screening refusal form that includes a waiver can be found elsewhere (9). The release or waiver should entail the following: acknowledgment that a preparticipation screening was provided, that the participant has been informed of the inherent risks of exercise participation, that the participant has chosen not to be screened, that the participant assumes personal responsibility, and that the participant releases the facility from any claims or suits arising from exercise participation. ACSM also recommends that prospective participants who sign the waiver or release have the opportunity to exercise in the facility. If someone chooses not to sign the waiver or release, the facility has the option of denying participation to the extent permitted by law (3). Lastly, it is recommended that a facility consult with a competent lawyer to establish policies and procedures regarding refusal for participation and the use of a waiver or release.

MR. PLEASE: Make Certain the Participant is a Current, Regular Exerciser

The first step in evaluating health status is addressed in section 2 of the preparticipation HSQ and entails determining whether the individual currently participates in regular exercise. A participant should be classified as a current exerciser if he or she has been performing planned, structured physical activity of at least moderate intensity (i.e., 40%-59% $\dot{V}O_2R$) for at least 30 min a day on 3 or more days a wk during the past 3 mo. This classification helps identify those individuals unaccustomed to regular physical activity and for whom exercise may place unwarranted demands on the CV system and increase the risk of complications (e.g., myocardial infarction; 1, 2, 24).

MR. PLEASE: Review Medical History for Diagnosis of CV, Metabolic, or Renal Disease

The next step is addressed in section 3 of the preparticipation HSQ and involves identifying if the participant has been previously diagnosed with CV, metabolic, or renal disease, which are specified as follows:

- Cardiovascular disease (CVD): coronary heart disease (CHD), congestive heart failure (CHF), peripheral vascular disease (PVD), and cerebrovascular disease (i.e., stroke)
- Metabolic disease: diabetes mellitus (type 1 or 2 diabetes)
- Renal disease: chronic kidney disease

The fitness professional should ask the participant if a physician or other qualified healthcare provider has ever diagnosed them with any of these diseases. Prior diagnosis of one of these diseases alone does not warrant medical clearance; that decision should also consider whether the participant is a regular exerciser, the participant's medical history, and the participant's desired aerobic exercise intensity (1, 2, 24).

MR. PLEASE: Pertinent Signs and Symptoms Indicative of CV, Metabolic, or Renal Disease

The main objective of section 3 of the preparticipation HSQ is to identify major signs and symptoms indicative of undiagnosed CV, metabolic, or renal disease (see table 2.1). According to the ACSM, people who mark in the affirmative any of the statements in this section would be considered to be symptomatic and should receive medical clearance from an appropriate health care provider before pursuing a regular exercise program, even if they are currently participating in regular exercise (1, 2, 24). Conversely, participants who don't present with the conditions in table 2.1 would be considered to be asymptomatic. Note that just because participants have one of these signs or symptoms, it does not mean that they have cardiovascular, metabolic, or renal disease. The fitness professional should evaluate the signs and symptoms within the context of the participant's recent medical history and seek additional information to further qualify the participant's responses. For instance, a participant may present with a resting heart rate (RHR) greater than 100 beats · min^{-1} but have no other symptoms suggestive of CVD. Upon further inquiry, the fitness professional finds that the participant has rushed to make the appointment and recently consumed a large dose of caffeine. Thus, the elevated heart rate (HR) may be the result of these recent events rather than an indication of possible CVD. This scenario demonstrates the importance of the fitness professional asking additional questions in order to interpret the preparticipation HSQ properly (1, 2, 24).

KEY POINT

Evaluation of sections 2 through 4 of the preparticipation HSQ helps the fitness professional determine whether a participant (1) is a current, regular exerciser, (2) has established CV, metabolic, or renal disease, and (3) shows signs or symptoms suggestive of these diseases. These criteria help determine whether it is appropriate for the participant to undergo fitness testing or begin regular physical activity or if medical clearance is recommended before doing so (2). This information is protected by HIPAA.

Table 2.1 Major Signs or Symptoms of Cardiovascular, Metabolic, and Renal Diseases

Sign or symptom	Clarification and significance
Angina (i.e., heart pain) in the chest, neck, jaw, arms or other areas; women may also present with unusual nausea	Angina is a hallmark of heart disease, especially CHD, and indicates the blood supply to the heart is insufficient (i.e., ischemia). Key features of angina include a constricting or heavy feeling in the middle of the chest, shoulders, or arms. These sensations may be provoked by exercise or exertion and other forms of stress.
Palpitations or tachycardia (i.e., RHR >100 beats · min^{-1})	A palpitation is the unpleasant awareness of a forceful or rapid heartbeat, which may indicate an irregular heartbeat. The fitness professional may be able to sense the palpitation by taking the HR manually at the carotid or radial artery. Palpitations can originate from unusual stress, fever, anemia, or a high cardiac output. **Tachycardia** is a common palpitation, and it can be due to recent actions (e.g., caffeine ingestion) or a sign of other cardiovascular problems.
Shortness of breath at rest or with mild exertion	Dyspnea is an abnormally uncomfortable awareness of breathing and is a principal symptom of cardiac and pulmonary disease. It occurs naturally during heavy exertion in individuals with high CRF and during mild exertion in untrained individuals. Dyspnea may be considered abnormal when it occurs at an atypical (e.g., low-intensity) level of exertion.
Dizziness or syncope	Syncope is the loss of consciousness and occurs most often due to lack of blood flow to the brain. Dizziness and especially syncope during exercise can be the product of cardiac disorders that prevent the normal increase or decrease in cardiac output. These cardiac output disorders are potentially life threatening. Dizziness or syncope can occur in healthy individuals after completing an exercise bout and should be addressed. These symptoms may occur because of reduced blood flow to the heart.
Ankle edema	Ankle edema is an unnatural accumulation of fluid surrounding the ankles and is characteristic of congestive heart failure (CHF), a common form of CVD. Individuals with CHF may exhibit generalized edema, whereas swelling in one limb may result from a venous thrombosis or blockage in the lymphatic system.
Intermittent claudication	Intermittent claudication is a burning or cramping pain (typically in the gluteal region) that is exacerbated by exertion. It occurs in a muscle with inadequate blood supply secondary to localized atherosclerosis. The pain should be consistent at a given exertion level and should resolve within 1-2 min after exercise cessation. Intermittent claudication is more prevalent in individuals with CHD and type 1 or 2 diabetes.

Based on American College of Sports Medicine 2014, *ACSM's guidelines for exercise testing and prescription*, 9th ed. (Philadelphia: PA: Lippincott, Williams, & Wilkins).

MR. PLEASE: Level of Desired Exercise Intensity

Determining the desired aerobic exercise intensity level is the final aspect of the preparticipation screening process and is noted in section 2 of the HSQ. The fitness professional should consider the participant's proposed exercise intensity, properly classify it (i.e., light, moderate, or vigorous), and compare it to his or her prior exercise level. Aerobic exercise intensity is commonly classified as follows: light (i.e., ≤40% $\dot{V}O_2R$), moderate (i.e., 40% to 59% $\dot{V}O_2R$), and vigorous (i.e., ≥ 60% $\dot{V}O_2R$) (1, 2, 24). Thus, the fitness professional can readily discern if the participant plans to make changes to the exercise volume or to the aerobic exercise intensity that will be performed. Compared to light-to-moderate intensity aerobic exercise, vigorous-intensity aerobic exercise is more likely to initiate acute cardiovascular events in selected individuals (27). Thus, the desired level of aerobic exercise intensity should be considered before recommending medical clearance prior to exercise participation. The fitness professional should consult chapter 11 for additional insight regarding how to calculate %$\dot{V}O_2R$ and further information concerning the classification of exercise intensity.

KEY POINT

Analyzing sections 2 through 4 of the preparticipation of HSQ combined with the participant's desired activity level determines whether a participant requires medical clearance before exercising, undergoing fitness testing, or progressing the intensity or volume of his or her exercise regimen.

MR. PLEASE: Establish if Medical Clearance is Recommended

At this juncture, the fitness professional should consider the individual's current exercise status, the presence of diagnosed CV, metabolic, or renal disease, signs or symptoms indicative of these diseases, and the participant's desired aerobic intensity level. The ACSM has provided a preparticipation screening algorithm (see tables 2.2a and 2.2b) to help fitness professionals make this decision. The starting point of the new logic model is based on the subject's participation in regular exercise, then decisions are broken down by disease and symptom status. This algorithm is specifically designed to identify those participants with underlying CV and metabolic disease who want to perform aerobic exercise at a vigorous intensity to which they are not accustomed (2, 27). It may help the fitness professional to consider these three caveats to determine if medical clearance is recommended.

1. Participants who have not been diagnosed with CV, metabolic, or renal disease and who don't demonstrate signs or symptoms of these diseases do not require medical clearance, regardless if they are current, regular exercisers or not.
2. Participants with signs and symptoms indicative of CV, metabolic, or renal disease are always recommended to receive medical clearance, regardless of their disease status or whether they are current, regular exercisers.
3. Participants with established CV, metabolic, or renal disease who are asymptomatic need medical clearance prior to aerobic exercise participation if they are not regular exercisers. In contrast, participants with these same characteristics who are regular exercisers only need medical clearance if they plan to pursue vigorous intensity aerobic exercise.

These guidelines, combined with the fitness professional's sound judgment, help determine whether a participant requires medical clearance prior to exercise participation (1, 2, 4, 24). It is important to note that the last portion of the algorithm addresses aerobic exercise progression.

Most exercise facilities offer vigorous-intensity exercises and thus the fitness professional should consult chapters 11-14 for recommendations regarding appropriate exercise progression. Also, it is important to note that pregnant women always require medical clearance before exercise testing or participation (1-4).

The AHA and ACSM offer specific recommendations regarding medical clearance before exercise participation. Fitness facilities should determine their preparticipation screening policy based on personnel qualifications, emergency preparedness, and target population (1-5). The type of medical clearance (e.g., verbal communications, ECG monitoring during a graded exercise test, and so forth) should be determined by the healthcare provider to whom the participant is referred, as there is no universally recommended screening test (1, 2).

MR. PLEASE: Administration of Fitness Tests and Evaluation of Results

The next step of the health appraisal involves administering and evaluating fitness tests. When combined with

Table 2.2a ACSM Preparticipation Screening Algorithm for Subjects Who Do Not Exercise Regularly

	MEDICAL CLEARANCE		FOLLOW EXERCISE PRESCRIPTION GUIDELINES ON PROGRESSION*		
Health status	**Recommended**	**Not necessary**	**Light-intensity exercise (30-<40% HRR)**	**Moderate-intensity exercise (40-<60% HRR)**	**Vigorous-intensity exercise (≥60% HRR)**
No CV, metabolic, or renal disease and no signs or symptoms of these		x →	Recommended →	Recommended →	May progress to this intensity*
Known CV, metabolic, or renal disease and asymptomatic	x →	→	Recommended, after medical clearance →	Recommended, after medical clearance →	May progress to this intensity*
Any sign or symptom of CV, metabolic, or renal disease	x →	→	Recommended, after medical clearance →	Recommended, after medical clearance →	May progress to this intensity*

Adapted from Riebe et al. 2015.

Table 2.2b ACSM Preparticipation Screening Algorithm for Subjects Who Exercise Regularly

	MEDICAL CLEARANCE		FOLLOW EXERCISE PRESCRIPTION GUIDELINES ON PROGRESSION*		
Health status	Recommended	Not necessary	Light-intensity exercise (30-<40% HRR)	Moderate-intensity exercise (40-<60% HRR)	Vigorous-intensity exercise (≥60% HRR)
No CV, metabolic, or renal disease and no signs or symptoms of these		x →	→	May continue at this intensity →	May continue or progress to this intensity *
Known CV, metabolic, or renal disease and asymptomatic		x →	→	May continue at this intensity	
	x →	→	→	→	May continue this intensity after medical clearance
Any sign or symptom of CV, metabolic, or renal disease	x → Stop exercising	→	May resume after medical clearance →	May resume after medical clearance →	May resume after medical clearance

CV = Cardiac, peripheral vascular, or cerebrovascular disease. Metabolic disease = type 1 and 2 diabetes mellitus. Regular exercise is defined as performing planned, structured physical activity for ≥30 min at a moderate or higher intensity for at least 3 days per wk over the past 3 mo or longer. *See chapter 11 for details on exercise prescription.

Adapted from Riebe et al. 2015.

the preparticipation HSQ, the test results provide greater insight into an individual's current level of physical fitness. Common measurements obtained before fitness testing are RHR (resting heart rate) and BP (blood pressure), percent body fat, waist circumference, and flexibility. Next, a submaximal graded exercise test is conducted to determine how the participant's HR, BP, and rating of perceived exertion (RPE) respond to gradually increasing exercise workloads. Additional fitness tests may be used to determine muscular strength and endurance and flexibility. Fitness testing procedures are included in chapters 7, 8, 9, and 10. If symptoms suggestive of CV disease occur during fitness testing, the fitness professional should seek medical clearance before conducting additional exercise testing or permitting the client to begin exercising in the facility. Signs and symptoms of these diseases that require medical clearance include the participant complaining of chest pain, experiencing a failure of SBP to rise appropriately with increases in exercise intensity, or indicating a pronounced shortness of breath at low exercise intensities. The results of the fitness tests should be compared with normative data based on the participant's age and sex (1). The classification of the fitness test values, combined with the participant's medical history and exercise goals, should serve as the framework for the exercise prescription.

MR. PLEASE: Setup of Exercise Prescription

At this point, the fitness professional should be prepared to address the next step in the health appraisal process: setting up the exercise prescription by following current guidelines (1-4). An appropriate exercise prescription considers a person's health status, personal goals, and fitness test results. Chapters 11 through 14 address exercise prescriptions for aerobic fitness, weight management, muscular strength and endurance, flexibility, and low-back function for generally healthy adults. In addition, chapters 16 through 22 provide information on prescribing exercise for special populations.

MR. PLEASE: Evaluation of Progress With Follow-Up Tests

The participant's exercise goals and health status are certain to change over time, which necessitates the last step in the health appraisal: evaluating progress with follow-up tests. Fitness tests should be periodically repeated and a preparticipation HSQ readministered. Follow-ups involving fitness tests and updates to the participant's health status serve several purposes: documenting the participant's health and fitness progress, identifying any changes in health status or response to activity, and indicating whether

Health Appraisal Overview

Make a classification regarding whether or not the individual currently exercises regularly using the standard of performing structured physical activity of at least moderate intensity (i.e., 40% to 59% $\dot{V}O_2R$) for at least 30 min on 3 or more days a wk during the past 3 months.

Review medical history for established CV, metabolic, or renal disease. When one or more of the diseases has been diagnosed and the participant is not a current, regular exerciser, then medical clearance is required before beginning an exercise program or fitness testing.

Pertinent signs and symptoms of CV, metabolic, or renal disease warrant medical clearance regardless of whether the participant is a current, regular exerciser or his or her disease status.

Level of physical activity desired. Determine the aerobic exercise intensity the participant plans to perform. This information should be considered along with the information in the prior three steps to help ascertain the necessity of medical clearance.

Establishing if medical clearance is necessary. Fitness professionals should use the information from the preparticipation HSQ, including current and expected exercise participation and a participant's medical history, to ascertain if medical clearance is recommended before pursuing an exercise program or fitness testing.

Administration of fitness tests and evaluation of results. Determine what fitness tests are appropriate given the participant's health status and compare the results with normative values based on age and sex.

Setup of exercise prescription. Consider the participant's medical history, past physical activity patterns, fitness results, and personal goals to prescribe an appropriate exercise program.

Evaluation of progress with follow-up tests. Determine if the participant's medical history or fitness level have changed.

changes in the exercise prescription or level of supervision are necessary. A follow-up fitness test may be conducted 3 mo after the participant has been exercising regularly, with biannual testing thereafter.

Fitness Program Decisions

This chapter has addressed the guidelines supported by the AHA and ACSM concerning when medical clearance is necessary before a participant undergoes fitness testing or begins an exercise program. The following section discusses additional criteria to consider as the fitness professional decides which of the following actions to pursue:

- Immediate referral for medical clearance
- Admission to one of the following fitness programs:
  - Clinic-based supervised exercise program
  - Appropriately prescribed exercise under the supervision of a fitness professional
  - Vigorous-intensity exercise program
  - Any unsupervised physical activity
- Educational information, seminars, or referral to other health professionals

Fitness professionals will encounter people who are on the verge of meeting the criteria for medical clearance. Do they require medical clearance? Should they possibly exercise in a supervised program? The following section helps resolve these dilemmas.

Determining If Referral to a Supervised Program Is Necessary

The fitness professional should consider the participant's health status and desired activity level to determine whether referral to a supervised exercise program is necessary. A supervised program, sometimes referred to as a *phase III program*, entails professionally qualified staff who have academic training in and clinical knowledge of monitoring special populations who are at a significantly higher risk for cardiac complications during exercise (e.g., people diagnosed with cardiovascular, metabolic, or renal disease) (1-4). These types of programs are also better suited for people with special conditions (e.g., emphysema, chronic bronchitis, cancer, epilepsy) that warrant additional supervision by medically qualified personnel (e.g., nurses or registered clinical exercise physiologists) who have experience with special populations.

Section 2 of the HSQ helps identify health conditions that require constant supervision. For example, the HSQ notes that a 65-yr-old male experiences unreasonable breathlessness at rest, and upon further inquiry it is noted that he has chronic bronchitis and typically requires supplemental oxygen when exercising. The participant has been walking regularly and independently but never monitors his blood oxygen levels (i.e., O_2 saturation levels). In this case, the pulmonary condition dictates that the participant's oxygen levels should be monitored before, during, and after exercise participation to ensure that O_2 saturation levels are maintained. This individual would benefit by initially exercising in a clinic-based supervised exercise program, such as a supervised pulmonary rehabilitation or cardiac rehabilitation program (e.g., phase III). As with medical clearance, there are no universal guidelines for referring an individual to supervised programs. Each exercise facility should have standards regarding the health conditions it considers itself qualified to supervise, and these standards should be based on the qualifications of its fitness professionals, the availability of medical equipment (e.g., supplemental O_2, automatic external defibrillator [AED]), and its emergency preparedness (5). As always, fitness professionals should use their personal experience, as well as consultation with a supervisor or physician, to determine whether referral to a supervised program is necessary.

Obtaining Medical Clearance

After determining that a person requires medical clearance, the fitness professional should immediately inform the participant of this requirement. The appropriate health care personnel, typically the participant's primary care physician, should provide the medical clearance and he or she will determine how the medical clearance will be granted (1, 2). A sample medical clearance form is presented in form 2.3. The form provides the healthcare professional with the option to refer the patient to a clinic-based supervised exercise facility. When the healthcare professional makes this recommendation, the fitness professional should contact the participant promptly and place him in contact with the nearest supervised exercise facility. In accordance with HIPAA regulations, the request for medical clearance must be accompanied by a notation indicating that the participant understands that personal health information will be shared with appropriate health care professionals. This permission is granted with the participant's signature in the medical release section of the HSQ (20).

Medical clearance can be sought in one of two ways. First, the participant can be given the paperwork to be signed by an appropriate health care professional. Afterwards, the participant can return the paperwork to the fitness professional for verification. Second, fitness professionals can contact the appropriate health care professional (e.g., fax the consent form to the physician's administrative office). Taking the initiative to obtain medical clearance has both benefits and challenges. The following are benefits of taking the initiative:

- Demonstrates recognition of conditions requiring medical clearance.
- Permits a relatively prompt reply from the health care professional.
- Acquires additional medical information so that the participant receives appropriate exercise testing and prescription.
- Builds rapport with local health care providers conducive to obtaining future exercise referrals from them.

The workload of many health care professionals does not allow them to quickly respond to each medical request they receive. Thus, it is recommended to wait 3 business days before sending a second medical clearance request. Thereafter, participants should be encouraged to contact the health care professional personally to expedite the return of the consent form. Participants requiring medical clearance should be informed of the facility's preparticipation screening protocol, so they understand that their clearance to begin exercising may take time. Although they may have to wait to exercise, participants should be assured that the steps taken in accordance with established protocols are serving their best health interests.

To prevent the delay of fitness tests for individuals requiring medical clearance, the preparticipation HSQ should be completed and submitted to the appropriate fitness professional for review 2 to 3 business days before a fitness test is scheduled. This will provide time to secure medical clearance and ensure that the appropriate paperwork is completed before the fitness test, allowing the participant to begin an exercise program shortly thereafter.

KEY POINT

The fitness professional should consider the participant's health status, desired activity level, and fitness test results, as well as the facility's preparticipation screening standards and emergency preparedness, to determine whether referral to a supervised exercise program is necessary. If necessary, medical clearance should be obtained or appropriate medical personnel contacted prior to exercise participation.

FORM 2.3 Sample Medical Clearance Form*

Dear ____:

Your patient ____ would like to begin an exercise program at our fitness facility, Fitness First. We would appreciate your medical opinion and recommendations concerning participation in regular exercise at our facility. The exercise program may include aerobic training, strength training, and flexibility exercises, which will be appropriately increased in duration and intensity over time. Please provide the following information and return this form to the fitness professional working with your patient.

Name: *JinAh Lee*

Address: *101 Healthy Street, City, State*

AUTHORIZATION

I consent to and authorize my health care professional to release health information, specifically concerning my ability to participate in an exercise program and fitness assessment, to Fitness First. By completing this form, the health care professional is not assuming any responsibility for the exercise and assessment program.

Participant's signature ______________________________ Date________________

Fitness professional's signature ________________________ Date________________

HEALTH CARE PROFESSIONAL RECOMMENDATIONS

Please identify any recommendations or restrictions for your patient regarding the following:

❍ I believe no contraindications to exercise exist and the client may begin an exercise program.

❍ I believe some contraindications to exercise may exist and the client may begin an exercise program with the following cautions: ______________________________.

❍ I believe contraindications to exercise exist and the following activities should be avoided: ____.

❍ I believe contraindications to exercise exist and the client should not begin an exercise program.

If this client has completed a graded exercise test, please provide a copy of the final exercise test report and interpretation.

Health care professional's signature ____

Health care professional's name ____

Address ____

Thank you for your consideration.

(Signature of fitness professional) ____

*Must be accompanied by a medical release form in accordance with HIPAA regulations.

From E.T. Howley and D.L. Thompson, 2017, *Fitness professional's handbook,* 7th ed. (Champaign, IL: Human Kinetics).

Education Regarding CVD Risk Factors

A thorough health risk appraisal includes a medical history and CVD risk factor assessment. Identifying and effectively controlling CVD risk factors is an important objective of overall CVD prevention and management even though it is no longer a part of the preparticipation screening process (16). Fitness professionals are encouraged to complete a CVD risk factor assessment with participants to ascertain if they meet the requirements for positive CVD risk factors (see table 2.3). Fitness professionals are encouraged to be conservative when identifying CVD risk factors. When a specific risk factor is unknown or unavailable, it is designated as a risk factor. It is common practice to sum the number of positive CVD risk factors. It is important to note that elevated high-density lipoprotein cholesterol (HDL-C) levels ≥HDL 60 mg · dl^{-1} (1.55 mmol · L^{-1}) are considered to be a negative CVD risk factor, as this provides a cardioprotective benefit. Participants with HDL-C levels ≥HDL 60 mg · dl^{-1} (1.55 mmol · L^{-1}) should have one positive CVD risk factor subtracted from the sum of his or her positive CVD risk factors (1, 2).

Fitness professionals should inform participants about their risk factors for CVD and the significance of those factors. Initially, they should explain the meaning of a risk factor (i.e., a clinical diagnosis or lifestyle behavior that increases the chances of developing heart disease). The fitness professional should then address which risk factors can be modified, which include all of the factors except family history and age. The participant should be informed that regular physical activity can have a positive influence on most risk factors for CHD and decrease the risk of developing new ones (1-4, 6). The fact that regular physical activity may help manage and prevent these risk factors can serve as powerful motivation for long-term exercise adherence.

The clinical significance of a given risk factor is predicated on its severity, and thus a risk-factor continuum should be considered (13, 14). Risk factors can simply be determined by noting the thresholds in table 2.3. A person who has a resting BP of ≥140/90 mmHg or is taking antihypertensive medication would simply be classified as hypertensive. Beginning at 115/75 mmHg, however, CVD risk doubles with each increment of 20/10 mmHg—the higher the BP, the higher the CVD risk (15). There is considerable research evidence that increasing levels of abdominal obesity, blood glucose, smoking, and LDL-C are associated with additional CVD risk (8, 12, 16, 25, 26). Therefore, the presence and magnitude of the risk factor should be considered in order to quantify the CVD risk. Furthermore, risk factors exert

Table 2.3 Atherosclerotic Cardiovascular Disease Risk-Factor Thresholds for Risk Classification

Positive risk factors	Defining criteria
Age	Men ≥45 yr; women ≥55 yr
Family history	Myocardial infarction (MI), coronary revascularization, or sudden death before age 55 in father or other male first-degree relative or before age 65 in mother or other female first-degree relative
Cigarette smoking	Current cigarette smoker, quit within previous 6 mo, or exposure to environmental tobacco smoke
Sedentary lifestyle	Not participating in at least 30 min of moderate-intensity (40%-59% $\dot{V}O_2$) aerobic physical activity on at least 3 days per wk for at least 3 mo
Obesity*	BMI ≥30 kg · m^{-2} or waist girth >40 in. (102 cm) for men and >35 in. (88 cm) for women
Hypertension	SBP ≥140 mmHg or DBP ≥90 mmHg confirmed by resting measurements on at least two separate occasions or on antihypertensive medications
Dyslipidemia	LDL-C ≥130 mg · dl^{-1} (3.37 mmol · L^{-1}), HDL-C <40 mg · dl^{-1} (1.04 mmol · L^{-1}); total serum cholesterol (if only measurement available) ≥200 mg · dl^{-1} (5.18 mmol · L^{-1}); or on lipid-lowering medication
Prediabetes**	Impaired fasting glucose (IFG) = fasting plasma glucose ≥100 mg · dl^{-1} (5.55 mmol · L^{-1}) and ≤125 mg · dl^{-1} (6.94 mmol · L^{-1}) or impaired glucose tolerance (IGT) = 2 hr values in oral glucose tolerance test (OGTT) ≥140 mg · dl^{-1} (7.77 mmol · L^{-1}) and ≤199 mg · dl^{-1} (11.04 mmol · L^{-1}) confirmed by measurements on at least two separate occasions
Negative risk factor	**Defining criteria**
High serum HDL-C***	≥60 mg · dl^{-1} (1.55 mmol · L^{-1})

MI = myocardial infarction, BMI = body mass index, SBP = systolic blood pressure, DBP = diastolic blood pressure, HDL = high density lipoprotein, LDL = low density lipoprotein, FBG = fasting blood glucose

* If the presence of or absence of a CVD risk factor is not disclosed or unavailable, that CHD risk factor should be counted as a risk factor.

**Recent ACSM guideline updates (1) move the risk factor criteria from prediabetes to diagnosed diabetes, with a higher cutoff value of fasting blood glucose at or above 126 mg · dl^{-1} (7.00 mmol · L^{-1}). Similarly, the OGTT value cutoff is higher at ≥ 200 mg · d^{-1} (11.1 mmol · dl^{-1}), and the guidelines place the overall glycated hemoglobin level of plasma glucose concentration risk level at 6.5%.

***It is common to sum risk factors in making clinical judgments. If HDL-C is high, subtract one risk factor from the sum of positive risk factors because high HDL-C decreases CVD risk.

Adapted, by permission, from American College of Sports Medicine, 2014, *ACSM's guidelines for exercise testing and prescription*, 9th ed. (Philadelphia, PA: Lippincott, Williams, & Wilkins), 27.

an independent effect on CVD risk and also interact with one another to further increase CVD risk. For instance, the presence of obesity alone increases CVD risk 15% to 25%, but when it is present with high cholesterol and elevated fasting blood glucose, CVD risk increases approximately 65% to 85% (21, 22, 31). The degree of increased risk for multiple risk factors is determined by their combination and severity. To do this, some fitness professionals quantify the severity of a participant's individual risk factors and overall relative risk for developing CVD by using the Framingham algorithm (18). Instructions for using this tool can be found in an article written by Wilson et al. (30), and an online version is available under the Risk Functions tab at www.framinghamheartstudy.org.

In addition, the fitness professional should discuss sensible lifestyle changes that participants can pursue to more readily control their CVD risk factors. However, information alone is unlikely to lead participants to make significant changes. Chapter 23 provides several approaches to changing behavior that fitness professionals can use to help the participant. In addition, the fitness professional can inform the participant of support groups, upcoming educational seminars, and other health professionals (e.g., dietitians) who can assist with healthy lifestyle choices.

Understanding Common Medications for CVD

Section 5 of the preparticipation HSQ requires the participant to document prescribed medications. The fitness professional should study chapter 19 of this book to be aware of common medications and their effects. Information on medication provides additional insight into the medical history and diagnosed CVD risk factors. For example, a participant may indicate that she does not have high cholesterol in section 3 but lists Lipitor as one of her medications in section 4. Reviewing chapter 19, the fitness professional can deduce that Lipitor is a class of drug known as a statin and is prescribed to treat high cholesterol. Some participants may indicate that they do not have a given medical condition because they are taking medication to treat it. However, taking a prescription medication to manage a chronic disease does not mean that the condition is absent, just that it is more likely to be effectively controlled. Thus, the participant still has the risk factor of high cholesterol and the fitness professional should note this accordingly.

In addition, the fitness professional should be able to determine whether a prescribed medication will alter the typical physiological responses to physical activity. For example, if a participant is taking a medication from the class of drugs known as beta-blockers, the fitness professional should be aware that the participant's HR will be substantially reduced (e.g., may not exceed 120 beats · min^{-1}) even though the participant is exercising vigorously. This response should not be considered abnormal; instead, it indicates the effectiveness of the medication and necessitates the use of a perceived exertion scale (see chapter 7) to monitor exercise intensity.

Changing Health or Fitness Status

People who regularly participate in physical activity are likely to experience positive changes in their fitness level (e.g., greater CRF) and more effectively manage their risk factors (e.g., lower resting BP). These changes can be readily observed by noting changes in participants' exercise duration or intensity and in resting BP measurements. Changes such as these improve quality of life and reduce the risk for chronic disease (see chapter 1).

However, new medical conditions may develop and not be readily apparent after a participant completes a preparticipation screening and fitness tests. Unless specifically asked about new conditions, participants may not reveal this information. For instance, a participant may begin to experience chest pain during exercise but may keep this information private. The preparticipation HSQ directs participants to contact the fitness director when they experience significant changes in their health status, but not all clients may understand the importance of this communication. Although some people will notify staff members when health changes occur, others will not. Therefore, semiannual fitness retesting and annual readministration of the HSQ are advisable to determine whether participants who are experiencing changes in health status should seek medical clearance or be assigned to a clinic-based supervised program (3).

If participants develop symptoms such as significant chest pain during exercise or other signs or symptoms suggestive of undiagnosed cardiovascular, metabolic, or renal disease, they should be required to obtain medical clearance. (1-4). Additional situations in which moderate- and vigorous-intensity exercise should be discontinued include musculoskeletal problems exacerbated with activity and severe psychological, medical, or drug or alcohol problems that are not responding to therapy (2). In addition, exercise should be deferred with major changes in resting BP (1). It is the responsibility of the fitness professional to determine the length of time between follow-up fitness tests or HSQ administrations to ensure participants are pursuing an appropriate exercise program.

KEY POINT

Fitness professionals should be aware of temporary or chronic conditions that alter a participant's health status and warrant medical clearance, additional supervision, or changes in exercise recommendations. These conditions can be identified with periodic readministration of the HSQ and follow-up fitness tests.

2

LEARNING AIDS

REVIEW QUESTIONS

1. What is the first step in the preparticipation screening process, and what is its main objective?
2. When is it appropriate to use the PAR-Q+ versus the preparticipation HSQ?
3. The categories of health appraisal can be recalled using the acronym *MR. PLEASE*. Provide a brief example of what each letter represents.
4. If a prospective exercise participant chooses not to complete a PAR-Q+ or preparticipation HSQ, what is the next course of action?
5. Explain a sign or symptom that may indicate a participant has CV, metabolic, or renal disease.
6. Patient education involves the identification of primary risk factors for CVD. Explain what a primary risk is and provide three examples, including the threshold for each.
7. Consider a 35-yr-old female who is 5 ft 6 in. (168 cm) and weighs 160 lb (72.6 kg), smokes occasionally on the weekends, and walks 3 days per wk for 35 min. Her HSQ indicates that she does not have high BP or cholesterol or type 2 diabetes. Her resting BP is 118/60 mmHg and her RHR is 85 beats $\cdot$ min^{-1}. What are her primary risk factors, and why did you designate them as such?
8. Why is it important to consider participants' HDL-C levels when determining the number of risk factors?
9. What is an example of a chronic disease that puts an individual at high risk for cardiovascular complications during exercise participation?
10. Provide an example of a medical condition that would require medical clearance prior to exercise testing or participation?
11. Why is it important to determine if a prospective exercise participant is a current, regular exerciser or not?
12. After obtaining fitness test results, what standards should the fitness professional compare them with?
13. Explain two scenarios in which a participant may be referred to a clinic-based supervised exercise program.

CASE STUDIES

1. Vikram is a 46-yr-old programmer who hasn't exercised regularly for 5 yr. He has not been diagnosed with CV, metabolic, or renal disease, nor does he report any major signs or symptoms suggestive of these diseases. He wants to begin a walking program. He is 5 ft 10 in. (178 cm), weighs 195 lb (88.5 kg), and thus has a BMI of 28.0 kg $\cdot$ m^{-2}. His father suffered a heart attack (MI) at 52 yr and takes BP medication. Additionally, Vikram's RHR is 74 beats $\cdot$ min^{-1}, with a BP of 122/78 mmHg, LDL-C of 115 mg $\cdot$ dl^{-1}, and HDL-C of 47 mg $\cdot$ dl^{-1}. He doesn't smoke and his fasting blood glucose level is 88 mg $\cdot$ dl^{-1}.
   a. Does the subject warrant medical clearance prior to exercise participation? Why or why not?
   b. Identify the subject's primary risk factors for CVD, including the clinical basis for each one.

2. Miriam is a 61-yr-old retired accountant who has been physically inactive for 15 yr. She wants to lose weight and is interested in using the elliptical trainer because she has heard that it burns the most calories. She was diagnosed with type 2 diabetes 12 yr ago and her last fasting blood glucose level was 145 mg · dl^{-1}. She does not smoke, nor does she report any major signs or symptoms suggestive of CVD, pulmonary disease, or metabolic disease. She is 5 ft 4 in. (163 cm) and weighs 169 lb (76.7 kg). Her waist circumference is 32 in. (81 cm) and hip circumference is 36 in. (92 cm). Her resting blood pressure is 124/74 mmHg, with a total cholesterol of 225 mg · dl^{-1} and an LDL-C level of 147 mg · dl^{-1}.
   a. Does the subject warrant medical clearance prior to exercise participation? Why or why not?
   b. Identify the subject's primary risk factors for CVD, including the clinical basis for each one.
3. Stephanie is a 23-yr-old graduate student who has been running 5 mi (8.0 km) 4 to 5 times per wk for the past 3 yr. She does not report any major signs or symptoms suggestive of CVD, metabolic, or renal disease. She is 5 ft 5 in. (165 cm) and weighs 125 lb (56.7 kg), and she is interested in performing high intensity interval training in order to improve her running speed. She has an RHR of 56 beats · min^{-1}, resting BP of 114/64 mmHg, and total cholesterol of 175 mg · dl^{-1} with an LDL-C level of 95 mg · dl^{-1} and an HDL-C level of 64 mg · dl^{-1}. Her mother was diagnosed with heart disease at 53 yr but underwent successful heart surgery.
   a. Does the subject warrant medical clearance prior to exercise participation? Why or why not?
   b. Identify the subject's primary risk factors for CVD, including the clinical basis for each one.
4. Daniel is a 57-yr-old sales representative who walks 3 days per wk for 30 min and wants to begin jogging 2 to 3 days per wk. He had a heart attack at 51 at has been exercising regularly ever since. He reports no major signs or symptoms suggestive of CVD, metabolic, or renal disease but has not seen a physician in 2 yr. He is 6 ft (183 cm), weighs 205 lb (93.0 kg), and has a waist circumference of 38 in. (97 cm). His resting BP is 124/80 mmHg, he is a nonsmoker, takes Atenolol to manage his blood pressure, and he does not know his cholesterol levels. His father died from a heart attack at 66 yr and his brother had heart surgery (coronary artery bypass graft) at 59 yr.
   a. Does the subject warrant medical clearance prior to exercise participation? Why or why not?
   b. Identify the subject's primary risk factors for CVD, including the clinical basis for each one.

Case Study Summaries

	Case study 1	Case study 2	Case study 3	Case study 4
Current, regular exerciser	No	No	Yes	Yes
Known cardiovascular, metabolic, or renal disease	No	Yes	No	Yes
Major signs or symptoms[1]	No	No	No	No
Desired aerobic intensity level	Light/moderate	Vigorous	Vigorous	Vigorous
Medical clearance warranted	No	Yes	No	Yes

(continued)

Case Study Summaries *(continued)*

	Case study 1	Case study 2	Case study 3	Case study 4
CHD risk factors[2]				
Age	Yes	Yes	No	Yes
Family history	Yes	No	Yes	No
Current cigarette smoker	No	No	No	No
Sedentary lifestyle	Yes	Yes	No	No
Obesity	No	Yes	No	No
Hypertension	No	No	No	Yes
Hyperlipidemia	No	Yes	No	Yes
Diabetes	No	Yes	No	No
Number of primary risk factors	3	5	1	4

[1]See table 2.1 for major signs and symptoms indicative of cardiovascular, metabolic, and renal diseases.

[2]See table 2.3 for clinical thresholds regarding risk factors for CVD.

Answers to Case Studies

1. For the case study of Vikram, consider the following:
   a. Vikram is not a regular exerciser but does not report established CV, metabolic, or renal disease, nor signs or symptoms suggestive of these diseases. He wants to pursue a light-to-moderate intensity aerobic exercise regimen and thus medical clearance isn't recommended prior to exercise participation.
   b. Vikram demonstrates three primary risk factors: age (≥45 yr), family history (first-degree male relative ≤55 yr with an MI), and a sedentary lifestyle (physically inactive for 5 yr).
2. For the case study of Miriam, consider the following:
   a. Miriam is nor a regular exerciser and she has been diagnosed with a metabolic disease (type 2 diabetes). She reports no signs and symptoms of CV or renal disease but wants to pursue a vigorous-intensity aerobic exercise program and thus medical clearance is recommended prior to exercise participation.
   b. She exhibits a series of primary risk factors, including age (≥55 yr), obesity (waist >35 in. [89 cm]), a sedentary lifestyle (physically inactive for 15 yr), high cholesterol (total cholesterol ≥200 mg $\cdot$ dl^{-1}; LDL-C ≥130 mg $\cdot$ dl^{-1}), and a diagnosis of type 2 diabetes (fasting BG ≥126 mg $\cdot$ dl^{-1}), a metabolic disease.
3. For the case study of Stephanie, consider the following:
   a. She is a current, regular exerciser with no history of CV, metabolic, or renal disease, nor signs and symptoms of these diseases. She is interested in performing higher-intensity aerobic exercise and medical clearance is not recommended prior to doing so.
   b. Although Stephanie does report one risk factor (family history—mother was diagnosed with heart disease ≤55 yr), she also demonstrates a negative risk factor (HDL ≥60 mg $\cdot$ dl^{-1}), which negates her positive risk factor. This results in a net of no primary risk factors.
4. For the case study of Daniel, consider the following:
   a. Although he is a current, regular exerciser, he has known CVD (e.g., heart attack) and wants to pursue vigorous-intensity aerobic exercise (e.g. jogging). Furthermore, he has not visited his physician in 2 yr, and thus needs to obtain medical clearance prior to his pursuit of a high-intensity aerobic exercise program.
   b. He presents with several risk factors, including age (≥55 yr), high cholesterol (because his cholesterol levels are unknown), and hypertension (takes Atenolol).

Scientific Foundations

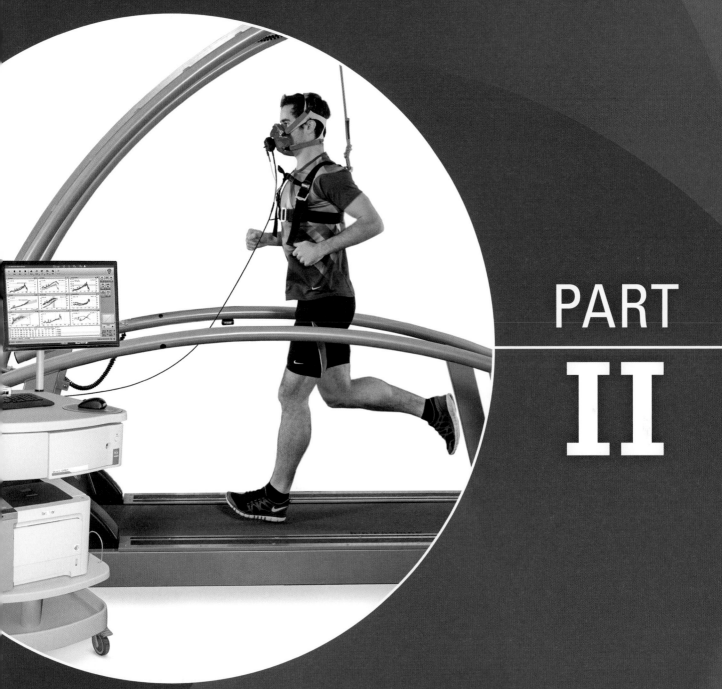

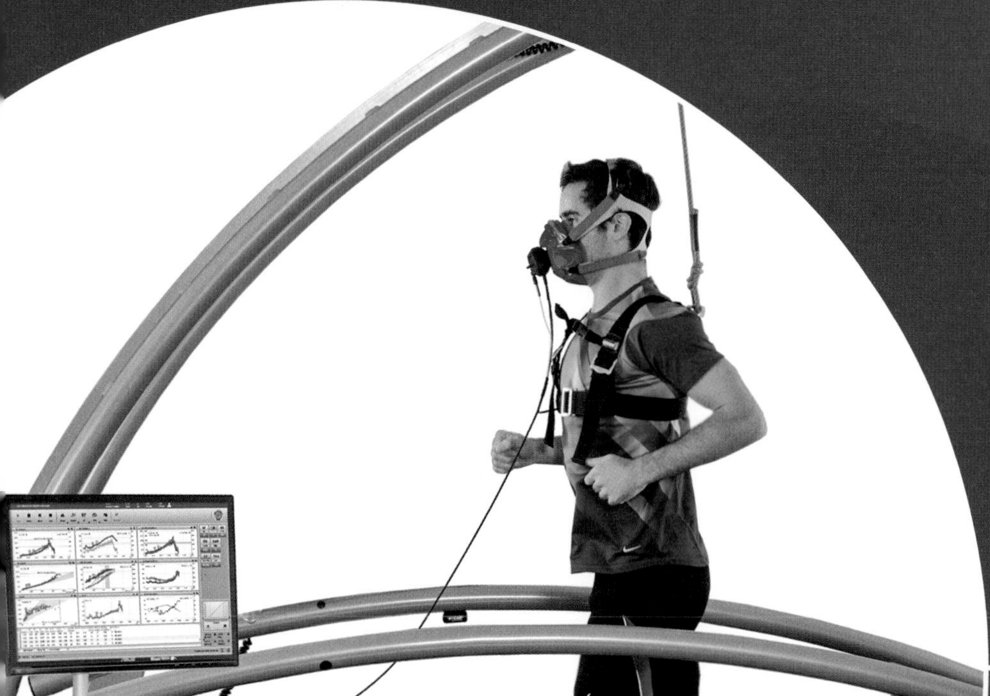

Courtesy of COSMED - Cardiopulmonary Diagnostics (www.cosmed.com)

PART II

Part II provides the basic scientific foundation for understanding the structure and function of the human body, nutrition, and energy expenditure. In chapter 3, we review the bones, joints, and muscles of the body and their biomechanical functions during common physical activities. In chapter 4, we cover the concepts of energy production, muscle function, and the physiological response to acute and chronic exercise. Differences due to gender, type of exercise, and temperature are described. In chapter 5, we discuss nutrition, and in chapter 6, we address how much energy (calories) we use doing physical activity.

3

Functional Anatomy and Biomechanics

Clare E. Milner

OBJECTIVES

The reader will be able to do the following:

1. Identify the major bones of the skeletal system and classify them by shape.
2. Name each synovial joint and demonstrate the movements possible.
3. Explain the differences among concentric, eccentric, and isometric muscle actions.
4. List the major muscles in each muscle group, and identify the major actions at the joints involved (shoulder girdle, shoulder joint, elbow joint, radioulnar joint, wrist joint, lumbosacral joint, vertebral column, hip joint, knee joint, ankle joint, and subtalar joint).
5. Cite common exercises involving the major muscle groups and point out potential errors in their execution.
6. Describe the three factors that determine stability and describe the relationships among them during physical activity.
7. Explain how contracting muscles produce torque at a joint.
8. Describe how an exerciser can change positions of body segments to alter the resistance torque.
9. Define the mechanical principles of *rotational inertia* and *angular momentum* as applied to human movement.
10. Describe the key muscle groups involved in locomotion, throwing, cycling, jumping, swimming, and carrying objects.
11. Discuss common errors seen in locomotion, throwing, and striking.

3

The fitness professional must have knowledge of the bones, joints, and muscles; must understand muscle forces and other forces (e.g., gravity); and must be able to apply biomechanical principles to human movement. With this knowledge, the fitness professional is better equipped to direct safe physical activity for participants seeking the health-related benefits of exercise. This knowledge also helps earn the respect of clients, who will view the instructor as a professional in the field rather than a technician who may know what to do but not why. This chapter is merely a summary; for greater detail on anatomy and biomechanics, see the reference list (1-7).

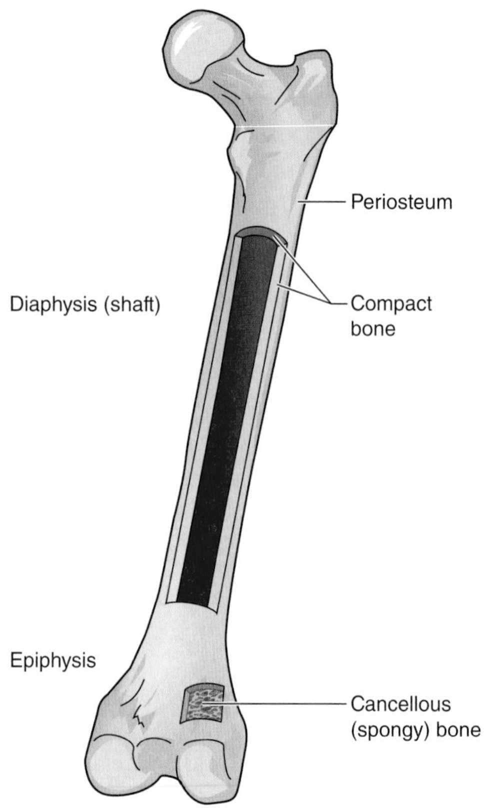

FIGURE 3.1 Structure of the femur, a long bone in the thigh.

Skeletal Anatomy

Most of the 200 distinct bones in the human skeleton are involved in movement. Their high mineral component gives them rigidity, while their protein component reduces their brittleness. The two types of bone tissue are cortical and trabecular bone. Cortical, or compact, bone is the dense, hard outer layer of a bone. Trabecular bone, also known as spongy or cancellous bone, has a lattice-like structure to provide greater internal strength along the lines of stress within a bone but with less overall weight than solid bone. Bones are living tissue and are constantly being remodeled in adaptation to the loading demands placed on them. Bones are divided into four classifications according to their shape: long, short, flat, and irregular.

Long Bones

The long bones, found in the limbs and digits, serve primarily as levers for movement. Each long bone has several distinct features. The **diaphysis**, or shaft, is made up of thick, compact bone surrounding the hollow medullary cavity. It is characteristic of long bones that the shaft is longer than it is wide. The **epiphyses**, or expanded ends, are composed of spongy bone with a thin outer layer of compact bone. The **articular cartilage** is a thin layer of hyaline cartilage covering the articulating surfaces (the surfaces of a bone that come into contact with another bone to form a joint) that provides a smooth, low-friction surface and helps absorb shock. The **periosteum** is a fibrous membrane covering the entire bone (except where the articular cartilage is present) to serve as an attachment site for muscles (see figure 3.1). Examples of long bones include the femur in the thigh, the ulna in the forearm, and the phalanges in the digits.

Short, Flat, and Irregular Bones

In addition to long bones, the skeleton is made up of short bones, flat bones, and irregularly shaped bones (see figure 3.2). The tarsals (in the ankle) and carpals (in the wrist) are the short bones, and they are approximately as wide as they are long. Their composition (internal trabecular bone covered with a thin outside layer of cortical bone) provides light weight and strength. Their roughly cubic shape decreases the potential for movement between adjacent bones. The flat bones, such as the ribs, ilia (wings of the pelvis), and scapulae (shoulder blades), serve primarily as broad sites for muscle attachments and, in the case of the ribs and ilia, to enclose cavities and protect internal organs. These bones have a broad, flattened structure. They are composed of trabecular bone covered with a thin layer of cortical bone. The ischium (inferior part of the pelvis), pubis (anterior part of the pelvis), and vertebrae are irregularly shaped bones that protect internal parts and support the body in addition to being sites for muscle attachments. An additional category of bone, sesamoid, is reserved for those few bones in the body that are embedded within a tendon. The role of these bones is to modify the way a tendon crosses a joint. The patella (kneecap) is a sesamoid bone embedded in the quadriceps tendon at the knee.

KEY POINT

Bones are living tissues that are light in weight but strong and stiff. The combination of solid cortical bone on the outside and a lightweight scaffold of trabecular bone inside provides strength with less weight than solid bone.

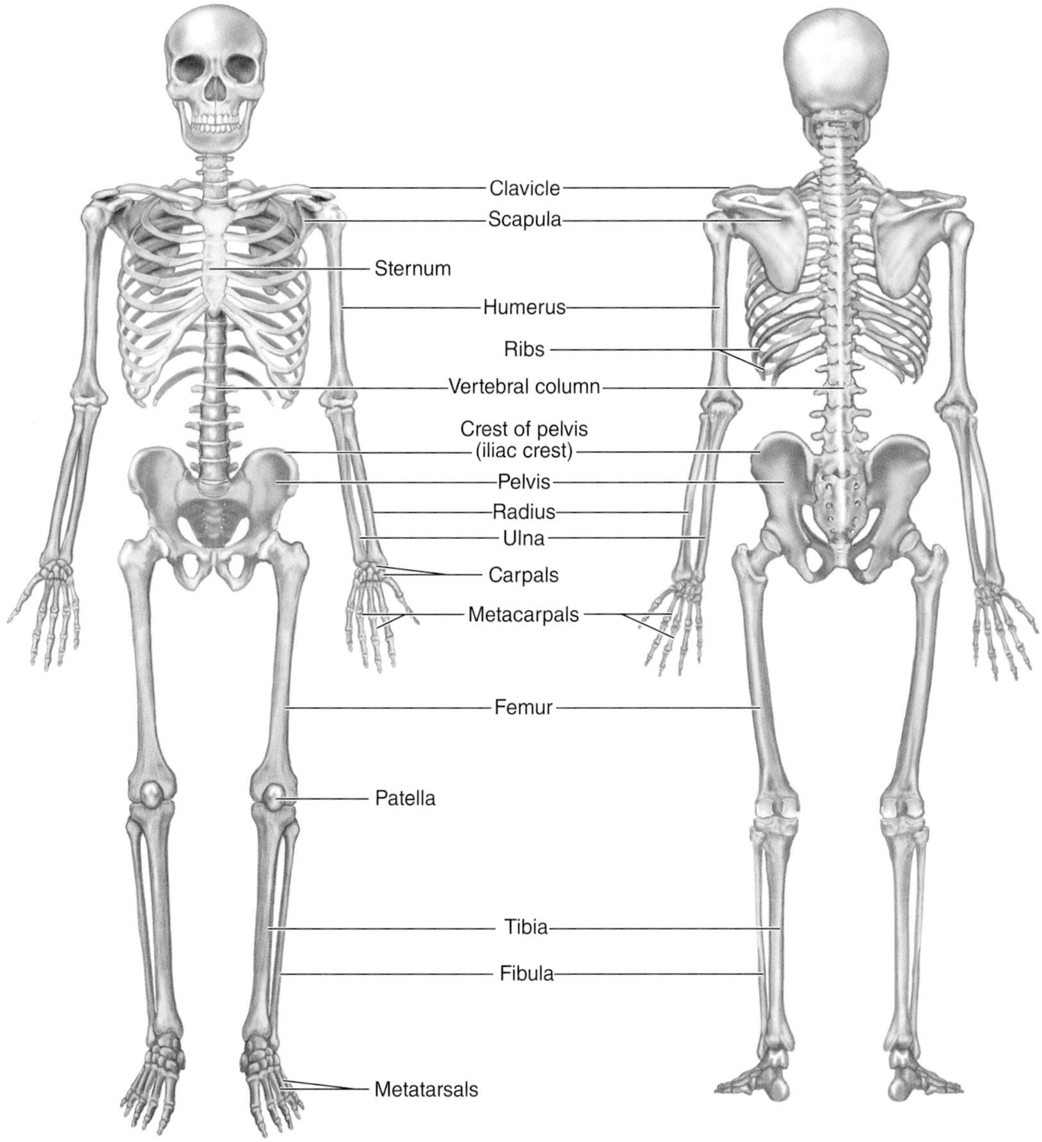

FIGURE 3.2 Anterior (front) and posterior (back) views of the human skeleton in the anatomical position.

Ossification of Bones

The skeleton begins as a cartilaginous structure that is gradually replaced by bone during growth and maturation in a process known as **ossification**. This process begins at the diaphysis of long bones (in centers of ossification) and spreads toward the epiphyses. The **epiphyseal plates** between the diaphyses and epiphyses are the growth areas where the cartilage is replaced by bone; bone growth continues in length and width until the epiphyseal plates are completely ossified. During growth, cartilage is added first and then eventually replaced by bone. When no further cartilage is produced and the cartilage has been replaced by bone, growth ceases. Secondary centers of ossification develop in the epiphyses and in some bony protuberances, such as the tibial tuberosity and the articular condyles of the humerus; however, short bones have one center of ossification. The age when growth plates close varies among individuals. Although bone fusion at some centers of ossification may occur by puberty or earlier, most of the long bones do not completely ossify until the late teens. Premature closing, which results in a shorter bone length, can be caused by trauma, abnormal stresses, or malnutrition.

KEY POINT

Ossification is the replacement of cartilage with bone during growth. Generally, bone growth is completed by the late teens.

Planes and Axes of Movement

Anatomical terminology enables the accurate description of position and movement of the human body. To describe joint movements, reference is made to rotation around one or more of three axes and to movement in one of three cardinal planes. These planes are perpendicular to each other and represent a side view (sagittal plane), front or back view (frontal or coronal plane), and top view, looking down from above (transverse plane). Movement observed in each plane is a rotation around an axis that is perpendicular to the plane. The reference position for describing movement is the anatomical position (standing erect, arms hanging at sides, palms facing forward, feet shoulder-width apart; see figure 3.3). The mediolateral axis is perpendicular to the sagittal plane, and joint rotations about this axis are flexion and extension. The anteroposterior axis is perpendicular to the frontal plane, and joint rotations about this axis are abduction and adduction. The longitudinal or vertical axis is perpendicular to the transverse plane, and rotations about this axis are internal and external rotation. Joint rotations are described according to how the distal segment (body part just below the joint) moves relative to the proximal segment (body part just above the joint).

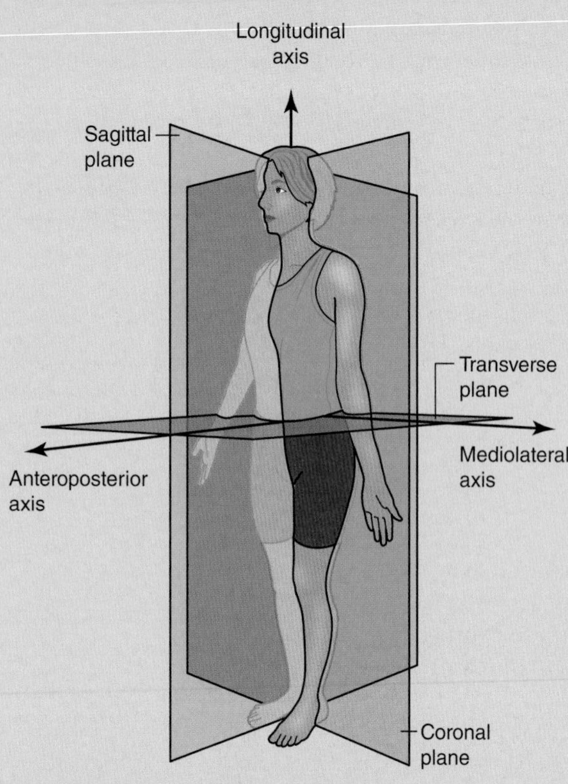

FIGURE 3.3 The anatomical position and the cardinal planes and axes of movement.

Structure and Function of Joints

Joints, which are the places where two or more bones meet, or articulate, are often classified according to the amount of movement that can take place at those sites. **Ligaments**, which are tough, fibrous bands of connective tissue, connect bones to each other across all joints. Joints are classified as synarthrodial, amphiarthrodial, or synovial based on how much they can move. **Synarthrodial joints** are immovable joints. The bones merge into each other and are bound together by fibrous tissue that is continuous with the periosteum. The sutures, or lines of junction, of the cranial (skull) bones are prime examples of this type of joint. **Amphiarthrodial joints**, or cartilaginous joints, allow only slight movement between bones. Usually a fibrocartilage disc separates the bones, and movement can occur only by deformation of the disc. Examples of these joints are the tibiofibular and sacroiliac joints and the joints between the bodies of the vertebrae in the spine.

Diarthrodial joints, more commonly known as synovial joints, are freely movable joints that allow greater movement direction and range; most of the joint movements during physical activity occur at these joints. The synovial joints are the most common type and include most joints of the extremities. Strong, inelastic ligaments, along with connective and muscle tissue crossing the joint, maintain their stability. Synovial joints have several distinguishing characteristics. The articulating surfaces of the bones are covered by articular cartilage, a type of hyaline cartilage that reduces friction and contributes to shock absorption between the bones. Each joint is completely enclosed by an **articular capsule**, whose thickness varies from thin and loose to thick and tight. The **synovial membrane** lines the inner surface of the capsule. It secretes synovial fluid into the **joint cavity**, the space enclosed by the articular capsule. Synovial fluid bathes the joint to nourish the articular cartilage and reduce friction when bones move. Normally, the joint cavity is small and, therefore, contains little synovial fluid, but an injury to the joint can increase the secretion of synovial fluid and cause swelling.

Some synovial joints, such as the sternoclavicular and knee joints, also have a partial or complete fibrocartilage disc between the bones to aid shock absorption and, in the case of the knee, to give greater stability to the joint. The partial, C-shaped discs between the femur and the tibia at the knee are called **menisci**. To reduce friction or rubbing as tendons move during muscle contraction, tendons often are surrounded by tendon sheaths—cylindrical, tunnel-like sacs lined with synovial membrane. For example, the two proximal tendons of the biceps brachii pass through these tunnels in the bicipital groove of the humerus. **Bursae**, or sacs of synovial fluid that lie between muscles, tendons, and bones, also reduce friction between the tissues and act as shock absorbers. Many bursae are found around the shoulder, elbow, hip, and knee. Bursitis, or the inflammation of a bursa, can result from repeated friction or mechanical irritation.

The primary movement at a joint is rotation about one or more axes. Some joints may exhibit a small amount of sliding (translation) between the bones. The limits to direction and range of motion (ROM) at a joint are determined primarily by the shape of the bones at their articulating ends. Depending on the bone shape, joints may rotate about one, two, or three axes.

The type of joint determines the movements that occur within that joint:

- Ball-and-socket joints, which are found at the hip and shoulder, allow a wide range of movement in all directions as the ball rotates within the socket.
- Hinge joints, such as the elbow and ankle joints, have only one axis of rotation due to the structure of the interlocking bones.
- Other types of joints include ellipsoidal joints, such as the wrist, and saddle joints, such as the sternoclavicular joint, whose shapes permit rotation about two axes.
- Pivot joints, such as the proximal radioulnar joint, permit rotation about one axis only, the longitudinal axis.
- Gliding joints, such as between the tarsal bones in the foot, have minimal sliding movement between the bones.

The length of the ligaments and to a lesser extent their **elasticity**, or ability to stretch passively and return to their normal length, also limit ROM. For example, the iliofemoral ligament at the anterior hip joint is a strong but short ligament that prohibits much hip extension.

KEY POINT

The moveable joints in the body are diarthrodial (synovial) joints. The bony surfaces are covered in smooth articular cartilage and the joint cavity is filled with synovial fluid, which lubricates the joint. The limits to range and direction of motion at a joint are determined by the shape of the articulating bones and the length of ligaments crossing the joint.

Joint Movements

Specific terminology is used to describe the direction of movement at the various joints. This ensures that movements are described accurately and can be immediately understood. The anatomical position (see figure 3.3) serves as a point of reference. Terminology generally relates to movements within planes and about axes. Flexion and extension are movements in the sagittal plane about a mediolateral axis. **Flexion** is moving the distal segment forward and upward from the anatomical position to bring two body segments closer together. **Extension** is the return from flexion, moving the segment in the opposite direction. Abduction and adduction are movements in the frontal plane about an anteroposterior axis. **Abduction** is moving the distal segment out to the side and away from the body from the anatomical position, whereas **adduction** is the return toward the anatomical position from abduction, moving the segment in the opposite direction. Internal and external rotation are movements in the transverse plane about a longitudinal axis. **Internal rotation** is turning a segment toward the midline of the body from the anatomical position. **External rotation** is the return toward the anatomical position, turning the segment in the opposite direction. Exceptions to these general descriptions are noted where they occur for specific joints.

The body can be divided into two regions: the axial skeleton and the appendicular skeleton. The axial skeleton forms the main axis of the body and consists of the bones and joints of the vertebral column. The appendicular skeleton consists of all four extremities, which are appended (attached) to the axial skeleton. We can further subdivide the appendicular skeleton into the upper extremities and lower extremities.

VIDEO

Watch **video 3.1**, which demonstrates joint movements and actions.

KEY POINT

Synovial joints rotate about one or more of the three primary axes of movement in the body, with some joints having additional movements (table 3.1). Anatomical terminology enables these movements to be described accurately and concisely.

Skeletal Muscle

Skeletal, or voluntary, muscles consist of thousands of muscle fibers (e.g., the brachioradialis has approximately 130,000 fibers; the gastrocnemius has more than 1 million) plus connective tissue. Each fiber is enclosed by the endomysium, a type of connective tissue. The **fascicles**, or bundles of fibers grouped together, are surrounded by the **perimysium**, and the entire muscle is enclosed by the **epimysium**. The **tendon** is the passive part of the muscle and is made up of elastic connective tissue. Each muscle attaches to bone at the periosteum or alternatively to deep, thick fascial tissue via tendons and the perimysium and epimysium connective tissues. The size and shape of tendons depend on the functions and shape of the muscles. Some tendons can be easily seen and palpated just under the surface of the skin, such as the hamstring muscle tendons at the sides of the posterior aspect of the knee and the Achilles tendon inserting into the posterior heel. Other muscles, such as the supraspinatus and infraspinatus (muscles of the rotator cuff in the shoulder), are attached directly to the bone with no observable tendon. Broad and flat tendons, such as the proximal tendinous sheath of the latissimus dorsi, are **aponeuroses**. Refer to figure 3.4 for anterior and posterior views of surface muscles. Other muscles lie underneath the surface muscles.

Forces That Cause Movement

Joint movement is caused primarily by either the shortening of a muscle or the action of gravity, although other forces, such as another person pushing or pulling on a body part, may cause joint movement. Whether a muscle contraction causes movement depends on the combined effect of the force developed and the amount of resistance from other forces.

Forces That Resist or Prevent Movement

The same forces that can cause movement may also resist or prevent movement. Joint movement caused by gravity can be resisted or decelerated by eccentric muscle action (which lengthens the muscle; see the section on eccentric action later in the chapter). Gravity always resists

Table 3.1 Movements at Main Synovial Joints

Joint	Movements
AXIAL SKELETON	
Vertebral column	Flexion, extension; lateral flexion; rotation
Lumbosacral joint	Anterior pelvic tilt, posterior pelvic tilt
APPENDICULAR SKELETON: UPPER EXTREMITY	
Shoulder girdle (scapulothoracic joint)	Elevation, depression; protraction (abduction), retraction (adduction); upward rotation, downward rotation
Shoulder joint (glenohumeral joint)	Flexion, extension; abduction, adduction; internal rotation, external rotation; horizontal adduction, horizontal abduction
Elbow joint	Flexion, extension
Radioulnar joint	Pronation, supination
Wrist joint	Flexion, extension; abduction (radial flexion), adduction (ulnar flexion)
Metacarpophalangeal joints	Flexion, extension; abduction, adduction
APPENDICULAR SKELETON: LOWER EXTREMITY	
Hip joint	Flexion, extension; abduction, adduction; internal rotation, external rotation
Knee joint	Flexion, extension
Ankle joint	Plantar flexion, dorsiflexion
Subtalar joint	Eversion, inversion

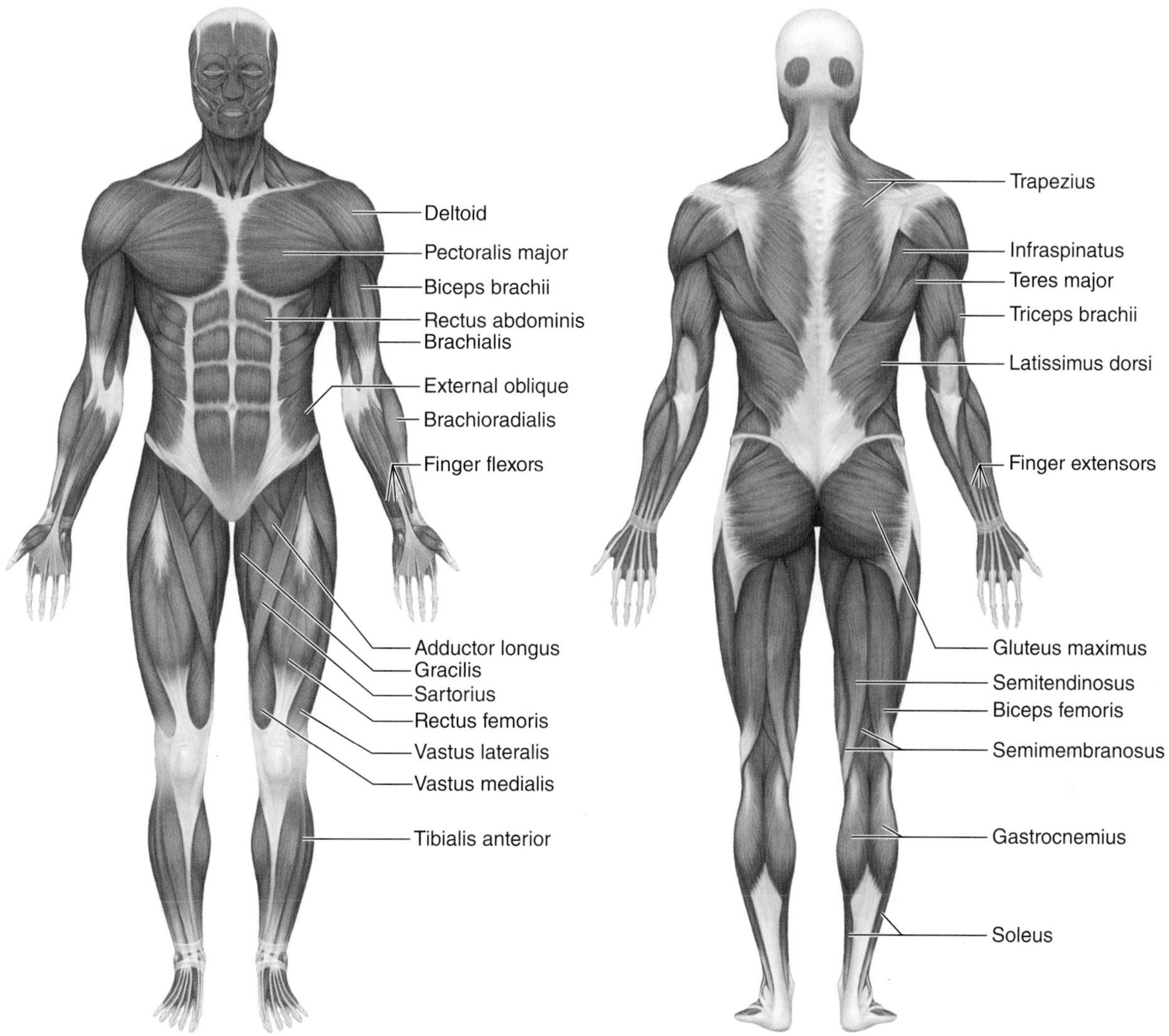

FIGURE 3.4 Anterior (front) and posterior (back) views of the human body in the anatomical position with surface muscles illustrated.

movement occurring in a direction away from the earth. Other forces that can resist movement include internal soft-tissue restriction by ligaments and tendons. Outside the body, exercise bands, hydraulic or air-pressure devices on resistance training equipment, and the drag provided by air and water against bodies moving through them can resist movement.

Muscle Action

Each muscle fiber is innervated, or receives stimuli, by a branch of a motor neuron. A **motor unit** consists of a single motor neuron, its branches, and all the muscle fibers that it innervates. With a sufficiently strong stimulus, each muscle fiber within that motor unit responds maximally; muscular tension increases as a result of the stimulation of more motor units (**recruitment**) or an increased rate of stimulation (summation). A muscle whose primary purpose is a strength or power movement (e.g., the gastrocnemius) rather than a delicate movement (e.g., the finger muscles) has a large number of muscle fibers and many muscle fibers per motor unit. When a muscle develops tension, it tends to shorten toward the middle, pulling on all of its bony attachments. Whether the attached bones move as a result of that muscle action depends on the amount of muscle force and the resistance to that movement from other forces. The three major muscle actions are concentric, eccentric, and isometric.

Concentric Action

Concentric action occurs when a muscle shortens under tension. This shortening pulls the points of attachment on each bone closer to each other, causing movement at the joint. Figure 3.5 illustrates elbow flexion moving a dumbbell against gravity as a result of a concentric action. The muscles responsible for flexion act with sufficient force to shorten, which pulls the forearm toward the humerus.

Although the pull is on all the bones of attachment, usually only the bone farthest from the trunk (i.e., more distal) moves during a concentric action. To stand up from a semisquat position, the body must extend at the hip joints and knee joints, but gravity resists that extension. The muscles must develop sufficient force to overcome the force of gravity as the muscle shortens in a concentric action, pulling on the bones to cause extension. Resistance training with free weights uses gravity as the resistance. The use of pulleys in resistance training machines changes the direction of the force needed to overcome gravity acting on the weight stack, offering resistance to movement in other directions. Water resists the movement of submerged body parts in all directions.

To exercise muscles by using gravity as the resisting force, the movements must be done in the direction opposite the pull of gravity (i.e., away from the earth). Shoulder abduction from a standing position occurs opposite the pull of gravity, so a concentric action is required by the muscles that will pull the humerus into the abducted position. Movements such as shoulder horizontal abduction and adduction executed from a standing position occur parallel to the ground and, therefore, are not resisted by gravity. During these movements, gravity is still trying to draw the upper limb toward the earth (requiring concentric action of the shoulder abductors to overcome it). To perform horizontal abduction and adduction against the resistance of gravity, the performer must get into a position in which these movements are away from the pull of gravity. To horizontally abduct the shoulder against gravity, the performer can lie prone on a bench or stand with the trunk flexed 90° at the hip. Horizontal adduction against gravity can be done from a supine position on a bench.

A concentric action is also necessary for a rapid movement, regardless of the direction of other forces. When an external force could cause the desired movement without any muscular action but would be too slow, concentric actions produce the desired speed. An example of this is seen in the upper-limb movements during the second count of a jumping jack, when the arms adduct from their abducted position. Gravity would adduct the arms, but concentrically acting muscles speed up the adduction.

A muscle that is very effective in causing a certain joint movement is a prime mover, or **agonist**. Assistant movers are muscles that are not as effective for the same movement. For example, the peroneus longus and brevis are prime movers for eversion of the foot, but they assist plantar flexion of the ankle joint only a little. During a concentric action, muscles that act opposite to the muscles causing the concentric action, the **antagonist** muscles, are mostly passive and lengthen as the agonists shorten. For example, for the elbow to flex against gravity, the muscles responsible for elbow flexion act concentrically, while the antagonists, or the muscles responsible for elbow extension, relax and lengthen passively.

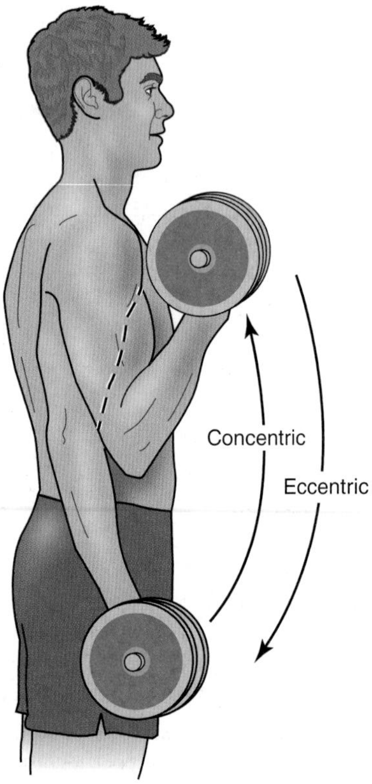

FIGURE 3.5 Concentric and eccentric action of the elbow flexors during a biceps curl.

VIDEO Watch **video 3.2**, which shows concentric and eccentric muscle actions as demonstrated in the biceps curl.

Eccentric Action

An **eccentric action** occurs when a muscle generates tension that is not great enough to cause movement but instead slows the speed of movement in the opposite direction caused by another force (see figure 3.5). The muscle exerts force, but its length increases while it is under tension. Shoulder abduction requires concentric action, but gravity will adduct the upper limb back to the side of the body. To adduct the upper limb more slowly than gravity does, the same muscles that acted concentrically to abduct the upper limb now act eccentrically to control the speed of the upper limb. Eccentric actions may also occur when the maximum effort of a muscle is not great enough to overcome the opposing force. Movement due to the opposing force will still occur despite the maximally activated muscle, which is lengthening under tension. An example of this may occur when a person with the elbow joint flexed to 90° is handed a heavy weight. The exerciser tries to flex the elbow joint or even maintain the 90° position but lacks the strength to do so. The elbow joint extends despite the efforts to flex it. Muscles that are antagonists to the eccentrically acting muscles will passively shorten during the movement.

Ballistic Movement

A **ballistic movement** is a fast movement that occurs when resistance is minimal, as in throwing a ball, and requires a burst of concentric action to initiate it. Once movement has begun, these initial muscles relax because any further action would slow the movement. Other muscles actively guide the movement in the appropriate direction. At the end of the movement, eccentric action of muscles that are antagonist to the initial muscles decelerates and stops the movement. For example, one of the most important movements in throwing is internal rotation of the shoulder joint. The muscles responsible for internal rotation act quickly and concentrically to begin the throwing motion. After the ball is released, the muscles responsible for external rotation act eccentrically to slow and stop the movement during the follow-through. The reverse is true for the windup, or preparation for the actual throw.

Jumping jacks require repeated ballistic movements in which opposing muscles come into play. The upper-limb movements require concentric action by the agonist muscles to initiate the rapid movement. Once the movement is initiated, these muscles relax. To stop the abduction movement and initiate the upper-limb movement in the opposite direction, muscles antagonistic to those that acted concentrically act eccentrically to decelerate the movement and then act concentrically to initiate the next movement (adduction).

Isometric Action

During an **isometric action**, or static action, the muscle exerts a force that is equal in magnitude to an opposing force. The muscle length does not change and the joint position is maintained: The contractile part of the muscle shortens, but the elastic connective tissue lengthens proportionately, so there is no overall change in the entire muscle length. Holding the upper limb in an abducted position or maintaining a semisquat position requires isometric action, producing just enough muscle force to counteract the pull of gravity and result in no movement. The effort involved in trying to move an immovable object (e.g., pushing against a wall) is another example of an isometric action; although the amount of muscular force can be maximal, the joint does not move (see figure 3.6).

The posterior pelvic tilt desired during some exercises is maintained by isometric action of the anterior trunk muscles after they have acted concentrically to tilt the pelvis backward. During all resistance exercises that involve the arms or legs, the trunk muscles should act isometrically to stabilize the trunk and help prevent injury.

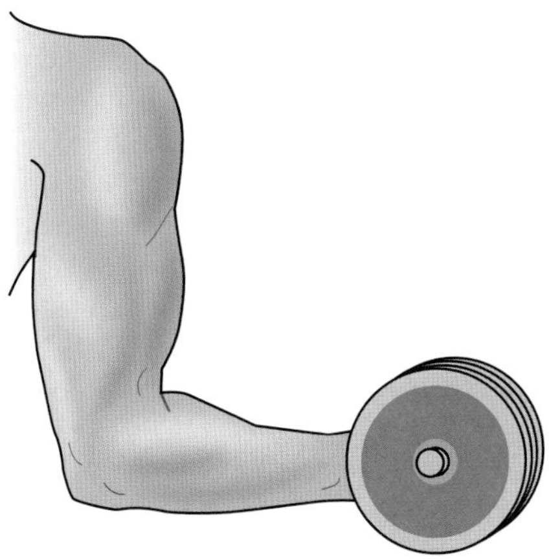

FIGURE 3.6 Isometric action of the elbow flexor muscles holding a dumbbell.

KEY POINT

During concentric muscle action, the muscle shortens and the joint moves in the direction the muscle is pulling. During eccentric muscle action, the muscle lengthens and the joint moves in the opposite direction than the muscle is pulling. During isometric muscle contraction, there is no change in length and the joint does not move.

Role of Muscles

Skeletal muscles can act in several ways and have a variety of effects on joint movement. They can cause movement via concentric action or decelerate movement caused by another force via eccentric action. Muscles may also act isometrically to stabilize or prevent undesirable movement. For example, during a push-up, gravity tends to cause the lumbar spine to hyperextend. Isometric action of the trunk muscles prevents this sagging and stabilizes the lumbar region in a neutral position.

Another function of muscle is to counteract an undesirable action caused by the concentric action of another muscle. The concentric action of many muscles causes more than one movement at the same joint or causes movement at more than one joint. If only one of those movements is intended, another muscle must act to prevent the undesirable movement. For example, concentric action of fibers in the upper trapezius both elevates and adducts the scapula. If only adduction is desired, fibers in the lower trapezius, which cause depression and adduction, neutralize the undesirable scapula elevation. In this example, different fibers of the same large trapezius muscle neutralize the unwanted action. As another example, the biceps brachii causes both elbow flexion and radioulnar supination, so for only flexion to occur, the pronator teres counteracts the supination movement.

Muscles can also guide movements caused by other muscles. During activities against a great resistance, such as lifting free weights, additional muscles help maintain balance and proper direction of the movement. After the force of a prime mover has initiated a ballistic movement, other muscles guide the movement in the proper direction.

KEY POINT

The major roles of the muscles are to cause movement (concentric action) regardless of an opposing force, decelerate or control the speed of movement (eccentric action) caused by another force, and prevent movement (isometric action). Other muscle functions include counteracting an undesirable action caused by the concentric action of another muscle and guiding movements caused by another muscle.

Muscle Groups

A **muscle group** includes all of the muscles that cause the same movement at the same joint. The group is named for the joint where the movement takes place and for the movement commonly caused by the concentric action of those muscles. The elbow flexors, for example, are a muscle group composed of the muscles responsible for flexion at the elbow joint when the muscles act concentrically. Table 3.2 lists the prime and assistant movers at each joint. A muscle group may also act eccentrically to control the opposite motion at the joint. For example, the elbow flexor muscle group flexes the elbow joint during an elbow curl. To return to the starting position, the pull of gravity extends the joint to the original position, but the elbow flexor muscle group is still exerting force to eccentrically control the speed of that movement. Maintaining the elbow in a flexed position requires an isometric action by those same elbow flexors (see figure 3.6). Specific muscles that cause more than one action at a joint or cause movement at more than one joint belong to more than one muscle group. For example, the flexor carpi ulnaris belongs in both the wrist flexor and wrist adductor muscle groups, and the biceps brachii is part of the elbow flexor and radioulnar supinator muscle groups.

Table 3.2 Muscle Groups at Each Joint

Joint	Prime movers (assistant movers)
	AXIAL SKELETON
Vertebral column (thoracic and lumbar areas)	Flexors—rectus abdominis, external oblique, internal oblique
	Extensors—erector spinae group
	Rotators—internal oblique, external oblique, erector spinae, rotatores, multifidus
	Lateral flexors—internal oblique, external oblique, quadratus, lumborum, multifidus, rotatores (erector spinae group)
Lumbosacral joint	Anterior pelvic tilters—iliopsoas (rectus femoris)
	Posterior pelvic tilters—rectus abdominis, internal oblique (external oblique, gluteus maximus)
	APPENDICULAR SKELETON: UPPER EXTREMITY
Shoulder girdle (scapulothoracic joint)	Protractors—serratus anterior, pectoralis minor
	Retractors—middle fibers of trapezius, rhomboids (upper and lower fibers of trapezius)
	Upward rotators—upper and lower fibers of trapezius, serratus anterior
	Downward rotators—rhomboids, pectoralis minor
	Elevators—levator scapulae, upper fibers of trapezius rhomboids
	Depressors—lower fibers of trapezius, pectoralis minor

Joint	Prime movers (assistant movers)
	APPENDICULAR SKELETON: UPPER EXTREMITY
Shoulder joint (glenohumeral joint)	Flexors—anterior deltoid, clavicular portion of pectoralis major (short head of biceps brachii)
	Extensors—sternal portion of pectoralis major, latissimus dorsi, teres major (posterior deltoid, long head of triceps brachii, infraspinatus, teres minor)
	Abductors—middle deltoid, supraspinatus (anterior deltoid, long head of biceps brachii)
	Adductors—latissimus dorsi, teres major, sternal portion of pectoralis major (short head of biceps brachii, long head of triceps brachii)
	External rotators—infraspinatus,* teres minor* (posterior deltoid)
	Internal rotators—pectoralis major, subscapularis,* latissimus dorsi, teres major (anterior deltoid, supraspinatus*)
	Horizontal adductors—both portions of pectoralis major, anterior deltoid
	Horizontal abductors—latissimus dorsi, teres major, infraspinatus, teres minor, posterior deltoid
Elbow joint	Flexors—brachialis, biceps brachii, brachioradialis (pronator teres, flexor carpi ulnaris and radialis)
	Extensors—triceps brachii (anconeus, extensor carpi ulnaris and radialis)
Radioulnar joint	Pronators—pronator quadratus, pronator teres, brachioradialis
	Supinators—supinator, biceps brachii, brachioradialis
Wrist joint	Flexors—flexor carpi ulnaris, flexor carpi radialis (flexor digitorum superficialis and profundus)
	Extensors—extensor carpi ulnaris, extensor carpi radialis longus and brevis (extensor digitorum)
	Abductors (radial flexors)—flexor carpi radialis, extensor carpi radialis longus and brevis (extensor pollicis)
	Adductors (ulnar flexors)—flexor carpi ulnaris, extensor carpi ulnaris
Metacarpophalangeal joint	Flexors—flexor digitorum superficialis, flexor digitorum profundus, flexor pollicis longus, flexor pollicis brevis, flexor digiti minimi, interossei, lumbricals
	Extensors—extensor digitorum, extensor indicis, extensor digiti minimi, extensor pollicis longus, extensor pollicis brevis, interossei
	Abductors—interossei
	Adductors—interossei
	APPENDICULAR SKELETON: LOWER EXTREMITY
Hip joint	Flexors—iliopsoas, pectineus, rectus femoris (sartorius, tensor fasciae latae, gracilis, adductor longus and brevis)
	Extensors—gluteus maximus, biceps femoris, semitendinosus, semimembranosus
	Abductors—gluteus medius (tensor fasciae latae, iliopsoas, sartorius)
	Internal rotators—gluteus maximus, the six deep external rotator muscles (iliopsoas, sartorius)
	External rotators—gluteus minimus, gluteus medius (tensor fasciae latae, pectineus)
Knee joint	Flexors—biceps femoris, semimembranosus, semitendinosus (sartorius, gracilis, gastrocnemius, plantaris)
	Extensors—rectus femoris, vastus medialis, vastus lateralis, vastus intermedius

(continued)

Table 3.2 *(continued)*

Joint	Prime movers (assistant movers)
	APPENDICULAR SKELETON: LOWER EXTREMITY
Ankle joint	Plantar flexors—gastrocnemius, soleus (peroneus longus, peroneus brevis, tibialis posterior, flexor digitorum, flexor hallucis longus)
	Dorsiflexors—tibialis anterior, extensor digitorum longus, peroneus tertius (extensor hallucis longus)
Subtalar joint	Invertors—tibialis anterior, tibialis posterior (extensor and flexor hallucis longus, flexor digitorum longus)
	Evertors—extensor digitorum longus, peroneus brevis, peroneus longus, peroneus tertius

*Rotator cuff muscles

KEY POINT

A muscle group includes all the muscles that act concentrically to cause a specific movement at a given joint.

Many errors that occur during exercise and movement activities result from a lack of knowledge of musculoskeletal anatomy rather than a lack of muscular strength or coordination. Applying basic knowledge allows exercisers to perform better and more safely. The following sections, from the axial through the appendicular skeleton, offer tips for exercising each major muscle group and avoiding common exercise mistakes.

Joints and Muscles of the Axial Skeleton

The axial skeleton forms the midline of the body. It consists of the skull, the vertebral column, and the rib cage, which attaches to the vertebral column.

Vertebral Column

The vertebral column contains 24 individual vertebrae and the sacrum. Although movement between adjacent vertebrae is just a few degrees, when combined over the whole vertebral column, the ROM of the trunk is substantial. Movements of the trunk occur in all three planes: flexion and extension, lateral flexion to the left and right, and rotation to the left and right (see figure 3.7).

Lumbosacral Joint

The pelvis (see figure 3.8) tilts mainly at the joint formed by the fifth lumbar vertebra and the sacrum. A reference for the direction of pelvic tilt is a line between the anterior and posterior superior iliac spines in the sagittal plane. When the pelvis tilts anteriorly, the angle between the horizontal and the line between the iliac spines increases. With posterior pelvic tilt, the angle of the line between the iliac spines becomes closer to the horizontal. Anterior pelvic tilt is accompanied by extension of the lumbar spine, whereas a backward tilt results in a flattening out of the lumbar spine.

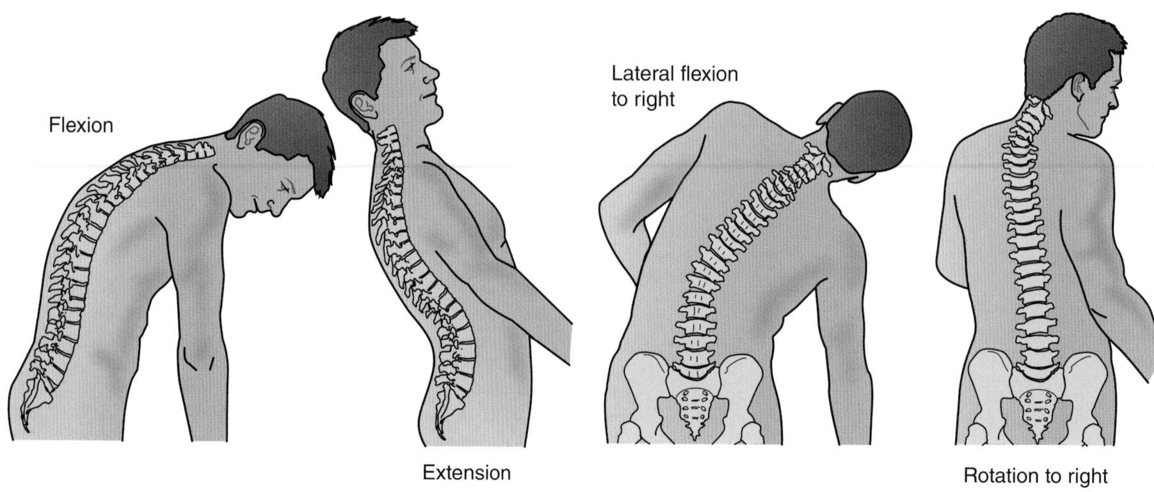

FIGURE 3.7 Movements of the vertebral column and trunk.

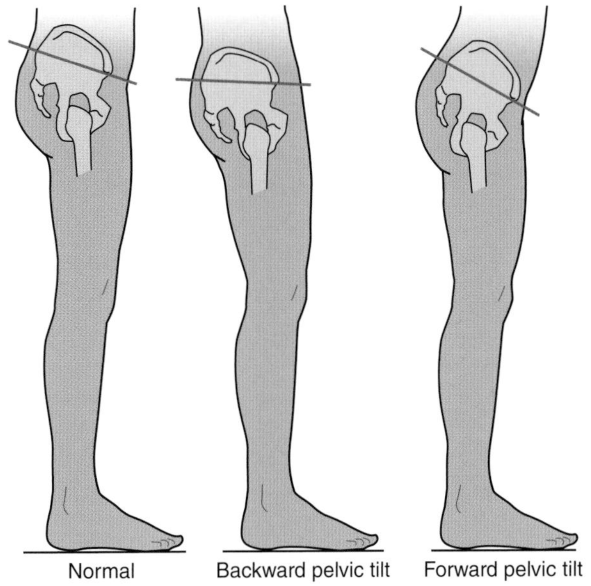

FIGURE 3.8 Movements of the lumbosacral joint and pelvis.

Exercise Tips

In general, neither neck hyperextension nor hyperflexion is desirable. The same pairs of muscles that act concentrically to cause flexion and extension can be strengthened or stretched, one side at a time, by cervical lateral flexion and rotation. Participants should tilt or turn the head from side to side rather than bend the neck forward or backward.

Many exercises require appropriate positioning of the lumbosacral joint and lumbar vertebrae and actions by the trunk muscles for either movement or stabilization. An abdominal curl-up or crunch should begin with a backward pelvic tilt that is maintained throughout the curl-up and return movement. If the backward pelvic tilt cannot be maintained or the exerciser feels tightness or an ache in the lumbar area, the exerciser should stop. If the problem is inadequate strength to maintain the backward tilt, the exercise should be modified to one that the exerciser has sufficient abdominal strength to perform correctly.

A full curl-up, in which the exerciser comes up to a sitting position, requires hip flexion by the hip flexor muscles during the last stages of the exercise. Initially, the abdominal muscles concentrically tilt the pelvis backward and then flex the vertebral column. Once flexion is achieved, these muscles act isometrically to keep the pelvis tilted backward and the trunk in a flexed position. During a full curl-up, the exerciser can feel a sticking point that occurs when the trunk flexion is complete and the hip flexors begin to bring the trunk to an upright position. Doing partial curl-ups or crunches helps eliminate the role of the hip flexors and maintain focus solely on strengthening the abdominal muscles.

The leg lift is considered an abdominal exercise, but often it is not taught correctly. From a supine position on the floor, the legs are lifted and held up by concentric and then isometric action of the hip flexors. Some of the hip flexors also pull the lumbosacral joint into a forward-tilted position. The abdominal muscles must prevent that forward tilt and maintain a flattened lumbar spine and posterior pelvic tilt. The backward pelvic tilt should precede the hip flexion, and, as in the case of the curl-up, if the proper tilt cannot be maintained, the exercise should not be done in that fashion.

The pelvis also tends to tilt forward during overhead upper-limb movements from a standing position. This can be prevented by keeping the arms in front of the ears and flexing the knees slightly.

When weights are lifted from a supine position, as in the bench press, there is a tendency to hyperextend the lumbar spine and tilt the pelvis forward. Although this tendency can allow the exerciser to lift a somewhat heavier weight, it does not increase the work of the upper limb and chest muscles, and it puts the low back into a compromising position. Bench presses are best done with the hips and knees in a flexed position and the feet on the bench or a bench extension to maintain a posterior pelvic tilt. Upright presses are best done seated with the back supported.

Joints and Muscles of the Appendicular Skeleton: Upper Extremity

The upper extremity begins at the shoulder girdle. It continues through the arm, elbow, forearm (including radioulnar joints), and wrist to the hand.

Shoulder Girdle

The primary articulation between the scapula (shoulder blade) and the thoracic cage (ribs) is not a traditional joint because there is no direct contact between the bones, which have several muscles between them. However, there is a large ROM of the scapula on the thoracic cage that has its own terminology. Vertical movements are *elevation* (upward movement) and *depression* (downward movement). Horizontal movements are *protraction* or *abduction* (out to the side) and *retraction* or *adduction* (in toward the spine). Rotational movements are *upward* and *downward rotation* (see figure 3.9). Movements of the shoulder girdle combine with movements of the shoulder joint to provide the large ROM found at the shoulder. The shoulder girdle also includes the sternoclavicular joint, between the sternum (breastbone) and clavicle (collarbone), and the acromioclavicular joint, between the scapula and clavicle. These joints move when the scapulothoracic joint moves.

Shoulder Joint

The glenohumeral joint is a ball-and-socket joint, so it can move in all directions—flexion, extension, abduction, adduction, internal and external rotation, and circumduction (tips of the fingers trace a circle in the sagittal plane). Horizontal adduction and horizontal abduction are additional movements of the upper limb toward and away from the midline when it is positioned in the transverse plane, or parallel to the ground (see figure 3.10).

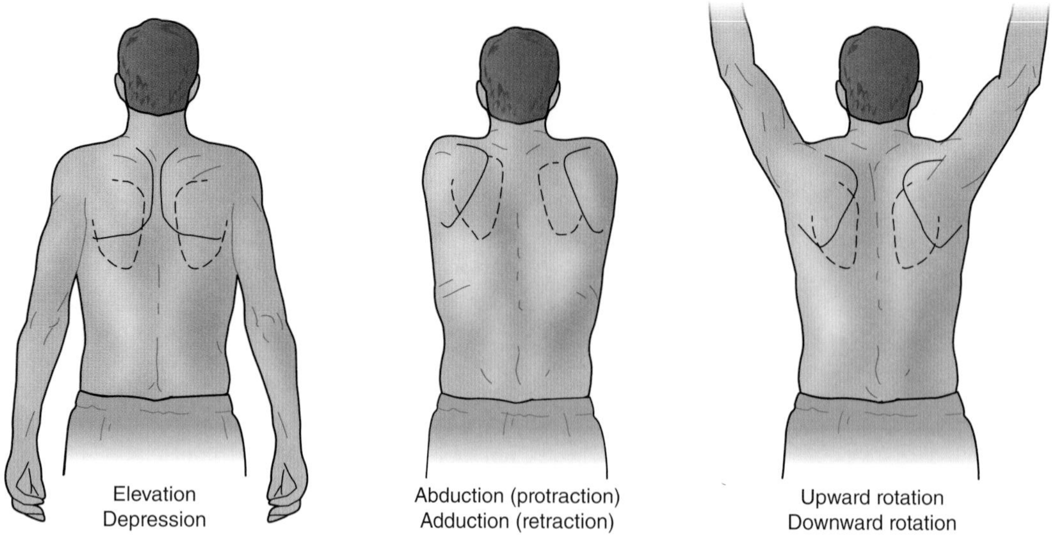

FIGURE 3.9 Movements of the scapulae (scapulothoracic joint).

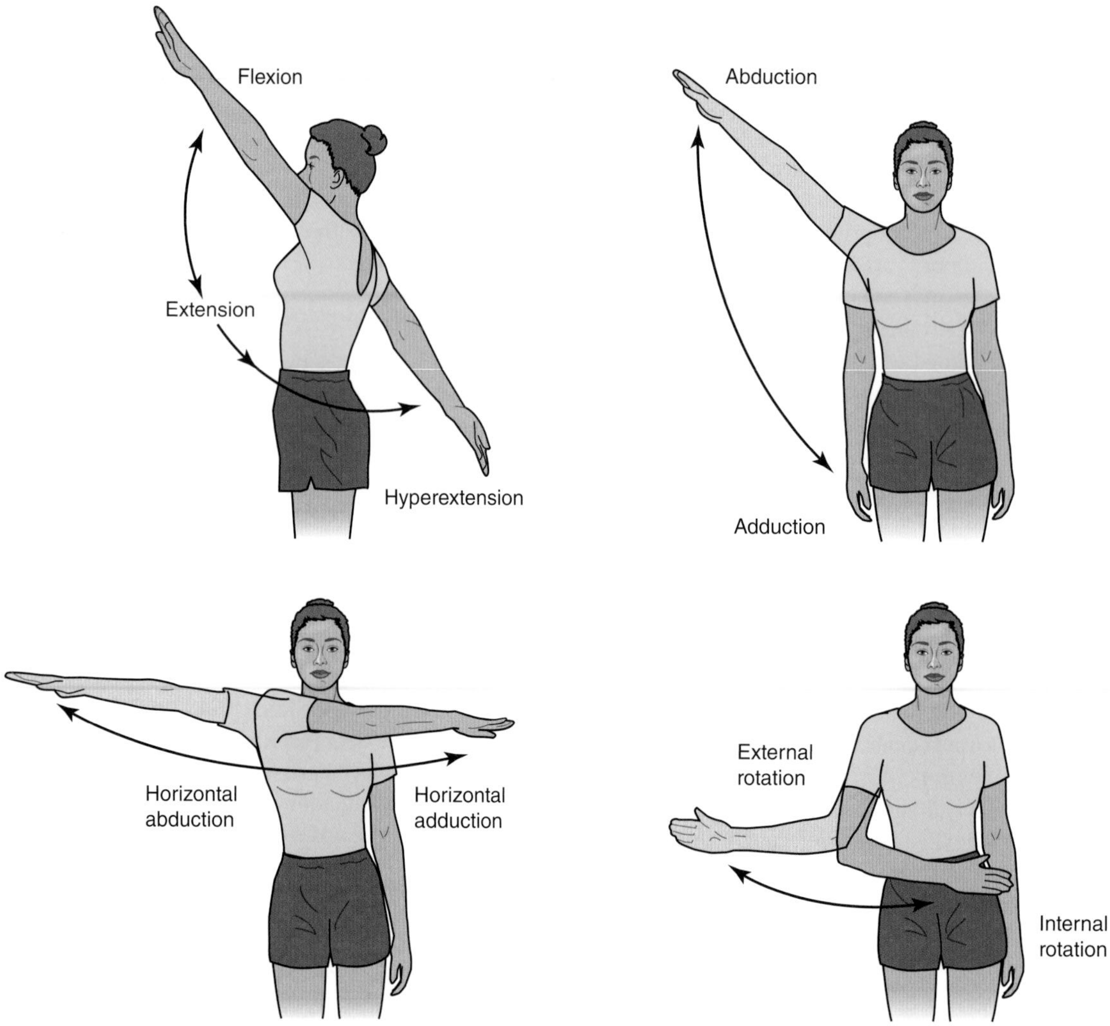

FIGURE 3.10 Movements of the shoulder (glenohumeral) joint.

The relationship between the scapulothoracic and shoulder joints is called *scapulohumeral rhythm*. The glenohumeral joint alone cannot reach the full ROM seen at the shoulder because it is restricted by the bone structure at the joint. However, the glenoid fossa that makes up part of the glenohumeral joint is part of the scapula, so if the scapula also moves, greater ROM can occur.

Elbow Joint

The elbow joint is the articulation between the humerus and the two forearm bones, the radius and ulna. The ulnohumeral joint is the primary joint, and as a hinge joint, it limits movements to flexion and extension (see figure 3.11). The radiohumeral joint is also part of the elbow joint, but it does not provide much bony stability. The ability of some people to hyperextend the elbow joint is due to differences in the shape of their articulating surfaces.

Radioulnar Joints

The radius and ulna articulate with each other both proximally and distally in the forearm. The joint movements are pronation and supination (see figure 3.12). Although the wrist is not involved in these movements, the position of the radioulnar joints can be identified by the direction the palms face. When the arms hang down alongside the trunk, the palms face forward in the supinated position and toward the back in the pronated position. In the supinated position, the radius and ulna are parallel with each other; in the pronated position, the radius lies across and on top of the ulna.

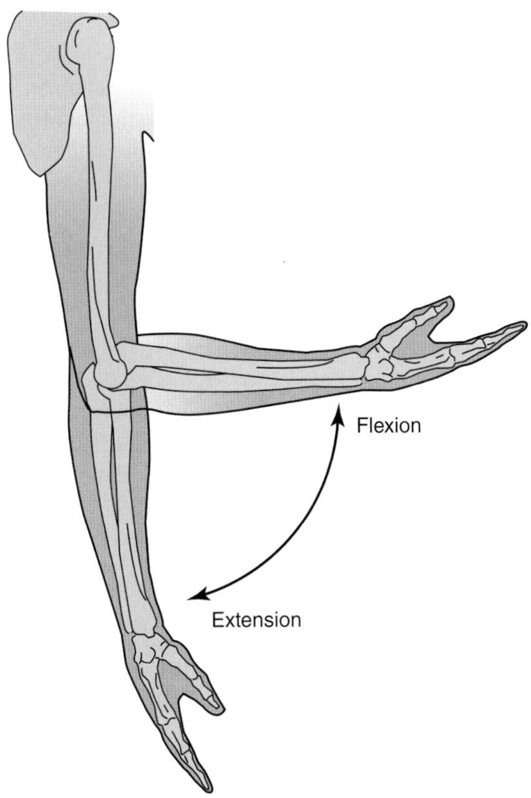

FIGURE 3.11 Movements of the elbow joint.

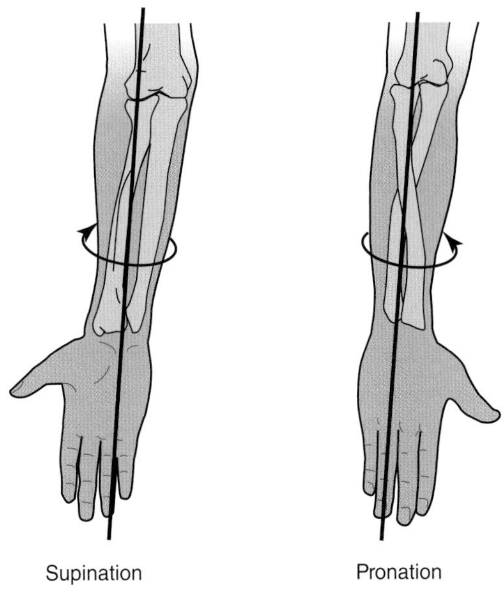

FIGURE 3.12 Movements of the radioulnar joints.

Wrist Joint

The wrist joint consists of the radiocarpal and ulnocarpal articulations between the forearm bones and the carpal bones of the wrist. Movements at the wrist include joint flexion, extension, abduction (radial flexion), and adduction (ulnar flexion) (see figure 3.13).

Metacarpophalangeal Joints of the Hand

The metacarpophalangeal joints are the knuckles of the hand. The second through the fifth joints move in flexion and extension as well as abduction and adduction of the fingers. The metacarpophalangeal joint of the thumb allows only flexion and extension. The ability of the opposable thumb to touch the tips of all the other digits comes from movement at the carpometacarpal joint. The interphalangeal joints of the fingers and thumb are hinge joints that flex and extend.

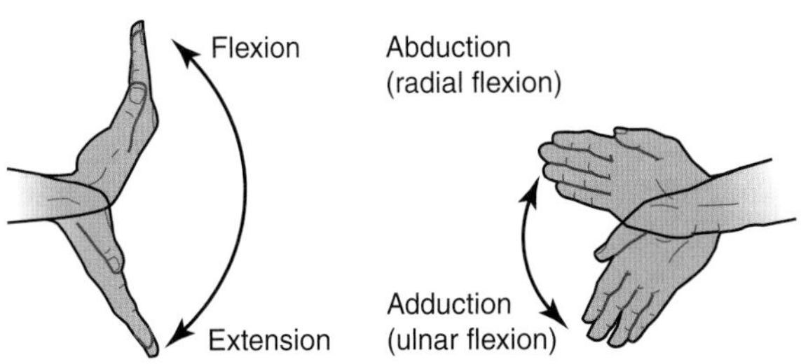

FIGURE 3.13 Movements of the wrist joint.

Exercise Tips

This section offers tips for exercising muscles of the upper extremity. Functional movements as well as exercises with weights are suggested.

Shoulder Girdle and Shoulder Joint Muscles Movement can be enhanced and more muscles involved if shoulder girdle movements are deliberately incorporated with shoulder joint movements. These muscles can be optimally involved in the following exercises and movements:

- Forward reaching. Glenohumeral joint flexion can be accompanied by scapular elevation and upward rotation if the exerciser reaches the fingertips as far forward as possible.
- Push-up. At the completion of a push-up, the scapulae can be protracted to raise the chest a bit more off the floor.
- Overhead reaching. Normally, some scapular elevation is involved when the upper limb is overhead. A conscious effort to reach as high as possible will involve the scapula elevators more. Conversely, a deliberate attempt to keep the shoulders down and the neck long requires concentric action by the scapula depressors.
- Sideward reaching. During horizontal abduction at the shoulder joint, the upper limb can be moved farther back with scapular retraction.

Elbow and Radioulnar Joint Muscles Flexion against resistance requires concentric action of the flexor muscles at the elbow joint. The degree to which these muscles are strengthened, however, is affected by supination and pronation—a good point to remember when instructing participants on how to perform curls. The biceps brachii attaches to the radius, and this bone rotates when the forearm pronates, stretching out the biceps and reducing its contribution to elbow flexion. Thus, elbow flexion with the radioulnar joint in a pronated position (a reverse curl) is a weaker movement than a traditional curl with the forearm in a supinated position. The brachialis muscle is not affected by the position of the radioulnar joint because it is attached to the ulna; therefore, its relationship to the humerus does not change with pronation and supination of the radius. Thus, a reverse curl puts more emphasis on the brachialis at the expense of the biceps. Further, the brachioradialis muscle can act with more force when the radioulnar joint is in a neutral position midway between pronation and supination. The elbow extensor muscles are not affected by the position of the radioulnar joint. Triceps push-downs, in which elbow extension occurs with the radioulnar joints in the pronated position, require the wrist flexors to stabilize the wrist joint, whereas triceps pull-downs (supinated position) utilize the wrist extensors, which are usually much weaker than the flexors. Exercisers who want to concentrate on building the elbow extensors should perform triceps push-downs.

Wrist Joint Muscles During wrist flexion and extension curls, the wrist muscles are affected by the position of the radioulnar joints. Gravity acts as resistance for wrist flexion when the radioulnar joints are in the supinated position and as resistance for extension when the radioulnar joints are in the pronated position.

Metacarpophalangeal Joint Muscles These gripping muscles can be strengthened in flexion by squeezing a small rubber ball. The extensor, adductor, and abductor muscles can be strengthened by placing a rubber band over the fingers and moving various combinations of fingers in adduction and abduction against the resistance of the band.

Joints and Muscles of the Appendicular Skeleton: Lower Extremity

The lower extremity begins at the pelvic girdle. It continues through the hip, thigh, knee, leg, and ankle to the foot.

Hip Joint

The hip joint is a ball-and-socket joint similar to the shoulder (glenohumeral joint), but the bony socket at the hip is much deeper compared with the shoulder. The deep socket makes the hip more stable than the shoulder at the expense of total ROM (see figure 3.14). For example, there is less extension at the hip than at the shoulder. Movements at the hip joint are flexion, extension, abduction, adduction, internal rotation, external rotation, and circumduction (a movement combining flexion, extension, abduction, and adduction that results in the foot moving in a circular motion).

Knee Joint

The tibiofemoral joint is the primary knee joint. The knee does not have good bony stability in flexion due to the flattened surface of the tibial plateau; therefore, it relies on ligaments to provide stability, making it vulnerable to injury. Flexion and extension are the major movements at the knee (see figure 3.15). When the knee is in a flexed position, limited rotation, abduction, and adduction are possible.

Ankle Joint

Also called the **talocrural joint**, the ankle joint is limited to movement in one plane only. Plantar flexion is pointing the foot downward and dorsiflexion is pulling the foot up toward the shin (see figure 3.16).

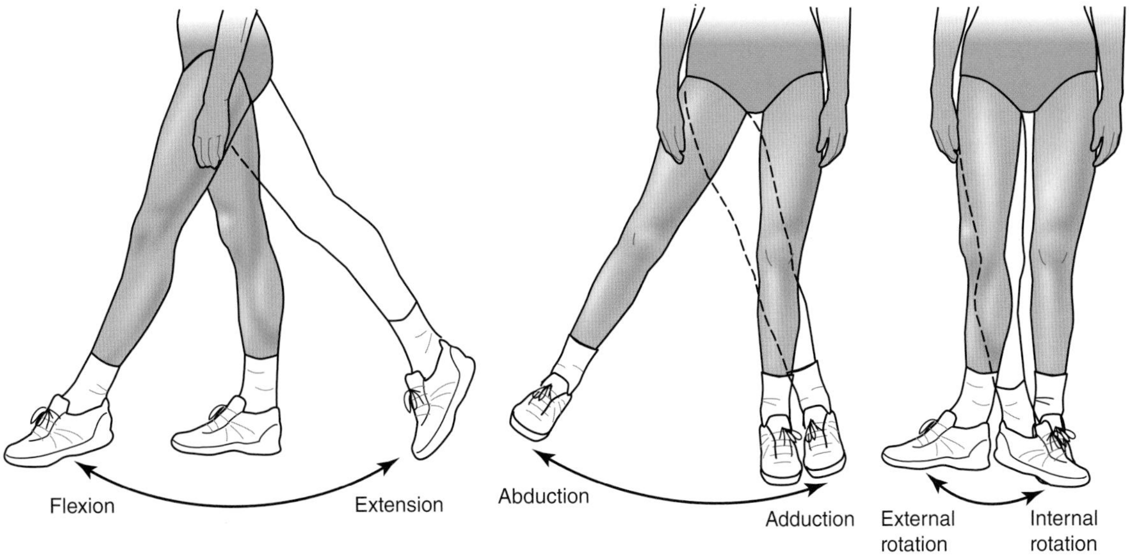

FIGURE 3.14 Movements of the hip joint.

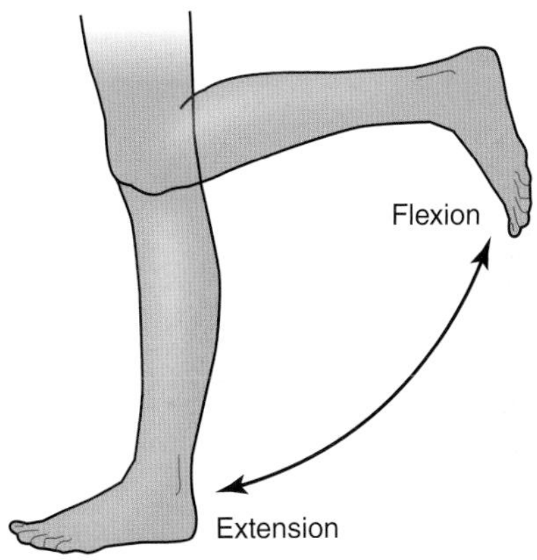

FIGURE 3.15 Movements of the knee joint.

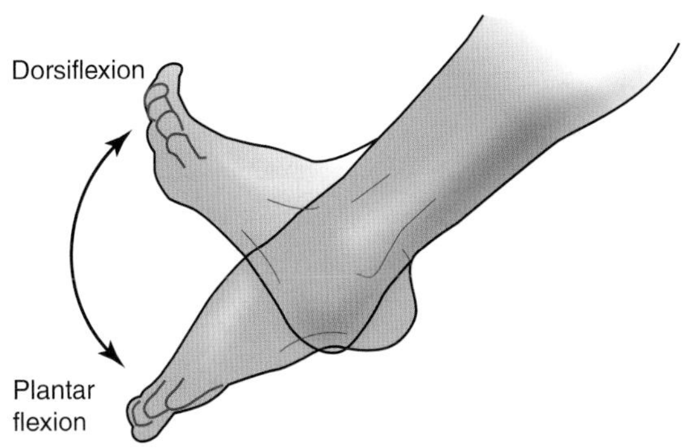

FIGURE 3.16 Movements of the ankle joint.

Subtalar Joint

The subtalar joint contributes to pronation and supination movements of the foot. In the frontal plane, these movements are eversion and inversion (see figure 3.17). In combination with other foot joints, the subtalar joint lowers the medial longitudinal arch (pronation) via a combination of eversion, dorsiflexion, and abduction. The opposite movement is supination, and it raises the arch via a combination of inversion, plantar flexion, and adduction.

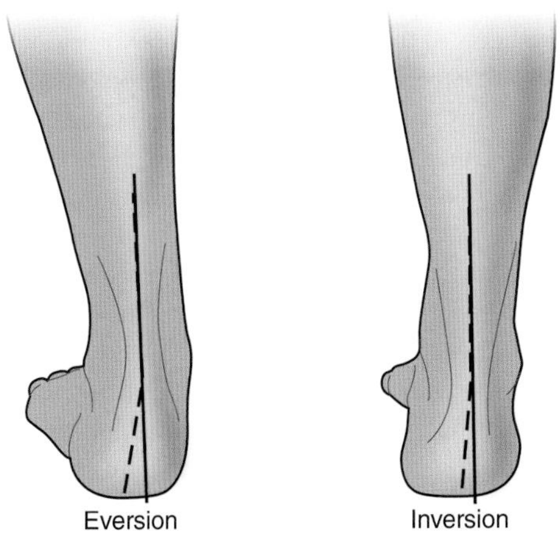

FIGURE 3.17 Movements of the subtalar joint. Left foot is everted and right foot is inverted.

Reprinted from J. Johnson, 2011, *Postural assessment* (Champaign, IL: Human Kinetics), 63.

Exercise Tips

This section offers tips for exercising muscles of the lower extremity. Functional movements as well as exercises with weights are suggested.

Hip Joint Muscles A common error during side-lying leg raises for the hip abductors is the attempt to move the foot as high as possible. Because the ROM for true abduction is limited (about 45°), the exerciser will externally rotate the top limb, which turns the foot out and allows it to go higher. However, this rotation changes the muscle involvement more to the hip flexors. To exercise the primary abductor muscles, the limb should not be rotated and the toes should face forward, not upward.

In backward lower-limb movements for strengthening the gluteus muscles, hip extension is limited primarily by the tightness of the hip ligaments. A limb can appear to be more extended if it is accompanied by a forward pelvic tilt. The exerciser should be cautioned to keep the pelvis in its neutral position in order to focus on the gluteal muscles, even though some apparent hip extension is lost.

Knee Joint Muscles Hyperflexion can strain and stretch knee ligaments and put pressure on the menisci. Therefore, a maximum squat depth to a 90° angle at the knee joint is recommended. During any lunging movements or forward–back stride positions in which the front knee is flexed, the knee should be over or in back of the foot and not in front. Any knee position that puts a twisting pressure on the knee joint should also be avoided. The hurdler position, with one limb out to the back and side with a flexed knee, should be avoided; instead, both legs should be out in front.

A common exercise position is standing with feet shoulder-width apart. The exerciser should have the feet turned slightly outward (7°-10°). The appropriate toe-out position is one that positions the kneecaps facing forward. During any squatting or standing movement, the knee should be in line directly above the foot (not moving to the outside or inside of the foot) to avoid straining the lateral and medial knee ligaments and to develop good lower-extremity positioning habits. Performing the exercise in front of a mirror is recommended to enable the exerciser to monitor the position of the knee relative to the foot.

Ankle Joint Muscles If the squat exercise is performed with the heels of the feet resting on a low block, the soleus muscles are exercised more than they would be if the feet were flat. This position with the heels up shortens the gastrocnemius muscles even more (they are already shortened by the flexed knee), limiting their ability to generate force. The soleus muscles, which do not cross the knees, aren't shortened to the same extent. To increase the force production of the gastrocnemius muscles, the squat could be done with the balls of the feet on the block. The mountain climber especially would benefit from this modification because it mimics the knee and ankle positions in climbing. Individual limits to ROM at the ankle joint should also be taken into consideration during the squat. Exercisers with limited dorsiflexion benefit from placing the heels on a low block to prevent them from going onto tiptoes at the bottom of the squat. This ensures they maintain a stable base and can perform the exercise safely.

Subtalar Joint Muscles The subtalar joint plays a role in adapting to uneven surfaces. One way of exercising the invertors and evertors is to walk across, instead of up and down, a ramp or hill.

KEY POINT

During exercises involving the vertebral column and lumbosacral joints, participants should remember to achieve a posterior (backward) pelvic tilt before initiating the exercise and should maintain the tilt throughout the exercise to protect the lumbar spine. For exercises involving the knee, participants should remember to keep the knee in line above the foot when observing themselves in a mirror. The knee should also stay behind or above the foot when observed from the side.

Basic Biomechanical Concepts for Human Movement

Biomechanics is the study of how the joints of the human body move and the forces that contribute to or hinder those movements. Understanding some key principles of biomechanics is necessary to fully understand human movement. Some of these concepts are described next.

Stability

Stability is a feature of the whole body and is influenced by the position of all parts of the body. It is the ability to maintain a stable, balanced position following a disruption such as being touched by an opposing player. In order to maintain balance, an individual's center of gravity must fall within the area of the base of support. In the simple case of standing on two feet with arms at the sides, there is a roughly rectangular base of support from the toes of each foot to the heels of each foot. With weight evenly distributed on both feet, the center of gravity will be in the middle of the base of support (see figure 3.18). Changing the foot position will change the shape and area of the base of support. Changing the position of the body or holding an object will alter the location of the center of gravity within the base of support.

Stability is proportional to the distance from the center of gravity to the edge of the base of support in the direction that an external force would propel the person. Figure

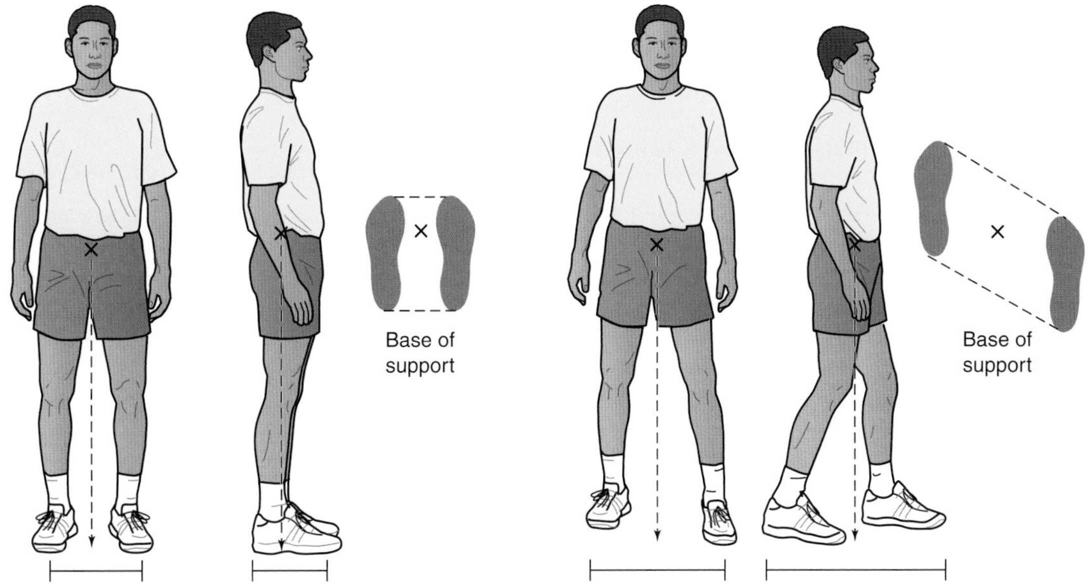

FIGURE 3.18 The relationships among center of gravity, body position, and base of support.

3.19 compares more and less stable positions relative to a force applied in a mediolateral direction. With the feet apart, if one leans so that the line of gravity falls directly over one foot and a pushing force is applied in the same direction of the lean, there is less stability than if the feet were together but with the line of gravity along the edge of the foot closer to the applied force. A wide base of support in the anticipated direction of perturbation typically provides greater stability. A lower body position and the accompanying lower center of gravity also contribute to a more stable position. For example, a football lineman may have a triangular base of support between one hand in contact with the ground and both feet. He will squat to lower his center of gravity and lean forward so that his center of gravity is as far as possible from the edge of the base of support in the direction he anticipates an opponent will try to move him. Stability is also directly proportional to body weight. With all other factors being equal, a heavy person is more stable than a lighter one. Thus, a 300 lb (136 kg) lineman in a three-point squat would be more stable than a 200 lb (91 kg) lineman in the same position.

Stability may be increased by moving the feet apart to widen the base of support and by flexing the knees and hips to lower the center of gravity. A wide base of support

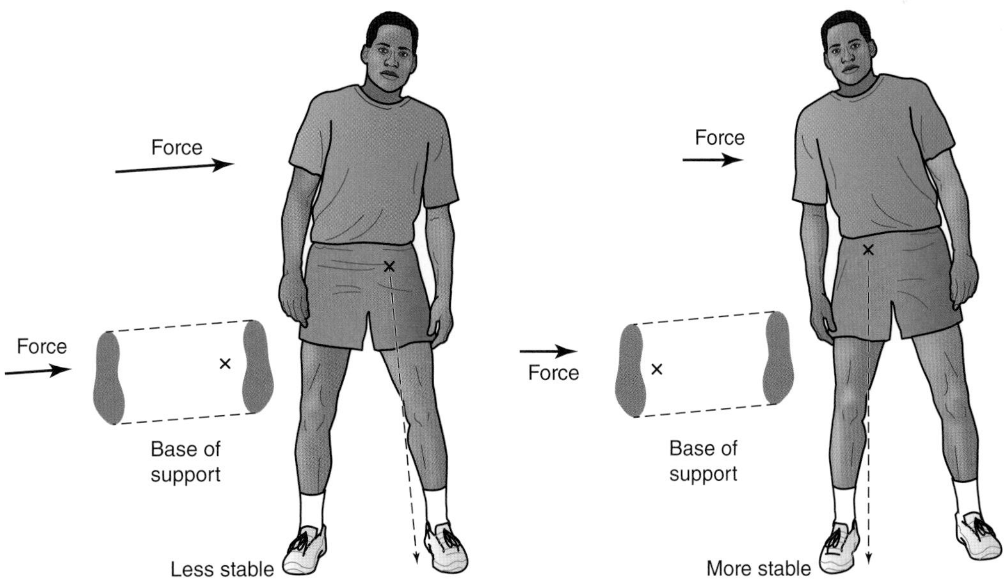

FIGURE 3.19 The relationships among the direction of a perturbing force, center of gravity, and base of support in more and less stable positions.

compromises the ability to respond quickly due to the large change in position required to initiate movement. During standing exercises that require balance, stability can also be aided by holding or pushing against a nearby object such as a wall or chair. Many exercises can be executed from a sitting position, which increases the base of support and lowers the center of gravity. To help maintain stability against a potentially upsetting force, the weight should be shifted toward that force. Just before walking begins, a position close to instability is attained by shifting the center of gravity in the direction of the intended movement, closer to the anterior limits of the base of support. During walking, as the line of gravity moves outside the base of support, a new base of support is established when the other foot makes contact and stability is restored. In basketball, a guard who takes a charge from a forward will fall quicker and easier if she is in an unstable position—standing erect with feet closer together and weight on the heels at the moment of the collision.

KEY POINT

Stability is directly proportional to the distance of the center of gravity from the edge of the base of support. It is inversely proportional to the height of the center of gravity above the base of support, and it is directly proportional to the weight of the body. For greater stability during standing, the knees should be flexed, the feet spread apart in the direction of an oncoming force, and body weight shifted toward the force.

Torque

A force is any push or pull that is applied to a person or object. In the body, when a force is applied at a distance from a joint, it produces a **torque (*T*)**, which will typically rotate the joint. Torque is the product of the magnitude of the force (*F*) and the **force arm (*FA*)**, which is the perpendicular distance from the axis of rotation to the direction of application of that force. Torque is also referred to as *moment*, and the torque arm is also called the *moment arm*. Torque can be expressed as follows:

$$T = F \times FA.$$

$$T_R = R \times RA.$$

When two opposing forces act to produce rotation in opposite directions, one of the forces is typically designated as the **resistance force (*R*)**, and its force arm is called the **resistance arm (*RA*)**, producing a resistance torque (T_R). In considering torque produced by a muscle to cause movement against gravity or some other external force, *F* and *FA* are designated for the muscle and *R* and *RA* are designated for gravity or other opposing forces.

Applying Torque to Muscle Action

Muscle action is a force. The force arm is the perpendicular distance from the axis of rotation of the joint to the direction of the force from its point of application (where the muscle attaches to the bone being moved). Figure 3.20 illustrates the direction of pull of the biceps brachii on the radius with the elbow flexed to 90°. The force arm is the perpendicular distance from the elbow joint to this line of force. If the muscle insertion were closer to the joint, the force arm would be smaller, and the same force would produce less torque, or more muscle force would be required to produce the same torque. Joint position also affects torque. Figure 3.21 shows the direction of pull of the biceps brachii with the elbow in a more extended position. Note that the force arm is not always parallel to the bone. This shortens the force arm, so the same muscle force produces less torque at that joint angle, or more muscle force is required to generate the same torque. This is why a dumbbell biceps curl feels harder at the start of the flexion movement compared with the middle of the flexion movement. It is crucial to remember that the force arm is the perpendicular distance from the line of action of the force to the axis of rotation, not the distance along the bone from the point of attachment of the muscle tendon on the bone to the joint axis.

Torque Resulting From Other Forces

The force of gravity directed vertically downward is treated as a resistance force. The resistance produced by gravity acting on a body part is the weight of the object.

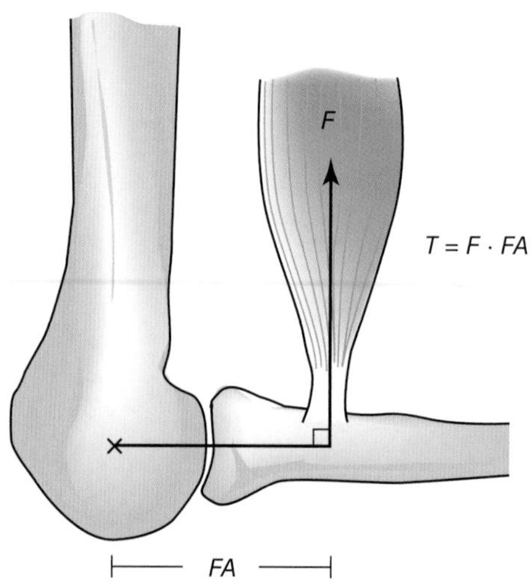

FIGURE 3.20 Muscle force (*F*) and force arm (*FA*) of the biceps brachii with the elbow joint flexed to 90°.

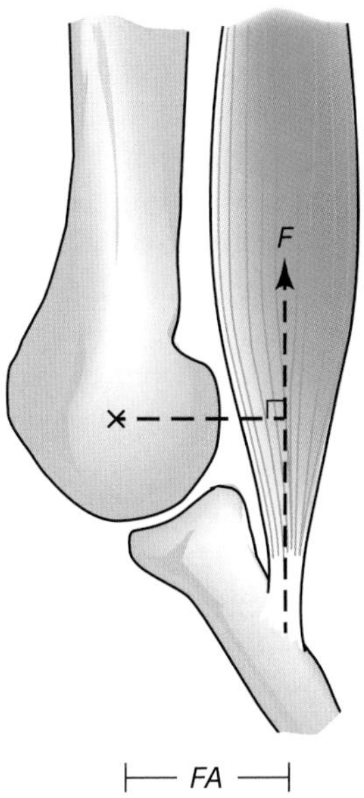

FIGURE 3.21 The influence of elbow flexion less than 90° at the elbow joint on the force arm (*FA*) of the biceps brachii. Note that *FA* is perpendicular to the muscle force (*F*).

The resistance arm is the perpendicular distance from the axis of rotation to the point of the object that represents its center of gravity. The torque is the product of the resistance and the resistance arm. Figure 3.22 illustrates the torque produced by gravity acting on the forearm and hand, which acts to extend the elbow. This torque can be increased by adding mass to increase both the magnitude of force (total weight of forearm and hand plus the added mass) and the length of the resistance arm if the mass is added farther from the axis of rotation. The resistance arm of a force applied by someone pushing or pulling on a limb is the perpendicular distance from the axis of rotation to the point of application of the push or pull.

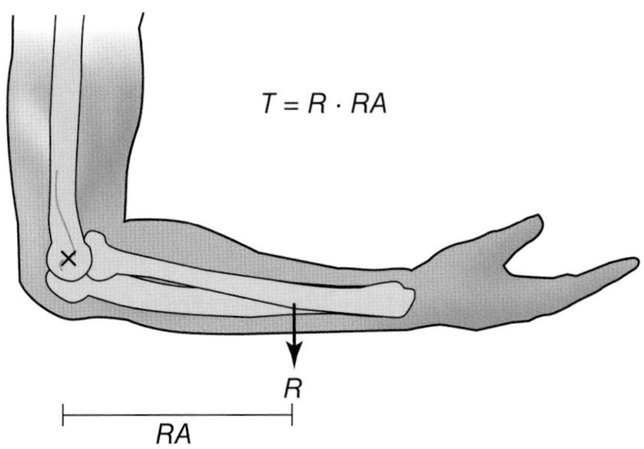

FIGURE 3.22 Extensor torque (*T*) is the product of resistance force (*R*), located at the center of gravity of the forearm and hand, and the resistance arm (*RA*).

For muscle contraction to move a bone, the muscle force generated must produce a torque greater than the opposing or resistance torque. In this case, the muscle action is concentric and the joint moves in the direction of the muscle torque. If the resistance torque is greater than the muscle torque, the muscle acts eccentrically and lengthens under tension. In this case, the joint moves in the opposite direction of the muscle torque (in the direction of the resistance torque). When the muscular torque equals the resistance torque, no movement occurs and the muscle acts isometrically.

KEY POINT

Torque at a joint is the product of the force and the perpendicular distance to the axis of rotation, known as the force arm. Torque due to muscle force is often resisted by a resistance torque due to gravity of another force. The direction of joint movement depends on whether muscle torque or resistance torque is greater.

Applying Torque to Exercising

Knowledge of torque can be used to modify exercises for individuals. The amount of muscle force required by the exercise can be tailored to a person's needs by altering the amount of resistance, the resistance arm, or both in order to change the resistance torque. For example, resistance torque can be increased by adding external weight so that greater muscle force is required to overcome it. The resistance torque also can be changed by altering the position of the body parts. Figure 3.23 shows an exerciser reducing the required muscle force by not holding added weight, thus decreasing both the resistance and the resistance arm, and then by flexing the elbow to shorten the resistance arm.

During an abdominal crunch, the position of the arms determines the length of the resistance arm and, therefore, the amount of resistance torque against which the abdominal muscles have to work to flex the trunk and lift the shoulders off the floor. The arms may be held at the sides of the body to bring the upper-body mass closer to the axis of rotation and reduce the required muscle force. To increase the challenge of this exercise, the arms can be raised with the hands on the back of the head. The resistance arm can be increased by holding the arms straight out overhead, which increases the resistance torque and therefore increases the muscle force required to perform the exercise.

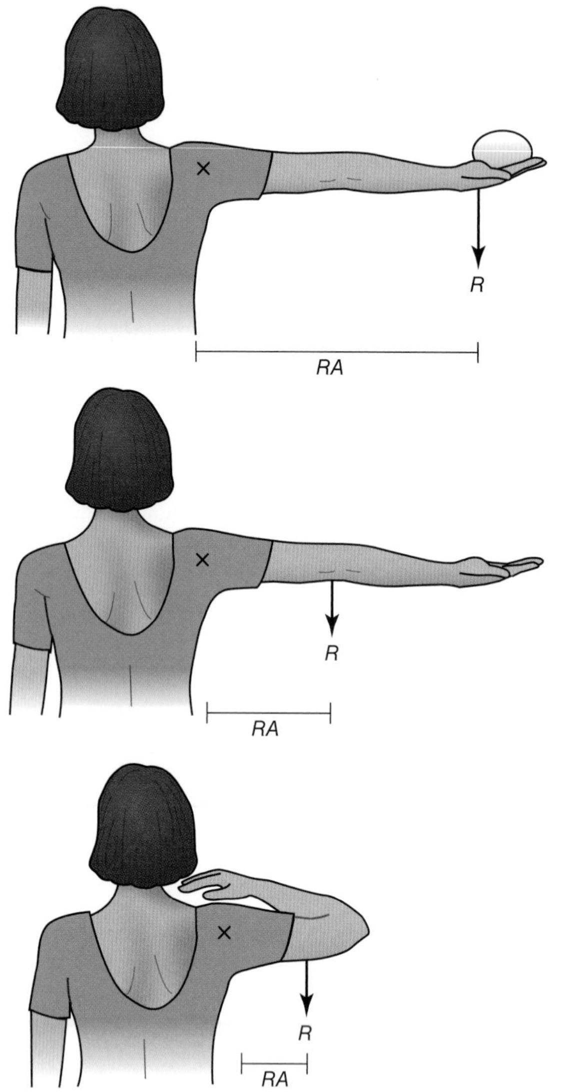

FIGURE 3.23 Modifying resistance torque by increasing the length of the resistance arm (*RA*) and by adding external mass in the form of an object to increase the resistance force *(R)*.

KEY POINT

The torque that resists limb movements can be altered by modifying the amount of the resistance force and by changing the length of the resistance arm.

Rotational Inertia

Rotational inertia, or the resistance to change in the rotation of a body segment around a joint axis, depends on the mass of the segment and its distribution around the joint. Rotational inertia is also referred to as the *moment of inertia*. A lower limb, for example, has more rotational inertia than an upper limb not only because it is heavier but also because its mass is concentrated a greater distance away from its axis of rotation. A swinging softball bat held by its striking end has less rotational inertia than when held at the handle. When holding the bat by the striking end, most of its mass is close to the axis of rotation, which reduces its rotational inertia and makes it easier to swing. However, with less mass at the striking end, the bat will not move the ball very far. Optimal weight and weight distribution of the bat is a trade-off against how quickly the bat can be swung.

The rotational inertia of body segments before or during movement depends on the mass of the segments, which cannot be changed, and on the distribution of the mass around the joints, which can be manipulated. For example, an upper limb with the elbow extended has a greater rotational inertia than with the elbow flexed. Similarly, a lower limb with an extended knee has more rotational inertia than with the knee flexed. The amount of muscle force necessary to cause rapid limb movement is proportional to the rotational inertia of the limb to be moved. During jogging, the knee of the recovery limb is partially flexed to reduce the rotational inertia around the hip joint. Less muscular force is needed to swing the recovery leg forward compared with a more extended knee, which reduces local fatigue of the hip flexors. In sprinting, on the other hand, the quicker the recovery limb is brought forward, the faster the running speed. Powerful actions of the hip flexors, along with maximal knee flexion, result in the recovery limb coming forward sooner and, thus, an increase in overall speed. Another example of rapid movement to which this principle can be applied is jumping jacks. Keeping the elbow flexed reduces the rotational inertia of the upper limb. This may reduce the amount of muscle force required from the shoulder abductor and adductor muscle groups to maintain a certain cadence, or, if greater muscle force is applied, it may result in faster movements.

Angular Momentum

Angular momentum, or the quantity of angular motion, is expressed as the product of angular velocity and rotational inertia. A moving body part possesses angular momentum; the faster it moves and the greater its rotational inertia, the greater the angular momentum. The amount of force necessary to change angular momentum is proportional to the amount of the momentum.

Applying Angular Momentum to Exercising

The concept of angular momentum can be applied to ballistic limb movements during exercise. A fast-moving body segment is decelerated by eccentric muscle actions; a faster movement, a greater mass, or a greater desired deceleration requires greater muscle force to decelerate the body segment. Care must be taken when performing rapid ballistic limb movements, especially when using added weight. The movements may generate great momentum, and considerable muscle strength may be required to decelerate and eventually stop them. This may result in damage to the muscle or the rotating joint.

Transfer of Angular Momentum

Transfer of angular momentum from one body segment to another can be achieved by stabilizing the initial moving body part at a joint, which causes angular movement of another body part. For example, when an exerciser performs an abdominal crunch to exercise the trunk flexors, flinging the arms forward from an overhead position transfers their momentum to the trunk. This decreases the amount of muscular force needed from the trunk flexors and makes the exercise easier. In another example, a jump with a turn in the air can be better achieved if, just before takeoff, the arms are swung forcibly across the body in the intended direction of the spin.

KEY POINT

Rotational inertia can be decreased by moving the mass of the limb closer to the joint axis and vice versa. The amount of eccentric force necessary to decelerate a moving body segment is proportional to its angular momentum (rotational inertia × angular velocity). Angular momentum can be transferred from one body segment to another.

Muscle Groups and the Mechanics of Physical Activity

Human movement is caused or controlled by muscle forces. The following sections briefly review the involvement of muscle groups in some common physical activities (see table 3.3). Success in physical activities depends in part on properly executing movement. Some of the more common errors are also discussed in the following sections.

Walking and Running

The phases and muscle groups involved in walking and running are similar. However, more forceful muscle actions are needed during running as speed increases and greater joint ROMs are observed.

Muscle Groups

The two phases of gait are the stance phase and the swing phase. The swing phase ends and the stance phase begins at foot contact; the stance phase ends at toe-off, when the swing phase begins. The key difference between walking and running is that during walking either one or both feet are on the ground at all times, but during running only one foot is on the ground at a time. In between foot contacts during running there is a flight phase when neither foot is in contact with the ground.

Just before foot contact, the hip extensors act eccentrically to decelerate the forward limb swing. At foot contact with the ground, the knee extensors act eccentrically to control knee flexion against gravity and cushion the

Table 3.3 Movements and Muscles Involved in Locomotion, Throwing, Cycling, Jumping, and Swimming

Major muscle group	Movement task
Hip extensors	Locomotion—push-off; cycling; jumping; swimming—front crawl, back crawl, sidestroke
Hip flexors	Locomotion—recovery; swimming—front crawl, back crawl, sidestroke
Hip abductors	Swimming—breaststroke; throwing
Hip adductors	Swimming—breaststroke
Hip external and internal rotators	Throwing
Knee extensors	Locomotion—landing; cycling; jumping
Knee flexors	Locomotion—recovery
Ankle plantar flexors	Locomotion—push-off, landing; jumping
Ankle dorsiflexors	Locomotion—recovery
Shoulder joint flexors	Underhand throwing
Shoulder joint extensors	Swimming—front crawl
Shoulder joint internal and external rotators	Throwing

(continued)

Table 3.3 *(continued)*

Major muscle group	Movement task
Anterior shoulder joint muscles	Swimming—back crawl, sidestroke lead arm; throwing
Posterior shoulder joint muscles	Swimming—sidestroke trail arm, breaststroke; throwing—windup
Shoulder girdle upward and downward rotators	Swimming—breaststroke, sidestroke lead arm, front crawl, back crawl
Shoulder girdle protractors	Swimming—back crawl; throwing
Shoulder girdle retractors	Swimming—front crawl, breaststroke
	Throwing—windup
Shoulder girdle elevators	Swimming—front crawl, back crawl, sidestroke lead arm, breaststroke
Elbow flexors	Throwing
Elbow extensors	Throwing
Trunk flexors	Throwing
Trunk rotators	Throwing

impact. The heel touches the ground first during walking and distance running. Following heel contact, the ankle dorsiflexors act eccentrically to lower the ball of the foot onto the ground. As running speed increases, the pattern of contact changes and the flat foot or the ball of the foot makes contact with the ground first. A small proportion of runners contact the ground with the flat foot or the ball of the foot at all speeds.

During the stance phase, the body moves forward over the stationary foot as the hip extends and the ankle dorsiflexes (see figure 3.24). Before push-off, the hip continues to extend as the knee extends and the ankle plantar flexes. At this point the swinging limb has moved forward in front of the body in preparation for the next foot contact. The push-off is accomplished by the concentric action of the hip extensors and ankle plantar flexors. The gluteus maximus assumes a greater role in hip extension as speed increases.

At the beginning of the swing phase, the hip flexors act concentrically to begin the forward limb swing. This is a ballistic movement, so the momentum initiated by the hip flexors continues the motion passively. Hip flexion is accompanied by pelvic rotation to bring the swinging limb in front of the body. The knee flexes at the beginning of the swing to reduce the rotational inertia of the swing limb. The knee extensors then initiate knee extension prior to foot contact, and the knee flexors work eccentrically to control knee extension at the end of the swing phase. The ankle joint is dorsiflexed to clear the foot from the ground and prepare for foot contact. Speed is a product of stride length and stride frequency; thus, one or both factors can be increased to increase speed. Greater hip ROM contributes to greater stride length. Rapid recovery of the swing leg via rapid hip flexion during the swing phase is vital to prepare for foot contact at the start of the next stance phase (see figure 3.25).

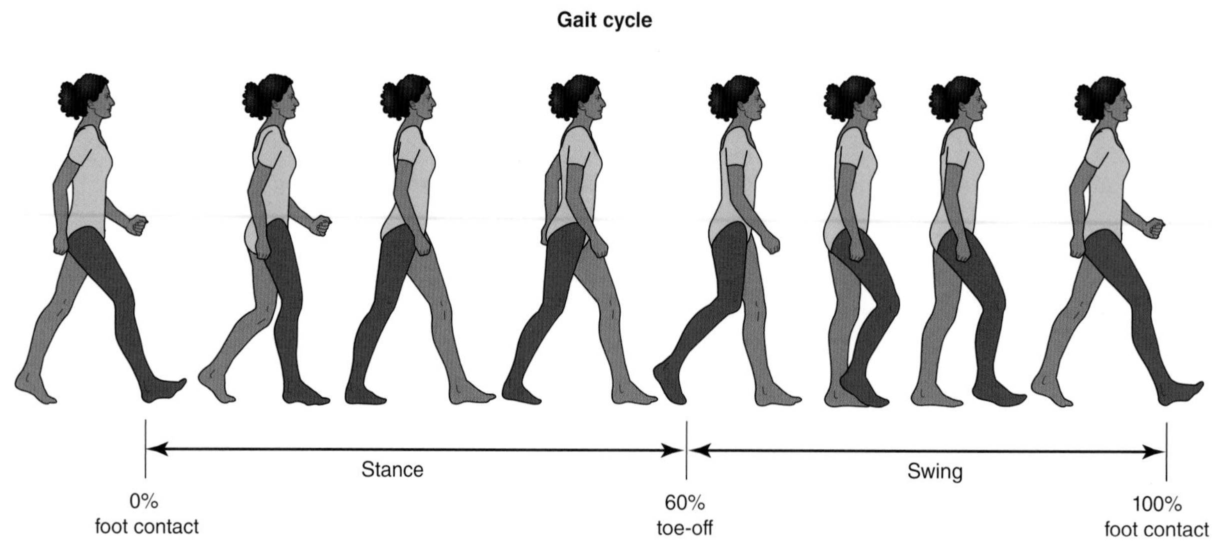

FIGURE 3.24 Stride cycle for walking.

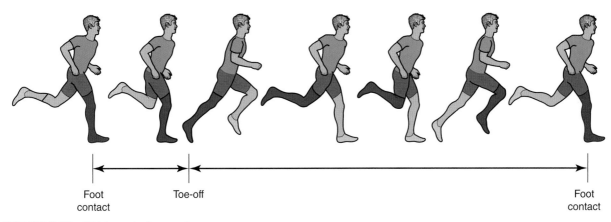

FIGURE 3.25 Stride cycle for running.

In the upper body, arm swing requires shoulder flexion and extension. As speed increases, the swing becomes more vigorous, and there is more elbow flexion. For the greatest efficiency, the arms should move in the sagittal plane. To increase the involvement of the upper limbs for exercise, a walker can exaggerate the shoulder flexion and extension movements.

Walking or running up an incline elicits greater action from the gluteus maximus muscle at the hip and from the knee extensors to raise the body against gravity. The ankle dorsiflexors are more active immediately before landing in order to match the position of the ankle joint to the angle of the incline. Because the ankle is in a more dorsiflexed position, the plantar flexors begin acting during push-off from a more stretched position. For these reasons, hill climbing requires greater flexibility in the plantar flexors, especially the soleus muscle, and greater strength in the dorsiflexors. During downhill running, there is more eccentric action by the knee extensors at foot contact compared with uphill running. As a result, these muscle groups are more apt to become fatigued and to be sore afterward.

Running in place requires the ankle plantar flexors to propel the body upward against gravity; thus, they work more than any of the other lower-extremity muscle groups in this activity. The knee extensors are primarily involved in eccentric action to cushion the landing at foot contact. During running in place, the ball of the foot touches the ground first. Therefore, the plantar flexors are active during the landing, acting eccentrically to control the speed and amount of ankle dorsiflexion. Additional muscles are involved in moving the limb immediately after push-off and before the foot lands again, including hip flexion and extension and knee flexion that brings the foot up to the front.

Common Mechanical Errors

Some novice runners have a tendency to run with stiff legs, or with insufficient knee flexion of the recovery limb. This results in a greater rotational inertia of the limb, which means the hip flexors must exert greater force than they would if the knee were more flexed. Keeping the knees stiff during foot contact can also expose the stance limb to greater forces and increase the potential for bone or soft-tissue injury.

Another potential error is the direction of upper- and lower-limb movements. All movements should be executed in the anterior and posterior directions. Excessively swinging the hands across the trunk rotates the upper trunk; in reaction, the lower trunk rotates in the opposite direction. This excess transverse-plane rotation does not contribute to forward motion of the runner. Excessive movements that do not contribute to forward motion are energetically wasteful.

Some joggers and runners propel themselves too high off the ground during the airborne phase. Again, excessive movement, this time in the vertical direction, does not contribute to forward motion of the runner. Typically, this bouncing style of running also shortens stride length. The runner must now increase stride frequency to maintain running speed.

Slapping the feet onto the ground in a noisy running style can increase the impact forces that the limbs are exposed to every time they strike the ground. The tactile and aural cues of running softly and quietly may enable runners to reduce their impact forces.

Cycling

Cycling is a predominantly lower-body activity. The upper body provides stable support for the lower limbs to generate force and transfer it to the pedal.

Muscle Groups

The main force in cycling comes from concentric contraction of the hip and knee extensors during the downward part of the pedal stroke. Ankle plantar flexors are also involved in maintaining the foot in a stable position to allow the transfer of forces to the pedal. With toe clips or clip-in shoes, riders can use the hip and knee flexors and ankle dorsiflexors on the upward part of the pedal stroke to help return the pedal to the top position. However, this technique requires conscious effort to develop.

Common Mechanical Errors

Good alignment of the lower limb in the frontal plane is important in reducing the risk of knee pain in cyclists. Allowing the knee to move into a varus or valgus position may change how forces are transmitted across the knee joint, potentially overloading tissues. Correct fit of the rider on the bicycle is essential in reducing such errors. Seat height and fore–aft position, as well as handlebar height and distance from the seat, have a large effect on body segment alignment and joint motions during cycling. Toe clips can help to maintain the ball of the foot over the pedal axis, creating a stable platform to push against on the downstroke.

Jumping and Landing

Jumping and landing are common in many team sports, such as basketball, volleyball, and soccer. Several individual sports also have jumping and landing components, including gymnastics and tennis.

Muscle Groups

The hip and knee extensors, followed by the ankle plantar flexors, forcibly propel the body upward against gravity. The amount of trunk flexion primarily determines the angle of takeoff. The trunk extends, and the arms flex from an extended position just before the lower-limb joints extend. If the reach height of the arms is important, as in a jump ball in basketball or in a tennis smash, the scapulae elevate. During the landing, the hip and knee extensors and the ankle plantar flexors act eccentrically to control the rate of flexion of the lower-body joints.

Common Mechanical Errors

Landing with an upright body position and stiff knees fails to take advantage of the shock-absorbing capabilities of the lower-extremity joints and results in high impact forces, which increase the risk of injury. In particular, landing from a jump in this extended position is a risk factor for knee ligament injury. Conversely, using a deep knee flexion reduces performance because the time taken to reverse the joint motions in preparation for takeoff is extended, and explosiveness is lost. In the frontal plane, landing from a jump with a valgus collapse of the knees has been associated with increased risk of noncontact knee injury, particularly in female athletes participating in sports with a jumping component, such as basketball.

Overarm Throwing

Overarm throwing is a component of many team sports. Examples include American football, baseball, softball, and cricket.

Muscle Groups

There are three phases in throwing: the windup, or preparation; the execution, or actual throw; and the follow-through, or recovery. Figure 3.26 illustrates the sequence of the execution phase.

In preparation for throwing, the weight shifts to the back foot, the back hip internally rotates (because the foot is fixed on the ground, rotation is seen at the pelvis), and the trunk rotates with some lateral flexion and extension. In the upper limb, the shoulder externally rotates, and there is some horizontal abduction of the throwing arm accompanied by retraction of the scapula, flexion of the elbow, and extension of the wrist. The movements of the throwing arm are ballistic. The external rotation at the shoulder is fast and powerful. Toward the end of the windup, the internal rotators begin to act eccentrically to decelerate the external rotation in preparation for the actual throw.

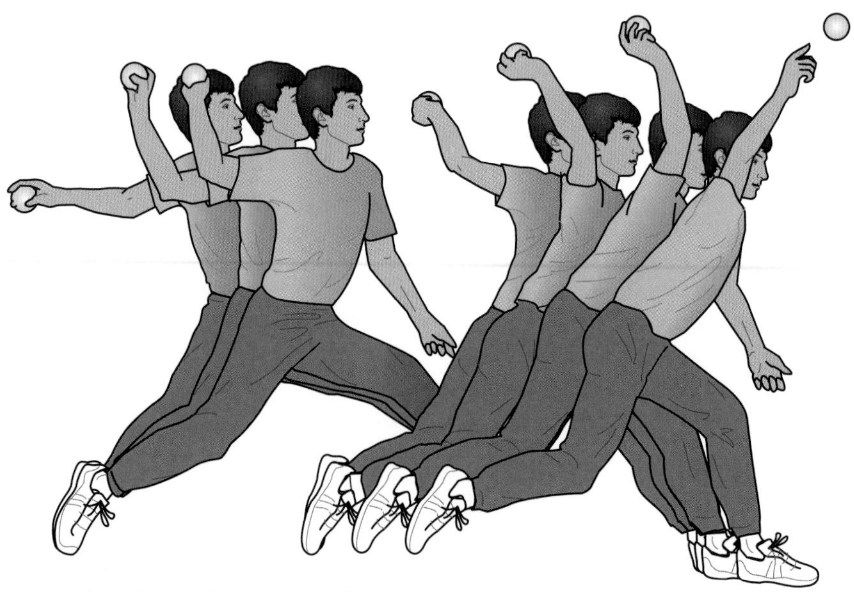

FIGURE 3.26 The execution phase of an overarm throw.

The weight shift forward is the initial movement in the execution of the throw. This is accomplished by the hip abductors, extensors, and external rotators; the ankle plantar flexors; and the subtalar evertors of the back limb. The front hip rotates externally. The trunk then flexes laterally in the direction opposite to that of the windup, rotates, and flexes. There is a forcible internal rotation of the shoulder, along with scapular protraction. Although there is some horizontal adduction, the contribution of the shoulder in an overhand throw mostly comes from this internal rotation. The elbow extends, and the wrist moves toward flexion. Depending on the desired spin on the ball, the forearm pronators and the wrist abductors or adductors also may be involved.

Because the actions at the shoulder and elbow joints are vigorous ballistic movements, the shoulder external rotators and horizontal abductors act eccentrically to decelerate the movements during the follow-through. The elbow flexors act eccentrically to prevent elbow hyperextension.

Common Mechanical Errors

The speed of the ball in the hand just before release is the speed of the ball immediately after it leaves the hand. The more joints involved in the throwing motion, the greater the ball speed when it is released. Most throwing problems that result in low velocity, such as pushing the ball rather than throwing it, stem from a lack of trunk rotation or from poor timing of this rotation with the movements of the shoulder joint. The thrower should rotate the trunk and hips during the windup so the pelvis is sideways to the intended direction of the throw and the shoulders are rotated even more to the back. As the hips and then the trunk rotate forward to begin the throw, the upper limb lags behind. This sets up a whipping action of the upper limb and allows adequate time for the important shoulder internal rotation. Without the trunk rotation, the resulting inadequate shoulder rotation produces a pushing motion during the throw.

Lifting and Carrying Objects

The object to be lifted from the ground should be located close to the lifter's spread feet or even between them. The lifter squats, keeping the trunk as erect as possible. The lift should be accomplished by the powerful lower limbs rather than the spine or arms.

Muscle Groups

Lifting begins by keeping the trunk in an upright position and then tilting the pelvis backward and keeping the abdominal muscles activated; the knee extensors along with the hip extensors then act concentrically. The lift should be slow and smooth, not jerky (see figure 3.27). The weight should be carried close to the body, with the trunk assuming a position that allows the center of gravity to fall within the area of the base of support. The trunk lateral flexors are more active when the weight is carried on one side, the extensors are more active when the weight is in front, and the abdominal muscles are more active when the weight is carried across the top of the back, as in backpacking.

Common Mechanical Errors

Insufficient lower-limb strength can result in poor lifting technique. In particular, emphasis shifts to the lumbar spine and trunk extensors to lift the object. The high forces generated at the lumbar spine can result in injury. Protect the lower back during lifting by using a wide lifting belt or activating the trunk musculature to provide support.

KEY POINT

Common mechanical errors in locomotion include running with stiff legs, swinging the arms across the trunk, lifting too high off the ground, and slapping the feet. Common errors in cycling and jumping relate to alignment of the lower extremities in the frontal plane. The most common mechanical errors in throwing are insufficient trunk rotation and poor timing among the trunk, hip, and upper-limb movements.

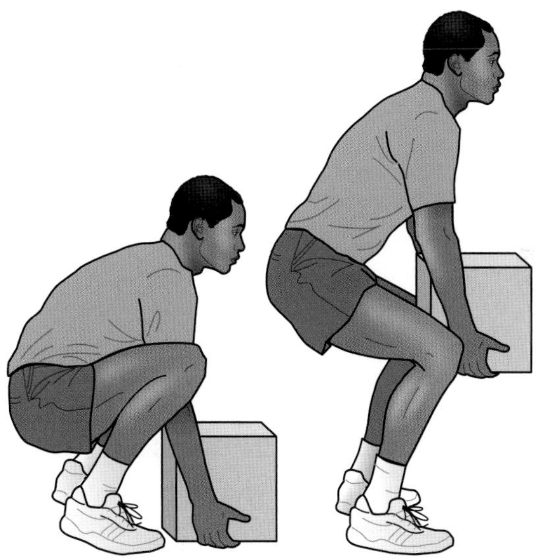

FIGURE 3.27 Lifting technique.

KEY POINT

The steps of proper lifting are to place the feet close to the object, keep the trunk upright, tilt the pelvis backward, and slowly extend the hips and knees while continuing to activate the abdominal muscles.

3

LEARNING AIDS

REVIEW QUESTIONS

1. Name the three cardinal planes and their associated axes.
2. Using the shoulder (glenohumeral) joint as an example, explain why a ball-and-socket joint is so mobile.
3. Explain how the trunk has such a large ROM even though each intervertebral joint within it has only a few degrees of motion.
4. Explain from an anatomical viewpoint why the knee is vulnerable to injury.
5. Identify the phase of a squat exercise in which quadriceps femoris is acting (a) concentrically and (b) eccentrically.
6. Explain in terms of torque how an abdominal crunch is more difficult when the arms are extended overhead compared with folded across the chest.
7. Using rotational inertia in your answer, explain why runners naturally flex the knee of the leg that is swinging forward.
8. Why is walking up an incline more challenging for the gluteal muscles than walking on level ground?
9. What type of muscle contractions are involved in exercises performed in water?
10. What is a common error made by novices when throwing a ball?

CASE STUDIES

1. You are supervising the resistance training area when you hear a lot of clanging noises coming from the vicinity of the seated leg press. You discover that the exerciser at that machine is not controlling the descent of the weights. You suggest that he slowly return the weights rather than letting them drop. He asks you why—he doesn't see any benefit in a controlled return other than reduced noise. What do you tell him?
2. Alice wants to know why she can move a heavier weight when she does wrist curls with her palms up than with her palms down and why she can do more pull-ups with her palms facing her than with her palms facing away. How do you answer her?
3. José complains that his lower back aches somewhat when he reaches overhead while standing in place during the cool-down portion of an aerobics class. What should he do during this movement to prevent the aching?

Answers to Case Studies

1. Explain to the exerciser that the hip and knee extensors that are used to push against the weights are also working to control the descent. The press requires concentric contraction; the return requires eccentric contraction. Both kinds of contractions lead to increased strength.
2. When she's doing the wrist curls with her palms down (radioulnar pronated position), the wrist extensors are the contracting muscles; when her palms are up (supinated position), the wrist flexors are the working muscles. The wrist flexors are usually stronger than the wrist extensors.

   The explanation is different for the pull-ups. The elbow flexor muscles are working regardless of the position of the radioulnar joint. However, when the palms are facing away (pronation), the distal tendon of the biceps brachii is wrapped around the radius bone and therefore this muscle cannot exert as much force as when the palms are facing toward the body (supinated position).
3. He should make a conscious effort to maintain a backward pelvic tilt. He should also keep his arms in front of his head instead of by his ears and his knees slightly flexed to help maintain the backward tilt.

4

Exercise Physiology

Edward T. Howley

OBJECTIVES

The reader will be able to do the following:

1. Explain how muscle produces energy aerobically and anaerobically, and evaluate the importance of aerobic and anaerobic energy production in fitness and sport.
2. Describe the structure of skeletal muscle and the sliding-filament theory of muscle contraction.
3. Describe the power, speed, endurance, and metabolism of the types of muscle fibers.
4. Identify the most important factor in generating muscular force, and describe the order in which the various muscle fiber types are recruited as exercise intensity increases.
5. Describe the various fuels for muscle work and how exercise intensity and duration affect the respiratory exchange ratio.
6. Describe how exercise tests, training, heredity, sex, age, altitude, carbon monoxide, and cardiovascular and pulmonary diseases influence $\dot{V}O_2$max.
7. Describe how ventilatory threshold (VT) and lactate threshold (LT) indicate fitness as well as predict performance in endurance events.
8. Describe how HR, stroke volume (SV), cardiac output, and oxygen extraction change during a graded exercise test (GXT) and the effect of endurance training on those responses, and link the variation in $\dot{V}O_2$max in the population to differences in maximal cardiac output.
9. Summarize the effects of endurance training on muscular, metabolic, and cardiorespiratory responses to submaximal work and on $\dot{V}O_2$max, and describe how reducing or ceasing training affects $\dot{V}O_2$max.
10. Describe how men and women differ in their cardiovascular responses to the same absolute work rate ($L \cdot min^{-1}$).
11. Contrast the importance of the various mechanisms for heat loss during heavy exercise and during submaximal exercise in a hot environment, and describe a program to improve one's heat tolerance.

Fitness professionals need to know basic exercise physiology to prescribe appropriate activities, deal with weight-loss concerns, and explain to participants what happens when training in a hot and humid environment. This chapter can't possibly cover the extensive detail found in texts devoted to exercise physiology; instead, we summarize major topics and, where possible, apply the discussion to exercise testing and prescription. We refer the interested reader to the texts on exercise physiology listed in the references (2, 8, 41, 42, 45, 50, 53, 55).

Energy and Work

Energy is essential for all bodily functions. Several kinds of energy exist in biological systems, including

- electrical energy in the nerves and muscles,
- chemical energy in the synthesis of molecules,
- mechanical energy in the contraction of muscle, and
- thermal energy, derived from all of these processes, that helps maintain body temperature.

The ultimate source of the energy found in biological systems is the sun. The radiant energy from the sun is captured by plants and used to convert simple atoms and molecules into carbohydrate, fat, and protein. The sun's energy is trapped within the chemical bonds of these food molecules.

For the cells to use this energy, they must break down the foodstuffs in a manner that conserves most of the energy contained in the bonds of the carbohydrate, fat, and protein. In addition, the final product of the breakdown must be a molecule the cell can use—adenosine triphosphate (ATP). Cells use ATP as the primary energy source for biological work, whether this work is electrical, mechanical, or chemical.

During muscular activity, ATP is constantly converted to adenosine diphosphate (ADP) and inorganic phosphate (P_i) in order to provide the energy needed for the work. The ATP must be replaced as fast as it is used if the muscle is to continue to generate force. Muscles have multiple systems for replacing ATP that allow athletes to run at high speeds for short periods of time (e.g., 100 m dash) or at slower speeds for longer distances (e.g., marathon). Two broad types of reactions are available to regenerate the ATP: anaerobic reactions for **anaerobic energy**, which can regenerate ATP rapidly and without oxygen, and aerobic reactions for **aerobic energy**, which are slower to activate but can sustain ATP regeneration for long periods of time using oxygen.

Anaerobic Energy Sources

One-enzyme reactions and one multiple-enzyme pathway can replace ATP at a fast rate. These energy systems allow muscle to continue to generate force during strenuous activities or help make the transition from rest to exercise as the slower aerobic system comes up to speed. In the most important of the one-enzyme reactions, **phosphocreatine (PC)** reacts with ADP to form ATP. The PC concentration in muscle is limited and can provide only about 5 s of energy during all-out activity.

$$\text{PC} + \text{ADP} \rightarrow \text{ATP} + \text{C}.$$

In the multiple-enzyme pathway called **glycolysis**, glucose is metabolized at a high rate and ATP is generated without oxygen. Lactic acid is produced in the process, leading to lactate and hydrogen ion (H^+) accumulation in the muscle and blood; the H^+ may interfere with the mechanism involved in muscle contraction. Glycolysis provides ATP at a high rate and is a substantial contributor to the ATP needed in all-out activities lasting less than 2 min. In contrast, when glucose is metabolized aerobically, it represents a long-lasting source of ATP, producing about 18 times more ATP per glucose molecule than when metabolized anaerobically.

Aerobic Energy Production

The oxidative metabolism of carbohydrate (muscle glycogen and blood glucose) and fat (from both adipose tissue and intramuscular sources) provides the long-term sources of ATP for physical activities and exercise that we typically associate with health-related outcomes. The complete oxidation of these fuels takes place in the **mitochondria** of the cell, which increase in number with endurance training. The larger number of mitochondria increases the capacity of the muscle to use fat as a fuel because fat can only be metabolized via aerobic pathways.

$$\text{Carbohydrate or fat} + O_2 \rightarrow \text{ATP}.$$

ATP production via aerobic mechanisms is slower than ATP production from anaerobic sources, and during submaximal work it may take 2 or 3 min before aerobic processes fully meet the ATP needs of the cell. One reason for this lag is the time it takes for the heart to increase the delivery of oxygen-enriched blood to the muscles at the rate needed to meet the ATP demands of the muscle. Another is the time it takes for the mitochondria to increase the rate of ATP production from resting levels to that needed to meet the exercise demand. Aerobic production of ATP is the primary means of supplying energy to the muscle in heavy exercise lasting more than 2 to 3 min and in all submaximal work.

Interaction of Exercise Intensity, Exercise Duration, and Energy Production

The proportion of energy coming from anaerobic sources is influenced by the intensity and duration of the activity.

Figure 4.1 shows that during an all-out activity lasting less than 1 min (e.g., a 400 m dash), the muscles obtain most of their ATP from anaerobic sources. In a 2 to 3 min maximal effort, approximately 50% of the energy comes from anaerobic sources and 50% comes from aerobic sources. In a 10 min maximal effort, the anaerobic component drops to 15%. For a 30 min all-out effort, the anaerobic component is about 5%, and it is even smaller in a submaximal 30 min training session.

KEY POINT

ATP is supplied at a high rate by the anaerobic processes of PC breakdown and glycolysis. Anaerobic energy is important in short, explosive events (e.g., shot put) and in athletic competitions requiring maximal effort for less than 2 min. ATP is supplied during prolonged exercise by the aerobic metabolism of carbohydrate and fat in the mitochondria of the muscle. This is the primary means of supplying energy to the muscle in maximal work lasting more than 2 min and in all submaximal work.

Understanding Muscle Structure and Function

Exercise me ans movement, and movement requires muscle action. To discuss human physiology related to exercise and endurance training, we must start with skeletal muscle, the tissue that converts the chemical energy of ATP to mechanical work. How does a muscle do this?

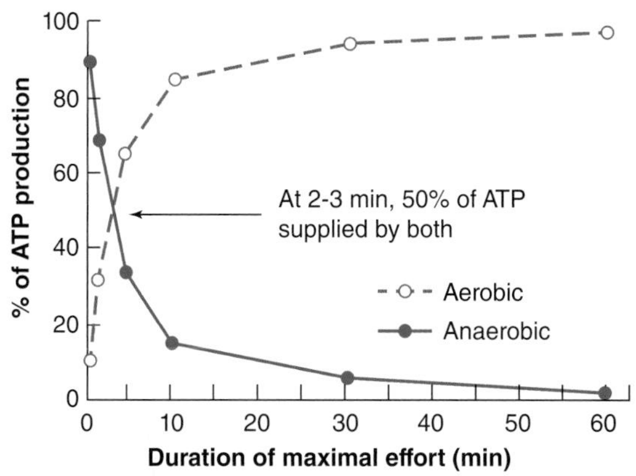

FIGURE 4.1 Percent of aerobic and anaerobic contributions to total energy supply during maximal work of various durations (53).

Skeletal muscle is a complex structure composed of a variety of tissues, including nerve, muscle, and connective tissue. Figure 4.2 shows the basic structure of muscle. The epimysium is the connective tissue that surrounds the whole muscle; the perimysium surrounds bundles of muscle fibers called fasciculi; and each muscle fiber is surrounded by the endomysium, which overlies the muscle fiber's membrane, the sarcolemma. The connective tissue transmits the force, generated by the muscle, to the bone so that movement can occur. Each **muscle fiber** is composed of a large number of the **myofibrils** which run the full length of the muscle, and give skeletal muscle its striated appearance. Figure 4.3 shows that a myofibril is composed of a series of **sarcomeres**, the fundamental units of muscle contraction. The sarcomere contains the thick

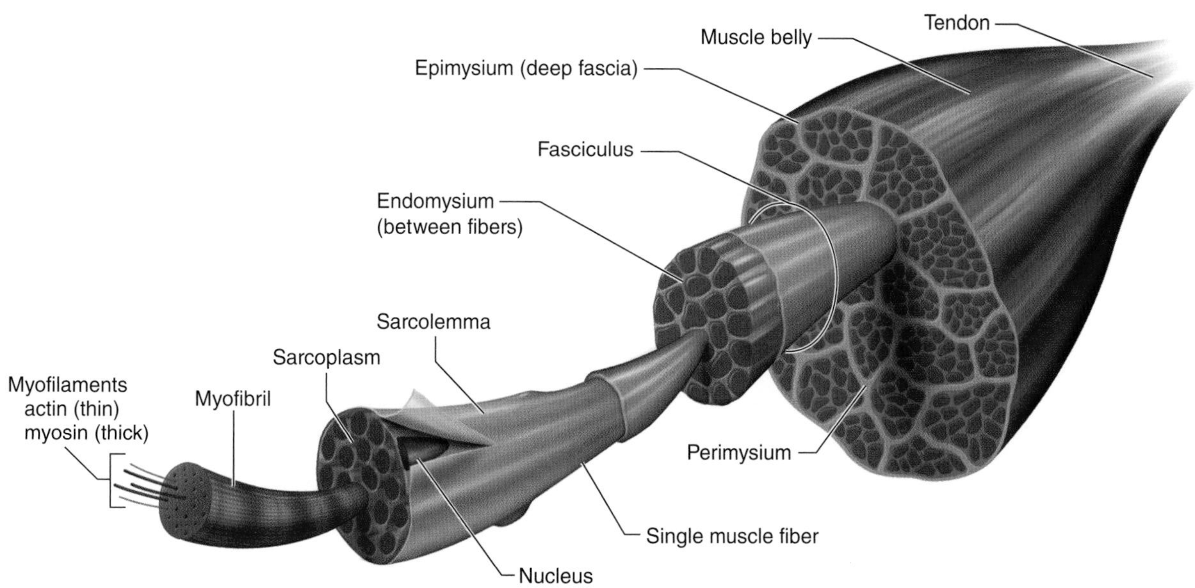

FIGURE 4.2 Basic structure of the muscle, including various types of connective tissue.

filament **myosin** and the thin filament **actin** and is bounded by connective tissue called the **Z line** (41, 53, 68).

An enlargement of two sarcomeres on the right side of figure 4.3 shows the **A band**, **I band**, and **H zone** and the changes that take place when the sarcomere moves from the resting state to the contracted state. The I band is composed of actin and is bisected by the Z line, and the A band is composed of myosin and actin. According to the **sliding-filament theory** of muscle contraction, the thin actin filaments slide over the thick myosin filaments, pulling the Z lines toward the center of the sarcomere. In this way the entire muscle shortens, but the contractile proteins do not change size. So how does the muscle release the energy in ATP for shortening?

If ATP is the energy supply, then an ATPase (an enzyme) must exist in muscle to split ATP and release the potential energy contained within its bonds. ATPase is found in an extension of the thick myosin filament, the myosin

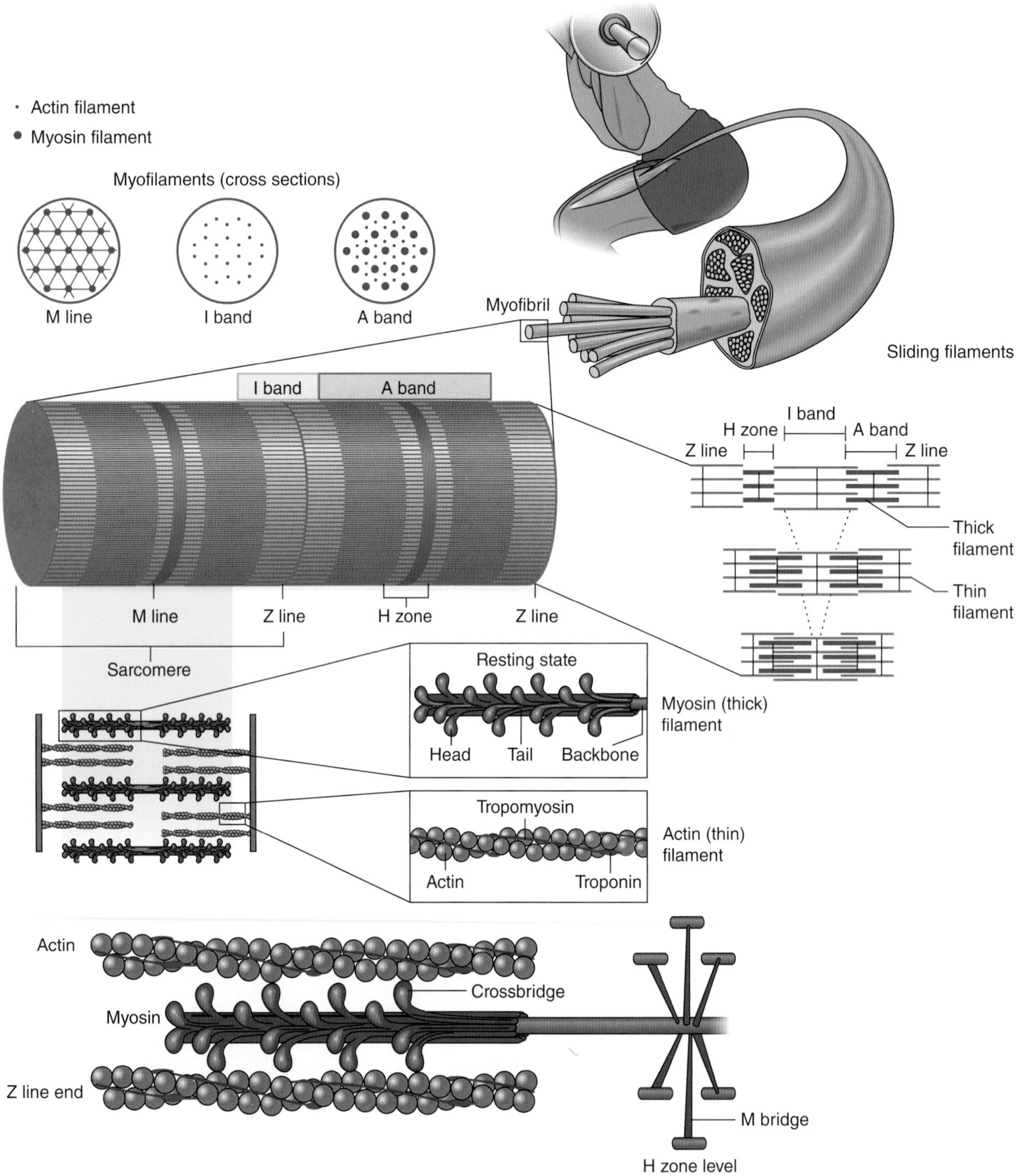

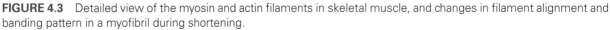

FIGURE 4.3 Detailed view of the myosin and actin filaments in skeletal muscle, and changes in filament alignment and banding pattern in a myofibril during shortening.

head, which also can bind to actin. The myosin head and its connection to the thick filament is called the **crossbridge**. Figure 4.4 shows how ATP, the crossbridge, and actin interact to shorten the sarcomere (41) through these steps:

1. At the end of a contraction cycle the myosin crossbridge is tightly bound to actin.
2. ATP binds to the myosin, allowing its release from actin.
3. ATP is broken down (hydrolyzed) to ADP and Pi (which remain bound to myosin) and the myosin head moves away from the actin.
4. The energized crossbridge binds to a new actin molecule.
5. It then releases Pi to initiate the power stroke, and pulls the thin filament (actin) toward the center of the sarcomere.
6. ADP is released from the myosin head and ATP must be available to initiate the event in step 1.

Why aren't the crossbridges always moving and the muscles always in contraction? At rest, two proteins that are associated with actin block the interaction of myosin with actin: **troponin**, which has the capacity to bind calcium, and **tropomyosin**. Figure 4.5 shows the myofibrils to be surrounded by a network of membranes called the **sarcoplasmic reticulum (SR)**. A portion of the SR, called the terminal cisternae, stores calcium and is in direct contact with the **transverse tubules**, communication channels running from the surface of the muscle fiber to its interior. Figure 4.6 shows that when a muscle fiber is depolarized (excited) by a motor neuron, the action potential spreads over the surface of the muscle fiber and enters the fiber through the transverse tubules. Once inside the muscle fiber, this wave of depolarization spreads over the SR and releases calcium (Ca^{2+}) into the sarcoplasm. When the calcium binds with troponin, the tropomyosin moves off the myosin binding site on actin so that the myosin head can interact with it. When the myosin head binds to actin, energy is released, the crossbridge moves, and the sarcomere

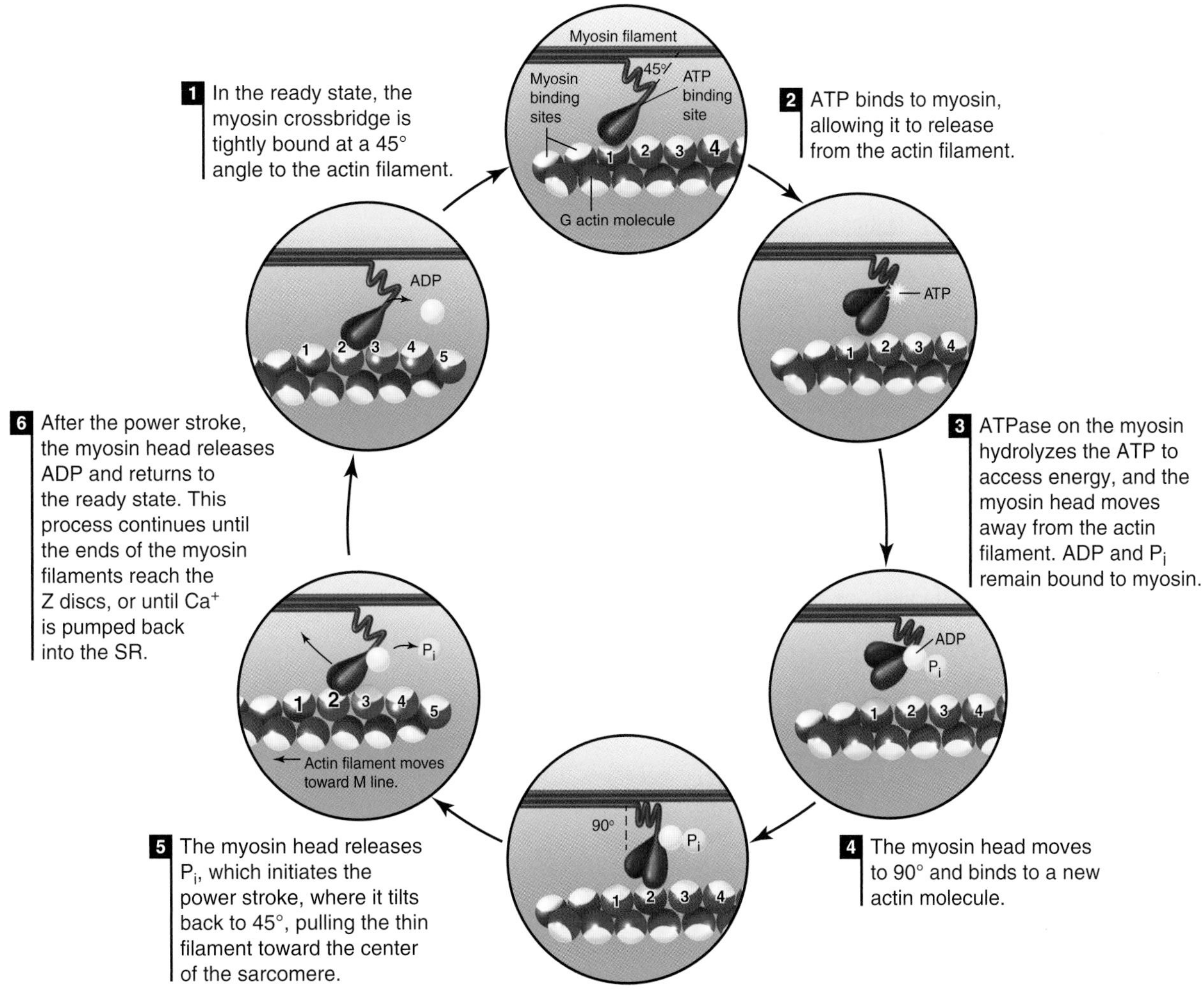

FIGURE 4.4 The molecular events of a contractile cycle illustrating changes in the myosin head during various phases of the power stroke.

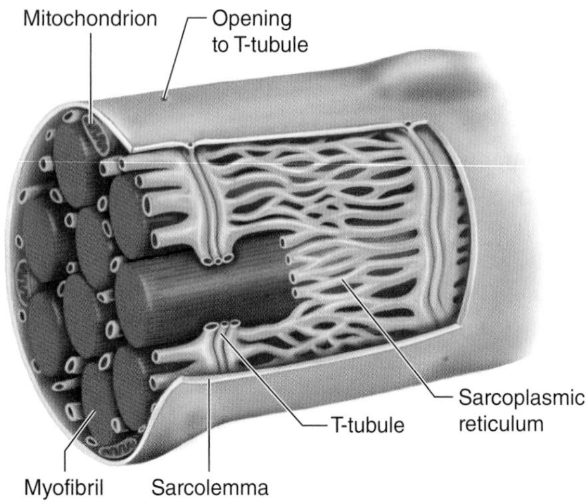

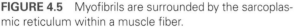

FIGURE 4.5 Myofibrils are surrounded by the sarcoplasmic reticulum within a muscle fiber.

shortens. This sequence of crossbridge cycling continues as long as calcium is present and the muscle can replace the ATP it uses. The muscle relaxes when the calcium is pumped back into the SR and troponin and tropomyosin can again block the interaction of actin and myosin (41). The two principal needs for ATP during exercise are for crossbridge cycling and pumping the calcium back to the SR, both of which increase with exercise intensity.

Muscle Fiber Types and Performance

Muscle fibers vary in their abilities to produce ATP by the aerobic and anaerobic mechanisms described earlier in the chapter. Some muscle fibers contract quickly and have an innate capacity to produce great force, but they fatigue quickly. These muscle fibers produce most of their ATP by PC breakdown and glycolysis, and they are called **fast glycolytic fibers** or **Type IIx fibers**. Other muscle fibers contract slowly and produce little force, but they have great resistance to fatigue. These fibers produce most of their ATP aerobically in the mitochondria and are called **slow oxidative fibers** or **Type I fibers**. These fibers have many mitochondria and a relatively large number of capillaries helping to deliver oxygen to the mitochondria. Last, there

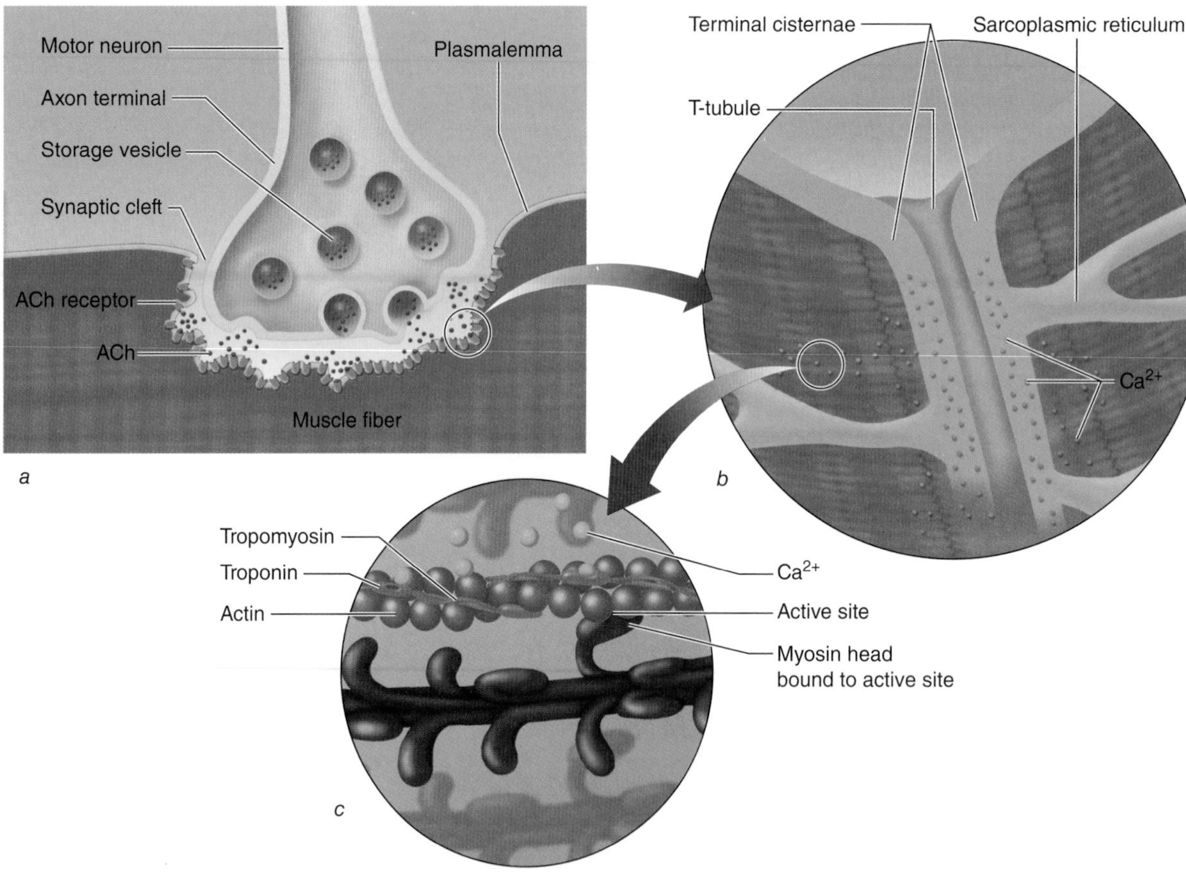

FIGURE 4.6 The sequence of events leading to tension development in a muscle. *(a)* When a motor neuron is depolarized, acetylcholine (Ach) is released, binds to receptors on the plasmalemma, and depolarizes the muscle fiber. *(b)* The wave of depolarization moves down the T-tuble to the sarcoplasmic reticulum, causing the release of calcium (Ca^{2+}). *(c)* This Ca^{2+} binds to troponin, which moves the tropomyosin off the binding sites on actin, and allows the myosin head to attach to the actin filament.

KEY POINT

A muscle contraction cycle begins when ATP binds to myosin, allowing it to be released from actin. After the ATP is split to form a high-energy myosin crossbridge, the myosin head binds to another actin and releases energy; the crossbridge moves and pulls actin toward the center of the sarcomere. ATP must bind to and release the crossbridge from actin to start the process again. Calcium from the SR blocks inhibitory proteins (troponin and tropomyosin) and allows the myosin head to bind to actin to begin moving the crossbridge. Relaxation occurs when calcium is pumped back into the SR.

is a fiber with both Type I and Type IIx characteristics. It is a fast-contracting muscle fiber that not only produces great force when stimulated but also resists fatigue because of its large number of mitochondria and capillaries. These fibers are called **fast oxidative glycolytic fibers** or **Type IIa fibers**.

KEY POINT

Muscle fibers differ in speed of contraction, force, and resistance to fatigue. Type I fibers are slow, generate low force, and resist fatigue. Type IIa fibers are fast, generate high force, and resist fatigue. Type IIx fibers are fast, generate high force, and easily fatigue.

Muscle Fiber Types: Genetics, Sex, and Training

In the average male and female, about 52% of the muscle fibers are Type I, with the fast-twitch fibers divided into approximately 33% Type IIa and 13% Type IIx (62, 63). However, the distribution of fiber types in the overall population is quite variable. Studies comparing identical and fraternal twins suggest that the distribution of fast and slow fibers is genetic. In addition, fast-twitch fibers cannot be converted to slow-twitch fibers, or vice versa, with endurance training (3). In contrast, the capacity of the muscle fiber to produce ATP aerobically (its oxidative capacity) seems to be easily altered by endurance training. In fact, Type IIx fibers can't be found in some elite endurance athletes; they have been converted to the oxidative version, Type IIa (62). The increase in mitochondria and capillaries in endurance-trained muscles allows a person to meet ATP demands aerobically, with less glycogen depletion and lactate formation (32).

The tension, or force, generated by a muscle depends on more than the fiber type. Tension increases with the frequency of stimulation, from a single twitch to a complete **tetanic contraction**, with the latter being the typical type of muscle fiber contraction. In addition, the force of contraction depends on the degree to which the muscle fibers contract simultaneously (synchronous firing) and the number of muscle fibers recruited for the contraction. The latter factor, muscle fiber recruitment, is the most important. Figure 4.7 shows the order in which the various muscle fiber types are recruited as the intensity of exercise increases. The order is from the most to the least oxidative, from the slowest to the fastest fiber (Type I to Type IIa to Type IIx) (60). Consequently, at higher work rates when the Type IIx fibers are recruited, there is a greater chance of producing lactate and hydrogen ions. Although chronic light exercise (less than 40% $\dot{V}O_2$max) only recruits and causes a training effect in Type I fibers, exercise beyond 70% $\dot{V}O_2$max involves all fiber types. This fact has important implications in the specificity of training and the potential for transferring training effects from one activity to another. Obviously, if you don't use a muscle fiber, it can't become trained.

When muscles work at high intensities for long periods of time, especially early in a training program, a condition called **rhabdomyolysis** (often called *rhabdo*) can develop. Such exercise causes the breakdown of muscle and the release of large proteins into the circulation that

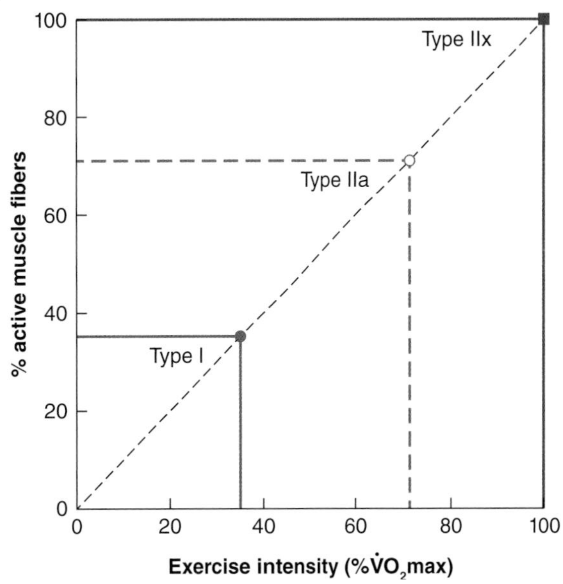

FIGURE 4.7 Recruitment of muscle fiber types in exercise of increasing intensity.

can cause kidney damage and death (41). In contrast, progressively increasing the difficulty of a workout from light to moderate to heavy over a long period of time minimizes the potential for such a problem. We use this approach throughout the text (see chapters 11 and 13). Legal implications for fitness instructors who cause rhabdomyolysis are addressed in chapter 26.

KEY POINT

Muscle tension depends on the frequency of the stimulation leading to a tetanus contraction, the synchronous firing of muscle fibers, and the recruitment of muscle fibers, with the latter being the most important. The order of recruitment of muscle fibers is from the most to the least oxidative. Light to moderate exercise uses Type I muscle fibers, whereas moderate to vigorous exercise requires Type IIa fibers in addition to the Type I fibers already involved. Both of these fibers favor the aerobic metabolism of carbohydrate and fat. Heavy exercise requires Type IIx fibers that favor anaerobic glycolysis, which increases the likelihood of lactate and hydrogen ion production.

Metabolic, Cardiovascular, and Respiratory Responses to Exercise

A primary task of the fitness professional is to recommend physical activities that increase or maintain cardiorespiratory function. Activities that demand aerobic energy (ATP) production automatically cause the circulatory and respiratory systems to deliver oxygen to the muscle to meet the demand. The selected aerobic activities must be strenuous enough to challenge and thus improve the cardiorespiratory system. This crucial link between aerobic activities and cardiorespiratory function provides the basis for much of exercise programming. The following sections summarize selected metabolic, cardiovascular, and respiratory responses to submaximal work and to a maximal graded exercise test (GXT). We begin by discussing how oxygen uptake is measured.

Measuring Oxygen Uptake

How does oxygen get to the mitochondria? First, oxygen enters the lungs during inhalation; it then diffuses from the alveoli of the lungs into the blood. Oxygen is bound to hemoglobin in the red blood cells, and the heart delivers the oxygen-enriched blood to the muscles. Oxygen then diffuses into the muscle cells and reaches the mitochondria, where it is used (consumed) in the production of ATP.

Oxygen consumption ($\dot{V}O_2$) during exercise is measured by subtracting the volume of oxygen exhaled from the volume of oxygen inhaled.

$$\dot{V}O_2 = \text{volume } O_2 \text{ inhaled} - \text{volume } O_2 \text{ exhaled.}$$

To measure $\dot{V}O_2$, the subject breathes through a two-way valve that allows the lungs to inhale room air (containing 20.93% O_2 and 0.03% CO_2) while directing exhaled air to a device that measures the number of liters of air exhaled per minute, which is called **pulmonary ventilation**. In addition, a sample of the exhaled air is directed to gas analyzers to determine its oxygen and carbon dioxide content (see figure 4.8). Oxygen consumption (uptake) is calculated by multiplying the volume of air breathed by the percentage of oxygen extracted. Oxygen extraction is the percentage of oxygen extracted from the inhaled air, the difference between the 20.93% of O_2 in room air and the percentage of O_2 in exhaled air.

The following is a simplified presentation of the steps used to calculate $\dot{V}O_2$. Note that computer-controlled oxygen uptake equipment (see figure 4.8) does all of the calculations and prints out the results of the test.

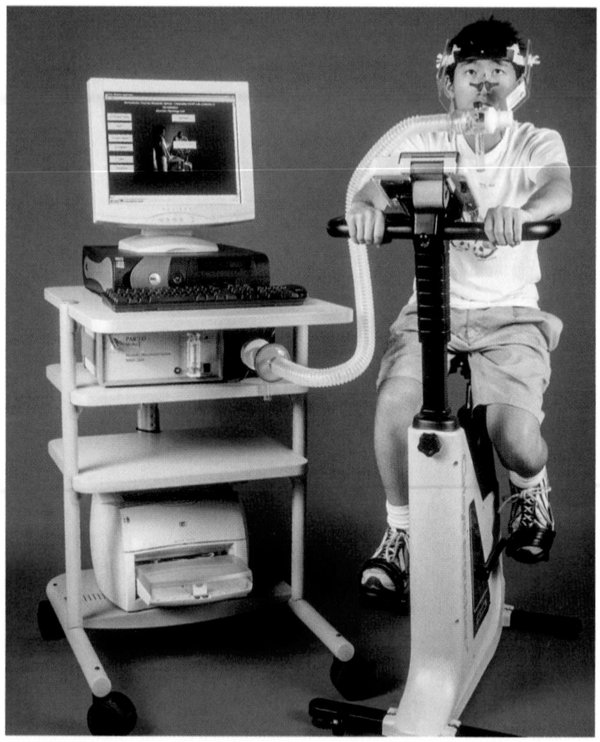

FIGURE 4.8 Computer-controlled equipment for measuring oxygen uptake and carbon dioxide production.
Photo courtesy of ParvoMedics.

$\dot{V}O_2$ = pulmonary ventilation ($L \cdot min^{-1}$) · O_2 extraction.

If ventilation = 60 $L \cdot min^{-1}$, and exhaled O_2 = 16.93%, then

$$\dot{V}O_2 = 60\ L \cdot min^{-1}\ (20.93\%\ O_2 - 16.93\%\ O_2), \text{ and}$$

$$\dot{V}O_2 = 60\ L \cdot min^{-1}\ (4.00\%\ O_2) = 2.4\ L \cdot min^{-1}.$$

CO_2 is produced in the mitochondria and diffuses out of the muscle into the venous blood, where it is carried back to the lungs. There it diffuses into the alveoli and is exhaled. CO_2 production ($\dot{V}CO_2$) can be calculated as described for the $\dot{V}O_2$:

If ventilation = 60 $L \cdot min^{-1}$, and exhaled CO_2 = 3.03%, then

$$\dot{V}CO_2 = 60\ L \cdot min^{-1}\ (3.03\%\ CO_2 - 0.03\%\ CO_2), \text{ and}$$

$$\dot{V}CO_2 = 60\ L \cdot min^{-1}\ (3.00\%\ CO_2) = 1.8\ L \cdot min^{-1}.$$

The ratio of CO_2 production ($\dot{V}CO_2$) to oxygen consumption ($\dot{V}O_2$) in the mitochondria of the cell is called the **respiratory quotient (*RQ*)**. Because $\dot{V}CO_2$ and $\dot{V}O_2$ are measured at the mouth rather than at the tissue, this ratio is called the **respiratory exchange ratio (*R*)**. This ratio can help us identify the type of fuel used during exercise (see the next section, Fuel Utilization During Exercise).

$$R = \dot{V}CO_2 \div \dot{V}O_2.$$

Using the values already calculated,

$$R = 1.8\ L \cdot min^{-1} \div 2.4\ L \cdot min^{-1} = 0.75.$$

Fuel Utilization During Exercise

In general, protein contributes less than 5% to total energy production during exercise, and for the purpose of our discussion it will be ignored (53). Ignoring protein leaves carbohydrate (muscle glycogen and blood glucose, which is derived from liver glycogen) and fat (adipose tissue and intramuscular fat) as the primary fuels for exercise. The ability of *R* to provide good information about the metabolism of fat and carbohydrate during exercise stems from the following observations about the metabolism of fat and glucose.

When *R* = 1.0, 100% of the energy is derived from carbohydrate and 0% from fat; when *R* = 0.7, the reverse is true. When *R* = 0.85, approximately 50% of the energy comes from carbohydrate and 50% comes from fat (see the *Respiratory Quotients for Carbohydrate and Fat* sidebar). For the *R* measurement to be correct, the subject must be in a steady state. If lactate and hydrogen ions (H^+) are increasing in the blood, the plasma bicarbonate (HCO_3^-) buffer store reacts with the acid (H^+) and produces CO_2. The exerciser is stimulated to hyperventilate and blow off the CO_2:

$$H^+ + HCO_3^- \rightarrow H_2CO_3 \rightarrow H_2O + CO_2.$$

This CO_2 does not come from the aerobic metabolism of carbohydrate and fat, so when it is exhaled it results in an overestimation of the true value of *R*. During strenuous work, H^+ are produced in great amounts, and *R* can exceed 1.0.

Effect of Exercise Intensity on Fuel Utilization

Figure 4.9 shows how *R* changes during increasing exercise intensity. The *R* increases at about 40% to 50% $\dot{V}O_2$max, indicating that Type IIa fibers are being recruited and carbohydrate is becoming a more important fuel source. Using carbohydrate provides an adaptive advantage—the muscle obtains about 6% more energy from each liter of O_2 when carbohydrate is used (5 $kcal \cdot L^{-1}$) compared with when fat is used (4.7 $kcal \cdot L^{-1}$).

Carbohydrate fuels for muscular exercise include muscle glycogen and liver glycogen, with the latter

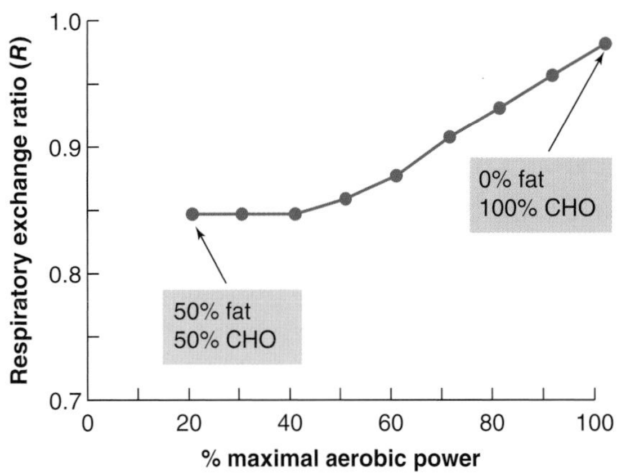

FIGURE 4.9 Changes in *R* (respiratory exchange ratio) with increasing exercise intensity (2).

Respiratory Quotients for Carbohydrate and Fat

For glucose ($C_6H_{12}O_6$),

$$C_6H_{12}O_6 + 6\ O_2 \rightarrow 6\ CO_2 + 6\ H_2O + \text{energy}$$

$$R = \frac{6\ CO_2}{6\ O_2} = 1.0$$

For palmitate ($C_{16}H_{32}O_2$, a fatty acid),

$$C_{16}H_{32}O_2 + 23\ O_2 \rightarrow 16\ CO_2 + 16\ H_2O + \text{energy}$$

$$R = \frac{16\ CO_2}{23\ O_2} = 0.7$$

maintaining the blood glucose concentration. Muscle glycogen is the primary carbohydrate fuel for heavy exercise lasting less than 2 hr, and inadequate muscle glycogen results in premature fatigue (11). As muscle glycogen is depleted during prolonged heavy exercise, blood glucose becomes more important in supplying the carbohydrate fuel. Toward the end of heavy exercise lasting 3 hr or more, blood glucose provides almost all the carbohydrate used by the muscles. Therefore, heavy exercise is limited by the availability of carbohydrate fuels, which must be either stored in abundance before exercise (muscle glycogen) or replaced through the ingestion of carbohydrate during exercise (blood glucose) (10).

Effect of Exercise Duration on Fuel Utilization

Figure 4.10 shows how *R* changes during a 90 min test performed at 65% of the subject's $\dot{V}O_2max$ (54). *R* decreases over time, indicating a greater reliance on fat as a fuel. The fat is derived from both intramuscular fat stores and adipose tissue, which releases free fatty acids into the blood to be carried to the muscle. Using more fat spares the remaining carbohydrate stores and extends the time to exhaustion.

Effect of Diet and Training on Fuel Utilization

The type of fuel used during exercise depends on diet. It has been demonstrated clearly that a diet high in carbohydrate (versus an average diet) increases the muscle glycogen content and extends the time to exhaustion (35). Further, the muscle gains a greater capacity to increase its glycogen store if a person performs strenuous exercise before eating high-carbohydrate meals (35, 66). Finally, during prolonged heavy exercise, carbohydrate beverages help to maintain the blood glucose concentration and extend the time to fatigue (10).

Endurance training increases the number of mitochondria in the muscles involved in the training program.

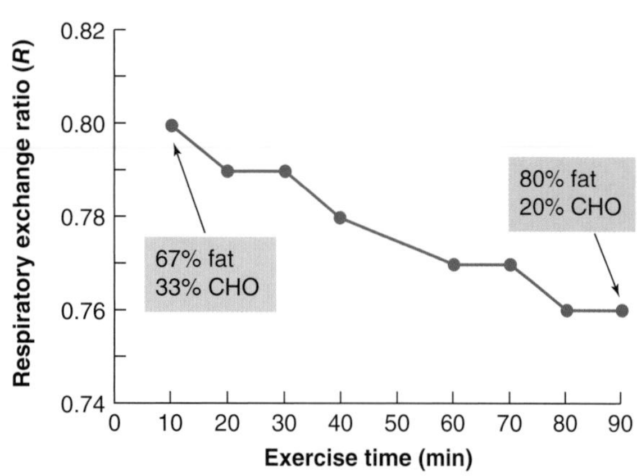

FIGURE 4.10 Changes in *R* (respiratory exchange ratio) during prolonged steady-state exercise (54).

Having more mitochondria increases the ability of the muscle to use fat as a fuel and to process the available carbohydrate aerobically. This ability spares the carbohydrate store and reduces lactate and H^+ production, both of which favorably influence performance (32).

KEY POINT

The respiratory exchange ratio (*R*) tracks fuel use during steady-state exercise. When *R* = 1.0, 100% of the energy is derived from carbohydrate; when *R* = 0.7, 100% of the energy is derived from fat. When hydrogen ions increase in the blood during heavy exercise, they are buffered by plasma bicarbonate. This buffering produces CO_2 and invalidates using *R* as an indicator of fuel use during exercise. As exercise intensity increases, *R* increases, indicating that carbohydrate plays a bigger role in generating ATP. During prolonged moderately strenuous exercise, *R* decreases over time, indicating that fat is being used more and carbohydrate is being spared.

Transition From Rest to Steady-State Work

Some readers might mistakenly assume from our discussion up to this point that anaerobic and aerobic sources of energy (ATP) are used in distinct activities and do not work together to allow the body to make the transition from rest to exercise. When a person steps onto a treadmill belt moving at a velocity of 200 m · min^{-1} (7.5 mi · hr^{-1}), the ATP requirement increases from the low level needed to stand alongside the treadmill to the new level required to run at 200 m · min^{-1}. This change in the ATP supply to the muscle must take place in the first step on the treadmill. If this change fails to occur, the person will drift off the back of the treadmill. What energy sources supply ATP during the first minutes of work?

Oxygen Uptake

The cardiovascular and respiratory systems cannot instantaneously increase the delivery of oxygen to the muscles to completely meet the ATP demands via aerobic processes. In the interval between the time a person steps onto the treadmill and the time the cardiovascular and respiratory systems deliver the required oxygen, anaerobic sources of energy supply the needed ATP. The volume of oxygen missing in the first few minutes of work is the **oxygen deficit** (figure 4.11). PC supplies some of the needed ATP, and the anaerobic breakdown of carbohydrate provides the rest until the oxidative mechanisms meet the ATP requirement. When the uptake of oxygen levels off during submaximal work, the oxygen uptake value represents the **steady-state oxygen requirement** for the activity. At this point, the ATP need of the cell is being met by the aerobic production of ATP in the mitochondria of the muscle on a pay-as-you-go basis.

When the person stops running and steps off the treadmill, the ATP need of the muscles that were involved in the activity suddenly drops toward the resting value. The oxygen uptake decreases quickly at first and then more gradually approaches the resting value. This elevated oxygen uptake during recovery from exercise is the **excess postexercise oxygen consumption (EPOC)**; it also has been called the *oxygen debt* and *oxygen repayment* (figure 4.11). In part, the elevated oxygen uptake is used to make additional ATP to bring the PC store of the muscle back to normal (remember that it was depleted somewhat at the onset of work). Some of the extra oxygen taken in during recovery is used to pay the ATP requirement for the higher HR and breathing during recovery (compared with rest). The liver uses a small part of the elevated oxygen consumption to convert some of the lactate produced at the onset of work into glucose (53).

If an individual reaches the steady-state oxygen requirement earlier during the first minutes of work, a smaller oxygen deficit is incurred. The body depletes less PC and produces less lactate and H^+. Endurance training speeds up the kinetics of oxygen transport; that is, it decreases the time needed to reach a steady state of oxygen uptake. People in poor condition, as well as people with cardiovascular or pulmonary disease, take longer to reach the steady-state oxygen requirement. They incur a larger oxygen deficit and must produce more ATP from the immediate and short-term sources of energy when beginning work or transitioning from one intensity to the next (28, 51).

Heart Rate and Pulmonary Ventilation

The link between the cardiorespiratory responses to work and the time it takes to reach the steady-state oxygen requirement should be no surprise. Figure 4.12 shows how HR and pulmonary ventilation typically respond to a submaximal run test. The shape of the curve in each case resembles the curve for oxygen uptake described earlier.

In addition, the muscle contributes to the lag in oxygen uptake at the onset of work. An untrained muscle has relatively few mitochondria available to produce ATP aerobically and relatively few capillaries per muscle fiber to bring the oxygen-enriched arterial blood to those mitochondria. Following endurance training, both of these factors increase so that the muscle can produce more ATP aerobically at the onset of work. In addition, less lactate and H^+ are produced at the onset of work and the blood lactate and H^+ concentrations are lower for a fixed submaximal work rate (28, 32, 51).

KEY POINT

At the onset of submaximal exercise, $\dot{V}O_2$ does not increase immediately (oxygen deficit), and some of the ATP must be supplied anaerobically by PC and glycolysis. At the end of exercise, $\dot{V}O_2$ remains elevated for some time (EPOC) to replenish PC stores, support the energy cost of the elevated HR and breathing, and synthesize glucose from lactate. Training reduces the oxygen deficit because $\dot{V}O_2$ increases more rapidly at the onset of work, allowing the steady-state oxygen requirement to be reached more quickly.

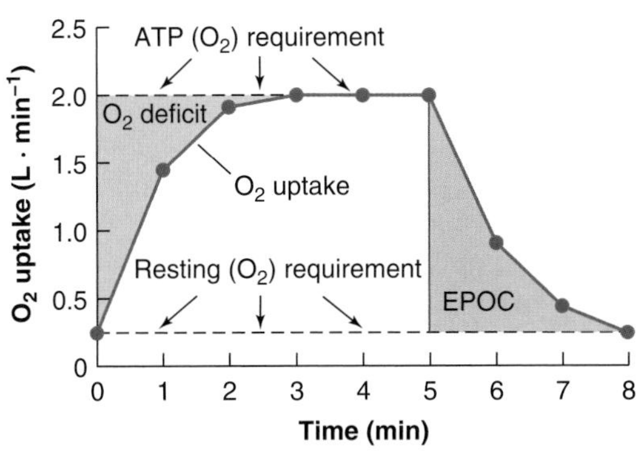

FIGURE 4.11 Oxygen (O_2) deficit and excess postexercise oxygen consumption (EPOC) during a 5 min run on a treadmill.

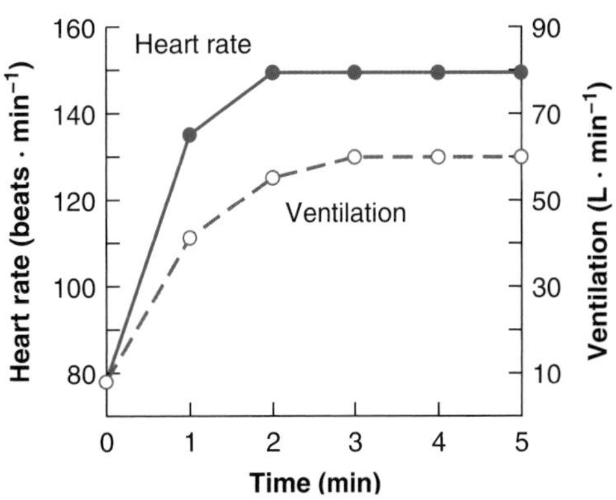

FIGURE 4.12 Response of HR and pulmonary ventilation during a 5 min run on a treadmill.

Graded Exercise Test

Oxygen consumption and CRF are clearly linked because oxygen delivery to tissue depends on lung and heart function. One of the most common tests used to evaluate cardiorespiratory function is a GXT, in which participants exercise at progressively increasing work rates until they reach maximum work tolerance. During the test the participant may be monitored for cardiovascular variables (ECG, HR, BP), respiratory variables (pulmonary ventilation, respiratory frequency), and metabolic variables (oxygen uptake, blood lactate level). The manner in which a person responds to the GXT provides important information about cardiorespiratory function and the capacity for prolonged work.

Oxygen Uptake and Maximal Aerobic Power

Oxygen uptake, measured as described earlier, is expressed per kilogram of body weight to facilitate comparisons between people or between tests for the same person over time. The $\dot{V}O_2$ value in liters per minute is simply multiplied by 1,000 to convert $\dot{V}O_2$ to $ml \cdot min^{-1}$, and that value is divided by the subject's body weight in kilograms to yield a value expressed in milliliters per kilogram per minute.

$$\dot{V}O_2 = 2.4\ L \cdot min^{-1} \cdot 1{,}000\ ml \cdot L^{-1} = 2{,}400\ ml \cdot min^{-1}.$$

For a 60 kg subject,

$$\dot{V}O_2 = 2{,}400\ ml \cdot min^{-1} \div 60\ kg = 40\ ml \cdot kg^{-1} \cdot min^{-1}.$$

Figure 4.13 shows a GXT conducted on a treadmill in which the speed is constant at 3 $mi \cdot hr^{-1}$ (4.8 $km \cdot hr^{-1}$) and the grade changes 3% every 3 min. With each stage of the GXT, oxygen uptake increases to meet the ATP demand of the work rate. Also, the participant incurs a small oxygen deficit at each stage as the cardiovascular system tries to adjust to the new demand of the increased work rate.

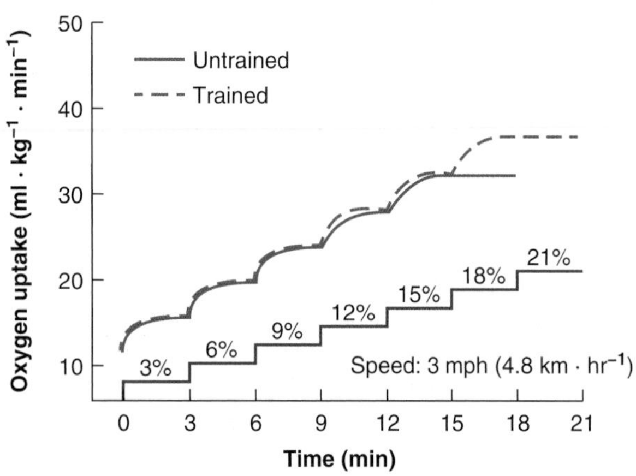

FIGURE 4.13 Oxygen uptake responses to a GXT (40).

Healthy individuals reach the steady-state oxygen requirement by 1.5 min or so of each GXT stage up to moderately heavy work (48, 49). People who have low CRF or who have cardiovascular and pulmonary diseases may not be able to reach the expected values in the same amount of time and might incur larger oxygen deficits with each stage of the test. Because these individuals do not reach the expected steady-state demands of the test at each stage, the oxygen uptake measured at various stages of the test is lower than expected.

Toward the end of a GXT, a point is reached at which the work rate changes (i.e., the grade on the treadmill increases) but the oxygen uptake does not. In effect, the cardiovascular system has reached its limits for transporting oxygen to the muscle. This point is called **maximal aerobic power**, or **maximal oxygen uptake ($\dot{V}O_2$max)**. A complete leveling off in oxygen consumption is not seen in many cases because the subject must work one stage past the actual point at which $\dot{V}O_2$max is reached, requiring high motivation. Over the years, a variety of approaches have been used to obtain evidence that the subject has achieved $\dot{V}O_2$max on the GXT (see Research Insight). Participation in a 10 to 20 wk endurance training program increases $\dot{V}O_2$max. When trained people retake the GXT, they typically reach the steady state sooner at light to moderate work rates and then go one or more stages further into the test, at which time the greater $\dot{V}O_2$max is measured.

Maximal aerobic power describes the greatest rate at which the body (primarily muscle) can produce ATP aerobically during dynamic exercise involving a large muscle mass (e.g., running, cycling). It is also the upper limit at which the cardiovascular system can deliver oxygen-enriched blood to the muscles. Thus, maximal aerobic power is not only a good index of CRF, it is also a good predictor of performance capability in aerobic events such as distance running, cycling, cross-country skiing, and swimming (4, 5). In the apparently healthy person, maximal aerobic power is the quantitative limit at which the cardiovascular system can deliver oxygen to tissues. This usual interpretation must be tempered by the mode of exercise (test type) used to impose the work rate on the subject.

Test Type

For the average person, the highest value for maximal aerobic power is measured when the subject completes a GXT involving uphill running. A GXT conducted at a walking speed usually results in a $\dot{V}O_2$max value 4% to 6% below the graded running value, and a test on a cycle ergometer may yield a value 10% to 12% lower than the graded running value (20, 46, 47). If a subject works to exhaustion using an arm ergometer, then the highest oxygen uptake value is less than 70% of that measured with the legs (23). Knowing these variations in maximal aerobic power is helpful in making recommendations about the intensity of various exercises needed to achieve the target or training HR. At any given submaximal work rate, most physiological responses (HR, BP, and blood lactate) are greater for arm work than for leg work (23, 65). Maximal aerobic power is influenced by more than the type of test used in its measurement. Other factors include endurance training, heredity, sex, age, altitude, pollution, and cardiovascular and pulmonary diseases.

Training and Heredity

Endurance training increases $\dot{V}O_2$max by 5% to 25%, with the magnitude of the change depending, in part, on the initial level of fitness. A person with a low $\dot{V}O_2$max sees the largest change, but there is considerable individual variation in response (see chapter 11 for more on this). Eventually, a point is reached where further training does not increase $\dot{V}O_2$max. Approximately 40% of the extremely high values of maximal aerobic power found in elite cross-country skiers and distance runners relates to a genetic predisposition to a superior cardiovascular system (6). Because typical endurance programs may increase $\dot{V}O_2$max by only 20% or so, it is unrealistic to expect a person with a $\dot{V}O_2$max of 40 ml · kg^{-1} · min^{-1} to increase to 80 ml · kg^{-1} · min^{-1}, a value measured in some elite cross-country skiers and distance runners (61). On the other hand, those who do severe interval training can achieve gains of 44% in $\dot{V}O_2$max (27).

Sex and Age

Women's $\dot{V}O_2$max values (ml · kg^{-1} · min^{-1}) are about 15% lower than men's, a difference that exists across ages 20 to 60. The primary reasons for the gender difference relate to differences in percent body fat and in hemoglobin levels (see later discussion). The 15% difference between men and women is an average value, and $\dot{V}O_2$max values overlap considerably in these populations (2). In most people, aging gradually but systematically reduces $\dot{V}O_2$max by about 1% each year. $\dot{V}O_2$max is influenced by physical activity and percent body fat, so people who remain active and maintain a healthy body weight (which is not the usual case) have higher $\dot{V}O_2$max values across the age span. In fact, endurance training by middle-aged people gives the appearance of reversing the aging effect because it elevates $\dot{V}O_2$max to a level consistent with that of a younger, sedentary person (37-39).

Altitude and Pollution

$\dot{V}O_2$max decreases with increasing altitude. At 7,400 ft (2,300 m), $\dot{V}O_2$max is only 88% of the sea-level value. This decrease in $\dot{V}O_2$max is attributable primarily to the reduction in arterial oxygen content that occurs as the oxygen pressure in the air decreases with increasing altitude. When the arterial oxygen content is lower, the heart must pump

RESEARCH INSIGHT

Criteria for $\dot{V}O_2$max

When a plateau in $\dot{V}O_2$ did not occur in a GXT, several investigators used an approach in which they observed how much the $\dot{V}O_2$ increased in the last stage of the GXT. If the increase was small, well below the expected increase in $\dot{V}O_2$ for the final stage, it was taken as evidence of a plateau and that $\dot{V}O_2$max was achieved. A classic plateau criterion established by Taylor, Buskirk, and Henschel (67) used an increase in $\dot{V}O_2$ in the last stage that was <2.1 ml · kg^{-1} · min^{-1} higher than the previous stage of the GXT, half the expected increase in $\dot{V}O_2$. In addition, other investigators identified a variety of secondary criteria (the plateau being the primary criterion) that could be used as evidence that the individual was working maximally when the highest $\dot{V}O_2$ was measured:

- An *R* greater than 1.10 (36). This indicated that lactate and H^+ levels were elevated and CO_2 was blown off in great amounts.
- A blood lactate concentration greater than 8 mmol · L^{-1}, about eight times the resting value (1). This also indicated that the individual was doing extreme work involving a sizable anaerobic component.
- An HR near that of the individual's age-predicted maximal HR. Given the error in estimating maximal HR, this approach has major problems as a criterion (see chapter 7).

These and other criteria have been used alone and in combination to establish whether or not the subject has achieved $\dot{V}O_2$max (34), but problems remain with this approach. The most recent approaches to confirming that a true $\dot{V}O_2$max has been reached in a GXT include doing a follow-up supramaximal test at an intensity higher than that achieved in the GXT! These follow-up tests have been used on the same day as the GXT (after a brief rest, the follow-up test begins) (18, 22), and on a different day (26, 57). These approaches have been very effective in confirming the $\dot{V}O_2$max value achieved on the GXT.

more blood per minute to meet the oxygen needs of any task. As a result, the HR response is higher at submaximal intensities performed at greater altitudes (33).

Carbon monoxide, produced from the burning of fossil fuel as well as from cigarette smoke, binds readily to hemoglobin and can decrease oxygen transport to muscles. The critical concentration of carbon monoxide in blood needed to decrease $\dot{V}O_2$max is about 4%. After that, $\dot{V}O_2$max decreases approximately 1% for every 1% increase in the carbon monoxide concentration in the blood (56).

Cardiovascular and Pulmonary Diseases

Cardiovascular and pulmonary diseases decrease $\dot{V}O_2$max by diminishing the delivery of oxygen from the air to the blood and reducing the capacity of the heart to deliver blood to the muscles. Patients with CVD have some of the lowest $\dot{V}O_2$max (functional capacity) values, but they also experience the largest changes in $\dot{V}O_2$max from endurance training. Table 4.1 shows common values for $\dot{V}O_2$max in a variety of populations (2, 41).

KEY POINT

Maximal oxygen uptake, $\dot{V}O_2$max, is the greatest rate at which O_2 can be delivered to working muscles during dynamic exercise. $\dot{V}O_2$max is influenced by heredity and training, decreases about 1% per year with age, and is about 15% lower in women compared with men. $\dot{V}O_2$max is lower at high altitudes, and carbon monoxide in the blood decreases $\dot{V}O_2$max because it binds to hemoglobin and limits oxygen transport. Cardiovascular and pulmonary diseases lower $\dot{V}O_2$max; however, people with CVD can attain large improvements in $\dot{V}O_2$max through endurance training.

Blood Lactate and Pulmonary Ventilation

Muscle produces lactate and H^+, which are released into the blood. Figure 4.14 shows that during a GXT, blood lactate concentration changes little or not at all at the lower work rates; lactate is metabolized as fast as it is produced (7). As the GXT increases in intensity, a work rate is reached at which the blood lactate concentration suddenly increases. This work rate is referred to as the **lactate threshold (LT)**, and it typically occurs between 50% and 80% $\dot{V}O_2$max. This sudden increase in the blood lactate concentration is sometimes called the *anaerobic threshold,* but because several conditions other than a lack of oxygen (hypoxia) at the muscle cell can result in lactate being produced and released into the blood, *lactate threshold* is the preferred term. Endurance training increases the number of mitochondria in the trained muscles, facilitating the aerobic metabolism of carbohydrate and the use of more fat as fuel. As a result, when the subject retakes the GXT following training, less lactate is produced and the lactate threshold occurs at a later stage of the test. LT is a good indicator of endurance performance and has been used to predict performance in endurance races (4, 5).

Pulmonary ventilation is the volume of air inhaled or exhaled per minute and is calculated by multiplying the frequency *(f)* of breathing by the tidal volume *(TV),* the volume of air moved in one breath. For example,

$$\text{Ventilation } (\text{L} \cdot \text{min}^{-1}) = TV\,(\text{L} \cdot \text{breath}^{-1}) \cdot f\,(\text{breaths} \cdot \text{min}^{-1}),$$

and

$$30\ \text{L} \cdot \text{min}^{-1} = 1.5\ \text{L} \cdot \text{breath}^{-1} \cdot 20\ \text{breaths} \cdot \text{min}^{-1}.$$

Pulmonary ventilation increases linearly with work rate until 50% to 80% of $\dot{V}O_2$max, at which point a relative **hyperventilation** results (see figure 4.15). The inflection point in the pulmonary ventilation response is the **ventilatory threshold (VT)**. The VT has been used as a noninvasive indicator of the LT and as a predictor of performance (17, 52). The increase in pulmonary ventilation

Table 4.1 Maximal Aerobic Power in Healthy and Diseased Populations

	$\dot{V}O_2$MAX (ML · KG^{-1} · MIN^{-1})	
Population	**Men**	**Women**
Elite cross-country skiers	75-85	65-75
Elite distance runners	70-80	65-75
College students	40-50	30-40
Middle-aged adults	30-40	25-35
Post-MI patients	~22	~18
Patients with severe pulmonary disease	~13	~13

Data compiled from Åstrand et al 2003; Fox, E.L., R.W. Bowers, and M.L. Foss. 1998, *Fox's the physiological basis for exercise and sport.* 6th ed. Dubuque, IA: Brown; J.H. Wilmore, D.L. Costill, and W.L. Kenney. 2008, *Physiology of sport and exercise.* 4th ed. Champaign, IL: Human Kinetics; the Fort Sanders Cardiac Rehabilitation Program; and J.T. Daniels (personal communication).

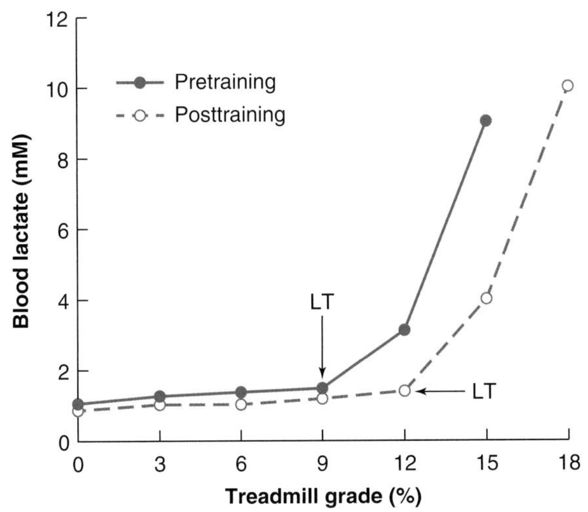

FIGURE 4.14 Training causes the LT to occur at a higher exercise intensity (19).

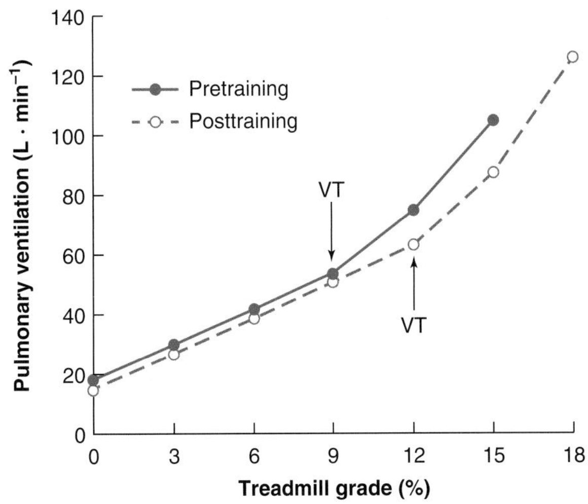

FIGURE 4.15 Following training, the VT occurs later in the GXT.

is mediated by changes in the frequency of breathing (from about 10-12 breaths · min^{-1} at rest to 40-50 breaths · min^{-1} during maximal work) and in the tidal volume (from 0.5 L · $breath^{-1}$ at rest to 2-3 L · $breath^{-1}$ in maximal work). Endurance training lowers pulmonary ventilation during submaximal work, so the VT occurs later in the GXT. The maximal value for pulmonary ventilation tends to change in the direction of $\dot{V}O_2$max.

KEY POINT

The points at which the blood lactate concentration and the pulmonary ventilation increase suddenly during a GXT are called the *lactate* and *ventilatory thresholds,* respectively. These typically occur between 50% and 80% $\dot{V}O_2$max. The LT and VT are good predictors of performance in endurance events (e.g., 10K runs, marathons).

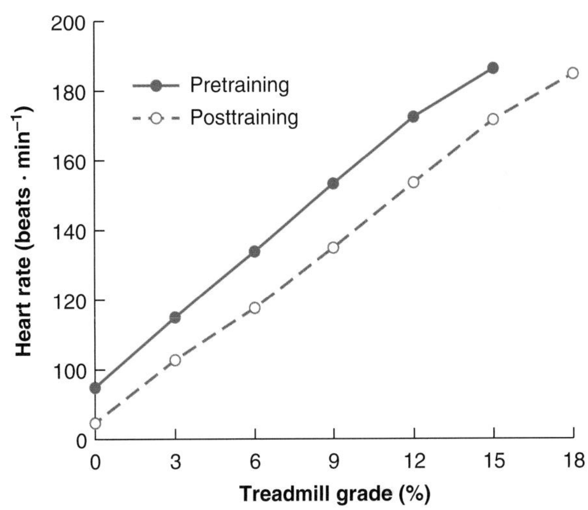

FIGURE 4.16 Training reduces the HR response to submaximal exercise (19).

Heart Rate

Once the HR reaches about 110 beats · min^{-1}, it increases linearly with work rate during a GXT until near-maximal efforts. Figure 4.16 shows how training influences the subject's HR response at the same work rates. The lower HR at submaximal work rates is a beneficial effect because it decreases the oxygen needed by the heart muscle. Maximal HR shows no change or is slightly reduced as a result of endurance training.

Stroke Volume

The volume of blood pumped by the heart per beat (ml · $beat^{-1}$) is the *stroke volume (SV).* For the typical person doing work in the upright position (cycling, walking), SV increases in the early stages of the GXT until about 40% $\dot{V}O_2$max is reached, and then it levels off (see figure 4.17) (2). Consequently, when $\dot{V}O_2$ is greater than 40% $\dot{V}O_2$max, HR is the sole factor responsible for the increased flow of blood from the heart to the working muscles. This is what makes HR a good indicator of the metabolic rate during exercise—it is linearly related to exercise intensity from light exercise to heavy exercise. One of the primary effects of endurance training is an increase in SV at rest and during work; this increase is due to a larger volume of the ventricle that is linked, in part, to a larger blood volume (19). This allows a greater **end-diastolic volume (EDV)**, the volume of blood in the heart just before contraction. So, following endurance training, even if the same fraction of blood in the ventricle is pumped per beat (**ejection fraction**), the heart pumps more blood per minute at the same HR.

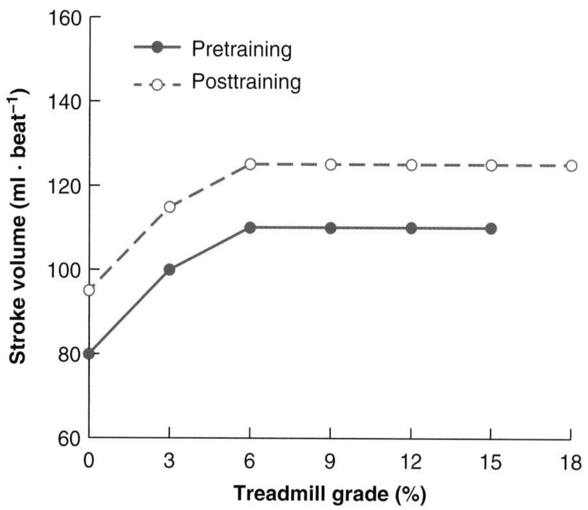

FIGURE 4.17 SV increases with training due to larger volume of the ventricle (19).

RESEARCH INSIGHT

Stroke Volume in Elite Athletes

For most people, SV levels off at about 40% $\dot{V}O_2max$, making HR the sole factor increasing blood flow to the muscles at higher exercise intensities. However, there is clear evidence that this is not the case for highly trained endurance athletes. Interestingly, in these athletes, SV increases systematically with exercise intensity up to $\dot{V}O_2max$. This appears to be due to both enhanced filling of the ventricle before contraction (EDV) and greater emptying of the ventricle during contraction (ejection fraction), in contrast to what is observed in people of average fitness (25, 69).

Cardiac Output

Cardiac output (*Q*) is the volume of blood pumped by the heart per minute and is calculated by multiplying the HR (beats · min $^{-1}$) by the SV (ml · beat^{-1}).

$$\text{Cardiac output} = \text{HR} \cdot \text{SV}$$
$$= 60 \text{ beats} \cdot \text{min}^{-1} \cdot 80 \text{ ml} \cdot \text{beat}^{-1}$$
$$= 4{,}800 \text{ ml} \cdot \text{min}^{-1}, \text{ or } 4.8 \text{ L} \cdot \text{min}^{-1}.$$

Cardiac output increases linearly with work rate. Generally, the cardiac output response to light and moderate work is not affected by endurance training. What changes is how the cardiac output is achieved: with a lower HR and higher SV.

Maximal cardiac output (highest value reached in a GXT) is the most important cardiovascular variable determining maximal aerobic power because the oxygen-enriched blood (carrying about 0.2 L of O_2 per liter of blood) must be delivered to the muscle for the mitochondria to use. If a person's maximal cardiac output is 10 L · min^{-1}, only 2 L of O_2 would leave the heart each minute (i.e., 0.2 L of O_2 per liter of blood times a cardiac output of 10 L · min^{-1} = 2 L of O_2 · min^{-1}). A person with a maximal cardiac output of 30 L· min^{-1} would deliver 6 L of O_2 · min^{-1} to the tissues. Endurance training increases the maximal cardiac output and thus the delivery of oxygen to the muscles (see figure 4.18). This increase in maximal cardiac output is matched by greater capillary numbers in the muscle to allow the blood to move slowly enough through the muscle to maintain the time needed for oxygen to diffuse from the blood to the mitochondria (62). The increase in maximal cardiac output accounts for 50% of the increase in maximal oxygen uptake that occurs in previously sedentary people who engage in endurance training (59).

Oxygen Extraction

Two factors determine oxygen uptake at any time: the volume of blood delivered to the tissues per minute (cardiac output) and the volume of oxygen extracted from each liter of blood. Oxygen extraction is calculated by subtracting the oxygen content of mixed venous blood (as it returns to the heart) from the oxygen content of the arterial blood. This is the **arteriovenous oxygen difference**, or the *(a – vō) O_2 difference.*

$$\dot{V}O_2 = \text{cardiac output} \cdot (a - v\bar{o})O_2 \text{ difference}.$$

At rest, cardiac output = 5 L · min^{-1},
arterial oxygen content = 200 ml of O_2 · L^{-1}, and
mixed venous oxygen content = 150 ml of O_2 · L^{-1}.

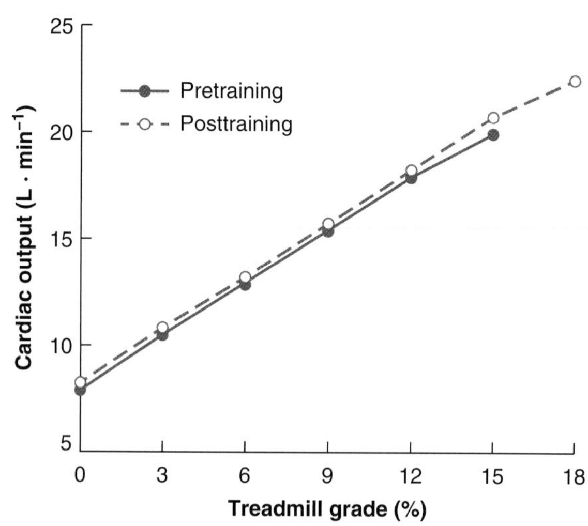

FIGURE 4.18 Maximal cardiac output increases following training (19).

$$\dot{V}O_2 = 5\ L \cdot min^{-1} \cdot (200 - 150\ ml\ of\ O_2 \cdot L^{-1})$$
$$= 5\ L \cdot min^{-1} \cdot 50\ ml\ of\ O_2 \cdot L^{-1}$$
$$= 250\ ml \cdot min^{-1}.$$

The $(a - v\bar{o})O_2$ difference reflects the ability of the muscle to extract oxygen, and it increases with exercise intensity (see figure 4.19). The ability of tissue to extract oxygen is a function of the capillary-to-muscle-fiber ratio and the number of mitochondria in the muscle fiber. Endurance training increases both of these factors, thus increasing the maximal capacity to extract oxygen in the last stage of the GXT (57). This increase in the $(a - v\bar{o})O_2$ difference accounts for about 50% of the increase in $\dot{V}O_2max$ that occurs with endurance training in previously sedentary individuals (59).

In the general population, SV is the major variable influencing maximal cardiac output. Differences in maximal cardiac output and maximal aerobic power that exist between females and males, between trained and untrained individuals, and between world-class endurance athletes and average fit individuals can be explained largely by differences in maximal SV. For example, in three groups of people who differed greatly in $\dot{V}O_2max$ (5.2 versus 3.2 versus 1.6 $L \cdot min^{-1}$), there was little difference in maximal HR (range 190-200 beats $\cdot$ min^{-1}) and oxygen extraction (range 160-170 ml $O_2 \cdot L^{-1}$). In contrast, SV differed greatly between the groups (160 versus 100 versus 50 ml $\cdot$ $beat^{-1}$) (58). Clearly, maximal SV is the primary factor related to the differences in $\dot{V}O_2max$ that exist from person to person.

Blood Pressure

BP is dependent on the balance between cardiac output and the resistance that blood vessels offer to blood flow (total peripheral resistance). The resistance to blood flow is altered by the constriction or dilation of **arterioles**, which are blood vessels located between the artery and the capillary.

BP = cardiac output · total peripheral resistance.

BP is sensed by **baroreceptors** in the arch of the aorta and in the carotid arteries. When BP changes, the baroreceptors send signals to the cardiovascular control center in the brain, which in turn alters cardiac output or the diameter of arterioles. For example, if a person who has been lying supine suddenly stands, blood pools in the lower extremities, SV decreases, and BP drops. If BP is not restored quickly, less blood flows to the brain and the person might faint. The baroreceptors monitor this decrease in BP, and the cardiovascular control center simultaneously increases the HR and reduces the diameter of the arterioles (to increase total peripheral resistance) to try to return BP to normal. During exercise, the arterioles dilate in the active muscle to increase blood flow and meet metabolic demands. This dilation is matched with a constriction of arterioles in the liver, kidneys, and gastrointestinal tract and an increase in HR and SV, as already mentioned. These coordinated changes maintain BP and direct most of the cardiac output to the working muscles.

BP is monitored at each stage of a GXT. Figure 4.20 shows how **systolic blood pressure (SBP)** increases with each stage until maximum work tolerance is reached. At that point, SBP might decrease. A fall in SBP with an increase in work rate is used as an indicator of maximal cardiovascular function and can aid in determining the end point for an exercise test. **Diastolic blood pressure (DBP)** tends to remain the same or decrease during a GXT. An increase in DBP toward the end of the test is another indicator that a subject has reached the limits of functional capacity. Endurance training reduces the BP responses at fixed submaximal work rates. See chapter 7 for criteria for terminating a GXT.

Two factors that determine the oxygen demand (work) of the heart during aerobic exercise are the HR and the SBP.

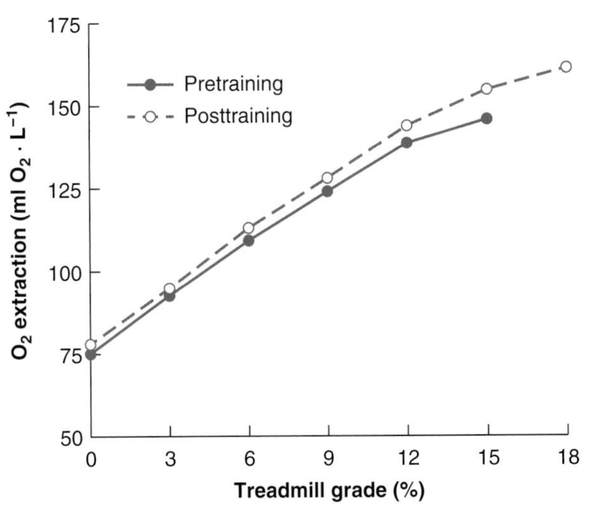

FIGURE 4.19 Following training, maximal O_2 extraction increases due to greater capillary and mitochondrial density in the trained muscles (19).

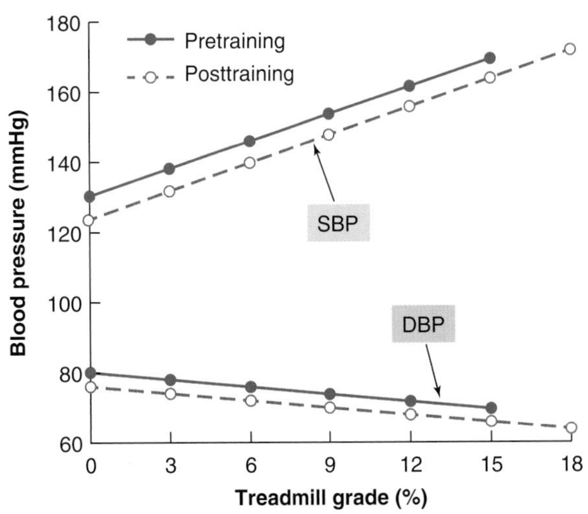

FIGURE 4.20 SBP increases until maximum work tolerance is reached. DBP remains steady or decreases.

KEY POINT

In people of average fitness, SV increases until about 40% $\dot{V}O_2$max, but both HR and cardiac output (HR · SV) increase linearly with work rate. Endurance training reduces HR and increases SV at rest and during exercise. In addition, maximal cardiac output is greater because maximal HR is generally unchanged. Variations in $\dot{V}O_2$max are primarily due to differences in maximal SV. Half of the increase in $\dot{V}O_2$max from endurance training is the result of an increase in maximal SV; the other half is due to an increase in oxygen extraction.

The product of these two variables is called the **rate–pressure product**, or the **double product**, and is proportional to the myocardial oxygen demand (i.e., the volume of oxygen the heart muscle needs each minute to function properly). Factors that decrease the HR and BP responses to work increase the chance that the coronary blood supply to the heart muscle will adequately meet the oxygen demands of the heart. Endurance training decreases the HR and BP responses to fixed submaximal work and protects against any diminished blood supply (ischemia) to the myocardium. Drugs are also used to lower HR and BP to reduce the work of the heart (see chapter 24).

When a person does the same rate of work with the arms as with the legs, the HR and BP responses are considerably higher during the arm work. Given that the load on the heart and the potential for fatigue are greater for arm work, fitness professionals should choose activities that use the large muscle groups of the legs. Such activities result in lower HR, BP, and perception of fatigue at the same work rate (23, 65), which allow one to accomplish more work in a fixed time period than with arm exercise. That said, if participants need to increase their capacity for arm work related to employment or sport, then structured progressive exercise programs should be implemented for that purpose.

KEY POINT

SBP increases with each stage of a GXT, whereas DBP remains the same or decreases. The work of the heart is proportional to the product of the HR and the SBP. Training lowers both, making it easier for the coronary arteries to meet the oxygen demand of the heart. HR and BP are higher during arm work compared with leg work at the same work rate.

Effects of Endurance Training and Detraining on Physiological Responses

Many observations have been made about the effects of endurance training on various physiological responses to exercise. In this section we show how some of these effects are connected.

- Endurance training increases the number of mitochondria and capillaries in muscle, causing all active fibers to become more oxidative. This effect is manifested by the increase in Type IIa fibers and decrease in Type IIx fibers. These changes boost the endurance capacity of the muscle by allowing fat to be used for a greater percentage of energy production, sparing the muscle glycogen store and reducing lactate production. The LT shifts to the right, and performance times in endurance events improve.
- Endurance training decreases the time it takes to achieve a steady state in submaximal exercise. This reduces the oxygen deficit and reliance on PC and anaerobic glycolysis for energy.
- Endurance training enlarges the volume of the ventricle. This accommodates an increase in the EDV such that more blood is pumped out per beat. The increased SV is accompanied by a decrease in HR during submaximal work, so the cardiac output remains the same. The heart works less to meet the oxygen needs of the tissues at the same work rate. Table 4.2 summarizes these changes that result from endurance training.
- Maximal aerobic power increases with endurance training, the increase being inversely related to the initial $\dot{V}O_2$max. In formerly sedentary people, about 50% of the increase in $\dot{V}O_2$max results from greater maximal cardiac output, a change brought about by an increase in maximal SV, given that maximal HR either remains the same or decreases slightly. The other 50% of the increase in $\dot{V}O_2$max is attributable to an increase in oxygen extraction at the muscle, shown by an increase in the $(a - \bar{v})$ O_2 difference. This occurs as a result of higher numbers of capillaries and mitochondria in the trained muscles.

Transfer of Training

The training effects that have been discussed are observed only when the trained muscles are the muscles used in the exercise test. Although this may appear obvious for the decrease in blood lactate that is attributable to, in part, the greater numbers of mitochondria in the trained

Table 4.2 Effects of Endurance Training on Cardiovascular Response to a Graded Exercise Test

Variable	Rest	At same relative $\dot{V}O_2 (ml \cdot kg^{-1} \cdot min^{-1})$	At maximal work
Cardiac output	Same	Same	Higher
SV	Higher	Higher	Higher
HR	Lower	Lower	No change or slightly lower

muscles, it is also linked to the changes that occur in the HR response to submaximal work following the training program. Figure 4.21 shows the results of repeated submaximal exercise tests conducted on subjects who trained only one leg on a cycle ergometer for 13 days. The HR response to a fixed submaximal work rate performed by the trained leg decreased as expected. At the end of the 13 days of training, the untrained leg was subjected to the same exercise test. The HR responded as if a training effect had not occurred. This indicates that part of the reason the HR response to submaximal exercise decreases following training is because of feedback from the trained muscles to the cardiovascular control center that, in turn, reduces sympathetic stimulation to the heart (9, 59). This finding has important implications for evaluating the effects of training programs. The expected training responses (lower lactate production, lower HR, greater fat use) are linked to testing the same muscle groups that were involved in the training. The probability of the training effect carrying over to another activity depends on the degree to which the new activity uses the muscles that were involved in the training program.

Detraining

How fast is a training effect lost? A number of investigations have explored this question by having subjects either reduce or completely cease training. Maximal oxygen uptake is typically used as the principal measure to evaluate physiological changes due to detraining, but an individual's response to a submaximal work rate also has been used to track these changes over time.

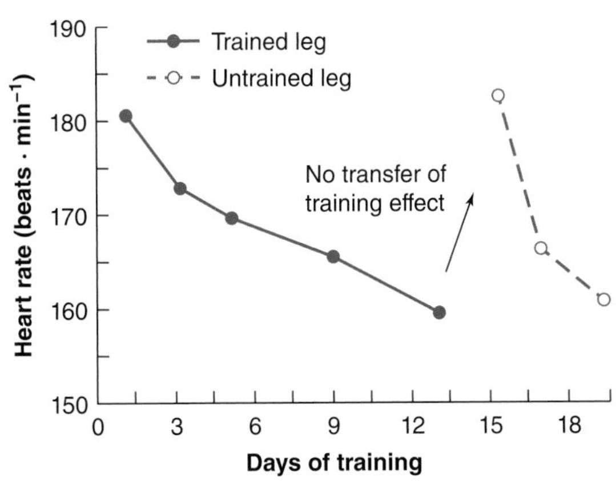

FIGURE 4.21 Lack of transfer of training effect (9).

Ceasing Training

The following study used subjects who had trained for 10 ± 3 yr and agreed to cease training for 84 days (15). They were tested on days 12, 21, 56, and 84 of detraining. Figure 4.22 shows how their $\dot{V}O_2$max decreased 7% within the first 12 days. Remember that $\dot{V}O_2$max = cardiac output · $(a - \bar{v})O_2$ difference. The decrease in $\dot{V}O_2$max was attributable entirely to a drop in maximal cardiac output because the maximal oxygen extraction, or $(a - \bar{v})O_2$ difference, was unchanged.

In turn, the lower maximal cardiac output was attributable entirely to a decrease in maximal SV, because maximal HR actually increased during detraining. A subsequent study showed that the reduced SV was caused by a reduction in plasma volume that occurred in the first 12 days of no training (13). In contrast, the drop in $\dot{V}O_2$max between days 21 and 84 was attributable to a decrease in the $(a - \bar{v})O_2$ difference because maximal cardiac output was unchanged (see figure 4.22). This lower oxygen extraction appeared to result from smaller numbers of mitochondria in the muscle, given that the number of capillaries surrounding each muscle fiber was unchanged (12).

The same subjects also completed a standard (fixed work rate) submaximal exercise test during the 84 days of no training (14). Figure 4.23 shows that HR and blood lactate responses to this work test increased throughout detraining. The higher responses relate to the fact that the same work rate required a greater percentage of $\dot{V}O_2$max because the latter variable decreased throughout the detraining. The magnitude of change in HR and blood lactate responses to this submaximal work, however, makes them sensitive indicators of a person's training state.

Reduced Training

To evaluate the effect of reduced training, Hickson and colleagues (29-31) trained subjects for 10 wk to increase $\dot{V}O_2$max. The training program was conducted 40 min per day, 6 days per wk. Three days involved running at near-maximum intensity for 40 min; the other 3 days required six 5-min bouts at near-maximum intensity on a cycle ergometer, with a 2 min rest between work bouts. Subjects expended about 600 kcal on each day of exercise,

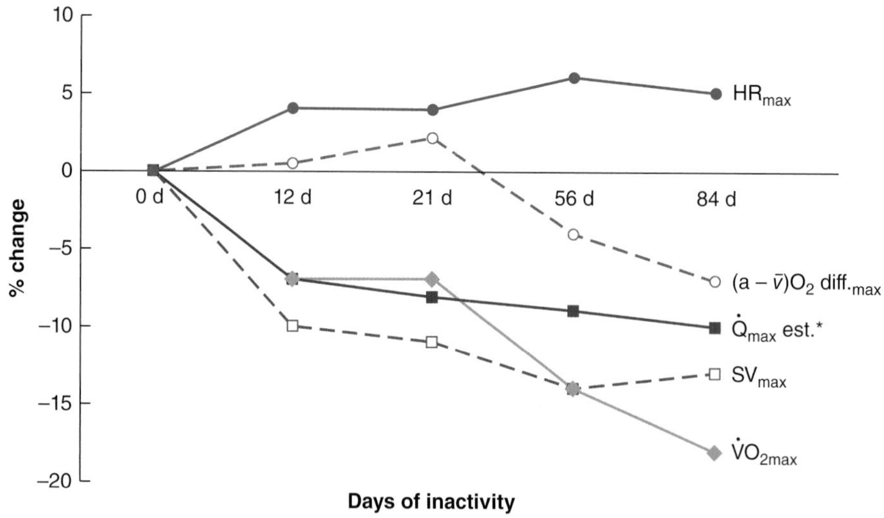

FIGURE 4.22 Effects of detraining on physiological responses during exercise. $\dot{V}O_2max$ = maximal oxygen uptake; $\dot{Q}max$ est. = maximal cardiac output; $(a - v\bar{o})O_2$ diff. max = maximal arteriovenous oxygen difference.
Data from Coyle 1984.

or 3,600 kcal each week. At the end of this 10 wk program, the subjects were divided into groups that trained at either a one-third or two-thirds reduction in the previous frequency (4 and 2 days per wk, respectively), duration (26 and 13 min per day, respectively), or intensity (a one-third or two-thirds reduction in work done or distance run per 40 min session).

Data collected on the maximal treadmill tests showed that cutting duration from 40 to 26 or 13 min or frequency from 6 to 4 or 2 days did not affect $\dot{V}O_2max$. In contrast, $\dot{V}O_2max$ clearly fell when the intensity of training was reduced by either one-third or two-thirds. The subjects were able to maintain $\dot{V}O_2max$ when the total exercise per week was cut from 3,600 to 1,200 kcal in the group whose exercise frequency and duration were reduced by two-thirds, but they were not able to maintain $\dot{V}O_2max$ when the intensity was reduced, even though the subjects were still expending about 1,200 kcal · wk^{-1}. This shows that exercise intensity is critical in maintaining $\dot{V}O_2max$ and that it takes less exercise to maintain than to achieve a specific level of $\dot{V}O_2max$.

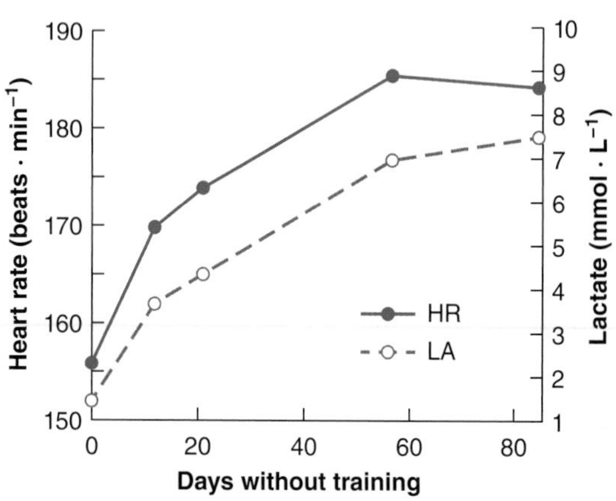

FIGURE 4.23 Changes in the HR and blood lactate responses to a standard exercise test taken during 84 days of detraining (14).

KEY POINT

Endurance training increases the ability of a muscle to use fat as a fuel and to spare carbohydrate, decreases the time it takes to achieve a steady state during submaximal work, increases the size of the ventricle, and increases $\dot{V}O_2max$ by increasing SV and oxygen extraction. Endurance training effects (lower HR, lower blood lactate) do not transfer when untrained muscles are used to perform the work. Maximal oxygen uptake decreases when training stops. The initial decrease is caused by a decrease in SV and, later, in oxygen extraction. Maximal oxygen uptake can be maintained by doing intense exercise, even when cutting exercise duration and frequency.

Cardiovascular Responses to Exercise

One of the physiological differences between men and women is that women require a higher body-fat percentage for good health (see chapter 8), and the additional mass attributed to fat affects performance. When performing activities such as running, the absolute energy demand depends upon weight. For anyone, extra fat weight will increase the total oxygen requirement at a given running pace. However, the energy demand of running at a given pace when expressed per kilogram of body weight is the same regardless of how much one weighs or how much is accounted for by fat mass (see chapter 6). For example, running at 180 m · min^{-1} requires a $\dot{V}O_2$ of 39.5 ml · kg^{-1} · min^{-1}. For a person who weighs 60 kg, this translates into a $\dot{V}O_2$ of 2.37 L · min^{-1}, but for a person who weighs 80 kg, the oxygen requirement would be 3.16 L · min^{-1}. Thus, extra fat mass will lead to a higher absolute oxygen demand and a higher HR at a given pace. Likewise, performance in the 12 min run test (used to evaluate maximal aerobic power) decreases by 89 m when body weight is experimentally increased to simulate a 5% gain in body fat (16). When a woman walks on a treadmill at a given grade and speed, her HR will be higher than that of a similarly trained man because of the additional fat weight she carries. Her lower hemoglobin concentration and smaller heart size also elevate the HR at the same oxygen uptake expressed per unit of body weight.

The differences between males and females in the cardiovascular response to submaximal work become more exaggerated when work is done on a cycle ergometer where a given work rate demands a similar $\dot{V}O_2$ in liters per minute, independent of sex or training. As previously mentioned, the average female has less hemoglobin and a smaller heart volume compared with the average male. To deliver the same volume of oxygen to the muscles, the woman must have a higher HR to compensate for the smaller SV and a slightly higher cardiac output to compensate for the slightly lower hemoglobin concentration (2). In addition, the average woman typically has a smaller muscle mass with which to accomplish the work, which increases the HR response (see arm versus leg work discussed previously). These differences between women's and men's cardiovascular responses to cycle ergometry are shown in figure 4.24. Table 4.3 summarizes the differences in cardiovascular responses between men and women in response to exercise.

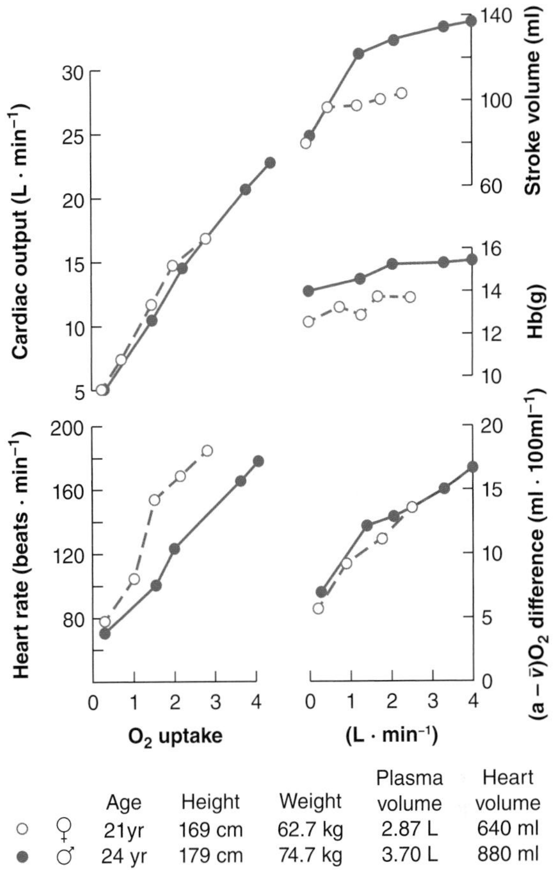

FIGURE 4.24 The cardiovascular responses of well-trained men and women to cycle ergometry. Hb = hemoglobin.

Reprinted, by permission, from P.-O. Åstrand and K. Rodahl, 2003, *Textbook of work physiology*, 4th ed. (Champaign, IL: Human Kinetics), 176.

KEY POINT

During submaximal exercise at the same relative $\dot{V}O_2$ (e.g., walking on a treadmill), women respond with a higher HR due to a higher percent fat, lower SV, and lower hemoglobin level. When exercising at the same work rate or absolute $\dot{V}O_2$(e.g., riding a cycle ergometer), women respond with a higher HR to compensate for a lower SV and a lower hemoglobin level (and oxygen content) in the arterial blood.

Table 4.3 Cardiovascular Responses of Women Compared With Men

Variable	Rest	At same absolute $\dot{V}O_2$ (L · min^{-1})	At same relative $\dot{V}O_2$ (ml · kg^{-1} · min^{-1})	At maximal work
Cardiac output	Lower	Slightly higher	—	Lower
SV	Lower	Lower	Lower	Lower
HR	Higher	Higher	Higher	Lower

Cardiovascular Responses to Isometric Exercise and Weightlifting

Most endurance exercise programs use dynamic activities involving large muscle masses to place loads on the cardiorespiratory system. The previous summary of the physiological responses to a GXT indicates that cardiovascular load is proportional to exercise intensity. But this is not necessarily the case for resistance training, in which a person can have a disproportionately high cardiovascular load relative to the exercise intensity. In a now classic study, a subject performed an isometric exercise test (sustained handgrip) at only 30% maximum voluntary contraction (MVC) strength while BP was monitored. In contrast to dynamic exercise, both the SBP and DBP increased over time, and SBP exceeded 220 mmHg. This kind of exercise puts a disproportionate load on the heart and is not recommended for older adults or people with heart disease (43). See chapter 13 for information on resistance training programs for patients with CVD.

Dynamic, heavy-resistance exercises can also cause extreme BP responses. Figure 4.25 shows the peak BP response achieved during exercise at 95% to 100% of the maximum weight that could be lifted one time (1RM). Both DBP and SBP are elevated, with average values exceeding 300/200 mmHg for the two-leg leg press done to fatigue. The elevation in pressure was believed to be caused by the compression of the arteries by the muscles, a reflex response attributable to the static component associated with near-maximal dynamic lifts, and by the Valsalva maneuver (trying to exhale forcefully against a closed airway), which can independently elevate BP (44). Another study reported peak values of about 190/140 mmHg for exercises of 50%, 70%, and 80% of 1RM done to fatigue in untrained lifters. Bodybuilders responded with lower BPs, indicating a cardiovascular adaptation to resistance training (21).

KEY POINT

Isometric exercise and heavy-resistance exercise elicit high BP responses compared with dynamic endurance exercise. Both SBP and DBP increase with isometric and dynamic resistance training.

Regulating Body Temperature

Under resting conditions, the body's core temperature is 37 °C, and heat production and heat loss are balanced. Mechanisms of heat production include the basal metabolic rate, shivering, work, and exercise. During exercise, mechanical efficiency is about 20% or less, which means that 80% or more of energy production ($\dot{V}O_2$) is converted to heat. For example, if you are working on a cycle ergometer at a rate requiring a $\dot{V}O_2$ of 2.0 L · min^{-1}, your energy production is about 10 kcal · min^{-1}. At 20% efficiency, 2 kcal · min^{-1} are used to do work and 8 kcal · min^{-1} are converted to heat. If most of this added heat is not lost, core temperature might quickly rise to dangerous levels. How does the body lose excess heat?

Heat-Loss Mechanisms

The body loses heat by four processes. In **radiation**, heat transfers from the surface of one object to the surface of another, with no physical contact between the objects.

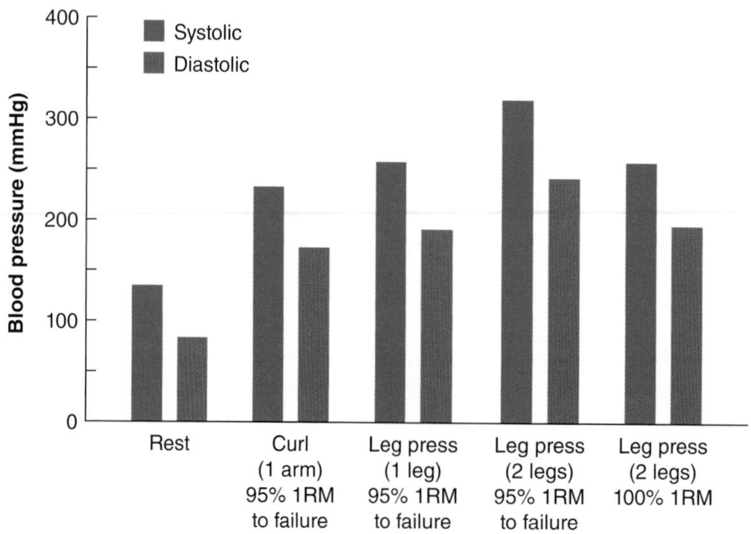

FIGURE 4.25 BP responses during weightlifting (44). RM = repetition maximum.

Heat loss depends on the temperature gradient; that is, the temperature difference between the surfaces of the objects. When a person is seated at rest in a comfortable environment (21-22 °C), about 60% of body heat is lost through radiation to cooler objects. **Conduction** is the transfer of heat from one object to another by direct contact, and, like radiation, it depends on a temperature gradient. A person sitting on a cold marble bench loses body heat by conduction. **Convection** is a special case of conduction in which heat is transferred to air (or water) molecules, which become lighter and rise away from the body to be replaced by cold air (or water). Heat loss can be enhanced by increasing the movement of the air (or water) over the surface of the body. For example, a fan stimulates heat loss by placing more cold air molecules into contact with the skin.

All of these heat-loss mechanisms can be heat-gain mechanisms as well. We gain heat from the sun by radiation across 93 million mi (150 million km) of space, and we gain heat by conduction when we sit on hot sand at the beach. Similarly, if a fan were to place more hot air (warmer than skin temperature) into contact with the skin, we would gain heat. Heat gained from the environment adds to that generated by exercise and puts an additional strain on heat-loss mechanisms.

The fourth heat-loss mechanism is the evaporation of sweat. **Sweating** is the process of producing a watery solution over the surface of the body, and **evaporation** is a process in which liquid water converts to a gas. This conversion requires about 580 kcal of heat per liter of sweat evaporated. The heat for this comes from the body, and thus the body is cooled. At rest, about 25% of heat loss is caused by evaporation, but during exercise evaporation becomes the primary mechanism for heat loss.

Evaporation depends on the **water vapor pressure gradient** between the skin and air and does not directly depend on temperature. The water vapor pressure of the air relates to the **relative humidity** and the **saturation pressure** at that air temperature. For example, the relative humidity can be 90% in winter, but because the saturation pressure of cold air is low, the water vapor pressure of the air is also low, and you can see water vapor rising from your body following exercise. In warm temperatures, however, the relative humidity is a good indicator of the water vapor pressure of the air. If the water vapor pressure of the air is too high, sweat will not evaporate, and sweat that does not evaporate does not cool the body (53).

Body Temperature Response to Exercise

Figure 4.26 shows that during exercise in a comfortable environment, the core temperature increases proportionally to the relative intensity (%$\dot{V}O_2$max) of the exercise and then levels off (64). The gain in body heat that occurs early in exercise triggers the heat-loss mechanisms discussed in

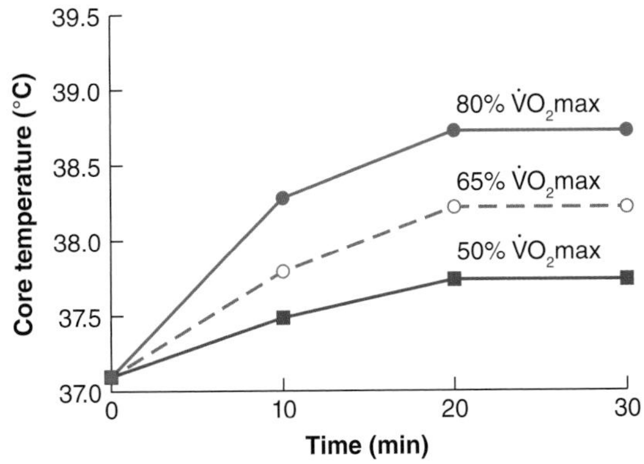

FIGURE 4.26 Core temperature increases over time as exercise intensity increases (2).

the preceding section. After 10 to 20 min, heat loss equals heat production, and the core temperature remains steady (24). What are the most important heat-loss mechanisms during exercise?

Heat Loss During Exercise

Exercise intensity and environmental temperature influence which heat-loss mechanism is primarily responsible for maintaining a steady core temperature during exercise. When a person participates in progressively difficult exercise tests in an environment that allows heat loss by all four mechanisms, the contribution that convection and radiation make to overall heat loss is modest. Because the temperature gradient between the skin and the room does not change much during exercise, the rate of heat loss is relatively constant. To compensate for this, evaporation picks up when heat losses by convection and radiation plateau, and evaporation is responsible for most of the heat loss in heavy exercise (figure 4.27).

When a person performs steady-state exercise in a warmer environment, the role that evaporation plays becomes even more important. Figure 4.28 shows that

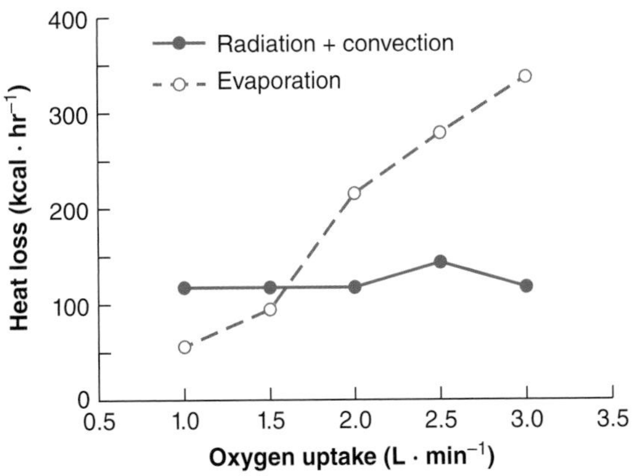

FIGURE 4.27 Importance of evaporation to relative work rate (64). Evaporation is more important at higher work rates.

as environmental temperature increases, the gradient for heat loss by convection and radiation decreases, and the rate of heat loss by these processes also decreases. As a result, evaporation must compensate to maintain core temperature.

In strenuous exercise or hot environments, evaporation is the most important process for losing heat and maintaining body temperature in a safe range. It should be no surprise, then, that factors affecting sweat production (such as dehydration) or sweat evaporation (such as impermeable clothing) are causes for concern. Chapter 11 provides details on dealing with heat and humidity when prescribing exercise, and chapter 25 discusses how to prevent and treat heat-related disorders.

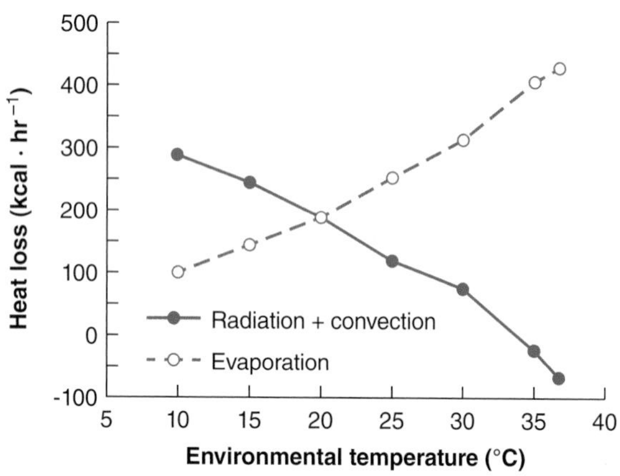

FIGURE 4.28 Importance of evaporation as a heat-loss mechanism during exercise as environmental temperature increases (2). At higher environmental temperatures, evaporation becomes more important.

Training in a hot and humid environment for as few as 7 to 12 days results in specific adaptations that improve heat tolerance and, as a result, lower the trained person's body temperature during submaximal exercise (24). Adaptations that improve heat tolerance include the following:

- Increased plasma volume
- Earlier onset of sweating
- Higher sweat rate
- Reduced salt loss through sweat
- Reduced blood flow to the skin

KEY POINT

Heat can be lost from the body by radiation and convection when a temperature gradient exists between the skin and the environment; however, evaporation is the primary mechanism of heat loss during high-intensity exercise or during exercise in a hot environment. Body temperature increases in proportion to the relative work rate (%$\dot{V}O_2$max) during submaximal exercise. Acclimatization to heat can be achieved in 7 to 12 days of training in a hot, humid environment and improves one's ability to exercise safely.

4

LEARNING AIDS

REVIEW QUESTIONS

1. What are the two anaerobic sources of energy?
2. In an all-out run lasting 10 min, which energy system provides the greatest amount of energy?
3. Name the three fiber types, and indicate the order in which they are recruited as exercise intensity increases.
4. As exercise intensity increases, which substrate provides more energy—carbohydrate or fat?
5. Following an endurance training program, what changes in muscle allow more fat to be used as fuel during exercise?
6. Draw a graph showing how oxygen uptake increases at the beginning of a submaximal exercise bout, and label the oxygen deficit.
7. Define or describe (graphically) the LT (lactate threshold). What happens to the LT as a result of an endurance training program?

8. Draw a graph of the HR response to a GXT, and show the effect of an endurance training program on the response.
9. For the average person, SV levels off at about 40% $\dot{V}O_2$max in a GXT. What causes the increase in cardiac output at higher exercise intensities?
10. Which cardiovascular variable (maximal HR, SV, or oxygen extraction) explains the large differences in $\dot{V}O_2$max observed across the population?
11. What happens to BP when the arms perform the same work rate as the legs?
12. What accounts for the decrease in $\dot{V}O_2$max with detraining?
13. Which is the most important training variable (intensity, frequency, duration) linked to maintaining $\dot{V}O_2$max when training level is reduced?
14. Why is the HR response of women higher at the same work rate compared with men?
15. What is the most important mechanism of heat loss during exercise?

CASE STUDIES

1. A female competitive distance runner took a GXT on a motor-driven treadmill in which the speed of the run increased 0.5 mi · hr^{-1} (0.8 km · hr^{-1}) each minute, with the test starting at 5 mi · hr^{-1}(8 km · hr^{-1}). Blood samples for lactate determination were obtained each minute, and the LT was found to occur at the 8 mi · hr^{-1}(13 km · hr^{-1}) stage of the test. Following an injury and a period of detraining, she repeated the test and found that the LT occurred at 6.5 mi · hr^{-1} (10.4 km · hr^{-1}). She wants to know what happened. What do you tell her?
2. A client with whom you have been working retakes a maximal GXT following 10 wk of endurance training and finds that his HR is lower at each stage of the test. He is bothered by this because he thought his heart would be stronger and beat more times per minute. How do you help him understand what happened?
3. A female client is bothered by the fact that elite female runners who train as hard as elite male runners don't achieve the same performance times in distance races, and she wants to know why this is the case. How do you respond?

Answers to Case Studies

1. The LT is the point during a GXT when the blood lactate concentration suddenly increases. Following a period of detraining, there are fewer mitochondria in muscle and a reduced capacity to use fat as a fuel. As a result, more carbohydrate is used as fuel in glycolysis, and the usual breakdown products begin to accumulate in the cytoplasm of the muscle rather than going to the mitochondria. This results in increased lactate formation, and the LT occurs at a lower running speed. As she increases her training, the number of mitochondria in muscle will increase and the LT will again occur later in the GXT.
2. You need to confirm your client's feeling that the heart is stronger after training and can pump more blood per beat (increased SV). As a result, the heart does not have to beat as many times to deliver the same amount of oxygen to the tissues. This is a more efficient way for the heart to pump blood, and the heart does not have to work as hard at this lower rate.
3. You might begin by briefly stating that running speed in distance races relates to the amount of oxygen the runner can deliver to the muscles. When more oxygen can be delivered, the running speed is faster. The elite female distance runner differs from the elite male distance runner in three ways that have a bearing on this issue: Her heart size is smaller and she cannot pump as much oxygen-rich blood to the muscles per minute, the oxygen content of her blood is lower due to the lower hemoglobin concentration, and she is carrying relatively more body fat, which negatively affects sustained running speed even at the same level of fitness.

5

Nutrition

Dixie L. Thompson

OBJECTIVES

The reader will be able to do the following:

1. List the six classes of essential nutrients and describe their role in the proper functioning of the body.
2. List the recommended percentage of calories from carbohydrate, fat, and protein.
3. Understand the importance of vitamins and minerals and how to optimize them in a typical diet.
4. Describe assessment of dietary intake for healthy adults.
5. Understand the role of the U.S. Dietary Guidelines in making healthy nutritional choices.
6. Explain the relationship between blood lipid profile and CVD, and explain the role of diet and exercise in modifying blood lipids.
7. Know how to maintain hydration during exercise.
8. Discuss the protein, vitamin, and mineral needs of a physically active person.
9. Understand the basic principles behind increasing glycogen storage before competition.
10. List the three components of the female athlete triad.

Good nutrition results from eating foods in the proper quantities and with the needed distribution of nutrients to maintain good health in the present and in the future. **Malnutrition**, on the other hand, is the outcome of a diet in which there is underconsumption, overconsumption, or unbalanced consumption of nutrients that leads to disease or increased susceptibility to disease. These definitions implicitly state that proper nutrition is essential to good health. A history of poor nutritional choices eventually leads to health consequences. Poor nutritional choices have been linked to chronic conditions including CVD and cancer.

The public is bombarded with messages about nutrition, and it is often difficult for the layperson to distinguish good information from bad. Fitness professionals can play an important role in conveying basic nutritional information. However, a registered dietitian is the appropriate health care professional to perform detailed dietary analysis and to counsel individuals with special nutrition needs.

Essential Nutrients

The body requires many **nutrients** for the maintenance, growth, and repair of tissues. Nutrients can be divided into six classes: carbohydrate, fat, protein, vitamins, minerals, and water. The IOM Food and Nutrition Board has established **dietary reference intakes (DRIs)** to help people achieve a healthy intake of nutrients (11). The DRIs consist of recommended intakes for nutrients based on age and sex, including the **recommended dietary allowances (RDAs)**, or the amounts found to be adequate for approximately 97% of the population; **adequate intakes (AIs)**, or the amounts considered adequate although insufficient data exist to establish the appropriate RDA; and **tolerable upper intake levels (ULs)**, or the highest intakes believed to pose no health risk. Additionally, **acceptable macronutrient distribution ranges (AMDRs)** have been established for fat, carbohydrate, and protein. The IOM reports can be accessed at the National Academies Press website (www.nap.edu).

Carbohydrate

Carbohydrate is a nutrient composed of carbon, hydrogen, and oxygen and is an essential source of energy in the body. It can be divided into three categories: monosaccharides, disaccharides, and polysaccharides. Examples of monosaccharides are glucose and fructose. Lactose and sucrose are two of the disaccharides, which are carbohydrate that forms when monosaccharides combine. The monosaccharides and disaccharides are sometimes called **simple sugars**. Simple sugars contribute significantly to the caloric content of foods such as fruit juices, soft drinks, and candy. The most important simple sugar in the human body is **glucose**. The molecular formula for glucose is $C_6H_{12}O_6$. Polysaccharides are **complex carbohydrate** formed by combining three or more sugar molecules. Starches and fiber are polysaccharides found in plants. Rice, pasta, and whole-grain breads are just a few examples of foods that are high in complex carbohydrate. When carbohydrate is stored in the body, glucose molecules join together to form large molecules called **glycogen**. Glycogen is stored in the liver and skeletal muscle.

Grains, vegetables, and fruits are excellent sources of carbohydrate. It is recommended that 45% to 65% of a person's daily calories come from carbohydrate (13) (see figure 5.1). The RDA for carbohydrate is 130 g · day^{-1} (13), but the average carbohydrate intake of Americans is well beyond this RDA. The majority of carbohydrate calories should come from complex carbohydrate; foods with added sugar should be limited (22). The reason for eating complex rather than simple carbohydrate is the higher **nutrient density** of complex carbohydrate. *Nutrient density* refers to the amount of essential nutrients in a food compared with the calories it contains. For example, a candy bar (containing simple sugars) has a low nutrient density, whereas a slice of whole-grain bread (containing complex carbohydrate and other essential nutrients) has a high nutrient density.

One of the benefits of consuming foods that are high in complex carbohydrate is that they also typically contain **dietary fiber**, a nonstarch polysaccharide that is found in plants and cannot be broken down by the human digestive system. Although fiber cannot be digested, it helps prevent hemorrhoids, constipation, and cancers of the digestive system because it helps food move quickly and easily through the digestive system. In addition, consuming water-soluble fiber has been shown to lower cholesterol levels (5). Unfortunately, the typical American diet is low

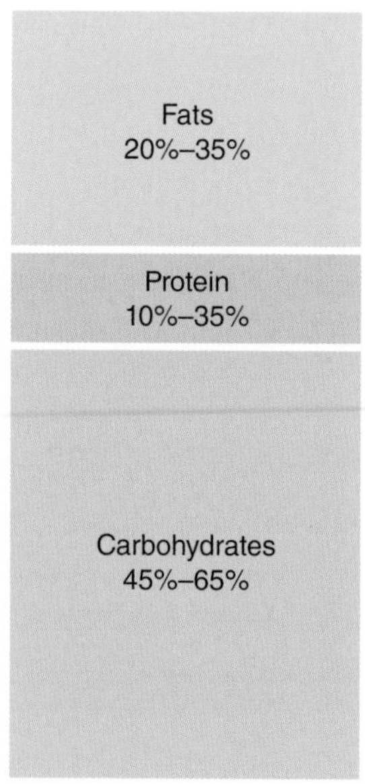

FIGURE 5.1 Acceptable macronutrient distribution for carbohydrate, fat, and protein (13).
Based on Food and Nutrition Board 2005.

in fiber, with the average intake being approximately 15 g · day^{-1} (22). The fiber AI for men and women aged 50 and younger is 38 g and 25 g · day^{-1}, respectively (13). For older men and women with lower calorie consumption, the daily recommended levels are 30 g and 21 g, respectively (13). *Dietary Guidelines for Americans, 2015-2020* (22) recommends that adults consume approximately 14 g of fiber for every 1,000 kcal consumed. Excellent sources of dietary fiber are grains, vegetables, legumes, and fruits.

As mentioned earlier, carbohydrate is a vital source of energy in the human body. During high-intensity exercise, carbohydrate is the primary fuel source for ATP production. When carbohydrate is broken down in the human body, it yields approximately 4 kcal of energy per gram. This means that a person who eats 10 g of carbohydrate gains approximately 40 kcal of energy to use or store.

KEY POINT

The six classes of nutrients are carbohydrate, fat, protein, vitamins, minerals, and water. The metabolism of 1 g of carbohydrate yields 4 kcal of energy. Carbohydrate should contribute 45% to 65% of one's daily calories, with limited calories coming from simple sugars.

Fat

Fat is essential to a healthy diet and contributes to vital functions in the human body. Among the functions performed by the body's fat stores are temperature regulation, protection of vital organs, distribution of some vitamins, hormone regulation, energy production, and formation of cell membranes. Similar to carbohydrate, fat is composed of carbon, hydrogen, and oxygen; however, the chemical structure is different. **Triglycerides** are the primary storage form of fat in the body. These large molecules are composed of three fatty acid chains connected to a glycerol backbone. The majority of triglycerides are stored in adipose cells (i.e., fat cells), but these stored fats can also be found in other tissues (e.g., skeletal muscle). The aerobic metabolism of triglycerides provides much of the energy needed during rest and low-intensity exercise. When metabolized, 1 g of fat yields 9 kcal of energy. **Phospholipids** are another type of fat found in the body. As the name implies, these fats have phosphate groups attached to them. Phospholipids are important constituents of cell membranes. **Lipoproteins** are large molecules that allow fat to travel through the bloodstream. **Cholesterol** is a sterol, or a fatty substance in which carbon, hydrogen, and oxygen atoms are arranged in rings. In addition to the cholesterol we consume in our diet, the body constantly produces cholesterol, which is used in forming cell membranes and making steroidal hormones. Meat and eggs are the major sources of cholesterol in the typical American

Focus on Glycemic Index and Glycemic Load

When carbohydrate is ingested, blood glucose rises and subsequently insulin is released from the pancreas. The rapidity with which blood glucose rises after food intake is represented by the **glycemic index (GI)**. Foods with a high GI cause a rapid spike in blood glucose, whereas foods with a low GI do not. A number of factors (e.g., biochemical composition, method of food preparation, fiber content) affect GI. Examples of foods with a high GI are baked potatoes, white rice, and soft drinks. Foods with a lower GI include apples, kidney beans, and milk. However, the change in blood glucose that occurs after eating a food depends both on the GI and on the quantity of carbohydrate in food. The **glycemic load (GL)** is a value that reflects the quality (i.e., the GI) and quantity of carbohydrate in a given f ood. To calculate GL, the GI of the food is multiplied by the grams of carbohydrate in the food, and the value is divided by 100. For example, a banana with a GI of 52 and 25 g of carbohydrate would produce a GL of 13 ($52 \times 25 / 100 = 13$). A food with a large GL will dramatically increase blood glucose levels. The University of Sydney maintains a website where the GI and GL of various foods can be determined (www.glycemicindex.com).

Controversy remains about the health impact of eating a diet low in GI foods. Though some argue that a low GI diet offers cardiovascular and metabolic benefits, the evidence is not strong. In fact, recent dietary guidelines from the American Diabetes Association (ADA) place only a minor emphasis on using the GI in making food choices. The ADA stresses attention to the total amount of carbohydrate rather than GI; however, when consuming foods with a high GI, it is wise to balance the meal with lower GI foods. The ADA acknowledges that a variety of eating patterns can be used to successfully manage blood glucose levels (5).

diet, but blood levels of cholesterol are influenced by factors other than consumption of dietary cholesterol. Thus, the U.S. Dietary Guidelines no longer emphasize cholesterol intake; instead the focus is on limiting saturated fat and trans fat.

Both animals and plants are sources of dietary fat. The AMDR for fat is 20% to 35% (13) (figure 5.1). Saturated fat comes primarily from animal sources and is typically solid at room temperature. Plant sources of saturated fat include palm oil, coconut oil, and cocoa butter. The chemical structure of saturated fat contains no double bonds between carbon atoms; in other words, the fat is saturated with hydrogen atoms. A high intake of saturated fat directly relates to increased CVD. Therefore, one should limit consumption of saturated fat to less than 10% of total calories (22). Unsaturated fat contains fewer hydrogen atoms because there are some double bonds between the carbon atoms. This type of fat is typically liquid at room temperature. Corn, peanut, canola, and soybean oil are sources of unsaturated fat. **Trans fat** is unsaturated fat that is common in many processed baked goods such as cookies and cakes. The intake of these fatty acids should be as low as possible because they are linked with negative health outcomes; in fact, the Food and Drug Administration (FDA) has mandated that food manufacturers phase out the use of trans fat (23). The effects of various kinds of fat on health risk are discussed later in the chapter (see Diet, Exercise, and the Blood Lipid Profile).

Monounsaturated fatty acids, found in olive and canola oil, have a single double bond between carbon atoms in the fatty acid chain. **Polyunsaturated fatty acids** (e.g., fish, corn, soybean, and peanut oils) have two or more double bonds between carbon atoms. Two polyunsaturated fatty acids, alpha-linolenic acid (a type of omega-3 fatty acid) and linoleic acid (an omega-6 fatty acid), cannot be made by the body and must be consumed in the diet. The AI for alpha-linolenic acid is 1.6 g $\cdot$ day^{-1} for men and 1.1 g $\cdot$ day^{-1} for women (13). Fish, walnuts, and canola oil are sources of this fatty acid. The AI for linoleic acid is 17 g and 12 g $\cdot$ day^{-1} for men and women, respectively (13). Sources include vegetable oils, nuts, avocados, and soybeans.

KEY POINT

The AMDR for fat is 20% to 35%, and less than 10% of calories should come from saturated fat. Intake of trans fat should be as low as possible. The breakdown of 1 g of fat yields 9 kcal of energy.

Protein

Protein is a substance composed of carbon, hydrogen, oxygen, and nitrogen. All forms of protein are combinations of **amino acids**. Amino acids are molecules composed of an amino group (NH_3), a carboxyl group (COO), a hydrogen atom, a central carbon atom, and a side chain. The differences in the side chains give unique characteristics to each amino acid. Amino acids can combine in innumerable ways to form proteins, and it is estimated that tens of thousands of protein types exist in the body. The order of the linked amino acids provides the unique structure and function of protein that allow it to serve many functions in the body. Some of the most common functions are the following:

- Carry oxygen (hemoglobin)
- Fight disease (antibodies)
- Catalyze reactions (enzymes)
- Allow muscle contraction (actin, myosin, and troponin)
- Act as connective tissue (collagen)
- Clot blood (prothrombin)
- Act as a messenger (protein hormones such as growth hormone)

Of the 20 amino acids required by the human body, most can be constructed from other substances in the body; however, there are eight **essential amino acids** (nine for children and some older adults) that the body cannot synthesize and so must be a part of one's regular diet. Eating a variety of protein-containing foods typically meets this need. Protein is found in both meat and plant products. Animal sources of protein such as meat, milk, and eggs contain the essential amino acids. Individual plant sources of protein such as beans, starchy vegetables, nuts, and grains do not always contain all essential amino acids when eaten in isolation. Because of this, vegetarians must consume a variety of protein-containing foods. Examples of foods that contain complementary proteins are legumes and grains, vegetables and nuts, and legumes and seeds (8). For more information on planning vegetarian diets, see the summary of the vegetarian food guide established by the American Dietetic Association (ADA; now the Academy of Nutrition and Dietetics) and Dietitians of Canada (16).

The AMDR for protein is 10% to 35% (figure 5.1). This amount ensures adequate protein for the growth, maintena nce, and repair of cells. The adult RDA is 0.8 g of protein for each kilogram of body weight (13). As discussed later in this chapter, people who are training intensely may have higher protein requirements. Additionally, children need more protein to support their continually growing bodies.

In addition to the functions listed previously, protein can be metabolized for energy production. The breakdown of 1 g of protein yields approximately 4 kcal of energy for the body. The contribution of protein to energy needs during exercise is usually quite small (<5%) in well-nourished individuals. However, during long bouts of exercise (>1 hr) or when a person is not well nourished, protein may supply up to 15% of the body's energy needs.

Vitamins

Vitamins are organic substances that are essential to the normal functioning of the human body. Although vitamins

KEY POINT

Protein is made of amino acids and serves numerous functions. To ensure that all needed amino acids are adequately available, people should eat a variety of protein-containing foods each day. The AMDR for protein is 10% to 35%. The breakdown of 1 g of protein yields 4 kcal of energy.

do not contain energy for the body, they are essential in the metabolism of fat, carbohydrate, and protein. The body needs 14 vitamins for numerous processes, including blood clotting, protein synthesis, and bone formation. Because of the critical role vitamins play, they need to exist in proper quantities in the body. Major functions, important dietary sources, and recommended intakes of vitamins are listed in table 5.1. There are two major classifications of vitamins: fat soluble and water soluble.

Table 5.1 Vitamins: Functions, Sources, and Dietary Reference Intakes

Vitamin	Function	Sources	Adult RDA[a]		UL[b]
			Men	Women	
Thiamin (B_1)	Functions as part of a coenzyme to aid utilization of energy	Whole grains, nuts, lean pork	1.2 mg	1.1 mg	ND
Riboflavin (B_2)	Involved in energy metabolism as part of a coenzyme	Milk, yogurt, cheese	1.3 mg	1.1 mg	ND
Niacin	Facilitates energy production in cells	Lean meat, fish, poultry, grains	16 mg	14 mg	35 mg
B_6	Absorbs and metabolizes protein, aids in red blood cell formation	Lean meat, vegetables, whole grains	1.3 mg	1.3 mg	100 mg
Pantothenic acid	Aids in metabolism of carbohydrate, fat, and protein	Whole-grain cereals, bread, dark green vegetables	5 mg*	5 mg*	ND
Folic acid	Functions as coenzyme in synthesis of nucleic acids and protein	Green vegetables, beans, whole-wheat products	400 µg	400 µg	1,000 µg
B_{12}	Involved in synthesis of nucleic acids, red blood cell formation	Only in animal foods, not plant foods	2.4 µg	2.4 µg	ND
Biotin	Functions as coenzyme in synthesis of fatty acids and glycogen	Egg yolk, dark green vegetables	30 µg*	30 µg*	ND
Choline	Important in cell membrane integrity and signaling, nerve transmission	Beef liver, chicken, codfish, wheat germ, cauliflower	550 mg*	425 mg*	3.5 g
C	Aids intracellular maintenance of bone, capillaries, and teeth	Citrus fruits, green peppers, tomatoes	90 mg	75 mg	2,000 mg
A	Aids vision, formation and maintenance of skin and mucous membranes	Carrots, sweet potatoes, butter, liver	900 µg	700 µg	3,000 µg
D	Aids growth and formation of bones and teeth, aids calcium absorption	Eggs, tuna, liver, fortified milk	15 µg	15 µg	100 µg
E	Protects polyunsaturated fat, prevents damage to cell membrane	Whole-grain cereals and breads, green leafy vegetables	15 mg	15 mg	1,000 mg
K	Important in blood clotting	Green leafy vegetables, peas, potatoes	120 µg*	90 µg*	ND

[a]Values are recommended daily allowance (RDA) for adults aged 19 to 50, unless marked with an asterisk. The requirements may vary for children, older adults, and pregnant or lactating women.

[b]Tolerable upper intake levels (UL) for adults aged 19 to 50. Intakes above the UL may lead to negative health consequences.

*Values are adequate intakes (AIs), indicating that sufficient data to set the RDA are unavailable.

ND = not yet determined.

Adapted from B.D. Franks and E.T. Howley, 1998, *Fitness leader's handbook*, 2nd ed. (Champaign, IL: Human Kinetics); and various reports of the Food and Nutrition Board.

The chemical structure of fat-soluble vitamins causes them to be transported and stored with lipids. The four fat-soluble vitamins are A, D, E, and K. Because these vitamins are stored in the body, it is not necessary to ingest large amounts daily; however, a small daily intake of each is recommended.

The B vitamins and vitamin C are water-soluble vitamins. These vitamins are not stored in large quantities in the body and therefore must be consumed daily. Deficiencies related to water-soluble vitamins such as scurvy (vitamin C deficiency) and beriberi (thiamin deficiency) may occur rather quickly. Overconsuming either fat-soluble or water-soluble vitamins can lead to toxic effects; however, because fat-soluble vitamins are stored in the body, the potential for overdose with these substances is greater (8).

Minerals

Minerals are inorganic elements that serve a variety of functions in the human body. The minerals that appear in the largest quantities (calcium, phosphorus, potassium, sulfur, sodium, chloride, and magnesium) are often called *macrominerals* or *major minerals*. Other minerals are also essential to normal functioning of the body, but because they exist in smaller quantities, they are called *microminerals* or *trace elements*. Functions, dietary sources, and recommended intakes of minerals are listed in table 5.2.

Table 5.2 Minerals: Functions, Sources, and Dietary Reference Intakes

Mineral	Functions	Sources	Adult RDA[a]		UL[b]
			Men	Women	
Calcium	Bones, teeth, blood clotting, nerve and muscle function	Milk, sardines, dark green vegetables, nuts	1,000 mg	1,000 mg	2,500 mg
Chloride	Nerve and muscle function, water balance (with sodium)	Salt	2.3 g*	2.3 g*	3.6 g
Magnesium	Bone growth, nerve, muscle, enzyme function	Nuts, seafood, whole grains, leafy green vegetables	420 mg	320 mg	350 mg[c]
Phosphorus	Bones, teeth, energy transfer	Meats, poultry, seafood, eggs, milk, beans	700 mg	700 mg	4,000 mg
Potassium	Nerve and muscle function	Fresh vegetables, bananas, citrus fruits, milk, meats, fish	4.7 g*	4.7 g*	ND
Sodium	Nerve and muscle function, water balance	Salt	1.5 g*	1.5 g*	2.3 g
Chromium	Glucose metabolism	Meats, liver, whole grains, dried beans	35 µg*	25 µg*	ND
Copper	Enzyme function, energy production	Meats, seafood, nuts, grains	900 µg	900 µg	10,000 µg
Fluoride	Bone and teeth growth	Fluoridated drinking water, fish, milk	4 mg*	3 mg*	10 mg
Iodine	Thyroid hormone formation	Iodized salt, seafood	150 µg	150 µg	1,100 µg
Iron	O_2 transport in red blood cells, enzyme function	Red meat, liver, eggs, beans, leafy vegetables, shellfish	8 mg	18 mg	45 mg
Manganese	Enzyme function	Whole grains, nuts, fruits, vegetables	2.3 mg*	1.8 mg*	11 mg
Molybdenum	Energy metabolism	Whole grains, organ meats, peas, beans	45 µg	45 µg	2,000 µg
Selenium	Works with vitamin E	Meat, fish, whole grains, eggs	55 µg	55 µg	400 µg
Zinc	Enzyme function, growth	Meat, shellfish, yeast, whole grains	11 mg	8 mg	40 mg

[a]Values are recommended daily allowance (RDA) for adults aged 19 to 50, unless marked with an asterisk. The requirements may vary for children, older adults, and pregnant or lactating women.

[b]Tolerable upper intake levels (UL) for adults aged 19 to 50. Intakes above the UL may lead to negative health consequences.

[c]Refers to pharmacological agents only and not to amounts contained in food and water. No evidence of ill effects from ingesting naturally occurring amounts in food and water.

*Values are adequate intakes (AIs), indicating that sufficient data to set the RDA are unavailable.

ND = not yet determined.

Adapted from B.D. Franks and E.T. Howley, 1998, *Fitness leader's handbook*, 2nd ed. (Champaign, IL: Human Kinetics); and various reports of the Food and Nutrition Board.

Calcium is often inadequately consumed by Americans. It is important in the mineralization of bone, in muscle contraction, and in transmission of nervous impulses. **Osteoporosis** is a disease characterized by a decrease in the total amount of bone mineral in the body and in the strength of the remaining bone. This condition is most common in the elderly but also may exist in younger people who have diets inadequate in calcium, vitamin D, or both. It is estimated that in the United States, osteoporosis results in approximately $22 billion in annual health care costs (7). Maximal bone density is achieved during the early adult years, and during older adult years, bone density declines in everyone. Those who achieve the highest bone density and maintain adequate intakes of calcium and vitamin D are most protected from osteoporosis. Recently, RDAs were released for calcium (see table 5.3) (15). The DRIs for vitamin D are contained in table 5.1. The calcium RDA for adults aged 19 to 50 is 1,000 mg $\cdot$ day^{-1}, with higher values for older adults and adolescents. Milk, dark green vegetables, and nuts are excellent sources of calcium. One cup (8 oz or 237 ml) of 1% milk has approximately 300 mg of calcium, which is almost one-third of the daily recommendation for a young adult.

Table 5.3 Guidelines for Daily Calcium Intake

Age	RDA (mg)
0-6 mo	200*
>6-12 mo	260*
1-3 yr	700
4-8 yr	1,000
9-18 yr	1,300
19-50 yr	1,000
51-70 yr men	1,000
51-70 yr women	1,200
71 yr and older	1,200
Pregnant or lactating 18 yr or younger	1,300
Pregnant or lactating 19 yr or older	1,000

*These values are AIs because insufficient evidence exists to clearly establish RDA for infants.

Data from Institute of Medicine 2011.

Iron is another mineral that is often underconsumed by Americans, particularly women and children. In fact, the most prevalent nutrient deficiency in the United States is iron deficiency (8). In addition to being a critical component of hemoglobin and myoglobin, iron is necessary for the functioning of the immune system, the formation of brain neurotransmitters, and the functioning of the electron transport chain (8). The oxygen-carrying properties of hemoglobin depend on iron. There is a continual turnover of red blood cells in the body, and much of the iron used to form new hemoglobin comes from old red blood cells. However, there is a daily need for iron, and if iron reserves (liver, spleen, bone marrow) and intake are inadequate, hemoglobin cannot be formed and **iron-deficiency anemia** results. In this condition, the amount of hemoglobin in red blood cells falls, which decreases the capacity of the blood to transport oxygen. The recommended intake of iron for males and postmenopausal women is 8 mg $\cdot$ day^{-1} (12). For females during the childbearing years, the recommended daily intake is 18 mg $\cdot$ day^{-1} (12). Red meat and eggs are excellent sources of iron. Additionally, spinach, lima

Focus on Antioxidant Vitamins

During metabolic processes, molecules or fragments of molecules form that can damage the body's tissues. These **free radicals** have at least one unpaired electron in their outer shells, and thus they are very chemically reactive. Lipid-rich cell membranes and DNA are highly susceptible to free radicals, and cell damage can occur when free radicals accumulate; for example, atherosclerosis is linked with free radicals. Some vitamins can react with free radicals and diminish the damage they cause. These **antioxidant vitamins** were hypothesized to counteract the effects of aging and decrease the likelihood of developing CVD and cancer. However, the scientific evidence finds that ingesting supplemental antioxidant vitamins does not play a prominent role in disease prevention, and in some cases there are negative side effects (17). For example, recent evidence suggests that high doses of **beta-carotene** (a precursor of vitamin A) may increase the risk of lung cancer in smokers, and high doses of vitamin E increase the risk of stroke and prostate cancer. However, studies continue to explore the potential health benefits and risks of these vitamins. Because of the toxic effects from an overdose of antioxidants, it is wise to avoid overconsuming these substances (see table 5.1).

and navy beans, and prune juice are excellent vegetarian sources of iron. Consuming vitamin C with meals increases the ability to absorb iron.

Sodium, on the other hand, is a mineral that many Americans overconsume. High sodium intake has been linked with hypertension. The adult AI for sodium is 1.5 g $\cdot$ day^{-1} (14). Adults should limit their daily sodium intake to no more than 2.3 g (14, 22). People can substantially reduce their sodium intake by consuming fewer processed foods and adding less salt to foods when cooking.

Water

Water is considered an essential nutrient because of its vital role in the normal functioning of the body. It constitutes approximately 60% of the total body weight (14) and is essential in creating the environment in which all metabolic processes occur. Water is necessary to regulate temperature and transport substances throughout the body.

AI for total water is 3.7 L $\cdot$ day^{-1} for men and 2.7 L $\cdot$ day^{-1} for women (14). Approximately 80% of this amount comes from beverages. As discussed later in this chapter, the amount needed for good health may be higher for individuals exercising intensely. Environmental conditions may also increase the need for water.

KEY POINT

Vitamins, minerals, and water do not provide energy but are essential to healthy functioning of the body. In general, most Americans would benefit from limiting sodium consumption (to decrease BP), increasing calcium intake (to improve bone strength), and increasing iron ingestion (to prevent anemia).

Examining Dietary Intake

The U.S. Dietary Guidelines (22) suggest engaging in regular physical activity and eating a balanced diet that contains the calories needed to achieve and sustain a healthy body weight. Keeping a food log (i.e., food diary or diet record) can help people reflect on their calorie intake and eating habits. For this activity to yield valid results, the client should record everything that is consumed over a certain period of time. These records typically are kept for 3 to 4 days (with at least 1 day being a weekend day) and provide a general idea of a person's nutritional habits (19). Once the records are completed, there are several software packages that can be used to analyze the diet. A free resource for analyzing one's diet, MyPlate, can be found at www.choosemyplate.gov. MyPlate provides dietary guidance based on age, sex, level of activity, and so on. This guide replaces MyPyramid and is designed to help people choose foods that promote health and assist with achieving and maintaining a healthy weight. The MyPlate website allows the user to enter foods eaten and receive an analysis that compares them with recommended intake levels. This useful tool can help people determine whether they are in caloric balance and consuming various nutrients in healthy amounts.

Although food diaries provide important information, they may pose some problems (24):

- People tend to underreport what they eat.
- People do not keep records that are specific enough to provide quality information.
- People often temporarily change how they eat when they record their food intake.

The fitness professional can take steps to minimize these problems. First, make sure that the clients understand the importance of completely and honestly recording what they eat. Emphasize to clients that the accuracy and usefulness of the food diary depend on the information provided. One of the most important results of completing a food record is that clients begin to become accountable for their food intake. By documenting the types and amounts of foods they eat, the clients begin to see for themselves opportunities to make healthier food choices. Additionally, provide clients with models or descriptions of how to accurately report food consumption. For more information on instructing clients on completing food diaries, see *ACSM's Resource Manual for Guidelines for Exercise Testing and Prescription* (19). Providing explicit instructions will allow the client to create a more useful and accurate record. Additionally, the food diary should be user friendly and include cues to elicit complete responses. A sample food log with instructions is provided on form 5.1. For the typical client, the following intakes should be included in a nutritional profile:

- Total calories
- Percentage of calories from fat, carbohydrate, and protein
- Saturated fat and trans fat
- Sodium
- Iron
- Calcium
- Fiber

It also can be useful to examine the food diary for emotional or social cues to eating behaviors. For example, some people eat when depressed or only eat when alone. Such information can be helpful in making behavior changes needed for weight loss and maintenance. More information on weight management is covered in chapter 12.

FORM 5.1 Sample Food Log

INSTRUCTIONS

1. Record everything you eat, including foods and beverages eaten at meals and snacks.
2. Record carefully how the food was prepared. Be as descriptive as possible (e.g., fried in corn oil, broiled in 1 tbsp of margarine).
3. Be sure to indicate the amount of food eaten. Use typical household measures when possible (tsp = teaspoon; tbsp = tablespoon; c = cup; oz = ounce; g = gram).
4. Provide brand names and labels for packaged foods.
5. For composite foods such as sandwiches, casseroles, and soups, indicate the ingredients contained in the food. For example, a turkey sandwich might be described as 2 slices of whole-wheat bread, 1 oz of baked turkey breast without skin, 1 slice of tomato, 2 leaves of iceberg lettuce, and 1 tbsp light mayonnaise.
6. Indicate where and with whom you were when you ate. Describe your feelings at the time—were you worried, content, lonely, stressed, hungry? (Be honest.)
7. Carry this form with you so that you can write down foods as you eat them. Do not wait until the end of the day to record your food intake.

Food and drink	Description (e.g., amount, cooking method, brand name)	Location (e.g., place, with people or alone)	Feelings (e.g., hunger, anger, joy)	Time

From E.T. Howley and D.L. Thompson, 2017, *Fitness professional's handbook,* 7th ed. (Champaign, IL: Human Kinetics).

It is important to consider what information fitness professionals can provide to clients who seek nutritional advice (21). The Dietary Guidelines for Americans (22) contain general nutrition information that can be shared with clients. The following section, Recommendations for Dietary Intake, provides more information about these guidelines. Additionally, it is within the scope of practice for fitness professionals to suggest healthy recipes, provide information about nutrients and their role in good health, and so on. Sass and colleagues (21) provide an overview of the scope of practice for fitness professionals and registered dietitians. Fitness professionals can serve an important role in helping clients think critically about what and how much they eat, with an ultimate goal of encouraging clients to make healthier food choices. Clients with special metabolic conditions such as diabetes mellitus should always be referred to a registered dietitian for nutrition advice.

KEY POINT

Accurate, detailed food diaries can be a useful tool in helping clients develop healthy dietary practices.

Key Components of the 2015-2020 Dietary Guidelines for Americans

1. **Follow a healthy eating pattern across the life span.** All food and beverage choices matter. Choose a healthy eating pattern at an appropriate calorie level to help achieve and maintain a healthy body weight, support nutrient adequacy, and reduce the risk of chronic disease.
2. **Focus on variety, nutrient density, and amount.** To meet nutrient needs within calorie limits, choose a variety of nutrient-dense foods across and within all food groups in recommended amounts.
3. **Limit calories from added sugar and saturated fat and reduce sodium intake.** Consume an eating pattern low in added sugar, saturated fat, and sodium. Cut back on foods and beverages higher in these components to amounts that fit within healthy eating patterns.
4. **Shift to healthier food and beverage choices.** Choose nutrient-dense foods and beverages across and within all food groups in place of less healthy choices. Consider cultural and personal preferences to make these shifts easier to accomplish and maintain.
5. **Support healthy eating patterns for all.** Everyone has a role in helping to create and support healthy eating patterns in multiple settings, from home to school to work to communities.

KEY RECOMMENDATIONS

Choose a healthy eating pattern that accounts for all foods and beverages within an appropriate calorie level. A healthy eating pattern includes the following:

- A variety of vegetables from all of the subgroups—dark green, red and orange, legumes (beans and peas), starchy, and other
- Fruits, especially whole fruits
- Grains, at least half of which are whole grains
- Fat-free or low-fat dairy, including milk, yogurt, cheese, and fortified soy beverages
- A variety of protein foods, including seafood, lean meats and poultry, eggs, legumes (beans and peas), nuts, seeds, and soy products
- Oils

A healthy eating pattern limits the following:

- Saturated fat and trans fat
- Added sugar
- Sodium

Quantitative key recommendations are provided for several dietary components that should be limited. These components are of particular concern to public health in the United States, and the specified limits can help people achieve healthy eating patterns within calorie limits:

- Consume less than 10% of calories per day from added sugar.
- Consume less than 10% of calories per day from saturated fat.
- Consume less than 2,300 mg per day of sodium.
- If alcohol is consumed, it should be consumed in moderation—up to one drink per day for women and up to two drinks per day for men—and only by adults of legal drinking age.

Adapted from U.S. Department of Agriculture and U.S. Department of Health and Human Services 2015.

Recommendations for Dietary Intake

Dietary Guidelines for Americans, 2015-2020 (22) is a joint effort of the U.S. Department of Health and Human Services (HHS) and the U.S. Department of Agriculture (USDA). These recommendations can help people make healthy food choices, and they focus on lowering the risk of chronic disease and promoting health. The guidelines acknowledge the complex interaction of factors (personal, social, and environmental) that influence food consumption and identify a variety of healthy eating patterns that may be adopted. They point out common nutritional inadequacies and suggest ways to improve health outcomes through nutritional changes. For example, most Americans are too sedentary and weigh too much; thus, the guidelines suggest increasing physical activity and reducing calorie intake to a level that will lead to a healthy weight. The guidelines provide both general and specific recommendations. For instance, general recommendations include limiting consumption of added sugars and saturated fat. An example of a specific recommendation is to limit sodium consumption to <2,300 mg per day. A complete copy of *Dietary Guidelines for Americans* can be found at http://health.gov/dietaryguidelines/2015/guidelines/.

These guidelines point out that many Americans fall short of healthy dietary practices. Commonly, Americans underconsume some foods (e.g., fruits, whole grains, calcium-containing foods) while overconsuming others (e.g., solid fat, added sugar, sodium-containing foods). The sidebar *Key Components of the 2015-2020 Dietary Guidelines for Americans* summarizes general dietary practices suggested in the guidelines.

People can choose a variety of eating plans to help achieve the goals set forward in the Dietary Guidelines for Americans. Table 5.4 outlines three viable approaches to healthy eating: the **Healthy U.S.-Style Eating Pattern**, the **Healthy Mediterranean-Style Eating Pattern**, and the **Healthy Vegetarian-Style Eating Pattern**. The Healthy U.S.-Style Pattern is based on the previously used USDA Food Patterns and the **DASH (Dietary Approaches to Stop Hypertension) diet**. This approach suggests daily amounts that people should consume from five major food groups (vegetables, fruits, grains, dairy products, and protein). These correspond with the five elements found in the MyPlate materials mentioned previously. Suggested limits on intake of certain products (e.g., solid fat) are also included. This plan is based on the established DRIs for nutrients and the Dietary Guidelines for Americans. It allows a great deal of flexibility in choosing foods and is adaptable to a vegetarian lifestyle.

Table 5.4 Comparison of Healthy Eating Patterns*

Food group	Healthy U.S.-Style Eating Pattern	Healthy Vegetarian-Style Eating Pattern	Healthy Mediterranean-Style Eating Pattern
Fruits (c)	2/day	2/day	2.5/day
Vegetables (c)	2.5/day	2.5/day	3/day
Dark green	1.5/wk	1.5/wk	2/wk
Red and orange	5.5/wk	5.5/wk	6/wk
Starchy	5/wk	5/wk	6/wk
Legumes	1.5/wk	1.5/wk	2/wk
Other	4/wk	4/wk	5/wk
Grains (oz)	6/day	6.5/day	7/day
Whole	≥3/day	3.5/day	3.5/day
Refined	≤3/day	3/day	3.5/day
Dairy (c)	3/day	3/day	2/day
Protein (oz)	5.5/day	3.5/day	7/day
Meats, poultry, eggs	26/wk	3/wk (eggs)	28/wk
Seafood	8/wk	—	16/wk
Nuts, seeds	4/wk	7/wk	5/wk
Soy products	4/wk	8/wk	5/wk
Oils (g)	27/day	27/day	29/day
Limit on calories from other sources	270/day	290/day	270/day

*Average daily intake at or adjusted to a 2,000-calorie level.

Reprinted from the Office of Disease Prevention and Health Promotion. Available: http://health.gov/dietaryguidelines/2015/guidelines/.

The DASH diet was originally designed to help people control their BP. This diet is characterized by sodium restriction; an emphasis on vegetables, fruits, low-fat milk products, whole grains, and lean meats; and elimination or minimization of added sugars and processed meats. Several studies have shown this dietary approach can be helpful in reducing BP and weight.

The Healthy Mediterranean-Style Pattern has become popular in the United States in recent years. The pattern varies somewhat based on region but generally emphasizes grains (particularly whole grains), fruits, vegetables, olive oil, and nuts. More monounsaturated fatty acids than saturated fatty acids are consumed in this pattern. Wine consumption with meals is also common. This eating pattern has been linked with a lower prevalence of CVD.

The FDA requires that all food be labeled with nutrition information. These labels, titled Nutrition Facts (see figure 5.2), list the serving size, total calories, fat (including saturated and trans fat), cholesterol, sodium, carbohydrate (including dietary fiber and added sugar), protein, and vitamins and minerals contained in the food. The FDA is currently considering a redesign of food labels to make them more user friendly and to reflect more realistic serving sizes. **Daily values (DVs)** are an important part of the label; they indicate the percentage of daily recommended levels of nutrients that are contained in a food. The DVs inform the public about the nutritional content of food and are based on a daily intake of 2,000 kcal. The nutrition label contains the percentage of the recommended DVs provided by nutrients found in the food. For example, the suggested DV for potassium is 4.7 g (4,700 mg); therefore, if a food contains 470 mg of potassium, it will constitute 10% of the recommended daily intake of potassium. Additional information on food labels can be found in the Food tab under the Ingredients, Packaging, and Labeling heading at www.fda.gov.

KEY POINT

The Dietary Guidelines for Americans (22) encourage most people to eat fewer calories, be more active, and make wiser food choices. The Healthy U.S.-Style Eating Pattern, Healthy Mediterranean-Style Eating Pattern, and Healthy Vegetarian-Style Eating Pattern are approaches to healthy food consumption. Food labeling allows consumers to evaluate the nutritional content of foods.

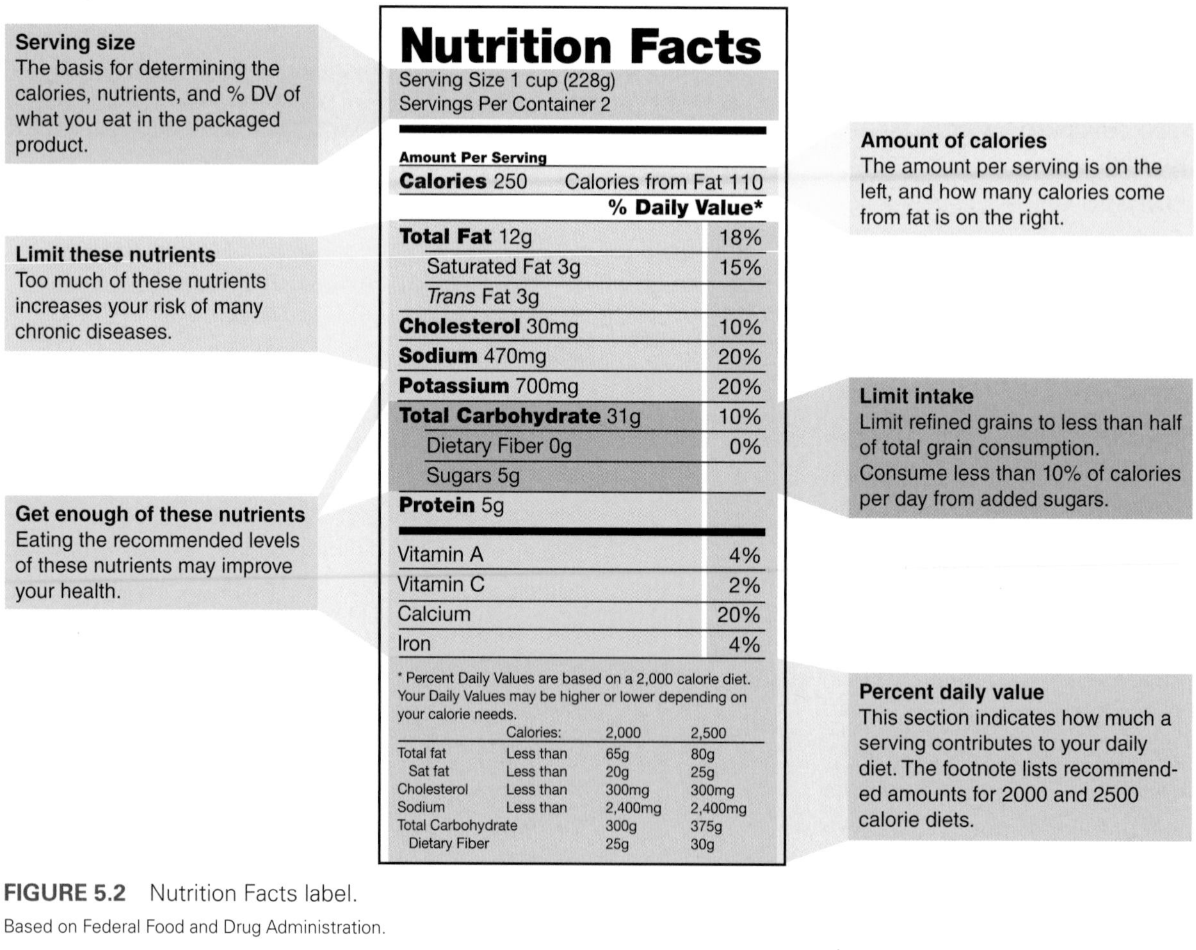

Serving size
The basis for determining the calories, nutrients, and % DV of what you eat in the packaged product.
Limit these nutrients
Too much of these nutrients increases your risk of many chronic diseases.
Get enough of these nutrients
Eating the recommended levels of these nutrients may improve your health.
Nutrition Facts
Serving Size 1 cup (228g)
Servings Per Container 2
Amount Per Serving
Calories 250 Calories from Fat 110
% Daily Value*
Total Fat 12g 18%
Saturated Fat 3g 15%
Trans Fat 3g
Cholesterol 30mg 10%
Sodium 470mg 20%
Potassium 700mg 20%
Total Carbohydrate 31g 10%
Dietary Fiber 0g 0%
Sugars 5g
Protein 5g
Vitamin A 4%
Vitamin C 2%
Calcium 20%
Iron 4%
* Percent Daily Values are based on a 2,000 calorie diet. Your Daily Values may be higher or lower depending on your calorie needs.
Calories: 2,000 2,500
Total fat Less than 65g 80g
Sat fat Less than 20g 25g
Cholesterol Less than 300mg 300mg
Sodium Less than 2,400mg 2,400mg
Total Carbohydrate 300g 375g
Dietary Fiber 25g 30g
Amount of calories
The amount per serving is on the left, and how many calories come from fat is on the right.
Limit intake
Limit refined grains to less than half of total grain consumption.
Consume less than 10% of calories per day from added sugars.
Percent daily value
This section indicates how much a serving contributes to your daily diet. The footnote lists recommended amounts for 2000 and 2500 calorie diets.

FIGURE 5.2 Nutrition Facts label.

Based on Federal Food and Drug Administration.

Diet, Exercise, and the Blood Lipid Profile

CVD is the leading cause of death in the United States. One of the primary risk factors for CVD is a poor blood lipid profile. Both diet and exercise can have a positive effect on this crucial risk factor.

Lipoproteins and Risk of Cardiovascular Disease

Because lipids are hydrophobic (i.e., not water soluble), they need to bind with some other substance to be transported in the blood. Lipoproteins are macromolecules composed of cholesterol, triglycerides, protein, and phospholipids. Classifications for these molecules are based on their size and makeup. The two classes of lipoproteins most closely linked with CVD are low-density lipoprotein (LDL) and high-density lipoprotein (HDL). LDL transports cholesterol and triglycerides from the liver to be used in various cellular processes. HDL retrieves cholesterol from the cells and returns it to the liver to be metabolized.

Elevated levels of **total cholesterol** (the sum of all forms of cholesterol) and **low-density lipoprotein cholesterol (LDL-C)** are linked with the development of atherosclerotic plaque in the arteries. Increased levels of **high-density lipoprotein cholesterol (HDL-C)** help prevent the atherosclerotic process. According to the 2001 National Cholesterol Education Program (NCEP) guidelines, total cholesterol levels below 200 mg · dl^{-1} and LDL-C values below 100 mg · dl^{-1} are desirable (10). Total cholesterol levels of 240 mg · dl^{-1} or higher and LDL-C values of 160 mg · dl^{-1} or higher are considered high and are associated with greater risk of CVD (see table 5.5). In addition, HDL-C values below 40 mg · dl^{-1} are considered too low, and levels of 60 mg · dl^{-1} or higher are considered ideal (10).

Table 5.5 Blood Lipid Classifications

Lipid level	Level rating
Total cholesterol	
<200	Desirable
200-239	Borderline high
≥240	High
HDL-C	
<40	Low
≥60	High
LDL-C	
<100	Optimal
100-129	Near or above optimal
130-159	Borderline high
160-189	High
≥190	Very high
Triglycerides	
<150	Normal
150-199	Borderline high
200-499	High
≥500	Very high

All values are mg · dl^{-1}.

Expert Panel on Detection, Evaluation, and Treatment of High Blood Cholesterol in Adults 2001.

Effects of Diet and Exercise on the Blood Lipid Profile

Consuming a diet low in saturated fat and cholesterol, losing weight, and participating in regular aerobic exercise all have been linked to positive changes in the blood lipid profile. The 2001 NCEP guidelines (10) recommend the Therapeutic Lifestyle Changes (TLC) diet to improve the blood lipid profile. The TLC diet includes the following dietary practices:

- Limiting total fat intake to 25% to 35% of calories (if at the higher end of the range, care should be taken to ensure that most fat is monounsaturated)
- Limiting saturated fat to 7%, polyunsaturated fat to 10%, and monounsaturated fat to 20% of calories
- Limiting cholesterol intake to <200 mg · day^{-1}, although more recent recommendations put less emphasis on dietary consumption of cholesterol (22)
- Limiting intake of trans fat

Consuming certain types of fat, such as omega-3 fatty acids, appears to benefit health. Omega-3 fatty acids are found in canola oil as well as in fish such as salmon and tuna. Omega-3 fatty acids are a polyunsaturated fat that get their name from the site of the first double bond in the fatty acid chain. American diets are typically low in omega-3 fatty acids and higher in omega-6 fatty acids (e.g., peanut, corn, and soybean oils). Bringing the intake of these two types of fat into better balance appears to improve the lipoprotein profile and lower the risk of CVD.

People who engage in regular aerobic exercise and maintain a healthy weight typically have a better blood lipid profile compared with their sedentary counterparts. It is difficult to ascertain which of these changes are attributable to the exercise and which relate to a healthy body weight. It appears that the primary blood lipid changes resulting from aerobic exercise are increases in HDL-C and decreases in blood levels of triglycerides (9). Weight loss has been linked with lower total cholesterol, LDL-C, and triglycerides as well as with higher HDL-C.

KEY POINT

Elevated total cholesterol and LDL-C and depressed HDL-C are risk factors for CVD. Aerobic exercise, weight loss, and low intake of saturated fat, trans fat, and cholesterol improve the blood lipid profile. A diet high in omega-3 fatty acids also has cardioprotective benefits.

Nutrition for Physically Active Individuals

Nutrition plays an important role in health, and it is also essential for optimal performance during physical activity. ACSM, the ADA, and Dietitians of Canada released an updated position statement in 2009 that addresses the dietary needs of physically active adults (3). Additionally, ACSM released a position stand on exercise and fluid replacement in 2007 (1). Fitness professionals should be familiar with these guidelines to provide basic nutritional advice to clients who exercise regularly.

Hydration Before, During, and After Exercise

Sweating is the primary mechanism for heat dissipation during exercise. The amount of sweat lost during exercise depends on environmental heat and humidity, the type and intensity of exercise, and the characteristics of the exerciser. Dehydration reduces the capacity for sweating and can impair performance by decreasing strength, endurance, and coordination. In addition, dehydration increases the risk of heat cramps, heat exhaustion, and heatstroke (see chapter 25).

Athletes should consume 5 to 7 $ml \cdot kg^{-1}$ body weight of water or a sport beverage at least 4 hr prior to competition (1, 3). If this fluid consumption does not yield urine output (or urine is dark), consume additional water (3-5 $ml \cdot kg^{-1}$) 2 hr before the event (1). Fluid replacement during exercise is essential in activities that last an hour or longer, especially if they take place in hot, humid environments. Preventing excessive dehydration (>2% of body weight) should be the goal during exercise (practice or competition). Sweat rates vary dramatically based on environmental conditions, intensity of exercise, and individual characteristics; thus, fluid consumption must be based on each specific case. Consuming 400 to 800 ml of water during endurance exercise is adequate for many people (1).

In activities where large amounts of sweat are lost, fluid should be fully replaced. Weighing oneself before and after these types of activities is recommended. The participant should drink approximately 16 to 24 oz (450-675 ml) of water for each pound (0.5 kg) of weight lost (3). If body weight has not returned to normal in the following days, additional water should be consumed before beginning exercise.

Protein Intake for Athletes

Athletes who are training intensely may benefit from increasing their protein intake above the level recommended for a sedentary person (i.e., 0.8 $g \cdot kg^{-1}$). An athlete training intensively in primarily endurance activities may benefit from consuming 1.2 to 1.4 g of protein per kilogram of body weight. For athletes engaging in high-intensity, high-volume resistance training, a protein intake of 1.2

Focus on Trans Fat

Recent attention has focused on the health risks of trans-fatty acids (i.e., trans fat). Although small amounts of trans fat are found in animal products, the majority of this hydrogenated fat is found in processed foods produced from fat in plants. The hydrogenation process chemically transforms the spatial orientation of hydrogen atoms in the fat. This hardens the liquid plant oil and leads to a more stable product that is better suited for cooking. Consequently, many processed foods (e.g., cookies, chips, doughnuts, french fries) are prepared with trans fat. Foods high in trans fat have partially hydrogenated vegetable oils as a primary ingredient on their food label. The problem with trans fat is that, as saturated fat, it can harm the blood lipid profile. Trans fat elevates LDL-C and lowers HDL-C; therefore, it should be avoided in order to improve the lipid profile (22, 23). One of the early public battles against trans fat occurred in New York City, where city government officials voted to ban trans fat from foods served in the city's restaurants. Although many restaurant owners fought this ordinance, the ban was successfully implemented. Now, the FDA is requiring that food manufacturers phase out the use of trans fat in U.S. food.

to 1.7 g · kg^{-1} may be needed (3). To this point, most of the studies in this area have focused on male athletes, so little is known about the protein needs of female athletes.

Athletes should generally meet additional protein requirements through food choices, not through supplements. There is an upper limit to the rate at which muscle mass can be increased; therefore, excessive protein intake (i.e., above the recommendations) does not enhance performance or increase muscle mass (3). Because intensively training athletes have a higher caloric intake, a diet with the normal distribution of macronutrients typically contains adequate amounts of protein, so purposefully consuming additional protein is usually not necessary (3, 25).

Another issue that sometimes arises is the adequacy of protein intake for vegetarian athletes. Because plant protein is not digested as well as animal protein, it is suggested that athletes following a strict vegetarian diet consume 1.3 to 1.8 g of protein per kilogram of body weight (3). The unique nutritional needs of the vegetarian athlete mean that consultation with a registered dietitian or sports dietitian may be needed (3).

Ergogenic Aids

The search for nutritional and pharmacological agents that improve performance has led to the marketing of numerous products touted as **ergogenic aids**. Some of these products (e.g., bee pollen, brewer's yeast) provide no scientifically proven physiological advantage. Other products, such as caffeine, may improve performance in some instances (25) and have been regulated by various sporting agencies such as the International Olympic Committee (IOC). Some ergogenic aids must be strictly avoided, such as anabolic steroids, because of severe and sometimes fatal side effects (20). For more information on rules regarding the use of ergogenic aids during competition, see the websites of the United States Anti-Doping Agency (www.usada.org) and the World Anti-Doping Agency (www.wada-ama.org). Additionally, ACSM (www.acsm.org) has released a number of Current Comments (official statements concerning topics of interest) on potential ergogenic aids.

Athletes often consume vitamins and minerals in amounts higher than the RDA in an attempt to improve performance. There is no evidence that this practice enhances performance; however, if an athlete's diet provides inadequate amounts of any nutrient, health and performance could suffer (25). The two minerals that often need to be increased in the diet are iron and calcium (6), and the most common mineral deficiency among athletes is iron deficiency (25). For athletes with anemia, increased iron consumption is advised and in many cases will improve performance (25). For female athletes with menstrual cycle irregularities, calcium supplementation often is prescribed to promote bone health. See chapter 18 for more information on issues specific to female athletes.

KEY POINT

Adequate hydration is essential to performance. Water should be consumed before, during, and after extended bouts of exercise. The typical protein RDA for adults (0.8 g · kg^{-1}) may be inadequate for athletes. People who are training intensely should consume additional protein. Ergogenic aids are pharmacological or nutritional agents thought to improve athletic performance. Although some products may enhance performance, there are many highly touted products with unproven results. In healthy, well-nourished athletes, extra vitamins and minerals (i.e., above the RDAs) do not improve performance.

Carbohydrate Loading and Intake During Exercise

Adequate intake of carbohydrate is necessary for optimal athletic performance in endurance events. Glucose is the major source of energy during exercise; when blood glucose levels decline, the ability to continue exercise is limited. A physically active person should routinely consume a diet in which 60% to 65% of the calories are from carbohydrate. For an athlete who trains heavily on consecutive days or who engages in frequent exhaustive exercise bouts, a diet providing 6 to 10 g of carbohydrate per kilogram of body weight is recommended (3).

Carbohydrate loading is used to maximize glycogen storage before competition. This practice is most beneficial for athletes who compete in events requiring continuous activity lasting longer than an hour, such as marathon running. The ADA and Canadian Dietetic Association recommend the following practices to enhance glycogen storage (4):

- Consume a diet in which 65% to 70% of the total calories are from carbohydrate.
- Decrease the duration of exercise bouts during the week before competition.
- Rest completely on the day before competition.

During events that involve continuous vigorous activity, it is beneficial to consume easily absorbed forms of carbohydrate. In events lasting up to an hour, a solution containing 6% to 8% carbohydrate is recommended to balance the need for blood glucose maintenance and fluid replacement (3). The solution should be consumed in small to moderate amounts (150-350 ml) every 15 to 20 min. In events beyond an hour, it is even more important to consume carbohydrate. Beverages, gels, and easily digested foods (e.g., bananas) can be used.

KEY POINT

Intake of adequate carbohydrate is necessary for optimal performance. Carbohydrate loading benefits extended bouts of exercise. Glucose intake during vigorous-intensity exercise can be beneficial, especially when exercise lasts 60 min or more.

Female Athlete Triad

The **female athlete triad** is a condition characterized by inadequate calorie intake, menstrual irregularities, and loss of bone mineral density (BMD) (2). As discussed in chapter 18, disordered eating is more common in female athletes than in the general population. It is thought that the pressure to succeed and the drive to be thin lead many female athletes to begin unhealthy eating practices such as severe caloric restriction (anorexia), purging food after eating (bulimia), and compulsive overexercising. These unhealthy patterns interfere with normal hormone secretion and eventually can lead to **oligomenorrhea** (irregular menses) or **amenorrhea** (lack of menses altogether). Because estrogen is essential in maintaining strong bones in women, the low estrogen levels observed in athletes with menstrual irregularities can lead to bone loss. Weakening of the bones makes athletes more susceptible to stress fractures and can lead to an early and severe onset of osteoporosis.

Fitness professionals should encourage all physically active people to consume adequate calories and nutrients to support their energy expenditure. Active females who begin to miss menstrual periods should be referred to a physician. Some signs of disordered eating are listed in chapter 12. Athletes who exhibit these signs should be referred to a nutritionist or psychologist (or both) who is qualified to counsel people with eating disorders. See chapter 18 for a more detailed discussion of the female athlete triad.

KEY POINT

The female athlete triad (disordered eating, amenorrhea, and osteoporosis) can lead to serious health consequences. Athletes who exhibit signs of an eating disorder should be referred to a qualified nutritionist, psychologist, or both.

Focus on Creatine Supplementation

Phosphocreatine, a high-energy compound found in skeletal muscle, is a critical source of energy during bursts of high-intensity exercise. Athletes use creatine supplementation (particularly in combination with carbohydrate) to increase the amount of phosphocreatine in muscle in an effort to enhance high-intensity exercise performance. Creatine supplementation has been touted as a remedy for a wide variety of conditions, including CHF, some vision problems, and various neurologic and musculoskeletal disorders (18). Studies demonstrate that creatine supplementation does improve high-intensity exercise performance, particularly repeated bouts of high-intensity cycling, under laboratory conditions. Less is known about its effect on performance under competitive conditions. Creatine supplementation also is associated with weight gain (~1 kg) as a result of water retention. It is unclear if this extra weight could impede performance in weight-bearing activities such as sprinting. Muscle cramping and gastrointestinal distress with creatine use are sometimes reported. Moderate ingestion of creatine is likely safe, but well-controlled, long-term studies are lacking (18). Potential damage to the kidneys and liver is a concern with high doses of creatine. For more information, refer to the review provided by the U.S. National Library of Medicine (18).

LEARNING AIDS

REVIEW QUESTIONS

1. What three nutrients provide energy for the body? How many calories come from the breakdown of each gram of these nutrients?
2. What is the acceptable macronutrient distribution range for carbohydrate, protein, and fat?
3. What is the AI for dietary fiber? How does this compare to the typical American intake?
4. What are trans-fatty acids? Why should they be avoided?
5. What is the RDA for iron for women of childbearing age? For men?
6. What nutrients do Americans typically overconsume? Underconsume?
7. According to NCEP, what are desirable values of HDL-C, LDL-C, and total cholesterol?
8. What are general recommendations regarding fluid intake during exercise?
9. What is the protein need for an intensely training endurance athlete? Strength athlete?
10. What are general recommendations to ensure adequate glycogen storage before competition?

CASE STUDIES

1. A male college basketball player (weight = 190 lb, or 86.4 kg) with a daily caloric intake of 3,500 kcal is considering additional protein supplements. Approximately 15% of his calories currently come from protein. Is his protein intake adequate? Would you recommend that he increase his protein intake?
2. Mr. Flanagan, a healthy 35-yr-old male, recently became your client for fitness training. He is gradually improving his fitness and is becoming more interested in his overall wellness. He is beginning to ask questions about how he should eat. What advice do you provide to Mr. Flanagan?
3. Mrs. Ortez is an obese 55-yr-old female with type 2 diabetes. She recently received physician clearance to join your fitness center. Her goals are to become regularly active, lose weight, and manage her diabetes with as little medication as possible. What dietary advice, if any, do you provide to Mrs. Ortez?

Answers to Case Studies

1. This athlete weighs 86.4 kg. The ACSM, ADA, and Dietitians of Canada position statement (4) suggests that such an athlete may benefit from ingesting 1.2 to 1.4 g of protein for each kilogram of body weight. This athlete is consuming approximately 525 kcal of protein each day (3,500 kcal · 0.15 = 525 kcal). This amount roughly equals 131 g of protein (525 kcal ÷ 4 kcal $\cdot$ g^{-1} = 131.25 g), or approximately 1.5 g $\cdot$ kg^{-1} (131.25 g ÷ 86.4 kg = 1.52 g $\cdot$ kg^{-1}). Additional protein intake appears unwarranted. If the athlete is unable to maintain weight, endurance, or strength with his current eating habits, a registered dietitian or sports dietitian should be consulted.
2. Mr. Flanagan is asking important questions about his overall wellness, and as a fitness professional, you are positioned to help him in several ways. First, point out to Mr. Flanagan the general recommendations contained in the Dietary Guidelines for Americans, which outline healthy eating practices that Americans should incorporate into their daily lives. The information contained in the sidebar *Key Components of the 2015-2020 Dietary Guidelines for Americans* summarizes some of these recommenda-

tions. Second, encourage Mr. Flanagan to begin tracking his dietary habits (see form 5.1). Tell him about the MyPlate website and encourage him to examine how his food intake matches recommended levels. Third, provide Mr. Flanagan with recipes for healthy and easy-to-cook meals.

3. Because Mrs. Ortez has a metabolic disease, type 2 diabetes, it is important that she seek out advice from a number of medical professionals, including her physician and a registered dietitian. However, as a fitness professional, you are a critical member of her overall wellness team. Here are things that you should do: (1) Encourage Mrs. Ortez to carefully follow the instructions of her physician regarding medications, weight loss, and any exercise limitations; (2) encourage Mrs. Ortez to consult a registered dietitian about her dietary habits (if necessary, point her to registered dietitians in your area); (3) provide general recommendations from the Dietary Guidelines for Americans about healthy eating habits; (4) provide examples of easy, low-calorie recipes; and (5) help her track her progress with exercise goals and weight loss and monitor her response to exercise for any unhealthy signs.

6

Energy Costs of Physical Activity

Edward T. Howley

OBJECTIVES

The reader will be able to do the following:

1. Describe how measurements of oxygen consumption can be used to estimate energy production, and list the number of calories derived per liter of oxygen and per gram of carbohydrate, fat, and protein.
2. Express energy expenditure as $L \cdot min^{-1}$, $kcal \cdot min^{-1}$, $ml \cdot kg^{-1} \cdot min^{-1}$, METs, and $kcal \cdot kg^{-1} \cdot hr^{-1}$.
3. Estimate the oxygen cost of walking, jogging, and running, including the cost of walking and running 1 mi (1.6 km).
4. Estimate the oxygen cost of cycle ergometry for both arm and leg work.
5. Estimate the oxygen cost of bench stepping.
6. Identify the approximate energy cost of recreational activities, sport, and other activities, and describe the effect of environmental factors on the HR response to a fixed work rate.

It's not uncommon to come across an advertisement such as: Expend up to 1,400 kcal in an hour by doing a one-on-one workout with a fitness professional. Really? Two fit people combined couldn't expend 1,400 kcal in an hour! That, of course, is not the only example of false promises about energy expenditure to lure people into joining a fitness program or buying a piece of exercise equipment. How can you help your clients make good judgments about what is real and what is not regarding energy expenditure? This chapter provides the background and examples to help answer those questions. Let's begin with how energy expenditure is measured.

Measuring Energy Expenditure

The most common way to measure energy expenditure is **indirect calorimetry**. In this procedure, described in the chapter 4 section *Measuring Oxygen Uptake*, oxygen consumption is measured and energy expenditure is calculated using simple conversion factors. These factors (constants) are derived in a two-step process:

1. First, we know from bomb calorimeter measurements that the heat given off from the combustion of carbohydrate, fat, and protein yields approximately 4.0, 9.0, and 5.6 kcal of heat per gram, respectively. Because the nitrogen in protein cannot be completely oxidized in the body and is excreted as urea, the physiological value for protein is actually 4.0 kcal · g^{-1}.
2. Knowing how much oxygen is required to oxidize 1 g of carbohydrate, fat, and protein allows one to calculate the number of calories of energy produced per liter of oxygen consumed. This is the **caloric equivalent of oxygen**. Values for carbohydrate, fat, and protein are listed in table 6.1.

Table 6.1 Measurements Associated With Oxidation of Carbohydrate, Fat, and Protein

Measurement	Carbohydrate	Fat	Protein[a]
Caloric density (kcal · g^{-1})	4.0	9.0	4.0
Caloric equivalent of 1 L of O_2 (kcal · L^{-1})	5.0	4.7	4.5
Respiratory quotient	1.0	0.7	0.8

[a]Does not include energy derived from the oxidation of nitrogen in the amino acids because the body excretes this as urea.

Based on Koebel 1984.

The table shows that carbohydrate gives about 6% more energy per liter of oxygen than fat gives (5.0 versus 4.7 kcal · L^{-1}), whereas fat gives more than twice as much energy per gram than carbohydrate gives (9 versus 4 kcal · g^{-1}). If a person is deriving energy from a 50–50 mixture of carbohydrate and fat during exercise, the caloric equivalent is approximately 4.85 kcal · L^{-1}, halfway between the value of 4.7 for fat and 5.0 for carbohydrate (19). However, a value of 5.0 kcal · L^{-1} may be used to convert oxygen uptake to kilocalories with little loss of accuracy. The ratio of carbon dioxide produced to oxygen consumed at the cell is called the *respiratory quotient (RQ)*. The same ratio, when measured by conventional gas exchange procedures, is called the *respiratory exchange ratio (R)* and is used to indicate fuel use (carbohydrate versus fat) during exercise (see chapter 4).

VIDEO Watch **video 6.1**, which demonstrates measuring oxygen consumption.

KEY POINT

Oxygen consumption $\dot{V}O_2$ is a measure of how much energy (calories) is produced by the body. The bomb calorimeter provides the number of calories gained per gram of food: 4 kcal · g^{-1} for carbohydrate, 9 kcal · g^{-1} for fat, and 4 kcal · g^{-1} for protein. Knowing how much oxygen is used to metabolize the food, we know that we obtain 4.7 kcal · L^{-1} when fat is oxidized and 5.0 kcal · L^{-1} when carbohydrate is oxidized. When a 50–50 mixture of carbohydrate and fat is used for energy, we obtain 4.85 kcal · L^{-1}. However, a value of 5.0 kcal · L^{-1} may be used to convert oxygen uptake to kilocalories, with little loss of accuracy.

RESEARCH INSIGHT

Accuracy of Wearable Fitness Trackers

Most people are familiar with pedometers that use simple technology to track the number of steps taken and the total distance moved throughout the day. In contrast, accelerometer-based devices can track both steps and the intensity of activities to generate an estimate of energy expenditure. Many have a simple computer interface that can generate a record of a client's activity pattern over time—great feedback for both the client and fitness professional (11). The newest accelerometers automatically transfer data to cell phones or to a website to simplify the tracking of physical activity and energy expenditure. The question is, how accurate are these estimates of energy expenditure? In a recent study of several devices (BodyMedia FIT, DirectLife, Fitbit One, Fitbit Zip, Jawbone UP Band, Nike FuelBand, and Basis B1 Band), all of the devices estimated energy expenditure within 9% to 13% of an indirect calorimetry measurement of energy expenditure, except for the Basis B1 Band (23%) (20). These results are promising and provide additional support for using these devices to help establish and maintain a regular pattern of physical activity.

Expressing Energy Expenditure

The energy requirement for an activity is calculated from the subject's steady-state oxygen uptake ($\dot{V}O_2$) measured during an activity. Once the subject reaches steady-state oxygen uptake, we know that the energy (ATP) supplied to the muscles is derived from aerobic metabolism. (See chapter 4 for more information on steady-state oxygen uptake.) The measured oxygen uptake then can be used to express energy expenditure in various ways. The five most common expressions follow.

1. $\dot{V}O_2$ ($L \cdot min^{-1}$). The calculation of oxygen uptake (see chapter 4) yields a value expressed in liters of oxygen used per minute, sometimes called the *absolute* $\dot{V}O_2$. For example, the following data were collected for an 80 kg man performing a submaximal run on a treadmill:

Ventilation (STPD) = $60\ L \cdot min^{-1}$, inspired O_2 = 20.93%, and expired O_2 = 16.93%, and

$$\dot{V}O_2\,(L \cdot min^{-1}) = 60\ L \cdot min^{-1}\,(20.93\%\ O_2 - 16.93\%\ O_2) = 2.4\ L \cdot min^{-1}.$$

2. Kilocalories per minute ($kcal \cdot min^{-1}$). Oxygen uptake can be expressed in kilocalories used per minute. The caloric equivalent of 1 L of O_2 ranges from 4.7 $kcal \cdot L^{-1}$ for fat to 5.0 $kcal \cdot L^{-1}$ for carbohydrate. For practical reasons, and with little loss in precision, 5 kcal per liter of O_2 is used to convert the oxygen uptake to kilocalories per minute. Energy expenditure is calculated by multiplying the kilocalories expended per minute ($kcal \cdot min^{-1}$) by the duration of the activity in minutes. For example, if the 80 kg man mentioned previously ran on the treadmill for 30 min at a $\dot{V}O_2$ of 2.4 $L \cdot min^{-1}$, the total energy expenditure can be calculated as follows.

$$\frac{2.4\ L\ O_2}{min} \cdot \frac{5\ kcal}{L\ O_2} = \frac{12\ kcal}{min}$$

$$\frac{12\ kcal}{min} \cdot 30\ min = 360\ kcal$$

3. $\dot{V}O_2$ ($ml \cdot kg^{-1} \cdot min^{-1}$). If the measured oxygen uptake, expressed in liters per minute, is multiplied by 1,000 to yield milliliters per minute and then divided by the subject's body weight in kilograms, the value is expressed in milliliters of O_2 per kilogram of body weight per minute, or $ml \cdot kg^{-1} \cdot min^{-1}$. This expression, sometimes called the *relative* $\dot{V}O_2$, helps in comparing values for people of varying body sizes. For example, for the 80 kg man with a $\dot{V}O_2$ of 2.4 $L \cdot min^{-1}$,

$$\frac{2.4\ L}{min} \cdot \frac{1000\ ml}{L} \div 80\ kg = 30\ ml \cdot kg^{-1} \cdot min^{-1}$$

4. METs. *MET* is a term used to describe a standard or reference resting metabolic rate. Because the actual resting metabolic rate varies with age and gender, being smaller in females than in males and decreasing with age (19), the MET is taken, by convention, to be $3.5\ ml \cdot kg^{-1} \cdot min^{-1}$. This is called *1 MET*. Activities are expressed in terms of multiples of the MET unit, which is nothing more than an alternative way of expressing oxygen uptake in $ml \cdot kg^{-1} \cdot min^{-1}$. For example, using the $\dot{V}O_2$ values presented previously in number 3,

$$30\ ml \cdot kg^{-1} \cdot min^{-1} \div 3.5\ ml \cdot kg^{-1} \cdot min^{-1} = 8.6\ METs.$$

5. Kilocalories per kilogram per hour ($kcal \cdot kg^{-1} \cdot hr^{-1}$). The MET expression of energy expenditure carries a special bonus: It also indicates the number of calories the subject uses per kilogram of body weight per hour. In the example mentioned previously, the subject is working at 8.6 METs, or about $30\ ml \cdot kg^{-1} \cdot min^{-1}$. When this value is multiplied by $60\ min \cdot hr^{-1}$, it equals $1{,}800\ ml \cdot kg^{-1} \cdot hr^{-1}$, or $1.8\ L \cdot kg^{-1} \cdot hr^{-1}$. If the person is using a mixture of carbohydrate and fat as fuel, then this oxygen consumption is multiplied by 4.85 kcal per liter of O_2 to give $8.7\ kcal \cdot kg^{-1} \cdot hr^{-1}$. The following steps show the details of this calculation.

$$8.6\ METs \cdot \frac{3.5\ ml \cdot kg^{-1} \cdot min^{-1}}{MET} = 30\ ml \cdot kg^{-1} \cdot min^{-1}$$

$$30\ ml \cdot kg^{-1} \cdot min^{-1} \cdot 60\ min \cdot hr^{-1} = 1{,}800\ ml \cdot kg^{-1} \cdot hr^{-1} = 1.8\ L \cdot kg^{-1} \cdot hr^{-1}$$

$$1.8\ L \cdot kg^{-1} \cdot hr^{-1} \cdot 4.85\ kcal \cdot L\ O_2^{-1} = 8.7\ kcal \cdot kg^{-1} \cdot hr^{-1}$$

As indicated in chapter 1, the volume of physical activity is linked to numerous health outcomes. The volume or amount of physical activity is easily calculated from the rate of energy expenditure and the duration of the activity. For example, if someone is exercising at an energy expenditure of 10 $kcal \cdot min^{-1}$ for 30 min, 300 kcal of energy are expended. The MET scale can also be used to calculate the volume of energy expenditure. If a person is exercising at 7 METs for 30 min, 210 MET-min of energy expenditure is accomplished. The Physical Activity Guidelines for Americans indicate that when people regularly accomplish 500 to 1,000 MET-min of physical activity per week, they realize substantial health benefits. In the case of the person working at 7 METs for 30 min sessions, only three sessions a week would be needed to meet the low end of that physical activity range (3 × 210 = 630 MET-min), and five sessions (5 × 210 = 1,050 MET-min) would allow the person to reach the top end of the range, where more health benefits are realized (28).

KEY POINT

Energy expenditure can be expressed in $L \cdot min^{-1}$, $kcal \cdot min^{-1}$, $ml \cdot kg^{-1} \cdot min^{-1}$, METs, and $kcal \cdot kg^{-1} \cdot hr^{-1}$:

- To convert $L \cdot min^{-1}$ to $kcal \cdot min^{-1}$, multiply by $5.0\ kcal \cdot L^{-1}$.
- To convert $L \cdot min^{-1}$ to $ml \cdot kg^{-1} \cdot min^{-1}$, multiply by 1,000 and divide by body weight in kilograms.
- To convert $ml \cdot kg^{-1} \cdot min^{-1}$ to METs or $kcal \cdot kg^{-1} \cdot hr^{-1}$, divide by $3.5\ ml \cdot kg^{-1} \cdot min^{-1}$.

Equations for Estimating the Energy Cost of Activities

In the mid-1970s, ACSM identified some simple equations to estimate the steady-state energy requirement associated with common modes of activities used in GXTs, including walking, stepping, running, and cycle ergometry (2). Over the years, the equations have been modified to reflect the best information available, and this chapter discusses the current thinking in estimating energy costs (3). The oxygen uptake calculated from these equations is an estimate, and a typical **standard deviation (SD)** associated with the actual measured average value is about 10% (3, 10). Remember this normal variation in the energy costs of activities when using these equations in prescribing exercise.

The ACSM equations have been applied to GXTs to estimate maximal aerobic power. This application gives reasonable estimates when the subjects are healthy and the rate at which the GXT progresses is slow enough to allow the subject to achieve steady-state oxygen uptake at each stage (23, 24). When the increments between the stages of the GXT are large or the person is somewhat unfit, oxygen uptake will not keep pace with each stage of the test. In these cases, the equations overestimate the actual measured oxygen uptake (17) because the equations are designed to estimate steady-state energy requirements. This overestimation is more likely to happen in populations with disease (e.g., cardiac patients), suggesting that the GXTs used to test these populations may be too aggressive (see Research Insight on how investigators have dealt with this problem). A test that progresses at a slower rate and allows the subject to reach the steady-state $\dot{V}O_2$ at each stage reduces the chance of overestimating functional capacity (see chapter 11).

RESEARCH INSIGHT

Specialized Equations for Graded Exercise Tests

All of the equations presented in this chapter estimate the energy cost of activities based on steady-state considerations. However, when a person completes a maximal GXT to volitional exhaustion (see chapter 7), the person is clearly *not* in a steady state in the last stage of the test. It has been shown that when $\dot{V}O_2max$ is estimated based on the steady-state equations, it is systematically higher than what is actually measured. To deal with this, investigators have developed unique equations for predicting $\dot{V}O_2max$ for the treadmill (14) and cycle (27). Additionally, if the patient or client holds onto the treadmill railing during the test, the overestimation is even greater (15) because the patient is off-loading some of the work by holding onto the railing and can complete more stages of the test. Thus, investigators have developed specialized equations to account for holding onto the railing (22). An interesting approach was taken by Foster et al. (15) in which they used the steady-state equations (presented in this chapter) to predict the oxygen cost of the last stage of the treadmill test and then developed a prediction equation to estimate $\dot{V}O_2max$. It worked both for patients who held onto the treadmill railing and those who did not.

When the ACSM equations were developed, an attempt was made to use a true physiological oxygen cost for each type of work. Each activity is broken down into the energy components. That is, in estimating the total oxygen cost of walking up a grade, you add the net oxygen cost of the horizontal walk (one component) to the net oxygen cost of the vertical (grade) walk (one component) to the resting metabolic rate (one component), which is taken to be 1 MET (3.5 ml · kg^{-1} · min^{-1}).

$$\text{Total } O_2 \text{ cost} = \text{net oxygen cost of activity} + 3.5 \text{ ml} \cdot \text{kg}^{-1} \cdot \text{min}^{-1}.$$

For the equations to properly estimate the oxygen cost of the activity, the subject must follow instructions carefully (e.g., not hold onto the treadmill railing, maintain the pedal cadence), and the work instruments (i.e., treadmill, cycle ergometer) must be calibrated so the settings are correct (see chapter 7).

Energy Requirements of Walking, Running, Cycle Ergometry, and Stepping

The following sections provide equations to estimate the energy cost of walking, running, cycle ergometry, and stepping. These activities are common in cardiac rehabilitation and adult fitness programs. Examples are provided to show how the equations are used in designing exercise programs.

Oxygen Cost of Walking

The oxygen cost of walking is determined by walking speed and whether the walker is on a horizontal or a graded surface. Prediction equations address all of these factors.

Horizontal Surface

One of the most common activities in exercise programs and GXTs is walking. The following equation can be used to estimate the energy requirement between the walking speeds of 50 and 100 $m \cdot min^{-1}$, or 1.9 and 3.7 $mi \cdot hr^{-1}$. (Multiply miles per hour by 26.8 to obtain meters per minute. Divide meters per minute by 26.8 to obtain miles per hour.) Dill (13) showed that the net cost of walking 1 $m \cdot min^{-1}$ on a horizontal surface is about 0.1 $ml \cdot kg^{-1} \cdot min^{-1}$, and this value is used in the ACSM equation. The ACSM equation for calculating the oxygen cost ($ml \cdot kg^{-1} \cdot min^{-1}$) of walking on a flat surface is as follows:

$$\dot{V}O_2 = 0.1\ ml \cdot kg^{-1} \cdot min^{-1}\ (\text{horizontal velocity}) + 3.5\ ml \cdot kg^{-1} \cdot min^{-1}.$$

QUESTION:

What are the estimated steady-state $\dot{V}O_2$ and METs for a walking speed of 90 $m \cdot min^{-1}$ (3.4 $mi \cdot hr^{-1}$)?

ANSWER:

$$\dot{V}O_2 = 90\ m \cdot min^{-1} \cdot \frac{0.1\ ml \cdot kg^{-1} \cdot min^{-1}}{m \cdot min^{-1}} + 3.5\ ml \cdot kg^{-1} \cdot min^{-1}$$

$$\dot{V}O_2 = 9.0\ ml \cdot kg^{-1} \cdot min^{-1} + 3.5\ ml \cdot kg^{-1} \cdot min^{-1} = 12.5\ ml \cdot kg^{-1} \cdot min^{-1}$$

$$12.5\ ml \cdot kg^{-1} \cdot min^{-1} \div 3.5\ ml \cdot kg^{-1} \cdot min^{-1} = 3.6\ \text{METs or } 3.6\ kcal \cdot kg^{-1} \cdot hr^{-1}$$

The equations also can be used to predict the level of activity required to elicit a specific energy expenditure.

QUESTION:

An unfit participant is told to exercise at 11.5 $ml \cdot kg^{-1} \cdot min^{-1}$ to achieve the proper exercise intensity. What walking speed would you recommend?

ANSWER:

$$11.5\ ml \cdot kg^{-1} \cdot min^{-1} = ?\ m \cdot min^{-1} \cdot \frac{0.1\ ml \cdot kg^{-1} \cdot min^{-1}}{m \cdot min^{-1}} + 3.5\ ml \cdot kg^{-1} \cdot min^{-1}$$

Subtract the resting metabolic rate of 3.5 $ml \cdot kg^{-1} \cdot min^{-1}$ from both sides of the equation. Subtracting 3.5 $ml \cdot kg^{-1} \cdot min^{-1}$ from 11.5 $ml \cdot kg^{-1} \cdot min^{-1}$ gives the net oxygen cost of the activity (8.0 $ml \cdot kg^{-1} \cdot min^{-1}$):

$$8\ ml \cdot kg^{-1} \cdot min^{-1} = ?\ m \cdot min^{-1} \cdot \frac{0.1\ ml \cdot kg^{-1} \cdot min^{-1}}{m \cdot min^{-1}}$$

The net cost (8 $ml \cdot kg^{-1} \cdot min^{-1}$) is divided by 0.1 $ml \cdot kg^{-1} \cdot min^{-1}$ per $m \cdot min^{-1}$ to yield 80 $m \cdot min^{-1}$. To obtain miles per hour, divide meters per minute by 26.8 to get 3 $mi \cdot hr^{-1}$:

$$80\ m \cdot min^{-1} = 8\ ml \cdot kg^{-1} \cdot min^{-1} \div \frac{0.1\ ml \cdot kg^{-1} \cdot min^{-1}}{m \cdot min^{-1}}$$

$$3.0\ mi \cdot hr^{-1} = 80\ m \cdot min^{-1} \div \frac{26.8\ m \cdot min^{-1}}{mi \cdot hr^{-1}}$$

Walking Up a Grade

The oxygen cost of walking up a grade is the sum of the oxygen cost of horizontal walking, the oxygen cost of the vertical component of walking on a grade, and the resting metabolic rate of 3.5 $ml \cdot kg^{-1} \cdot min^{-1}$. Studies have shown that the oxygen cost of moving (walking or stepping) 1 $m \cdot min^{-1}$ vertically is 1.8 $ml \cdot kg^{-1} \cdot min^{-1}$ (7, 25). The vertical component (vertical velocity) is calculated by multiplying the grade (expressed as a fraction) times the speed in meters per minute. A person walking at 80 $m \cdot min^{-1}$ on a 10% grade is walking 8 $m \cdot min^{-1}$ vertically ($0.10 \cdot 80\ m \cdot min^{-1}$). The equation for calculating the oxygen cost ($ml \cdot kg^{-1} \cdot min^{-1}$) of walking on a grade is as follows:

$$\dot{V}O_2 = 0.1\ ml \cdot kg^{-1} \cdot min^{-1}(\text{horizontal velocity}) + 1.8\ ml \cdot kg^{-1} \cdot min^{-1}(\text{vertical velocity}) + 3.5\ ml \cdot kg^{-1} \cdot min^{-1}.$$

QUESTION:
What is the total oxygen cost of walking 90 m · min^{-1} up a 12% grade?

ANSWER:
The horizontal component is calculated as in the preceding equation for walking on a horizontal surface and equals 9 ml · kg^{-1} · min^{-1}. The following equations show how to calculate the vertical component and finally the total oxygen cost for walking 90 m · min^{-1} up a 12% grade:

$$\dot{V}O_2 = 0.12\ (\text{grade}) \cdot 90\ m \cdot min^{-1} \cdot \frac{1.8\ ml \cdot kg^{-1} \cdot min^{-1}}{m \cdot min^{-1}} = 19.4\ ml \cdot kg^{-1} \cdot min^{-1}$$

$$\dot{V}O_2\ (ml \cdot kg^{-1} \cdot min^{-1}) = 9.0\ (\text{horizontal}) + 19.4\ (\text{vertical}) + 3.5\ (\text{rest}) = 31.9\ ml \cdot kg^{-1} \cdot min^{-1} \text{ or } 9.1 \text{ METs or } 9.1\ kcal \cdot kg^{-1} \cdot hr^{-1}$$

As indicated earlier, the equations can be used to estimate the treadmill settings needed to elicit a specific oxygen uptake.

QUESTION:
How would you set the treadmill grade to achieve an energy requirement of 6 METs (21.0 ml · kg^{-1} · min^{-1}) when walking at 60 m · min^{-1}?

ANSWER:
The net oxygen cost of the activity is 21 – 3.5, or 17.5 ml · kg^{-1} · min^{-1}. Now we must calculate the vertical and horizontal energy components to reach the final answer:

$$\text{Horizontal component} = 60\ m \cdot min^{-1} \cdot \frac{0.1\ ml \cdot kg^{-1} \cdot min^{-1}}{m \cdot min^{-1}} = 6.0\ ml \cdot kg^{-1} \cdot min^{-1}$$

$$\text{Vertical component} = 17.5 - 6.0 = 11.5\ ml \cdot kg^{-1} \cdot min^{-1}$$

$$11.5\ ml \cdot kg^{-1} \cdot min^{-1} = \text{fractional grade} \cdot 60\ m \cdot min^{-1} \cdot \frac{1.8\ ml \cdot kg^{-1} \cdot min^{-1}}{m \cdot min^{-1}}$$

$$11.5\ ml \cdot kg^{-1} \cdot min^{-1} = \text{fractional grade} \cdot 108\ ml \cdot kg^{-1} \cdot min^{-1}$$

$$\text{Fractional grade} = 11.5 \div 108 = 0.106 \cdot 100\% = 10.6\%\ \text{grade}$$

Walking at Various Speeds

The preceding equations are useful for walking speeds of 50 to 100 m · min^{-1} (1.9-3.7 mi · hr^{-1}); beyond that, the oxygen requirement for walking increases curvilinearly (10). Because many people choose to walk quickly rather than jog, knowing the energy requirements for walking at these higher speeds is useful in prescribing exercise. Values for the energy requirements for walking horizontally and at various grades at these faster speeds (4.0-5.0 mi · hr^{-1}, or 107-134 m · min^{-1}) are included in table 6.2.

One of the most common and useful ways to express the energy cost of walking is in kilocalories per minute. In this way, the fitness professional can simply locate the walking speed in a table, identify the number of calories used per minute, and calculate the total energy expenditure based on the duration of the walk. Table 6.3 presents the energy cost (in kcal · min^{-1}) for walking speeds of 2 to 5 mi · hr^{-1} (54-134 m · min^{-1}) and includes values for various body weights. The energy cost of walking increases with the speed of the walk; however, the rate of increase is larger at higher speeds. For example, when a 170 lb (77.3 kg) participant increases walking speed from 2 to 3 mi · hr^{-1} (from 54 to 80 m · min^{-1}), the energy cost increases from 3.2 to 4.2 kcal · min^{-1}. But going from 4 to 5 mi · hr^{-1} (from 107 to 134 m · min^{-1}), the energy cost increases from 6.3 to 10.2 kcal · min^{-1}. A sedentary person can walk at slow speeds and achieve the desired exercise intensity, and a relatively fit person can walk at higher speeds at which the elevated energy requirement provides the necessary stimulus for a training effect.

Table 6.2 Energy Requirement in METs for Walking at Various Speeds and Grades

	SPEED (MI · HR^{-1}/M · MIN^{-1})						
Grade (%)	2.0/54	2.5/67	3.0/80	3.5/94	4.0/107	4.5/121	5.0/134
0	2.5	2.9	3.3	3.7	4.9	6.2	7.9
2	3.1	3.6	4.1	4.7	5.9	7.4	9.3
4	3.6	4.3	4.9	5.6	7.1	8.7	10.6
6	4.2	5.0	5.8	6.6	8.1	9.9	12.0
8	4.7	5.7	6.6	7.5	9.3	11.1	13.4
10	5.3	6.3	7.4	8.5	10.4	12.4	14.8
12	5.8	7.1	8.3	9.5	11.4	13.6	16.6
14	6.4	7.7	9.1	10.4	12.6	14.9	17.5
16	6.9	8.4	9.9	11.4	13.6	16.1	18.9
18	7.5	9.1	10.7	12.4	14.8	17.4	20.3
20	8.1	9.8	11.6	13.3	15.9	18.6	21.7
22	8.6	10.3	12.4	14.3	17.0	19.9	23.1
24	9.1	11.1	13.2	15.3	18.1	21.1	
26	9.7	11.9	14.0	16.2	19.2	22.3	
28	10.3	12.5	14.9	17.2	20.3	23.6	
30	10.8	13.2	15.7	18.2	21.4		

Based on American College of Sports Medicine 2014, *ACSM's guidelines for exercise testing and prescription*, 9th ed. (Philadelphia: PA: Lippincott, Williams, & Wilkins); Bubb et al. 1985.

Table 6.3 Energy Costs of Walking (k cal · min^{-1})

BODY WEIGHT		SPEED (MI · HR^{-1}/M · MIN^{-1})						
kg	lb	2.0/54	2.5/67	3.0/80	3.5/94	4.0/107	4.5/121	5.0/134
50.0	110	2.1	2.4	2.8	3.1	4.1	5.2	6.6
54.5	120	2.3	2.6	3.0	3.4	4.4	5.6	7.2
59.1	130	2.5	2.9	3.2	3.6	4.8	6.1	7.8
63.6	140	2.7	3.1	3.5	3.9	5.2	6.6	8.4
68.2	150	2.8	3.3	3.7	4.2	5.6	7.0	9.0
72.7	160	3.0	3.5	4.0	4.5	5.9	7.5	9.6
77.3	170	3.2	3.7	4.2	4.8	6.3	8.0	10.2
81.8	180	3.4	4.0	4.5	5.0	6.7	8.4	10.8
86.4	190	3.6	4.2	4.7	5.3	7.0	8.9	11.4
90.9	200	3.8	4.4	5.0	5.6	7.4	9.4	12.0
95.4	210	4.0	4.6	5.2	5.9	7.8	9.9	12.6
100.0	220	4.2	4.8	5.5	6.2	8.2	10.3	13.2

Multiply value by duration of the activity to obtain total calories expended.

Based on American College of Sports Medicine 2014, *ACSM's guidelines for exercise testing and prescription*, 9th ed. (Philadelphia: PA: Lippincott, Williams, & Wilkins); Bubb et al. 1985.

How Body Weight Affects Energy Expenditure

Body weight is important when calculating how much energy a client may expend during exercise. You can see in table 6.3 that a person weighing 220 lb (100 kg) expends twice as many kcal per minute as a person weighing only 110 lb (50 kg) when walking at the same speed (i.e., 6.2 versus 3.1 kcal · min^{-1} at 3.5 mi · hr^{-1}). Consequently, if you set energy expenditure goals for your clients in kilocalories, a lighter person will need to exercise for a longer time compared with a heavier person. Consistent with that, as a client loses weight, the energy cost of walking at a certain speed decreases because the energy cost depends on body weight. The participant can compensate for the lower energy cost by walking for a longer duration at that speed or by walking for the same duration at a higher speed. This example involves clients doing submaximal exercise; however, the same point can be made when predicting energy expenditure for clients working at their maximal aerobic power ($\dot{V}O_2max$). If two clients have the same $\dot{V}O_2max$ of 12 METs (12 kcal · kg^{-1} · hr^{-1}), and one weighs 50 kg and the other weighs 100 kg, the amount of energy that they can expend if they work for 1 hr at that maximum (which they cannot!) is 600 and 1,200 kcal, respectively. Going back to the advertisement mentioned at the beginning of this chapter, you can see that neither could expend 1,400 kcal in an hour, even working at 100% of $\dot{V}O_2max$. We will see more on this at the end of this chapter.

Oxygen Cost of Jogging and Running

Jogging and running are common in fitness programs for apparently healthy people. It is possible to use the ACSM equations to estimate the oxygen cost of these activities for a broad range of speeds, generally from 130 to 350 m · min^{-1}. The equations are also useful at speeds below 130 m · min^{-1} as long as the person is actually jogging. The fact that a person can walk or jog at speeds below 130 m · min^{-1} complicates the issue. The oxygen cost of walking is less than that of jogging at slow speeds; however, at approximately 140 m · min^{-1} (5.2 mi · hr^{-1}), the oxygen costs of jogging and walking are about the same. Above this speed, the oxygen cost of walking exceeds that of jogging (5).

Jogging and Running on a Horizontal Surface

The net oxygen cost of jogging or running 1 m · min^{-1} on a horizontal surface is about twice that of walking, 0.2 ml · kg^{-1} · min $^{-1}$ per m · min^{-1} (6, 9, 21). Remember that the equation gives reasonable estimates of the oxygen cost of running for the average person. However, it is well known that trained runners are more economical (in terms of energy expenditure) than the average person and that running economy varies within any group, trained or untrained (9, 12, 24). The equation for estimating the oxygen cost (ml · kg^{-1} · min^{-1}) of running on a flat surface is as follows:

$$\dot{V}O_2 = 0.2 \text{ ml} \cdot \text{kg}^{-1} \cdot \text{min}^{-1} \text{ (horizontal velocity)} + 3.5 \text{ ml} \cdot \text{kg}^{-1} \cdot \text{min}^{-1}.$$

QUESTION:
What is the oxygen requirement for running a 10K (10,000 m) race on a track in 60 min?

ANSWER:

$$10{,}000 \text{ m} \div 60 \text{ min} = 167 \text{ m} \cdot \text{min}^{-1}$$

$$\dot{V}O_2 = 167 \text{ m} \cdot \text{min}^{-1} \cdot \frac{0.2 \text{ ml} \cdot \text{kg}^{-1} \cdot \text{min}^{-1}}{\text{m} \cdot \text{min}^{-1}} + 3.5 \text{ ml} \cdot \text{kg}^{-1} \cdot \text{min}^{-1}$$

$$= 36.9 \text{ ml} \cdot \text{kg}^{-1} \cdot \text{min}^{-1} \text{ or } 10.5 \text{ METs or } 10.5 \text{ kcal} \cdot \text{kg}^{-1} \cdot \text{hr}^{-1}$$

QUESTION:
A 20-yr-old female distance runner with a $\dot{V}O_2max$ of 50 ml · kg^{-1} · min^{-1} wants to run intervals at 90% of $\dot{V}O_2max$. At what speed should she run on a track given that 1 mi equals 1,610 m?

ANSWER:

90% of 50 = 45 $ml \cdot kg^{-1} \cdot min^{-1}$, and the net cost of the run equals 45 $ml \cdot kg^{-1} \cdot min^{-1}$ – 3.5 $ml \cdot kg^{-1} \cdot min^{-1}$, or 41.5 $ml \cdot kg^{-1} \cdot min^{-1}$.

$$41.5\ ml \cdot kg^{-1} \cdot min^{-1} \div \frac{0.2\ ml \cdot kg^{-1} \cdot min^{-1}}{m \cdot min^{-1}} = 207\ m \cdot min^{-1}$$

$$1610\ m \cdot mi^{-1} \div 207\ m \cdot min^{-1} = 7.78\ min, \text{ or } 7{:}47\ (min{:}s) \text{ mile pace}$$

Jogging and Running Up a Grade

There is not as much information about the oxygen cost of running up a grade as there is about the cost of walking up a grade or running on a flat track. But one thing is clear—the oxygen cost of running up a grade is about half that of walking up a grade (8, 21). Some of the vertical lift associated with running on a flat surface is used to accomplish some of the grade work during inclined running, lowering the net oxygen requirement for the vertical work. The oxygen cost of running 1 $m \cdot min^{-1}$ vertically is about 0.9 $ml \cdot kg^{-1} \cdot min^{-1}$. As in the calculations for uphill walking, the vertical velocity is calculated by multiplying the fractional grade times the horizontal velocity. The following equation is used for calculating the oxygen cost of running up a grade.

$$\dot{V}O_2 = 0.2\ ml \cdot kg^{-1} \cdot min^{-1}\ (\text{horizontal velocity}) +$$
$$0.9\ ml \cdot kg^{-1} \cdot min^{-1}\ (\text{vertical velocity}) + 3.5\ ml \cdot kg^{-1} \cdot min^{-1}.$$

QUESTION:

What is the oxygen cost of running 150 $m \cdot min^{-1}$ up a 10% grade?

ANSWER:

Horizontal component:

$$\dot{V}O_2 = 150\ m \cdot min^{-1} \cdot \frac{0.2\ ml \cdot kg^{-1} \cdot min^{-1}}{m \cdot min^{-1}} = 30\ ml \cdot kg^{-1} \cdot min^{-1}$$

Vertical component:

$$\dot{V}O_2 = 0.10\ (\text{fractional grade}) \cdot 150\ m \cdot min^{-1} \cdot \frac{0.9\ ml \cdot kg^{-1} \cdot min^{-1}}{m \cdot min^{-1}}$$
$$= 13.5\ ml \cdot kg^{-1} \cdot min^{-1}$$
$$\dot{V}O_2 = 30.0\ (\text{horizontal}) + 13.5\ (\text{vertical}) + 3.5\ (\text{rest}) = 47\ ml \cdot kg^{-1} \cdot min^{-1}$$
$$= 13.4\ \text{METs or } 13.4\ kcal \cdot kg^{-1} \cdot hr^{-1}$$

QUESTION:

The oxygen cost of running 350 $m \cdot min^{-1}$ on a flat surface is about 73.5 $ml \cdot kg^{-1} \cdot min^{-1}$. What grade should be set on a treadmill for a speed of 300 $m \cdot min^{-1}$ to achieve the same $\dot{V}O_2$?

ANSWER:

Horizontal component:

$$\dot{V}O_2 = 300\ m \cdot min^{-1} \cdot \frac{0.2\ ml \cdot kg^{-1} \cdot min^{-1}}{m \cdot min^{-1}} = 60\ ml \cdot kg^{-1} \cdot min^{-1}$$

Vertical component:

$$\text{Net } \dot{V}O_2 = 73.5\ (\text{total}) - 60\ (\text{horizontal}) - 3.5\ (\text{rest}) = 10.0\ ml \cdot kg^{-1} \cdot min^{-1}$$
$$10.0\ ml \cdot kg^{-1} \cdot min^{-1} = \text{fractional grade} \cdot 300\ m \cdot min^{-1} \cdot \frac{0.9\ ml \cdot kg^{-1} \cdot min^{-1}}{m \cdot min^{-1}}$$
$$\text{Fractional grade} = 10\ ml \cdot kg^{-1} \cdot min^{-1} \div 270\ ml \cdot kg^{-1} \cdot min^{-1}$$
$$= .037, \text{ or } 3.7\% \text{ grade}$$

Table 6.4 summarizes oxygen costs of running on a level surface and up a grade.

Jogging and Running at Various Speeds

In contrast to the energy cost of walking, the energy cost of jogging and running increases linearly with increasing speed. Table 6.5 shows the caloric cost of running, in kilocalories per minute, for runners of various body weights. For the 170 lb (77.3 kg) participant, the energy cost increases from 7.2 to 11.2 $kcal \cdot min^{-1}$ when speed jumps from 3 to 5 $mi \cdot hr^{-1}$ (from 80 to 134 $m \cdot min^{-1}$); the increase is also 4 $kcal \cdot min^{-1}$ when speed increases from 7 to 9 $mi \cdot hr^{-1}$ (from 188 to 241 $m \cdot min^{-1}$). As with walking, the energy cost is higher for heavier individuals.

Table 6.4 Energy Requirement in METs for Jogging or Running at Various Speeds and Grades

	SPEED ($MI \cdot HR^{-1}/M \cdot MIN^{-1}$)							
Grade (%)	3/80	4/107	5/134	6/161	7/188	8/215	9/241	10/268
0	5.6	7.1	8.7	10.2	11.7	13.3	14.8	16.3
1	5.8	7.4	9.0	10.6	12.2	13.8	15.4	17.0
2	6.0	7.7	9.3	11.0	12.7	14.4	16.0	17.7
3	6.2	7.9	9.7	11.4	13.2	14.9	16.6	18.4
4	6.4	8.2	10.0	11.9	13.7	15.5	17.3	19.1
5	6.6	8.5	10.4	12.3	14.2	16.1	17.9	19.8
6	6.8	8.8	10.7	12.7	14.6	16.6	18.5	20.4
7	7.0	9.0	11.0	13.1	15.1	17.1	19.1	21.1
8	7.2	9.3	11.4	13.5	15.6	17.7	19.7	21.8
9	7.4	9.6	11.7	13.9	16.1	18.3	20.3	22.5
10	7.6	9.9	12.1	14.3	16.6	18.8	21.0	23.2

Based on American College of Sports Medicine 2014, *ACSM's guidelines for exercise testing and prescription*, 9th ed. (Philadelphia: PA: Lippincott, Williams, & Wilkins).

Table 6.5 Energy Costs of Jogging and Running ($kcal \cdot min^{-1}$)

BODY WEIGHT		SPEED ($MI \cdot HR^{-1}/M \cdot MIN^{-1}$)							
kg	lb	3.0/80	4.0/107	5.0/134	6.0/161	7.0/188	8.0/215	9.0/241	10.0/268
50.0	110	4.7	5.9	7.2	8.5	9.8	11.1	12.3	13.6
54.5	120	5.1	6.4	7.9	9.3	10.6	12.1	13.4	14.8
59.1	130	5.5	7.0	8.6	10.0	11.5	13.1	14.6	16.1
63.6	140	5.9	7.5	9.2	10.8	12.4	14.1	15.7	17.3
68.2	150	6.4	8.1	9.9	11.6	13.3	15.1	16.8	18.5
72.7	160	6.8	8.6	10.5	12.4	14.2	16.1	17.9	19.8
77.3	170	7.2	9.1	11.2	13.1	15.1	17.1	19.1	21.0
81.8	180	7.6	9.7	11.8	13.9	15.9	18.1	20.2	22.2
86.4	190	8.1	10.2	12.5	14.7	16.8	19.1	21.3	23.5
90.9	200	8.5	10.8	13.2	15.4	17.7	20.1	22.4	24.7
95.4	210	8.9	11.3	13.8	16.2	18.6	21.1	23.5	25.9
100.0	220	9.3	11.8	14.5	17.0	19.5	22.2	24.7	27.2

Multiply value by duration of the activity to obtain total calories expended.

Oxygen Cost of Walking and Running a Mile

Despite the vast amount of information regarding the costs of walking and running, a good deal of misunderstanding still exists. We hear claims that the energy cost of walking 1 mi (1.6 km) is equal to that of running the same distance. In general, this is not the case (18). The equations for estimating the energy cost of walking and running can be used to estimate the caloric cost of walking and running 1 mi (1.6 km)—information that is useful in achieving energy expenditure goals.

If a person walks at 3 mi · hr^{-1} (80 m · min^{-1}), he completes 1 mi (1.6 km) in 20 min. The caloric cost for walking 1 mi (1.6 km) for a 70 kg person is calculated as follows:

$$\dot{V}O_2 = 80\ \text{m} \cdot \text{min}^{-1}\ (0.1\ \text{ml} \cdot \text{kg}^{-1} \cdot \text{min}^{-1}) + 3.5\ \text{ml} \cdot \text{kg}^{-1} \cdot \text{min}^{-1} = 11.5\ \text{ml} \cdot \text{kg}^{-1} \cdot \text{min}^{-1},$$

$$\dot{V}O_2\ (\text{ml} \cdot \text{mile}^{-1}) = 11.5\ \text{ml} \cdot \text{kg}^{-1} \cdot \text{min}^{-1} \cdot 70\ \text{kg} \cdot 20\ \text{min} \cdot \text{mile}^{-1} = 16{,}100\ \text{ml} \cdot \text{mi}^{-1},$$

and so

$$\dot{V}O_2\ (\text{L} \cdot \text{min}^{-1}) = 16{,}100\ \text{ml} \cdot \text{mi}^{-1} \div 1{,}000\ \text{ml} \cdot \text{L}^{-1} = 16.1\ \text{L} \cdot \text{mi}^{-1}.$$

At about 5.0 kcal per liter of O_2, the gross caloric cost per mile of walking is 80.5 kcal (5 kcal · L^{-1} · 16.1 L · mi^{-1}). The net caloric cost for the mile walk can be calculated by subtracting the oxygen cost of 20 min of rest from the gross cost of the 3 mi · hr^{-1} walk. For this person,

- resting oxygen uptake = 3.5 ml · kg^{-1} · min^{-1} · 70 kg = 245 ml · min^{-1};
- 20 min of rest (20 min · 245 ml · min^{-1}) = 4,900 ml, or 4.9 L O_2;
- at 5 kcal · L^{-1}, 4. 9 L O_2 equals 24.5 kcal for 20 min of rest; and
- the net cost of the mile walk is 80.5 kcal – 24.5 kcal, or 56 kcal for each mile.

If the same 70 kg man ran the mile at 6 mile · hr^{-1} (161 m · min^{-1}), his oxygen cost could be calculated by the following method.

$$\dot{V}O_2 = 161\ \text{m} \cdot \text{min}^{-1}\ (0.2\ \text{ml} \cdot \text{kg}^{-1} \cdot \text{min}^{-1}) + 3.5\ \text{ml} \cdot \text{kg}^{-1} \cdot \text{min}^{-1} = 35.7\ \text{ml} \cdot \text{kg}^{-1} \cdot \text{min}^{-1},$$

$$\dot{V}O_2\ (\text{ml} \cdot \text{mi}^{-1}) = 35.7\ \text{ml} \cdot \text{kg}^{-1} \cdot \text{min}^{-1} \cdot 70\ \text{kg} \cdot 10\ \text{min} \cdot \text{mi}^{-1} = 25{,}000\ \text{ml} \cdot \text{mi}^{-1},$$

and so

$$\dot{V}O_2\ (\text{L} \cdot \text{min}^{-1}) = 25{,}000\ \text{ml} \cdot \text{mi}^{-1} \div 1{,}000\ \text{ml} \cdot \text{L}^{-1} = 25\ \text{L} \cdot \text{mi}^{-1}.$$

At about 5 kcal per liter of O_2, 125 kcal are used to jog or run 1 mi (5 kcal · L^{-1} · 25 L · mi^{-1}). The gross caloric cost per 1 mi (or per 1.6 km) is about 50% higher for jogging than for walking (125 versus 80 kcal). The net caloric cost of jogging or running 1 mi or 1.6 km (calories used above resting), however, is independent of speed and is about twice that of walking. For example, when we subtract the caloric cost for 10 min of rest (12 kcal) from the gross caloric cost of the run (125 kcal), the net cost is 113 kcal, or twice that for the walk (56 kcal). This follows from the net cost of running versus walking: 0.2 ml · kg^{-1} · min^{-1} per m · min^{-1} versus 0.1 ml · kg^{-1} · min^{-1} per m · min^{-1}. Table 6.6 lists values for the net and gross caloric costs of walking and running 1 mi (1.6 km) for a variety of body weights, with the values expressed in kilocalories per mile.

For weight control, it is important to use the net cost of the activity because it measures the energy used above that used for sitting. When a person walks at slow to moderate speeds (2-3.5 mi · hr^{-1}, or 54-94 m · min^{-1}), the net cost of walking a mile (1.6 km) is about half that of jogging or running the mile. This means that a person who jogs a mile at 3 mi · hr^{-1} (80 m · min^{-1}) expends twice as many calories as someone who walks at the same speed. Because many people walk at these slower speeds, it is important to remember that the net energy cost of the mile is half that of running. If we look at high walking speeds such as 5 mi · hr^{-1} (134 m · min^{-1}), or 1 mi in 12 min, however, we see that the net energy cost of walking 1 mi is similar to that of running.

Table 6.6 shows that the net cost of running a mile (1.6 km) is independent of speed. It does not matter whether participants jog at 3 mi · hr^{-1} (80 m · min^{-1}) or run at 6 mi · hr^{-1} (161 m · min^{-1})—the net caloric cost for running a mile is the same. At 6 mi · hr^{-1}, the participant expends energy at about twice the rate measured at 3 mi · hr^{-1} (161 m · min^{-1}), but because the mile is finished in half the time, the net energy expenditure is about the same. HR will, of course, be higher in the 6 mi · hr^{-1} (161 m · min^{-1}) run in order to deliver oxygen to the muscles at the higher rate.

Table 6.6 Gross and Net (Gross/Net) Cost for Walking and Running One Mile (kcal · mi^{-1})

WALKING

BODY WEIGHT		SPEED (MI · HR^{-1}/M · MIN^{-1})						
kg	lb	2.0/54	2.5/67	3.0/80	3.5/94	4.0/107	4.5/121	5.0/134
50.0	110	64/39	58/39	54/39	53/39	60/48	68/57	79/67
54.5	120	69/42	63/42	59/42	57/42	66/52	75/63	86/81
59.1	130	75/45	68/45	64/45	62/45	71/57	81/68	93/81
63.6	140	80/49	73/49	69/49	67/49	77/61	87/73	100/88
68.2	150	87/52	79/52	74/52	72/52	82/65	93/78	108/94
72.7	160	92/56	84/56	79/56	76/56	88/70	100/84	115/100
77.3	170	98/59	90/59	84/59	81/59	93/74	106/89	122/107
81.8	180	104/63	95/63	89/63	86/63	99/78	112/94	139/113
86.4	190	110/66	100/66	94/66	91/66	104/83	118/99	136/119
90.9	200	115/70	105/70	99/70	95/70	110/87	124/104	144/125
95.4	210	121/73	111/73	104/73	100/73	115/92	131/110	151/132
100	220	127/77	116/77	109/77	105/77	121/96	137/115	158/138

RUNNING

BODY WEIGHT		SPEED (MI · HR^{-1}/M · MIN^{-1})						
kg	lb	4.0/107	5.0/134	6.0/161	7.0/188	8.0/215	9.0/241	10.0/268
50.0	110	89/77	86/77	84/77	84/77	82/77	82/77	81/77
54.5	120	97/83	94/83	92/83	92/83	89/83	89/83	89/83
59.1	130	105/90	102/90	100/90	99/90	97/90	97/90	96/90
63.6	140	113/97	110/97	108/97	107/97	104/97	104/97	104/97
68.2	150	121/104	118/104	115/104	114/104	112/104	112/104	111/104
72.7	160	129/111	125/111	123/111	122/111	119/111	119/111	119/111
77.3	170	137/118	133/118	131/118	130/118	127/118	127/118	126/118
81.8	180	146/125	141/125	138/125	137/125	134/125	134/125	133/125
86.4	190	154/132	149/132	146/132	145/132	141/132	141/132	141/132
90.9	200	162/139	157/139	154/139	153/139	149/139	149/139	148/139
95.4	210	170/146	165/146	161/146	160/146	156/146	156/146	155/146
100	220	178/153	173/153	169/153	168/153	164/153	164/153	163/153

Multiply value by the number of miles walked or run to obtain the total (gross/net) calories expended.

KEY POINT

The oxygen cost of walking increases linearly between the speeds of 50 and 100 m · min^{-1}; it increases faster at higher walking speeds. The oxygen cost of jogging or running increases linearly with speed from slow jogging (3 mi · hr^{-1}, or 80 m · min^{-1}) to fast running. The net caloric cost of jogging or running a mile (1.6 km) is twice that of walking a mile at a moderate pace.

Oxygen Cost of Cycle Ergometry

Cycle ergometry is a popular exercise done at a sport club, at home, or as part of a rehabilitation program. Generally, cycle ergometry expends energy while causing less trauma to the ankle, knee, and hip joints compared with jogging. Cycle ergometers are used for conventional leg-exercise programs, but they are also adapted for arm exercise (by placing the ergometer on a table). The following sections describe how to estimate the energy costs of leg and arm cycle ergometry.

Leg Ergometry

In the previous activities the participants were carrying their body weight, and the oxygen requirement was therefore proportional to body weight ($ml \cdot kg^{-1} \cdot min^{-1}$). This is not the case in cycle ergometry, in which body weight is supported by the cycle seat and the work rate is determined primarily by the pedal rate and the resistance on the wheel. The oxygen requirement, in liters per minute, is approximately the same for people of all sizes for the same work rate. Thus, when a light person is doing the same work rate as a heavy person, the relative $\dot{V}O_2$ ($ml \cdot kg^{-1} \cdot min^{-1}$), or MET level, is higher for the lighter person.

The work rate is set on the simple, mechanically braked cycle ergometers by varying the force (weight, or load) on the wheel and the number of pedal revolutions per minute ($rev \cdot min^{-1}$). On the Monark cycle ergometer, the wheel travels 6 m per pedal revolution. At a pedal rate of 50 $rev \cdot min^{-1}$, the wheel moves a distance of 300 m (6 m · 50 $rev \cdot min^{-1}$). If a 1 kg weight (force) is applied to the wheel, the work rate is 300 $kgm \cdot min^{-1}$ (kilogram-meters per minute). Work rates also are expressed in watts (W), where 6.1 $kgm \cdot min^{-1}$ equals 1 W; the 300 $kgm \cdot min^{-1}$ work rate would be expressed as 50 W. The work rate can be doubled by changing the force from 1 to 2 kg or by changing the pedal rate from 50 to 100 $rev \cdot min^{-1}$. In contrast, some cycle ergometers are electronically controlled to deliver a specific work rate somewhat independent of pedal rate; as the pedal rate decreases, the load on the wheel increases proportionally to maintain the work rate (4).

The total oxygen cost of leg cycle ergometry is the sum of the resting oxygen uptake, the cost of unloaded cycling (movement of the legs against no resistance), and the cost of the work itself. The oxygen cost of doing 1 kgm of work is 1.8 ml. The energy required to move the pedals against no resistance has been estimated to be 1 MET, or 3.5 $ml \cdot kg^{-1} \cdot min^{-1}$. As with the other equations, resting oxygen uptake is 3.5 $ml \cdot kg^{-1} \cdot min^{-1}$ (3). The latter two terms are combined in the equation to yield 7 $ml \cdot kg^{-1} \cdot min^{-1}$. The estimates from the following equations are reasonable for work rates between approximately 150 and 1,200 $kgm \cdot min^{-1}$ (see table 6.7). The equations for work rates expressed in $kgm \cdot min^{-1}$ and watts follow.

$$\dot{V}O_2\ (ml \cdot kg^{-1} \cdot min^{-1}) = (kgm \cdot min^{-1} \cdot 1.8\ ml\ O_2 \cdot kgm^{-1}) \div \text{body weight (kg)} + 7\ ml \cdot kg^{-1} \cdot min^{-1},$$

and

$$\dot{V}O_2\ (ml \cdot kg^{-1} \cdot min^{-1}) = (W \cdot 10.8\ ml\ O_2 \cdot W^{-1}) \div \text{body weight (kg)} + 7\ ml \cdot kg^{-1} \cdot min^{-1}.$$

Table 6.7 Energy Expenditure in METs for Cycle Ergometry for Legs and Arms

BODY WEIGHT		WORK RATE ($KGM \cdot MIN^{-1}$/W)						
kg	lb	300/50	450/75	600/100	750/125	900/150	1,050/175	1,200/200
50	110	5.1(6.1)	6.6(8.7)	8.2(11.3)	9.7(13.9)	11.3(–)	12.8(–)	14.3(–)
60	132	4.6(5.3)	5.9(7.4)	7.1(9.6)	8.4(11.7)	9.7(–)	11.0(–)	12.3(–)
70	154	4.2(4.7)	5.3(6.5)	6.4(8.3)	7.5(10.2)	8.6(12.0)	9.7(–)	10.8(–)
80	176	3.9(4.2)	4.9(5.8)	5.9(7.4)	6.8(9.0)	7.8(10.6)	8.8(12.3)	9.7(–)
90	198	3.7(3.9)	4.6(5.3)	5.4(6.7)	6.3(8.1)	7.1(9.6)	8.0(11.0)	8.9(12.4)
100	220	3.5(3.6)	4.3(4.9)	5.1(6.1)	5.9(7.4)	6.6(8.7)	7.4(10.0)	8.2(11.3)

Values in ( ) are for arm work.

Based on American College of Sports Medicine 2014, *ACSM's guidelines for exercise testing and prescription*, 9th ed. (Philadelphia: PA: Lippincott, Williams, & Wilkins).

QUESTION:
What is the oxygen cost of doing 600 kgm · min^{-1} (100 W) on a cycle ergometer for 50 kg and 100 kg subjects?

ANSWER:
For the 50 kg subject:

$$\dot{V}O_2\ (\text{ml} \cdot \text{kg}^{-1} \cdot \text{min}^{-1}) = (600\ \text{kgm} \cdot \text{min}^{-1} \cdot 1.8\ \text{ml}\ O_2 \cdot \text{kgm}^{-1}) \div 50\ \text{kg} + 7\ \text{ml} \cdot \text{kg}^{-1} \cdot \text{min}^{-1}$$
$$= 28.6\ \text{ml} \cdot \text{kg}^{-1} \cdot \text{min}^{-1}, \text{ or } 8.2\ \text{METs}\ (8.2\ \text{kcal} \cdot \text{kg}^{-1} \cdot \text{hr}^{-1}).$$

For the 100 kg subject:

$$\dot{V}O_2\ (\text{ml} \cdot \text{kg}^{-1} \cdot \text{min}^{-1}) = (600\ \text{kgm} \cdot \text{min}^{-1} \cdot 1.8\ \text{ml}\ O_2 \cdot \text{kgm}^{-1}) \div 100\ \text{kg} + 7\ \text{ml} \cdot \text{kg}^{-1} \cdot \text{min}^{-1}$$
$$= 17.8\ \text{ml} \cdot \text{kg}^{-1} \cdot \text{min}^{-1}, \text{ or } 5.1\ \text{METs}\ (5.1\ \text{kcal} \cdot \text{kg}^{-1} \cdot \text{hr}^{-1}).$$

In some exercise programs, a participant might use a variety of exercise equipment to achieve a training effect and might want to set about the same intensity on each machine. The equation for the cycle ergometer can be used to set the load to achieve a particular MET value on the cycle ergometer and bring it in balance with what is done during walking or jogging.

QUESTION:
A 70 kg participant must work at 6 METs (21 ml · kg^{-1} · min^{-1}) to match the intensity of his walking program. What force (load) should be set on a Monark cycle ergometer at a pedal rate of 50 rev · min^{-1}?

ANSWER:

$$21\ \text{ml} \cdot \text{kg}^{-1} \cdot \text{min}^{-1} = (?\ \text{kgm} \cdot \text{min}^{-1} \cdot 1.8\ \text{ml}\ O_2 \cdot \text{kgm}^{-1}) \div 70\ \text{kg} + 7\ \text{ml} \cdot \text{kg}^{-1} \cdot \text{min}^{-1}.$$
$$\text{Net cost of cycling} = 21 - 7\ \text{ml} \cdot \text{kg}^{-1} \cdot \text{min}^{-1} = 14\ \text{ml} \cdot \text{kg}^{-1} \cdot \text{min}^{-1}.$$
$$14\ \text{ml} \cdot \text{kg}^{-1} \cdot \text{min}^{-1} = (?\ \text{kgm} \cdot \text{min}^{-1} \cdot 1.8\ \text{ml}\ O_2 \cdot \text{kgm}^{-1}) \div 70\ \text{kg}.$$

Multiply each side by 70 kg.

$$980\ \text{ml} \cdot \text{min}^{-1} = ?\ \text{kgm} \cdot \text{min}^{-1} \cdot 1.8\ \text{ml}\ O_2 \cdot \text{kgm}^{-1}.$$

Divide each side by 1.8 ml O_2 · kgm^{-1} to obtain the work rate.

$$\text{Work rate} = 544\ \text{kgm} \cdot \text{min}^{-1}.$$

Because the Monark wheel travels 300 m · min^{-1} at 50 rev · min^{-1}, the load on the wheel should be 544 kgm · min^{-1} ÷ 300 m · min^{-1}, or 1.8 kg.

Arm Ergometry

A cycle ergometer can be used to exercise the muscles of the arms and shoulder girdle by modifying the pedals and placing the cycle on a table. Arm ergometry is used on a limited basis as a GXT to evaluate cardiovascular function. It is used more generally as a routine exercise in rehabilitation programs (16). There are a variety of factors to keep in mind when considering arm ergometry:

- $\dot{V}O_2$max for the arms is only 70% of that measured with the legs in a normal healthy population and is less in individuals who are unfit or elderly or in those with chronic diseases.
- The natural endurance of the muscles used in this work is less than that of the legs.
- The HR and BP responses are higher for arm work compared with leg work at the same $\dot{V}O_2$.
- There is no need to account for unloaded arm cycling, but the oxygen cost of doing 1 kgm is about 3 ml O_2 · kgm^{-1} for arm work because of the inefficiency of the action (3).

The equations for estimating the oxygen cost of arm work for work rates expressed in kgm · min^{-1} or watts are as follows:

$$\dot{V}O_2\ (\text{ml} \cdot \text{kg}^{-1} \cdot \text{min}^{-1}) = (\text{kgm} \cdot \text{min}^{-1} \cdot 3\ \text{ml}\ O_2 \cdot \text{kgm}^{-1}) \div \text{body weight (kg)} + 3.5\ \text{ml} \cdot \text{kg}^{-1} \cdot \text{min}^{-1},$$
and
$$\dot{V}O_2\ (\text{ml} \cdot \text{kg}^{-1} \cdot \text{min}^{-1}) = (\text{W} \cdot 18\ \text{ml}\ O_2 \cdot \text{W}^{-1}) \div \text{body weight (kg)} + 3.5\ \text{ml} \cdot \text{kg}^{-1} \cdot \text{min}^{-1}.$$

See table 6.7 for estimates of the oxygen cost of arm work on a cycle ergometer.

QUESTION:

What is the oxygen requirement for a 70 kg man doing 150 kgm · min^{-1} on an arm ergometer?

ANSWER:

$$\dot{V}O_2\ (\text{ml} \cdot \text{kg}^{-1} \cdot \text{min}^{-1}) = (150\ \text{kgm} \cdot \text{min}^{-1} \cdot 3\ \text{ml}\ O_2 \cdot \text{kgm}^{-1}) \div 70\ \text{kg} + 3.5\ \text{ml} \cdot \text{kg}^{-1} \cdot \text{min}^{-1}$$
$$= 9.9\ \text{ml} \cdot \text{kg}^{-1} \cdot \text{min}^{-1}\text{, or } 2.8\ \text{METs}\ (2.8\ \text{kcal} \cdot \text{kg}^{-1} \cdot \text{hr}^{-1}).$$

KEY POINT

The oxygen cost of cycle ergometry primarily depends on the work rate because body weight is supported. The net oxygen cost of leg ergometry is 1.8 ml · kgm^{-1} versus 3 ml · kgm^{-1} for arm ergometry. Physiological responses (HR, BP) are exaggerated for arm work compared with leg work at the same work rate because the oxygen cost is higher and represents a higher percentage of the arm $\dot{V}O_2$max.

Oxygen Cost of Bench Stepping

One of the most useful and inexpensive forms of exercise is bench stepping; it can be done at home and requires little or no equipment. The work rate is easily adjusted by simply increasing step height or cadence (number of lifts per minute). The total oxygen cost of this exercise is the sum of the costs of (a) stepping up, (b) stepping down, (c) moving back and forth on a level surface at the specified cadence, and (d) resting oxygen uptake (3.5 ml · kg^{-1} · min^{-1}). The oxygen cost of stepping up is 1.8 ml · kg^{-1} · min^{-1} per m · min^{-1}, as in walking (25). The oxygen cost of stepping down is a third of the cost of stepping up; therefore, the oxygen cost of stepping up and down is 1.33 times the cost of stepping up. The oxygen cost of stepping back and forth on a flat surface is equal to 0.2 ml O_2 per kilogram of body mass for each four-cycle step (3). The number of meters moved up or down per minute is calculated by multiplying the number of lifts per minute by the height of the step; for example, if the step height is 0.2 m (20 cm) and the cadence is 30 steps · min^{-1}, then the total lift or descent per minute is 30 times 0.2 m, or 6 m · min^{-1}. To determine step height, multiply inches by 2.54 to obtain centimeters, and divide centimeters by 100 to obtain meters. The equation for estimating the energy requirement for stepping follows:

$$\dot{V}O_2\ (\text{ml} \cdot \text{kg}^{-1} \cdot \text{min}^{-1}) = (0.2 \cdot \text{step rate}) + (1.8 \cdot 1.33 \cdot \text{step rate} \cdot \text{step height in meters}) + 3.5\ \text{ml} \cdot \text{kg}^{-1} \cdot \text{min}^{-1}.$$

QUESTION:

What is the oxygen requirement for stepping at a rate of 20 steps · min^{-1} on a 20 cm bench?

ANSWER:

$$\dot{V}O_2 = \left(\frac{0.2\ \text{ml} \cdot \text{kg}^{-1} \cdot \text{min}^{-1}}{\text{steps} \cdot \text{min}^{-1}} \cdot 20\ \text{steps} \cdot \text{min}^{-1}\right) +$$
$$\left(\frac{1.8\ \text{ml}}{\text{kgm}} \cdot 1.33 \cdot \frac{0.2\ \text{m}}{\text{step}} \cdot \frac{20\ \text{steps}}{\text{min}}\right) + 3.5\ \text{ml} \cdot \text{kg}^{-1} \cdot \text{min}^{-1}$$
$$= 4.0\ \text{ml} \cdot \text{kg}^{-1} \cdot \text{min}^{-1} + 9.6\ \text{ml} \cdot \text{kg}^{-1} \cdot \text{min}^{-1} + 3.5\ \text{ml} \cdot \text{kg}^{-1} \cdot \text{min}^{-1}$$
$$= 17.1\ \text{ml} \cdot \text{kg}^{-1} \cdot \text{min}^{-1}\text{, or } 4.9\ \text{METs}\ (4.9\ \text{kcal} \cdot \text{kg}^{-1} \cdot \text{hr}^{-1})$$

Table 6.8 summarizes the energy requirement of stepping at various rates.

KEY POINT

The oxygen cost of bench stepping includes the cost of stepping up and down, moving horizontally back and forth, and resting oxygen uptake. The oxygen cost of stepping up is the same as in walking. The oxygen cost of stepping up and down is 1.33 times the cost of stepping up. The oxygen cost of stepping back and forth is 0.2 ml · kg^{-1} · min^{-1} times the step rate.

Table 6.8 **Energy Expenditure in METs During Stepping at Various Rates and Step Heights**

STEP HEIGHT		STEPS · MIN^{-1}			
cm	in.	12	18	24	30
0	0.0	1.7	2.0	2.4	2.7
4	1.6	2.0	2.5	3.0	3.5
8	3.2	2.3	3.0	3.7	4.4
12	4.7	2.7	3.5	4.3	5.2
16	6.3	3.0	4.0	5.0	6.0
20	7.9	3.3	4.5	5.7	6.8
24	9.4	3.7	5.0	6.3	7.6
28	11.0	4.0	5.5	7.0	8.5
32	12.6	4.3	6.0	7.6	9.3
36	14.2	4.6	6.5	8.3	10.1
40	15.8	5.0	7.0	8.9	10.9

Based on American College of Sports Medicine 2014, *ACSM's guidelines for exercise testing and prescription*, 9th ed. (Philadelphia: PA: Lippincott, Williams, & Wilkins).

Energy Requirements of Other Activities

Clients have a wide variety of interests when it comes to the physical activities they use to achieve health and fitness goals. Fitness professionals now have a great tool to help clients understand the energy cost associated with physical activities. Scientists have provided a detailed summary of the energy cost of numerous activities that can be readily accessed online in the easily located Google Site: Compendium of Physical Activities (https://sites.google.com/site/compendiumofphysicalactivities/).

Using the Compendium of Physical Activities

The Compendium of Physical Activities is an excellent source of information about the energy cost of many physical activities, including leisure and occupational activities (1). Dr. Bill Haskell of Stanford University conceptualized the compendium and developed a prototype that was used in studies examining physical activity, exercise, and fitness patterns in populations. In this way, investigators could link the energy expenditure of physical activity to various health outcomes and determine, for example, the relationship of physical activity to the risk of type 2 diabetes. In 1993, the first complete version of the compendium was published, followed by an update in 2000. Both articles offered a long list of activities that included specific codes to identify the activity and energy cost values expressed in METs, where 1 MET is equal to 3.5 ml · kg^{-1} · min^{-1} or 1 kcal · kg^{-1} · hr^{-1}. In 2011, an update of the compendium was published, but this time the list of activities, codes, and MET values were published on a website that will be updated more regularly.

The following examples show how to use the information on the website to estimate the energy cost of activities. Keep in mind that the energy cost values in the compendium are measured or estimated values of a group; large interindividual variation in energy cost may exist for some activities.

EXAMPLE 1

Your client, who weighs 60 kg, bicycles to and from work each day (1 hr round trip) and wants to know how much energy she is using each day.

1. On the home page of the website, choose Activity Categories in the top menu bar.
2. Select Bicycling and scroll down to "bicycling to and from work, self-selected pace." The MET value is 6.8.
3. 6.8 kcal · kg^{-1} · hr^{-1} · 1 hr · day^{-1} · 60 kg = 408 kcal · day^{-1}.

EXAMPLE 2

Your client, who weighs 80 kg, does a 30 min brisk walk 5 days per wk and wants to know how much energy he is using per wk with this activity.

1. On the home page of the website, choose Activity Categories in the top menu bar.
2. Select Walking and scroll down to "walking, 3.5 mph, level, brisk, firm surface, walking for exercise." The MET value is 4.3.
3. $4.3\ kcal \cdot kg^{-1} \cdot hr^{-1} \cdot 2.5\ hr \cdot wk^{-1} \cdot 80\ kg = 860\ kcal \cdot wk^{-1}$.

Estimation of Energy Expenditure Without Equations

You also can estimate energy expenditure using information about your client's HR response to exercise and $\dot{V}O_2$max. The fitness professional selects activities that cause participants to exercise at 40% to 84% of their $\dot{V}O_2$max, the intensity range needed to improve or maintain CRF and realize health benefits (see chapter 11). It should be possible, therefore, to estimate the energy expenditure for each subject on the basis of the subject's $\dot{V}O_2$max and the portion of the THR range at which the subject is working. If a person has a $\dot{V}O_2$max of 10 METs, energy expenditure can be estimated in the following way.

- 10 METs = $10\ kcal \cdot kg^{-1} \cdot hr^{-1}$.
- If a person exercises at the low end of the vigorous-intensity range, at about 60% $\dot{V}O_2$max, then the energy expenditure should be about $6\ kcal \cdot kg^{-1} \cdot hr^{-1}$ (60% of 10 METs).
- If the person weighs 70 kg, then 420 kcal are expended per hour ($70\ kg \cdot 6\ kcal \cdot kg^{-1} \cdot hr^{-1}$).
- A 30 min workout expends half this amount, or about 210 kcal.

These simple calculations assume that the person is performing an activity that uses large muscle groups. Table 6.9 shows the estimated calorie expenditure for a 30 min workout at 70% $\dot{V}O_2$max for a variety of fitness levels ($\dot{V}O_2$max expressed as METs) and body weights (26). To return briefly to the advertisement at the beginning of the chapter and the possibility of expending 1,400 kcal in an hour, you can see in table 6.9 that it is possible—*if* the person has an incredibly high $\dot{V}O_2$max (20+ METs) *and* weighs more than 198 lb (90 kg). On the other hand, for the typical adult with a $\dot{V}O_2$max of 10 to 12 METs, an energy expenditure of 600 to 700 kcal would be a more reasonable expectation. This assumes that the client can work at 70% $\dot{V}O_2$max for that full hour—a reasonable proposition for someone who has been systematically involved in a strenuous exercise program for some time.

Table 6.9 Estimated Gross Energy Expenditure for a 30 Min Workout at 70% Functional Capacity for People of Various Fitness Levels ($\dot{V}O_2$max) and Body Weights

$\dot{V}O_2$max in METs ($kcal \cdot kg^{-1} \cdot hr^{-1}$)	70% max in METs ($kcal \cdot kg^{-1} \cdot hr^{-1}$)	50 kg/110 lb	70 kg/154 lb	90 kg/198 lb
20	14.0	350	490	630
18	12.6	315	441	567
16	11.2	280	392	504
14	9.8	245	343	441
12	8.4	210	294	378
10	7.0	175	245	315
8	5.6	140	196	252
6	4.2	105	147	189

MET = metabolic equivalent.

Environmental Concerns

Although changes in temperature, relative humidity, pollution, and altitude do not change the energy requirements for submaximal exercise, they do change the participant's response to the exercise. Remember that a person's HR response is the best indicator of the relative stress being experienced due to the interaction of exercise intensity, exercise duration, and environmental factors. The participant should cut back on the intensity of the activity when environmental factors increase the HR response. The duration of the activity can be increased to accommodate any energy expenditure goal.

KEY POINT

The Compendium of Physical Activities is an excellent source of information about the energy cost of many physical activities, including leisure and occupational activities. Energy expenditure also can be estimated without equations. If a person works at 60% of $\dot{V}O_2$max and has a $\dot{V}O_2$max of 10 METs, the energy expenditure is 6 METs, or 6 kcal · kg^{-1} · hr^{-1}. If the person weighs 80 kg, 480 kcal are expended per hour. Environmental factors such as heat, humidity, altitude, and pollution can increase the HR response to work while not affecting the energy cost. HR should be monitored more frequently in these settings to adjust the intensity of the activity downward to keep the person in the appropriate HR range (see chapter 11).

LEARNING AIDS

REVIEW QUESTIONS

1. What can an accelerometer measure that a pedometer cannot when monitoring physical activity?
2. How do you convert oxygen uptake in L · min^{-1} to kcal · min^{-1}?
3. What is a MET equal to in ml · kg^{-1} · min^{-1} and kcal · kg^{-1} · hr^{-1}?
4. How much greater is the net oxygen cost of running 1 m · min^{-1} on a flat surface compared with walking?
5. When a 50 kg person and an 80 kg person exercise at 600 kgm · min^{-1} on a cycle ergometer, how do the oxygen uptakes compare in L · min^{-1} and ml · kg^{-1} · min^{-1}?
6. If a woman has a $\dot{V}O_2$max of 10 METs and is working at 70% $\dot{V}O_2$max, how many calories is she expending in kcal · kg^{-1} · hr^{-1}?

CASE STUDIES

1. A 75 kg man walks at 3.5 mi · hr^{-1} for 30 min. How many calories does he expend?
2. A 60 kg woman rides a cycle ergometer at a work rate of 100 W. What is her oxygen uptake?
3. A 70 kg college student runs 3 mi (4.8 km) in 24 min. How many calories does he expend?
4. An 85 kg man with a $\dot{V}O_2$max of 12 METs works at 70% $\dot{V}O_2$max for 30 min. How many calories does he expend?

5. A client mentions he has read that he can expend the same number of calories per mile whether he walks at 3 mi · hr^{-1} (4.8 km · hr^{-1}) or jogs at 6 mi · hr^{-1} (9.7 km · hr^{-1}). How do you respond?

Answers to Case Studies

1. $3.5\text{ mi}\cdot\text{hr}^{-1}\cdot 26.8\text{m}\cdot\text{min}^{-1} = 93.8\text{m}\cdot\text{min}^{-1}$

$$93.8\text{m}\cdot\text{min}^{-1}\left(\frac{0.1\text{ml}\cdot\text{kg}^{-1}\cdot\text{min}^{-1}}{\text{m}\cdot\text{min}^{-1}}\right) +$$

$$3.5\text{ml}\cdot\text{kg}^{-1}\cdot\text{min}^{-1} = 12.9\text{ml}\cdot\text{kg}^{-1}\cdot\text{min}^{-1}$$

$$12.9\text{ml}\cdot\text{kg}^{-1}\cdot\text{min}^{-1}\cdot 75\text{kg} =$$

$$968\text{ml}\cdot\text{min}^{-1}\text{, or } 0.97\text{L}\cdot\text{min}^{-1}$$

$$0.97\text{L}\cdot\text{min}^{-1}\cdot 5\text{kcal}\cdot\text{L}^{-1} = 4.85\text{kcal}\cdot\text{min}^{-1}$$

$$4.85\text{kcal}\cdot\text{min}^{-1}\cdot 30\text{min} = 146\text{kcal}$$

2. $100\text{ W} = 600\text{ kpm}\cdot\text{min}^{-1}$

$$\dot{V}O_2 = \frac{(600\text{ kpm}\cdot\text{min}^{-1}\cdot 1.8\text{ ml } O_2\cdot\text{min}^{-1})}{60\text{ kg} + 7\text{ ml}\cdot\text{kg}^{-1}\cdot\text{min}^{-1}}$$

$$25\text{ ml}\cdot\text{kg}^{-1}\cdot\text{min}^{-1} =$$

$$18\text{ ml}\cdot\text{kg}^{-1}\cdot\text{min}^{-1} + 7\text{ ml}\cdot\text{kg}^{-1}\cdot\text{min}^{-1}$$

3. $3\text{ mi}\cdot 1{,}610\text{ m}\cdot\text{mi}^{-1} = 4{,}830\text{ m}\div 24\text{ min} = 201\text{ m}\cdot\text{min}^{-1}$

$$201\text{ m}\cdot\text{min}^{-1}\left(\frac{0.2\text{ ml}\cdot\text{kg}^{-1}\cdot\text{min}^{-1}}{\text{m}\cdot\text{min}^{-1}}\right) +$$

$$3.5\text{ ml}\cdot\text{kg}^{-1}\cdot\text{min}^{-1} = 43.7\text{ ml}\cdot\text{kg}^{-1}\cdot\text{min}^{-1}$$

$$43.7\text{ ml}\cdot\text{kg}^{-1}\cdot\text{min}^{-1}\cdot 70\text{ kg} =$$

$$3{,}059\text{ ml}\cdot\text{min}^{-1}\text{, or } 3.06\text{ L}\cdot\text{min}^{-1}$$

$$3.06\text{ L}\cdot\text{min}^{-1}\cdot 5\text{ kcal}\cdot\text{L}^{-1} =$$

$$15.3\text{ kcal}\cdot\text{min}^{-1}\cdot 24\text{ min} = 367\text{ kcal}$$

4. 12 METs = 12 kcal · kg^{-1} · hr^{-1} · 70% = 8.4 kcal · kg^{-1} · hr^{-1}
5. You might indicate that the cost of jogging 1 m · min^{-1} (0.2 ml · kg^{-1} · min^{-1}) is about twice that for walking (0.1 ml · kg^{-1} · min^{-1}) due to the extra energy needed to propel the body off the ground and absorb the force of impact on each step. You might provide a summary table he can use describing the caloric cost of walking and running 1 mi (1.6 km).

Fitness Assessment

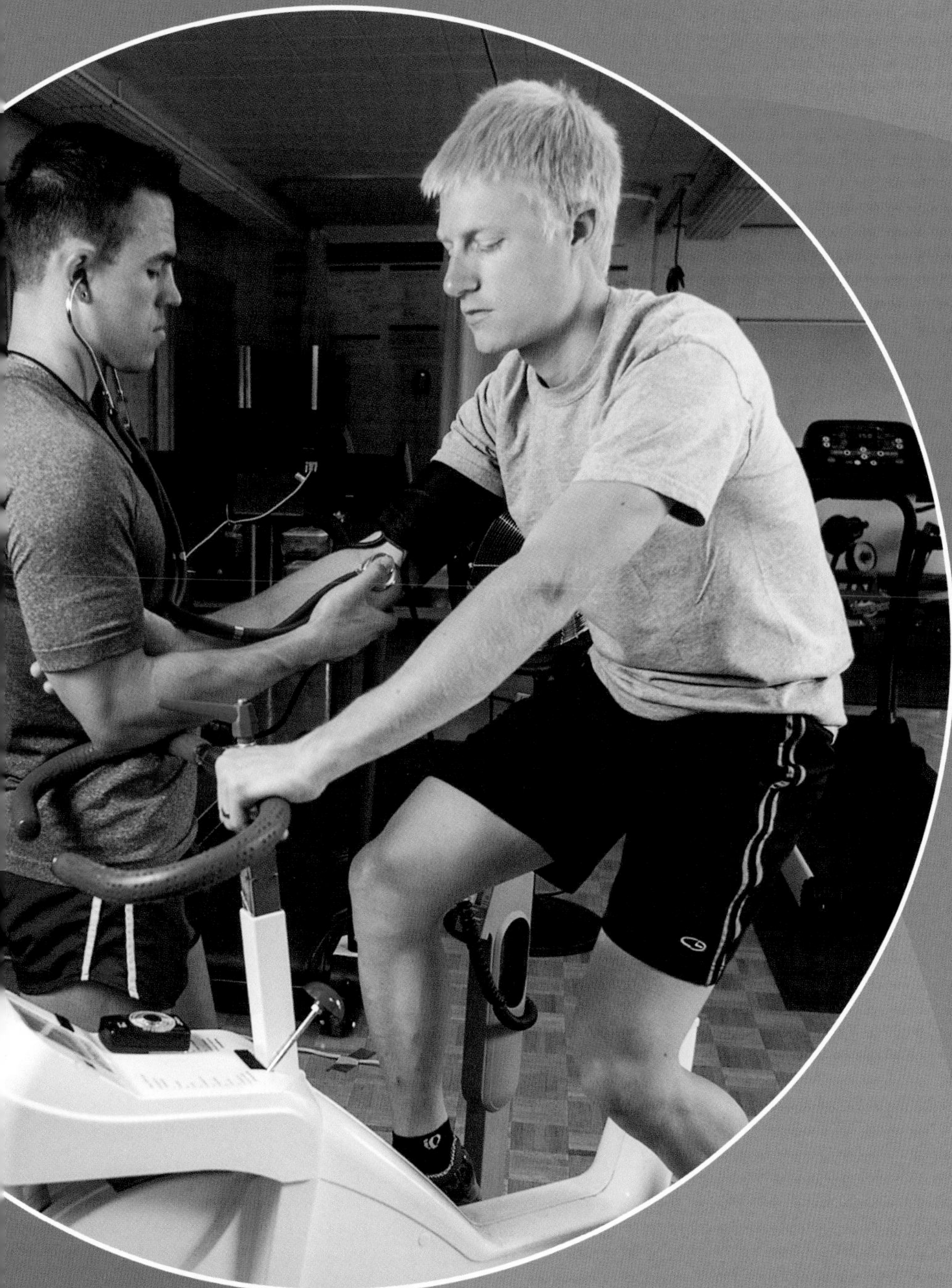

PART III

Fitness professionals must know how to measure the components of fitness and interpret the scores for the clients. In the chapters in part III, we examine the assessment of cardiorespiratory fitness (CRF) (chapter 7), body composition (chapter 8), muscular strength and endurance (chapter 9), and flexibility and low-back function (chapter 10).

Before you begin, you may want to review the general principles of fitness testing. How do you select appropriate tests? How can you obtain more accurate results? For a more complete introduction to the topic of fitness assessment, please see appendix B.

7

Assessment of Cardiorespiratory Fitness

Edward T. Howley

OBJECTIVES

The reader will be able to do the following:

1. Describe how CRF relates to health and list reasons for testing CRF as well as risks associated with CRF testing.
2. Present a logical sequence of testing.
3. Describe procedures for walking and jogging or running field tests to estimate CRF.
4. Contrast the treadmill, cycle ergometer, and bench step as instruments for GXTs.
5. List variables measured during a GXT.
6. Describe procedures used before, during, and after testing.
7. Contrast submaximal and maximal GXTs.
8. Describe the HR extrapolation procedures to estimate $\dot{V}O_2$max using submaximal treadmill, cycle, and bench-step GXTs.
9. Calibrate a treadmill, a Monark cycle ergometer, and a sphygmomanometer.

As described in chapter 1, there is no question that higher levels of physical activity and cardiorespiratory fitness (CRF) are associated with reduced risks of chronic diseases and death. Consequently, it is important to focus on a healthy level of CRF as a lifelong goal that makes life more enjoyable as well as healthy. Those benefits alone merit the inclusion of CRF in any discussion about positive health. CRF, also called *cardiovascular* or *aerobic fitness*, is a good measure of the heart's ability to pump oxygen-rich blood to the muscles. Although the terms *cardio* (heart), *vascular* (blood vessels), *respiratory* (lungs and ventilation), and *aerobic* (working with oxygen) differ technically, they all reflect aspects of CRF. A person with a healthy heart that can pump great volumes of blood with each beat has a high level of CRF. CRF values are expressed in the following ways (see chapter 6):

- Liters of oxygen used by the body per minute ($L \cdot min^{-1}$)
- Milliliters of oxygen used per kilogram of body weight per minute ($ml \cdot kg^{-1} \cdot min^{-1}$)
- METs, multiples of resting metabolic rate, where 1 MET = 3.5 $ml \cdot kg^{-1} \cdot min^{-1}$

A person with the ability to use 35 $ml \cdot kg^{-1} \cdot min^{-1}$ during maximal exercise is said to have a CRF equal to 10 METs ($35 \div 3.5 = 10$). Aerobic training programs increase the heart's ability to pump blood, so it is no surprise that such programs improve CRF.

Chapter 4 describes how a wide variety of physiological variables (HR, BP, and so on) respond to acute or short-term exercise and how endurance training affects those responses. Chapter 11 explains how to recommend activities to clients to improve their CRF. This chapter emphasizes how to evaluate CRF. The reader is referred to other resources for additional details (2, 3).

Historically, HR, BP, and electrocardiogram (ECG) measurements taken at rest were used to evaluate CRF. In addition, some static pulmonary function tests (e.g., vital capacity) were used to characterize respiratory function. It became clear, however, that measurements taken at rest reveal little about the way a person's cardiorespiratory system responds to physical activity. We are now familiar with using GXTs to evaluate HR, ECG, BP, ventilation, and oxygen uptake responses during work and using those responses in the assessment of CRF.

Results from CRF tests are used to write exercise recommendations and allow the fitness professional or physician to evaluate positive or negative changes in CRF resulting from physical conditioning, aging, illness, or inactivity. Given the current increase in obesity and inactivity in people of all ages, it makes sense to evaluate CRF throughout life, from early childhood to old age. This information can indicate where individuals stand on health-criterion tests, and it alerts them to subtle lifestyle changes that may compromise positive health. The nature of the tests and the level of monitoring should vary across age groups to reflect the information that is needed.

CRF testing depends on the purposes of the test, the type of person to be evaluated, and the work tasks available. Reasons for testing include

- determining physiological responses at rest and during **submaximal** or maximal work,
- providing a basis for exercise programming,
- evaluating the effectiveness of a training program,
- screening for CHD, and
- determining a person's ability to perform a specific work task.

Choosing an appropriate test depends on several factors. People differ in age, fitness level, known health problems, and risks of CHD. Also, financial considerations determine the amount of time that can be devoted to each person (e.g., physician versus fitness professional administering the test) and the work tasks available.

As indicated in chapters 1 and 2, the risks associated with exercising and taking exercise tests are quite low. Health professionals should emphasize that the overall CHD risk is greater for those who remain sedentary than for those who take an exercise test and then embark on a regular exercise program (2). This is consistent with evidence showing that low CRF directly relates to a higher risk of heart disease and death (13).

KEY POINT

CRF is an important aspect of quality of life as well as a risk factor for CHD. The ability to use oxygen during exercise is the basis for CRF and can be expressed in $L \cdot min^{-1}$, $ml \cdot kg^{-1} \cdot min^{-1}$, and METs. CRF testing is used for programming exercise, screening for heart disease, and determining a person's ability to do a specific task. The risk of death attributable to exercise testing is very low.

Testing Sequence

A logical sequence for fitness testing (and activities) can be followed when people attend the same fitness center over time. This sequence progresses from the initial screening to fitness testing and programming, with opportunities for periodic retesting and revision of the program as fitness gains are made. The sequence of testing and activity prescription is shown in the sidebar *Sequence of Testing and Activity Prescription*. The rest of this section details the process. In addition to CRF, flexibility and muscular strength and endurance are often measured in this sequence (see chapters 9 and 10). For people who request fitness testing but are not continually involved with the fitness center, the submaximal and maximal tests are usually part of the same GXT protocol.

Informed Consent

Fitness participants should be informed volunteers. The informed-consent form should clearly describe all of the procedures and potential risks and benefits. Participants should understand that their data are confidential and that they can terminate any test or activity at any time should they feel uncomfortable. They should sign a written informed-consent form after reading a description of the program and having all questions answered. A sample consent form is included in the appendix at the end of this chapter.

Health History

Chapter 2 describes procedures for conducting a health screening prior to participation in exercise and exercise testing. The need for medical clearance is based on the individual's current level of physical activity, existence of signs or symptoms or known CV, metabolic, or renal disease, and the desired exercise intensity (2). If you have not already done so, please read chapter 2 to become familiar with the methods of obtaining information from your clients that are essential in making appropriate judgments.

Screening

On the basis of the health screening information collected from your client, decisions can be made regarding participation in physical activity and exercise testing, or the need for referral.

Guidance is provided by both the ACSM and the Canadian Society of Exercise Physiology in this regard—see chapter 2 for details. The emphasis in the screening process is on the safety of the client. In the sidebar *American Heart Association's Contraindications to Exercise Testing* we list the conditions (absolute contraindications) that have been identified in which the risk of testing outweighs the possible benefits. Other conditions (relative contraindications) may increase the risk of exercise testing; people with these conditions should only be tested if a doctor determines that the need for the test outweighs the potential risk. Note that the ACSM interprets these contraindications as being for symptom-limited maximal exercise testing.

Resting Measurements

Typical resting tests may include CRF measures (e.g., 12-lead ECG, HR, BP, blood chemistry profile) as well as other fitness variables such as body composition. Evaluation of the ECG by a physician determines whether any abnormalities require further medical attention.

Submaximal Tests to Estimate Cardiorespiratory Fitness

If the resting tests reflect normal values, then a submaximal test is administered. The submaximal test usually provides the HR and BP responses to various intensities of work ranging from light intensity up to a predetermined point (usually 85% of predicted maximum HR). This test can use a bench step, cycle ergometer, or treadmill. Once again, if unusual responses to the submaximal test appear, the person is referred for further medical tests. If the results appear normal, then the person begins an activity program at intensities less than those reached on the test (e.g., a person goes to 85% of maximum HR on the test and starts

Sequence of Testing and Activity Prescription

1. Informed consent
2. Health history
3. Screening
4. Resting cardiovascular tests (e.g., BP) and body composition assessment
5. Submaximal CRF tests
6. Tests for low-back function and flexibility
7. Beginning of moderate-intensity physical activity program
8. Tests for muscular strength and endurance
9. Maximal CRF tests
10. Activity program revision (including games and sports)
11. Periodic retest and activity revision

the fitness program at 70%). After the person has become accustomed to regular exercise and appears to be adjusting to fitness activities, a maximal test can be administered.

Submaximal tests also can be used to estimate maximal oxygen uptake by extrapolating HR to a predicted maximum and then using the linear relationship between HR and oxygen uptake to estimate maximal oxygen uptake. Although this estimated maximum is useful for evaluating a person's current CRF status and prescribing or revising exercise, the estimation involves considerable error (±15%).

Maximal Tests to Estimate or Measure Cardiorespiratory Fitness

If no problems occur up to this point, a maximal test can be administered. Two types of maximal tests are used to estimate CRF: laboratory tests that measure physiological responses (e.g., HR, BP, $\dot{V}O_2$) to increasing workloads and field tests that measure all-out endurance performance (e.g., time on a 1 mi, or 1.6 km, run). The results of the maximal test can be used to revise the activity program (e.g., the person's maximal oxygen uptake provides a new basis for selecting fitness activities). The person's measured maximal HR (instead of an age-predicted estimate) should be used to determine the target or training HR when it is available (see chapter 11).

Program Modification and Periodic Retests

After the program participant achieves a minimum level of fitness, a wider variety of activities (e.g., games and sports) can be included in the fitness program. All of the fitness tests should be readministered periodically to determine the progress being made and to revise the program in areas where the gains are not as great as desired.

American Heart Association's Contraindications to Exercise Testing

Absolute Contraindications

- Acute myocardial infarction (MI), within 2 days
- Ongoing unstable angina
- Uncontrolled cardiac arrhythmia with hemodynamic compromise
- Active endocarditis
- Symptomatic severe aortic stenosis
- Decompensated heart failure
- Acute pulmonary embolism, pulmonary infarction, or deep vein thrombosis
- Acute myocarditis or pericarditis
- Acute aortic dissection
- Physical disability that precludes safe and adequate testing

Relative Contraindications

- Known obstructive left main coronary artery stenosis
- Moderate to severe aortic stenosis with uncertain relation to symptoms
- Tachyarrhythmias with uncontrolled ventricular rates
- Acquired advanced or complete heart block
- Hypertrophic obstructive cardiomyopathy with severe resting gradient
- Recent stroke or transient ischemic attack
- Mental impairment with limited ability to cooperate
- Resting hypertension with systolic or diastolic blood pressures >200/110 mm Hg
- Uncorrected medical conditions, such as significant anemia, important electrolyte imbalance, and hyperthyroidism

Reprinted, by permission, from G.F. Fletcher et al., 2013, "Exercise standards for testing and training: A scientific statement from the American Heart Association," *Circulation* 128(8): 873-934.

RESEARCH INSIGHT

Error Involved in Estimating $\dot{V}O_2max$

Estimating $\dot{V}O_2max$ by any of the methods described in this chapter is associated with an inherent error compared with the directly measured $\dot{V}O_2max$. To determine the validity of an exercise test to estimate $\dot{V}O_2max$, investigators must first test large numbers of subjects in the laboratory to measure each subject's $\dot{V}O_2max$. On another day, the investigators may have the subjects complete a distance run for time or a standardized graded treadmill or cycle ergometer test to determine the highest percent grade and speed or work rate that the subject can achieve. That information is then used to develop an equation to predict the measured $\dot{V}O_2max$ from the time of the distance run, the last grade and speed achieved on a treadmill test, or the final work rate on the cycle ergometer test.

The predicted value will not usually equal the measured $\dot{V}O_2max$ value, and the standard error of estimate (SEE) describes how far off (higher or lower) the predicted value might be from the true value when using the prediction equation. One SEE describes where 68% of the estimates are compared with the true value. If the SEE were 1 $ml \cdot kg^{-1} \cdot min^{-1}$, then 68% of the predicted $\dot{V}O_2max$ values would fall within ±1 $ml \cdot kg^{-1} \cdot min^{-1}$ of the true value. Typically, the SEE is larger than that, approaching 5 $ml \cdot kg^{-1} \cdot min^{-1}$ in some cases (44).

The relatively large standard errors might suggest that these exercise tests have little value, but that is not the case. The tests are reliable, and when the same person takes the same test over time, the change in estimated $\dot{V}O_2max$ monitored by the test is a reasonable reflection of improvements in CRF. This can serve as both a motivational and an educational tool when working with fitness clients.

Field Tests

A variety of field tests can be used to estimate CRF. They are called *field tests* because they require little equipment, can be done just about anywhere, and use the simple activities of walking and running. Because these tests involve running or walking as fast as possible over a set distance, they are not recommended at the start of an exercise program. Instead, participants should complete the graduated walking program before taking the walking test and the graduated jogging program before taking the running test. The walking and jogging programs are found in chapter 11. The graduated nature of the fitness programs allows participants to start at a low, safe level of activity and gradually improve. It is then appropriate to administer an endurance run test to evaluate fitness status.

Field tests rely on the observation that for a person to walk or run at high speeds over long distances, the heart must pump great volumes of oxygen to the muscles. In this way, the average speed maintained in these walk or run tests gives an estimate of CRF. The higher the CRF score, the greater the heart's capacity to transport oxygen. An endurance run of a set distance for a given time or of a set time for a given distance provides information about a person's cardiorespiratory endurance as long as the run is 1 mi (1.6 km) or longer. The advantages of an endurance run test include its moderately high correlation to maximum oxygen uptake, the use of a natural activity, and the large numbers of participants who can be tested in a short time. The disadvantages of endurance running are that it is difficult to monitor physiological responses, and other factors influence the outcome (e.g., motivation, environment).

Mile Walk Test

A 1 mi (1.6 km) walk test to predict CRF accommodates individuals of different ages and fitness levels. In this test, the person walks as fast as possible on a measured track, and HR is measured at the end of the mile. Use the following steps to administer the mile walk test. Note that these directions were written for a class setting; however, the test can be used in a one-on-one setting as well.

Steps to Administering the Mile Walk Test

Before Test Day

1. Arrange to have the following elements at the test site:
   - A person to start and read the time from a stopwatch
   - A partner with a watch (with a second hand) for each walker (perhaps with a sheet to mark off laps)

(continued)

Steps to Administering the Mile Walk Test *(continued)*

- A stopwatch for the timer (with a spare ready)
- A score sheet or scorecard

2. Explain the purpose of the test (i.e., to determine how fast the participants can walk 1 mi [1.6 km], which reflects the endurance of the cardiovascular system).
3. Select and mark off (if needed) a level area for the walk.
4. Explain to the participants that they are to walk the mile in the fastest time possible. Only walking is allowed, and the goal is to cover the distance as fast as possible.

Test Day

1. Participants warm up with stretching and slow walking.
2. Several people will walk at the same time.
3. Explain the procedure again. Remind the participants not to speed up at the end of the walk but to maintain a fast, steady pace throughout.
4. The timer says, "Ready, go," and starts the stopwatch.
5. Each participant has a partner standing at the start and finish line with a watch with a second hand.
6. The partner counts the laps and tells the participant at the end of each lap how many more laps to walk.
7. The timer calls out the minutes and seconds as each person finishes the mile walk.
8. The partner listens for the time when the walker finishes the mile and records it (to the nearest second) immediately on a scorecard.
9. The walker takes a 10 sec HR immediately after the end of the mile walk, with the partner timing it. Using an HR watch simplifies this measurement.

You can then manually calculate an estimated $\dot{V}O_2max$ (ml $\cdot$ kg^{-1} $\cdot$ min^{-1}) using the data collected in the mile walk test in the following equation:

$$\dot{V}O_2max = 132.853 - 0.0769\,(weight) - 0.3877\,(age) + 6.315\,(sex) - 3.2649\,(time) - 0.1565\,(HR),$$

where weight is body weight in pounds, age is in years, sex equals 0 for females and 1 for males, time is in minutes and hundredths of minutes, and HR is in beats per minute. The formula was developed and validated on men and women aged 30 to 69 yr (32), and the SEE is about 5 ml $\cdot$ kg^{-1} $\cdot$ min^{-1} (2, 32).

QUESTION:

What is the CRF of a 25-yr-old, 170 lb (77.1 kg) man who walks the mile in 20 min and has an immediate postexercise HR of 140 beats $\cdot$ min^{-1}?

ANSWER:

$$\begin{aligned}\dot{V}O_2max &= 132.853 - 0.0769\,(weight) - 0.3877\,(age) + 6.315\,(sex) - 3.2649\,(time) - 0.1565\,(HR)\\ &= 132.853 - 0.0769\,(170) - 0.3877\,(25) + 6.315\,(1) - 3.2649\,(20.0) - 0.1565\,(140)\\ &= 29.2\ ml \cdot kg^{-1} \cdot min^{-1}.\end{aligned}$$

To simplify the calculations for this 1 mi (1.6 km) walk test, table 7.1 was generated on the basis of the preceding formula for men weighing 170 lb (77.1 kg) and women weighing 125 lb (56.7 kg). For each 15 lb (6.8 kg) above (or below) these weights, subtract (or add) 1 ml $\cdot$ kg^{-1} $\cdot$ min^{-1}.

To use table 7.1, find the part of the table for the person's sex and age, go across the top until you find the time (to the nearest minute) that person took to walk a mile (1.6 km), and then go down that column until it intersects with the person's postexercise HR (listed on the left side). The number at which the mile time and postexercise HR meet is the CRF value in terms of ml $\cdot$ kg^{-1} $\cdot$ min^{-1}. For example, a 25-yr-old man who walked the mile in 20 min and had a postexercise HR of 140 has an estimated maximal oxygen uptake of 29.2 ml $\cdot$ kg^{-1} $\cdot$ min^{-1}.

You can evaluate CRF by comparing that number with the standards presented in table 7.2 on page 139, which lists percentile values for maximal aerobic power with age and sex considerations. In the example of the 25-yr-old man, his maximal oxygen uptake of 29.2 ml $\cdot$ kg^{-1} $\cdot$ min^{-1} is below the 10th percentile, indicating a considerable need for improvement. This low value places him at a much higher risk for heart disease. The percentile values in table 7.2 provide reference points for comparison with members of a group. However, the client is best served by using the value as a reference point for personal change when an exercise program is introduced. See chapter 17 for a special 6 min walk test to assess CRF in seniors.

Jog or Run Test

One of the most common CRF field tests is the 12 min or 1.5 mi (2.4 km) run popularized by Cooper (19). This test is similar to the walk test mentioned previously: Participants jog or run as fast as possible for 12 min or for 1.5 mi (2.4 km). This test is based on work by Balke (10), who showed that 10 to 20 min running tests could be used to estimate $\dot{V}O_2max$. Balke found the optimal duration for the run test to be 15 min. The test relies on the relationship between running velocity and the oxygen uptake required to run at that velocity (see figure 7.1 on page 139). The greater the running speed, the greater the oxygen uptake required. The reason for the duration of 12 to 15 min is that the running test has to be long enough to diminish the contribution of anaerobic sources of energy to the average velocity. The average velocity that can be maintained in a 5 or 6 min run overestimates $\dot{V}O_2max$ because anaerobic energy sources contribute substantially to total energy production in a 5

Table 7.1 Estimated Maximal Oxygen Uptake (ml · kg⁻¹ · min⁻¹) for Men and Women Aged 20 to 69

	MIN · MI⁻¹										
HR	10	11	12	13	14	15	16	17	18	19	20
MEN (20-29)											
120	65.0	61.7	58.4	55.2	51.9	48.6	45.4	42.1	38.9	35.6	32.3
130	63.4	60.1	56.9	53.6	50.3	47.1	43.8	40.6	37.3	34.0	30.8
140	61.8	58.6	55.3	52.0	48.8	45.5	42.2	39.0	35.7	32.5	29.2
150	60.3	57.0	53.7	50.5	47.2	43.9	40.7	37.4	34.2	30.9	27.6
160	58.7	55.4	52.2	48.9	45.6	42.4	39.1	35.9	32.6	29.3	26.1
170	57.1	53.9	50.6	47.3	44.1	40.8	37.6	34.3	31.0	27.8	24.5
180	55.6	52.3	49.0	45.8	42.5	39.3	36.0	32.7	29.5	26.2	22.9
190	54.0	50.7	47.5	44.2	41.0	37.7	34.4	31.2	27.9	24.6	21.4
200	52.4	49.2	45.9	42.7	39.4	36.1	32.9	29.6	26.3	23.1	19.8
WOMEN (20-29)											
120	62.1	58.9	55.6	52.3	49.1	45.8	42.5	39.3	36.0	32.7	29.5
130	60.6	57.3	54.0	50.8	47.5	44.2	41.0	37.7	34.4	31.2	27.9
140	59.0	55.7	52.5	49.2	45.9	42.7	39.4	36.1	32.9	29.6	26.3
150	57.4	54.2	50.9	47.6	44.4	41.1	37.8	34.6	31.3	28.0	24.8
160	55.9	52.6	49.3	46.7	42.8	39.5	36.3	33.0	29.7	26.5	23.2
170	54.3	51.0	47.8	44.5	41.2	38.0	34.7	31.4	28.2	24.9	21.6
180	52.7	49.5	46.2	42.9	39.7	36.4	33.1	29.9	26.6	23.3	20.1
190	51.2	47.9	44.6	41.4	38.1	34.8	31.6	28.3	25.0	21.8	18.5
200	49.6	46.3	43.1	39.8	36.5	33.3	30.0	26.7	23.5	20.2	16.9
MEN (30-39)											
120	61.1	57.8	54.6	51.3	48.0	44.8	41.5	38.2	35.0	31.7	28.4
130	59.5	56.3	53.0	49.7	46.5	43.2	39.9	36.7	33.4	30.1	26.9
140	58.0	54.7	51.4	48.2	44.9	41.6	38.4	35.1	31.8	28.6	25.3
150	56.4	53.1	49.9	46.6	43.3	40.1	36.8	33.5	30.3	27.0	23.8
160	54.8	51.6	48.3	45.0	41.8	38.5	35.2	32.0	28.7	25.5	22.2
170	53.3	50.0	46.7	43.5	40.2	36.9	33.7	30.4	27.1	23.9	20.6
180	51.7	48.4	45.2	41.9	38.6	35.4	32.1	28.8	25.6	22.3	19.1
190	50.1	46.9	43.6	40.3	37.1	33.8	30.5	27.3	24.0	20.8	17.5
WOMEN (30-39)											
120	58.2	55.0	51.7	48.4	45.2	41.9	38.7	35.4	32.1	28.9	25.6
130	56.7	53.4	50.1	46.9	43.6	40.4	37.1	33.8	30.6	27.3	24.0
140	55.1	51.8	48.6	45.3	42.1	38.8	35.5	32.3	29.0	24.7	22.5
150	53.5	50.3	47.0	43.8	40.5	37.2	34.0	30.7	27.4	24.2	20.9
160	52.0	48.7	45.4	42.2	38.9	35.7	32.4	29.1	25.9	22.6	19.3
170	50.4	47.1	43.9	40.6	37.4	34.1	30.8	27.6	24.3	21.0	17.8
180	48.8	45.6	42.3	39.1	35.8	32.5	29.3	26.0	22.7	19.5	16.2
190	47.3	44.0	40.8	37.5	34.2	31.0	27.7	24.4	21.2	17.9	14.6

(continued)

Table 7.1 *(continued)*

	MIN · MI⁻¹										
HR	10	11	12	13	14	15	16	17	18	19	20
MEN (40-49)											
120	57.2	54.0	50.7	47.4	44.2	40.9	37.6	34.4	31.1	27.8	24.6
130	55.7	52.4	49.1	45.9	42.6	39.3	36.1	32.8	29.5	26.3	23.0
140	54.1	50.8	47.6	44.3	41.0	37.8	34.5	31.2	28.0	24.7	21.4
150	52.5	49.3	46.0	42.7	39.5	36.2	32.9	29.7	26.4	23.1	19.9
160	51.0	47.7	44.4	41.2	37.9	34.6	31.4	28.1	24.8	21.6	18.3
170	49.4	46.1	42.9	39.6	36.3	33.1	29.8	26.5	23.3	20.0	16.7
180	47.8	44.6	41.3	38.0	34.8	31.5	28.2	25.0	21.7	18.4	15.2
WOMEN (40-49)											
120	54.4	51.1	47.8	44.6	41.3	38.0	34.8	31.5	28.2	25.0	21.7
130	52.8	49.5	46.3	43.0	39.7	36.5	33.2	29.9	26.7	23.4	20.1
140	51.2	48.0	44.7	41.4	38.2	34.9	31.6	28.4	25.1	21.8	18.6
150	49.7	46.4	43.1	39.9	36.6	33.3	30.1	26.8	23.5	20.3	17.0
160	48.1	44.8	41.6	38.3	35.0	31.8	28.5	25.2	22.0	18.7	15.5
170	46.5	43.3	40.0	36.7	33.5	30.2	26.9	23.7	20.4	17.2	13.9
MEN (50-59)											
120	53.3	50.0	46.8	43.5	40.3	37.0	33.7	30.5	27.2	23.9	20.7
130	51.7	48.5	45.2	42.0	38.7	35.4	32.2	28.9	25.6	22.4	19.1
140	50.2	46.9	43.7	40.4	37.1	33.9	30.6	27.3	24.1	20.8	17.5
150	48.6	45.4	42.1	38.8	35.6	32.3	29.0	25.8	22.5	19.2	16.0
160	47.1	43.8	40.5	37.3	34.0	30.7	27.5	24.2	20.9	17.7	14.4
170	45.5	42.2	39.0	35.7	32.4	29.2	25.9	22.6	19.4	16.1	12.8
WOMEN (50-59)											
120	50.5	47.2	43.9	40.7	37.4	34.1	30.9	27.6	24.3	21.1	17.8
130	48.9	45.6	42.4	39.1	35.8	32.6	29.3	26.0	22.8	19.5	16.2
140	47.3	44.1	40.8	37.5	34.3	31.0	27.7	24.5	21.2	17.9	14.7
150	45.8	42.5	39.2	36.0	32.7	29.4	26.2	22.9	19.6	16.4	13.1
160	44.2	40.9	37.7	34.4	31.1	27.9	24.6	21.3	18.1	14.8	11.5
170	42.6	39.4	36.1	32.8	29.6	26.3	23.0	19.8	16.5	13.2	10.0
MEN (60-69)											
120	49.4	46.2	42.9	39.6	36.4	33.1	29.8	26.6	23.3	20.0	16.8
130	47.9	44.6	41.3	38.1	34.8	31.5	28.3	25.0	21.7	18.5	15.2
140	46.3	43.0	39.8	36.5	33.2	30.0	26.7	23.4	20.2	16.9	13.6
150	44.7	41.5	38.2	34.9	31.7	28.4	25.1	21.9	18.6	15.3	12.1
160	43.2	39.9	36.6	33.4	30.1	26.8	23.6	20.3	17.0	13.8	10.5
WOMEN (60-69)											
120	46.6	43.3	40.0	36.8	33.5	30.2	27.0	23.7	20.5	17.2	13.9
130	45.0	41.7	38.5	35.2	31.9	28.7	25.4	22.2	18.9	15.6	12.4
140	43.4	40.2	36.9	33.6	30.4	27.1	23.8	20.6	17.3	14.1	10.8
150	41.9	38.6	35.3	32.1	28.8	25.5	22.3	19.0	15.8	12.5	9.2
160	40.3	37.0	33.8	30.5	27.2	24.0	20.7	17.5	14.2	10.9	7.7

Calculations assume 170 lb (77.1 kg) for men and 125 lb (56.7 kg) for women. For each 15 lb (6.8 kg) beyond these values, subtract 1 ml · kg⁻¹ · min⁻¹. HR = heart rate.

Based on Kline et al. 1987.

min run compared with a 12 to 15 min run. If the run lasts too long, the person is not able to run close to 100% of $\dot{V}O_2max$ and the estimate is too low (figure 7.2).

The $\dot{V}O_2$ associated with a specific running speed can be calculated from the following formula (see chapter 6 for details):

$$\dot{V}O_2 = \text{horizontal velocity } (m \cdot min^{-1}) \cdot \frac{0.2\ ml \cdot kg^{-1} \cdot min^{-1}}{(m \cdot min^{-1})} + 3.5\ ml \cdot kg^{-1} \cdot min^{-1}$$

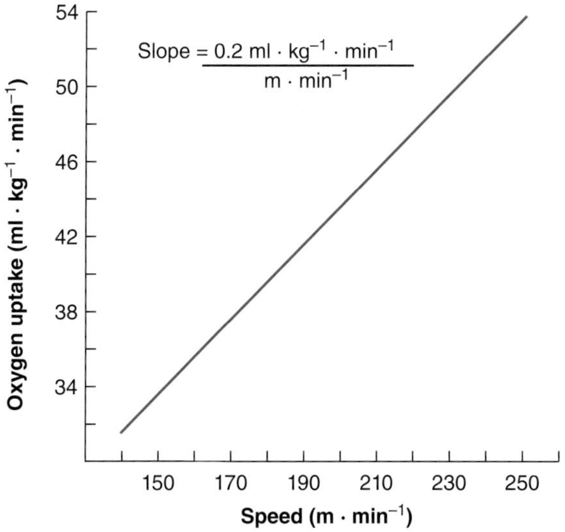

FIGURE 7.1 Relationship between steady-state oxygen uptake and running speed (15).

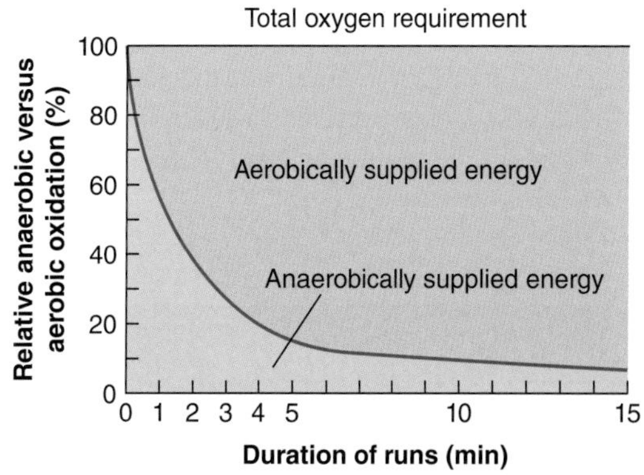

FIGURE 7.2 The relative role of aerobic and anaerobic energy sources in best-effort runs of various durations.

Adapted from Balke 1963.

Table 7.2 Percentile Values for Maximal Oxygen Uptake

	Age 20-29		Age 30-39		Age 40-49		Age 50-59		Age 60-69		Age 70-79	
Rating (percentile)	M	W	M	W	M	W	M	W	M	W	M	W
95	66.3	56.0	59.8	45.8	55.6	41.7	50.7	35.9	43.0	29.4	39.7	24.1
90	61.8	51.3	56.5	41.4	52.1	38.4	45.6	32.0	40.3	27.0	36.6	23.1
85	59.3	48.3	54.2	39.3	49.3	36.0	43.2	30.2	38.2	25.6	35.5	22.2
80	57.1	46.5	51.6	37.5	46.7	34.0	41.2	28.6	36.1	24.6	31.4	21.3
75	55.2	44.7	49.2	36.1	45.0	32.4	39.7	27.6	34.5	23.8	30.4	20.8
70	53.7	43.2	48.0	34.6	43.9	31.1	38.2	26.8	32.9	23.1	28.4	20.5
65	52.1	41.6	46.6	33.5	42.1	30.0	36.3	26.0	31.6	22.0	27.6	19.9
60	50.2	40.6	45.2	32.2	40.3	28.7	35.1	25.2	30.5	21.2	26.9	19.4
55	49.0	38.9	43.8	31.2	38.9	27.7	33.8	24.4	29.1	20.5	25.6	19.2
50	48.0	37.6	42.4	30.2	37.8	26.7	32.6	23.4	28.2	20.0	24.4	18.3
45	46.5	35.9	41.3	29.3	36.7	25.9	31.6	22.7	27.2	19.6	24.0	17.8
40	44.9	34.6	39.6	28.2	35.7	24.9	30.7	21.8	26.6	18.9	22.8	17.0
35	43.5	33.6	38.5	27.4	34.6	24.1	29.5	21.2	25.7	18.4	22.4	16.8
30	41.9	32.0	37.4	26.4	33.3	23.3	28.4	20.6	24.6	17.9	21.2	15.9
25	40.1	30.5	35.9	25.3	31.9	22.1	27.1	19.9	23.7	17.2	20.4	15.6
20	38.1	28.6	34.1	24.1	30.5	21.3	26.1	19.1	22.4	16.5	19.2	15.1
15	35.4	26.2	32.7	22.5	29.0	20.0	24.4	18.3	21.2	15.6	18.2	14.6
10	32.1	23.9	30.2	20.9	26.8	18.8	22.8	17.3	19.8	14.6	17.1	13.6
5	29.0	21.7	27.2	19.0	24.2	17.0	20.9	16.0	17.4	13.4	16.3	13.1

Values are in $ml \cdot kg^{-1} \cdot min^{-1}$; M = men; W = women. Fitness categories (percentile): Superior = 95; Excellent = 80-90; Good = 60-75; Fair = 40-55; Poor = 20-35; Very Poor = 5-15.

CRF Registry Advisory Board.

These estimates are reasonable for adults who jog or run the entire 12 min or 1.5 mi (2.4 km). The formula underestimates $\dot{V}O_2max$ in children because they have a higher oxygen cost of running (22). In contrast, the formula overestimates $\dot{V}O_2max$ in trained runners because of their better running economy (21) and in those who walk the test because the net oxygen cost of walking is half that of running (see chapter 6).

The 1 mi (1.6 km) run is used in many youth fitness programs (20, 45). These steps can be used for other endurance runs (e.g., 1.5 mi or 12 min run). Note that these directions were written for a class setting; however, the test can be used in a one-on-one setting as well.

Steps to Administering the Mile Run

Before Test Day

1. Arrange to have the following elements at the test site:
    - A person to start and read the time from a stopwatch
    - A partner for each runner (perhaps with a sheet to mark off laps)
    - A stopwatch for the tester (with a spare ready)
    - A score sheet or scorecard
2. Explain the purpose of the test (i.e., to determine how fast participants can run 1 mi [1.6 km], which reflects the endurance of the cardiovascular system).
3. Do not administer the test until participants have had several fitness sessions, including some with running.
4. Have participants practice running at a set submaximal pace for 1 lap, then 2, and so on several times before the test day.
5. Select and mark off (if needed) a level area for the run.
6. Explain to people being tested that they are to run the mile in the fastest time possible. Walking is allowed, but the goal is to cover the distance as quickly as possible.

Test Day

1. Participants warm up with stretching, walking, and slow jogging.
2. Several people will run at the same time.
3. Explain the procedure again.
4. The timer says, "Ready, go," and starts the stopwatch.
5. Each participant has a partner with a watch with a second hand.
6. The partner counts the laps and tells the participant at the end of each lap how many more laps to run.
7. The timer calls out the minutes and seconds as the runner finishes the mile run.
8. The partner listens for the time when the runner finishes the mile and records it (to the nearest second) immediately on a scorecard.
9. The runner continues to walk 1 lap after finishing the run.

QUESTION:

A 20-yr-old woman takes the Cooper 12 min run test following a 15 wk walk and jog program and completes 6 laps on a 440 yd (402.3 m) track. What is her $\dot{V}O_2max$?

ANSWER:

$$402.3\ m \cdot lap^{-1} \cdot 6\ laps = 2{,}414\ m, \text{ and } 2{,}414\ m \div 12\ min = 201\ m \cdot min^{-1}, \text{ so}$$

$$\dot{V}O_2 = 201\ m \cdot min^{-1} \cdot \frac{0.2\ ml \cdot kg^{-1} \cdot min^{-1}}{(m \cdot min^{-1})} + 3.5\ ml \cdot kg^{-1} \cdot min^{-1}$$

$$\dot{V}O_2max = 40.2 + 3.5 = 43.7\ ml \cdot kg^{-1} \cdot min^{-1}.$$

Table 7.2 shows that for this 20-yr-old woman, a value of 43.7 ml · kg^{-1} · min^{-1} is above the 70th percentile, consistent with good CRF. Encourage participants to achieve and maintain healthy levels of CRF. Blair et al. (13) found that values of 9 METs (31.5 ml · kg^{-1} · min^{-1}) for women and 10 METs (35 ml · kg^{-1} · min^{-1}) for men were associated with low risks of chronic disease and death from all causes. If people are not at that level, help them make small, systematic progress toward that goal by using the walking and jogging programs in chapter 11.

The advantage of the 12 min run is that it can be used to regularly evaluate CRF without expensive equipment. It is easily adapted to cyclists and swimmers, who can evaluate their CRF progress by determining how far they can ride or swim in 12 min. Although no equations exist that relate cyclists' and swimmers' respective performances to $\dot{V}O_2max$, participants can personally judge their current CRF and improvement attributable to training by monitoring the distance they can cover in 12 min.

As Cooper (19) and others agree, an endurance run should not be used for testing CRF at the beginning of an exercise program. A person new to exercise should progress through the walking and jogging programs (see chapter 11) to make fitness improvements before taking an endurance run test.

KEY POINT

A 1 mi (1.6 km) walking test can be used to estimate CRF. The time of the walk and the HR measured at the end of the walk are used to calculate $\dot{V}O_2max$. A 1.5 mi (2.4 km) run test also can be used to estimate CRF. The time for the 1.5 mi (2.4 km) is used to determine average velocity, and a formula (see chapter 4) is used to calculate $\dot{V}O_2max$.

Modified Canadian Aerobic Fitness Test

In contrast to the Cooper 1.5 mi (2.4 km) run test and the 1 mi (1.6 km) walk test, which require an all-out effort, the Canadian Aerobic Fitness Test (CAFT) is a submaximal field test. Originally called the *Canadian Home Fitness Test*, it used two 8 in. (20.3 cm) steps found in a conventional staircase in a home (9). This truly was a field test that could be done at home, and millions of people performed the CAFT with few problems (49). However, concerns were raised about the accuracy of the test as an estimate of $\dot{V}O_2max$, especially in fit subjects (54). In 1993, Weller et al. (56) provided a modified version of the CAFT (mCAFT) to address these concerns. One of the primary changes was to have the subjects work until they achieved an HR of 85% of age-predicted maximal HR (220 – age). The other was to add two more stages (using a single 16 in. (40.6 cm) step with a 4-step cadence) to challenge the fittest subjects. A stepping platform with two 8 in. (20.3 cm) steps accommodates both needs because the back of the platform is 16 in. (40.6 cm) high.

A stepping cadence of 6 counts per step cycle is used for the two 8 in. (20.3 cm) steps (step-step-up, step-step-down) and is maintained using a recording. Before the test, participants complete the PAR-Q+ (see chapter 2) to determine if they should proceed. In the mCAFT, the first stage of the test requires the person to step for 3 min at a rate equivalent to 65% to 70% of the average $\dot{V}O_2max$ of the next oldest age group (remember, $\dot{V}O_2max$ generally decreases with age) (17). Consequently, the first 3 min stage of the mCAFT is based on the age of the subject, with each stage having a specified cadence (steps per min) for males and females (see table 7.3):

- Males aged 60 to 69 yr and females 50 to 69 yr should begin at stage 1.
- Males 50 to 59 yr and females 40 to 49 yr should begin at stage 2.
- Males 30 to 49 yr and females 15 to 39 yr should begin at stage 3.
- Only males aged 15 to 29 yr should begin the test at stage 4.

An HR monitor (preferred) is used to obtain an HR at the end of each 3 min stage, but an immediate 10 sec recovery pulse, counted between 5 and 15 sec postexercise, can be used. If the HR does not exceed the maximum allowable (85% of age-predicted maximal HR), another 3 min step

Progressive Aerobic Cardiovascular Endurance Run

An alternative CRF field test is the Progressive Aerobic Cardiovascular Endurance Run, or PACER. This test, developed by Leger et al. (34, 35), is a 20 m shuttle run test done to the sound of a beep as the individual moves between the boundary lines. The speed required at the start is 5.3 mi · hr^{-1} (8.5 km · hr^{-1}), and it increases 0.3 mi · hr^{-1} (0.5 km · hr^{-1}) each minute. Three rapid beeps signal progression to the next level, where the time between beeps becomes shorter. The test is terminated when the individual cannot keep up with the beeps, and the number of 20 m laps completed is used to estimate CRF. The PACER test is part of the fitness testing battery in the Fitnessgram, developed by the Cooper Institute (see www.fitnessgram.net for more information) (20). In a recent study of 10- to 15-yr-old youth (46), the average $\dot{V}O_2max$ measured (not estimated) on the PACER test was identical to that measured on a standard treadmill test. In addition, there were no differences in the maximal HR or the respiratory exchange ratio (RER) values, lending additional validity to the PACER test as an excellent indicator of CRF in children. Criterion-referenced standards for CRF (see chapter 16) have been validated for this test (18). This protocol has also been used to estimate $\dot{V}O_2max$ in adults (39, 52); however, a practice trial may be needed to establish a stable baseline to use as a reference for monitoring changes over time (33). In another version, called the *square shuttle run*, subjects run around a 15 m square in a gym. Based on directly measured $\dot{V}O_2$ during the run, it has been shown to have good validity and reliability when testing adults (24).

Table 7.3. Stepping Cadence and Oxygen Cost of the Modified Canadian Aerobic Fitness Test (mCAFT)

mCAFT stage	Stepping cadence	O_2 cost	Stepping cadence	O_2 cost
	Women		Men	
1	66	15.9	66	15.9
2	84	18.0	84	18.0
3	102	22.0	102	22.0
4	114	24.5	114	24.5
5	120	26.3	132	29.5
6	132	29.5	144	33.6
7	144	33.6	118*	36.2
8	118*	36.2	132*	40.1

*Single step test with 4 counts per step cycle. The O_2 cost is in ml · kg^{-1} · min^{-1}.

From: the Canadian Society of Exercise Physiology: Physical Activity Training for Health, 2013

test is completed at the next higher intensity or until the last stage is completed. $\dot{V}O_2$max can be estimated from these results using the following equation (55), with a SEE of 6 ml · kg^{-1} · min^{-1}.

$$\text{Estimated } \dot{V}O_2\text{max} = 17.2 + (1.29 \times \dot{V}O_2) - (0.09 \times \text{mass}) - (\ 0.18 \times \text{age}),$$

where $\dot{V}O_2$ = oxygen cost of the final stage in ml · kg^{-1} · min^{-1} (see table 7.3), mass is in kg, and age is in yr.

As with all submaximal GXTs, the simple HR response to the last stage of the test, independent of its conversion to a $\dot{V}O_2$max value, can be used to educate and motivate clients, one of the original intents of the CAFT (48, 49, 50, 51). Details and materials for the administration of this test can be obtained from the Canadian Society of Exercise Physiology (CSEP; see www.csep.ca) (17).

Graded Exercise Tests

Many fitness programs use **graded exercise tests (GXTs)** to evaluate CRF. These multilevel tests can be administered with a bench, cycle ergometer, or treadmill.

Bench Step

Bench stepping is economical and can be used for both submaximal and maximal testing. The disadvantages include the limited number of stages for any one bench height and individual fitness level and the difficulty of taking certain measurements during the test (e.g., BP). The oxygen costs for stepping at various rates on steps of various heights are presented in chapter 6.

Cycle Ergometer

Cycle ergometers are portable, moderately priced work instruments that allow easy measurement of HR and BP because the participant's upper body is essentially stationary. Their disadvantages, however, are that the exercise load is self-paced and that fatigued leg muscle may be a limiting factor. On mechanically braked cycle ergometers such as the Monark models, altering the pedal rate or the resistance on the flywheel changes the work rate. Generally, the pedal rate is constant during a GXT at a rate appropriate to the person being tested: 50 to 60 rev · min^{-1} for those of low to average fitness and 70 to 100 rev · min^{-1} for highly fit and competitive cyclists (28). A metronome or some other source of feedback such as a speedometer helps the person maintain the pedal rate. The resistance (load) on the wheel is increased sequentially to systematically overload the cardiovascular system. The starting work rate and the increment from one stage to the next depend on the fitness of the person being tested and the purpose of the test. $\dot{V}O_2$ can be estimated from a formula (2) that gives reasonable estimates of $\dot{V}O_2$ up to work rates of about 1,200 kgm · min^{-1} or 200 W (see chapter 6 for details):

$$\dot{V}O_2\ (\text{ml} \cdot \text{kg}^{-1} \cdot \text{min}^{-1}) = (\text{work rate [kgm} \cdot \text{min}^{-1}] \cdot 1.8\ \text{ml } O_2 \cdot \text{kgm}^{-1}) \div \text{body weight (kg)} + 7\ \text{ml} \cdot \text{kg}^{-1} \cdot \text{min}^{-1},$$

or

$$\dot{V}O_2\ (\text{ml} \cdot \text{kg}^{-1} \cdot \text{min}^{-1}) = (\text{work rate [W]} \cdot 10.8\ \text{ml } O_2 \cdot \text{W}^{-1}) \div \text{body weight (kg)} + 7\ \text{ml} \cdot \text{kg}^{-1} \cdot \text{min}^{-1}.$$

The cycle ergometer differs from the treadmill in that the seat supports the body weight and the work rate depends primarily on pedal rate and the load on the wheel. This means that the relative $\dot{V}O_2$ at any work rate is higher for a smaller person than for a bigger person.

QUESTION:

What is the MET value for two individuals, one weighing 60 kg and the other 90 kg, who exercise at the same work rate (900 kgm · min^{-1}) on a cycle ergometer?

ANSWER:

For the 60 kg subject,

$$\dot{V}O_2\ (ml \cdot kg^{-1} \cdot min^{-1})$$
$$= (900\ kgm \cdot min^{-1} \cdot 1.8\ ml\ O_2 \cdot kgm^{-1})$$
$$\div\ 60\ kg + 7\ ml \cdot kg^{-1} \cdot min^{-1},$$
and $\dot{V}O_2\ (ml \cdot kg^{-1} \cdot min^{-1})$
$$= 34\ ml \cdot kg^{-1} \cdot min^{-1}, \text{ or } 9.7\ METs.$$

For the 90 kg subject,

$$\dot{V}O_2\ (ml \cdot kg^{-1} \cdot min^{-1})$$
$$= (900\ kgm \cdot min^{-1} \cdot 1.8\ ml\ O_2 \cdot kgm^{-1})$$
$$\div\ 90\ kg + 7\ ml \cdot kg^{-1} \cdot min^{-1}, \text{ and}$$
$$\dot{V}O_2\ (ml \cdot kg^{-1} \cdot min^{-1})$$
$$= 25\ ml \cdot kg^{-1} \cdot min^{-1}, \text{ or } 7.1\ METs.$$

In addition, the increments in the work rate demand a fixed increase in the $\dot{V}O_2$ (e.g., an increment of 150 kgm · min^{-1} equals a $\dot{V}O_2$ change of 270 ml · min^{-1}), forcing the small or unfit subject to make cardiovascular adjustments greater than those of a large or highly fit subject. As we will see, these factors are considered in selecting work rates for a cycle ergometer test used to evaluate CRF. Table 7.4 summarizes how differences in body weight affect the metabolic responses to weight-supported (e.g., cycle ergometry) and weight-carrying (e.g., bench stepping, walking, jogging) work tasks. Thus, for tasks in which body weight provides the resistance (weight-carrying tasks), a larger person achieves a greater absolute $\dot{V}O_2$ (L · min^{-1}) than a smaller person achieves, but both work at the same MET level. In cycling (a weight-supported task), the two people achieve a similar absolute $\dot{V}O_2$, but the larger person has a lower MET level.

Treadmill

Treadmill protocols are very reproducible because they set the pace for the subject, whereas the subject may go too slow or too fast on the bench step or the cycle ergometer. Treadmill tests can accommodate people of any fitness level and use the natural activities of walking and running, with the running tests placing the greatest potential load on the cardiovascular system. Treadmills, however, are expensive, are not portable, and make some measurements (e.g., BP, blood sampling) difficult. The type of treadmill test influences the measured $\dot{V}O_2$max, with the graded running test giving the highest value, the running test at 0% grade giving the next highest value, and the walking test giving the lowest value (8, 38).

To estimate $\dot{V}O_2$ by varying grade and speed, the grade and speed settings on the treadmill must be calibrated correctly (see details on how to calibrate a treadmill in appendix 7.2 at the end of this chapter). Further, the subject cannot hold onto the treadmill railing during the test if the estimated $\dot{V}O_2$ values are going to be correct. For example, it was observed that HR decreased 17 beats · min^{-1} when a subject who was walking on a treadmill at 3.4 mi · hr^{-1} (5.5 km · hr^{-1}) and at a 14% grade held onto the treadmill railing (6). Holding onto the railing results in an overestimation of the $\dot{V}O_2$max because the HR is lower at any stage of the test and so the test lasts longer. With the treadmill test, there is no need to adjust the $\dot{V}O_2$ calculation for differences in body weight because the person being tested carries her own weight; therefore, the $\dot{V}O_2$ (ml · kg^{-1} · min^{-1}) is independent of body weight (40).

KEY POINT

CRF can be determined with bench stepping, cycle ergometers, or treadmills. The oxygen uptake values (expressed in ml · kg^{-1} · min^{-1}) are similar for most adults at specific stages of a treadmill or step test because the energy cost is proportional to body weight, which is carried by the test participant. In contrast, the absolute oxygen uptake (expressed in L · min^{-1}) is similar for most adults at each stage of a cycle ergometer test; however, the relative oxygen cost (ml · kg^{-1} · min^{-1}) is higher for lighter participants.

Table 7.4 Effect of Body Weight on Metabolic Responses to Various Work Tasks

	$\dot{V}O_2$MAX			
Work task	L · min^{-1}	ml · kg^{-1} · min^{-1}	Energy production (kcal)	METs
Bench	↑	=	↑	=
Walk	↑	=	↑	=
Jog	↑	=	↑	=
Body-weight-supported cycle	=	↓	=	↓

MET = metabolic equivalent. Symbols (↑ or ↓ or =) indicate how a heavier person responds compared with a lighter person.

Common Variables Measured During a Graded Exercise Test

The cardiovascular variables commonly measured for resting and submaximal tests include HR and BP; RPE is generally recorded to assess subjective effort. For maximal testing, the final stage achieved on a GXT is recorded, and $\dot{V}O_2max$ may be measured or may be estimated from the final stage of the test.

Heart Rate

Heart rate (HR) often is used as a fitness indicator at rest and during a standard submaximal-work task. Maximal HR is useful for determining the THR for fitness workouts (see chapter 11), but it is not a good fitness indicator because it changes little with training. Table 7.5 summarizes how endurance training affects HR in various situations.

When an ECG is recorded, the HR can be taken from the ECG strip (see chapter 24). Without an ECG, HR can be taken with an HR watch, a stethoscope, or manual palpation of an artery at the wrist or neck. HR watches are accurate and are the easiest way to measure HR. When palpating, fingers (not the thumb) should be used, preferably at the wrist (radial artery). Taking the HR at the neck (carotid artery) requires caution because applying too much pressure can trigger a reflex that slows the HR. Reliable measures are obtained, however, when people are trained in this procedure (43). The HR at rest or during steady-state exercise should be taken for 30 sec for higher reliability. When HR is taken after exercise, measurement should begin soon after exercise ends (e.g., within 5 sec) and should be taken for 10 or 15 sec because the HR changes so rapidly. The 10 or 15 sec rate is multiplied by 6 or 4, respectively, to calculate beats per minute. For example, if a 10 sec postexercise HR is 20 beats · min^{-1}, the HR is 120 beats · min^{-1} (6 · 20).

Blood Pressure

SBP and DBP are often determined at rest, during work, and after work. Proper cuff size (in which the bladder overlaps two-thirds of the arm) and a sensitive stethoscope are required to get accurate values at rest and during work. At rest, the person should have both feet flat on the floor and be in a relaxed position with the arm supported. The cuff should be wrapped securely around the arm at heart level, usually with the tube on the inside of the arm. The stethoscope should be below (not under) the cuff; placement depends on where the sound can be most easily heard, often toward the inside of the arm (25). The first and fourth Korotkoff sounds (the first sound heard and the sound when the tone changes or becomes muffled) should be used for SBP and DBP, respectively, during exercise. The fifth Korotkoff sound (disappearance of sound) is used to classify BP at rest (2).

Rating of Perceived Exertion

Borg introduced the **rating of perceived exertion (RPE)**—that is, how hard a person perceives exercise to be—using a scale from 6 to 20 (roughly based on resting to maximal HR, i.e., 60-200 beats · min^{-1}) (14). For many years the Borg RPE scale has been used to judge the degree of effort experienced during an exercise test or an exercise session. For example, using the classic scale of 6 to 20, level of effort can be classified in the following way (see also table 11.2):

- Very light <10
- Light 10-11
- Moderate 12-13
- Vigorous 14-16
- Very hard 17-19
- Maximal 20

The RPE scale can be used with a GXT to provide useful information during the test as the person approaches exhaustion and to serve as a reference for exercise prescription. In the latter case, RPE values of 12 to 13 are taken as moderate-intensity physical activity and 14 to 16 as vigorous or hard physical activity. We will see more on how to use the RPE scale in exercise prescriptions in chapter 11. When administering the RPE scale during a GXT, we recommend that fitness professionals provide the following instructions (1, p. 78):

Table 7.5 Effects of Endurance Training on Heart Rate

Condition	Effects of fitness on HR
Rest	↓
Standard submaximal work (same external work rate)	↓
Maximal work	No change
Set % of maximal	No change

HR = heart rate.

Adapted from Golding 2000.

> During the exercise test we want you to pay close attention to how hard you feel the exercise work rate is. This feeling should reflect your total amount of exertion and fatigue, combining all sensations and feelings of physical stress, effort, and fatigue. Don't concern yourself with any one factor such as leg pain, shortness of breath, or exercise intensity, but try to concentrate on your total, inner feeling of exertion. Try not to underestimate or overestimate your feelings of exertion; be as accurate as you can.

Estimating Versus Measuring Functional Capacity ($\dot{V}O_2$max)

Functional capacity is defined as the highest work rate (oxygen uptake) reached in a GXT during which HR, BP, and ECG responses are within the normal range for heavy work. For cardiac patients, the highest work rate normally does not reflect the maximal capacity of the cardiorespiratory system because the GXT might be stopped for ECG changes, angina, claudication pain, and so on. For the apparently healthy person, functional capacity can be called *maximal aerobic power* or *maximal oxygen uptake*, or $\dot{V}O_2$max (see chapter 4 for procedures for measuring oxygen uptake).

Oxygen uptake increases with each stage of the GXT until it reaches its upper limit. At that point, $\dot{V}O_2$ does not increase when the test moves to the next stage; the person's $\dot{V}O_2$max has been reached. Given the complexity and cost of procedures for directly measuring $\dot{V}O_2$max, it is usually estimated with equations relating the stage of the GXT to a specific oxygen uptake.

As discussed in chapter 6, many formulas may be used to estimate oxygen uptake from the stage reached in a GXT. In general, these formulas reasonably estimate $\dot{V}O_2$ if the GXT is suited to the individual. However, if the increments in the GXT stages are too large relative to the person's CRF, or if the time spent at each stage is too short, then the person might not reach the steady-state oxygen requirement associated with that stage (41). Failure to achieve the oxygen requirement for a GXT stage results in overestimating $\dot{V}O_2$ at each stage of the test, with the overestimation growing larger with each stage. The inability to reach the oxygen requirement is a common problem with people who are less fit (e.g., cardiac patients). This inability suggests that more conservative (i.e., smaller increments between stages) GXT protocols should be used to allow these individuals to reach the oxygen demand at each stage. This problem is explained more completely in chapter 4, and the use of non-steady-state formulas to deal with this concern is presented in chapter 6.

In contrast, shorter stages and larger increments between stages in a GXT can be used if the purpose of the test is to screen for ECG abnormalities (rather than to estimate $\dot{V}O_2$max). In addition, changes in a participant's CRF over time can be determined by periodically using the same GXT.

KEY POINT

Common variables measured during a submaximal GXT include HR, BP, and RPE. Oxygen uptake can be measured at each stage of a test and at maximal exertion; however, $\dot{V}O_2$max usually is estimated from the final stage achieved during a maximal GXT.

Procedures for Graded Exercise Tests

This section explains how to administer a GXT and uses examples of various testing protocols. Because HR, BP, and RPE responses to submaximal work are influenced by several factors, variation in each factor from test to test should be carefully minimized. Some of these factors include

- temperature and relative humidity of the room;
- number of hours of sleep before testing;
- emotional state;
- hydration state;
- medication;
- time of day;
- time since last meal, cigarette smoking, caffeine intake, and exercise; and
- psychological environment of the test (i.e., the participant's comfort level with the surroundings during testing).

Attention to these factors increases the likelihood that changes in HR, BP, or RPE from one test to the next actually reflect changes in physical fitness and physical activity habits. A form such as the Pretest Instructions for a Fitness Test (see form 7.1) helps ensure that the client is ready for testing.

Typical procedures to follow during GXTs are shown here in *Steps to Administer a Graded Exercise Text.* A series of end points should be used to stop a GXT (1). These guidelines are for nondiagnostic testing performed without direct physician involvement or ECG monitoring.

FORM 7.1 Pretest Instructions for a Fitness Test

Name ____________________________ Test date ______________ Time ______________

Report to ____

INSTRUCTIONS

Please observe the following:

1. Wear athletic shoes, shorts, and a loose-fitting shirt.
2. No food, drink (except water), tobacco, or caffeine for 3 hours before the test.
3. Do minimal physical activity on the day of the test.

CANCELLATION

If you cannot keep this appointment, please call _______ or _______.

From E.T. Howley and D.L. Thompson, 2017, *Fitness professional's handbook*, 7th ed. (Champaign, IL: Human Kinetics).

Steps to Administering a Graded Exercise Test

Before Test Day

1. Ensure that testing personnel have been trained to implement the emergency action plan (EAP; see chapters 25 and 26).
2. Calibrate the exercise equipment (e.g., treadmill, cycle ergometer).
3. Make sure a scale, stadiometer, HR monitor, and sphygmomanometer are available.
4. Check supplies and data forms and that the RPE chart is clearly visible.
5. Select the appropriate test protocol for the participant.

Test Day

1. Ensure that the testing room is clean, quiet, and comfortable (e.g., temperature between 20 and 25 °C, adequate ventilation).
2. Greet participant and verify that pretest instructions were followed.
3. Obtain informed consent (oral and written).
4. Record age and measure height and weight. Calculate and record estimated HRmax and 70% and 85% HRmax.
5. Obtain resting HR and BP.
6. Demonstrate how to do the step test and ask if there are any questions.
   - Have the participant practice the test protocol.
   - Make sure the participant can keep pace with the metronome or recording of step cadence.

OR

7. Teach the participant how to use the cycle ergometer.
   - Adjust the seat height so the participant's knee is slightly flexed when the foot is at the bottom of the pedal swing and parallel to the floor.
   - Instruct the participant to keep pace (e.g., 50 rpm) with the metronome, speedometer, or digital display of pedal rate.
   - Tell the participant to lightly hold onto the handlebars and to release hold when BP is taken.

OR

8. Demonstrate how to get on and off and how to walk on the treadmill.
   - Have the participant hold onto the railing while getting a feel for belt speed by putting one foot on the belt to practice keeping up with the belt.
   - Have the participant step onto the belt, keeping eyes ahead and back straight, and walk in a relaxed manner with first one arm and then both arms swinging.
   - To maintain balance, the participant can touch the railing lightly with just a finger or the back of the hand.
9. Follow test protocol exactly.
   - Ask how the participant feels during the test.
   - Follow the criteria for terminating the test (e.g., 85% HRmax).
   - For submaximal fitness tests, HR, BP, and RPE are the usual variables recorded at each stage of the test.

Based on American College of Sports Medicine 2014, *ACSM's guidelines for exercise testing and prescription*, 9th ed. (Philadelphia: PA: Lippincott, Williams, & Wilkins).

When to Use Submaximal and Maximal Tests

GXTs have been used to evaluate CRF in fitness programs for healthy populations and in the clinical assessment of ischemic heart disease, a condition in which an inadequate blood flow to the heart muscle can alter the ECG. Exercise is used to place a load on the heart to determine the cardiovascular response and to see if the ECG changes (23).

Some controversy has arisen concerning whether to use submaximal or maximal GXTs. On the basis of thousands of exercise stress tests conducted since the mid-1950s, a maximal or sign- and symptom-limited exercise test is generally recommended for finding ischemic heart disease in asymptomatic individuals. Although submaximal exercise tests are not as effective in identifying disease, they are appropriate for making activity recommendations, adjusting the medical regimen, and identifying the need for additional diagnostic tests (2).

When a fitness center is responsible for both fitness testing and the fitness program, the sequence of testing and activity recommended earlier provides the advantages of each while minimizing their disadvantages. The main objection to using maximal tests is that they require too much exertion for people who have been inactive. Although the health risk of a maximal GXT is very small with adequate screening and qualified testing personnel, the discomfort of performing at maximum exertion without previous conditioning may discourage some people from participating in a fitness program. Objections to the submaximal test include finding fewer abnormal responses to exercise and inaccurately estimating $\dot{V}O_2max$ from submaximal data. In a fitness program for apparently healthy people, the objections against giving either maximal or submaximal tests are overcome by administering the submaximal test early in the fitness program and the maximal test after the participant has been involved in regular exercise. Any of the GXT protocols can be used for submaximal or maximal testing—the only difference is the criteria for stopping the test. Either test is stopped if any of the abnormal responses listed in the sidebar *ACSM's General Indications for Stopping an Exercise Test* occur. In the absence of abnormal responses, the submaximal test is usually terminated when the person reaches a certain HR (often 85% of maximum HR), and the maximal test is stopped when the person reaches voluntary exhaustion.

KEY POINT

GXT protocols can be used for submaximal tests (early in the testing sequence) or maximal tests (for active people who have reached a minimal fitness level). Submaximal and maximal tests can use the same GXT protocol; however, their criteria for test termination differ. Maximal tests are more effective in identifying ischemic heart disease. Submaximal tests are useful in assessing fitness and are relatively inexpensive to administer. Although the $\dot{V}O_2max$ estimated from a submaximal test is not as accurate as that obtained from a maximal test, it is useful in evaluating changes in CRF due to an exercise program.

*ACSM's General Indications for Stopping an Exercise Test**

- Onset of angina or angina-like symptoms
- Drop in SBP of >10 mmHg with an increase in work rate or if SBP decreases below the value obtained in the same position prior to testing
- Excessive rise in BP: systolic pressure of >250 mmHg and/or diastolic pressure of >115 mmHg
- Shortness of breath, wheezing, leg cramps, or claudication
- Signs of poor perfusion: light-headedness, confusion, ataxia, pallor, cyanosis, nausea, or cold and clammy skin
- Failure of HR to increase with increased exercise intensity
- Noticeable change in heart rhythm by palpation or auscultation
- Request by subject to stop
- Physical or verbal manifestations of severe fatigue
- Failure of the testing equipment

*Assumes that testing is nondiagnostic and is being performed without ECG monitoring.

Reprinted, by permission, from American College of Sports Medicine, 2014, *ACSM's guidelines for exercise testing and prescription*, 9th ed. (Philadelphia, PA: Lippincott, Williams & Wilkins), 87.

Maximal Exercise Test Protocols

No one GXT protocol is appropriate for all people. The durations, starting points, and increments between stages vary from person to person. Young active people, normal sedentary people, and people with questionable health status should start at 6, 4, and 2 METs, respectively. The same three groups should increase by 2 to 3, 1 to 2, and 0.5 to 1 METs, respectively, for progressive stages of the test. If the test is for comparing CRF at different times, then 1 or 2 min per stage can be used. If it is for predicting $\dot{V}O_2max$, however, the time per stage should be 2 to 3 min.

The following testing protocols are examples of tests used for various populations. These protocols can be used for submaximal or maximal testing, remembering that the criteria for stopping the test will not be the same. The first protocol, shown in table 7.6, could be used with deconditioned subjects, who would start at a low MET level, walk slowly, and increase 1 MET per 3 min stage (42). The Balke standard protocol (11) could be used for typical inactive adults by having them start at a higher MET level and progress 1 MET per 2 min stage. More active or younger people could be tested on the Bruce protocol (16), which starts at a moderate MET level and goes up 2 or 3 METs per 3 min stage. Unfortunately, some testing centers use the same testing protocol for all people, with the result that the initial stage is often too high or too low and the work increments for each stage are too small or too large for the person being tested. Estimating $\dot{V}O_2max$

Table 7.6 Treadmill Protocols for Various Categories

Stage	METs	Speed (km · hr^{-1})	Grade (%)	Time (min)
		DECONDITIONED INDIVIDUALS[a]		
1	2.5	3.2	0.0	3
2	3.5	3.2	3.5	3
3	4.5	3.2	7.0	3
4	5.4	3.2	10.5	3
5	6.4	3.2	14.0	3
6	7.3	3.2	17.5	3
7	8.5	4.8	12.5	3
8	9.5	4.8	15.0	3
9	10.5	4.8	17.5	3
		NORMAL INACTIVE INDIVIDUALS[b]		
1	4.3	4.8	2.5	2
2	5.4	4.8	5.0	2
3	6.4	4.8	7.5	2
4	7.4	4.8	10.0	2
5	8.5	4.8	12.5	2
6	9.5	4.8	15.0	2
7	10.5	4.8	17.5	2
8	11.6	4.8	20.0	2
9	12.6	4.8	22.5	2
10	13.6	4.8	25.0	2
		YOUNG ACTIVE INDIVIDUALS[c]		
1	5.0	2.7	10.0	3
2	7.0	4.0	12.0	3
3	9.5	5.4	14.0	3
4	13.0	6.7	16.0	3
5	16.0	8.0	18.0	3

MET = metabolic equivalent.

[a]From Naughton and Haider 1973. [b]From Balke 1970. [c]From Bruce 1972.

from the final stage of a maximal GXT has a SEE of about 3 ml · kg^{-1} · min^{-1} (44).

Submaximal Exercise Test Protocols

Any GXT protocol can be used for submaximal or maximal testing. The fitness professional typically uses a submaximal GXT to estimate $\dot{V}O_2$max or to simply show how the exercise program changes selected variables. Predicting maximal oxygen uptake from any submaximal test involves substantial error. However, it can provide useful information for estimating a person's functional capacity and for determining the person's fitness category and what exercise programming is most appropriate. The only way to determine a participant's true functional capacity is to measure it during a maximal test. However, submaximal tests are reliable, and changes in HR, BP, and RPE resulting from exercise conditioning make submaximal tests a good mechanism for showing improvements in CRF. Estimation of $\dot{V}O_2$max from submaximal exercise tests has a SEE of about 5 ml · kg^{-1} · min^{-1} (44).

Submaximal Treadmill Test Protocol

The initial stage and rate of progression of the GXT should be selected using the guidelines mentioned earlier In the following example, a Balke protocol listed in table 7.6 for normal inactive individuals (3 mi · hr^{-1}, or 4.8 km · hr^{-1}, 2.5% grade increase every 2 min) was used; HR was monitored in the last 30 sec of each stage. The test was terminated at 85% of the age-predicted maximal HR (with the equation 220 – age). Maximal aerobic power was estimated by extrapolating the HR response to the person's estimated maximal HR. Figure 7.3 presents the results of this test with a graph showing the HR response at each work rate. The HR response is rather flat between the 0% and 5% grades. This is not uncommon (see the discussion that follows the YMCA test); perhaps the subject is too excited, or perhaps the SV changes are accounting for the changes in cardiac output at these low work rates. The HR response is usually quite linear between 110 beats · min^{-1} and the subject's 85% HRmax.

To estimate $\dot{V}O_2$max, the procedures of Maritz and colleagues (36) are followed. A line is drawn through the HR points from the 7.5% grade to the final work rate. This line is extended (extrapolated) to the person's estimated maximal HR (183 beats · min^{-1}). A vertical line is dropped from the last point to the baseline to estimate the subject's maximal aerobic power, which in this example is 11.8 METs, or 41.3 ml · kg^{-1} · min^{-1}. Any formula (e.g., 220 – age) used to estimate maximal HR has a SEE of about 10 beats · min^{-1}. Consequently, this possible inaccuracy influences any estimate of maximal oxygen uptake derived from extrapolating HR to an estimated maximal HR. If this person's true (measured) maximal HR is 173 or 193 beats · min^{-1}, the estimated maximal MET level is 11.0 METs or 12.6 METs, respectively.

Submaximal Cycle Ergometer Test Protocol

The steps in administering submaximal cycle ergometer tests are as follows.

Name: ______ Age: 37 Estimated HRmax: 183 85% HRmax: 155

Test type: Balke standard Ht: ______ Wt: ______ Sex: Male

Speed: 3 mph (4.8 kmh)

% grade	Time (min)	Heart rate
0	1	
	2	94
2.5	3	
	4	95
5	5	
	6	100
7.5	7	
	8	118
10	9	
	10	131
12.5	11	
	12	143
15	13	
	14	155

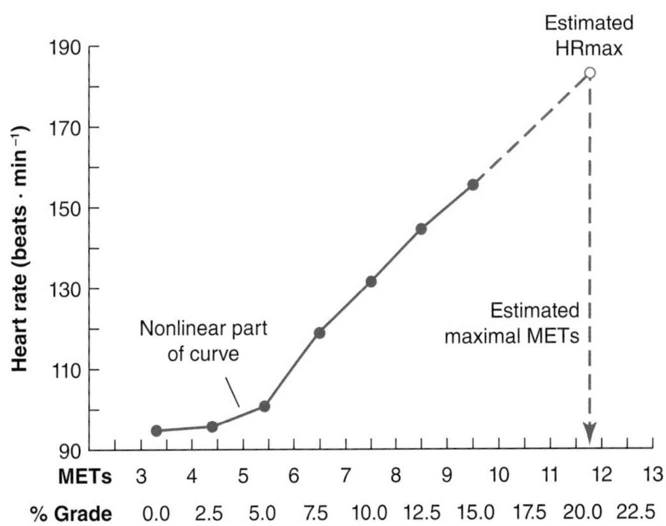

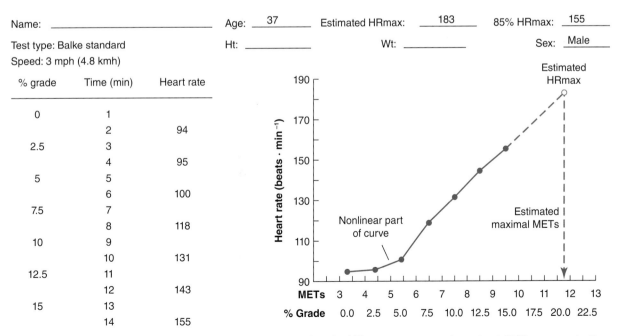

FIGURE 7.3 Maximal aerobic power estimated by measuring the HR response to a submaximal GXT on a treadmill.

Steps to Administering a Submaximal Cycle Ergometer Test

1. Complete the pretest items.
2. Select the test protocol.
3. Estimate the participant's HRmax (220 – age = HRmax in beats · min^{-1}).
4. Determine 85% of the participant's HRmax (HRmax · 0.85 = 85% HRmax).
5. Review the procedure with participant.
6. Set and record the seat height (the leg should be slightly bent at the knee when the foot is at the bottom of the pedaling stroke).
7. Start the metronome (set at 100 beats · min^{-1} so that one foot is at the bottom of the pedaling stroke on each beat, resulting in 50 complete rev · min^{-1}).
8. Have the participant begin pedaling in rhythm with the metronome.
9. As soon as the correct pace is achieved, set the resistance according to the protocol chosen.
10. Start the timer for the beginning of the 3 min stage.
11. Check the resistance setting (it may drift) and observe the participant for signs or symptoms that require termination of the test.
12. At 1:30 into the stage, measure and record BP and HR.
13. At 2:30, measure and record HR.
14. At 2:50, ask for and record the participant's RPE.
15. At 2:55, ask the participant, "How are you doing?"
16. At 3:00, if HR is less than 85% of HRmax, BP is responding normally, and the participant is all right, increase resistance to the next stage.
17. Repeat steps 10 through 16 until the participant reaches 85% of HRmax or there is another reason to stop the test. Go back to stage 1 (for cool-down) and repeat steps 10 through 15, stopping at 3:00 in the cool-down stage.
18. Talk with the participant and check for any problems.

Adapted, by permission, from B.D. Franks and E.T. Howley, 1998, *Fitness leader's handbook*, 2nd ed. (Champaign, IL: Human Kinetics), 73.

One of the most common submaximal cycle ergometer protocols (figure 7.4) originates from the *YMCA Fitness Testing and Assessment Manual* (27). This protocol relies on the linear relationship between HR and work rate ($\dot{V}O_2$) that occurs once an HR of approximately 110 beats · min^{-1} is reached. The test requires the person to complete one more stage beyond the one that induces an HR of 110 beats · min^{-1}. The line describing the HR–work rate relationship is extrapolated to the person's age-predicted maximal HR (as was done for the treadmill protocol) to estimate the person's $\dot{V}O_2$max. Each stage of the test lasts 3 min, unless a person's HR has not yet reached a steady state (there is >5 beats · min^{-1} difference between 2nd and 3rd min HR). In that case, an extra minute is added to that stage. The pedal rate is maintained at 50 rev · min^{-1} so that, on a Monark cycle ergometer, a 0.5 kg increase in load equals 150 kgm · min^{-1} (25 W). Seat height is adjusted so that the knee is slightly bent (7) when the pedal is at the bottom of the swing through 1 revolution. The seat height is recorded for future reference. HR is monitored during the latter half of the second and third minutes of each stage.

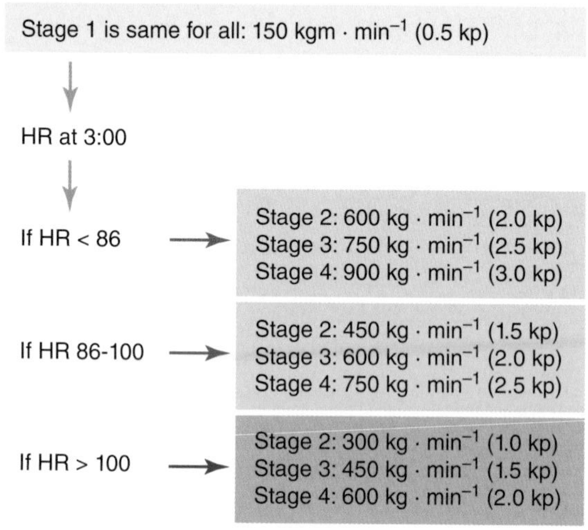

FIGURE 7.4 Guide for setting power outputs (workloads) on submaximal cycle ergometer tests.

VIDEO Watch **video 7.1**, which demonstrates the submaximal cycle ergometer test.

Selection of the initial work rate and the rate of progression on the cycle ergometer should consider body weight, sex, age, and physical activity level. In general,

- absolute $\dot{V}O_2$max (L · min^{-1}) is lower in smaller people,
- women have lower absolute $\dot{V}O_2$max values than men,

- $\dot{V}O_2$max decreases with age, and
- inactivity is associated with low $\dot{V}O_2$max values.

The YMCA test addresses body weight, fitness, and so on by starting everyone at 150 kgm · min^{-1} and using the HR response to that specified work rate to set subsequent stages in the test (see figure 7.4). Large or fit subjects would have a low HR response to this work rate and would use the most strenuous sequence of work rates (top box in the figure). A small or unfit subject would have a high HR response to the 150 kgm · min^{-1} work rate and would follow the sequence with the smallest increments in the power output (see bottom box in figure). Subjects should complete only one additional work rate beyond the one demanding an HR of 110 beats · min^{-1}.

The HR values for the second and third minutes of each work rate are recorded, and directions are followed to estimate $\dot{V}O_2$max in liters per minute. Figure 7.5 presents an example of a test for a 50-yr-old woman who weighs 59 kg. The stages followed the pattern dictated by the HR response to the initial work rate of 150 kgm · min^{-1}. A line was drawn through the last two HR values and extrapolated to the estimated maximal HR. A vertical line, dropped from the last point of the extrapolated line to the baseline, estimated the subject's maximal work rate to be 750 kgm · min^{-1}. With the formula described earlier (and in chapter 6) for the cycle ergometer, $\dot{V}O_2$max for this woman was estimated to be about 30 ml · kg^{-1} · min^{-1}, or 1.77 L · min^{-1}.

In contrast to the YMCA test, the Åstrand and Ryhming cycle ergometer test (7) requires the subject to complete only one 6 min work rate demanding an HR between 125 and 170 beats · min^{-1}. These investigators observed that for young (18-30 yr) subjects, the average HR was 128 beats · min^{-1} for males and 138 beats · min^{-1} for females at 50% $\dot{V}O_2$max, while at 70% $\dot{V}O_2$max the average HRs were 154 and 164 beats · min^{-1}, respectively. So if you know from an HR response that a person is at 50% $\dot{V}O_2$max at a work rate equal to 1.5 L · min^{-1}, then you know the estimated $\dot{V}O_2$max is twice that, or 3.0 L · min^{-1}. Table 7.7 is used to estimate $\dot{V}O_2$max from the subject's HR response to one 6 min work rate (5).

Using the data from the previous example of the woman taking the YMCA test, we can see how $\dot{V}O_2$max is estimated in the Åstrand and Ryhming protocol. The 50-yr-old woman had an HR of 140 beats · min^{-1} at a work rate of 450 kgm · min^{-1}. Using table 7.7, look down the leftmost column of values for women to an HR of 140, and look across to the second column of values (for a work rate of 450 kgm · min^{-1}). The estimated $\dot{V}O_2$max is 2.4 L · min^{-1}. Because maximal HR decreases with increasing age, however, and the data in table 7.7 were collected on young subjects, I. and P.-O. Åstrand (4, 5) established the following age-correction factors to correct for the lower maximal HR:

Age	Factor
15	1.10
25	1.00
35	0.87
40	0.83
45	0.78
50	0.75
55	0.71
60	0.68
65	0.65

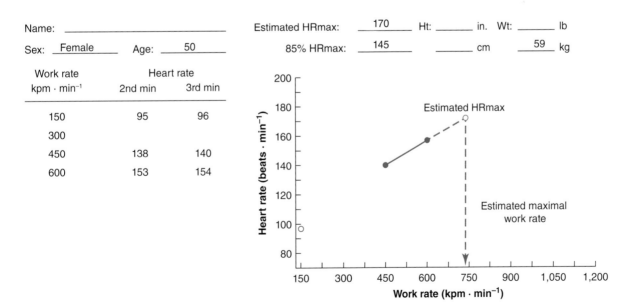

Name: ______ Estimated HRmax: 170 Ht: ______ in. Wt: ______ lb

Sex: Female Age: 50 85% HRmax: 145 ______ cm 59 kg

Work rate kpm · min^{-1}	Heart rate 2nd min	Heart rate 3rd min
150	95	96
300		
450	138	140
600	153	154

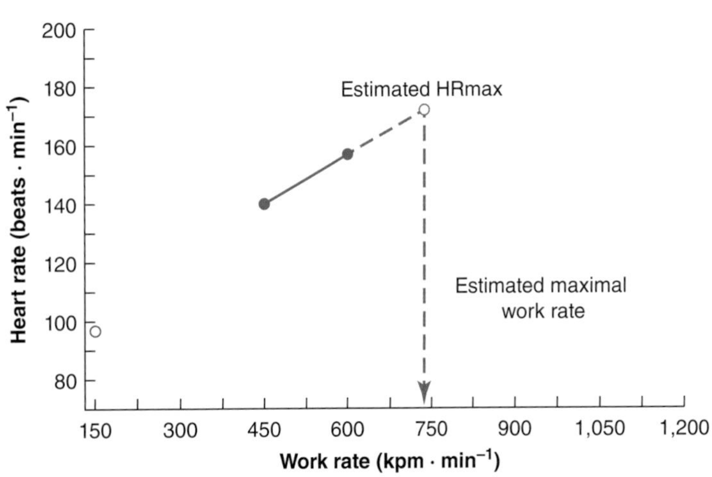

FIGURE 7.5 Maximal aerobic power estimated by measuring the HR response to a submaximal GXT on a cycle ergometer using the protocol from the *YMCA Fitness Testing and Assessment Manual.*

Table 7.7 Predicting Maximal Oxygen Uptake From Heart Rate and Workload During a 6 Min Cycle Ergometer Test

$\dot{V}O_2$MAX ($L \cdot MIN^{-1}$) VALUES FOR WOMEN						$\dot{V}O_2$MAX ($L \cdot MIN^{-1}$) VALUES FOR MEN					
HR	300 $kgm \cdot min^{-1}$	450 $kgm \cdot min^{-1}$	600 $kgm \cdot min^{-1}$	750 $kgm \cdot min^{-1}$	900 $kgm \cdot min^{-1}$	HR	300 $kgm \cdot min^{-1}$	600 $kgm \cdot min^{-1}$	900 $kgm \cdot min^{-1}$	1,200 $kgm \cdot min^{-1}$	1,500 $kgm \cdot min^{-1}$
120	2.6	3.4	4.1	4.8		120	2.2	3.5	4.8		
122	2.5	3.2	3.9	4.7		122	2.2	3.4	4.6		
124	2.4	3.1	3.8	4.5		124	2.1	3.3	4.5	6.0	
126	2.3	3.0	3.6	4.3		126	2.0	3.2	4.4	5.8	
128	2.2	2.8	3.5	4.2	4.8	128	2.0	3.1	4.2	5.6	
130	2.1	2.7	3.4	4.0	4.7	130	1.9	3.0	4.1	5.5	
132	2.0	2.7	3.3	3.9	4.5	132	1.8	2.9	4.0	5.3	
134	2.0	2.6	3.2	3.8	4.4	134	1.8	2.8	3.9	5.2	
136	1.9	2.5	3.1	3.6	4.2	136	1.7	2.7	3.8	5.0	
138	1.8	2.4	3.0	3.5	4.1	138	1.6	2.7	3.7	4.9	
140	1.8	2.4	2.8	3.4	4.0	140	1.6	2.6	3.6	4.8	6.0
142	1.7	2.3	2.8	3.3	3.9	142		2.5	3.5	4.6	5.8
144	1.7	2.2	2.7	3.2	3.8	144		2.5	3.4	4.5	5.7
146	1.6	2.2	2.6	3.2	3.7	146		2.4	3.3	4.4	5.6
148	1.6	2.1	2.6	3.1	3.6	148		2.4	3.2	4.3	5.4
150		2.0	2.5	3.0	3.5	150		2.3	3.2	4.2	5.3
152		2.0	2.5	2.9	3.4	152		2.3	3.1	4.1	5.2
154		2.0	2.4	2.8	3.3	154		2.2	3.0	4.0	5.1
156		1.9	2.3	2.8	3.2	156		2.2	2.9	4.0	5.0
158		1.8	2.3	2.7	3.1	158		2.1	2.9	3.9	4.9
160		1.8	2.2	2.6	3.0	160		2.1	2.8	3.8	4.8
162		1.8	2.2	2.6	3.0	162		2.0	2.8	3.7	4.6
164		1.7	2.1	2.5	2.9	164		2.0	2.7	3.6	4.5
166		1.7	2.1	2.5	2.8	166		1.9	2.7	3.6	4.5
168		1.6	2.0	2.4	2.8	168		1.9	2.6	3.5	4.4
170		1.6	2.0	2.4	2.7	170		1.8	2.6	3.4	4.3

Reprinted, by permission, from P.-O. Åstrand, 1979, *Work tests with the bicycle ergometer* (Varberg, Sweden: Monark Exercise AB), 24.

To calculate the corrected $\dot{V}O_2$max, the estimated $\dot{V}O_2$max is multiplied by the appropriate correction factor. For our 50-yr-old subject, the correction factor is 0.75, and the corrected $\dot{V}O_2$max is $0.75 \cdot 2.4\ L \cdot min^{-1} = 1.8\ L \cdot min^{-1}$. This value compares well with that estimated by the YMCA protocol. The Åstrand and Ryhming calculations can be simplified using formulas developed by Shephard (47).H

Submaximal Step-Test Protocol

A multistage step test can be used to estimate $\dot{V}O_2$max and to show changes in CRF resulting from training or detraining. As always, the initial stage and rate of progression of the stages must be suited to the individual. The subject must follow the metronome (4 counts per cycle, i.e., up-up-down-down) and step all the way up and all the way down. Each stage should last at least 2 min, with HR monitored in the last 30 sec of each 2 min. Using an HR watch simplifies the process of obtaining an accurate HR measure during a step test.

As in most submaximal GXT protocols, HR is plotted against work rate or $\dot{V}O_2$ for each stage, and a line is drawn through the points to the estimated maximal HR. A vertical line is then drawn to the baseline to estimate the step rate that would have been achieved if the subject had completed a ma ximal test. Figure 7.6 shows the results of a step test for a sedentary 55-yr-old man. His estimated maximal step rate was 40 steps · min^{-1}. The $\dot{V}O_2$max, calculated with the formula for stepping given in chapter 6, was 7.7 METs, or about 27 ml · kg^{-1} · min^{-1}. Please note that the mCAFT was presented earlier in the *Field Tests* section because it was originally designed for testing to be done in one's home. That said, the mCAFT is also well suited for a fitness setting.

KEY POINT

A plot of HR responses (>110 beats · min^{-1}) to a GXT on a treadmill, cycle ergometer, or bench step can be used to estimate $\dot{V}O_2$max. A line is drawn through the HR values and is extrapolated to the subject's age-predicted estimate of maximal HR. A vertical line is drawn to the x-axis to estimate the work rate and $\dot{V}O_2$the person would have achieved if the test had been a maximal test.

Posttest Procedures

When the test is over, the tester should conduct a cool-down, monitor test variables, and give posttest instructions. The tester should also organize the test data.

Posttest Protocol

1. Use an active cool-down procedure to help the participant transition back to rest:
   - Decrease intensity (e.g., grade on treadmill, load on cycle ergometer) and have participant do an active recovery for 3 min.
   - Monitor HR and BP during recovery and transition to sitting rest when the subject feels comfortable.
   - Monitor HR and BP at the end of 1 and 3 min of sitting rest.
   - Remove BP cuff and HR monitor when BP and HR are close to pretest values.
2. Provide instructions for showering:
   - The participant should wait about 30 min before showering.
   - The participant should move around in the shower and use warm (not hot) water.
   - Wait for the participant to return from the shower.
3. Have the participant make an appointment to discuss the results of all the fitness tests (e.g., body composition, muscular strength and endurance, CRF).

Name: ______ Age: 55 Estimated HRmax: 165 85% HRmax: 140

Step test protocol
Step height = 16 cm

Ht: ______
Wt: ______
Sex: Male

Step rate	Heart rate
12	100
18	115
24	128
30	142

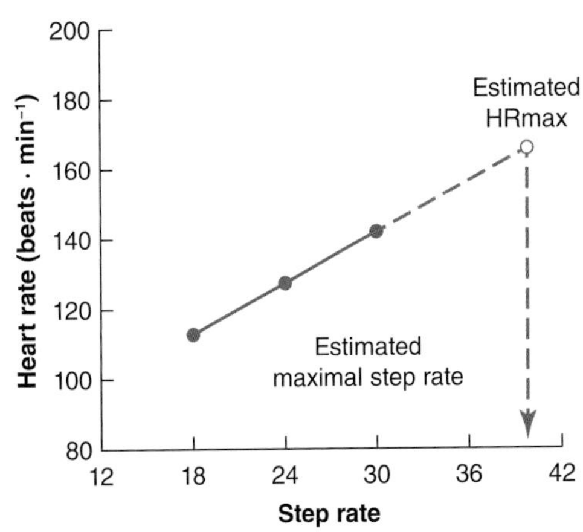

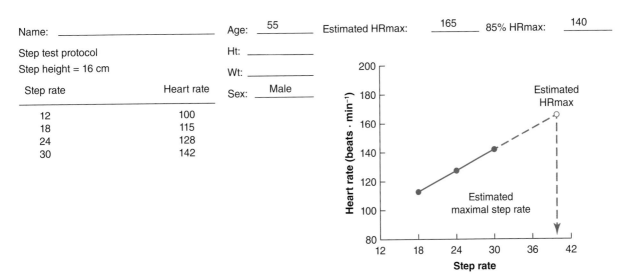

FIGURE 7.6 Maximal aerobic power estimated by measuring HR response to a submaximal graded exercise step test.

RESEARCH INSIGHT

Can $\dot{V}O_2$max Be Estimated Without Doing an Exercise Test?

This may seem like a strange question given the focus of this chapter on exercise testing. However, if it were possible, it would allow investigators (primarily epidemiologists) to easily classify large numbers of people into CRF categories (e.g., bottom 20%, middle 20%, and top 20%) and determine if CRF is linked to various chronic diseases. Doing exercise testing on such large populations would be impossible due to time, cost, personnel, and so on.

In one of the earliest investigations, Jackson and colleagues (31) showed that by using the simple variables of age, gender, body fatness or BMI, and self-reported physical activity, $\dot{V}O_2$max could be estimated with a SEE of ~5 ml · kg^{-1} · min^{-1}, an error similar to what we observe with field tests and submaximal GXT estimates of $\dot{V}O_2$max. The accuracy of the prediction (SEE ~4-6 ml · kg^{-1} · min^{-1}) has been confirmed in several other studies (26, 29, 37, 53, 57, 58). These models have been useful in placing subjects into fitness categories; however, the prediction is less accurate in the most and least fit subjects (53).

What does this say about doing exercise tests? As we mentioned at the outset, even though the SEE is relatively large for field tests and submaximal GXTs, the tests are reliable, and when the same person takes the same test over time, the change in estimated $\dot{V}O_2$max monitored by the test is a reasonable reflection of improvements in CRF. This can serve as both a motivational and an educational tool when working with fitness clients.

7

LEARNING AIDS

REVIEW QUESTIONS

1. What is the general relationship between CRF and chronic disease?
2. What is the logical sequence of steps to take leading up to a GXT?
3. You are using the 1 mi (1.6 km) walk test to track CRF over time, but you are not concerned with generating a $\dot{V}O_2$max value. If you wanted to provide good feedback to your client about fitness improvements being made, what two variables would you measure from this test? What would you expect to happen to them as fitness improves?
4. Why are running tests to estimate $\dot{V}O_2$max usually done for 12 min or so for adults? What would happen to the estimated $\dot{V}O_2$max value if an all-out 3 min run test were used?
5. What are some advantages and disadvantages of cycle ergometer tests compared with treadmill tests?
6. Why are clients asked to not eat, smoke, or drink caffeinated beverages in the hours before a submaximal GXT?
7. What is the difference between a submaximal and maximal GXT?
8. If submaximal GXT protocols have an inherent error associated with estimating $\dot{V}O_2$max, why do the test?
9. What investigators would be interested in estimating $\dot{V}O_2$max without exercise testing?

CASE STUDIES

1. You are contacted by a fitness club to review the test it uses to evaluate CRF in middle-aged participants. The club requires the participants to perform the 1.5 mi (2.4 km) run test during their first exercise session. The club director says he uses this test because, over the past decade, he has developed a good database to track clients. What is your reaction?

2. You conduct the 1 mi (1.6 km) walk test with a 45-yr-old male client and record the following information: Time = 15 min, HR = 140 beats · min^{-1}, and weight = 170 lb (77.1 kg). Calculate and evaluate his estimated $\dot{V}O_2$max.
3. A 50-yr-old male weighing 180 lb (81.7 kg) completes a submaximal GXT on a cycle ergometer, and the following data are obtained:

kgm · min^{-1}	**HR**
300	100
450	110
600	125
750	140

Estimate the subject's $\dot{V}O_2$max using the extrapolation procedure. Express the value in METs.

4. A 30-yr-old woman weighing 120 lb (54.4 kg) completes four stages of a submaximal Balke treadmill test at 3 mi · hr^{-1} (4.8 km · hr^{-1}), and the following data are obtained:

% Grade	**HR**
2.5	96
5.0	120
7.5	135
10.0	150

Estimate the subject's $\dot{V}O_2$max using the extrapolation method and express it in ml · kg^{-1} · min^{-1}, L · min^{-1}, and METs.

5. A Monark cycle ergometer is calibrated with 0.5, 1.0, 1.5, and 2.0 kg weights, and each of the values is 0.25 kg too high on the scale. What could have caused this?

Answers to Case Studies

1. Requiring sedentary middle-aged participants to take a maximal, unmonitored test at the beginning of their fitness program is inappropriate. You might suggest the club replace the 1.5 mi (2.4 km) run with the 1 mi (1.6 km) walk test, which should be used after the participants have demonstrated that they can comfortably walk 1 mi.
2. His estimated $\dot{V}O_2$max is 37.8 ml · kg^{-1} · min^{-1}. In terms of group comparisons, his level of CRF is "fair," and just short of "good" for his age group. However, his value indicates that he has a low risk of chronic disease and death from all causes.
3. The HR response of 100 beats · min^{-1} at the work rate of 300 kgm · min^{-1} should be ignored. The HR values are extrapolated to 170 beats · min^{-1}, and the vertical line dropped from that point indicates a work rate of about 1,050 kgm · min^{-1},

$$\dot{V}O_2 = \frac{(1050\ \text{kpm} \cdot \text{min}^{-1} \cdot 1.8\ \text{ml O}_2 \cdot \text{kpm}^{-1})}{81.7\ \text{kg}} + 7\ \text{ml} \cdot \text{kg}^{-1} \cdot \text{min}^{-1}$$

$$= \frac{30.1\ \text{ml} \cdot \text{kg}^{-1} \cdot \text{min}^{-1}}{3.5\ \text{ml} \cdot \text{kg}^{-1} \cdot \text{min}^{-1}} = 8.6\ \text{METs}$$

4. The HR value of 96 beats · min $^{-1}$ should be ignored. The line is extrapolated to 190 beats · min^{-1}, and the vertical line dropped from that point indicates a value of about 16.75% grade, which equals a $\dot{V}O_2$ of about 35.6 ml · kg · min^{-1}. This is 10.2 METs, or 1.94 L · min^{-1}.
5. The reference point for the scale is the zero point established when the free-swinging pendulum stops (with the cycle on a flat surface). All scale values are relative to this zero, and if the zero is off, all scale readings are off. If the pendulum does not rest at zero when no weight is attached, the entire scale is off by the amount the zero value is off by. For example, if the scale reads 0.25 kg when no weight is attached, each scale value shifts 0.25 kg upward when known weights are attached.

7

APPENDIX 7.1: CONSENT FORM

The following is an example of a general consent form for exercise testing. The consent form you use should be developed and approved by administrative personnel associated with the setting in which you work (see chapter 26).

Sample Informed Consent for Fitness Test Participation

Testing objectives: In order to more safely participate in an exercise program, I hereby consent, voluntarily, to a series of exercise tests. Each test will assist in the determination of my overall physical fitness and will assess the following: cardiorespiratory fitness, body composition, muscular strength and endurance, and flexibility. I shall perform a graded exercise test (GXT) by walking on a treadmill or riding a cycle ergometer. The GXT will begin at a low level and gradually increase in difficulty until my target heart rate is achieved. The test may be stopped at any time because of feelings of significant fatigue or for any other personal reason. Body composition will be determined using skinfold tests. Muscular strength and endurance will be assessed with proper resistance training equipment. A sit-and-reach test will ascertain the flexibility of the hip joint.

Risk and discomforts: I understand that the risks of the GXT or other test procedures may include abnormal heart rhythms, abnormal blood pressure response, fainting, and very rarely a heart attack. Every professional effort will be made to minimize these risks through proper administration of a completed health status questionnaire (HSQ) as well as assessment of relevant health questions and supervision during the tests.

Responsibilities of the participant: I acknowledge that I have completed the HSQ and answered any attendant health questions accurately. During the GXT or other tests, I will report any heart-related symptom (i.e., pain, pressure, tightness, or heaviness in the chest, neck, jaw, back, or arms) immediately. I have reported all medications (including nonprescription medications) taken on a regular basis, including today, to the appropriate staff member.

Benefits to be expected: I desire to pursue a GXT and additional fitness tests so that I may obtain better advice regarding my present level of cardiorespiratory fitness and overall physical fitness. This information will be used to prescribe an appropriate individualized exercise program. I understand that this test does not entirely eliminate risk in the proposed exercise program.

Inquiries: I understand that I can withdraw my consent or discontinue participation in any aspect of the fitness testing at any time without penalty or prejudice toward me. I have read the above statements and have had all of my questions answered to my satisfaction.

Use of medical records: I have been informed that the information obtained from the fitness tests is privileged and confidential as described in the Health Insurance Portability and Accountability Act of 1996 (HIPAA). It will not be disclosed to anyone other than my physician or individuals responsible for designing and supervising my exercise program without my express written permission.

______________________________ Signature of participant	______________________ Date
______________________________ Signature of witness	______________________ Date

From E.T. Howley and D.L. Thompson, 2017, *Fitness professional's handbook,* 7th ed. (Champaign, IL: Human Kinetics).

APPENDIX 7.2: TREADMILL SPEED AND ELEVATION SETTINGS

To calibrate a measuring device is to check its accuracy by comparing it with a known standard and adjusting the device so that it provides an accurate reading. These are suggestions only and should not be viewed as substitutes for the specific procedures recommended by the equipment manufacturers (30). The speed and grade settings on the treadmill must be calibrated because they determine physiological demand and are crucial in estimating CRF. These procedures should be used routinely to maintain test validity and reliability over time. A chart should be posted near each piece of equipment indicating when the calibration was done and by whom.

Calibrating Speed

An easy way to calibrate the speed on any treadmill is to measure the length of the belt and count the number of belt revolutions in a certain amount of time. To calibrate treadmill speed, follow these steps (30):

1. Measure the exact length of the belt in meters.
    - Place a meter stick on the belt surface and mark a starting point.
    - Advance the belt by hand, marking the belt 1 m at a time until you return to the starting point; record the value for belt length.
2. Place a small piece of tape near the edge of the belt surface.
3. Turn on the treadmill to a given speed by using the speed control.
4. Count 20 revolutions of the belt while tracking time with a stopwatch. Start your watch as the tape first moves past the fixed point, beginning the count with 0.
5. Convert the number of revolutions to revolutions per minute ($rev \cdot min^{-1}$). For example, if the belt made 20 complete revolutions in 35 sec, then

$$35 \text{ sec} \div 60 \text{ sec} \cdot \text{min}^{-1} = 0.583 \text{ min.}$$

$$20 \text{ rev} \div 0.583 \text{ min} = 34.3 \text{ rev} \cdot \text{min}^{-1}.$$

6. Multiply the calculated revolutions per minute (step 5) times the belt length (step 1). This gives the belt speed in meters per minute ($m \cdot min^{-1}$).

For example, if the belt length is 5.025 m, then

$$34.3 \text{ rev} \cdot \text{min}^{-1} \cdot 5.025 \text{ m} \cdot \text{rev}^{-}$$
$$= 172.35 \text{ m} \cdot \text{min}^{-1}.$$

7. To convert meters per minute to miles per hour, divide the answer in step 6 by 26.8 $(m \cdot min^{-1}) \cdot (mi \cdot hr^{-1})^{-1}$:

$$\frac{172.35 \text{ m} \cdot \text{min}^{-1}}{26.8\ ([\text{m} \cdot \text{min}^{-1}] \cdot [\text{mi} \cdot \text{hr}^{-1}]^{-1})} = 6.43 \text{ mi} \cdot \text{hr}^{-1}$$

8. The value obtained in step 7 is the actual treadmill speed in miles per hour. If the speed indicator does not agree with this value, adjust the dial to the proper reading. Check the instruction manual for the location of the speed adjustment.
9. Repeat for a number of speeds to ensure accuracy across the speeds used in test protocols.

Calibrating Elevation

Treadmill manuals describe how to calibrate the grade using a simple carpenter's level and a square edge:

1. Use a carpenter's level to make sure that the treadmill is level, and check the zero setting on the grade meter under these conditions (with the treadmill electronics turned on). If the meter does not read zero, follow instructions to make the adjustment (usually by using the small screw on the face of the dial).
2. Elevate the treadmill so that the percentage grade dial reads approximately 20%. Measure the exact incline of the treadmill as shown in figure 7.7. When the bubble is exactly in the center of the tube in the level, the rise measurement is obtained.
3. Calculate the grade from the rise over the run and adjust the treadmill meter to read that exact grade. For example, if the rise is 4.5 in. (11.4 cm) and the run is 22.5 in. (57.2 cm), the fractional grade is calculated as follows:

$$\text{Grade} = \text{tangent } \Theta = \text{rise} \div \text{run}$$
$$= 4.5 \text{ in.} \div 22.5 \text{ in.} = 0.20 = 20\%.$$

1. The rise-over-run method is a typical engineering method for calculating grade, giving the tangent of the angle (the opposite side divided by the adjacent side of the right triangle, as shown in figure 7.7). Although the sine of the

angle (opposite side divided by the hypotenuse) provides the most accurate setting of grade, table 7.8 shows that the tangent value is a good approximation of the sine value for grades less than 20%, or 12°. The rise-over-run method can also be used to calibrate steep grades: Obtain the tangent value as described previously and simply look across table 7.8 to obtain the correct sine value to set on the treadmill dial. For example, if the rise-over-run method yielded 0.268, or 26.8% (tangent), the correct setting would be 25.9% (sine). The latter value is set on the grade dial of the treadmill.

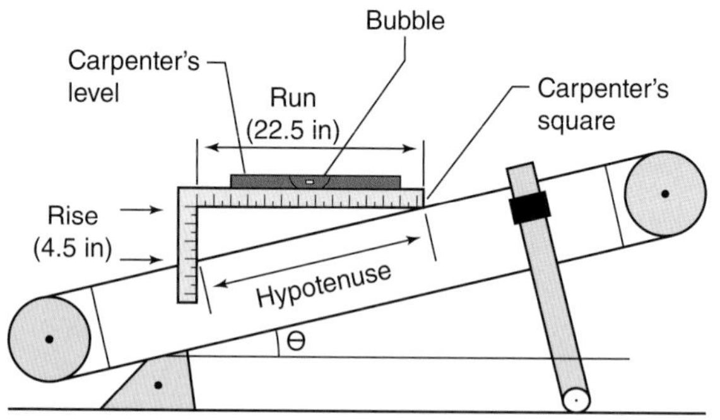

FIGURE 7.7 Calibrating grade using the tangent method (rise ÷ run) with a carpenter's square and level.

Adapted from Howley 1988.

Table 7.8 Natural Sines and Tangents

Degrees	Sine	Grade (%)	Tangent	Grade (%)
0	0.0000	0.0	0.0000	0.0
1	0.0175	1.7	0.0750	1.7
2	0.0349	3.5	0.0349	3.5
3	0.0523	5.2	0.0524	5.2
4	0.0698	7.0	0.0699	7.0
5	0.0872	8.7	0.0875	8.7
6	0.1045	10.4	0.1051	10.5
7	0.1219	12.2	0.1228	12.3
8	0.1392	13.9	0.1405	14.0
9	0.1564	15.6	0.1584	15.8
10	0.1736	17.4	0.1763	17.6
11	0.1908	19.1	0.1944	19.4
12	0.2079	20.8	0.2126	21.3
13	0.2250	22.5	0.2309	23.1
14	0.2419	24.2	0.2493	24.9
15	0.2588	25.9	0.2679	26.8
20	0.3420	34.2	0.3640	36.4
25	0.4067	40.7	0.4452	44.5

Reprinted, by permission, from E.T. Howley, 1988, The exercise testing laboratory. In *Resource manual for guidelines for exercise testing and prescription*, edited by S.N. Blair et al. (Philadelphia, PA: Lea & Febiger), 409.

APPENDIX 7.3: CALIBRATING THE CYCLE ERGOMETER

To calibrate a measuring device is to check its accuracy by comparing it with a known standard and adjusting the device so that it provides an accurate reading. These are suggestions only and should not be viewed as substitutes for the specific procedures recommended by the equipment manufacturers. The cycle ergometer must be calibrated routinely to ensure that the work rate is accurate. Altering either the pedal rate or the load on the wheel varies the work rate on the mechanically braked cycle ergometer. Work equals force times the distance through which the force acts: $w = f \cdot d$. The kilopond (kp), defined as the force acting on a mass of 1 kg at the normal acceleration of gravity, is the proper unit for force. However, the kilopond and the kilogram typically are used interchangeably in exercise testing.

On a mechanically braked cycle ergometer, the force (kilograms of weight on the wheel) is moved through a distance (in meters), so work is expressed in kilogram-meters (kgm). Because work is accomplished over time (e.g., minutes), the activity is referred to as a *work rate* or *power output* ($\text{kgm} \cdot \text{min}^{-1}$), not a *workload.* On the Monark cycle ergometer, a point on the rim of the wheel travels 6 m per pedal revolution, so at 50 $\text{rev} \cdot \text{min}^{-1}$, the wheel travels 300 $\text{m} \cdot \text{min}^{-1}$. If a weight of 1 kg is hanging from that wheel, the work rate, or power output, is 300 $\text{kgm} \cdot \text{min}^{-1}$. From these simple calculations you can see the importance of maintaining a correct pedal rate during the test—if the subject pedals at 60 $\text{rev} \cdot \text{min}^{-1}$, the work rate is actually 20% higher (360 versus 300 $\text{kgm} \cdot \text{min}^{-1}$) than it appears to be. The force setting (resistance on the wheel) also must be carefully set and checked because it tends to drift as the test progresses. It is crucial that the force (resistance) values on the scale are correct. The following four steps outline the procedure for calibrating the Monark cycle ergometer scale (5) (refer to figure 7.8).

1. Disconnect the belt at the spring.
2. Loosen the lock nut and use the adjusting screw on the front of the bike against which the force scale rests so that the vertical mark on the pendulum weight matches with 0 kp on the weight scale (see figure 7.8*a).* The pendulum must be swinging freely. Lock the adjustment screw with the lock nut. To keep the calibration weights from touching the flywheel, it may be easier to elevate the rear of the ergometer (with a 2×4 board on edge), set the zero as described previously, and proceed to the next step.
3. Suspend a 4.0 kg weight from the spring so that it's not in contact with the flywheel, and see if the pendulum moves to the 4.0 kp mark (see figure 7.8*b).* If it doesn't, alter the position or size of the adjusting weight in the pendulum (see figure 7.8*c).* By loosening the lock screw on the back of the pendulum weight, the adjusting weight can be lowered, raised, or replaced. Check the force scale again and calibrate the ergometer through the range of values used in your tests. If you used the 2×4 to elevate the rear of the ergometer, remove it and reset the zero as described in step 2.
4. Reassemble the cycle ergometer.

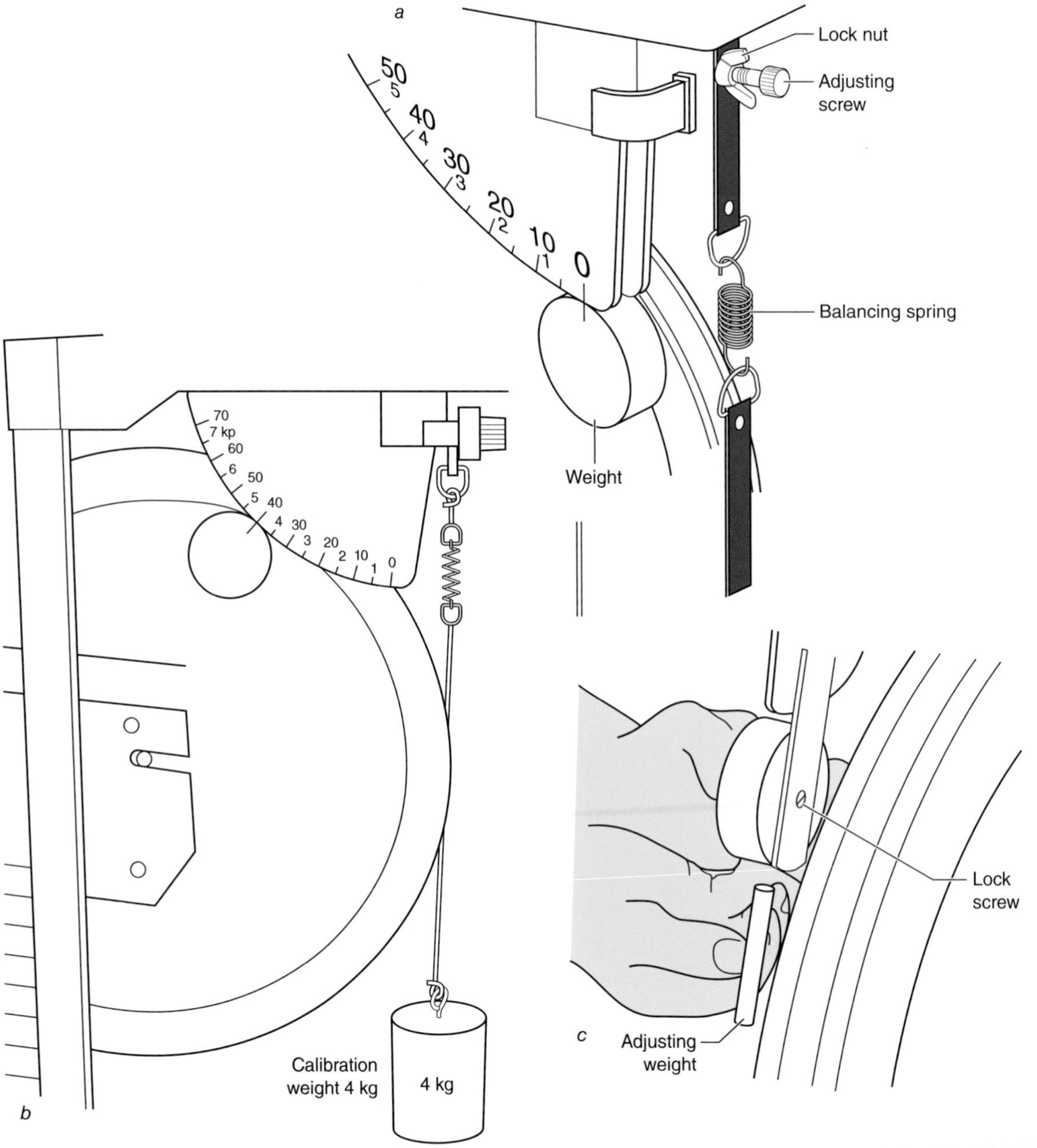

FIGURE 7.8 Calibrating the Monark cycle ergometer. *(a)* Adjust the pendulum to align with zero, *(b)* suspend a 4.0 kg weight from the spring, and *(c)* adjust the position or size of the weight in the pendulum.

Adapted, by permission, from Monark Sports and Medical, *Instruction manual, Monark model 818E* (Varberg, Sweden: Monark Exercise AB), 18.

APPENDIX 7.4: CALIBRATING THE SPHYGMOMANOMETER

To calibrate a measuring device is to check its accuracy by comparing it with a known standard and adjusting the device so that it provides an accurate reading. These are suggestions only and should not be viewed as substitutes for the specific procedures recommended by the equipment manufacturers. A **sphygmomanometer** is a BP measurement system composed of an inflatable rubber bladder, an instrument that indicates the applied pressure, an inflation bulb that creates pressure, and an adjustable valve that deflates the system. The cuff and the measuring instrument are the most important for measurement accuracy. The cuff should be about 20% wider than the diameter of the limb to which it is applied, and when inflated, the bladder should not cause a bulging or displacement. If the bladder is too wide, BP will be underestimated; if it is too narrow, BP will be overestimated. Consequently, it is important to match cuff size to the subject being measured.

The device measuring the pressure, the manometer, can be a mercury or an aneroid type. The mercury type is the standard, and its calibration is easily maintained. The mercury column should rise and fall smoothly, form a clear meniscus, and read zero when the bladder is deflated. If the mercury sticks in the tube, remove the cap and swab out the inside. If it is very dirty, the tube should be removed and cleaned (with detergent, a water rinse, and alcohol for drying). If the mercury column falls below zero, add mercury to bring the meniscus exactly to the zero mark (12, 25, 30). Special care must be taken when handling toxic materials such as mercury; follow your institution's guidelines.

The aneroid gauge uses a metal bellows assembly that expands when pressure is applied, and the expansion moves the pointer on the indicator dial. A spring attached to the pointer moves the pointer downscale to zero when the bladder is deflated. This gauge should be calibrated at least once every 6 mo in a variety of settings using the mercury column just described. A simple Y tube (from the stethoscope) is used to connect the two systems (see figure 7.9). Readings should be taken with pressure falling to simulate the readings taken during an actual measurement (30).

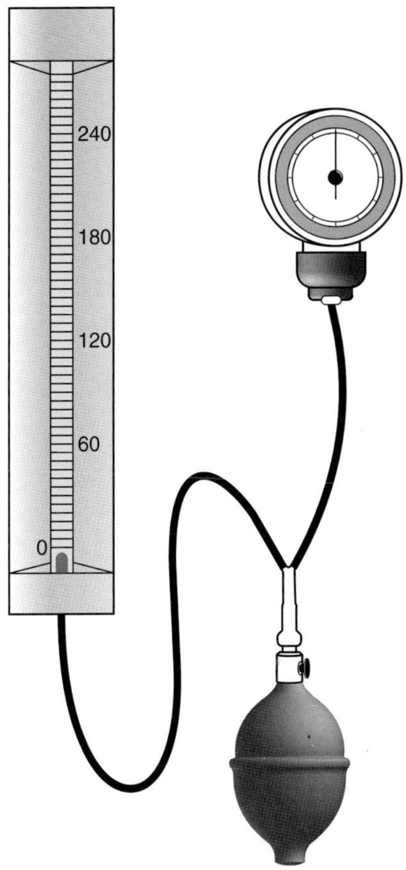

FIGURE 7.9 Calibrating an aneroid manometer with a mercury manometer.

8

Assessment of Body Composition

Dixie L. Thompson

OBJECTIVES

The reader will be able to do the following:

1. Discuss how body composition affects health and describe the health implications of various patterns of body-fat distribution.
2. Compare and contrast hydrostatic weighing, air displacement plethysmography, bioelectrical impedance analysis (BIA), and skinfold measurement as means for estimating body composition.
3. Identify common measurement sites for skinfolds and girths.
4. Calculate and interpret BMI.
5. Assess body composition using a variety of techniques and describe the advantages and disadvantages of these techniques.

American media are filled with advertisements for programs designed to help people improve their health and fitness. Often the primary focus of these programs is weight loss. A healthy body weight and an appropriate amount of body fat are important aspects of physical fitness, and fitness professionals need to understand the importance of appropriate body composition, become aware of the various means for assessing body fat, and become proficient at estimating body fat through skinfold and girth measurements. As with other aspects of fitness assessment, paying attention to detail and gaining experience with the techniques are necessary in order to become proficient at estimating body fatness. This chapter is meant to assist fitness professionals in acquiring these skills.

Health and Body Composition

Body composition describes the component tissues of the body and is most often used to refer to the relative percentages of fat and fat-free tissues. **Fat-free mass (FFM)**, **fat mass (FM)**, and **percent body fat (%BF)** are the most frequently reported values in a body composition assessment. *Percent body fat* refers to the percentage of the total body mass that is composed of fat:

$$\%BF = (\text{fat mass} \div \text{body mass}) \cdot 100\%.$$

Fat-free mass refers to the mass of the fat-free tissues of the body and often is used synonymously with the term **lean body mass**. Table 8.1 lists suggested age-based %BFs (23). Body composition is a vital aspect of overall fitness because of the ill effects related to excessively low or high body fatness. Various techniques are used to assess body composition, and fitness professionals should be skilled in their use.

Table 8.1 Age-Based Body-Fat Percentage Standards for Adults

Men	Recommended range[a]
18-34 yr	8-22
35-55 yr	10-25
56 yr or older	10-25
Women	**Recommended range[a]**
18-34 yr	20-35
35-55 yr	23-38
56 yr or older	25-38

[a]Values are %BF levels considered generally healthy.

Based on Ratamess 2014.

Obesity is a condition in which a person has excess **adipose tissue**, or fat tissue. It may be classified either by %BF or by the relationship of height and weight (see the section on BMI later in the chapter). Although there are no uniform standards for body-fat percentages, a %BF of >38% for females and >25% for males generally is considered in the obese range (23). According to BMI standards, obesity is a value ≥30 kg · m^{-2} (3). **Overweight**, a BMI between 25 and 29.9 kg · m^{-2}, is the condition in which a person is above the recommended weight range but is not yet in the obese category. The **prevalence** of obesity and overweight among American adults and children increased dramatically during the latter half of the 20th century. Estimates from 2011 to 2012 show that approximately 35% of American adults and 17% of American children are obese (20). This is in sharp contrast with statistics from the 1960s, when less than 15% of American adults were obese (5).

Obesity has been causally linked with numerous negative health consequences, including coronary artery disease (CAD), hypertension, stroke, type 2 diabetes, increased risk of various cancers, osteoarthritis, sleep apnea, and dyslipidemia (3). In 2008, nearly $150 billion in health care spending was attributed to overweight and obesity (7). A recent review of previous studies concluded that obesity, particularly extreme obesity, is linked with a higher all-cause mortality (8). Because of the link between obesity and poor health, fitness professionals must provide clients with an accurate assessment of this important fitness component.

When people gain excess fat, genetics determines where the adipose tissue accumulates. Researchers are quite interested in learning how **body-fat distribution**, or **fat patterning**, affects health. **Android-type obesity** (i.e., male-pattern obesity, apple shape) refers to the excessive storage of fat in the trunk and abdominal areas. Excessive fat in the hips and thighs is labeled **gynoid-type obesity** (i.e., female-pattern obesity, pear shape). In terms of negative health consequences, android-type obesity appears to be the most dangerous, and it is closely linked with disease (3). **Waist-to-hip ratio (WHR)** can be a useful tool for differentiating gynoid-type and android-type obesity. Waist circumference also is used to classify excessive trunk fat. Descriptions of how to take these measurements are presented later in this chapter.

Just as excessive body fat can be unhealthy, too little body fat also can compromise health. Among the many important roles of fat in human health are providing energy, helping with temperature regulation, and cushioning the joints. The minimum level of body fat needed to maintain health varies among individuals and depends on sex and genetics. The %BF thought to be necessary for good health, also known as **essential fat**, is 8% to 12% for women and 3% to 5% for men (23). Infertility, depression, impaired temperature regulation, and early death are among the outcomes of excessive weight loss. Extreme fat loss results from starvation imposed by internal or external forces. Eating disorders that result in self-starvation are discussed in chapter 12. Because of the important link between health and body composition, a client's body fat should be analyzed during physical fitness assessments.

KEY POINT

The prevalence of obesity in the United States is 35% for adults and 17% for children. Significant health consequences (e.g., CVD, type 2 diabetes) may result from obesity. Disease risk is linked more closely with android-type obesity (apple shape) than with gynoid-type obesity (pear shape). Too little body fat also can lead to negative health outcomes.

Methods for Assessing Body Composition

Numerous techniques have been used to estimate body composition. None of the methods currently used actually measures %BF; the only way to truly measure the volume of fat in the body would be to dissect and chemically analyze tissues in the body. The techniques routinely used to estimate %BF are based on the relationship between %BF and other factors that can be accurately measured, such as skinfold thicknesses or underwater weight. Because of the predictable relationship between the measured value and body composition, %BF can be estimated through these indirect methods.

Each of the techniques described in the following sections has advantages and disadvantages. Knowing these characteristics will help you decide wisely when choosing the method for body composition assessment. A comparison of important considerations can be found in table 8.2. For fitness professionals, ease of measurement, relative accuracy, and cost are the primary considerations when choosing a technique. In other situations (for research or clinical applications), the accuracy of the measurement may outweigh other considerations. A recent review of techniques endorsed by the AHA provides greater detail about assessment of body composition (3).

Body Mass Index

A widely used clinical assessment of the appropriateness of a person's weight is the anthropometric calculation of the **body mass index (BMI)**, or Quetelet index. This value is calculated by dividing the weight in kilograms by height in meters squared. BMI is a quick and easy method for determining if body weight is appropriate for body height. Table 8.3 lists the adult BMI categories. In the past, height–weight charts were used for this purpose, but BMI is currently the accepted method for interpreting the height–weight relationship. BMI does not differentiate between fat and fat-free weight, which is problematic when testing athletic individuals with a large lean mass. For example, a football linebacker who is 6 ft 2 in. (1.9 m) and weighs 220 lb (100 kg) is considered overweight according to BMI standards (BMI = 28.3 $kg \cdot m^{-2}$), when in fact he may have a very low %BF. On the other hand, an inactive person with a similar height and weight is probably carrying excess adipose tissue. Additionally, although BMI standards are applied to adults without regard to age, race, sex, or ethnicity, the relationship between BMI and body-fat percentage varies among groups (3). For example, African American women have a lower body-fat percentage

Table 8.2 Comparison of Common Body Composition Techniques

	Equipment cost	Time required	Technician expertise	Day-to-day variation	Accuracy
Skinfold measurement	*	**	**	*	**
Hydrostatic weighing	***	***	***	*	***
BIA	* to **	*	*	**	**
Dual-energy X-ray absorptiometry	***	*	***	*	***
Air displacement plethysmography	***	*	*	*	***

* = low; ** = moderate; *** = high.

at a given BMI than similarly aged white American women do. Because of group differences in the relationship between BMI and body-fat percentage, some have argued that a different BMI standard should be applied to Asian adults, but this has not been universally accepted.

Even with its limitations, for most adults there is a clear correlation between elevated BMI and negative health consequences (3). The recommended BMI range is 18.5 to 24.9 kg · m^{-2}. Overweight is classified as a BMI of 25 to 29.9 kg · m^{-2}, and a BMI of 30 kg · m^{-2} or higher is considered obese (1, 3, 23). In screening situations where estimating body fat is impossible or impractical, BMI can be useful for providing feedback to people about the appropriateness of their body weight. It is important to note that BMI standards for children are age and sex specific (21, 22). Children at the 95th percentile or greater for their age and sex are considered obese. Consult the CDC growth charts for BMI standards for children (22).

Girth Measurements

Several girth measurements (body and limb circumferences) are used to either estimate body composition or describe body proportions. Girth measurements provide quick and reliable information. They are sometimes used in equations to predict body composition and may also be used to track changes in body shape and size during weight loss. The major disadvantage is that they provide little information about the fat and fat-free components of the body. For example, a bodybuilder's thigh can have a larger circumference yet less fat than that of a person who is obese. A list of several commonly measured girths follows; refer to *ACSM's Guidelines for Exercise Testing and Prescription* (1) for additional circumference sites.

- Waist—narrowest part of the torso between the xiphoid process and the umbilicus
- Abdomen—circumference of the torso at the height of the iliac crest
- Hips—maximal circumference of the buttocks above the gluteal fold
- Thigh—largest circumference of the right thigh below the gluteal fold

WHR is a frequently used clinical application of girth measurements. This value is often used to reflect the degree of abdominal, or android-type, obesity. A WHR greater than 0.95 for young men or 0.86 for young women is associated with elevated health risks. For men and women 60 to 69 yr old, a WHR of >1.03 and >0.9, respectively, is linked with disease risk (1). There have been mixed findings on the use of ratios, such as WHR, for predicting disease risk; thus, the use of waist circumference (WC) is often preferred (3).

WC alone can also provide valuable information about disease risk (1, 3). A WC of greater than 102 cm (40 in.) in men or 88 cm (35 in.) in women significantly increases the risk of obesity-related disease (1). ACSM now uses BMI and WC as the techniques for establishing obesity risk classification (1).

When assessing girths, use the following procedures to standardize the measurements:

- Make sure the measuring tape is horizontal when measuring trunk circumference and is perpendicular to the long axis of the limb when measuring limbs. Use either a mirror or an assistant to help ensure that the tape is placed properly.
- Apply constant pressure to the tape without pinching the skin. Use a tape measure fitted with a handle that indicates the amount of tension exerted.
- When measuring limbs, measure on the right side of the body. Alternatively, measure on both sides and record the values for both right and left.
- Ensure that the person stands erect, relaxed, and with feet together.
- When measuring girths of the trunk, take the measurement after the person exhales and before the next breath begins.

Table 8.3 Body Mass Index Classification

Classification	BMI (kg · m^{-2})
Underweight	<18.5
Normal	18.5-24.9
Overweight	25.0-29.9
Obesity	
Grade 1	30.0-34.9
Grade 2	35.0-39.9
Grade 3 (extreme obesity)	≥40.0

Based on National Heart, Lung, and Blood Institute 1998; Cornier et al. 2011.

Skinfold Measurements

Measuring skinfold thickness is one of the most frequently performed tests to estimate %BF. This quick, noninvasive, inexpensive method can provide a fairly accurate assessment of %BF. The value obtained by skinfold measurement is typically within 3.5% of the value measured with underwater weighing (23). Skinfold measurement is based on the assumption that, as a person gains adipose tissue, the increase in skinfold thickness is proportional to the additional fat weight.

Because of the widespread use of skinfold measurement, fitness professionals should master the skills involved. Accurately assessing skinfold thickness requires the correct performance of several steps: locating the skinfold site, pinching the skinfold away from the underlying tissue, measuring with the caliper, and choosing the proper equation. The following sections address these concerns.

VIDEO Watch **videos 8.1** through **8.7**, which demonstrate skinfold measurements.

Locating the Skinfold Site

It is critical to accurately determine the site of the skinfold measurement. To increase the accuracy of the measurement, especially for the inexperienced technician, the site should be located and then marked with a washable marker. This helps ensure that the calipers are placed in the correct position each time the skinfold is measured. All skinfold measurements should be taken on the right side of the body unless otherwise specified. Refer to table 8.4 and figure 8.1 for some of the most commonly used measurement sites. For a more complete description of determining skinfold sites, refer to the *Anthropometric Standardization Reference Manual* (18) or ACSM resources (1, 23). Measuring skinfolds immediately after exercise should be avoided because exercise can shift fluid volume, leading to inaccurate results.

Pinching the Skinfold

Once the correct location for the skinfold measurement is determined, the tester gently but firmly pinches and lifts the skinfold away from the underlying muscle in order to measure it. The following are guidelines for measuring skinfolds correctly:

1. Place the fingers perpendicular to the skinfold approximately 1 cm from the site to be measured.
2. Gently yet firmly pinch the skinfold between the thumb and the first two fingers and lift away from the underlying tissues. Place the jaws of the caliper perpendicular to the skinfold at the measurement site. The jaws of the caliper should be halfway between the bottom and top of the fold. Maintain the pinch while taking the measurement.
3. Read the measurement on the caliper 1 to 2 sec after the jaws contact the skin.
4. Wait at least 15 sec before taking a subsequent measurement. To allow time for the fold to return to normal, take one measurement at each site and then repeat measurements. If the second measurement varies by more than 1 to 2 mm, repeat the measurement a third time.

Measuring the skinfolds of people who are obese can be difficult, if not impossible. If the jaws of the caliper will not open wide enough to measure the skinfold, use an alternative method for assessing body composition. Girth measurements for predicting %BF (26, 27) along with BMI, WC, and WHR may be used instead for people who are obese.

Measuring With the Caliper

Skinfold thickness is measured with a skinfold caliper. The numerous commercially available calipers vary in price and accuracy. Lange and Harpenden calipers are the ones most

Table 8.4 Commonly Used Skinfold Sites

Skinfold site	Description
Abdomen	Measure the vertical fold 2 cm to the right of and level with the umbilicus. Make sure the head of the caliper is not in the umbilicus.
Triceps	Measure the vertical fold over the belly of the triceps muscle. The arm should be relaxed. The specific site is the posterior midline of the upper arm, half the distance between the acromion and olecranon processes.
Chest	Measure a diagonal fold along the natural line of the skin one-half (men) or one-third (women) the distance between the anterior axillary line and the nipple.
Midaxillary	Measure the vertical fold at the level of the xiphoid process on the midaxillary line.
Subscapular	Measure 2 cm below the inferior angle of the scapula along the diagonal fold at a 45° angle.
Suprailiac	Measure the diagonal fold in line with the natural angle of the iliac crest. Measure along the anterior axillary line just above the iliac crest.
Thigh	Measure the vertical fold over the quadriceps muscle on the midline of the thigh. Measure half the distance between the top of the patella and the inguinal crease. The leg should be relaxed.

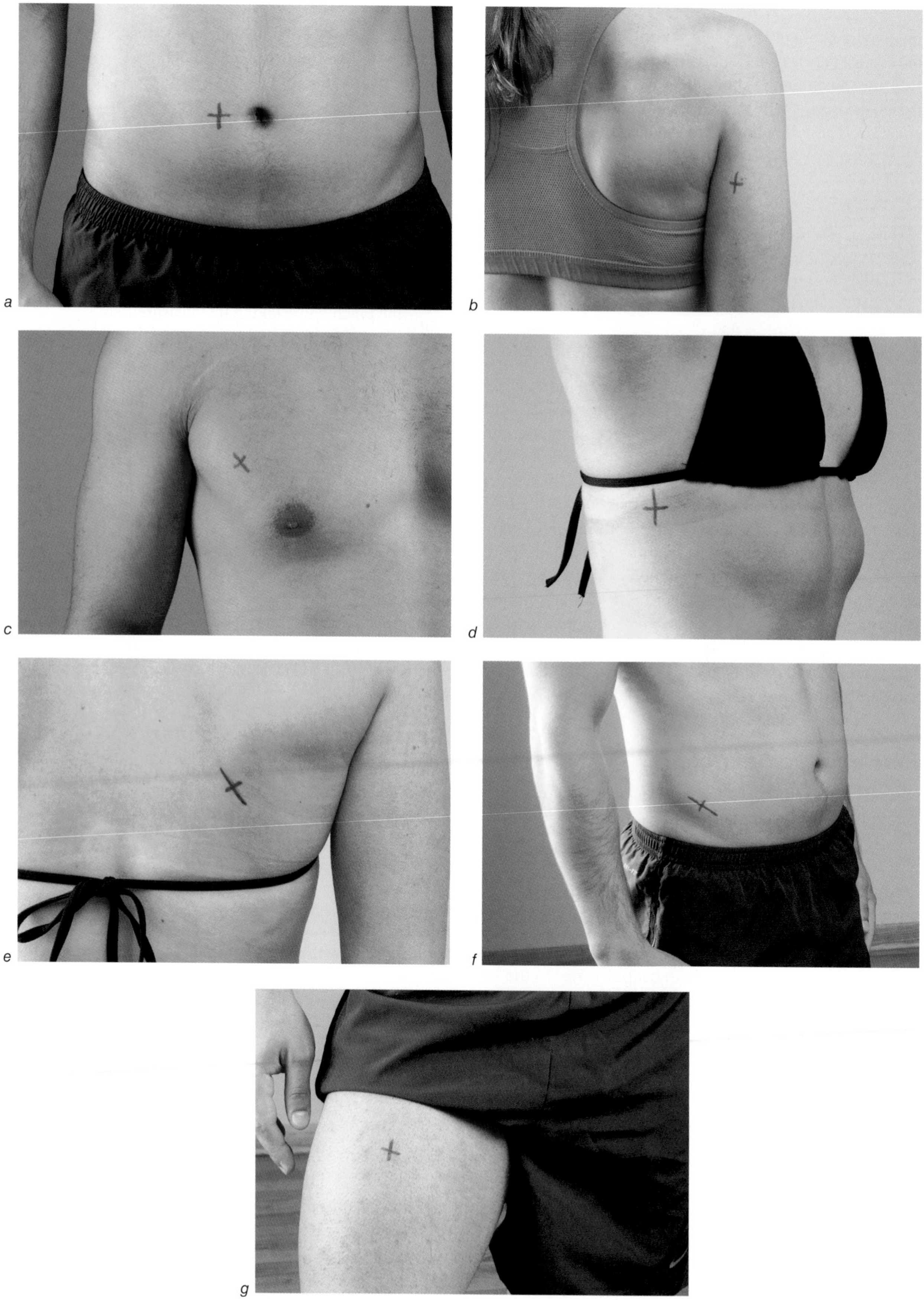

FIGURE 8.1 Common skinfold testing sites include the *(a)* abdomen, *(b)* triceps, *(c)* chest, *(d)* midaxillary, *(e)* subscapular, *(f)* suprailiac, and *(g)* thigh.

often used in research settings because of their precision and reliability; however, other calipers may also be used effectively (2). Obviously, if the calipers do not measure skinfolds accurately, they will compromise the estimate of body fat. Measure with calipers that closely match those used in the development of the equation you are using.

Choosing the Proper Equation

Most skinfold equations were developed using underwater weighing as the criterion method and actually are designed to estimate body density. To develop skinfold equations, the body density of many people was measured (typically using hydrostatic weighing), and these values were compared with skinfold thickness through a statistical method called *regression analysis*. This statistical technique results in the development of an equation that reflects the relationship between skinfolds and body density. Inserting a client's skinfold measurements (and sometimes other information such as age) into these equations produces an estimate of the client's body density. Body density then is converted to %BF by using a two-compartment model equation such as the Siri equation, described later in this chapter.

Both generalized and population-specific skinfold equations have been developed (13, 23). Generalized equations estimate body composition in groups of people who vary greatly in age, body composition, and fitness. An advantage of these equations is that they can be used to estimate body composition in most people; however, the equations lose accuracy when testing individuals who are dissimilar to those used to develop the equations. These equations are also less accurate for people at either end of the fatness continuum.

Population-specific equations predict body composition in a particular subgroup of the population, such as female runners. The advantage of using population-specific equations is that they tend to have higher accuracy when testing people who fit the physical profile of those in the subgroup of interest.

Because sex influences the areas where fat is stored, separate skinfold equations for men and women have been developed. The Jackson and Pollock (12) equations for men and the Jackson, Pollock, and Ward (14) equations for women are generalized equations that are used widely. Note that the client's age is used in these equations. This

Equations for Estimating Body Density From Skinfold Thicknesses

Women: Three Sites

$$D_b = 1.0994921 - 0.0009929\ (X1) + 0.0000023\ (X1)^2 - 0.0001392\ (X2).$$

$$D_b = 1.089733 - 0.0009245\ (X3) + 0.0000025\ (X3)^2 - 0.0000979\ (X2).$$

X1 = sum of triceps, suprailiac, and thigh skinfolds.
X2 = age in years.
X3 = sum of triceps, suprailiac, and abdominal skinfolds.

Women: Seven Sites

$$D_b = 1.097 - 0.00046971\ (X4) + 0.00000056\ (X4)^2 - 0.00012828\ (X2).$$

X4 = sum of triceps, abdominal, suprailiac, thigh, chest, subscapular, and midaxillary skinfolds.

Men: Three Sites

$$D_b = 1.10938 - 0.0008267\ (X1) + 0.0000016\ (X1)^2 - 0.0002574\ (X2).$$

$$D_b = 1.1125025 - 0.0013125\ (X3) + 0.0000055\ (X3)^2 - 0.0002440\ (X2).$$

X1 = sum of chest, abdomen, and thigh skinfolds.
X2 = age in years.
X3 = sum of chest, triceps, and subscapular skinfolds.

Men: Seven Sites

$$D_b = 1.112 - 0.00043499\ (X4) + 0.00000055\ (X4)^2 - 0.00028826\ (X2).$$

X4 = sum of triceps, abdominal, suprailiac, thigh, chest, subscapular, and midaxillary skinfolds.

From Jackson and Pollock, 1978; Jackson and Pollock, 1985; Jackson, Pollock, and Ward 1980.

is because the relationship between total body fat and subcutaneous fat changes with age; as a person ages, proportionally less fat is stored subcutaneously. Equations from these authors that require three or seven skinfold sites are listed in the sidebar *Equations for Estimating Body Density From Skinfold Thicknesses*. In addition, tables 8.5 and 8.6 provide quick references for estimating body fatness from skinfold thicknesses for men and women. To use these tables, total the sum of your client's skinfolds (chest, abdominal, and thigh sites for men; triceps, suprailiac, and thigh sites for women) and locate the corresponding value in the far left column. Then, locate the client's age in the top row. The intersection of the row and column is the client's estimated %BF.

Table 8.5 Estimating Body-Fat Percentage for Men Using Age and the Sum of Chest, Abdominal, and Thigh Skinfolds

	AGE TO THE LAST YEAR								
Sum of skinfolds (mm)	Under 22	23-27	28-32	33-37	38-42	43-47	48-52	53-57	Over 57
8-10	1.3	1.8	2.3	2.9	3.4	3.9	4.5	5.0	5.5
11-13	2.2	2.8	3.3	3.9	4.4	4.9	5.5	6.0	6.5
14-16	3.2	3.8	4.3	4.8	5.4	5.9	6.4	7.0	7.5
17-19	4.2	4.7	5.3	5.8	6.3	6.9	7.4	8.0	8.5
20-22	5.1	5.7	6.2	6.8	7.3	7.9	8.4	8.9	9.5
23-25	6.1	6.6	7.2	7.7	8.3	8.8	9.4	9.9	10.5
26-28	7.0	7.6	8.1	8.7	9.2	9.8	10.3	10.9	11.4
29-31	8.0	8.5	9.1	9.6	10.2	10.7	11.3	11.8	12.4
32-34	8.9	9.4	10.0	10.5	11.1	11.6	12.2	12.8	13.3
35-37	9.8	10.4	10.9	11.5	12.0	12.6	13.1	13.7	14.3
38-40	10.7	11.3	11.8	12.4	12.9	13.5	14.1	14.6	15.2
41-43	11.6	12.2	12.7	13.3	13.8	14.4	15.0	15.5	16.1
44-46	12.5	13.1	13.6	14.2	14.7	15.3	15.9	16.4	17.0
47-49	13.4	13.9	14.5	15.1	15.6	16.2	16.8	17.3	17.9
50-52	14.3	14.8	15.4	15.9	16.5	17.1	17.6	18.2	18.8
53-55	15.1	15.7	16.2	16.8	17.4	17.9	18.5	19.1	19.7
56-58	16.0	16.5	17.1	17.7	18.2	18.8	19.4	20.0	20.5
59-61	16.9	17.4	17.9	18.5	19.1	19.7	20.2	20.8	21.4
62-64	17.6	18.2	18.8	19.4	19.9	20.5	21.1	21.7	22.2
65-67	18.5	19.0	19.6	20.2	20.8	21.3	21.9	22.5	23.1
68-70	19.3	19.9	20.4	21.0	21.6	22.2	22.7	23.3	23.9
71-73	20.1	20.7	21.2	21.8	22.4	23.0	23.6	24.1	24.7
74-76	20.9	21.5	22.0	22.6	23.2	23.8	24.4	25.0	25.5
77-79	21.7	22.2	22.8	23.4	24.0	24.6	25.2	25.8	26.3
80-82	22.4	23.0	23.6	24.2	24.8	25.4	25.9	26.5	27.1
83-85	23.2	23.8	24.4	25.0	25.5	26.1	26.7	27.3	27.9
86-88	24.0	24.5	25.1	25.7	26.3	26.9	27.5	28.1	28.7
89-91	24.7	25.3	25.9	26.5	27.1	27.6	28.2	28.8	29.4
92-94	25.4	26.0	26.6	27.2	27.8	28.4	29.0	29.6	30.2
95-97	26.1	26.7	27.3	27.9	28.5	29.1	29.7	30.3	30.9
98-100	26.9	27.4	28.0	28.6	29.2	29.8	30.4	31.0	31.6
101-103	27.5	28.1	28.7	29.3	29.9	30.5	31.1	31.7	32.3
104-106	28.2	28.8	29.4	30.0	30.6	31.2	31.8	32.4	33.0

	AGE TO THE LAST YEAR								
Sum of skinfolds (mm)	Under 22	23-27	28-32	33-37	38-42	43-47	48-52	53-57	Over 57
107-109	28.9	29.5	30.1	30.7	31.3	31.9	32.5	33.1	33.7
110-112	29.6	30.2	30.8	31.4	32.0	32.6	33.2	33.8	34.4
113-115	30.2	30.8	31.4	32.0	32.6	33.2	33.8	34.5	35.1
116-118	30.9	31.5	32.1	32.7	33.3	33.9	34.5	35.1	35.7
119-121	31.5	32.1	32.7	33.3	33.9	34.5	35.1	35.7	36.4
122-124	32.1	32.7	33.3	33.9	34.5	35.1	35.8	36.4	37.0
125-127	32.7	33.3	33.9	34.5	35.1	35.8	36.4	37.0	37.6

Percentage of fat is calculated using equations by Jackson and Pollock (12) and Siri (25).

Adapted, by permission, from M.L. Pollock, D.H. Schmidt and A.S. Jackson, 1980, "Measurement of cardiorespiratory fitness and body composition in a clinical setting," *Comprehensive Therapy* 6(9): 12-27.

Table 8.6 Estimating Body-Fat Percentage for Women Using Age and the Sum of Triceps, Suprailiac, and Thigh Skinfolds

	AGE TO THE LAST YEAR								
Sum of skinfolds (mm)	Under 22	23-27	28-32	33-37	38-42	43-47	48-52	53-57	Over 57
23-25	10.8	11.1	11.4	11.7	12.0	12.3	12.6	12.9	13.2
26-28	11.9	12.2	12.5	12.8	13.1	13.4	13.7	14.0	14.3
29-31	13.1	13.4	13.7	14.0	14.3	14.6	14.9	15.2	15.5
32-34	14.2	14.5	14.8	15.1	15.4	15.7	16.0	16.3	16.6
35-37	15.2	15.6	15.9	16.2	16.5	16.8	17.1	17.4	17.7
38-40	16.3	16.6	16.9	17.2	17.6	17.9	18.2	18.5	18.8
41-43	17.4	17.7	18.0	18.3	18.6	18.9	19.2	19.6	19.9
44-46	18.4	18.8	19.1	19.4	19.7	20.0	20.3	20.6	20.9
47-49	19.5	19.8	20.1	20.4	20.7	21.0	21.4	21.7	22.0
50-52	20.5	20.8	21.1	21.4	21.8	22.1	22.4	22.7	23.0
53-55	21.5	21.8	22.1	22.5	22.8	23.1	23.4	23.7	24.0
56-58	22.5	22.8	23.1	23.5	23.8	24.1	24.4	24.7	25.0
59-61	23.5	23.8	24.1	24.4	24.8	25.1	25.4	25.7	26.0
62-64	24.5	24.8	25.1	25.4	25.7	26.1	26.4	26.7	27.0
65-67	25.4	25.7	26.1	26.4	26.7	27.0	27.3	27.7	28.0
68-70	26.4	26.7	27.0	27.3	27.6	28.0	28.3	28.6	28.9
71-73	27.3	27.6	27.9	28.2	28.6	28.9	29.2	29.5	29.8
74-76	28.2	28.5	28.8	29.1	29.5	29.8	30.1	30.4	30.8
77-79	29.1	29.4	29.7	30.0	30.4	30.7	31.0	31.3	31.7
80-82	29.9	30.3	30.6	30.9	31.2	31.6	31.9	32.2	32.5
83-85	30.8	31.1	31.5	31.8	32.1	32.4	32.8	33.1	33.4
86-88	31.6	32.0	32.3	32.6	33.0	33.3	33.6	33.9	34.3
89-91	32.5	32.8	33.1	33.5	33.8	34.1	34.4	34.8	35.1
92-94	33.3	33.6	33.9	34.3	34.6	34.9	35.3	35.6	35.9
95-97	34.1	34.4	34.7	35.1	35.4	35.7	36.1	36.4	36.7
98-100	34.8	35.2	35.5	35.8	36.2	36.5	36.8	37.2	37.5
101-103	35.6	35.9	36.3	36.6	36.9	37.3	37.6	37.9	38.3

(continued)

Table 8.6 *(continued)*

	AGE TO THE LAST YEAR								
Sum of skinfolds (mm)	Under 22	23-27	28-32	33-37	38-42	43-47	48-52	53-57	Over 57
104-106	36.3	36.7	37.0	37.3	37.7	38.0	38.3	38.7	39.0
107-109	37.1	37.4	37.7	38.1	38.4	38.7	39.1	39.4	39.7
110-112	37.8	38.1	38.4	38.8	39.1	39.4	39.8	40.1	40.5
113-115	38.5	38.8	39.1	39.5	39.8	40.1	40.5	40.8	41.1
116-118	39.1	39.5	39.8	40.1	40.5	40.8	41.1	41.5	41.8
119-121	39.8	40.1	40.4	40.8	41.1	41.5	41.8	42.1	42.5
122-124	40.4	40.7	41.1	41.4	41.8	42.1	42.4	42.8	43.1
125-127	41.0	41.4	41.7	42.0	42.4	42.7	43.1	43.4	43.7
128-130	41.6	41.9	42.3	42.6	43.0	43.3	43.7	44.0	44.3

Percentage of fat is calculated using Jackson, Pollock, and Ward (14) and Siri (25) equations.

Adapted, by permission, from M.L. Pollock, D.H. Schmidt and A.S. Jackson, 1980, "Measurement of cardiorespiratory fitness and body composition in a clinical setting," *Comprehensive Therapy* 6(9): 12-27.

KEY POINT

Skinfold measurements are a quick and relatively accurate method for estimating %BF; however, care must be taken in making these measurements if the values are to be reliable. Girth measurements, particularly WC, can be useful in assessing risk of obesity-related disease, and BMI is useful for classifying people into overweight and obese categories. The recommended BMI range is 18.5 to 24.9 kg · m^{-2}.

Densitometry

The density of an object is defined as the ratio of its weight to its volume (density = weight ÷ volume). Two common procedures that estimate body composition based on densitometry are hydrostatic weighing and air displacement plethysmography. The foundation of these techniques is that different types of tissues in the body have different and consistent densities. For example, fat tissue has a density far less than either muscle or bone. Each of these techniques results in the assessment of total body volume and subsequently the calculation of body density.

Once the body density is calculated, it must be converted into %BF. To make this conversion, a **two-compartment model** is used. In a two-compartment model, all body tissues are classified as either fat or fat free. One of the most commonly used equations for this procedure is the Siri (25) equation: %BF = (495 ÷ D_b) – 450. In this model, the fat-free portion of the body is composed of all tissues except lipids and is assumed to have a density of 1.1 kg · L^{-1}. Fat is assumed to have a density of 0.9 kg · L^{-1}. It has been suggested that the inherent error (caused by variations in hydration or bone density) of this method is 2% to 2.8% in young Caucasian adults (17).

Fat density is fairly consistent among individuals; however, there are situations in which the density of the fat-free body is different from the assumed 1.1 kg · L^{-1}. For example, if a person's bone density is different from the standard used by Siri, then the assumption that the fat-free body density equals 1.1 kg · L^{-1} becomes invalid. This is the case for African Americans, who typically have a higher bone density than their Caucasian counterparts, and Schutte and colleagues (24) proposed that a different equation be used to calculate %BF for African American men. Many equations have been proposed to convert body density into %BF. Some of these are listed in table 8.7. For more equations and information on converting body density into %BF, see *ACSM's Guidelines for Exercise Testing and Prescription* (1). Researchers sometimes use techniques more advanced than two-compartment models. Although these techniques are currently impractical for nonresearch settings, they are briefly described in the sidebar *Multicompartment Models in Body Composition Assessment.*

Hydrostatic Weighing

Hydrostatic (underwater) **weighing** is one of the most common means for estimating body composition in research settings and is often used as the **criterion method** for assessing %BF. A criterion method provides the standard against which other methodologies are compared. In this procedure, the participant is submerged in a tank of warm water and then exhales fully while technicians record the body mass (figure 8.2). The body mass while submerged and the body mass on land are used to calculate %BF.

Table 8.7 Equations Used to Convert Body Density Into Body-Fat Percentage

Group	Sex	Equation
African American	Male	%BF = (437 ÷ D_b) – 393
	Female	%BF = (485 ÷ D_b) – 439
Caucasian	Male	%BF = (495 ÷ D_b) – 450
	Female	%BF = (501 ÷ D_b) – 457

%BF = body-fat percentage; D_b = body density.

Based on Heymsfield et al. 1990.

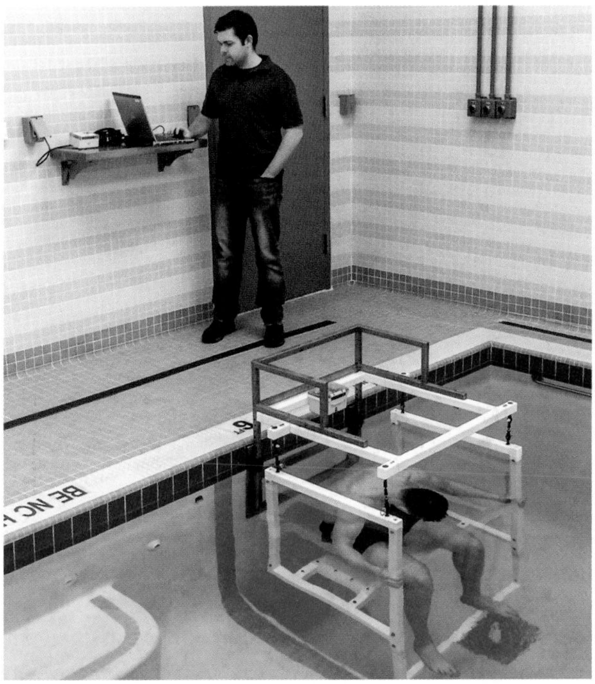

FIGURE 8.2 Hydrostatic weighing.

Photo courtesy of Meghan Perry.

Hydrostatic weighing is based on Archimedes' principle, which states that a submerged object is buoyed up by a force equal to the volume of water it displaces. This buoyant force causes the object to weigh less underwater than it does on land. The difference between land mass and underwater mass is used to calculate the volume of the object. Because the density of an object is calculated by dividing mass by volume, body density (D_b) can be calculated using the following formula.

$$D_b = \frac{M}{\frac{(M - M_{UW})}{D_{H_2O}} - RV - GV}$$

In addition to body mass (M) and mass underwater (M_{UW}), the density of the water (D_{H_2O}) in the hydrostatic tank, the residual lung volume (RV), and the gastrointestinal air volume (GV) are needed for this calculation. Water density depends on water temperature and is necessary to convert mass into volume; therefore, accurate measurement of the water temperature is essential. Also, this equation corrects for the residual lung volume because any air in the lungs creates an additional buoyant effect that reduces underwater mass. The oxygen dilution technique described by Wilmore (28) is one of the most frequently used methods for assessing residual lung volume. Estimating instead of measuring residual lung volume dramatically decreases the accuracy of hydrostatic weighing. Because sex, age, and height correlate with residual lung volume, it can be estimated with a formula that incorporates the client's age and height (9). Formulas for males and females are shown in the sidebar *Formulas to Calculate Residual Lung Volume From Height and Age*. Because the volume of air trapped in the gastrointestinal tract cannot be measured, an estimate of 0.1 L is typically used.

Hydrostatic weighing accurately estimates body composition for most adults, and it remains a standard of comparison for other methods. Major disadvantages to this procedure are the time, expense, and technical expertise required. Also, many people are unable to undergo this procedure because of their discomfort with being underwater. Following are guidelines that will help ensure accurate assessment of body composition with hydrostatic weighing:

- The participant should not eat within 4 hr of testing.
- The participant should urinate and defecate before testing.
- The participant should wear as little clothing as possible. Remove any trapped air bubbles from clothing before weighing.
- Instruct the participant to exhale completely while submerged. (This will take practice for most individuals.)

Formulas to Calculate Residual Lung Volume From Height and Age

Females

(0.009 · age in yr) + (0.08128 · height in in.) – 3.9 = RV in L.

Males

(0.017 · age in yr) + (0.06858 · height in in.) – 3.447 = RV in L.

From Goldman and Becklake 1959.

- The participant should remain as motionless as possible while submerged.
- Perform several (5-10) trials to obtain consistent measurements.
- Measure, rather than estimate, residual volume.

Air Displacement Plethysmography

Another technique for determining %BF that uses the concept of density as the ratio of body mass to body volume is **air displacement plethysmography**. The Bod Pod is a commercially available air displacement plethysmograph (see figure 8.3). In this method, body volume is estimated while the subject sits in a sealed chamber. During testing, a computer-controlled diaphragm moves, changing the volume of the chamber. Pressure changes in the chamber are related to the size of the person being measured. By examining the pressure–volume relationship, body volume and, subsequently, body density are calculated (4, 19). Once body density is known, the two-compartment equations listed in table 8.7 can be used to estimate %BF.

The primary advantage of air displacement plethysmography compared with hydrostatic weighing is that it is quicker and is less anxiety-inducing for many people. Although researchers continue to gather data on this device in an attempt to determine if it can be considered a criterion measurement technique (6), the high reliability, validity, and ease of use make it the technique of choice for many (3). The SEE for this technique varies among studies but is typically between 2% and 4% (23). The major disadvantage is the cost of the highly technical equipment needed to make the measurements. A major consideration for obtaining accurate measurements with the Bod Pod is that subjects must dress according to the manufacturer's specifications (i.e., in a tight-fitting swimsuit and swim cap).

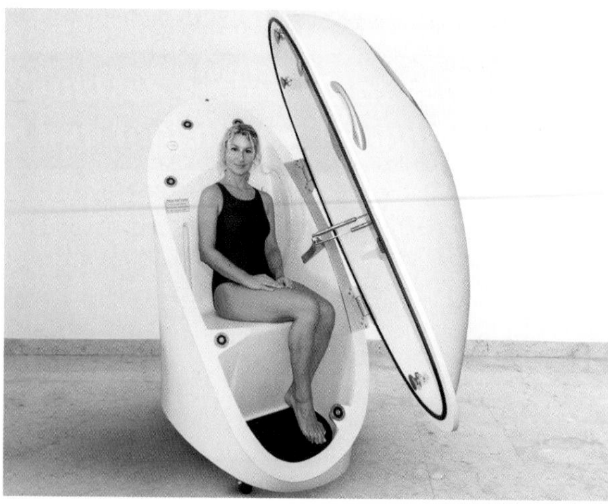

FIGURE 8.3 Bod Pod.

Photo courtesy of COSMED USA, Inc.

Dual-Energy X-Ray Absorptiometry

A technique that has gained wide acceptance in clinical settings is dual-energy X-ray absorptiometry (DXA or DEXA). DXA was developed for measuring the density of bones. Although bone density measurement remains the primary use of this methodology, software has been developed that can estimate total and regional %BF from DXA scans (see figure 8.4). To estimate %BF from DXA, a total-body X-ray is performed with extremely low-dosage energy beams. As the X-rays pass through the subject, the density of all parts of the body is determined. Because fat, bone, and nonbone lean tissue have different densities, these three compartments can be identified (15).

Although DXA requires a full-body X-ray, the radiation exposure is minimal and is only a small fraction of the radiation exposure of a chest X-ray. Some researchers claim DXA as the new criterion method for body composition assessment; however, there are still unresolved issues for this technology (3). For example, differences in DXA software packages may result in varied body fat outcomes. Also, variations in body-segment thicknesses tend to alter DXA results (15). Studies investigating the error associated with this technique have reported errors ranging from 1.2% to 4.8% (17).

This procedure is relatively quick (approximately 15 min) and has the potential for accurate results regardless of the age, sex, or race of the subject. The major prohibitive factors for using this procedure are cost and access to the equipment. Because of the radiation exposure involved, DXA equipment is housed in hospitals or clinically oriented research centers. At present, DXA is used most frequently as a research tool and in the clinical assessment of body composition.

Computed Tomography and Magnetic Resonance Imaging

Magnetic resonance imaging (MRI) and computed tomography (CT) are also imaging techniques that provide important information to clinicians and researchers. One of the common uses of these techniques is to determine the amount of fat, particularly deep fat, found in the trunk. Because deep fat (visceral fat) is highly associated with disease, researchers use these techniques to quantify its distribution pattern. CT scans use X-rays to produce images of the fat and nonfat tissues, whereas MRI uses a strong magnetic field. The equipment necessary for this type of imaging is expensive and is found in clinical settings. These techniques provide criterion measurement for regional fat distribution and deep versus superficial fat depots (3).

Bioelectrical Impedance Analysis

Bioelectrical impedance analysis (BIA) is a simple, quick, noninvasive method that can be used to estimate

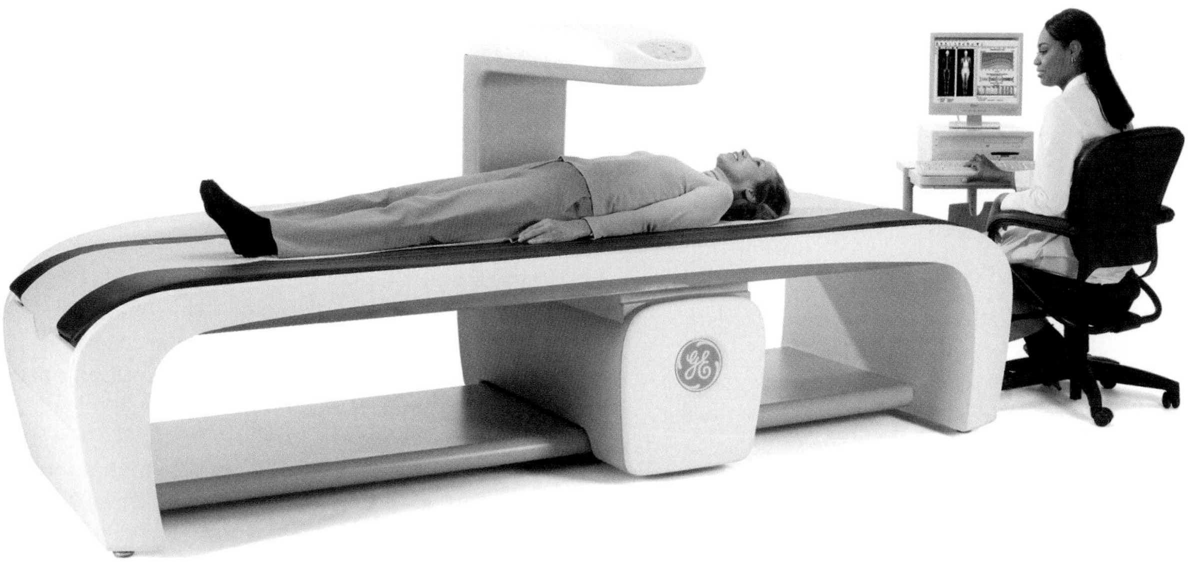

FIGURE 8.4 Dual-energy X-ray absorptiometry.
Courtesy GE Healthcare

%BF. This technique is based on the assumption that tissues high in electrolyte-rich water content conduct electrical currents with less resistance than those with little water do (3). Because adipose tissue contains little water, fat impedes the flow of electrical current; muscle, on the other hand, conducts electrical current very well.

BIA requires that a small electrical current be sent through the body. This current is undetectable to the person being tested. There are several types of commercially available BIA devices. Some place electrodes on the hand and foot, some are handheld, and others have contact points for the bottom of the feet and look similar to bathroom scales. Whatever the design of the machine, as the introduced current passes through the body, voltage decreases. This voltage drop (impedance) is used to calculate %BF. Typically, other information such as sex, height, and age (and sometimes race) are used in conjunction with impedance to predict %BF.

BIA has gained wide acceptance in the fitness industry because it is easy, inexpensive, and noninvasive, and there are versions of these devices designed for in-home use by consumers. The accuracy of this technique depends on the type of equipment and equations used; however, a standard error of 2.7% to 6.3% commonly is reported (23). An issue that complicates the application of BIA is that the relationship between impedance and %BF varies among populations. In other words, for an accurate estimate of %BF, one must take into account age, gender, and other factors. Most commercially available devices have programmed equations to account for many of these factors. BIA estimates are based on the principle that water makes up 73% of the body's fat-free mass. Thus, BIA does not produce accurate results for individuals with amputations, significant muscular atrophy, severe obesity, or diseases that alter the state of hydration. In addition, it is recommended that people with implanted defibrillators avoid BIA assessment until the safety of BIA for these individuals has been determined (3).

A person's state of hydration can greatly alter BIA results; therefore, it is essential to follow standardized procedures with this assessment technique (23). Following is a list of these suggested procedures.

- Remove oil and lotions from the skin with alcohol before placing electrodes.
- Place electrodes precisely as directed by the manufacturer of the impedance device. Incorrect electrode placement greatly reduces the accuracy of BIA.
- If required to measure height, mass, or both, measure height to the nearest 0.5 cm and body mass to the nearest 0.1 kg.
- Ask clients to avoid any substance that alters the body's hydration state, such as alcohol or diuretics, for at least 48 hr before BIA. (Diuretics being taken under a doctor's direction should not be stopped.)
- Inform clients that during the 4 hr before assessment, they should avoid eating and should drink only enough water to maintain normal hydration.
- Instruct clients to avoid exercise for 12 hr preceding BIA.
- Note the phase of the menstrual cycle because of its ability to alter hydration levels.

KEY POINT

Two-compartment models divide the body into fat and fat-free components. Although the Siri two-compartment model is often used, other models are available. Both hydrostatic weighing and air displacement plethysmography use a two-compartment model. BIA is based on the principle that electrical currents flow more easily through more hydrated tissues (muscle) than through less hydrated tissues (fat). Although BIA is useful in body composition screening, steps should be taken to ensure that the client's hydration is normal at the time of testing. Multicompartment modeling and imaging techniques are used in research to assess body composition.

RESEARCH INSIGHT

Multicompartment Models in Body Composition Assessment

A disadvantage to using two-compartment models in calculating body composition is the need to make broad generalizations about the composition and density of various body tissues. To avoid this problem, researchers sometimes use models that combine measurements to estimate body composition. Although these techniques must still rely on some basic assumptions about the body's makeup, fewer broad generalizations about its component parts are made. Therefore, these multicompartment models more accurately assess body composition.

An example of a multicompartment model is Siri's three-compartment model, in which the body is divided into fat, water, and solids (protein and mineral) (25). This model requires measuring total body density and total body water. Measurements of total body water are typically determined by having the participant ingest an isotope of hydrogen such as deuterium or tritium. After the ingested isotope spreads through the body's water, a fluid sample (e.g., urine, blood) can be used to calculate total body water. This model is particularly useful in clinical situations when patients have significantly altered body water. In cases where the bone mineral varies from what is assumed in a two-compartment model (e.g., in an osteoporotic patient), a technique requiring bone measurement is needed. Lohman (16) presented a model that divides the body into fat, protein and water, and mineral components. Both body density and bone mineral measurement (obtained via X-ray imaging) are needed for this technique. Sometimes bone and water measurements are added separately to body density to provide a four-compartment model (i.e., protein, mineral, fat, and water) (10).

Multicompartment models provide important criterion measures of body composition for researchers. Data from these methodologies are used to develop better field methods for assessing body composition in diverse populations. However, the cost, time, and technical expertise required for these processes make them impractical in nonresearch settings.

Calculating Target Body Weight

As shown in table 8.1, healthy %BF ranges are quite different for females and males and cover a wide range. One of the important tasks of fitness professionals is helping clients determine an appropriate weight goal. Once an estimate of %BF has been obtained and %BF goals have been determined, the fitness professional can calculate an appropriate target weight. As discussed in chapter 12, setting reasonable goals for weight loss is a major factor in maintaining compliance. To calculate target body weight, you must know body weight, %BF, and the desired level of body fatness. The following equations are needed for these calculations:

$$\text{Fat mass (FM)} = \text{body mass} \cdot (\%\text{BF} \div 100\%).$$

$$\text{Fat-free mass (FFM)} = \text{body mass} - \text{FM}.$$

$$\text{Target body weight} = \frac{\text{FFM}}{1 - \left(\dfrac{\text{desired \% BF}}{(100)}\right)}$$

QUESTION:

A 40-yr-old woman weighs 155 lb (70 kg) and has a %BF of 30. Her goal is to reach 23% body fat. What is her target weight?

ANSWER:

$$\text{FM} = 155 \text{ lb} \cdot (30 \div 100) = 46.5 \text{ lb (21 kg)}.$$

$$\text{FFM} = 155 \text{ lb} - 46.5 \text{ lb} = 108.5 \text{ lb (49 kg)}.$$

$$\text{Target body weight} = \frac{108.5}{1 - \left(\dfrac{23}{(100)}\right)} = 140.9 \text{ lb, or } 63.9 \text{ kg}$$

LEARNING AIDS

REVIEW QUESTIONS

1. What is the recommended BMI range? What is the BMI range for overweight? For obesity?
2. What are other names for the android-type obesity pattern? What conditions are linked to this obesity pattern?
3. Hydrostatic weighing and air displacement plethysmography use a two-compartment model for body composition. What are the two compartments assumed by this model?
4. Which technique applies a small electrical current to estimate %BF? What are ways that you can improve the accuracy of this technique?
5. What are important considerations when using skinfold measurements to estimate %BF that will help reduce measurement errors?
6. What are some advantages to using air displacement plethysmography?
7. What body composition technique is also used to measure bone density?
8. Why are multicompartment models of body composition assessment generally limited to research settings?

CASE STUDIES

1. Ms. Anderson is a 30-yr-old female who comes into your fitness facility wanting to lose weight. What are appropriate measurements and calculations for a fitness professional to make to assist Ms. Anderson with her goal?
2. Mr. Johnson is a 48-yr-old male who recently joined your fitness facility. At his initial evaluation you take the following measurements:
   - Height: 70 in. (178 cm)
   - Weight: 215 lb (97.5 kg)
   - Hip circumference: 39 in. (99 cm)
   - WC: 41 in. (104 cm)
   - Skinfolds: chest 35 mm, abdomen 49 mm, thigh 20 mm

Calculate and interpret Mr. Johnson's BMI, WHR, and %BF.

3. Mr. Johnson sets his initial %BF goal at 28%. Calculate the target body weight that will allow Mr. Johnson to achieve this goal.

Answers to Case Studies

1. Height, weight, BMI, %BF, and waist and hip circumference are appropriate.
2. First calculate Mr. Johnson's BMI and WHR:

$$\text{BMI} = 97.7\text{ kg} \div (1.778\text{ m} \cdot 1.778\text{ m}) = 30.9\text{ kg} \cdot \text{m}^{-2}\text{, which is in the obese range.}$$

$$\text{WHR} = 41\text{ in.} \div 39\text{ in.} = 1.05\text{, which is considered high risk.}$$

To calculate %BF, first calculate body density using the three-site formula:

$$D_b = 1.10938 - 0.0008267\text{ (sum of skinfolds)} + 0.0000016\text{ (sum of skinfolds)}^2 - 0.0002574\text{ (age)} = 1.10938 - 0.0008267\text{ (104)} + 0.0000016\text{ (104)}^2 - 0.0002574\text{ (48)} = 1.0283.$$

Next, use the Siri equation to convert the density into %BF:

$$\%\text{BF} = (495 \div D_b) - 450 = (495 \div 1.0283) - 495 = 31.4\%\text{, which is in the obese range.}$$

3. First calculate fat mass and fat-free mass:

$$\text{FM} = \text{weight} \cdot \%\text{BF} = 215 \cdot 31.4\% = 67.5 \text{ lb } (30.6 \text{ kg}).$$

$$\text{FFM} = \text{total weight} - \text{FM} = 215 - 67.5 = 147.5 \text{ lb } (66.9 \text{ kg}).$$

Now calculate target weight:

$$\text{Target weight} = \text{FFM} \div (1 - \text{desired } \%\text{BF}) = 147.5 \div (1 - 0.28) = 205 \text{ lb } (93.0 \text{ kg}).$$

9

Assessment of Muscular Fitness

Avery Faigenbaum

OBJECTIVES

The reader will be able to do the following:

1. Explain purposes of assessing muscular fitness.
2. Discuss precautions that enhance participant safety during muscular fitness assessments.
3. Describe various methods of assessing muscular fitness, including repetition maximum tests, push-up and abdominal curl-up tests, the YMCA bench press test, and others.
4. Identify methods for standardizing testing protocols to increase accuracy and reproducibility of test results.
5. Describe how to interpret the results from various muscular fitness tests.
6. Describe how to assess muscular strength and local muscular endurance in older adults.
7. Describe safety procedures and precautions for assessing muscular fitness in clients who are at elevated risk for adverse cardiovascular responses (e.g., people with high blood pressure or CHD).
8. Describe the benefits, safety, and precautions for assessing muscular fitness in children and adolescents.

Muscular fitness is a term that refers to the integrated status of **muscular strength** (maximal force a muscle or muscle group can generate), **muscular endurance** (ability of a muscle to make repeated contractions or to resist muscular fatigue), and muscular **power** (the rate of performing work) (6, 27, 51). Muscular fitness is important in promoting and maintaining both health- and skill-related components of physical fitness. Accordingly, in ACSM's position stand on the recommended quantity and quality of exercise to achieve and maintain fitness (30) and in public health recommendations from HHS (57) and the World Health Organization (WHO) (63), people are encouraged to participate regularly in structured activities that enhance muscular fitness. ACSM recommends that resistance training at a moderate intensity, sufficient to develop and maintain muscular fitness, be performed 2 to 3 days per wk as part of a well-rounded exercise program (see chapter 13).

This chapter describes tests commonly used in the health and fitness setting to assess muscular strength and local muscular endurance. Particular emphasis is given to measures of muscular fitness that are valid, reliable, safe, and relatively easy to administer in the fitness setting. Tests that are indicative of a client's health and fitness and those that do not require specialized equipment or sophisticated procedures are highlighted. Assessments of muscular fitness and functional capabilities in special populations, such as older adults, people at increased cardiovascular risk, and children or adolescents, are also described.

Preliminary Considerations

Muscular fitness refers to the parameters of muscular strength, local muscular endurance, and muscular power. Although each component of muscular fitness can improve with an appropriately designed resistance training program, this chapter focuses on the assessment of muscular strength and local muscular endurance. Power training may be beneficial for some participants (5), but assessment of muscular power is not typically performed in general exercise programs that focus on health and fitness.

Assessments in this chapter may be viewed along a continuum with maximal strength at one end of the assessment scale and local muscular endurance at the other (figure 9.1) (6). According to ACSM (6), tests allowing few repetitions (<3) before momentary muscle fatigue measure muscular strength, whereas those that require high numbers of repetitions (>12) measure local muscular endurance. However, the performance of a maximal repetition range (e.g., 4, 6, or 8 repetitions at a given resistance) also can assess muscular strength (6). Performing fitness tests to assess muscular strength and local muscular endurance before commencing exercise training or as part of a fitness screening can provide valuable information about a client's baseline fitness. For example, results from a muscular strength test can be compared with established standards and can help identify weaknesses in certain muscle groups or muscle imbalances that exercise programs could target. The information obtained during baseline muscular fitness assessments also can serve as a basis for designing individualized exercise programs and educating participants about the importance of resistance training. An equally useful application of fitness testing is to motivate participants by evaluating their progress over time. Note that there is no single best test for assessing muscular strength, local muscular endurance, or muscular power.

For safety purposes, all participants who undergo fitness testing should first complete a medical history questionnaire and, if necessary, consult with a qualified health care provider to obtain advice on modifying exercise participation. This includes people with known cardiovascular or orthopedic conditions. The ACSM procedures for administering a careful health risk assessment have been described in detail in this textbook (see chapter 2) and elsewhere (6).

- Standardization of testing protocols. According to ACSM (6), people should participate in familiarization (practice) sessions, follow a standardized testing protocol, and perform a proper warm-up in order to obtain a reliable score that can be used to track physiologic adaptations over time. Other standardized conditions that promote safe muscular fitness tests that yield valid and reproducible results include reviewing safety measures with each participant and ensuring that the participant uses proper exercise technique throughout the full ROM at a predetermined speed of movement. The same equipment (free weight versus weight machine) should be used for pre- and posttesting, and multiple tests should be organized so the same muscle groups are not repeatedly stressed. Additionally, the muscular fitness tests should be specific to the training program.
- Familiarization. To obtain a reliable test score that can be used to track physiological adaptations over time, people should become familiar with the testing equip-

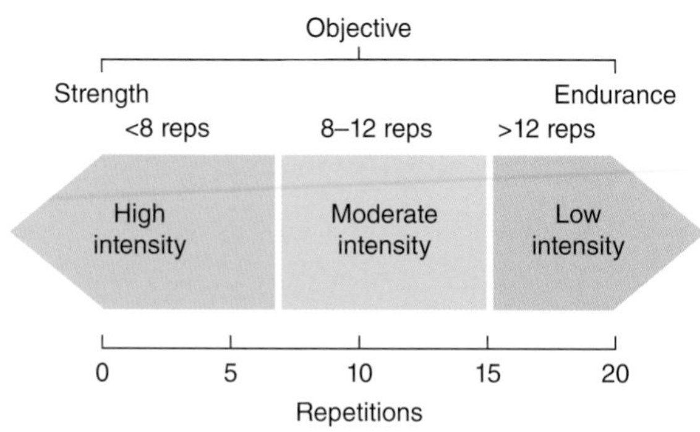

FIGURE 9.1 Intensity of resistance exercise for training and assessment. Weight loads allowing few reps (<8) test for muscular strength, and weight loads that can be repeatedly lifted (>12 reps) assess local muscular endurance.

Adapted from American College of Sports Medicine 2014, *ACSM's guidelines for exercise testing and prescription*, 9th ed. (Philadelphia: PA: Lippincott, Williams, & Wilkins).

ment and protocol by participating in several practice sessions with qualified instruction (40). Without adequate familiarization, strength testing may not provide a stable, reproducible value. A lack of familiarization prior to testing will result in relatively large increases in strength over a short-term training period. Participants with resistance training experience require little familiarization, but untrained participants may need two or three practice sessions to become familiar with testing procedures and exercise technique.

- Warm-up. A 5 to 10 min general warm-up, including low-intensity cardiorespiratory exercise, calisthenics, and several light repetitions of the specific testing exercise, should precede muscular fitness testing. This increases muscle temperature and localized blood flow, and it promotes appropriate cardiovascular responses to exercise (5, 6). Warm-up procedures that include dynamic movements for the upper and lower body may be particularly useful when assessing muscular fitness (9). Do not use static stretching as the sole warm-up activity prior to strength testing (56).
- Specificity. Muscular strength and local muscular endurance are specific to the muscle or muscle group, the type of muscular action (static or dynamic, concentric or eccentric), the speed of muscular action (slow or fast), and the joint angle being tested (40). Accordingly, muscular fitness tests should be similar to the exercises used during the training program.
- Safety. Safety measures related to the testing equipment, testing environment and quality of supervision, spotting, and instruction should be employed before testing. Review safety measures with all participants before testing, and ensure that the environment is comfortable (68-72 °F or 20-22 °C), with humidity less than 60%.
- Interpretation of results. The availability of health criteria or normative data should be considered when choosing a test, particularly when classifying a participant's test data, such as when performing a health and fitness screening. However, norms are less of a concern when the test is used primarily to detect improvements in muscular strength, where the absolute strength values (e.g., kilograms lifted) or relative scores (e.g., kilograms lifted per kilogram of body weight) can be compared during repeated testing.

Muscular Strength

Muscular strength refers to the maximal force that can be generated by a specific muscle or muscle group. Isometric or static strength (constant muscle length during muscle activation) can be measured conveniently with a variety of devices, including cable tensiometers and handgrip dynamometers, which measure strength at one specific point in the ROM. The peak force achieved in such tests is called the **maximum voluntary contraction (MVC)**. Although the handgrip test has been found to be a reliable measure of grip strength in adults (31, 50), dynamic tests are used more commonly. Testing procedures for using handgrip dynamometers are described in detail elsewhere (17).

Isokinetic testing involves the assessment of maximal muscle tension throughout a range of joint motion at a constant angular velocity (e.g., $60° \cdot sec^{-1}$). Isokinetic testing devices measure peak rotational force, or torque, and data are obtained with specialized equipment that allows the tester to control the speed of rotation (degrees per second) around various joints (e.g., knee, hip, shoulder, elbow). Although the data collected from isokinetic strength assessments may be useful to health and fitness professionals, the necessary computerized equipment is expensive and therefore limits isokinetic testing almost entirely to rehabilitation and research settings. Consequently, isokinetic strength evaluations may not be practical for most health and fitness practitioners.

The most common type of strength assessment performed by fitness professionals is **dynamic testing**, which involves movement of the body (e.g., push-up) or an external load (e.g., bench press). Dynamic testing is typically inexpensive because it does not require specialized equipment. Moreover, dynamic assessments can be performed with a variety of equipment, such as free weights (barbells and dumbbells) or weight-stack machines, and they can test any major muscle or muscle group through a variety of exercises. Exercises typically used for dynamic strength testing in fitness centers include the bench press and leg press.

Repetition Maximum Testing

The gold standard of dynamic strength testing is the **1-repetition maximum (1RM)**, the heaviest weight that can be lifted only once in a specific exercise using proper form (5, 6). If appropriate testing guidelines are followed, a 1RM test is a reliable measure of maximal strength and can be performed safely in the health and fitness setting with qualified supervision, for example, by fitness professionals who adhere to current guidelines of exercise leadership such as those described in this chapter and by ACSM (6, 43, 55). Although a 1RM can be performed for various exercises, multijoint exercises such as the bench press and leg press are typically used for this type of testing. The fitness professional should ensure proper positioning of the client (e.g., grip position and foot stance) and must be readily available to assist in case of a failed repetition. Spotting is particularly important for free-weight exercises such as the bench press and squat. Also, beginners must learn how to exert maximal effort by participating in several familiarization sessions with each strength testing protocol prior to testing. Untrained clients tend to misinterpret submaximal effort for maximal effort due to lack of training experience.

Components of Muscular Fitness Related to Promoting or Maintaining Good Health, Fitness, and Athletic Performance

Health Aspects of Muscular Fitness

- Preservation or enhancement of fat-free mass and resting metabolic rate
- Preservation or enhancement of bone mass with aging
- Improved glucose tolerance and insulin sensitivity
- Reduced HR and BP response while lifting any submaximal load (which reduces myocardial oxygen demand during activities requiring muscular force)
- Lowered risk of musculoskeletal injury, including low-back pain
- Improved ability to carry out daily activities (ADLs) in older age
- Improved balance and decreased risk of falls in older age
- Improved self-esteem

Performance Aspects of Muscular Fitness

- Enhanced muscular strength and local muscular endurance
- Enhanced speed and power
- Improved agility and balance
- Reduced risk for musculoskeletal injuries
- Improved body composition for various events and activities
- Improved confidence for performing certain athletic events and activities involving high levels of muscular fitness
- Enhanced performance in most athletic activities

From American College of Sports Medicine 2014, *ACSM's guidelines for exercise testing and prescription*, 9th ed. (Philadelphia: PA: Lippincott, Williams, & Wilkins).

Familiarization and the presence of experienced spotters who can recognize potentially hazardous situations (e.g., poor exercise technique) will enhance the safety and reliability of strength testing procedures.

Maximal or near-maximal strength tests have also been shown to be safe and reliable for clinical populations, including those with CHD and type 2 diabetes (1, 8, 23). Nonetheless, caution should be used when testing older adults, patients with clinical conditions, and people with certain orthopedic concerns (6). In some cases, it may be prudent to delay or even avoid testing until a qualified health care provider has determined the person to be clinically stable.

Multiple **repetition maximum (RM)** tests (e.g., 4RM, 8RM) can also safely and effectively assess muscular strength in healthy adults, although a more conservative approach may be needed for patients with health conditions, such as CVD, pulmonary disease, and diabetes (6). For patients at high risk for or with known disease, the assessment of a 10- to 15RM that is consistent with resistance training recommendations may be prudent (6, 59). When the purpose of testing is to define an initial training load, multiple RM testing minimizes the potential error compared with extrapolating the exercise intensity as a percentage of 1RM. For example, the maximum weight a person can lift 10 times during testing can be used to identify an appropriate weight load for this number of repetitions performed during training and to provide an index of strength changes over time.

The procedures for assessing 1RM can be modified to test any given number of repetitions. It is possible to estimate the 1RM when multiple RM tests are used. For example, a 10RM is the most weight a person can lift with proper form for 10 repetitions but not 11. The 10RM weight has been shown to be approximately 75% of the 1RM weight (59). Although a fair amount of individual variability can be expected when extrapolating 1RM from 10RM, this testing protocol may be desirable in some cases. Also, researchers have developed 1RM prediction equations based on the number of repetitions performed using a submaximal load (e.g., 70%-80% 1RM) (12, 45, 46). Because most researchers use the bench press to predict 1RM strength values, the error rate will likely increase if these equations are used with other strength exercises such as the leg press or squat. Regardless of the testing protocol, fitness professionals must communicate with the client to determine a progression pattern of loading that is consistent with the client's capacity. Asking questions (e.g., "Can you lift five more pounds?" or "Are you close to your max?"), offering encouragement, and showing concern for the client during the testing session can help to ensure maximal performance.

Procedures for 1RM Testing

1. The subject performs a light warm-up set of 5 to 10 repetitions at 40% to 60% of perceived maximum (e.g., light to moderate exertion).
2. After a 1 min rest, the subject performs 3 to 5 repetitions at 60% to 80% of perceived maximum (e.g., moderate to hard exertion).
3. The subject attempts a 1RM lift. If the lift is successful, the subject rests 3 min and repeats the test with a heavier load. This process continues until a failed attempt occurs. The goal is to find the 1RM within 3 to 5 attempts to avoid excessive fatigue.
4. The 1RM is reported as the weight of the last successfully completed lift with proper exercise technique.

Adapted, by permission, from W. Kraemer et al., 2006, Strength training: Development and evaluation of methodology. In *Physiological assessment of human fitness,* edited by P.J. Maud and C. Foster (Champaign, IL: Human Kinetics), 119-150.

KEY POINT

Muscular strength is best assessed using a resistance that requires maximum or near-maximum resistance with few repetitions, whereas local muscular endurance is assessed using lighter loads with a greater number of repetitions. In either case, muscular fitness can be assessed safely in the health and fitness setting to provide important information for individualized exercise prescription. An ideal application of these tests is to evaluate changes in muscular fitness over time using standardized testing procedures that ensure valid and reproducible results.

Interpreting Results

It is best to express strength as a ratio of weight lifted during a single or multiple RM test relative to body weight when comparing strength assessments of people who differ in body mass, such as when comparing men and women. The following procedure describes how to determine a strength ratio from a 10RM test:

1. Determine the heaviest weight the client can lift for 10 good repetitions (10RM weight load).
2. Convert the 10RM weight load to a 1RM estimation by dividing the weight load by 0.75.
3. Divide the estimated 1RM by the client's body weight to obtain the strength ratio.

For example, a client who weighs 140 lb (63.5 kg) and completes 10 leg presses with 120 lb (54.4 kg) has an estimated 1RM of 120 ÷ 0.75, or 160 lb (72.6 kg). Her leg press weight ratio is 1.14 (160 ÷ 140).

Normative Data

Normative strength scores for various age and sex categories have been published in *ACSM's Guidelines for Exercise Testing and Prescription* (6). However, most normative data have been derived from a relatively homogeneous sample of subjects using only certain types of resistance training equipment, which limits interpretation of test scores. For example, because equipment design can vary significantly from one manufacturer to another and because of inherent differences in using free weights versus machine weights, strength scores can vary using different testing equipment. Thus, client scores can only be compared with norms generated from tests performed with the same type of equipment. Valid measures of upper-body strength include 1RM values for the bench press and shoulder press, and corresponding indices of lower-body strength include the leg press and leg extension (6). Future research is needed to provide norms for a variety of resistance training equipment as well as norms for diverse races, ethnicities, and age groups.

Comparing Pretraining and Posttraining

Often, the primary purpose of a muscular fitness test is to evaluate changes in strength over the course of a fitness program. Periodic muscle fitness testing is particularly appealing because it eliminates the need to compare individual data with data provided in normative tables. The frequency of follow-up testing depends on the quality and quantity of exercise training by the client as well as the client's desire and the availability of the fitness staff. When multiple tests are performed over time, useful feedback to the client should include the *percentage improvement of strength or local muscular endurance* (i.e., percentage change between tests). This is obtained by dividing the change in strength (posttraining minus pretraining score) by the pretraining score and multiplying by 100%. For example, if your client performs a 10RM baseline of 40 lb (18.1 kg) on the chest press and improves to 60 lb (27.2 kg) during follow-up testing, she has demonstrated a 50% strength gain ([60 − 40) ÷ 40] · 100%) on that lift. This information can provide positive reinforcement about the efficacy of the training program. In cases when the client does not improve, recommendations for altering the exercise program can be made based on the client's goals and adherence to the exercise program.

RESEARCH INSIGHT

Obtaining Accurate 1RM Baseline Measures

The purpose of a study by Amarante do Nascimento et al. (2) was to determine the number of practice sessions required to achieve consistent 1RM strength measures in untrained older women (>60 yr). All subjects were apparently healthy and were not involved in any structured resistance training program for 6 mo preceding the study. Forty-five women performed a 1RM test for the leg extension, bench press, and arm curl exercises on 3 nonconsecutive days. The performance of each exercise was standardized and monitored by qualified professionals. Each 1RM trial was preceded by a warm-up set that familiarized the subjects with the testing equipment and lifting technique. Analysis of the data revealed that differences in 1RM strength were reduced to nonsignificant levels by the third trial for all exercises. These data indicate that several familiarization sessions are needed to establish consistent 1RM baseline measures in older untrained women.

Local Muscular Endurance

Local muscular endurance is the ability of a muscle group to repeatedly contract against a fixed resistance until muscular fatigue is experienced or the ability to maintain a specific percentage of the MVC for a prolonged time (6). Equipment (e.g., free weights or machines) for measuring strength can be used to assess **local muscular endurance.** In addition, a simple field test such as the maximum number of push-ups that can be performed without rest (8) can be used to evaluate the local muscular endurance of the upper-body muscles. This field test can be used either independently or in combination with other methods of strength or endurance assessment, such as RM testing. Tests such as the push-up can screen for muscle weaknesses related to various health indicators. Moreover, the muscles of the upper body are used in many daily activities such as raking or gardening, carrying luggage, or painting. Thus, this test is a practical way to evaluate a client's muscular fitness and can provide useful feedback to the client about how muscular conditioning affects many common activities.

Push-Up Test

The procedures of the push-up test as described by ACSM (6) are presented here and shown in figures 9.2 and 9.3. The push-up test evaluates muscular strength and local muscular endurance of the upper body, including the triceps, deltoid, and pectoral muscles. There are two standard push-up positions: one with the hands and toes in contact with the floor and the other with the hands and knees in contact with the floor (the modified push-up position). Regardless of the push-up position, the hand position should be standardized because varied hand placements elicit varied responses from the pectoralis major and triceps (18). The procedures for administering the test are similar, and either position may be used for men or women because the position should be based on strength, not sex. However, the norms for the standard push-up are for men and the norms for the modified push-up are for women. When women perform the standard push-up and men perform the modified push-up, pre- and posttraining scores can be compared to evaluate improvement over time; however, the table of norms should not be used in these circumstances. As with RM testing, the push-up test should be used with caution when testing older adults and people at heightened cardiac risk.

Push-Up Test Procedures

1. Explain the purpose of the test to the client (to determine how many push-ups can be completed in order to reflect upper-body muscular strength and local muscular endurance). Demonstrate the test and allow the client to practice if desired.
2. Inform the client of proper breathing technique (to exhale with the effort, which occurs when pushing away from the floor).
3. The push-up test usually is administered with male subjects in the standard down position with hands shoulder-width apart, back straight, and head up, using the toes as the pivotal point. For female subjects, the modified knee push-up

(continued)

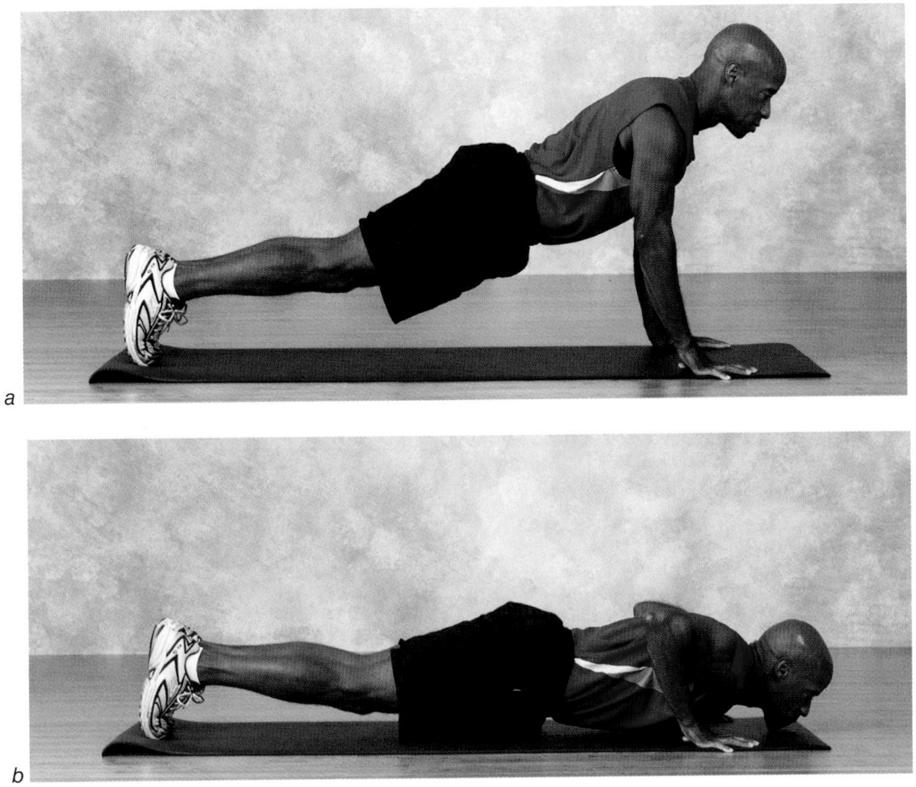

FIGURE 9.2 Proper form for the *(a)* starting position and *(b)* finishing position of the standard push-up test, as described by ACSM.

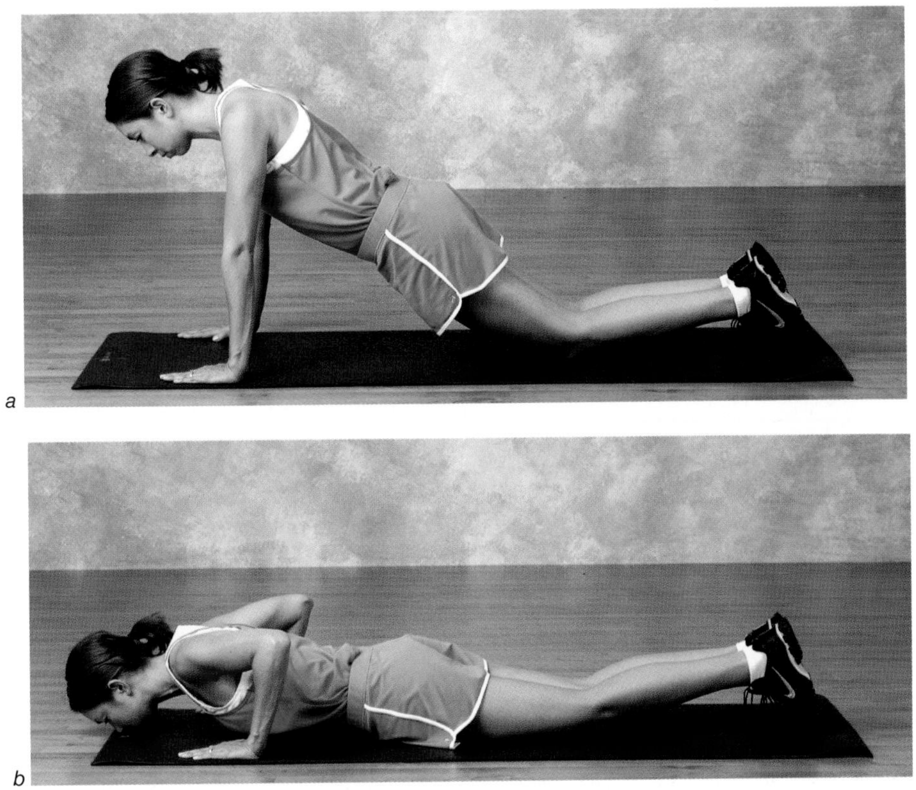

FIGURE 9.3 Proper form for the *(a)* starting position and *(b)* finishing position of the modified push-up test, as described by ACSM.

Push-Up Test Procedures *(continued)*

position often is used, with legs together, lower legs in contact with mat, ankles plantar flexed, back straight, hands shoulder-width apart, and head up. Some males will need to use the modified position, and some females can use the full-body position.

4. The subject must raise the body by straightening the elbows and then return to the down position until the chin touches the mat. The stomach should not touch the mat.
5. For both men and women, the back must be straight at all times and the subject must push up to a straight-arm position.
6. Stop the test when the client strains forcibly or is unable to maintain the appropriate exercise technique for 2 consecutive repetitions. The score is the maximal number of push-ups performed consecutively without rest.

Adapted from American College of Sports Medicine 2014, *ACSM's guidelines for exercise testing and prescription*, 9th ed. (Philadelphia: PA: Lippincott, Williams, & Wilkins).

VIDEO Watch **video 9.1**, which demonstrates the push-up test.

The push-up test is a relatively simple, inexpensive method for assessing local muscular endurance, and it can be used for men and women of various ages. Results of the standard push-up test for men and modified push-up test for women can be compared with the standards in table 9.1. As with RM testing, the push-up test can be performed on multiple occasions over time to reliably assess changes in local muscular endurance that occur with training. Finally, very deconditioned people, especially those who are overweight or obese, may find these tests difficult, and poor results obtained during testing may discourage them from exercise participation. Thus, the fitness professional must carefully consider whether these tests are appropriate and likely to yield useful information. In such circumstances where relatively low strength prohibits performance of the test with proper exercise technique, the push-up test is not adequate to assess muscular strength or local muscular endurance.

YMCA Bench Press Test

There are alternatives to the push-up test. The fitness professional can adapt resistance training equipment to measure local muscular endurance by selecting an appropriate submaximal level of resistance and measuring the number of repetitions or the duration of static contraction before fatigue. For example, the YMCA bench press test involves performing standardized repetitions at a rate of 30 repetitions per min to test local muscular endurance of the upper body (33, 39). Men use an 80 lb (36.3 kg) barbell and women use a 35 lb (15.9 kg) barbell, and subjects are scored by the number of successful repetitions completed. The main disadvantage of the test is that it uses a fixed weight, which favors larger clients over smaller clients. Also, the fixed weight may be too heavy for deconditioned or older clients to lift repeatedly. On the other hand, the load may be too light for very fit subjects, who may perform significantly more repetitions than typically used during training.

Despite these limitations, this test can be used independently or in combination with other tests in the overall assessment of muscular fitness in clients who have experience using free weights. The procedures for this test are summarized next, and norms are shown in tables 9.2 and 9.3.

Table 9.1 Fitness Categories by Age and Sex for Push-Up Test Using Number Completed

	20-29 YR		30-39 YR		40-49 YR		50-59 YR		60-69 YR	
Fitness	M	F	M	F	M	F	M	F	M	F
Excellent	≥36	≥30	≥30	≥27	≥25	≥24	≥21	≥21	≥18	≥17
Very good	29-35	21-29	22-29	20-26	17-24	15-23	13-20	11-20	11-17	12-16
Good	22-28	15-20	17-21	13-19	13-16	11-14	10-12	7-10	8-10	5-11
Fair	17-21	10-14	12-16	8-12	10-12	5-10	7-9	2-6	5-7	1-4
Needs improvement	≤16	≤9	≤11	≤7	≤9	≤4	≤6	≤1	≤4	≤1

Canadian Standardized Test of Fitness Operations Manual, 3rd ed., Health Canada, 2003. Reproduced with permission from the Minister of Public Works and Government Services Canada, 2011.

Table 9.2 YMCA Bench Press Norms for Number of Repetitions Completed for Men Using 80 lb (36.3 kg)

	AGE (YR)					
Fitness	**18-25**	**26-35**	**36-45**	**46-55**	**56-65**	**66+**
Excellent	44-64	41-61	36-55	28-47	24-41	20-36
Good	34-41	30-37	26-32	21-25	17-21	12-16
Above average	29-33	26-29	22-25	16-20	12-14	9-10
Average	24-28	21-24	18-21	12-14	9-11	7-8
Below average	20-22	17-20	17-14	9-11	5-8	4-6
Poor	13-17	12-16	9-12	5-8	2-4	2-3
Very poor	<10	≤9	≤6	≤2	≤1	≤1

Adapted from Golding 2000.

Table 9.3 YMCA Bench Press Norms for Number of Repetitions Completed for Women Using 35 lb (15.9 kg)

	AGE (YR)					
Fitness	**16-25**	**26-35**	**36-45**	**46-55**	**56-65**	**65+**
Excellent	42-66	40-62	40-62	29-50	24-42	18-30
Good	30-38	29-34	29-34	20-24	17-21	12-16
Above average	25-28	24-28	24-28	14-18	12-14	8-10
Average	20-22	18-22	18-22	10-13	8-10	5-7
Below average	16-18	14-17	14-17	7-9	5-6	3-4
Poor	9-13	9-13	9-13	2-6	2-4	0-2
Very poor	≤6	≤6	≤4	≤1	≤1	0

Adapted from Golding 2000.

YMCA Bench Press Test Procedures

1. Use a 35 lb (15.9 kg) straight barbell for women or an 80 lb (36.3 kg) straight barbell for men. A spotter should be present during the test.
2. Set a metronome to 60 beats $\cdot$ min^{-1}.
3. Have the subject begin with the bar in the down position touching the chest, with the elbows flexed and hands shoulder-width apart.
4. Count 1 repetition when the elbows fully extend. After each extension, the participant should lower the bar to touch the chest.
5. Instruct the client to complete up or down movements in time to the 60 beats $\cdot$ min^{-1} rhythm, which should be 30 lifts $\cdot$ min^{-1}.
6. Count the total number of repetitions completed in good form.

VIDEO

Watch **video 9.2**, which demonstrates the YMCA bench press test.

KEY POINT

The most common type of muscle fitness assessment in the fitness setting is dynamic strength testing with a single or multiple RM protocol. Although lack of adequate normative data often limits the evaluation of individual test data, such tests are valuable for tracking strength and local muscular endurance improvement. Field tests such as the push-up test provide a practical approach for evaluating local muscular endurance, either alone or together with other types of muscular fitness evaluations.

RESEARCH INSIGHT

Predicting Assistance Exercise Training Loads From Bench Press Test Results

Because the bench press is a common exercise in resistance training programs, Wong and colleagues (62) investigated whether loads for assistance exercises could be predicted from loads on the bench press exercise. Assistance exercises involve movement at one primary joint and recruit smaller muscle groups or only one large muscle group. Physically active adults performed a 6RM test on the bench press, barbell biceps curl, overhead dumbbell triceps extension, hammer curl, and dumbbell shoulder press. An analysis of the data revealed that the bench press load was significantly correlated with loads on the assistance exercises. The nonsignificant differences between the actual 6RM load and prediction equations developed by the researchers for each assistance exercise ranged between 6.5% and 8.5%. These findings suggest that health and fitness professionals can use the 6RM bench press load as an accurate method to predict training loads for upper-body assistance exercises.

Testing Older Adults

The number of older adults in the United States is expected to increase exponentially over the next several decades. For instance, in 2010 there were 18.6 million U.S. adults aged 75 or older, and this number is expected to double by the year 2050 (28). Further, the number of adults aged 85 and older is growing the fastest, with numbers expected to reach 19.5 million by 2040 (28). Because people are living longer, it is becoming increasingly important to find ways to extend active, healthy lifestyles and moderate the effects of sarcopenia and physical frailty in later years (4, 13, 28, 35). Assessing muscular strength and local muscular endurance as well as other aspects of physical fitness in older adults can reveal physical weaknesses and be used to design exercise programs that improve strength before serious functional limitations occur.

Senior Fitness Test

In response to the need for improved assessment for older adults, Rikli and Jones (52, 53) developed a functional fitness test battery, the Senior Fitness Test (SFT). This test evaluates the key physiological parameters (i.e., strength, endurance, agility, and balance) needed to perform everyday physical activities that are often difficult in later years. The SFT is used by researchers as well as health and fitness professionals who work with older men and women. In addition to evaluating a participant's strengths and identifying areas of physical weakness, data gathered from the SFT can provide evidence of outcome measures to document the effectiveness of an exercise program (54). Test items in the SFT are the 30 sec chair stand, 30 sec arm curl test, 6 min walk test, 2 min step test, chair sit-and-reach test, back-scratch test, 8 ft (2.4 m) up-and-go test, and height and weight (54). One of the most popular aspects of the SFT is the 30 sec chair stand test (38) (see Research Insight). This test, as well as others of the SFT, meets scientific standards for reliability and validity, is simple and easy to administer in the field setting, and has performance norms for men and women aged 60 to 94 based on a study of more than 7,000 older Americans (52). This test also has been shown to correlate well with other strength tests such as the 1RM. The fitness professional can use the SFT to safely and effectively assess functional ability in most older adults.

Before testing, all participants should warm up and follow other preliminary procedures as described earlier. In addition, the following instruction is recommended as a standardization procedure for administering the chair stand test and the arm curl test to all clients:

> Do the best you can on each test item, but never push yourself to a point of overexertion or beyond what you think is safe for you.

30 Sec Chair Stand Test

The 30 sec chair stand test, which reflects lower-body strength, involves counting the number of times within 30 sec that the participant can rise to a full stand from a seated position on a chair with a seat height of 17 in. (43 cm) with arms folded across the chest (see figure 9.4) (54). Studies have shown that chair stand performance, a common method of assessing lower-body strength in older adults, correlates well with major criterion indicators of lower-body strength (e.g., isokinetic-measured knee extensor and knee flexor strength), stair-climbing ability, walking speed, and risk of falling (10), and it has been found to detect normal age-related declines in strength (20). Further, the chair stand has been found to be safe and sensitive in detecting the effects of physical training in older adults (34, 47). Table 9.4 summarizes the normal range of scores of participants aged 60 to 94 yr. The normal range is defined as the middle 50% of the population tested for each age group, with the lower limits being equivalent to the 25th percentile rank and the upper limits equivalent to the 75th percentile rank within each 5 yr age group.

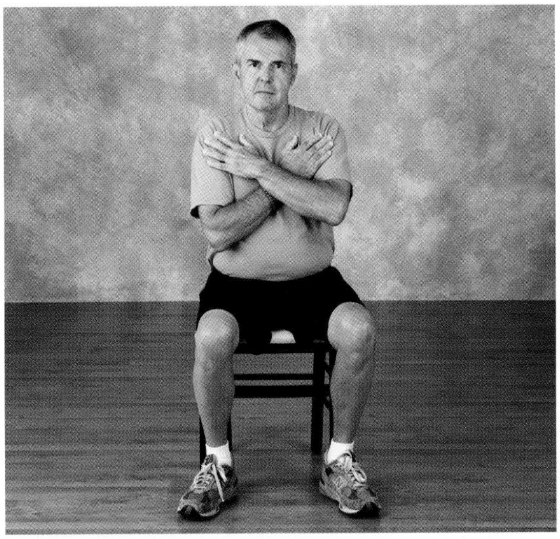

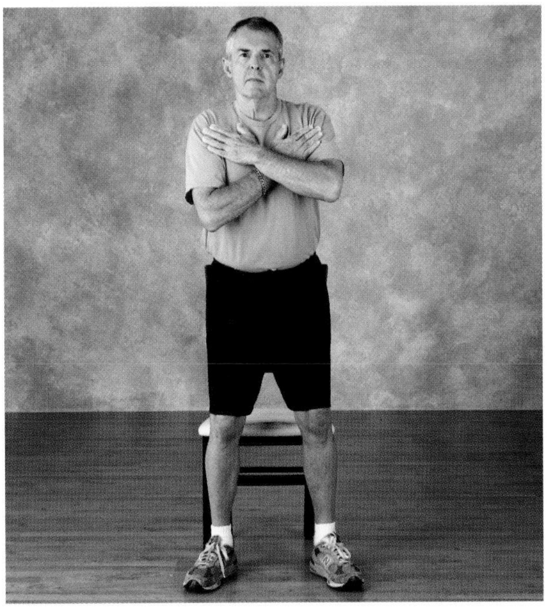

FIGURE 9.4 The 30 sec chair stand test.

RESEARCH INSIGHT

Influence of Seat Height on Chair Stand Performance

The 30 sec chair stand is a useful measure of lower-body strength and performance in seniors. Kuo (41) examined the influence of chair seat height on 30 sec chair stand performance in older adults (age 70 ± 6.3 yr). Participants performed the test from the standard height of 17 in. (43 cm) and from five randomly ordered seat heights from 80% to 120% of each participant's lower-leg length. Analysis of the data revealed that seat height significantly influenced the performance of older adults. The average score for standard conditions was significantly lower than those at 100%, 110%, and 120% conditions. These findings indicate that seat height can influence performance on the 30 sec chair stand test in older adults. Although a standard seat height of 17 in. (43 cm) is recommended for the 30 sec chair stand, health and fitness professionals should consider the influence of seat height on performance when interpreting test results.

Arm Curl Test

Upper-body function, including arm strength and local muscular endurance, is important in executing many everyday activities such as carrying groceries, lifting a suitcase, and picking up grandchildren. The 30 sec single-arm curl test, a measure of upper-body strength and local muscular endurance, determines the number of times a dumbbell

Table 9.4 Normal Range of Scores on the 30 Sec Chair Stand and 30 Sec Arm Curl Tests for Older Adults

	AGE (YR)						
	60-64	65-69	70-74	75-79	80-84	85-89	90-94
CHAIR STAND (NUMBER OF STANDS)							
Women	12-17	11-16	10-15	10-15	9-14	8-13	4-11
Men	14-19	12-18	12-17	11-17	10-15	8-14	7-12
ARM CURL (NUMBER OF REPS)							
Women	13-19	12-18	12-17	11-17	10-16	10-15	8-13
Men	16-22	15-21	14-21	13-19	13-19	11-17	10-17

Normal is defined as the middle 50% of the population. Participants scoring above or below these ranges would be considered above normal or below normal for their age.

Reprinted, by permission, from R.E. Rikli, and C.J. Jones, 2013, *Senior fitness test manual*, 2nd ed. (Champaign, IL: Human Kinetics), 89-90.

(5 lb [2.3 kg] for women and 8 lb [3.6 kg] for men) can be curled through a full ROM in 30 sec while sitting on a chair with back straight and feet flat (54). The prescribed protocol includes holding the weight in the dominant hand in a handshake grip at full extension (to the side of the chair) and then supinating during flexion so that the palm of the hand faces the biceps at full flexion (figure 9.5). The score is the total number of arm curls performed in 30 sec. Studies indicate that the 30 sec arm curl test is a good predictor of both biceps and overall upper-body strength and local muscular endurance (52). Results obtained from the 30 sec arm curl test can be compared with the norms presented in table 9.4.

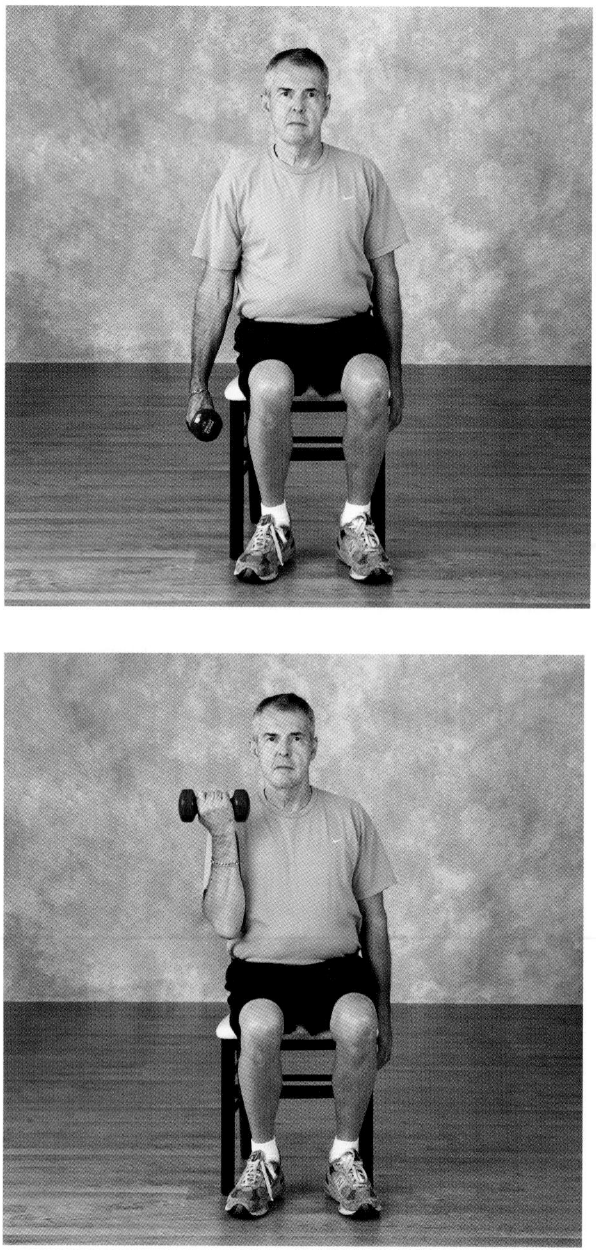

FIGURE 9.5 The 30 sec arm curl test.

Testing Clients With Cardiovascular Disease

Moderate resistance training performed 2 days per wk improves muscular fitness, prevents and manages a variety of chronic medical conditions, modifies coronary risk factors, and enhances psychosocial well-being for people with CVD, including high BP (hypertension) and CHD (32, 58, 64). Resistance training could benefit most adults living with heart disease and its associated risk factors, including dyslipidemia, hypertension, and prediabetes. This is because many adults with and without cardiovascular conditions do not regularly participate in muscular strengthening exercises and lack the physical strength and self-confidence to perform common daily activities that require muscular effort (16, 29, 35). Consequently, authoritative professional medical organizations, including the AHA (29), ACSM (6), and American Association of Cardiovascular and Pulmonary Rehabilitation (AACVPR) (3), support resistance training as an adjunct to endurance exercise in their current recommendations and guidelines for exercise for people with CVD.

Moderate-intensity (e.g., 10 to 15 repetitions) resistance testing and training can be performed safely by cardiac patients deemed low risk (e.g., patients with absence of angina, ST-segment changes on the ECG, or complex ventricular dysrhythmias) (6, 29). Moreover, despite concerns that resistance exercise elicits abnormal cardiovascular pressor responses, such as severely elevated BP in patients with CHD or controlled hypertension, studies have found that strength tests and resistance training in these individuals typically elicit clinically acceptable HR and BP responses (24, 36, 60, 61) Data on the benefits and safety of resistance training in patients with poor left ventricular function, such as those with CHF, are increasing, but additional study is warranted (42). According to ACSM, absolute contraindications for resistance training and testing include uncontrolled hypertension (>180/110 mmHg); unstable CHD; uncontrolled arrhythmias; severe pulmonary hypertension; severe and symptomatic aortic stenosis; acute myocarditis, endocarditis, or pericarditis; aortic dissection; Marfan syndrome; and decompensated CHF (6). Also, patients with active proliferative retinopathy or moderate or worse nonproliferative diabetic retinopathy should avoid high-intensity resistance training (80%-100% 1RM) (6).

As with GXTs, the risk of a serious cardiac event during strength testing can be minimized by preparticipation screening and close supervision by fitness professionals, particularly those with specialized training and certification regarding people who have special health concerns. When testing patients with known or suspected CHD or hypertension, the fitness professional should do preliminary work to establish appropriate weight loads and instruct the participant on proper lifting techniques. This should include demonstrating proper ROM and speed of movement for each exercise as well as correct breathing patterns to avoid the Valsalva maneuver. The monitoring of resting and recovery BP (e.g., every few min) and identification and evaluation of abnormal signs and symptoms should be standard protocol during the initial evaluation of the cardiovascular response during testing. Exaggerated BP responses, clinical signs or symptoms of CHD, or any other abnormal findings as previously described by ACSM that occur during resistance testing or training indicate termination of the activity until further evaluation by a qualified health care provider (6). Because BP measured immediately after exercise tends to underestimate values during contractions, the fitness professional should act conservatively when evaluating cardiovascular responses to testing in this population (26).

Studies have shown no adverse hemodynamic responses in low-risk cardiac patients who perform 1RM or multiple RM testing for upper- and lower-body exercises (23, 26, 59). Moreover, there is no scientific evidence suggesting that 1RM testing is riskier than 10RM testing for low-risk cardiac patients. However, multiple RM testing (e.g., 10RM) is a more conservative and, therefore, sensible approach to testing clients with a history of CVD. Thus, multiple RM testing that includes higher repetitions (i.e., 10 to 15) rather than single or low repetitions is a recommended practice for the fitness professional to assess strength and endurance in people with stable CHD. Regardless of the number of repetitions used during testing, the initial resistance or weight should be moderate to allow the participant to achieve the proper repetition range by working at a level that is strong, or heavy (i.e., 5-6 on Borg's 10-grade RPE scale; see chapters 7 and 11) (11). Furthermore, the procedures for strength assessment previously described in this chapter can be applied safely to clients with a history of known or occult CHD who are clinically stable and to clients with controlled hypertension, diabetes, or other cardiovascular high risk factors. Careful screening and astute monitoring of abnormal signs or symptoms, such as angina, dizziness, or light-headedness, are paramount to minimize any potential risks while simultaneously maximizing the benefits of resistance testing or training for people with and without known CVD.

Testing Children and Adolescents

Along with CRF, flexibility, and body composition, muscular strength is an important component of health-related fitness in children and adolescents (21, 49). Enhancing muscular strength helps young people develop proper posture, reduce the risk of injury, improve body composition, and enhance motor skills such as sprinting and jumping (44). Assessing muscular strength and endurance with the push-up test is common in most physical education programs and YMCA recreation programs, whereas maximal load lifting (e.g., 1RM and 10RM) is often used to evaluate training-induced changes in performance in youth sport centers and pediatric research facilities (44).

Although standardized 1RM strength and power testing procedures have been developed for children and adolescents (24, 25), RM testing is time consuming and requires close supervision. Therefore, a standardized field test program, such as the Fitnessgram (19), is a time-efficient method for assessing muscular fitness in a group or class of school-aged youth. Performance on field-based tests such as the long jump is strongly associated with upper- and lower-body muscular strength tests in youth (15), although the long jump is not included in the standard Fitnessgram assessment (see Research Insight). Normative data for children and teenagers are available in the Fitnessgram test manual and fitness testing resources (19, 37). A variety of fitness measures can be used to assess a child's strength and local muscular endurance, develop a personalized fitness program, track progress, and motivate participants. Generally, when children are ready to participate in sport activities (about age 7 or 8), they are also ready for structured testing and training (44).

Unsupervised or poorly administered strength assessments may not only discourage young people from participating in fitness activities but also result in injury (48). Qualified fitness professionals should demonstrate how to properly perform each exercise, allow the child to practice a few repetitions of each exercise, and offer guidance when necessary. In order to assess muscular strength in a safe and efficacious manner with a focus on proper exercise technique, some youth health and fitness professionals use an approach called *criterion repetition maximum testing (CRM)* instead of RM (22). CRM testing focuses on the quality of the movement and the physical effort needed to perform the lift, which requires testers to carefully assess the technical performance of every repetition. Although all strength testing requires proper exercise technique and qualified supervision, the perception of a CRM as opposed to an RM may help to reinforce the importance of proper exercise technique. This approach may be particularly important when testing untrained youth, who may not be aware of the inherent risks associated with resistance training. All participants must understand that the amount of weight lifted or number of repetitions completed is not as important as how the exercise was performed.

When assessing fitness in young people, avoid the pass–fail mentality that may discourage some boys and girls from participating. Instead, refer to the assessment as a *challenge* in which all participants can feel good about their performance and get excited about monitoring their progress. Fitness professionals should also understand that children are not simply miniature adults. Because children are physically and psychologically less mature than adults, evaluating any measure of physical fitness requires special considerations. Fitness professionals should develop a friendly rapport with each child, and the exercise area should be nonthreatening. Because most children have limited experience performing at maximum exertion, fitness professionals should reassure children that they can safely perform exercise at a high exertion. Moreover, positive encouragement can motivate children to help ensure a valid test outcome. Following the strength assessment, cool down afterward with gentle calisthenics and stretching exercises.

KEY POINT

Muscular fitness testing is useful for a variety of special populations, including older adults, people at increased cardiovascular risk, and children and adolescents. Although strength tests, particularly those involving maximal exertion, were once thought to evoke unsafe physiological responses in these populations, scientific evidence shows that such tests are safe and can provide valuable information for the resistance training prescription if properly administered and performed. For older adults and people at elevated cardiovascular risk, proper screening by a physician or other qualified health care professional is warranted to promote safe and effective muscular fitness evaluations.

RESEARCH INSIGHT

Field Tests Versus Repetition Maximum Testing in Children

Although RM testing has been found to be safe and reliable for assessing muscular strength in children, it may not be practical for large groups when time is limited. Artero and colleagues (7) analyzed the association between isokinetic strength and field-based muscular fitness tests in 126 adolescents. Upper- and lower-body isokinetic strength were measured at preset angular velocities, and muscular fitness was assessed with various field tests, including handgrip strength, arm hang, standing long jump, squat jump, and countermovement jump tests. Analysis of the data found that all field-based tests were significantly associated with isokinetic peak torque and power, but handgrip strength and standing long jump were the most valid field-based muscular fitness tests when compared with isokinetic strength. Health and fitness professionals who work with youth should consider using these field tests to assess muscular fitness when RM testing methods are not feasible.

9

LEARNING AIDS

REVIEW QUESTIONS

1. Define *muscular strength*, *local muscular endurance*, and *muscular power*.
2. What would you include in a standardization procedure to improve the safety and reliability of a strength test?
3. Describe the procedures for measuring a 1RM on the leg press exercise for an adult.
4. Describe two tests for measuring local muscular endurance, one using weights and one using body weight as the resistance.
5. How you would compare the 1RM strength of two people who differ markedly in body weight?
6. Describe a lower-body and an upper-body muscular fitness test for seniors.
7. How would you assess muscular strength in a low-risk cardiac patient?
8. What field-based tests can be used to assess muscular fitness in school-aged youth?

CASE STUDIES

1. A 32-yr-old healthy male (height 70 in. [178 cm], weight 190 lb [86.2 kg]) has been resistance training on weight machines at a fitness center for 2 mo. Although he did not have an initial strength assessment when he joined the center, he wants an evaluation of his upper- and lower-body strength. Outline a 1RM testing protocol for this client and discuss safety procedures. How would you use the test results to provide meaningful feedback to this client?
2. A middle-aged female who recently joined your fitness facility would like to participate in an initial fitness assessment and receive advice about beginning a general fitness program to improve her muscular fitness. She has not participated in a structured exercise program for several years, although she reports that she leads an active lifestyle and often achieves moderate amounts of physical activity throughout the day. Her preparticipation health history questionnaire reveals that she is without signs, symptoms, or diagnosis of any cardiovascular, metabolic, or musculoskeletal conditions. With a classmate playing the role of this client, practice the following procedures presented in this chapter:

    a. Explain, demonstrate, and perform the procedures for the push-up test.

    b. Using the client information just described, explain, demonstrate, and perform the procedures for the 1RM bench press test.

Answers to Case Studies

1. Because this healthy adult has 2 mo of resistance training experience, he does not need to participate in familiarization sessions. However, the exercises used for strength testing (e.g., chest press and leg press) should be part of his resistance training program. After a proper warm-up and explanation of testing procedures (e.g., proper exercise technique, full ROM, and predetermined speed of movement), follow standard 1RM testing guidelines. Begin with a light set of 5 to 10 repetitions at 50% perceived maximum. After a 1 min rest, perform 3 to 5 repetitions at 60% to 80% perceived maximum. Then begin the 1RM tests with a 3 min rest interval between trials. Continue the process until a failed attempt, ideally within 3 to 5 trials. To determine his relative strength on each exercise, divide the 1RM weight by his body weight. Fitness categories for upper- and lower-body strength are available (6). Percentile values (very poor to superior) can be used to assess his performance and provide meaningful feedback.
2. For this exercise:

    a. Please see pages 184 and 186 for a summary of the push-up test.

    b. Please see page 183 for a summary of the 1RM test.

10

Assessment of Flexibility and Low-Back Function

Laura Horvath Gagnon

I am pleased to have been able to build on the work of Dr. Wendell Liemohn.

OBJECTIVES

The reader will be able to do the following:

1. List factors that influence low-back function and flexibility.
2. Identify relative flexibility compensations that affect flexibility testing.
3. Describe and demonstrate tools used in assessing flexibility and ROM.
4. Describe the pros and cons of the sit-and-reach test.
5. Recognize when referral to a medical professional is needed.

Flexibility is an important component of overall physical fitness because many activities require good joint motion and muscular extensibility (1). Impaired flexibility negatively affects low-back function. The fitness professional will likely come in contact with clients who have a history of or who are currently experiencing **low-back pain (LBP)**. LBP has a lifetime prevalence of 80% (54, 58) and a 1 yr prevalence ranging from 22% to 65% (66). About one-fourth of U.S. adults have reported experiencing LBP in the past 3 mo (22). Estimates of recurrence at 1 yr range from 24% to 80% (34). This high incidence of low-back dysfunction places a burden on economic, social, and medical resources. Any positive impact that fitness professionals can have on their clients' back function in LBP prevention or rehabilitation can have a large benefit to both individuals and society. Multiple tools may be used in addressing low-back function and flexibility, some used by fitness professionals and some by the medical community.

As the fitness professional assesses a client, it is essential to consider the factors that may be influencing flexibility and low-back function. The assessment tools need to be well understood and appropriately applied to create an effective and safe individualized program. A solid understanding of basic spine anatomy related to ROM (range of motion) and flexibility are important in choosing the correct assessment tool. (A more thorough discussion of spinal anatomy and biomechanics related to core stability is presented in chapter 14.) In addition, the fitness professional may be in a position to suggest that a client seek medical intervention, and the parameters that guide this decision need to be clear. The complexity of the spine can cause anxiety among fitness professionals; however, the importance of low-back function in everyday life makes it an important area in which to gain confidence.

Basics of Flexibility

Flexibility relates to the ability to bend without breaking; **flexion** is the act of bending or being bent. In applied anatomy, *flexion* denotes a bending movement that occurs in the sagittal plane as two body segments are brought together (see chapter 3). **Flexibility** is defined as the capacity to move joints freely through their normal ROM. As one assesses the flexibility of a region, all the components influencing the ROM need to be considered, including (1) which joints are involved with the motion; (2) the shapes and positions of the joints (i.e., correct alignment of joints); (3) the muscles, tendons, ligaments, and joint capsules of the involved joints; and (4) whether the muscle stretch reflex is being activated in the assessment process. For example, a person reaching to touch the floor from a standing position flexes both the spine and the hips. The movement pattern that occurs is called the *lumbopelvic rhythm* and is a combination of flexion of the lower intervertebral joints of the spine, lumbosacral motion, and iliofemoral (hip) flexion in varying ratios (14, 25, 47). Therefore, when using the toe-touch test to assess flexibility, one needs to take into account all of the joints involved, the muscles crossing these joints, and the position of each of these joints.

Consider another example in which hamstring flexibility is assessed with the subject lying on his back. If the spine is flexed as the leg is lifted, the assessment includes some spine ROM as well as hamstring extensibility. If this assessment is performed quickly, the stretch reflex may be activated and the true length of the hamstring may not be apparent. Sometimes, in an attempt to obtain a greater ROM in an area, the joint is compromised by poor positioning. This may overstretch the ligaments instead of stretching the appropriate muscles, leading to hypermobility of that joint. Awareness of these flexibility components will make the assessment, and the prescription of stretching exercises, more effective.

Having functional ROM at all joints of the musculoskeletal system ensures efficient body movement, which is one reason why flexibility is a key component of physical fitness. Assessing which joints are involved in a particular movement is pivotal in the assessment of flexibility in that region. If a flexibility test involves more than one joint, a person may have a good overall score for ROM but still have stiffness across one of the joints or regions tested. For example, a person may seem flexible because she touches her toes easily from a standing position (see figure 10.1). But which structure is more flexible in the person in figure 10.1*a*, the hamstrings or low back? Clearly, the hamstrings are more flexible; there is little curvature in the back in contrast with the spinal curvature in figure 10.1*b*.

According to Sahrmann (61), *relative flexibility* is demonstrated when a person can touch his toes yet exhibits decreased low-back flexibility. Stiffness across one joint or in one muscle group creates compensatory movements at neighboring joints and muscles. These structures may then have to increase flexibility or become hypermobile to meet the goal of the overall movement. In other words, the body will follow the path of least resistance or the most flexible route to accomplish the overall movement. If the fitness professional prescribes the toe-touch exercise as a low-back stretch for the person in figure 10.1*a*, it will likely improve hamstring flexibility but not back flexibility because the body will choose the easiest way to get to the floor—using the hamstrings. Caution should be used in interpreting this exercise as a flexibility test due its inclusion of many joints (intervertebral, lumbosacral, and iliofemoral) and relative flexibility when multiple joints are involved.

Another example of relative flexibility is performing a squat with the feet in a flattened or overpronated position due to a lack of ankle dorsiflexion (see figure 10.2). The forefoot and midfoot can become more flexible to compensate for the lack of ankle dorsiflexion. The increased flexibility or laxity of the arch or midfoot allows flattening of the arch, and thus the ankle is not required to move as much in dorsiflexion. The whole lower-extremity position changes based on the position of the foot. This lack of ankle flexibility can have a profound impact on the health of the lower extremity; for instance, injuries to the medial knee structures have been reported (45). If the fitness professional prescribes an ankle dorsiflexion stretch to address the gastrocnemius and soleus but does not block overpronation

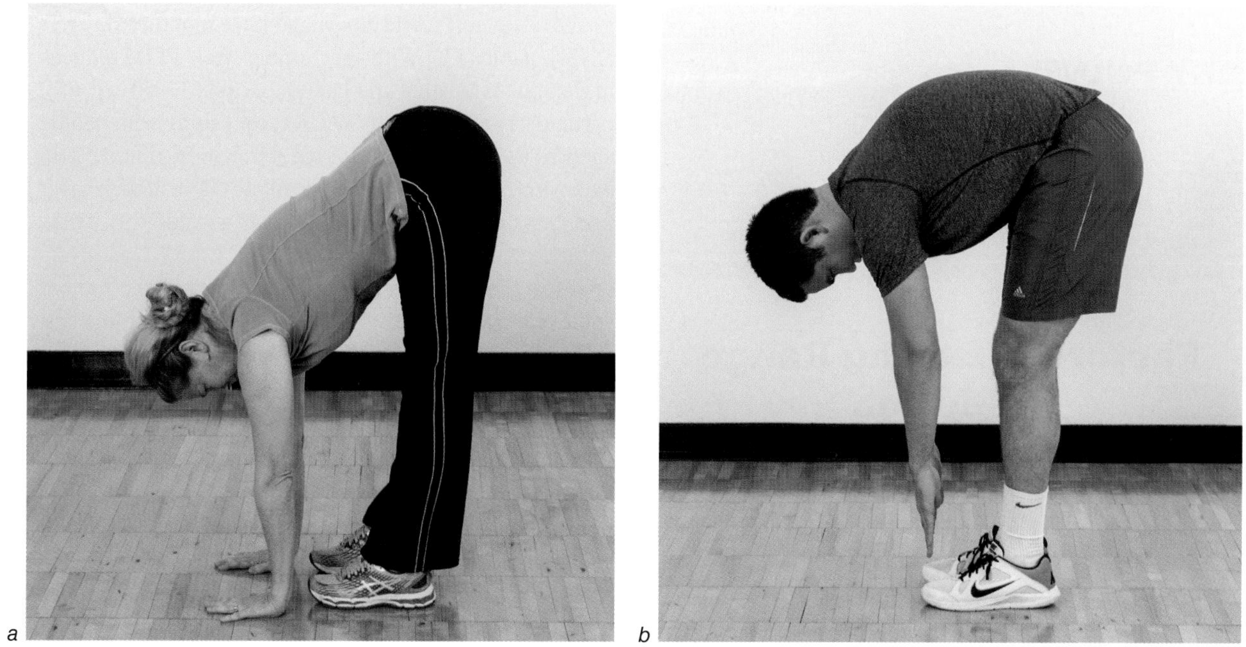

FIGURE 10.1 Relative flexibility demonstrated by the toe-touch test. In *(a)* the lumbar spine is relatively flat and in *(b)* the lumbar spine has a greater curve. The person in *(a)* has good hamstring flexibility but limited lumbar spine ROM. In *(b)* the person has good lumbar spine ROM and moderate hamstring flexibility.

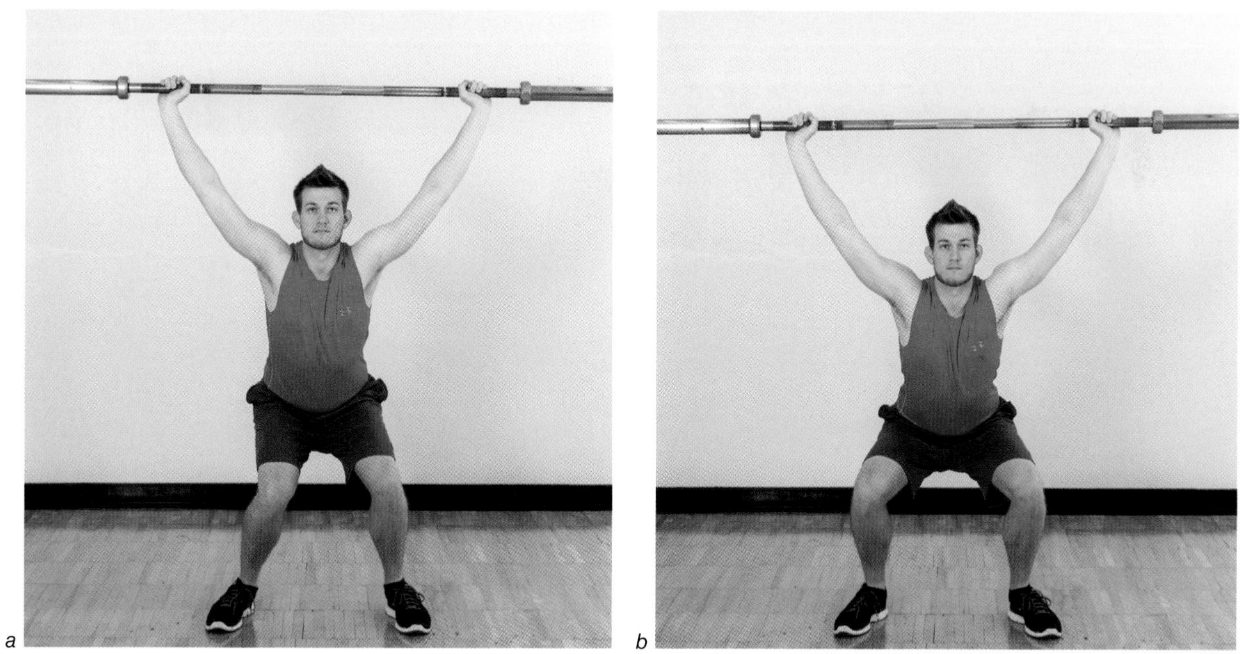

FIGURE 10.2 Relative flexibility demonstrated by the position of the squat *(a)* obtained through the already flexible midfoot (flatfoot) rather than by acquiring more calf flexibility and ankle dorsiflexion. To perform the squat correctly, *(b)* the excessive midfoot motion needs to be controlled with orthotics or foot position changes.

of the mid- and forefoot, the stretch will not only be ineffective but might actually increase the hypermobility in the foot. Relative flexibility needs to be considered in all flexibility assessment tests because compensatory patterns need to be identified and addressed either by the fitness professional or by physical therapy.

KEY POINT

Having good ROM at all joints reduces the risk of injury. Noting and addressing relative flexibility compensations can decrease pain and dysfunction.

Factors Affecting Range of Motion

When evaluating a client for ROM limitations, it is helpful to consider factors that may lead to restrictions in flexibility. Some of the most common factors include demographics such as age and sex, postural stressors, diseases such as arthritis and osteoporosis, and previous injuries. A good baseline questionnaire or interview of the client should provide this useful information.

Age and Sex

Flexibility can be affected by several demographic variables. For example, ROM typically decreases in adulthood; however, it is unknown how much of this diminution is attributable to aging or to the reduction in physical activity related to aging. Overall joint flexibility has been shown to decrease at a rate of 0.6% per year for females and 0.8% for males (seven joints included in the study) (51). In general, the shoulders and trunk show less flexibility as age advances, while elbow and knee mobility stay relatively stable (51). With age, lumbar spine ROM reduces in flexion, extension, and lateral flexion (37, 50, 51, 65), particularly after age 40 (37). A recent study with people aged 20 to 75 showed a 31% reduction in flexion, 12% in extension, and 20% in lumbar lordotic curve in those over age 50 as compared with the 20- to 29-yr-olds (23). There is little change in lumbar rotation (37, 65). One group of researchers reports that the lower part of the lumbar spine retains its mobility and lordosis, but the middle part flattens and becomes less mobile as we age (23).

Posture

If people do not use the full ROM at a joint, tissues may compensate by shortening. It then becomes difficult to perform some of the movements needed in ADLs. For example, a person sitting at a computer desk several hours each day might develop a greater thoracic curve (i.e., dorsal kyphosis) and rounded shoulders (see figure 10.3*a*). If this posture becomes habitual and no countermeasures are taken to change it, tissue that previously permitted good movement can shorten (31), and correction of this posture may become difficult, if not impossible. A much better posture to assume at a desk is seen in figure 10.3*b*.

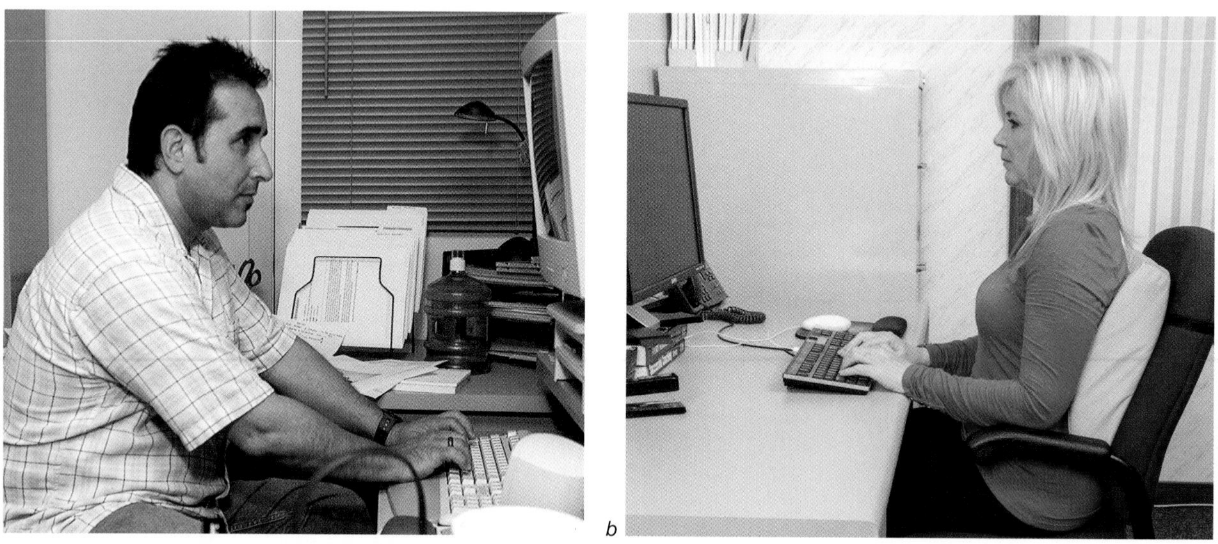

a *b*

FIGURE 10.3 Connective-tissue structures (e.g., ligaments and tendons) adapt to *(a)* habitual poor sitting posture (e.g., rounding of the upper back or less lordotic curve in the lumbar region) by lengthening in response to stress. Without an attempt to remove these stresses or to develop counterbalancing ones, poor sitting postures can transfer to poor standing postures. The person in *(b)* demonstrates a properly balanced sitting posture.

Disease

A wide variety of diseases can negatively affect ROM. Two of the most common diseases that have an impact on joint mobility are arthritis and osteoporosis.

Arthritis

Arthritis can have a debilitating effect on ROM because it affects articular cartilage. Articular cartilage, also called *hyaline cartilage,* is **avascular** (i.e., it does not have a blood supply), which means its healing capability is poor. Because articular cartilage does not repair itself well, fibrocartilage and bony spicules may replace the cartilage, diminishing joint movement (57). Two common types of arthritis are **rheumatoid arthritis (RA)** and **osteoarthritis (OA)**. RA occurs more frequently in females than males and can appear any time in life. This autoimmune condition is a chronic inflammatory polyarthritis, an arthritis that affects five or more joints (19). The inflammatory process primarily affects the lining of the joints (synovial membrane). The inflamed synovium leads to erosion of the cartilage and bone, and sometimes joint deformity results, causing joint stiffness and decreased ROM (19). Chronic low-back dysfunction has been associated with RA (10).

OA is a much more prevalent condition, accounting for 90% to 95% of arthritis cases, and it usually begins after the age of 40. OA is a disease of the entire joint involving the cartilage, joint lining, ligaments, and underlying bone (17). The breakdown of these tissues eventually leads to pain and joint stiffness and has a significant impact on the incidence of low-back dysfunction and loss of ROM. The causes of OA are complex and often are the result of both mechanical (injuries or overuse) and cellular (inflammation) events in the affected joint (3, 17). More than 27 million people in the United States have OA, with women more likely to have it than men (4). It can occur in any joint, including those in the spine, hands, ankles, feet, hips, and knees, but the knees and the spine are the most commonly affected areas. Arthritis can decrease mobility in the spine if the site is a facet joint (see figure 10.4) that helps guide motion in the spine (57). Facet joint OA is a common cause of low-back dysfunction (30), and it seems to follow lumbar disc degeneration (29) due to the increased forces on the facet joints (see figure 10.4). Because articular cartilage is avascular, it depends on the diffusion of nutrients from tissue fluid, and so further deterioration can result from lack of movement. Thus, it is desirable for people with arthritis to maintain as much movement and ROM as possible. (See also chapter 14.)

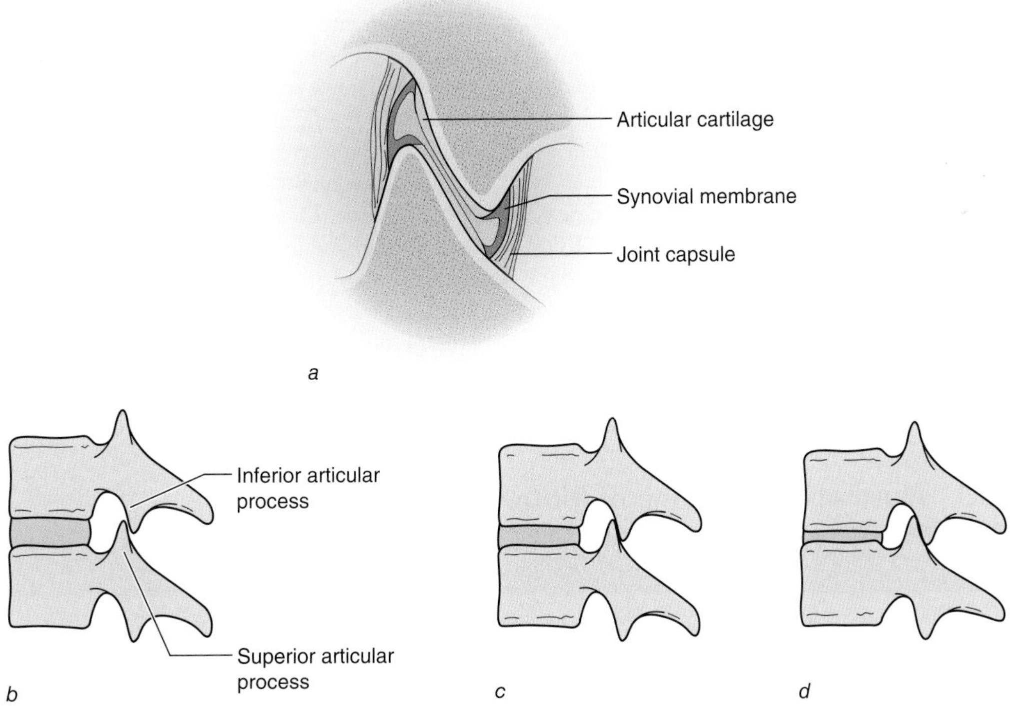

FIGURE 10.4 Posterior junctions between two vertebrae often are referred to as *facet joints.* Facet joints are synovial joints and have articular cartilage, as seen here in the *(a)* sagittal view and *(b)* vertebral column with normal disc thickness. *(c)* Reduction of the disc thickness adds stress to the facet joint. *(d)* Further disc degeneration leads to impingement at the tips of both the superior articulate process and inferior articulate process.

Osteoporosis

Osteoporosis is characterized by a loss in BMD (bone mineral density) or bone mass. Risk factors include being female, postmenopausal, or older; having a small body size; eating a diet low in calcium; and being physically inactive (18). Common osteoporotic sites include the hip, wrist, and vertebrae—all sites where cancellous bone predominates (see chapter 3). In the spine, osteoporosis can cause buckling and compression of vertebrae. A person with this condition may show extreme curves in the spine as well as loss of ROM. Fortunately, cancellous bone can become denser through weight-bearing activities and resistance training. (See also chapter 17.)

Previous Injury

Previous injury can create either decreased flexibility in injured tissue or increased joint motion (hypermobility). Muscle that has been disrupted due to an injury may show decreased extensibility and loss of endurance and strength (57). For example, a hamstring strain can significantly decrease the capacity of the muscle to lengthen as one reaches to touch the floor. However, ligaments that run bone to bone and guide joint motion may be overstretched if injured and allow too much joint motion (hypermobility) (57). A common example is the case of an inversion ankle sprain. If the sprain disrupts the supporting ligaments sufficiently, the ankle typically becomes more mobile. Some low-back injuries may also have both immediate and long-term impacts on ROM, including herniated discs (all planes of motion possibly limited), spinal stenosis (extension), ankylosing spondylitis (decreased spinal curves), spondylolisthesis (extension), lumbar facet syndrome (usually extension and rotation), muscle strain (can be decreased in any plane) (31), and degenerative disc disease and hypermobility (may have increased or decreased ROM changes) (42). A history of LBP is predictive of low-back dysfunction (64). Some injuries may not show any change in low-back ROM but will affect overall function and strength. Having a complete history of the client's injuries is ideal in assessing flexibility and low-back function.

KEY POINT

Factors relating to ROM include age, sex, posture, disease, and injury history. If the ROM of a joint is not used, it may be lost. Although declines in ROM often relate to increased age, some result from a decline in physical activity or from injury. Habitual poor posture also can decrease ROM. Arthritis is a disease of the joints and thus tends to decrease joint ROM. Osteoporosis can reduce spine ROM because of its destructive effect on vertebral bodies. Injury changes the extensibility of soft tissue.

Hip, Knee, Ankle, and Shoulder Flexibility Testing

Flexibility can be assessed at each joint using both quantitative and qualitative approaches. For example, the ROM available at the knee can be measured in degrees with a goniometer or noted in terms of full motion or exhibiting mild, moderate, or significant limitations. Most fitness professionals do not need the specificity of goniometric measures; however, recognizing the extent (i.e., mild, moderate, significant) to which a joint is limited will help identify areas where flexibility is compromised. The fitness professional can then select stretches appropriate for that client's needs. Common joints that should be assessed include the shoulders, elbows, wrists, hips, knees, and ankles. Table 10.1 presents the normal ROM for the major joints. Again, the assessment of joint flexibility in a fitness center is not likely to require a goniometer, but knowledge of the full ROM possible at each joint is necessary in order to assess limitations in flexibility (mild, moderate, or sig-

Table 10.1 Normal Joint Range of Motion

Area	Flexion	Extension	Abduction	Adduction	External rotation	Internal rotation
Shoulder	167-180°	60°	180°		90°	70°
Hip	140°	15°	30°	25°	90°	70°
Knee	140°	0°			45° max at 90°	35° max at 90°
Ankle	PF* 40-55°	DF** 10-20°				

*PF=plantar flexion; **DF=dorsiflexion

nificant). Flexibility can also be considered by investigating the length of specific muscles that cover two joints, such as the hamstrings or hip flexors (iliopsoas). The next section covers tests addressing the flexibility of the hamstrings, hip flexors, iliotibial band (ITB), quadriceps, gastrocnemius, soleus, piriformis, and shoulders. A postural assessment can suggest which muscles may be tight.

Some postural deviations to note are as follows:

- A client with rounded, forward-placed shoulders may have tight pectoralis muscles and limited shoulder motion.
- A client with a posteriorly tilted pelvic girdle may have tight hamstrings.
- A client with an anteriorly tilted pelvic girdle may have tight hip flexors and lumbar musculature.
- A client with overpronated feet or fallen arches may have tight calves and ITBs.

The tight musculature identified through these assessments can be listed in a chart in the client's file to recheck as the fitness program progresses.

Iliofemoral Range of Motion

There is some evidence showing that hip muscle imbalance is associated with LBP and dysfunction (55, 56). The muscles crossing the hip joint are sometimes viewed as guy-wires because they can limit pelvic motion (see figure 10.5). If any of these guy-wires are too tight, the trunk musculature may have difficulty controlling pelvic position. Because the sacrum (in the pelvis) is the foundation of the 24 vertebrae stacked on it, pelvic positioning plays an important role in the integrity of the spine. For example, tightness in the hip flexors, such as the psoas, can produce an anterior or forward pelvic tilt, and tightness in the hip extensors, such as the hamstrings, can produce a backward or posterior pelvic tilt (see figure 10.5). Thus, if either of these muscle groups is tight, the abdominal muscles are less able to control pelvic positioning. People who cannot control their pelvic positioning with their abdominal muscles are predisposed to LBP, which is one of the reasons why ROM at the iliofemoral joint is important.

Biering-Sorensen's study revealed that weak trunk musculature and poor flexibility of the back and hamstrings

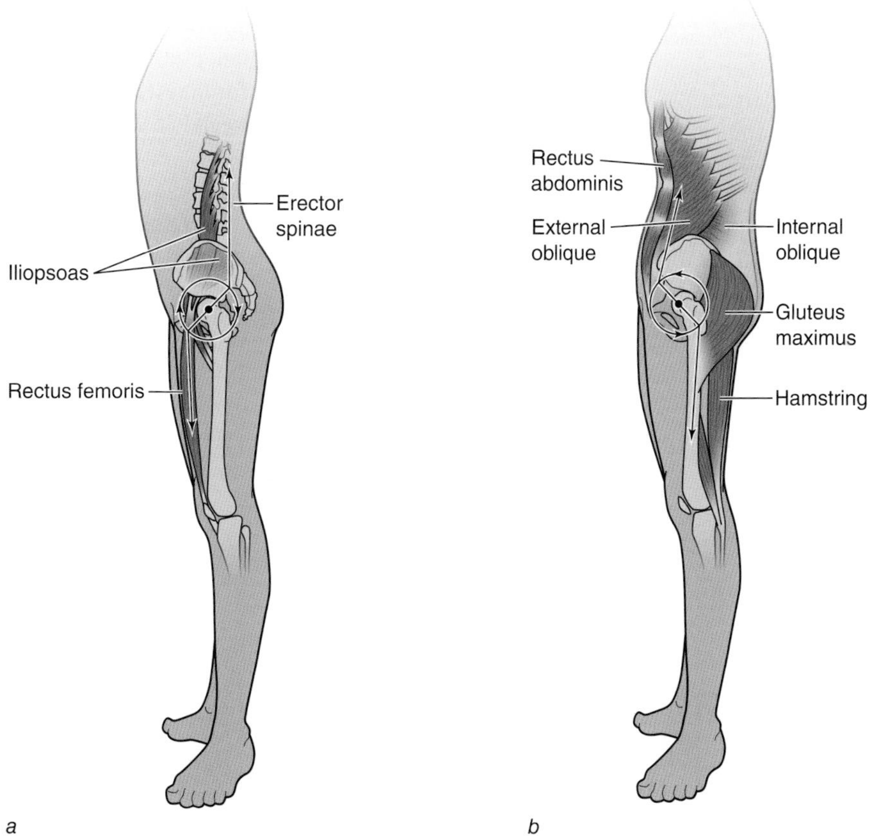

FIGURE 10.5 The muscles crossing the hip joint can be viewed as guy-wires. If, for example, the erector spinae guy-wires are too tight, *(a)* they will tend to anteriorly rotate the pelvis. If the hamstring guy-wires are too tight, *(b)* they will tend to posteriorly rotate the pelvis, making it difficult for the rectus abdominis to control pelvic positioning. Inability to control pelvic positioning with the abdominal musculature predisposes a person to low-back problems.

were present in those with recurrent or persistent LBP (12). There also may be tightness in the ITB, which can limit thigh adduction. Tightness in the piriformis muscle can limit movement in the transverse plane, but this is a little more complex because such tightness can limit outward or inward rotation of the femur depending on the angle between hip and thigh (60). Healthy subjects were compared with patients with LBP in terms of their hip ROM patterns (24). The results suggest an association between hip rotation ROM imbalance (internal and external ROM) and the presence of LBP.

Correct assessment of the musculature crossing the hip is essential to creating an effective flexibility program. The following tests of the ITB, iliopsoas, hamstring, piriformis, gastrocnemius, soleus, and shoulder girdle musculature can be used in the fitness setting.

Thomas Test

The Thomas test measures tightness in the hip flexors (31), including the iliopsoas, rectus femoris, and ITB (see figure 10.6). The reliability between testers has been shown to be high for this test (28). The client starts by sitting on the edge of a surface and leaning back to the supine position. The client then brings both knees toward the chest. The left leg is released so that extends and touches the surface. The left thigh should remain in contact with the testing surface (26, 31). If it does not, the degree of elevation indicates the tightness of the left hip flexors (iliopsoas). If the knee is bent 70° or less, the rectus femoris is tight. If the left leg abducts or angles outward, the ITB is tight. The pelvic girdle and low back need to remain in a neutral position to avoid a false negative or positive. The low back should be against the surface but not in a posteriorly tilted position.

VIDEO Watch video **10.1**, which demonstrates the Thomas test.

Active Knee Extension Test

Two popular tests that measure tightness of the hamstrings are the knee extension test, which is an active test, and the straight leg raise test, which is a passive test. The active knee extension (AKE) test has been shown to have excellent intra- and inter-rater reliability for assessing hamstring length in healthy individuals (32). The client lies supine with the hip held at 90° flexion while the angle between the femur and tibia is measured with a goniometer as the knee is actively extended (figure 10.7). In this test, sometimes referred to as the *90–90 test*, the thigh of one leg is raised perpendicular (i.e., 90°) to the testing surface with the lower leg 90° to the thigh (the tester will have to hold the thigh in this position). The subject then actively extends the lower leg. A measure of zero indicates that the leg moved 90° (i.e., perpendicular to the table and in line with the thigh); a measure of 10 indicates that the leg moved 80°.

A fully extended leg would measure 0°, and a leg extended 10° shy of fully straight (180°) would measure an angle of 10°. Normal angles for the AKE hamstring assessment are 37.7° ± 7.7° for males and 25.2° ± 12° for females (21).

VIDEO Watch **video 10.2**, which demonstrates the active knee extension (AKE) test.

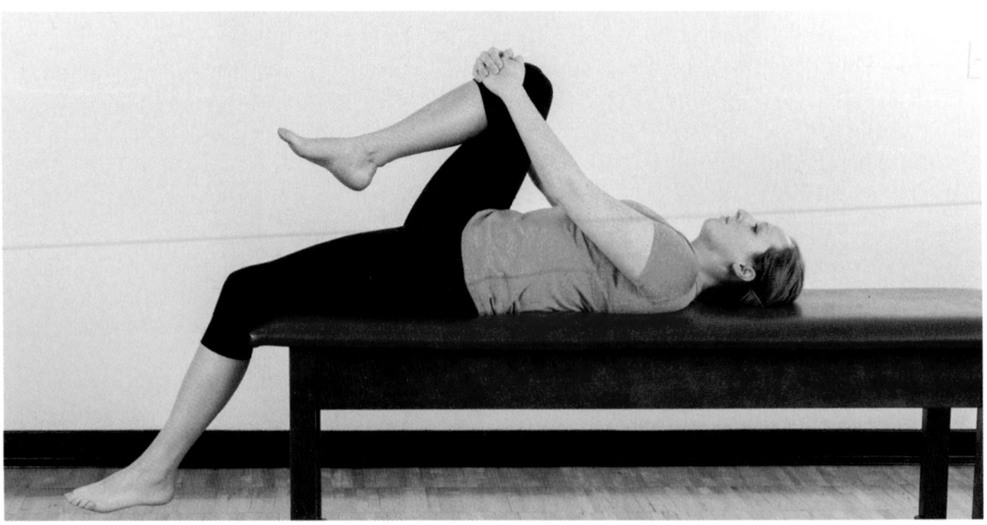

FIGURE 10.6 Thomas test.

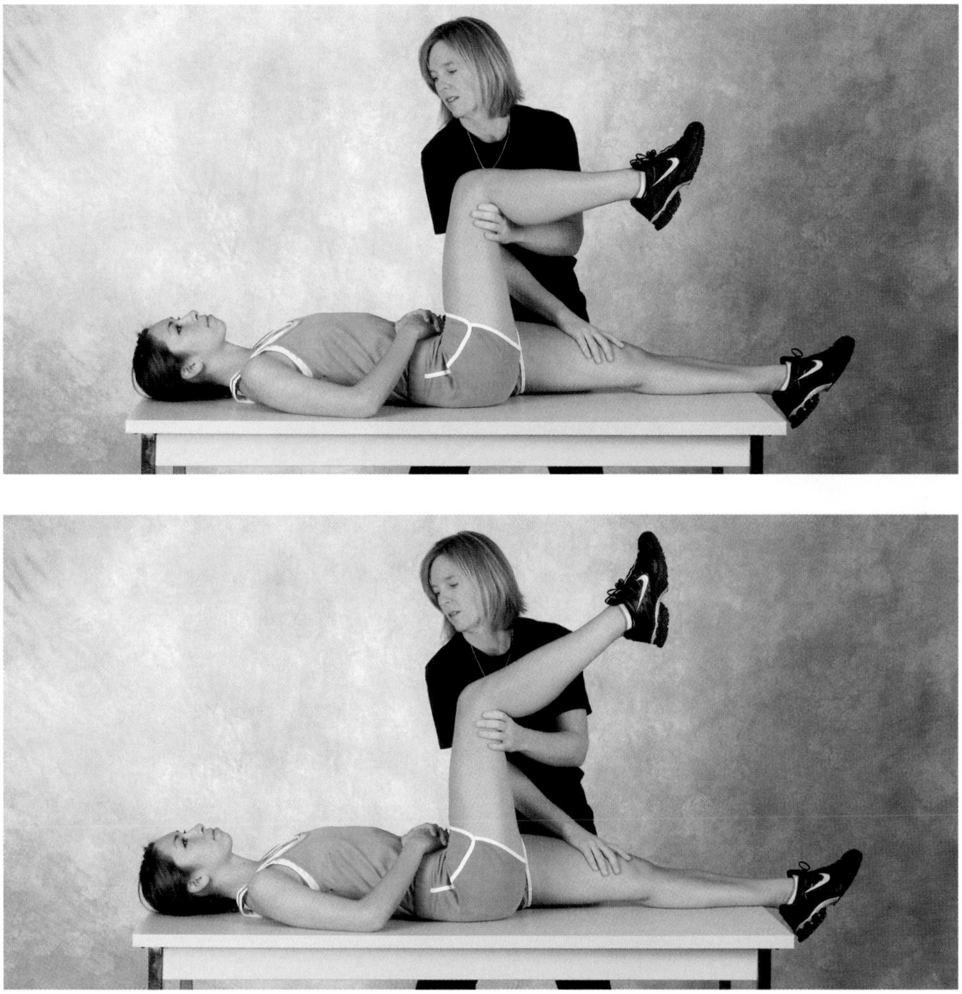

FIGURE 10.7 Active knee extension (AKE) test.

Straight Leg Raise Test

The other common test for hamstring flexibility is the passive straight leg raise (PSLR; figure 10.8) (6). The leg is passively lifted while the back is held in a normal lordotic curve (7). The pelvic girdle may tip posteriorly as the leg is lifted, especially when the hamstrings reach their full stretch (13). Therefore, properly stabilizing the pelvis is of utmost importance to obtain an accurate measure of hamstring length. A goniometer (with its axis on the greater trochanter) can provide a specific measurement of the angle from the surface to the passively lifted leg. The normal range for this test is ≥80° for adults (6, 26).

VIDEO Watch **video 10.3**, which demonstrates the passive straight leg raise (PSLR) test.

Ober's Test

ITB tightness is common in both the athlete and nonathlete. It frequently contributes to knee dysfunction and is affected by alignment challenges such as overpronation of the feet. Ober's test is performed to assess ITB tightness. The client is in a side-lying position so that the involved hip is upward. The pelvis is in the neutral position with the hips stacked. The hip is passively extended and then allowed to adduct toward the surface. The test is positive if the upper leg remains abducted and does not move toward the table surface (figure 10.9) (31). The inter-rater reliability has been shown to be very high for this test (28).

Piriformis Test

The piriformis muscle is frequently involved in both low-back and hip dysfunctions and can be tested in at least two ways. A common clinical test is the supine version (figure 10.10, *a* and *b*, on page 205); however, the seated version (figure 10.10*c* on page 205) may be easier to use in the

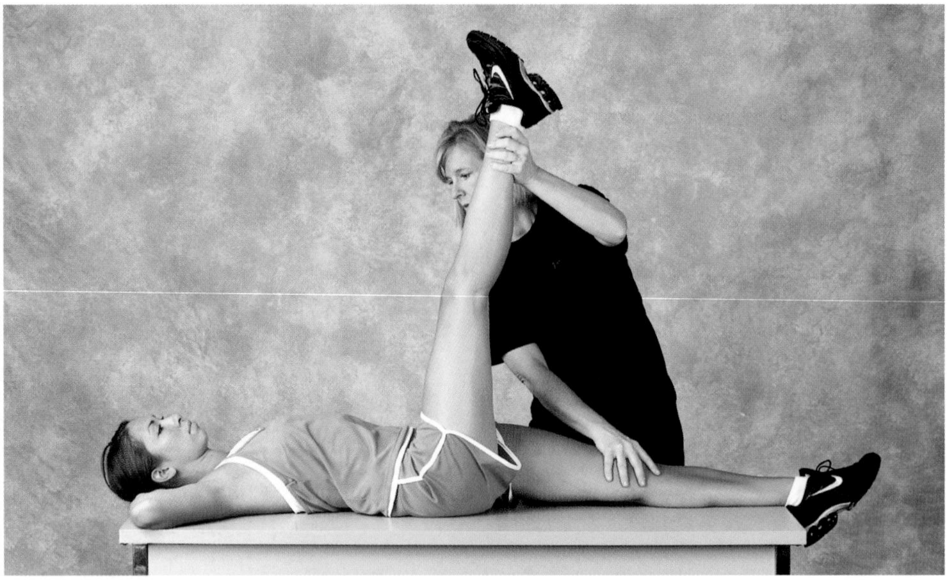

FIGURE 10.8 Passive straight leg raise test (PSLR).

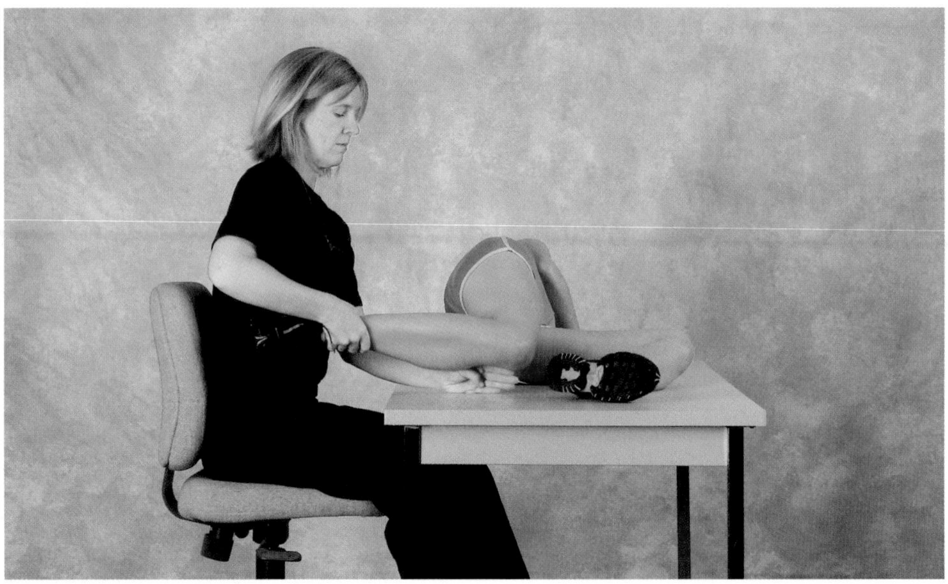

FIGURE 10.9 Ober's test.

fitness setting. The client is supine with the hip flexed 70° to 80° and maximally adducted. The test is positive if pain is produced. Internal rotation stretches the superior fibers and external rotation stretches the inferior fibers (31).

As mentioned, the seated version of the piriformis flexibility test may be more applicable to the fitness setting. It is easily performed in a chair instead of on a table. The spine should stay straight as the body leans forward at the hips. Compare the ease of opening of the top leg with the other side. A tight piriformis can lead to the inability to open or externally rotate the top leg easily. If either test elicits pain, refer the client to a physical therapist for a medical evaluation.

Ely's Test

Ely's test measures quadriceps flexibility, specifically the rectus femoris, and is performed in the prone position (figure 10.11). Atamaz et al. (5) measured from the heel to the back of the leg and hip as the knee was maximally flexed to document quadriceps flexibility. They concluded that this measurement of flexibility is reliable. It is important to keep the hips on the surface because a tight rectus femoris may tilt the pelvis anteriorly or laterally, resulting in an inaccurate measurement. The test may be performed in either a side-lying or prone position. The heel should touch the posterior leg or buttocks. The distance from the

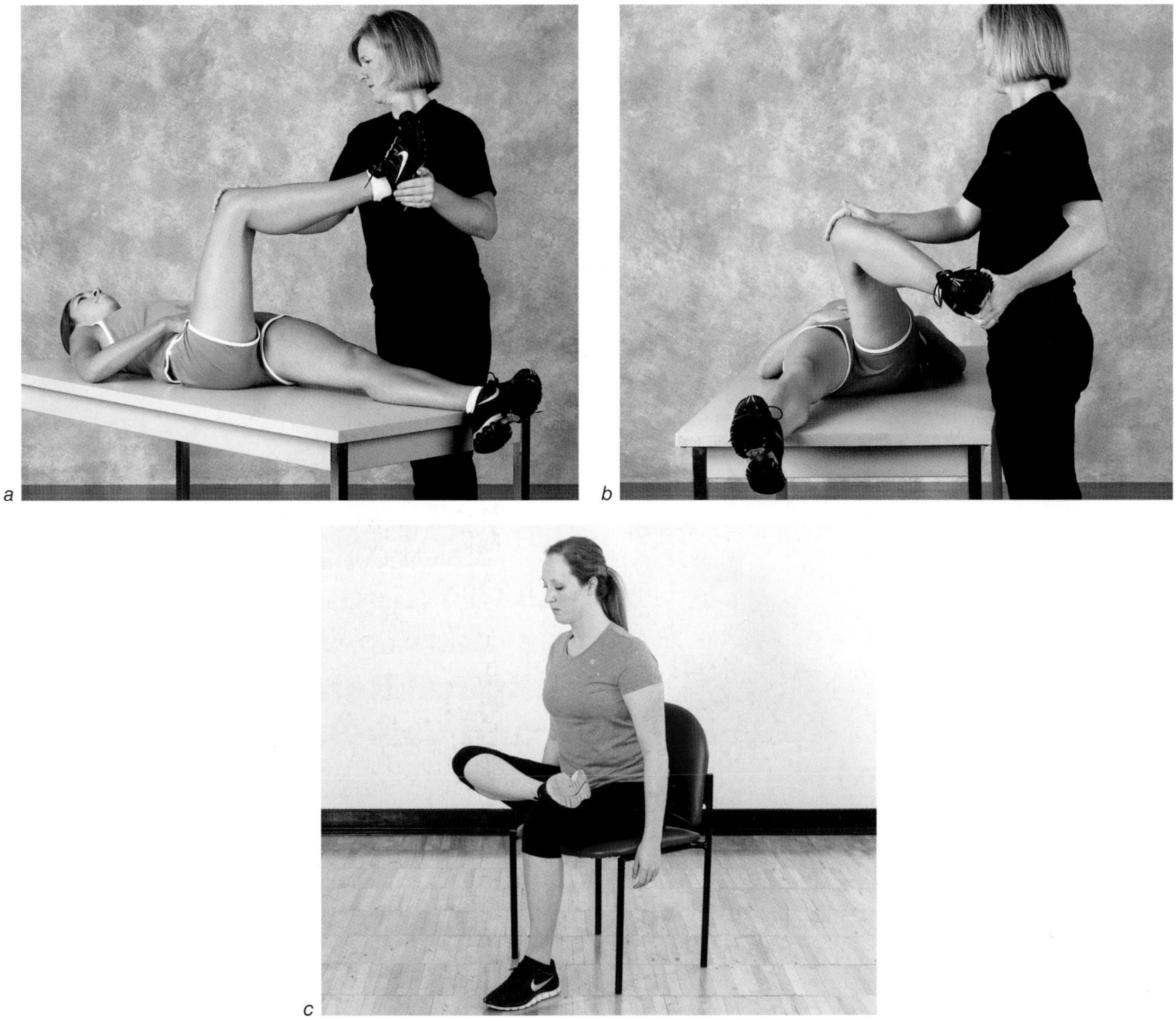

a *b* *c*

FIGURE 10.10 Piriformis test performed *(a, b)* supine and *(c)* seated.

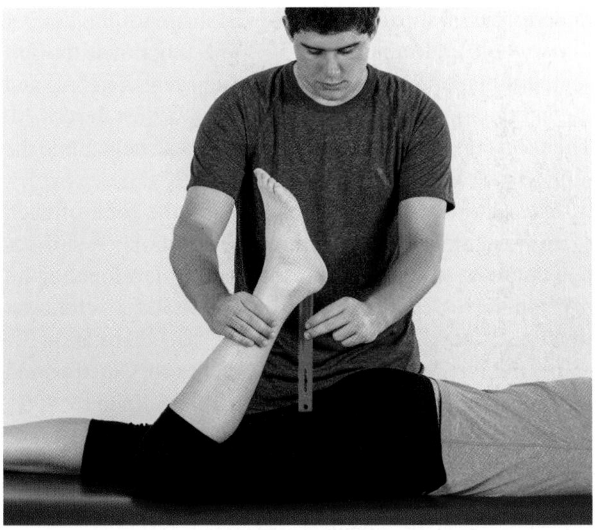

FIGURE 10.11 Prone quadriceps test (Ely's test).

buttocks or leg to the heel can be used as a measurement guide to assess progress in quadriceps flexibility.

Ankle Range of Motion

Motion at the ankle can be measured with a goniometer, or it can be assessed using active tests that are appropriate for a fitness setting, such as the straight-leg or bent-knee foot raise tests. The gastrocnemius is tested for tightness in the straight-leg test because the muscle crosses both the posterior knee and ankle (figure 10.12). Measure the distance from the foot to the floor. The ankle joint needs to move 10° for normal walking without compensations and 15° for running. The test may be adapted (bent-knee foot raise test) to target the soleus by having the subject sit, raising the toes while keeping the heel on the surface and the lower leg vertical.

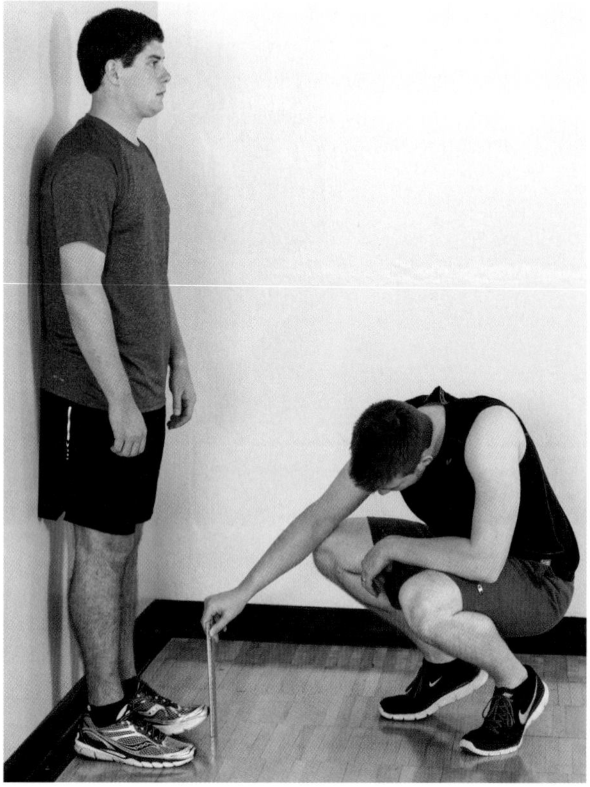

FIGURE 10.12 Straight-leg foot raise test.

Shoulder Flexibility

A quick test of upper-extremity flexibility is the back-scratch test (figure 10.13). It is relatively easy to perform and document objectively (38). If the fingertips touch, then the score is zero. If they do not touch, measure the distance between the fingertips (a positive score); if they overlap, measure by how much (a negative score). Practice two times and then test two times. Stop the test if there is pain. The scores can be compared over time as the fitness program progresses.

KEY POINT

Flexibility of the hip musculature (ITB, iliopsoas, piriformis, hamstrings) needs to be accurately assessed and addressed. Good ROM at the hip joint is necessary for good biomechanics of the spine (55, 56). Although tightness in the hip flexors is not as common as tightness in the hip extensors, both are important in maintaining a healthy spine. Tightness in the muscles crossing the hip joint may predispose a person to low-back problems (55, 56).

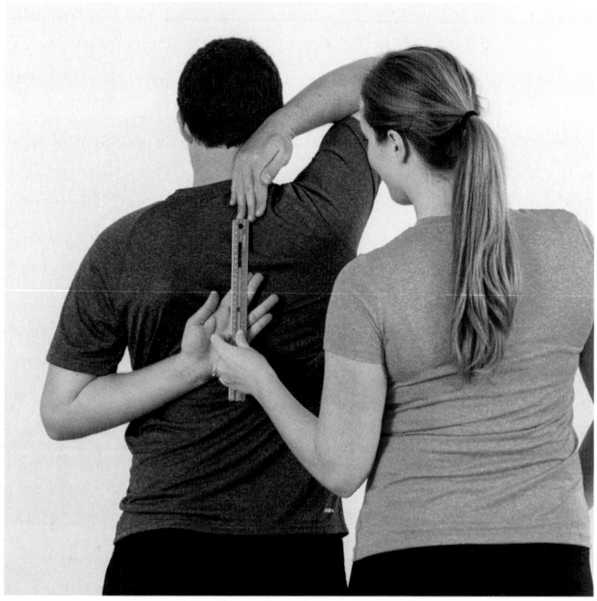

FIGURE 10.13 Back-scratch test.

Spinal Range of Motion and Low-Back Function

Most movements emanate from or have an impact on the spine. Good spinal mobility and muscle control are essential for normal function without predisposition to LBP. Spinal (intervertebral) ROM will be addressed first, followed by the interaction of the spine and hips in bending forward, termed *lumbopelvic motion*.

If a person were to bend forward at the waist from an upright standing position (with the movement occurring primarily in the lumbar spine), the nuclei of lumbar intervertebral discs would drift posteriorly in the direction of the spinous processes of the lumbar vertebrae. If this person were to resume an upright posture and then hyperextend at the lumbar spine, the nuclei of the lumbar discs would drift anteriorly (57). The functional **motion segment** of the spine consists of two adjacent vertebrae and the intervening disc whose movement was just described. The facets on the upper and lower vertebrae help guide the motion (see figure 10.4) (57).

Overall spine flexibility or ROM is the total of each motion segment's contribution to the whole. A normative database of lumbar spine ROM was developed in an asymptomatic population aged 16 to 90 yr and is as follows: flexion 73° to 40°, lateral flexion 28° to 14°, rotation 7°, and extension 29° to 6° (65). The larger ranges are reported for the younger ages; over time flexion declined by 45%, lateral flexion by 48%, and extension by 79%. The average rotation did not decline with age.

Tests to assess spine flexibility range from goniometric measures typically done in a physical therapist's office (see the Research Insight) to overall flexibility tests that include both spine and hip measures, such as the sit-and-reach and toe-touch tests that are more appropriate for the fitness setting. A discussion of the combination tests will follow later in this chapter.

When assessing spine ROM, the fitness professional may note a rib hump as shown in figure 10.14. This is indicative of scoliosis, which is a curvature of the thoracic and lumbar spine that includes both a lateral curve and a rotatory component. If a client might have scoliosis, the professional can use the Adam's test to get a better perception of its presence (figure 10.14). Depending on the degree of scoliosis, a person with this condition may present with a different posturing of the rib cage during abdominal strengthening exercises because of the spinal rotation that occurs with scoliosis. The fitness professional should obtain advice from an appropriate medical professional before prescribing trunk exercises for any client with suspected scoliosis.

Trunk extension can be measured with the inclinometer technique (see the Research Insight called *Reliability of Lumbar Spine Flexibility Assessments*); however, this is typically performed in a physical therapist's office. There are a few tests that may be appropriately used in a fitness setting. It is important to note that normal lumbar spine extension ROM ranges from 20°–25° (31) to 6°–29° (65) because many adults have lost the capacity to extend due to prolonged activities in a flexed posture (i.e., desk work).

RESEARCH INSIGHT

Reliability of Lumbar Spine Flexibility Assessments

Dual and single inclinometer techniques (8, 47, 62) have been shown to be reliable and have no significant difference from radiographic determination of lumbar spine ROM. The dual technique requires one inclinometer placed over the sacrum and the other over T12 to L1 spinous processes while the client is standing in a relaxed position. Angular readings are taken while standing and then in the fully flexed position. The upper inclinometer represents the total motion, and the lower one represents the hip or pelvic motion. The difference between the two represents the true lumbar spine motion. The single technique is similar but measurements are taken separately. Both flexion and extension can be measured in this manner. There are even goniometer applications for smart phones or tablets that have been shown to have high intra-rater reliability and moderate inter-rater reliability (11).

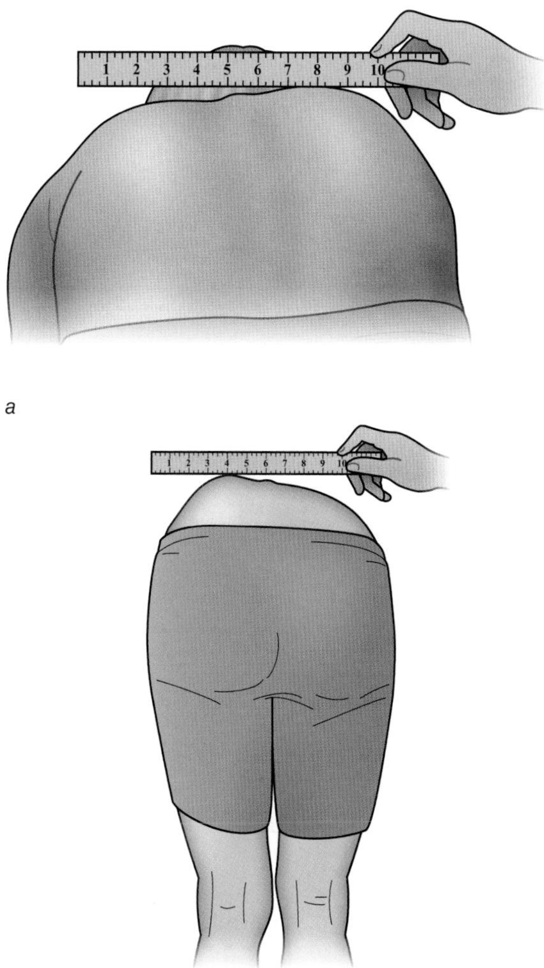

a

b

FIGURE 10.14 Adam's test. Viewing the spinous processes as the subject stands does not always clearly reveal a scoliotic curve. However, if you watch from behind as the subject bends forward, *(a)* a rib hump may be noted (placing a straight edge on the latter magnifies its presence). Scoliosis in the lumbar region *(b)* can be seen if the subject bends further down.

Passive Extension Test

In Imrie and Barbuto's (36) test for back extension, the back musculature is not actively used. This is a passive test of back ROM because the hyperextension movement in the spine results from arm and shoulder muscle contraction (see figure 10.15). While keeping the anterior part of the pelvis (i.e., anterior superior iliac spine) in contact with the floor, the subject elevates the torso with the arm and shoulder muscles; the muscles of the back are not used (36). The score is the perpendicular distance from the suprasternal notch to the floor. People with longer trunks tend to perform better on this test, which should be considered when interpreting scores. Scoring 30 cm (12 in.) or more is excellent, 20 cm (8 in.) is good, and 10 cm (4 in.) is fair.

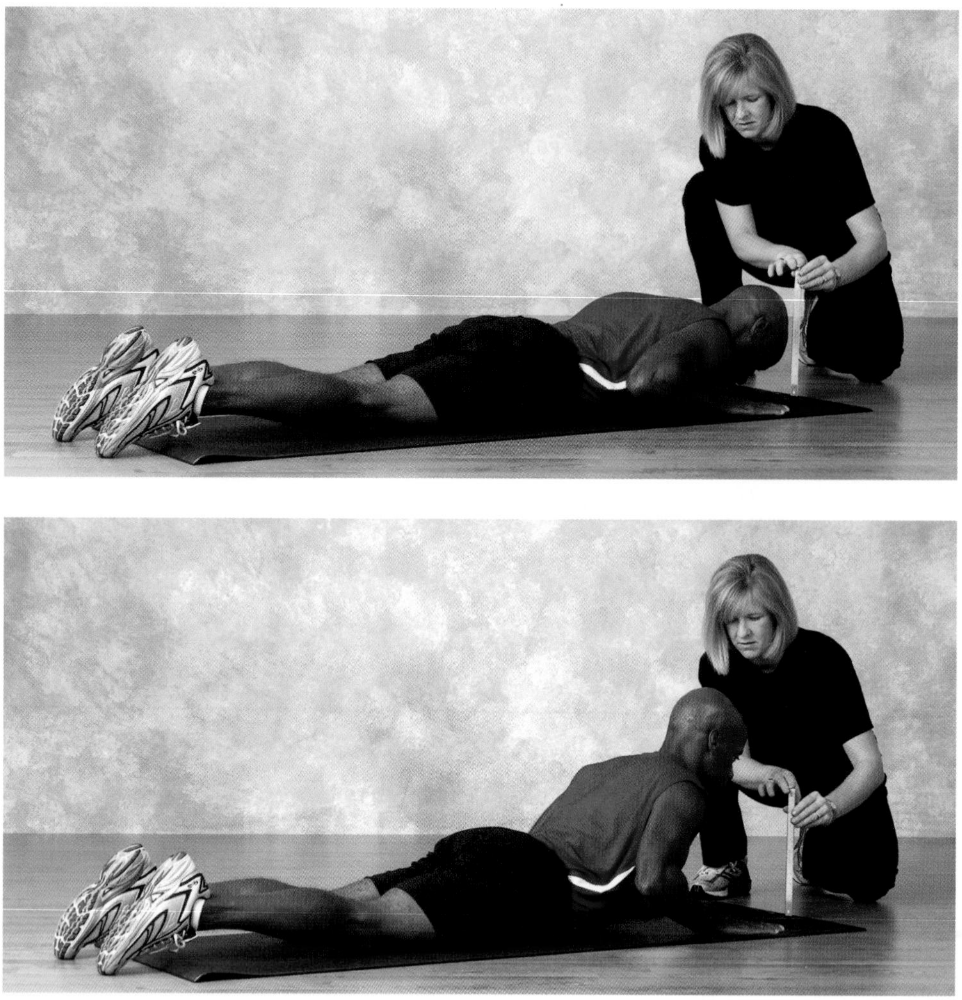

FIGURE 10.15 Passive back ROM test.

Watch **video 10.4**, which demonstrates the passive back ROM test.

Active Extension Test

An active test of spine extension ROM, called the *trunk lift,* was developed by the Cooper Institute for Aerobics Research (20). It is an active test because muscles of the spine (i.e., erector spinae and multifidus) hyperextend the spine (see figure 10.16). In this test, the subject slowly lifts the torso by contracting the erector spinae and multifidus muscle groups until the chin is a maximum of 30 cm (12 in.) from the mat. Although the Cooper Institute for Aerobics Research did not present norms, most people should be able to raise the chin at least 15 cm (6 in.). People with longer trunks tend to perform better on this test, which should be considered when interpreting scores.

Because both trunk extensor strength and ROM contribute to performance in the trunk lift and only ROM contributes to performance in the passive test, Liemohn et al. (44) used multiple regression analyses to further study performance on these tests by university students. Somewhat to their surprise, they found that the two tests measured the same construct (44); thus, this area could benefit from further research. However, because the passive test only measures ROM, and strength is not a factor, there are advantages to its use.

Watch **video 10.5**, which demonstrates the active back ROM and strength test.

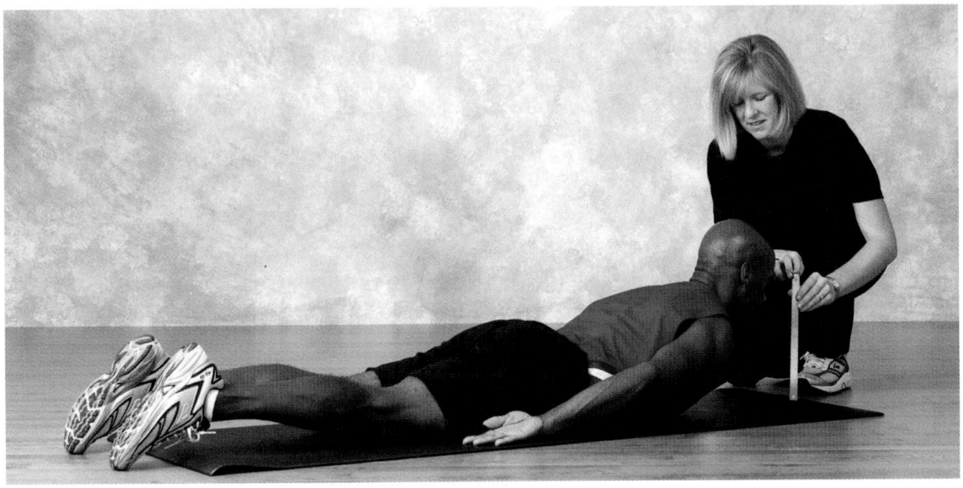

FIGURE 10.16 Active back ROM and strength test.

Lumbopelvic Rhythm

When a person reaches toward the floor, both the spine and the hips flex. The pattern that occurs is called the *lumbopelvic rhythm* and is a combination of both spine and hip flexion in varying ratios. This pattern can be affected by tightness in both the lower extremities and areas of the spine. A recent study (25) divided the forward bending range into three segments—early (0°-30°), middle (30°-60°), and late (60°-90°)—to investigate the pattern of motion in more detail. This revealed that the lumbar spine had a greater contribution to early bending, the hips and lumbar spine contributed roughly equally to the middle phase, and the hips had a greater contribution to the late phase (25). Therefore, a person with a healthy spine who bends over to touch the floor uses spine flexibility throughout the beginning and middle phases and stretches the hamstrings close to the floor. Subjects with a history of LBP tended to use their lumbar range earlier in the forward bending pattern, reaching the end of their lumbar flexibility earlier than those without LBP. The authors suggest that the earlier lumbar spine motion used by those with a history of LBP predisposes them to a higher risk of recurrence because they have an earlier tensile stress to the posterior elements of the spine.

Hamstring tightness has been thought to significantly affect the lumbopelvic rhythm (39). When investigators compared the lumbopelvic patterns and hamstring length in healthy people, it was apparent that flexible hamstrings were associated with a pelvic-dominant pattern and tight hamstrings led to a lumbar-dominant pattern, possibly creating more load on the spine (33). Why does this matter? Tight hamstrings may prevent people from unloading their L5-S1 junction as well as the posterior elements of the spine, creating a higher risk for LBP. Researchers found that healthy subjects demonstrated the same pattern that diminishes the L5-S1 forces during forward bending, and they suggested that the LBP subjects who use lumbar flexion in a higher ratio early on have larger compressive and shear forces at L5-S1 (63). The lumbopelvic rhythm during a stooping activity was analyzed in subjects with tight hamstrings (39). The investigators found that an increase in hamstring length translated into a change in the stooping form with less lumbar flexion, potentially taking some of the load off the lower spine. Consequently, hamstring flexibility testing needs to be a priority in the fitness professional's assessment of clients.

KEY POINT

Tight hamstrings may alter the lumbopelvic rhythm and place an increased load on the L5-S1 junction. The principle of relative flexibility is apparent in this situation, with the hamstring tightness creating compensation in the lumbar spine with earlier flexion and an increased load. Improving hamstring flexibility changes this compensation and lessens the load to the posterior elements of the spine, thus decreasing the risk for LBP.

Combined Tests of Range of Motion in Trunk and Hip Flexion

The fingertips-to-floor (or toe-touch) and sit-and-reach tests have often been used under the belief that they measure flexibility in the low back as well as at the hip joint. However, although both can be used to measure hip joint flexibility (i.e., hamstring length), neither effectively measures low-back ROM in conventional use (5, 46, 48).

The toe-touch test is performed with the client standing and bending forward, reaching for the floor with straight legs. As previously noted, this may be performed with little spine motion (figure 10.1). Both the sit-and-reach and the toe touch were found to have moderate validity and acceptable reproducibility (5, 7, 41) as hamstring tests. Several sit-and-reach variations have been found to be reliable (5, 9, 35, 52). These variations include the chair sit-and-reach and the modified back-saver sit-and-reach.

Using the sit-and-reach movement pattern as an exercise has been questioned. For example, if the hamstrings are tight and the sitting stretch is performed ballistically, the spine may be obligated to absorb these stresses, and over time these repetitive motions may have serious consequences for low-back function. Moreover, even if the sit-and-reach is done slowly, the static postures resulting during the stretching phase can place high compressive forces on the intervertebral discs (49, 53), and this movement might damage ligaments of the spine, particularly if the hamstrings are tight (15).

Sit-and-Reach Test

A traditional sit-and-reach test requires a solid box about 30 cm tall. Fix a meter stick on top of the box so that 26 cm of the ruler extend over the front edge of the box toward the subject. The 26 cm mark should be at the edge of the box. The client removes his shoes and sits on the floor with his legs stretched out in front with knees straight and feet flat against the front end of the test box. Instruct the client to move forward at the hips at a slow, steady pace, keeping the knees straight. The hands slide up the ruler as far as they can go (figure 10.17).

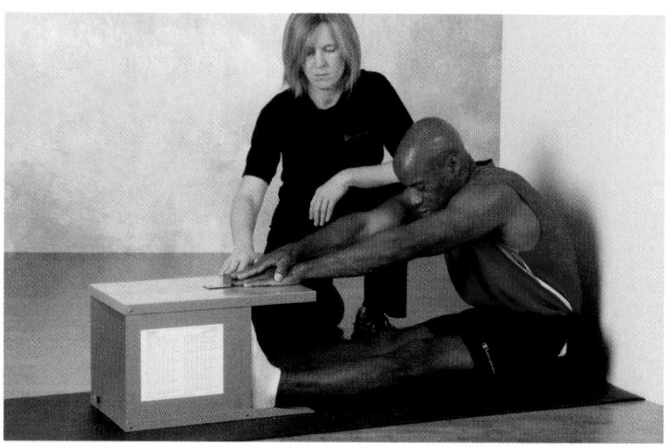

FIGURE 10.17 Traditional sit-and-reach test.

The client should exhale and drop the head between the arms while reaching, to facilitate the best score possible. This position should be held for 2 sec. Record the result in centimeters, rest, and repeat two times. Chose the best result for the final score (2). The scores are categorized from excellent to poor by decades as noted in table 10.2. The fitness professional can set goals and reassess based on these norms as the flexibility program progresses.

Even though the sit-and-reach test has medical contraindications and a host of factors can affect performance, it still has value as a field test provided that users are aware of its shortcomings. Following are suggestions that can make the sit-and-reach a better test.

- It is argued that the number of centimeters reached is not the most valid indicator of performance. The test administrator is better advised to examine the subject's quality of movement. Look for the angle of the sacrum (see figure 10.18) and the smoothness of the spinal curve. These relatively simple determinations can make the sit-and-reach a measure of low-back mobility as well as of hamstring length. These and other quality points are delineated in figure 10.18.
- It is recommended that the subject extend only one leg during the sit-and-reach test. Although this technique doubles the number of measurements required, the tester will also be able to evaluate symmetry. As stated previously, lower-extremity symmetry is desirable with respect to strength and flexibility because imbalance may have an untoward effect on the spine.
- If a sit-and-reach box is used to make measurements, it should be altered to permit passive plantar flexion at the ankle joint; however, normative data are not available for this modification. To alter the standard sit-and-reach box, simply replace the vertical surface under the cantilever extension with a 4 cm rod, which permits plantar flexion into the box but restrains the heel. This adjustment is not necessary if the protocol of Hui and Yuen (35) is followed.

Chair Sit-and-Reach Test

In the chair sit-and-reach, the client sits in a chair about 17 in. (43 cm) tall with one foot flat on the ground. The other leg is extended as straight as possible in front of the hip with the heel on the floor and with the foot dorsiflexed. The client reaches to touch the toes and the distance from the fingertips to the middle toe is measured (figure 10.19 on page 212). Norms are listed in table 10.3 on page 212 (38, 59) and can help the fitness professional assess the client, set goals, and reassess the client in the future.

Modified Back-Saver Sit-and-Reach Test

The modified back-saver sit-and-reach is a reliable test for low-back and hamstring flexibility (35). There are two versions of the test: a variation with one leg bent while reaching

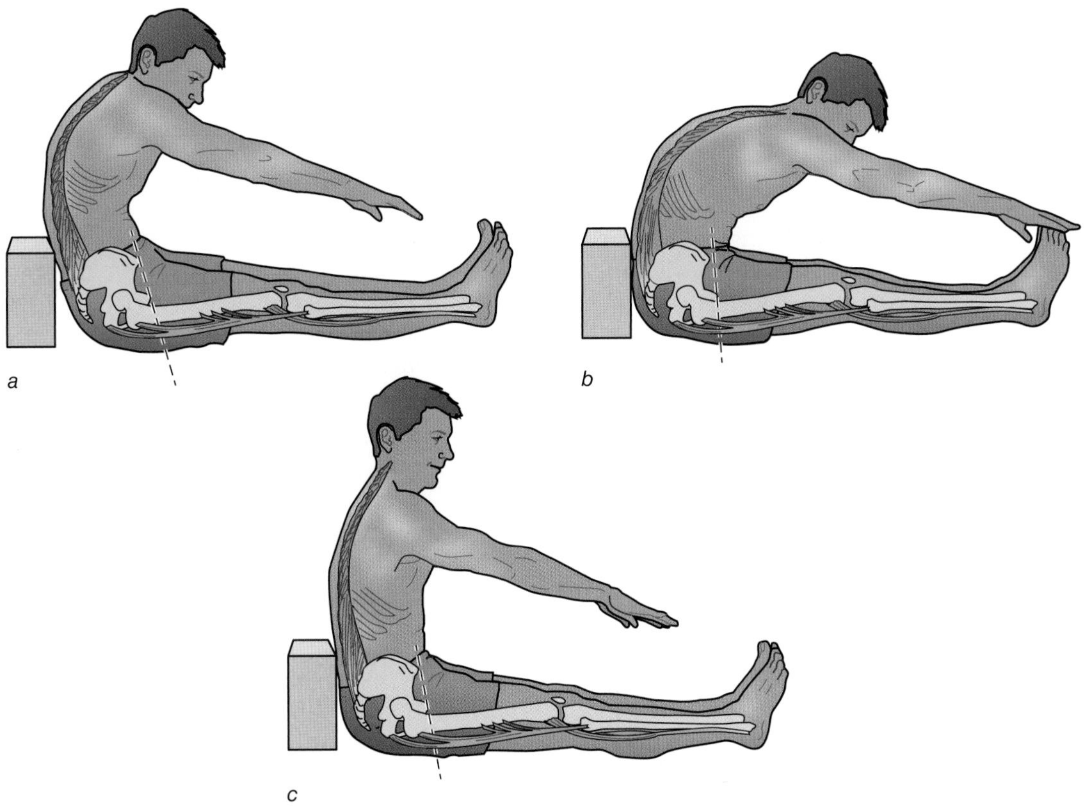

FIGURE 10.18 Sit-and-reach test. Quality points to look for include *(a)* tight hamstrings (note tilt of pelvis), tight low back, and stretched upper back; *(b)* normal length of hamstrings and low back; and *(c)* tight hamstrings (note tilt of pelvis) and tight low back.

Table 10.2 Sit-and-Reach Test Scores

Age	Zone	Male	Female	Age	Zone	Male	Female
20-29	Excellent	≥40	≥41	50-59	Excellent	≥35	≥39
	Very good	34-39	37-40		Very good	28-34	33-38
	Good	30-33	33-36		Good	24-27	30-32
	Fair	25-29	28-32		Fair	16-23	25-29
	Poor	<24	<27		Poor	<15	<24
30-39	Excellent	≥38	≥41	60-69	Excellent	≥33	≥35
	Very good	33-37	36-40		Very good	25-32	31-34
	Good	28-32	32-35		Good	20-24	27-30
	Fair	23-27	27-31		Fair	15-19	23-26
	Poor	<22	<26		Poor	<14	<22
40-49	Excellent	≥35	≥38				
	Very good	29-34	34-37				
	Good	24-28	30-33				
	Fair	18-23	25-29				
	Poor	<17	<24				

Note: All measurements are in centimeters.

Data from the Canadian Society for Exercise Physiology; *Physical activity training for Health Ottawa* 2013.

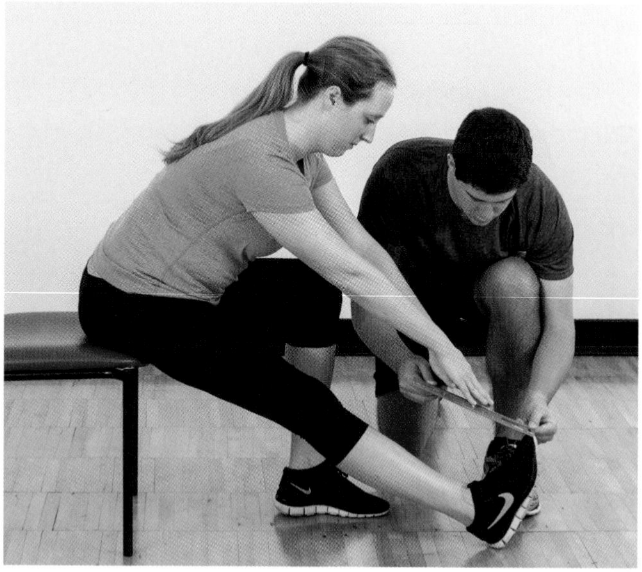

FIGURE 10.19 The chair sit-and-reach test.

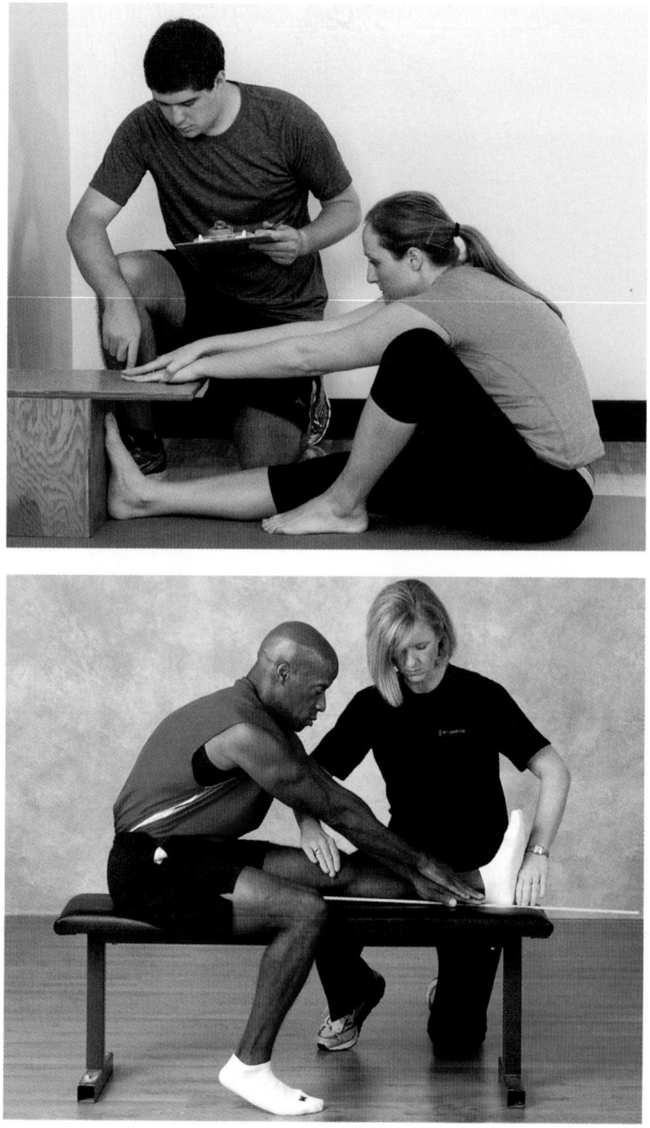

a

b

FIGURE 10.20 Variations of the modified back-saver sit-and-reach test: *(a)* one leg bent while reaching forward and *(b)* using meter stick and bench.

forward (use the same testing procedure as the SRT; see figure 10.20*a*) and a variation with only a meter stick and a bench (figure 10.20*b*). The client sits with a single straight leg on a bench and reaches for the toes. The distance reached is the score. Because the ankle is permitted to passively plantar flex, connective-tissue tightness behind the knee, as well as other factors such as sciatic nerve tension, does not affect performance.

An important consideration in any of the SRT tests is foot position. The ankle position for the SRT tests makes a difference, with higher flexibility scores for the plantar-flexed position (43, 52). Limohn's research (43) suggests that factors such as tightness in the connective-tissue structures located behind the knee and tension on the **sciatic nerve** can affect performance on the sit-and-reach. More recently Hui and Yuen (35) reported on a test that also permits plantar flexion of the foot of the tested leg and does not require a sit-and-reach box.

Table 10.3 Chair Sit-and-Reach Test Norms

Percentile rank	Age						
	60-64	65-69	70-74	75-79	80-84	85-89	90-94
WOMEN'S NORMS (IN. [CM])							
75	4.8 (12.2)	4.4 (11.2)	3.9 (9.9)	3.7 (9.4)	3.0 (7.6)	2.4 (6.1)	1.0 (2.5)
50	2.1 (5.3)	2.0 (5.1)	1.4 (3.6)	1.2 (3.0)	0.5 (1.3)	−0.1 (−0.3)	−1.7 (−4.3)
25	−0.6 (−1.5)	−0.4 (−1.0)	−1.1 (−2.8)	−1.3 (−3.3)	−2.0 (−5.1)	−2.6 (−6.6)	−4.4 (−11.2)
MEN'S NORMS (IN. [CM])							
75	3.8 (9.7)	3.1 (7.9)	3.0 (7.6)	2.0 (5.1)	1.4 (3.6)	0.4 (1.0)	−0.7 (−1.8)
50	0.6 (1.5)	0.0	0.0	−1.1 (−2.8)	−2.0 (−5.1)	−2.4 (−6.1)	−3.6 (−9.1)
25	−2.6 (−6.6)	−3.1 (−7.9)	−3.1 (−7.9)	−4.2 (−10.7)	−5.3 (−13.5)	−5.2 (−13.2)	−6.5 (−16.5)

Reprinted, by permission, from R.E. Rikli and C. J. Jones, 2013, *Senior fitness test manual*, 2nd ed. (Champaign, IL: Human Kinetics), 158.

Other Assessment Tools for Low-Back Function

Surveys (questionnaires) are frequently used to assess beginning level of dysfunction, disability, and outcomes in those with LBP. These tools may or may not be appropriate for all fitness settings; however, they are used widely in health care settings. They are typically simple and give a general idea of the current functional level. There may be opportunities to use these tools to guide the direction of the fitness program and to help the instructor and client realize what progress has been made. A common survey is the Oswestry Disability Index (ODI). It has shown to be valid (27), is easy to score, and gives a percent disability score that can be compared over time. A newer test, the Self-Reported Fitness Survey (SRFit), has been shown to be valid and reliable (40). This survey estimates muscular fitness and flexibility as well as other areas of fitness and may be helpful in assessing new clients.

LEARNING AIDS

REVIEW QUESTIONS

1. Some of the tests presented in this chapter require a thorough understanding of the nuances of human movement capability (for example, relative flexibility). Why could it be a mistake to administer these tests if you do not understand these nuances?
2. Why are sitting postures often detrimental to low-back function and flexibility?
3. Differentiate between RA and OA. Discuss which factors appear to have an impact on ROM.
4. Demonstrate flexibility tests for the ITB, hamstrings, iliopsoas, gastrocnemius, soleus, piriformis, quadriceps, and general mobility of the upper extremities.
5. Why is hip mobility important for a healthy back?
6. Movement capability in the lumbar spine is often misunderstood. Describe the movements and the factors that limit each one.
7. Define and differentiate between active and passive ROM in the spine extension test.
8. A prime reason for using the sit-and-reach test is that it is easy to administer. Discuss the limitations of this test. What are some modifications that can improve the test?

CASE STUDIES

1. A participant in your physical fitness program was told that his hamstrings were tight, so you administer the sit-and-reach test to get some baseline data. To your surprise, he can reach beyond his toes. What quality factors (other than centimeters reached) in his sit-and-reach performance might you further examine to explain this disparity? What other hamstring length test might you administer?
2. According to a client's record, previous Thomas tests show she has tight hip flexors. However, when you administer the Thomas test, you do not find evidence of tightness in the hip flexors. Assume that this person has done nothing to increase her ROM and you are confident that you administered the Thomas test correctly. Explain how the previous administrator of the test might have erred.
3. You note a definite scoliosis in a client with whom you are planning exercise activities. Why is it important to obtain good advice before prescribing exercises of the axial skeleton for this person? Whom might you ask for this advice?

Answers to Case Studies

1. The sacral angle should be at least 80° (a book or board on edge placed against the sacrum would be snug if the angle were 90°). Next examine the curvature of the spine; it should be smooth with no evident flatness or hypermobility in any one particular area. Discrepancy in arm–leg length might also be a factor (e.g., long arms in relation to legs). You might administer the PSLR or AKE test to assess hamstring flexibility.
2. Most false positives in the Thomas test result when the subject brings the thigh too close to the chest. This can result in excessive posterior rotation of the pelvis, which can make it appear that the hip flexors are tight.
3. As with most conditions, a scoliosis may be minor and not necessitate any special consideration. In some cases a client's scoliosis might benefit from a few specific exercise routines; however, the cause of a scoliosis can be complex, so it would be inappropriate for a fitness professional to prescribe exercises involving spinal movement in an attempt to correct a scoliosis without discussing this with the client and consulting an expert. Has the client been under the care of an orthopedist, physiatrist, chiropractor, or other medical personnel for the condition? Have any specific exercises or activities been recommended for the scoliosis? Are there any contraindicated exercises or activities?

Exercise Prescription for Health, Fitness, and Performance

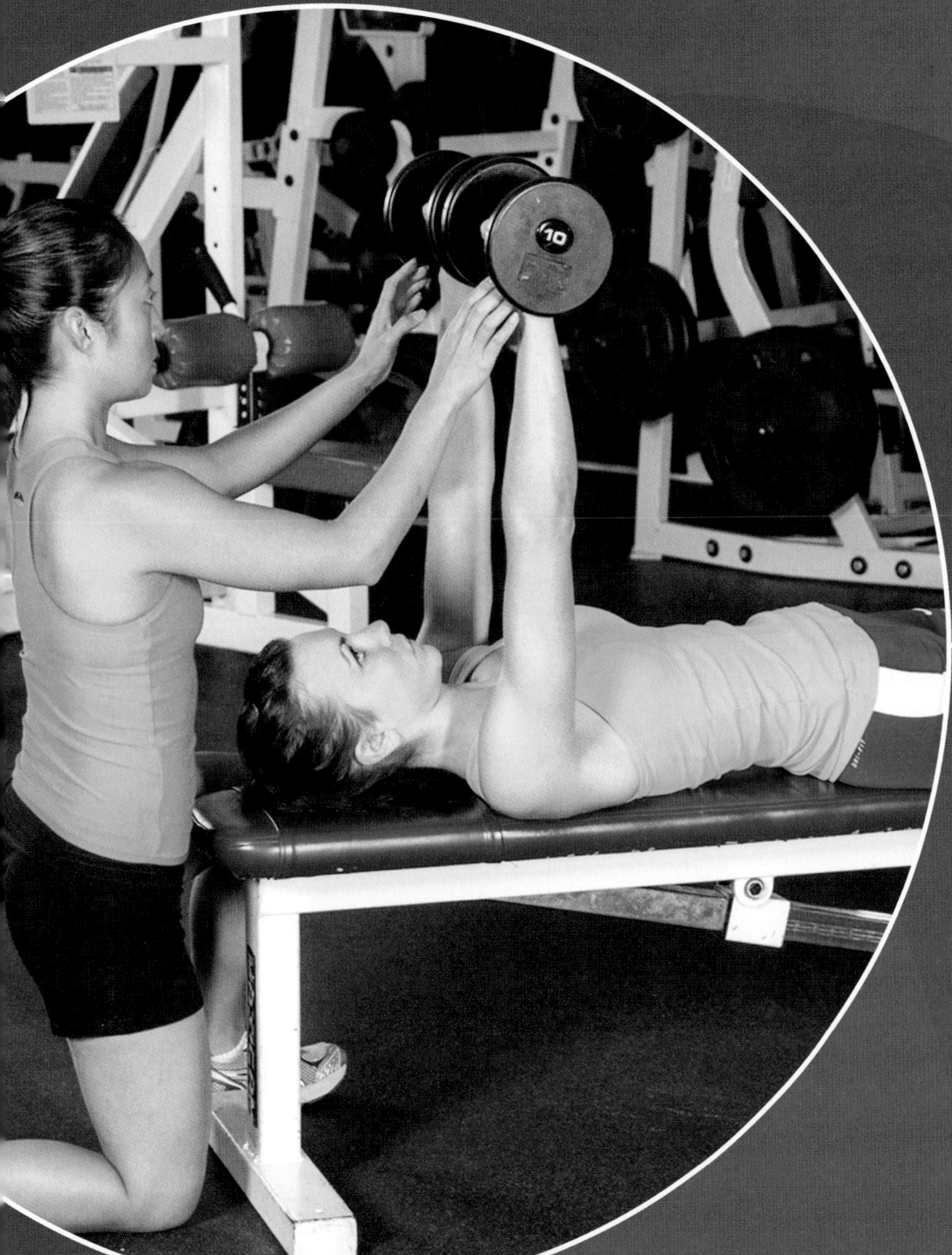

PART IV

In part IV we provide guidelines for exercise programming for cardiorespiratory fitness (CRF) (chapter 11), weight management (chapter 12), muscular strength and endurance (chapter 13), flexibility and low-back function (chapter 14), and training for performance (chapter 15). The degree to which a tissue such as bone, skeletal muscle, or cardiac muscle functions depends on the activity to which it is exposed. This statement summarizes the two major principles underlying training programs: overload and specificity.

The principle of overload describes a dynamic characteristic of living creatures: Use increases functional capacity. If a tissue or organ system is required to work against a load to which it is not accustomed, it becomes stronger. The corollary of the overload principle is the principle of reversibility, which indicates that physiological gains are lost when a tissue or organ system is not used. The common adage for this principle is "Use it or lose it." The variables that contribute to overload in an exercise program include intensity, duration, and frequency of exercise. As we will see, it is the combination of these elements that results in a sufficient volume of exercise or energy expenditure that increases the functional capacity of the cardiorespiratory system.

The principle of specificity states that the training effects derived from an exercise program are specific to the exercise performed and the muscles involved. For example, a person who runs for exercise shows little change in the arm muscles. A person who exercises at a low intensity that recruits only slow-twitch muscle fibers will see little or no training effect in the fast-twitch fibers. If muscle fibers are not used, they cannot adapt, and thus they will not become trained. The type of adaptation that occurs as a result of training is specific to the type of training taking place (e.g., endurance versus heavy resistance training). Running increases the number of capillaries and mitochondria in the muscle fibers involved in the exercise, which makes them more resistant to fatigue. Resistance training causes hypertrophy of the muscles involved due to an increase in the amount of contractile proteins, actin and myosin, in the muscle.

11

Exercise Prescription for Cardiorespiratory Fitness

Edward T. Howley

OBJECTIVES

The reader will be able to do the following:

1. Characterize the dose of exercise in an exercise prescription and identify means by which a health-related effect might occur.
2. Describe the public health recommendation for physical activity.
3. Explain the concepts of overload and specificity as they relate to training programs.
4. Describe general guidelines related to CRF programs, including those related to the warm-up and cool-down.
5. Develop an exercise prescription with the exercise intensity, duration, and frequency needed to achieve and maintain CRF goals.
6. Express exercise intensity in terms of energy production, HR, and RPE.
7. Contrast the approaches used for developing exercise prescriptions for the general public, for the fit population, and for people whose complete GXT results are available.
8. Describe the differences between a supervised and an unsupervised program.
9. Describe how temperature and humidity, altitude, and pollution affect exercise prescriptions.

There is no question that higher levels of physical activity, exercise, and CRF are linked to reduced risk of many chronic diseases and death from all causes (13, 25, 41, 62, 64, 65). Of the hundreds of health objectives for the United States, *Healthy People 2020* (63) selected physical activity as one of the top 10 health indicators. Figure 11.1 from Myers et al. (40) shows that as CRF increases, the risk of death decreases. There are two important takeaways from this figure. First, the greatest decrease in risk occurs when moving from the lowest 20% (quintile) of CRF to the next level, and second, the risk continues to decrease with increases in fitness (more is better). The results from this study were consistent with those in the classic study of Blair et al. (5), which found that risk levels off at a CRF level of only 9 METs for women and 10 METs for men.

As we move through this chapter, it will become clear that it is not difficult to achieve levels of physical activity and CRF consistent with a lower risk of chronic disease. This knowledge forms the basis for the public health physical activity recommendations. Consequently, the primary purpose of this chapter is to show how to prescribe physical activity and exercise to improve CRF in adults. Later chapters present additional information on prescribing physical activity and exercise for children, older adults, and people with known diseases.

Prescribing Exercise

There is a close parallel between the fitness professional's desire to know the proper **dose** of exercise needed to bring about a desired **effect** (response) and the physician's need to know the type and quantity of a drug needed to cure a disease. In fact, the ACSM–AMA program called *Exercise is Medicine* speaks to that connection, and materials are available to help fitness professionals interact with medical personnel (http://exerciseismedicine.org/support_page.php?p=12). If we think about prescriptions from a medical perspective, there is a difference between what is needed to cure a headache and what is needed to cure tuberculosis. In the same way, there is no question that the dose of physical activity required to achieve a high level of performance is different from that required to improve a health-related outcome (e.g., lower BP, lower risk of CHD). Similarities can be drawn between the dose–response relationship for medications and that for exercise, which is shown in figure 11.2 (18).

- *Potency.* The potency of a drug is a relatively unimportant characteristic in that it makes little difference whether the effective dose is 1 mg or 100 mg as long as the drug can be administered in an appropriate dosage (18). Likewise in exercise prescriptions, walking 4 mi (6.4 km) at a moderate pace is as effective in expending calories as running 2 mi (3.2 km)—see chapter 6.
- *Slope.* The slope of the curve describes how much of an effect comes from a change in dose (18). Some physiological measures (e.g., HR and lactate response to a fixed exercise task) change quickly (in days) for a dose of exercise, whereas some health-related effects (e.g., changes in serum cholesterol) are realized only after many months of exercise.
- *Maximal effect.* The maximal effect (efficacy) of a drug varies with the type of drug. For example, morphine can relieve pain of all intensities, whereas aspirin is effective against only mild to moderate pain (18). Similarly, strenuous exercise can increase $\dot{V}O_2$max and modify risk factors, whereas light to moderate exercise can improve risk factors but cause only a small increase in $\dot{V}O_2$max.
- *Variability.* The effect of a drug varies among and within individuals depending on the circumstances (18). In terms of exercise, gains in $\dot{V}O_2$max attributable to endurance training show considerable variation, even when the initial $\dot{V}O_2$max value is controlled for (11).

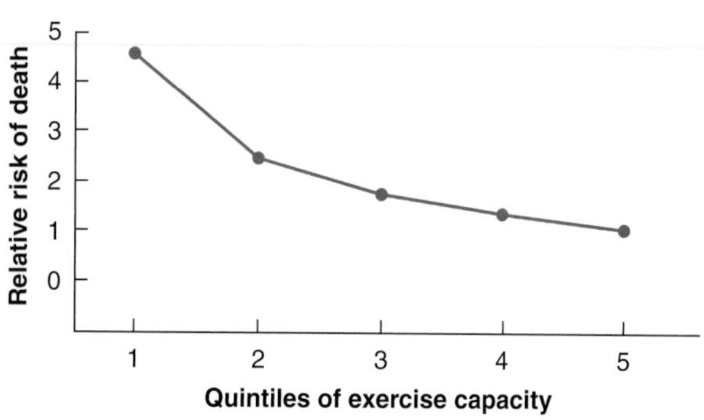

FIGURE 11.1 Relative risk of all-cause mortality to quintiles of exercise capacity (METs) among normal subjects.
Data from Myers et al. 2002.

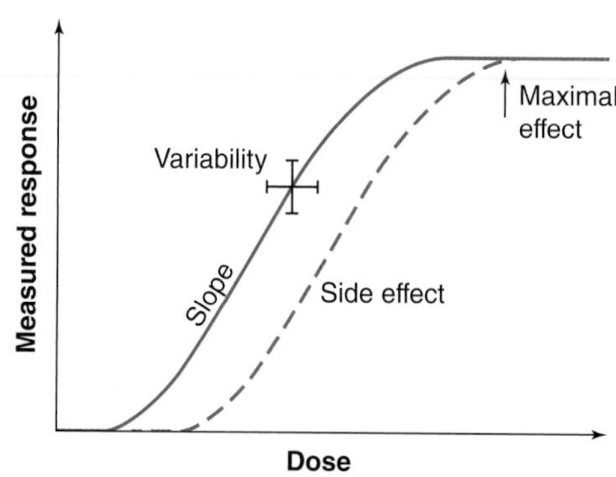

FIGURE 11.2 Representative dose–effect curve with four characterizing parameters.
Adapted from Goodman 1975.

- *Side effect.* No drug produces a single effect (18), and the effects might include adverse (side) effects that limit the usefulness of the drug. For exercise, the side effects might include an increased risk of injury.

Unlike most drugs, which people stop taking when a disease is cured, physical activity is needed throughout life to promote its health-related and fitness effects. What factors make up the dose of exercise?

The dose of physical activity and exercise is described in the FITT principle, which contains the following factors introduced in chapter 1:

- Frequency—how often an activity is done. This can be expressed in days per week or number of times per day.
- Intensity—how hard the activity is. Intensity can be described in terms of %$\dot{V}O_2$max, % maximal HR, RPE, and LT.
- Time—the duration of the activity. This is typically expressed as the number of minutes of activity.
- Type—the mode or kind of activity done. This could simply refer to whether the exercise is resistance versus cardiorespiratory endurance, or within the latter, swimming versus running versus rowing.

The FITT principle is useful because it allows the major elements of an exercise intervention to be altered to suit a given person. In addition, the product of frequency × intensity × time yields the volume (V) of exercise, which is directly related to health benefits (see the next section for more details). Another element of an exercise prescription, progression (P), describes the manner in which a person transitions from easier to harder exercise over the course of an intervention; we will address that in the context of general guidelines for exercise later in the chapter. Lastly, the *ACSM Guidelines for Exercise and Prescription* (4) incorporates all of these variables to yield the acronym *FITT-VP* as a reminder of what to address in an exercise prescription.

Over the past two decades, we have learned a great deal about how much physical activity is needed to achieve a variety of health outcomes. As mentioned in chapter 1, the health-related benefits of physical activity are not dependent on an increase in CRF. That said, there is no question that an increase in $\dot{V}O_2$max is associated with a decrease in the risk of many chronic diseases and death from all causes. A detailed review of the effects of physical activity on health and disease that was carried out before the development of the first U.S. Physical Activity Guidelines (64) supported and added to the findings of earlier reports (13). The following Research Insight provides excellent information on the health benefits associated with regular physical activity in adults and older adults.

RESEARCH INSIGHT

Physical Activity and Health Outcomes

The following information provides the level of evidence (strong, moderate, weak) that supports the connection between physical activity and various health outcomes in adults and older adults. An impressive amount of research has been done over the past four decades to allow us to make such statements (64, 65).

Strong Evidence

- Lower risk of early death
- Lower risk of CHD
- Lower risk of stroke
- Lower risk of high BP
- Lower risk of adverse blood lipid profile
- Lower risk of type 2 diabetes
- Lower risk of metabolic syndrome
- Lower risk of colon and breast cancer
- Prevention of weight gain
- Weight loss, particularly when combined with a reduced caloric intake
- Improved CRF and muscular strength
- Prevention of falls
- Reduced depression
- Better cognitive function (for older adults)

Moderate to Strong Evidence

- Better functional health (older adults)
- Reduced abdominal obesity

Moderate Evidence

- Lower risk of hip fracture
- Lower risk of lung and endometrial cancer
- Weight maintenance after weight loss
- Increased bone density
- Improved sleep quality

KEY POINT

An exercise dose reflects the interaction of the intensity, frequency, duration, and type of exercise. Many health-related benefits are derived from participation in physical activity and exercise, and within limits, more is better. These benefits are not dependent on an increase in CRF, but there is no question that a higher level of CRF is related to a lower risk of chronic disease.

Short- and Long-Term Responses to Exercise

Haskell has indicated that in addition to understanding the cause-and-effect connection between physical activity and specific outcomes, we need to distinguish between short-term (acute) and long-term (training) responses (23, 24). The responses in the days and weeks following the initiation of a dose of exercise can vary substantially, depending on the variable being measured:

- Acute responses—responses occur with one or several exercise bouts but do not improve further.
- Rapid responses—benefits occur early and plateau.
- Linear responses—gains are made continuously over time.
- Delayed responses—responses occur only after weeks of training.

The need for such distinctions can be seen in figure 11.3 (34), which shows proposed dose–response relationships between physical activity, defined as minutes of exercise per week at 60% to 70% of maximal work capacity, and a variety of physiological responses:

- BP and insulin sensitivity are most responsive to exercise, as shown by the blue line in figure 11.3.
- Changes in $\dot{V}O_2$max and resting HR are intermediate, as shown by the green line in figure 11.3.
- Serum lipid changes such as increases in HDL are delayed, as shown by the purple line in figure 11.3.

The dose–response relationship of exercise has important implications when exercise is used alone or in concert with medication to control disease; we discuss this further in chapter 24.

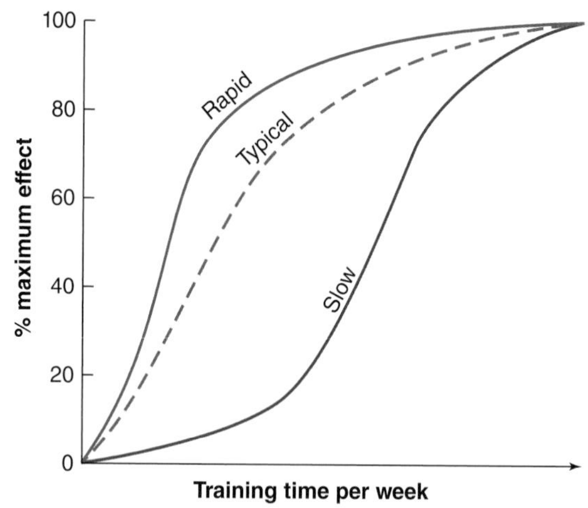

FIGURE 11.3 Proposed dose–response relationships between amount of exercise performed per week at 60% to 70% maximum work capacity and changes in BP and insulin sensitivity (curve on left), which appear most sensitive to exercise; maximum oxygen consumption ($\dot{V}O_2$max) and resting HR, which are parameters of physical fitness (middle curve); and lipid changes, such as increases in HDL (curve on right).

Public Health Recommendations for Physical Activity

Given the previous discussion, it should be no surprise that it is difficult to provide a single exercise prescription that addresses all the issues related to preventing and treating various diseases. Despite this, there has been a great need to provide a general physical activity recommendation to improve the health status of all adults in the United States. ACSM and the CDC responded to this need by publishing public health guidelines for physical activity in 1995 (42): *Every U.S. adult should accumulate 30 min or more of moderate-intensity physical activity on most, preferably all, days of the week.*

In 2007, ACSM and the AHA released an update to this 1995 public health guideline for physical activity (25), and in 2008 the first U.S. Physical Activity Guidelines were released (64). Both guidelines supported the original statement but attempted to provide more clarity about the roles of moderate versus strenuous (vigorous) exercise in meeting the recommendation (25, 64). Because of the similarity between the two, we will present only the U.S. Physical Activity Guidelines.

- People can realize the health-related benefits of physical activity by doing 150 to 300 min of moderate-intensity activity per wk, 75 to 150 min of vigorous-intensity activity per wk, or some combination of the two (e.g., walking briskly for 30 min on 3 days per wk and jogging for 30 min on 2 days per wk would meet the minimum goal).
- The minimum goal is 150 min of moderate-intensity activity or 75 min of vigorous-intensity activity.
- The range of physical activity is given because more health-related benefits can be realized by doing additional activity (i.e., more is better).
- Doing the activity in multiple intermittent bouts (e.g., 10 min each) is an alternative way of meeting the goals.

In addition, the new guidelines recommend resistance training on at least 2 days per wk to improve or maintain muscular strength and endurance (25, 64). Note that these new guidelines spell out the number of minutes per week but not the number of days per week to exercise. That does not mean that one should do 150 min of moderate-intensity activity in 1 day and rest for 6 days. For reasons that will be discussed later, spreading out exercise over the course of the week makes it easier to schedule and reduces the risk of injury (64).

The health-related gains associated with physical activity are realized when the volume of physical activity is between 500 and 1,000 MET-min · wk^{-1} (64). *Moderate-intensity activity* is defined as absolute intensities of 3.0 to 5.9 METs, and *vigorous-intensity activity* is defined as intensities of 6.0 METs or more.

- For example, walking at 3 mi · hr^{-1}(4.8 km · hr^{-1}) requires 3.3 METs, at the low end of the moderate-intensity range. If the person walks at this speed for 30 min, an energy expenditure of 99 MET-min (3.3 METs × 30 min) is achieved. If done 5 days per wk, the weekly volume of activity is 495 MET-min.
- If a person were to jog at 5 mi · hr^{-1} or 8 km · hr^{-1} (8 METs) for 25 min, the volume would be 200 MET-min. If done 3 days per wk, the weekly energy expenditure would be 600 MET-min.
- The fact that it takes about twice the time when doing moderate-intensity activity to achieve the same energy expenditure as when doing vigorous-intensity activity leads to the 2:1 ratio when comparing the time it takes to meet the guidelines for these intensities (150 versus 75 min).

Those who meet the upper end of the activity guidelines (1,000 MET-min · wk^{-1}) have a greater chance of achieving and maintaining a normal body weight (see chapters 12 and 20). How do we convert MET-min to kcal of energy expended? If a person is 75 kg and walks 150 min · wk^{-1} at 3.0 mi · hr^{-1} (4.8 km · hr^{-1}), which requires an energy expenditure of 3.3 METs, the number of kcal expended can be computed as described in chapter 6 (remember, 1 MET = 1 kcal · kg^{-1} · hr^{-1}):

$$75\ kg \cdot 3.3\ kcal \cdot kg^{-1} \cdot hr^{-1} = 248\ kcal \cdot hr^{-1} \cdot 2.5\ hr = 620\ kcal \cdot wk^{-1}.$$

Table 11.1 shows the number of MET-min and kcal expended at various exercise intensities for those meeting the 150 and 300 min goals. Obviously, someone who is fit has a greater capacity to work at a higher intensity and meet the

Table 11.1 Energy Expenditure of Walk, Jog, and Run Speeds for 150 min and 300 min of Weekly Physical Activity

Speed mi · hr^{-1} (km · hr^{-1})	METs	150 min · wk^{-1} MET-min†	150 min · wk^{-1} kcal†	300 min · wk^{-1} MET-min†	300 min · wk^{-1} kcal†
Rest	1.0	150	190	300	380
2.5 (4.0)	3.0	450	565	900	1,130
3.0 (4.8)	3.3	495	620	990	1,240
4.0 (6.4)	5.0	750	940	1,500	1,880
4.3 (6.9)	6.0	900	1,125	1,800	2,250
5.0 (8.0)	8.0	1,200	1,500	2,400	3,000
6.0 (9.7)	10.0	1,500	1,875	3,000	3,750
7.0 (11.3)	11.5	1,725	2,155	3,450	4,310
8.0 (12.9)	13.5	2,025	2,530	4,050	5,060
10.0 (16.1)	16.0	2,400	3,000	4,800	6,000

2.5 to 4.3 mi · hr^{-1} (4.0-6.9 km · hr^{-1}) = walk; 5 to 10 mi · hr^{-1} (8.0-16.0 km · hr^{-1}) = jog or run.

†Kilocalories for 75 kg (165 lb) adult when exercising at the given intensity for either 150 or 300 min. These are gross energy expenditure values during exercise; thus, they include the energy expenditure at rest and not just the additional energy expenditure due to the activity. Kilocalories calculated using 1 MET = 1 kilocalorie per kilogram per hour and rounded to nearest 5 kilocalories.

U.S. Department of Health and Human Services 2008.

KEY POINT

To achieve the physical activity energy expenditure associated with substantial health benefits, either moderate-intensity or vigorous-intensity physical activity can be used. The goal is to achieve between 500 and 1,000 MET-min · wk^{-1} of energy expenditure in physical activity.

goal in a shorter time. Consequently, benefits are gained not only when a sedentary person becomes active but also when a moderately active person engages in more vigorous exercise that increases energy expenditure and functional capacity ($\dot{V}O_2$max). This chapter provides the steps for developing an exercise prescription to improve CRF in apparently healthy people.

General Guidelines for Cardiorespiratory Fitness Programs

To apply the principles of overload and specificity in exercise programs (see the introduction to part IV), activities that overload the heart and respiratory system need to be used. Activities that involve the large muscle groups contracting in a rhythmic and continuous manner can overload the cardiorespiratory system. Activities that involve a small muscle mass or resistance training exercises are less appropriate because they tend to generate high cardiovascular loads relative to energy expenditure (see chapter 4). Activities that improve CRF are high in caloric cost and therefore help to achieve a goal of relative leanness. So, how does a fitness professional help someone start a CRF program?

Screen Participants

If the person has not already done so, have her fill out a preparticipation health screening questionnaire (e.g., PAR-Q+). Chapter 2 provides guidelines for who should and should not seek medical clearance before exercising.

Encourage Regular Participation

Physical activity and exercise must become a valuable part of a person's lifestyle. It should not be done sporadically, nor will doing it for only a few months or years build up a fitness reserve. Dramatic gains accomplished through fitness activities are lost quickly with inactivity (see chapter 4). Only people who continue activity as a way of life enjoy its long-term benefits (see chapter 23 for more on how to help clients establish healthy behaviors).

Provide a Variety of Activities

A fitness program starts with easily quantified activities, such as walking or cycling, so that the proper exercise

Walking Program Progression

Guidelines

- Start at a level that feels comfortable.
- Stretch before each session.
- Be aware of aches and pains.
- Progress one stage when comfortable.
- Monitor HR, but do not be concerned about being in the THR zone.
- Walk at least 5 days per wk.

Stage	Time (min)	Comments
1	10	Walk at a comfortable pace.
2	15	
3	20	Split into two 10 min walks if needed.
4	25	
5	30	Do two 15 min walks if preferred.
6	35	
7	40	Two 20 min walks will meet goal.
8	45	
9	50	You can do 25 min in the morning and afternoon.

intensity can be achieved. After establishing a regular routine of physical activity and achieving some gains in fitness, a variety of activities (e.g., games, sports) may be included in the program, with attention on progressing from easier to more difficult activities.

Program for Progression

Given the importance of helping sedentary people become active, the emphasis in any health-related fitness program for such participants should be to start slowly and, when in doubt, do too little rather than too much. A 10% increase in the number of minutes per week is a reasonable increase in the quantity of activity to minimize injury risk. One should gradually increase the number of minutes per session and the number of days per week before increasing the intensity (64). For example, sedentary participants who are interested in jogging should begin a training program by walking a distance that they can complete without feeling fatigued or sore. With time, the participants will be able to walk farther and faster without discomfort. After they can walk several miles briskly without stopping, they can gradually work up to jogging continuously during each workout. When the participants are first ready to begin jogging, introduce the interval workout (walking, jogging, walking, jogging). As they adapt to the interval workouts, they will be able to gradually increase the amount of jogging while decreasing the distance walked (see the walking and running programs as examples of progression). The importance of progression cannot be overemphasized, whether the client is a child, adult, or older adult (64).

Adhere to Format for a Fitness Workout

The main body of the fitness workout consists of dynamic activities using large muscle groups at an intensity high enough and a duration long enough to accomplish enough total work to specifically overload the cardiorespiratory system. Stretching and light endurance activities are included before the workout (warm-up) and after the workout (cool-down) for safety and for improving low back function.

There are physiological, psychological, and safety reasons for including the warm-up and cool-down. In general, the warm-up and cool-down should consist of the following:

- Activities similar to those in the main body of the workout but at a lower intensity (e.g., walking, jogging, or cycling below THR)
- Stretching exercises for the muscles involved in the activity as well as for those in the core (see chapter 14)
- Muscular endurance exercises, especially for the muscles in the abdominal region (see chapter 14)

Running Program Progression

Guidelines

- Complete a walking program first.
- Walk and stretch before each session.
- Be aware of aches and pains.
- Progress one stage when comfortable.
- Stay at the low end of the THR zone by varying the time of the walk–jog interval or jogging pace.
- Do the program every other day.

Stage	Time (min)	Comments
1	20-30	Jog 10 steps, walk 10 steps; repeat 5 times and check HR.
2	20-30	Jog 20 steps, walk 10 steps; repeat 5 times and check HR.
3	20-30	Jog 30 steps, walk 10 steps; repeat 5 times and check HR.
4	20-30	Jog 1 min, walk 10 steps; repeat 5 times and check HR.
5	20-30	Jog 2 min, walk 10 steps; repeat 5 times and check HR.
6	x	Jog 1 lap and check HR. Walk briefly and complete 4-6 laps.
7	x	Jog 2 laps and check HR. Walk briefly and complete 4-6 laps.
8	x	Jog 1 mi (1.6 km) and check HR. Walk briefly and do 1.5-2 mi (2.4-3.2 km).
9	20-40	Jog continuously and check HR.

These activities help participants ease into and out of a workout and promote a healthy low back. If a workout is going to be shorter than usual, the main body of the workout should be shortened so that 5 to 10 min are retained for the warm-up and cool-down.

Conduct Periodic Fitness Tests

Routine health-related fitness testing to determine a participant's progress can be motivational and may help alter programs that are not achieving desired results. The fitness professional can help by setting realistic goals for the next testing session when discussing test results. A general rule would be a 10% improvement in 3 mo in the test scores that need to change. Once the person has reached a desirable fitness level, the goal is to maintain that level.

KEY POINT

People interested in a fitness program should be screened prior to participation and encouraged to exercise regularly. The program should provide a variety of activities that use large muscle groups and overload the heart and respiratory system, and the participant should start slowly and progress gradually to higher levels of work. The workout should have a warm-up and a cool-down, including stretching and muscular endurance exercises for the core. Periodic CRF tests can be used to alter the exercise prescription.

Formulating the Exercise Prescription

The CRF training effect depends on the degree to which the systems are overloaded; that is, it depends on the following variables in the FITT principle: frequency, intensity, time (duration), and type of exercise. The interaction of intensity (low to high), duration (short to long), and frequency (seldom to often) should result in a total energy expenditure (volume of exercise) of 500 to 1,000 MET-min · wk^{-1} (64).

Frequency

The recommended frequency of exercise is higher for moderate-intensity exercise (≥5 days per wk) than vigorous-intensity exercise (≥3 days per wk) in order to achieve the recommended volume of exercise. Figure 11.4 shows that improvements in CRF increase with the frequency of vigorous exercise sessions, with two sessions being the minimum and the gains in CRF leveling off after three to four sessions per week (43, 44). Gains in CRF can be achieved in 2 days per wk, but the intensity has to be higher than a program with 3 days per wk, and weight-loss goals might be difficult to achieve (43). The long-recommended routine of working a day and then resting a day has been validated by improvements in CRF, low incidence of injuries, and achievement of weight-loss goals. Figure 11.4 shows that exercising for more than 4 days per wk at a vigorous intensity seems to be too much for previously sedentary people, resulting in more dropouts and injuries and less psychological adjustment to the exercise (10, 43). This figure demonstrates the increasing risk of orthopedic problems attributable to exercise sessions that are too long or conducted too many times per week. The probability of cardiac complications increases with exercise intensity beyond that recommended for improving CRF.

Intensity

How hard does a person have to work to sufficiently overload the cardiovascular and respiratory systems to increase CRF? To answer this question, we must first define the various expressions of exercise intensity and show how they relate to each other.

- **Percentage of maximal oxygen uptake (% $\dot{V}O_2$max).** Across a broad range of CRF levels, many physiological responses are normalized (i.e., made similar between individuals) when the intensity of exercise is expressed as a percentage of $\dot{V}O_2$max (%$\dot{V}O_2$max). A person who is working at 24.5 ml · kg^{-1} · min^{-1} and has a $\dot{V}O_2$max of 35 ml · kg^{-1} · min^{-1} is working at 70% $\dot{V}O_2$max. This approach has been used extensively to develop exercise guidelines, as can be seen in the *ACSM's Guidelines for Exercise Testing and Prescription* and ACSM position stands. However, in recent updates of these documents, the relative intensity is expressed as percentage of oxygen uptake reserve (%$\dot{V}O_2$R) (3, 4).

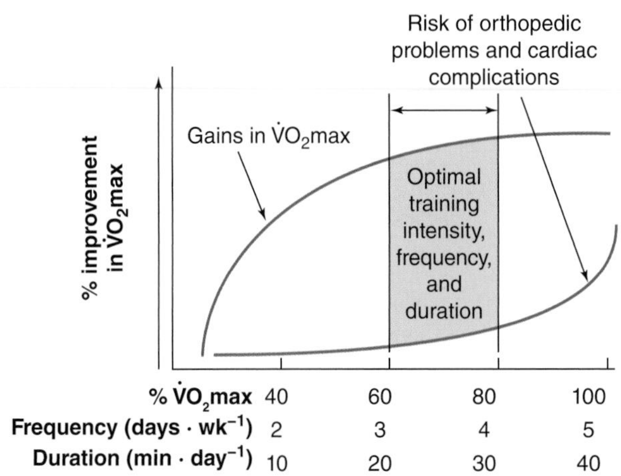

FIGURE 11.4 Effects of increased frequency, duration, and intensity of exercise on $\dot{V}O_2$max.

- **Percentage of oxygen uptake reserve (%$\dot{V}O_2R$).** $\dot{V}O_2R$ is calculated by subtracting 1 MET (3.5 ml · kg^{-1} · min^{-1}) from the subject's $\dot{V}O_2$max. For example, if a subject's $\dot{V}O_2$max is 35 ml · kg^{-1} · min^{-}, the $\dot{V}O_2R$ is 35 – 3.5 ml · kg^{-1} · min^{-1} = 31.5 ml · kg^{-1} = · min^{-1}. The %$\dot{V}O_2R$ is calculated by subtracting 1 MET from the exercise oxygen uptake, dividing by the subject's $\dot{V}O_2R$, and multiplying by 100%. For instance, if this person is exercising at 24.5 ml · kg^{-1}· min^{-1}, the exercise intensity is 67% $\dot{V}O_2R$: (24.5 – 3.5 ml · kg^{-1} · min^{-1}) ÷ (35 – 3.5 ml · kg^{-1} · min^{-1}) · 100% = 67% $\dot{V}O_2R$. The %$\dot{V}O_2R$ equals the HR response when HR is expressed as a percentage of the heart rate reserve (HRR) (58, 59).
- **Percentage of HRR (%HRR).** The HRR is calculated by subtracting resting HR from maximal HR. The %HRR is a percentage of the difference between resting and maximal HR and is calculated by subtracting resting HR from exercise HR, dividing by HRR, and multiplying by 100%.
  1. A 20-year-old man is exercising at 160 beats · min^{-1}.
  2. He has a maximal HR of 200 beats · min^{-1} and a resting HR of 60 beats · min^{-1}.
  3. Consequently, he is working at 71% of the HRR: (160 – 60 beats · min^{-1}) ÷ (200 – 60 beats · min^{-1}) · 100%.

For many years, %HRR was believed to be linked to %$\dot{V}O_2$max on a one-to-one basis; that is, 70% HRR = 70% $\dot{V}O_2$max. However, Swain and colleagues (58, 59) pointed out that although this is the case when fit people exercise vigorously, it is not the case for low intensities of exercise, especially when they are performed by people with low fitness levels. For example, a 3 MET activity for someone with a 5 MET maximal aerobic power is 60% $\dot{V}O_2$max but only 50% $\dot{V}O_2R$: (3 – 1 MET) ÷ (5 METs – 1 MET) · 100%. An advantage of expressing exercise intensity as %HRR is that % $\dot{V}O_2R$ is numerically identical to %HRR across the fitness continuum.

- **Percentage of maximal HR (%HRmax).** Because of the linear relationship between HR (above 110 beats · min^{-1}) and $\dot{V}O_2$ during dynamic exercise, investigators and clinicians have long used a simple percentage of maximal HR (%HRmax) to estimate %$\dot{V}O_2$max in setting exercise intensity. This method of expressing exercise intensity is easier to teach than is %HRR.
- **Rating of perceived exertion (RPE).** The RPE is not viewed as a substitute for prescribing exercise intensity by HR, but once the relationship between the HR and RPE has been established for an individual, RPE can be used in its place (3). However, the RPE may not consistently translate to the same intensity for different modes of exercise, so do not expect the RPE to exactly match a %HRmax or %HRR (4).

Table 11.2 shows the categories of exercise intensity as described in the 2008 report of the U.S. Physical Activity Guidelines Advisory Committee (65), with %$\dot{V}O_2R$ and

Table 11.2 Classification of Physical Activity Intensity

	RELATIVE INTENSITY			INTENSITY (METS AND %$\dot{V}O_2$MAX) IN HEALTHY ADULTS DIFFERING IN $\dot{V}O_2$							
Intensity	%HRR %$\dot{V}O_2R$*	%HRmax[y]	RPE‡	$\dot{V}O_2$max = 12 METs		$\dot{V}O_2$max = 10 METs		$\dot{V}O_2$max = 8 METs		$\dot{V}O_2$max = 5 METs	
				METs	%$\dot{V}O_2$max	METs	%$\dot{V}O_2$max	METs	%$\dot{V}O_2$max	METs	%$\dot{V}O_2$max
Very light	<20	<50	<10	<3.2	<27	<2.8	<28	<2.4	<30	<1.8	<36
Light	20-39	50-63	10-11	2.3-5.3	27-44	2.8-4.5	28-45	2.4-3.7	30-47	1.8-2.5	36-51
Moderate	40-59	64-76	12-13	5.4-7.5	45-62	4.6-6.3	46-63	3.8-5.1	48-64	2.6-3.3	52-67
Hard/vigorous	60-84	77-93	14-16	7.4-10.2	63-85	6.4-8.6	64-86	5.2-6.9	65-86	3.4-4.3	68-87
Very hard	≥85	≥94	≥17-19	≥10.3	≥86	≥8.7	≥87	≥7.0	≥87	≥4.4	≥88
Maximal	100	100	20	12.0	100	10.0	100	8.0	100	5.0	100

*%$\dot{V}O_2R$ = percentage of oxygen uptake reserve; %HRR = percentage of heart rate reserve.

[y]%HRmax = 0.7305 (%$\dot{V}O_2$max) + 29.95 (Londeree and Ames 1976); values based on 10 MET group.

‡Borg rating of perceived exertion 6-20 scale (Borg 1998).

%$\dot{V}O_2$max = [(100% – %$\dot{V}O_2R$) MET max^{-1}] + %$\dot{V}O_2R$ (personal communication, Dave Swain, 2000).

Adapted from American College of Sports Medicine 2014, *ACSM's guidelines for exercise testing and prescription*, 9th ed. (Philadelphia: PA: Lippincott, Williams, & Wilkins); Howley 2001.

%HRR used to set the standard for the other expressions of exercise intensity. These are shown on the left side of the table, with intensities ranging from very light to maximal. Note that in the 2011 ACSM position stand on the quantity and quality of exercise for developing and maintaining CRF (3), the number of categories was reduced from six to five, shrinking the light-exercise classification to 30%-39% HRR (from 20%-39%) and stretching out the vigorous-intensity classification to 60%-89% HRR (from 60%-84%). Because we believe these new classifications have little impact on developing an exercise prescription, we have chosen to maintain the classification cut points from the U.S. Physical Activity Guidelines Advisory Committee (65).

The RPE values are based on the Borg RPE scale (6). The values in table 11.2 for %HRmax and $\%\dot{V}O_2max$ accurately reflect the relationship between them and $\%\dot{V}O_2R$ (%HRR) (32). Further, table 11.2 provides the absolute exercise intensities (in METs) for each of the intensity classifications for four groups that vary in $\dot{V}O_2max$. Looking across the table from the 12 MET to the 5 MET column, there is little difference between $\%\dot{V}O_2max$ and $\%\dot{V}O_2R$ at higher $\dot{V}O_2max$ values, especially at higher exercise intensities; however, the differences are more obvious for the very light to moderate intensities and lower $\dot{V}O_2max$ values.

For people with $\dot{V}O_2max$ values of 12 METs, $\%\dot{V}O_2max$ is similar to $\%\dot{V}O_2R$:

- Moderate intensity equals 40% to 59% $\dot{V}O_2R$ and 45% to 62% $\dot{V}O_2max$.
- Hard (vigorous) intensity equals 60% to 84% $\dot{V}O_2R$ and 63% to 85% $\dot{V}O_2max$.

For people with $\dot{V}O_2max$ values of 5 METs, $\%\dot{V}O_2max$ is higher than $\%\dot{V}O_2R$:

- Moderate intensity equals 40% to 59% $\dot{V}O_2R$ and 52% to 67% $\dot{V}O_2max$.
- Hard (vigorous) intensity equals 60% to 84% $\dot{V}O_2R$ and 68% to 87% $\dot{V}O_2max$.
- Consequently, for people of average or higher CRF, the difference between $\%\dot{V}O_2max$ and $\%\dot{V}O_2R$ is small, and these expressions will be used interchangeably except where noted otherwise.

The %HRmax values listed in table 11.2 were derived from an equation by Londeree and Ames (36).

$$\%HRmax = 0.7305\ (\%\dot{V}O_2max) + 29.95.$$

This equation is similar to those of Swain and colleagues (57) and of Hellerstein and Franklin (27). There was little difference in the %HRmax values across the four fitness groups for each of the intensity classifications, so the $\%\dot{V}O_2max$ values for the 10 MET fitness group were used to provide the %HRmax values for table 11.2. Table 11.2 allows the fitness professional to consistently classify data on exercise intensity, whether they are expressed in oxygen uptake (METs), HR, or RPE.

A broad range of exercise intensities, from 40% to 84% of HRR, can be used to achieve CRF goals. However, the lower end of this range (i.e., 40%-59% HRR) is appropriate for people who are extremely deconditioned. That is consistent with the need of this group to focus on moderate-intensity physical activity that can be carried out long enough to achieve health-related benefits and perhaps gains in CRF.

- For the average sedentary person, an appropriate range of exercise intensities for achieving CRF goals is 50% to 84% HRR.
- For adults who are physically active and at the high end of the fitness scale, intensities greater than 80% HRR are appropriate.
- However, for most people who are cleared to participate in a structured exercise program, 60% to 80% HRR seems to be the optimal range of exercise intensities.

Figure 11.4 shows that exercise at the high end of the scale has been associated with more cardiac complications (10, 27). Exercise intensity must be balanced against duration so that the person can exercise long enough to expend 500 to 1,000 MET-min · wk^{-1}, the higher volume being consistent with greater improvements in CRF and greater reductions in chronic disease risk factors (64, 65). If the exercise intensity is too high, the person may not be able to exercise long enough to achieve the desired energy expenditure.

Time (Duration)

How many minutes of exercise should a person do per session? Figure 11.4 shows that improvements in $\dot{V}O_2max$ increase with the **duration** of the exercise session. However, the optimal duration of an exercise session depends on the intensity. The **total work** or volume of exercise accomplished in a session is the most important variable determining CRF gains once the minimal intensity **threshold** is achieved (4). If the goal were to accomplish 300 kcal of total work in an exercise session in which the participant works at 10 kcal · min^{-1} (2 L of oxygen per min), the duration of the session would have to be 30 min. If the person were working at half that intensity, 5 kcal · min^{-1}, the duration would have to be twice as long. A half hour of exercise can be taken as one 30 min session, two 15 min sessions, or three 10 min sessions. Figure 11.4 also shows that when the duration of hard exercise (75% $\dot{V}O_2max$) exceeds 30 min, the risk of orthopedic injury increases (43).

KEY POINT

CRF improves across a broad range of exercise intensities: 40% to 84% HRR. The intensity threshold for a training effect is lower (40%-59% HRR) for people who are sedentary, and it is higher (>80% HRR) for people who are physically active and have high CRF. The optimal range of training intensities for the average person is approximately 60% to 80% HRR. The duration of an exercise session should balance the exercise intensity to result in an energy expenditure of 500 to 1,000 MET-min · wk^{-1}, the higher volume being consistent with greater improvements in health benefits and CRF. The optimal frequency of training, based on improvement in CRF and a low risk of injuries, is 3 to 4 days a wk for exercise intensities rated as *hard*.

Determining Intensity

How is exercise intensity set for a particular client? This section reviews direct and indirect methods to determine appropriate exercise intensity, with a focus on the typically sedentary individual cleared for participation in this type of program.

Metabolic Load

The most direct way to determine the appropriate exercise intensity is to use a percentage of the measured maximal oxygen consumption. Remember, the optimal range of exercise intensities associated with improved CRF in people who are ready to move from moderate-intensity physical activity to a vigorous-intensity exercise program is 60% to 80% $\dot{V}O_2$max. The advantage of measuring oxygen consumption to determine exercise intensity is that the method is based on the criterion test for CRF—maximal oxygen consumption. The major disadvantages are the expense and difficulty of measuring oxygen consumption for each person and trying to suit specific fitness activities to meet the specific metabolic demand for each person.

QUESTION:

A 75 kg man completes a maximal GXT, and his $\dot{V}O_2$max is 3.0 L · min^{-1}. This equals 15 kcal · min^{-1} (5 kcal · L^{-1} · 3 L · min^{-1}), 40 ml · kg^{-1} · min^{-1}, and 11.4 METs. At what exercise intensities should he work in order to be at 60% to 80% $\dot{V}O_2$max?

1. 60% of 3.0 L · min^{-1} = 1.8 L · min^{-1};
   80% of 3.0 L · min^{-1} = 2.4 L · min^{-1}
2. 60% of 15 kcal · min^{-1} = 9 kcal · min^{-1};
   80% of 15 kcal · min^{-1} = 12 kcal · min^{-1}
3. 60% of 40 ml · kg^{-1} · min^{-1} = 24 ml · kg^{-1} · min^{-1};
   80% of 40 ml · kg^{-1} · min^{-1} = 32 ml · kg^{-1} · min^{-1}
4. 60% of 11.4 METs = 6.8 METs;
   80% of 11.4 METs = 9.1 METs

Consequently, he should use activities that require the following:

1.8 to 2.4 L · min^{-1}

9 to 12 kcal · min^{-1}

24 to 32 ml · kg^{-1} · min^{-1}

6.8 to 9.1 METs

At what exercise intensities does he work in order to be at 60% and 80% $\dot{V}O_2R$?

ANSWER:

Using the preceding data, we find that $\dot{V}O_2R$ = 40 ml · kg^{-1} · min^{-1} – 3.5 ml · kg^{-1} · min^{-1} = 36.6 ml · kg^{-1} · min^{-1}. For 60% $\dot{V}O_2R$:

Target $\dot{V}O_2$ = 0.6 (36.5 ml · kg^{-1} · min^{-1}) + 3.5 ml · kg^{-1} · min^{-1}, and

Target $\dot{V}O_2$ = 21.9 + 3.5 = 25.4 ml · kg^{-1} · min^{-1} = 7.3 METs.

For 80% $\dot{V}O_2R$:

Target $\dot{V}O_2$ = 0.8 (36.5 ml · kg^{-1} · min^{-1}) + 3.5 ml · kg^{-1} · min^{-1}, and

Target $\dot{V}O_2$ = 29.2 + 3.
= 32.7 ml · kg^{-1} · min^{-1}= 9.3 METs.

He should use activities that require the following:

25.4 to 32.7 ml · kg^{-1} · min^{-1}

7.3 to 9.3 METs

When these exercise intensity values are known, appropriate exercises can be selected from tables listing the energy costs of various activities (e.g., Compendium of Physical Activities—see chapter 6). However, this is a cumbersome method for prescribing exercise. Prescribing on the basis of the caloric cost of the activity does not take into consideration the effect that environmental (e.g., heat, humidity, altitude, cold, pollution), dietary (e.g., hydration state), and other variables have on a person's response to some absolute exercise intensity. The ability of participants to complete a workout depends on their physiological responses and perception of effort rather than the metabolic cost of the activity itself. Fortunately, by using specific HR values that are approximately equal to 60% to 80% $\dot{V}O_2$max, it is possible to formulate an exercise prescription that takes many of these factors into consideration. These HR values form the **target heart rate (THR)** range. How is the THR range determined?

Target Heart Rate: Direct Method

As described in chapters 4 and 7, HR increases linearly with the metabolic load. In the direct method for determining THR, HR is monitored at each stage of a maximal GXT. HR is then plotted on a graph against the $\dot{V}O_2$ (or MET) equivalents of each stage of the test. The fitness professional determines the THR range by taking the percentages of $\dot{V}O_2$max (%$\dot{V}O_2$max) at which the person should train and finding what the HR responses were at those points. Figure 11.5 shows this method being used for a subject with a functional capacity of 10.5 METs. Work rates of 60% to 80% of maximal METs demanded HR responses of 132 to 156 beats · min–1. The HR values become the intensity guide for the subject and represent the THR range (3).

Target Heart Rate: Indirect Methods

In contrast to the direct method, which requires the participant to complete a maximal GXT, two indirect methods have been developed to estimate an appropriate THR. These are the HRR method and the %HRmax method.

Heart Rate Reserve Method

HRR is the difference between resting and maximal HR. For a maximal HR of 200 beats · min^{-1} and a resting HR of 60 beats · min^{-1}, the HRR is 140 beats · min^{-1}. As shown in figure 11.6, the percentage of the HRR equals the percentage of $\dot{V}O_2$R across the range of exercise intensities (58, 59). For participants with average to high levels of CRF, %HRR approximately equals %$\dot{V}O_2$max.

The HRR method of determining the THR range, made popular by Karvonen, requires a few simple calculations (35):

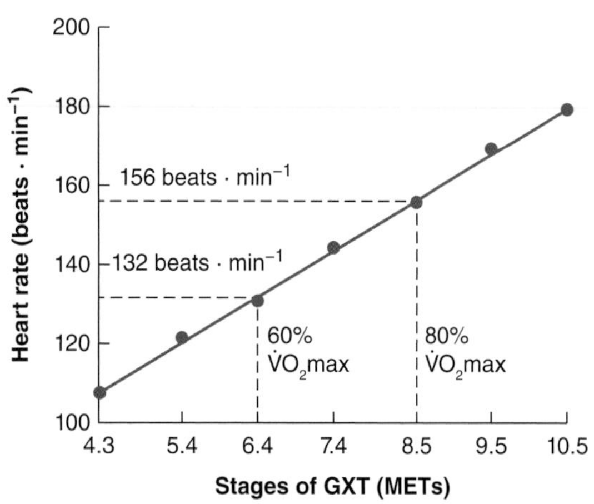

FIGURE 11.5 Direct method of determining the THR zone when maximal aerobic power (functional capacity) is measured during a GXT.

1. Subtract the resting HR from the maximal HR to obtain the HRR.
2. Calculate 60% and 80% of the HRR.
3. Add each value to the resting HR to obtain the THR range.

QUESTION:

A 40-yr-old male participant has a measured maximal HR of 175 beats · min^{-1} and a resting HR of 75 beats · min $^{-1}$. What is his THR range as calculated by the Karvonen (HRR) method?

ANSWER:

HRR = 175 beats · min^{-1} – 75 beats · min^{-1}
= 100 beats · min^{-1}.

60% of 100 beats · min^{-1} = 60 beats · min^{-1},
and 80% of 100 beats · min^{-1} = 80 beats · min^{-1}.

60 beats · min^{-1} + 75 beats · min^{-1} = 135 beats · min^{-1}
for 60% $\dot{V}O_2$max, and

80 beats · min^{-1} + 75 beats · min^{-1} = 155 beats · min^{-1}
for 80% $\dot{V}O_2$max.

The advantages of using this procedure to determine exercise intensity are that the recommended THR is always between the person's resting and maximal HRs and the %HRR equals the %$\dot{V}O_2$R across the entire range of CRF. Although the resting HR varies and can be influenced by factors such as caffeine, lack of sleep, dehydration, emotional state, and training, this variation does not introduce serious errors into calculating the THR by the Karvonen method (22). Consider the following example.

QUESTION:

The 40-yr-old subject mentioned previously participates in an endurance training program, and his resting HR decreases by 10 beats · min^{-1}. Because maximal HR (175 beats · min^{-1}) is not affected by training, what happens to his THR range?

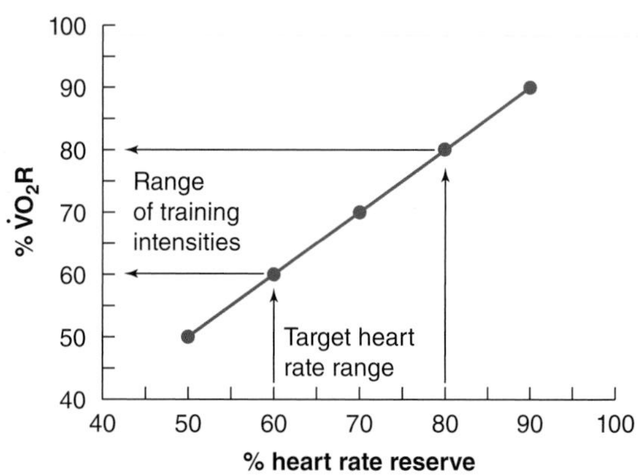

FIGURE 11.6 Relationship of %HRR and %$\dot{V}O_2$R.

Adapted from Swain et al. 1998.

ANSWER:

The HRR now equals 175 beats · min^{-1} – 65 beats · min^{-1} = 110 beats · min^{-1},

60% of 110 beats · min^{-1} = 66 beats · min^{-1} + 65 beats · min^{-1} = 131 beats · min^{-1}, and

80% of 110 beats · min^{-1} = 88 beats · min^{-1} + 65 beats · min^{-1} = 153 beats · min^{-1}.

Consequently, the change in resting HR had only a minimal effect on the THR range.

Percentage of Maximal Heart Rate Method

Another method of determining THR range is to use a fixed percentage of the maximal HR (%HRmax). The advantage of this method is its simplicity and the fact that it has been validated across many populations (27, 37, 57). Figure 11.7 shows the relationship between %HRmax and %$\dot{V}O_2$max.

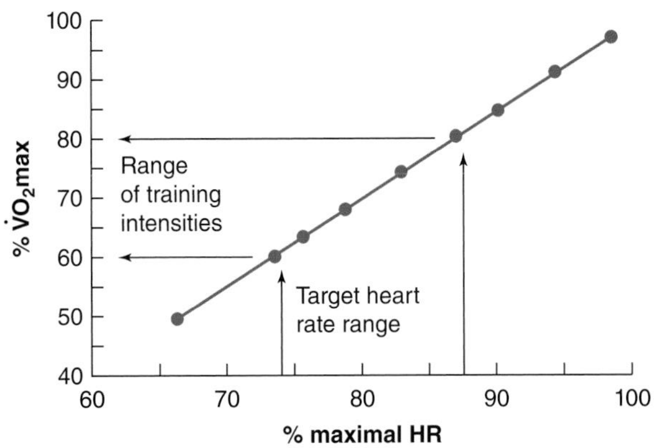

FIGURE 11.7 Relationship of %HRmax and %$\dot{V}O_2$max.
Adapted from Londeree and Ames 1979.

It is clear that %HRmax and %$\dot{V}O_2$max are linearly related and that %HRmax can be used to estimate the metabolic load in training programs. The usual guideline to estimate reasonable exercise intensity for the typically sedentary person is 70% to 85% HRmax. This THR range equals approximately 55% to 75% $\dot{V}O_2$max and results in an intensity prescription that is slightly more conservative than that generated by the HRR method when 60% to 80% of HRR is used. The range of 75% to 90% HRmax is more similar to 60% to 80% $\dot{V}O_2$max and HRR. The following example shows how to use the %HRmax method to calculate the THR range.

QUESTION:

How can you calculate a THR range if you don't know what the resting HR is? Use the data from the 40-yr-old subject mentioned previously, who had a measured maximal HR of 175 beats · min^{-1}.

ANSWER:

Take 75% and 90% of the maximal HR:

75% of 175 beats · min^{-1} = 131 beats · min^{-1},

and

90% of 175 beats · min^{-1} = 158 beats · min^{-1}.

These values are similar to those calculated using the HRR method described earlier. Table 11.3 shows the relationship between %$\dot{V}O_2$max and %HRmax across the range of exercise intensities from 50% to 85% $\dot{V}O_2$max. Using this table simplifies the process of making specific intensity recommendations by using the %HRmax method.

Table 11.3 Relationship of %HRmax and %$\dot{V}O_2$max

$\dot{V}O_2$max	%HRmax
50	66
55	70
60	74
65	77
70	81
75	85
80	88
85	92

Adapted from Londeree and Ames 1976.

Threshold

As mentioned earlier, the intensity of exercise that provides an adequate stimulus for cardiorespiratory improvement varies with activity level and age and spans the range of 40% to 84% $\dot{V}O_2$R and $\dot{V}O_2$max. In a systematic review of the literature, Swain and Franklin verified the low end of the threshold range. They found that the threshold for improvement in $\dot{V}O_2$max was only 30% HRR for people with $\dot{V}O_2$max values less than 40 ml · kg^{-1} · min^{-1} and only 46% HRR for people with higher $\dot{V}O_2$max values; however, higher intensities more effectively increased $\dot{V}O_2$max (60). Consequently, for most of the population, the optimal intensity threshold is in the following ranges:

- 60% to 80% of $\dot{V}O_2$max, HRR, and $\dot{V}O_2$R
- 75% to 90% of HRmax

As we discussed at the beginning of this section, the threshold is toward the lower part of the range (50%-60% HRR) for older, sedentary populations and toward the upper part of the range (>80% HRR) for younger, fitter populations. The middle of the range (70% HRR, 70% $\dot{V}O_2$max, or 80% HRmax) is an *average* training intensity and is appropriate for the typical apparently healthy person who wishes to be involved in a regular fitness program. Participating in activities at these intensities constitutes an overload on the cardiorespiratory system, resulting in adaptation over time.

Maximal Heart Rate

The indirect methods for determining exercise intensity use HRmax, and it is recommended that the HRmax be measured directly (by maximal GXT) when possible. If HRmax cannot be measured, then any estimation must consider the effect of age on it. Previously, HRmax had been estimated by subtracting age from 220. However, this formula underestimates HRmax for older adults. Tanaka, Monahan, and Seals (61) evaluated the validity of the classic formula of 220 – age for estimating HRmax. They analyzed 351 published studies and cross-validated these findings with a well-controlled laboratory study. They found almost identical results for both studies: HRmax = 208 – 0.7 · age. This new formula yields HRmax values that are 6 beats · min^{-1} lower for 20-yr-olds and 6 beats · min^{-1} higher for 60-yr-olds. Although the new formula yields better estimates of HRmax on average, the investigators emphasize that the estimated HRmax for a given individual is still associated with an SD (standard deviation) of 10 beats · min^{-1}.

Any estimate of HRmax is a potential source of error for both the HRR and the %HRmax methods of calculating a THR. For example, given that 1 SD of this estimate of HRmax is about 10 beats · min^{-1}, a 45-yr-old's true HRmax may be anywhere between 145 and 205 beats · min^{-1} (3 SD) rather than the estimated 175. However, 68% (1 SD) of the population would be between 165 and 185 beats · min^{-1}. If the HRmax is known (e.g., from a GXT), the fitness professional should use this measured HRmax to determine THR rather than using the estimate with its potential error (37). Estimating HRmax is another reason for using caution when relying solely on the THR range as an indicator of exercise intensity. The potential for error exists both in the estimate of HRmax and in the equations in which various percentages of HRmax are used to predict %$\dot{V}O_2$max. The intensity levels should only be considered as guidelines (see the sidebar *Error Involved in Estimating %$\dot{V}O_2$max from HR*).

Use of Target Heart Rate

The concept of an intensity threshold provides the basis for regular fitness workouts. The THR can be used as an intensity guide for large-muscle-group, continuous, whole-body activities such as walking, running, swimming, rowing, cycling, skiing, and dancing. However, the same training results may not occur from activities using small muscle groups or resistance exercises, because these exercises elevate the HR much higher for the same metabolic load.

The THR range associated with improvements in CRF and health-related outcomes is 40 to 84 %HRR; however, for people who are less active and have more risk factors, the lower end of the THR range should be used. For example, moderate-intensity activity, equal to only 40% to 59% HRR, is well within the capabilities of most people and carries a low risk of injury or complications (64). That is why it is the best starting place for most sedentary deconditioned people. Further, many clients may wish to continue doing moderate-intensity activity and not move to vigorous-intensity activity, because it suits them and they can work it into their schedule. More active people with fewer risk factors can use the upper end of the THR range. The THR can be divided by 6 to provide the desired 10 sec THR. If the person's HRmax is unknown, the estimated THR for 10 sec, by age and activity level, can be found in table 11.4. People can learn to exercise at their THRs by walking or jogging for several minutes and then stopping and immediately taking a 10 sec HR. If their HR is not within the target range, they should adjust the intensity by going slower or faster for a few minutes and then taking another 10 sec count. Using the THR to set exercise intensity has many advantages:

Error Involved in Estimating %$\dot{V}O_2$max from HR

The two indirect HR methods (%HRR and %HRmax) for estimating exercise intensity are simply guidelines to use in an exercise program, and small differences between methods are not important. Both approaches must be used as guidelines because, as for any prediction equation, an error is involved in estimating the %$\dot{V}O_2$max value. For example, even though we estimate that a person is at 70% $\dot{V}O_2$max when the HR is 81% HRmax (see table 11.3), in reality, 68% (1 SD) of the true values are between 64% and 76% $\dot{V}O_2$max for that HR value, and we don't know exactly where in that range any individual is (36). Because of this uncertainty, the calculated THR values should be used as guidelines in helping clients increase or maintain CRF. The fitness professional needs other indicators of exercise intensity to compensate for some of the inherent uncertainty in the THR prescription (see later in this chapter).

- It has a built-in individualized progression (i.e., as people increase their fitness, they have to work harder to achieve the THR).
- It accounts for environmental conditions (e.g., a person decreases the intensity while working in hot temperatures).
- It is easily determined, learned, and monitored.

These recommendations are appropriate for most people, but individuals differ in terms of the threshold needed for a training effect, the rate of adaptation to the training, and how exercise feels to them. The fitness professional must use subjective judgment, based on observations of the person exercising, to determine whether the intensity should be higher or lower. If the work is so easy that the person experiences little or no increase in ventilation and is able to work without effort, then the intensity should be increased. At the other extreme, if a person shows signs of working very hard and is still unable to reach THR, then a lower intensity should be chosen. In this case, the top part of the THR range might be above the person's true HRmax because the 220 – age formula only roughly estimates the true value. The fitness professional should not rely on the THR as the only method of judging whether the participant is exercising at the correct intensity; attention should be paid to other signs and symptoms of overexertion. The Borg RPE scale might be useful in this regard.

Rating of Perceived Exertion

The Borg RPE scale that is used to indicate the subjective sensation of effort experienced during a GXT (see chapter 7) can be used in prescribing exercise for the apparently healthy person (6). Exercise perceived as just below somewhat hard to just above hard, a rating of 12 to 16 on the original RPE scale, approximates 40% to 84% of HRR and 60% to 90% of HRmax (65). As mentioned earlier, the RPE is not a substitute for prescribing exercise intensity by HR (4). However, if the HRmax is not known and the THR range is perceived as too low or too high, an RPE rating can estimate the overall effort experienced by the person, and the exercise intensity can then be adjusted accordingly. Further, as a participant becomes accustomed to the physical sensations experienced when exercising at the THR range, there will be less need for frequently measuring the pulse rate. In the Physical Activity Guidelines for Americans, a 10-point relative intensity (level-of-effort) scale was recommended, with 5 to 6 being moderate intensity and 7 to 8 being vigorous intensity (64).

KEY POINT

The exercise intensity for a CRF training effect can be described in a variety of ways: 40% to 84% $\dot{V}O_2R$ (HRR), 60% to 90% HRmax, and 12 to 16 on the original RPE scale.

Exercise Recommendations for the Untested Masses

Certain general recommendations can be made for anyone wanting to begin a fitness program. Although the fitness professional might wish to have each client undergo a complete testing protocol before beginning exercise, that simply is not realistic. In addition, people without known health problems who follow these general guidelines can begin to exercise at low risk. In fact, the CHD risks of continuing not to exercise are greater than those of beginning a moderate-intensity exercise program.

Table 11.4 Estimated 10 Sec Target Heart Rate for People Whose Maximal Heart Rate Is Unknown

	INTENSITY	AGE (YR)						
Population	% $\dot{V}O_2max$	20	30	40	50	60	70	80
Inactive with several risk factors	50	22	21	20	18	17	16	15
	55	23	22	21	19	18	17	16
Normal activity with few risk factors	60	24	23	22	20	19	18	17
	65	25	24	23	21	20	19	18
	70	26	25	24	22	21	20	18
	75	28	26	25	24	22	21	19
	80	29	28	26	25	23	22	20
Very active with low risk	85	30	29	27	26	24	23	21
	90	31	30	28	27	25	24	22

Data from Londeree and Ames 1976.

When Moderate-Intensity Exercise May Be Hard

The U.S. Physical Activity Guidelines (64) recommend 150 min · wk^{-1} or more of moderate-intensity (3-5.9 METs) physical activity. The fitness professional must recognize that the range of 3 to 5.9 METs may be moderate exercise for some but hard exercise for others. Figure 11.8 shows that the relative intensity for a fixed exercise varies considerably across the range of $\dot{V}O_2$max values (32, 65). Consequently, some people with low $\dot{V}O_2$max values would function in the intensity range consistent with achieving gains in $\dot{V}O_2$max, whereas those with higher CRF values would not. This example emphasizes the need to consider the THR range and RPE when following recommendations that specify absolute exercise intensities (e.g., METs).

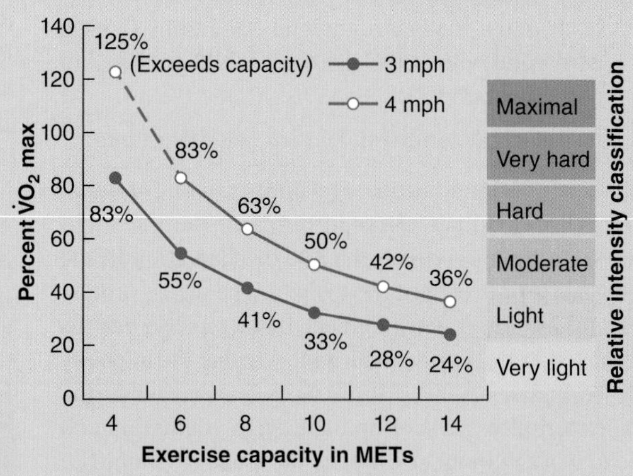

FIGURE 11.8 Relative exercise intensity for walking at 3.0 mi · hr^{-1} (4.8 km · hr^{-1} or 3.3 METs) and 4.0 mi · hr^{-1} (6.4 km · hr^{-1} or 5.0 METs) expressed as a percent of $\dot{V}O_2$max for adults with an exercise capacity ranging from 4 to 14 METs.

From U.S. Department of Health and Human Services (DHHS), 2008, *Physical Activity Guidelines Advisory Committee report 2008*, Fig, D.1, page D-7.

Figure 11.9 summarizes the recommendations for achieving health, fitness, and performance goals. On the left side we see the U.S. Physical Activity Guidelines for adults, the starting place for most sedentary deconditioned individuals (64). We want to emphasize that there is no structural barrier between what is needed for health and what is needed for fitness. The high end of moderate intensity (59% HRR) is clearly not different from the low end of vigorous intensity (60% HRR); think of the two categories as a continuum to realize much of the same benefits that we have discussed throughout the text. The fitness professional's challenge is to match the starting point to the client's status and progress the client through a program in a manner that is safe and consistent with the client's goals, which may change as fitness improves.

Exercise Programming for the Fit Population

Exercise recommendations for people who are regularly active and have achieved a reasonable level of physical fitness tend to be associated with less risk, and these participants require less supervision. People who become fit can simply continue their program using the guidelines in the middle box of figure 11.9. As fitness improves, higher

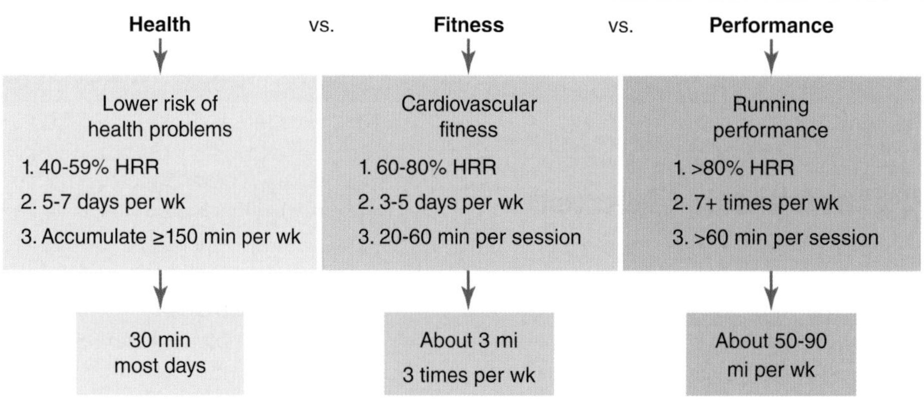

FIGURE 11.9 Contrasting recommendations for achieving health, fitness, and performance goals.

absolute intensities of exercise (e.g., faster jogging speeds) will be needed for the HR to stay in the THR range. Some people in this group may want to focus on performance, in contrast to health and fitness, as the primary goal. A wide variety of programs, activities, races, and competitions are available to address the needs of this group.

The THR range will be calculated as described before, but very fit individuals can work at the top part of the range (≥85% of $\dot{V}O_2$max or >90% of HRmax). As mentioned earlier, individuals who are less fit can start working out at the low end of the range and still experience a training effect. Those who are fitter need to work at the top end of the range to maintain a high level of fitness. Training for competition demands more than the training intensity needed for CRF. Individuals who do interval-type training programs have peak HRs close to maximum during the intervals. The recovery period between the intervals should include some work at a lower intensity (near 40%-50% $\dot{V}O_2$max) to help metabolize the lactate produced during the interval (12) and to reduce the chance of cardiovascular complications that can occur when a person comes to a complete rest at the end of a strenuous exercise bout (44) (see chapter 15 for more on training for performance).

For people who participate in sports that are intermittent in nature but that still require high levels of aerobic fitness, a running and jogging program is a good way to maintain general conditioning when not participating in the primary sport. However, given the specificity of training, there is no substitute for the real activity when conditioning for a sport.

As figure 11.9 shows, people interested in performance who work at the top end of the THR range, exercise 5 to 7 or more times each week, and exercise for longer than 60 min each exercise session are doing much more than those interested in fitness, and it should be no surprise that they tend to experience more injuries (64) (see chapter 1 for information about adverse events). When the risk of injury during exercise is coupled with the inherent risks associated with competitive activities, it is clear that alternative activities should be planned that can be done when participation in the primary activity is not possible. This planning reduces the chance of becoming detrained when injuries do occur. Further, the alternative activities can be used as a part of the regular activity program to reduce the chance of an injury in the first place.

Exercise Prescriptions Using Complete Graded Exercise Test Results

In the previous sections, the exercise recommendations were based on little or no specific information about the people involved. In many adult fitness programs, potential participants have had a general medical exam or a maximal GXT with appropriate monitoring of HR, BP, and possibly ECG responses. Unfortunately, this information is not always used in designing the exercise program; instead, the measured HRmax is used in the THR formulas and the rest of the data are ignored. This section outlines the steps that should be followed when the fitness professional assists in making the exercise recommendation using information about the person's functional capacity and cardiovascular responses to graded exercise. The fitness professional is not generally involved in the clinical evaluation of a GXT, but understanding the procedures used to make clinical judgments clearly enhances communication with the program director, exercise specialist, and physician. The following information on using GXTs for exercise prescription and programming was written with this intent.

Program Selection

Exercise program options include exercising alone, in small groups, in fitness clubs, and in clinically oriented settings. The fitness professional must consider a variety of factors before recommending participation in a supervised or an unsupervised program.

Supervised Program

The risk factors, the response to the GXT, the health and activity history, and personal preference influence the type of program in which a client should participate. Generally, the higher the risk, the more important it is that the person participate in a supervised program. People at high risk for CHD and those who have diseases such as diabetes, hypertension, asthma, and CHD should be encouraged to participate under supervision, at least at the beginning of an exercise program. The personnel in the supervised program are trained to provide the necessary instruction in the appropriate activities, to help monitor the participant's response to the activity, to provide encouragement, and to administer appropriate first aid or emergency care.

Supervised programs run the gamut from those conducted within a hospital for patients with CHD and other diseases to programs conducted in fitness clubs for people at low risk for CHD. In general, as a person moves along the continuum from inpatient to outpatient, less formal monitoring is required. In addition, the background and training of the personnel tend to vary. Exercise programs aimed at maintaining the fitness level of CHD patients who have gone through a hospital-based program have medical personnel and emergency equipment appropriate for the population being served. Supervised fitness programs for the apparently healthy have a fitness professional who can focus more on the appropriate exercise, diet, and other lifestyle behaviors needed to improve health.

The supervised program offers a socially supportive environment for people to become and stay active. This is important, given the difficulty of changing lifestyle behaviors (see chapter 23). The group program allows for more variety in activities (e.g., group games) and reduces

Using Graded Exercise Tests for Exercise Prescription and Programming

Analyzing a Graded Exercise Test for Exercise Prescription

1. Analyze the person's history and list the known risk factors for CHD; also, identify those factors that might have a direct bearing on the exercise program, such as orthopedic problems, previous physical activity, and current interests.
2. Determine if the functional capacity is a true maximum or if it is limited by a sign or symptom. Express the functional capacity in METs, and record the highest HR and RPE achieved without significant signs or symptoms.
3. If ECG was monitored, itemize the person's ECG changes as indicated by the physician.
4. Examine the HR and BP responses to see if they are normal.
5. List the symptoms reported at each stage.
6. List the reasons why the test was stopped (e.g., ECG changes, falling SBP, dizziness).

Designing an Exercise Program From a Graded Exercise Test

1. Given the overall response to the GXT, decide to either refer for additional medical care or initiate an exercise program.
2. Identify the THR range and approximate MET intensities of selected activities needed to be within that THR range.
3. Specify the frequency and duration of activity needed to meet the goals of increased CRF and weight loss.
4. Recommend that the person (a) participate in either a supervised or an unsupervised program, (b) be monitored or unmonitored, and (c) do group or individual activities.
5. Select a variety of activities at the appropriate MET level that allow the person to achieve THR. Consider environmental factors, medication, and any physical limitations of the participant when making this recommendation.

RESEARCH INSIGHT

Supervised Exercise and Phase II Cardiac Rehabilitation Programs

Shipe (55) assessed whether the provision of a pedometer and exercise diary could increase the activity levels of phase II cardiac rehabilitation program (CRP) patients on the days they did not attend the 12 wk program (Tuesday, Thursday, Saturday, and Sunday). Members of the control group were given a blinded pedometer, and the physical activity information stored on the pedometer was downloaded at regular weekly intervals when the subjects came to class. Members of the experimental group received a pedometer that they could view as well as an exercise diary to record their daily step counts (the information on their pedometers also was downloaded each week). Control patients wore the pedometer during all of their waking hours and were encouraged to increase their overall activity levels in accordance with the standard level of care. Patients in the experimental group were encouraged to gradually increase their step counts on the days they did not attend phase II CRP (i.e., non-CRP days) until they were accumulating 2,000 steps a day above their baseline levels for those days. Over the 12 wk program, the experimental group increased its daily step count on non-CRP days from 3,763 at wk 1 to 5,772 at wk 5 and maintained that level (i.e., 6,400 steps each day at wk 12); the control group remained virtually unchanged (3,175 at wk 1 versus 3,364 at wk 12). Clearly, the use of pedometers and an exercise diary helped these phase II CRP patients be more active.

the chance of boredom. For the program to be effective in the long run, the program leader should try to wean the participants from the group in a way that encourages them to maintain their activity patterns when they are no longer in the program. See the following Research Insight for information about how pedometers were effective in increasing the physical level of patients in a cardiac rehabilitation program.

Unsupervised Program

Despite the risks just described, the vast majority of people at risk for or already having CHD participate in unsupervised exercise programs. Reasons for this include the limited number of supervised programs, the level of interest of the participant and physician in such programs, and the financial resources required to participate in such programs.

Participation in an unsupervised exercise program requires the fitness professional or physician to clearly communicate how to begin and maintain the exercise program. The emphasis in beginning an unsupervised exercise program is on low to moderate intensity (i.e., 40%-50% $\dot{V}O_2R$), because the threshold for a training effect is lower in deconditioned people. The goal is to increase the duration of the activity, with exercise frequency approaching every day. This reduces the chance of muscular, skeletal, or cardiovascular problems caused by the exercise intensity and increases muscle function with the expenditure of a relatively large number of calories. In addition, the regularity of the exercise program encourages a positive habit. The outcome of such programs results in participants being able to conduct their daily affairs with more comfort and sets the stage for people who would like to exercise at higher levels.

In an unsupervised exercise program, the client should be provided explicit information about the intensity (THR), duration, and frequency of exercise so that no doubt remains about what should be done. For example, the exercise recommendation might read, "Walk 1 mile (1.6 km) in 30 minutes each day for 2 weeks. Monitor and record your heart rate." The person must be told how to take the pulse rate and be encouraged to follow through on the recording.

KEY POINT

Exercise recommendations for the general public emphasize moderate intensity (40%-59% HRR) and regular participation. Exercise performed at 60% to 80% HRR for 20 to 40 min 3 or 4 days per wk increases and maintains CRF. Exercise recommendations for very fit individuals emphasize the top end of the training intensity (>80% $\dot{V}O_2R$) and frequent (almost daily) participation. The potential for injury is greater for such performance-driven workouts. For people who undergo a comprehensive diagnostic GXT with ECG monitoring, all test results are used to select an optimal and safe exercise prescription. Participants with multiple risk factors for CHD and those with existing diseases benefit from participating in a supervised program. However, most of these individuals will participate in an unsupervised program, necessitating clear communication about the exercise prescription and safety concerns.

Updating the Exercise Program

During participation in an endurance training program, the capacity for work increases. The best sign of this is that the recommended exercise is no longer sufficient to reach THR; clearly the person is adapting to the exercise. Taking the HR during a regular activity session provides a sound basis for upgrading the intensity or duration of the exercise session.

The exercise program, including the THR, should be updated periodically. The need to update is greater for those with a lower initial level of fitness and a greater number of risk factors. A person who has a low functional capacity because of heart disease, orthopedic limitations, or chronic inactivity (which might include prolonged bed rest) has difficulty reaching a true maximum on a first treadmill test. Further, he experiences the greatest improvements in the shortest time during the fitness program. This person benefits from frequent retesting because the test allows progress (or the lack thereof) to be monitored, and it may give new information that influences the exercise prescription.

If the client has had a change in medication that influences the HR response to exercise, the exercise program must be reevaluated, especially if the exercise prescription was originally based on the initial HR response. These issues are found more in clinical rehabilitation programs, but as Exercise is Medicine initiatives (www.exerciseismedicine.org) come into place, fitness professionals will have to become more aware of how to help patients make a transition to fitness facilities.

For people who reach a true maximum in the first test, actual THR will change little during a fitness program because the HRmax is affected very little by regular endurance exercise. However, these people still benefit from regular evaluation of the overall exercise program because their activity interests may change or they may develop orthopedic problems that did not exist before. The reevaluation allows fitness professionals to probe for information that may enable them to refer the person for treatment at a time when treatment will do the most good. Such contact increases the chance that the person will stay involved in an activity program—the most important factor in maintaining aerobic fitness.

Environmental Concerns

THR is used to indicate the proper exercise intensity in health-related fitness programs. However, environmental factors such as heat, humidity, pollution, and altitude can elevate HR and RPE during an exercise session, which may shorten the session and reduce the participant's chance of expending sufficient calories to meet energy balance goals. Fortunately, by decreasing the exercise intensity, the fitness professional can work around these environmental problems to provide a safe and effective exercise prescription. This section discusses the effects of various environmental factors on the exercise prescription and what the fitness professional can do about them.

Heat and Humidity

Chapter 4 describes the increases in body temperature that occur with exercise, the mechanisms of heat loss called into play, and the benefits of becoming acclimatized to the heat. Our core temperature (37 °C, or 98.6 °F) is within a few degrees of a value that could lead to death by heat injury. As described in chapter 25, to prevent a progression from the least to the most serious heat injury, people should recognize and attend to a series of stages from heat cramps to heatstroke. Preventing the problem in the first place is a better approach than treating the problem after it has occurred.

Each of the following factors influences susceptibility to heat injury and can alter the HR and metabolic responses to exercise (45):

- *Fitness.* Fit people have a lower risk of heat injury (1, 17), can tolerate more work in the heat (14), and acclimatize to heat faster (8).
- *Acclimatization.* Exercising for 7 to 14 days in the heat increases the capacity to sweat, initiates sweating at a lower body temperature, and reduces salt loss. Body temperature and HR responses are lower during exercise, and the chance of salt depletion is reduced (1, 4, 8).
- *Hydration.* Inadequate hydration reduces sweat rate and increases the chance of heat injury (1, 8, 51, 52). In general, during exercise the focus should be on replacing water, not salt or carbohydrate stores.
- *Environmental temperature.* Exercising in temperatures greater than skin temperature results in a heat gain by convection and radiation. Evaporation of sweat must compensate for this gain if body temperature is to remain at a safe level.
- *Clothing.* As much skin surface as possible should be exposed in order to encourage evaporation, although the skin should be protected from the sun by using sunblock. Materials should be chosen that wick sweat to the surface for evaporation; materials impermeable to water increase the risk of heat injury and should be avoided.
- *Humidity (water vapor pressure).* Evaporation of sweat depends on the water vapor pressure gradient between skin and environment. In warm and hot environments, relative humidity is a good index of the water vapor pressure, with a lower relative humidity facilitating the evaporation of sweat.
- *Metabolic rate.* During times of high heat and humidity, decreasing the exercise intensity decreases the heat load as well as the strain on the physiological systems that must deal with it.
- *Wind.* Wind places more air molecules in contact with the skin and can influence heat loss in two ways: If there is a temperature gradient for heat loss between the skin and the air, wind will increase the rate of heat loss by convection. In a similar manner, wind increases the rate of evaporation, assuming the air can accept moisture.

Recommendations for Fitness

Members of a fitness program should be educated about all of the heat-related factors just mentioned. The fitness professional might suggest the following:

- Learning about the symptoms of heat illness (e.g., cramps, light-headedness) and how to deal with them (see chapter 25)
- Exercising in the cooler parts of the day to avoid heat gain from the sun or from building or road surfaces heated by the sun
- Gradually increasing exposure to high heat and humidity over 7 to 14 days to safely acclimatize to the environmental conditions
- Drinking water before, during, and after exercise and weighing in each day to monitor hydration
- Wearing only shorts and a tank top in order to expose as much skin as possible while being careful to use sunblock to reduce the chance of skin cancer
- Taking HR measurements several times during the activity and reducing exercise intensity to stay in the THR zone

The last recommendation is most important: HR is a sensitive indicator of dehydration, environmental heat load, and acclimatization, and variation in any of these factors will modify the HR response to any fixed submaximal exercise. It is therefore important for fitness participants to monitor HR regularly and slow down to stay within the THR zone. RPE also can be used in extreme heat to provide an index of the overall physiological strain that the participant is experiencing.

Implications for Performance

Any athlete performing in an environment that is not conducive to heat loss is at an increased risk of heat injury. Traditionally this has been a major problem for American football, where clothing and equipment prevent heat loss, but the increased number of people participating in 10K races, marathons, and triathlons has shifted our focus to them (1, 20, 33). In the latter cases, the athlete has a high metabolic rate while exercising in direct exposure to the sun. In response to this problem and on the basis of sound research, ACSM developed position stands on exercise-related thermal injuries (1). The elements in this position stand are consistent with the information presented at the beginning of this section.

Environmental Heat Stress

The preceding discussion mentioned high temperature and relative humidity as important factors increasing the risk of heat injuries. To quantify the overall heat stress associated with an environment, a **wet-bulb globe temperature (WBGT)** guide has been developed (1). This overall heat stress index is composed of the following measurements (see figure 11.10):

- **Dry-bulb temperature (T_{db})**—ordinary measure of air temperature taken in the shade
- **Black-globe temperature (T_g)**—measure of the radiant heat load in direct sunlight; temperature is measured inside a copper globe (15 cm diameter) painted flat black
- **Wet-bulb temperature (T_{wb})**—measurement of air temperature with a thermometer whose mercury bulb is covered with a wet cotton wick, which makes it sensitive to the relative humidity (water vapor pressure) and provides an index of the ability to evaporate sweat

The formula used to calculate the WBGT temperature shows the importance of the wet-bulb temperature, which makes up 70% (0.7) of the WBGT index, in determining heat stress (1). This is related to the role the wet-bulb temperature plays in estimating the ability to evaporate sweat, the most important heat-loss mechanism in most situations. The formula is as follows:

$$WBGT = 0.7\ T_{wb} + 0.2\ T_g + 0.1\ T_{db}$$

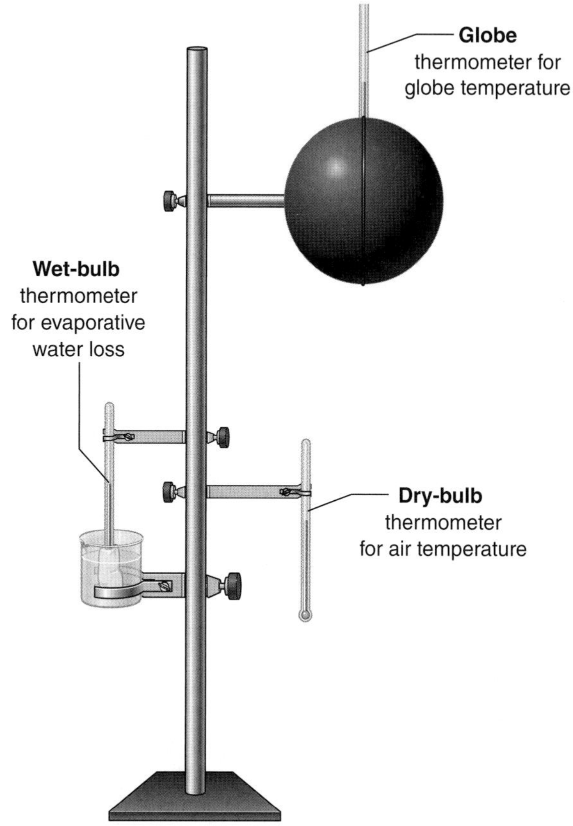

FIGURE 11.10 A WBGT stand, which provides valuable information on humidity and solar radiation that should be factored into heat stress calculations.

The risk of **hyperthermia** (heat illness), including **exertional heat stroke (EHS)**, attributable to environmental stress while wearing shorts, socks, shoes, and a T-shirt is rated on the following scale (1, 50):

WBGT EXCEEDS 27.9 °C (>82.1 °F)

Extreme risk of hyperthermia; cancel or postpone

WBGT = 25.7 TO 27.8 °C (78.1-82 °F)

Extreme caution; high risk for unfit, nonacclimatized

WBGT = 22.3 TO 25.6 °C (72.1-78 °F)

Extreme caution; risk of hyperthermia increased for all

WBGT = 18.4 TO 22.2 °C (65.1-72 °F)

Caution: moderate risk of hyperthermia; high-risk people monitored or not compete

WBGT 10 TO 18.3 °C (50-65 °F)

Low risk of hyperthermia and hypothermia, but EHS can occur

The risk of **hypothermia** while wearing shorts, socks, shoes, and a T-shirt also must be considered in distance running. A WBGT index of <10 °C (<50 °F) is associated with an increased risk of hypothermia, especially in wet and windy conditions, but EHS can still occur (1).

Cold Exposure

Exercising in the cold can create problems if certain precautions are not taken. As mentioned previously, a WBGT of less than 10 °C (50 °F) is associated with hypothermia. Hypothermia is a decrease in body temperature that occurs when heat loss exceeds heat production, and it is clinically defined as a core temperature below 35 °C (95 °F). In cold air, there is a larger gradient for convective heat loss from the skin; cold air also is dryer (has a low water vapor pressure) and facilitates the evaporation of moisture from the skin to further cool the body. The combined effects can be deadly, as shown in Pugh's report of three deaths during a walking competition of 45 mi (72 km) that was performed in very cold temperatures (46).

Factors related to hypothermia include environmental variables, such as temperature, water vapor pressure, wind, and whether air or water are involved; personal characteristics, such as age and sex; insulating factors, such as clothing and subcutaneous fat; and the capacity for sustained energy production (45). Each of these factors is discussed in the following paragraphs.

Environmental Factors

Conduction, convection, and radiation depend on a temperature gradient between the skin and the environment; the larger the gradient, the greater the rate of heat loss. What surprises many is that the environmental temperature does not have to be below freezing to cause hypothermia. Other environmental factors interact with temperature to facilitate heat loss, namely, wind and water (2).

Windchill Index The rate of heat loss at any given temperature is influenced directly by wind speed. Wind increases the number of cold air molecules coming into contact with the skin, increasing the rate of heat loss. The **windchill index** indicates the temperature equivalent (under calm air conditions) for any combination of temperature and wind speed (see figure 11.11). This index allows the fitness professional to properly gauge the cold stress associated with a variety of wind velocities and temperatures. Keep in mind that for activities such as running, riding, or cross-country skiing into the wind, the speed of the activity must be added to the wind speed to evaluate the full impact of the windchill. For example, cycling at 20 mi · hr^{-1} (32 km · hr^{-1}) into calm air at 0 °F (−17.8 °C) has a windchill value of −22 °F (−30.0 °C)! However, wind is not the only factor that can increase the rate of heat loss at any given temperature.

Water Heat is lost 25 times faster in water than in air of the same temperature. Unlike air, water offers little or no insulation where it meets the skin, so heat is lost rapidly from the body. Movement in cold water increases heat loss from the arms and legs (29), so it is better to stay as still as possible in long-term unplanned immersions or to wear a wetsuit for anticipated activities in cold water.

Personal Characteristics

Both age and sex influence the ability to respond to a cold environment. The fitness professional should give special attention to those at greater risk of hypothermia.

Temperature (°F)

Wind (mph) / Calm	40	35	30	25	20	15	10	5	0	−5	−10	−15	−20	−25	−30	−35	−40	−45
5	36	31	25	19	13	7	1	−5	−11	−16	−22	−28	−34	−40	−46	−52	−57	−63
10	34	27	21	15	9	3	−4	−10	−16	−22	−28	−35	−41	−47	−53	−59	−66	−72
15	32	25	19	13	6	0	−7	−13	−19	−26	−32	−39	−45	−51	−58	−64	−71	−77
20	30	24	17	11	4	−2	−9	−15	−22	−29	−35	−42	−48	−55	−61	−68	−74	−81
25	29	23	16	9	3	−4	−11	−17	−24	−31	−37	−44	−51	−58	−64	−71	−78	−84
30	28	22	15	8	1	−5	−12	−19	−26	−33	−39	−46	−53	−60	−67	−73	−80	−87
35	28	21	14	7	0	−7	−14	−21	−27	−34	−41	−48	−55	−62	−69	−76	−82	−89
40	27	20	13	6	−1	−8	−15	−22	−29	−36	−43	−50	−57	−64	−71	−78	−84	−91
45	26	19	12	5	−2	−9	−16	−23	−30	−37	−44	−51	−58	−65	−72	−79	−86	−93
50	26	19	12	4	−3	−10	−17	−24	−31	−38	−45	−52	−60	−67	−74	−81	−88	−95
55	25	18	11	4	−3	−11	−18	−25	−32	−39	−46	−54	−61	−68	−75	−82	−89	−97
60	25	17	10	3	−4	−11	−19	−26	−33	−40	−48	−55	−62	−69	−76	−84	−91	−98
Frostbite occurs in:							30 min		10 min		5 min							

$$\text{Windchill (°F)} = 35.74 + 0.6215T - 35.75(V^{0.16}) + 0.4275T(V^{0.16})$$

T = air temperature (°F) V = wind speed (mph)

FIGURE 11.11 Windchill index.

Courtesy of the NOAA National Weather Service. www.nws.noaa.gov

Age Adults older than 60 yr may be less responsive to cold stress due to a reduced capacity to vasoconstrict the skin blood vessels and conserve body heat. In addition, from a behavioral standpoint, they respond later to a drop in environmental temperature than younger people. Because of their higher body surface area-to-mass ratios and lower body fat, children may experience a greater drop in body temperature when exposed to the same cold environment as adults (2).

Sex Sex differences exist in the ability to respond to a cold-water challenge. These are primarily related to sex differences in body fatness, subcutaneous fat, and muscle mass (2).

Insulating Factors

The rate at which heat is lost from the body is related inversely to the insulation between the body and the environment. The insulating quality is related to the thickness of subcutaneous fat, the ability of clothing to trap air, and whether the clothing is wet or dry.

Body Fat Subcutaneous fat thickness is an excellent indicator of total body insulation per unit surface area through which heat is lost (26). For example, in one report an obese man was able to swim for 7 hr in 16 °C water with no change in body temperature, but a thinner man had to leave the water in 30 min with a core temperature of 34.5 °C (47). For this reason, long-distance swimmers tend to have more body fat than short-distance swimmers; the higher body fatness provides more buoyancy, requiring less energy to swim at any set speed (28).

Clothing Clothing can extend our natural subcutaneous fat insulation, allowing us to endure very cold environments. The insulation quality of clothing is given in clo units, where 1 clo unit is the insulation needed at rest (1 MET) to maintain core temperature when the environmental temperature is 21 °C (70 °F), the relative humidity is 50%, and the air movement is 6 mi · hr^{-1} (9.7 km · hr^{-1}) (7). As the air temperature falls, clothing with a higher clo value must be worn to maintain core temperature because the gradient between skin and environment is increasing. Figure 11.12 shows the insulation needed at various energy expenditures across a broad range of environmental temperatures, from −60 to 80 °F (−51.1 to 26.7 °C) (7). As energy production increases, insulation must decrease to maintain core temperature. When clothing is worn in layers, insulation can be removed as needed to maintain core temperature. By following these steps, the sweat rate will be reduced and the clothing will retain more of its insulating value.

If the clothing becomes wet, its insulating quality decreases because the water can now conduct heat away from the body about 25 times better than air can (29). A primary goal, then, is to avoid wetness caused by either

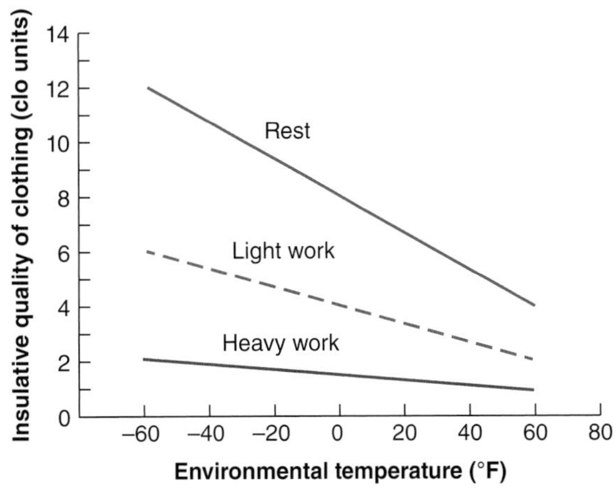

FIGURE 11.12 As work intensity increases, less insulation is needed to maintain core temperature.
Data from Burton and Edholm 1955.

sweat or weather. This problem is exacerbated by the very dry air of the cold environment, which causes a greater evaporation of moisture. When this problem of cold, dry air and wet clothing is coupled with windy conditions, the risk is even greater. The wind not only provides for greater convective heat loss, as described in the windchill section, but it also accelerates evaporation (21).

Energy Production

Energy production can modify the amount of insulation needed to maintain core temperature and prevent hypothermia (see figure 11.12). When thin (>16.8% body fat) male subjects were immersed in cold water, the drop in body temperature that occurred at rest was prevented when they exercised at an energy expenditure of about 8.5 kcal · min^{-1} (38, 39). Although being physically fit does not affect the thermoregulatory responses to cold, a fit person can exercise for a longer time at a higher metabolic rate, which can help maintain core temperature (2).

Table 11.5 shows the progression of signs and symptoms of hypothermia that occur as body temperature decreases (2, 56). It is important to deal with these problems on-site rather than wait until the person can be taken to an emergency room. According to Sharkey (54), do the following to help a person with hypothermia:

- Get the person out of the cold, wind, and rain.
- Remove all wet clothing.
- Provide warm drinks, dry clothing, and a warm, dry sleeping bag for a mildly impaired person.
- Keep the person awake; if semiconscious, undress the person and put him in a sleeping bag with another person.
- Find a heat source, such as a campfire.

Table 11.5 Clinical Symptoms of Hypothermia

Core temperature (°C)	Symptoms and signs
35	Maximal shivering
34	Amnesia, poor judgment
33	Ataxia, apathy
30	Cardiac arrhythmias
26	No response to pain
23	No corneal reflexes
18-19	EEG silence, asystole

Adapted from American College of Sports Medicine 2006.

Air Pollution

Air pollution includes gases and particulates that are products of the combustion of fossil fuels. The smog that results when these pollutants are highly concentrated can have detrimental effects on health and performance. The gases can affect performance by decreasing the capacity to transport oxygen, increasing airway resistance, and altering the perception of effort required when the eyes burn and the chest hurts.

Physiological responses to these pollutants are related to the amount, or dose, received. Several factors determine the dose:

- Concentration of the pollutant
- Duration of exposure to the pollutant
- Volume of air inhaled

The volume of air inhaled is large during exercise, and this is one reason why physical activity should be curtailed during times of peak pollution (15). The following discussion focuses on the major air pollutants: particulate matter, ozone, sulfur dioxide, and carbon monoxide.

Particulate Matter

The air is full of microscopic and submicroscopic particles, many of which can be tied to motor vehicles (especially diesel vehicles) and industrial sources. Over the past several years, more attention has been directed on the very small particles because of their potential to promote pulmonary infection and to cross the epithelium to enter the blood circulation (16). Fine-particle pollution elevates BP in people with preexisting CVD and may contribute to an increased risk of cardiac mortality and morbidity (53, 66).

Ozone

The **ozone** in the air we breathe is generated by the reaction between ultraviolet (UV) light and emissions from internal combustion engines. There is evidence that a single 2 hr exposure to a high ozone concentration, 0.75 parts per million (PPM), decreases $\dot{V}O_2$max; further, recent studies show that a 6 to 12 hr exposure to a concentration of only 0.12 PPM (the U.S. air quality standard) decreases lung function and increases respiratory symptoms. Interestingly, people can adapt to ozone exposure, showing diminished responses to subsequent exposures during the ozone season. Concern about long-term lung health suggests, however, that it would be prudent to avoid heavy exercise during the time of day when ozone and other pollutants are highest (15).

Sulfur Dioxide

Sulfur dioxide (SO_2) is produced by smelters, refineries, and electrical utilities that use fossil fuel for energy generation. SO_2 does not affect lung function in most people, but it causes bronchoconstriction in people who have asthma—a response influenced by the temperature and humidity of the inspired air. Nose breathing is encouraged to scrub the SO_2, and drugs such as cromolyn sodium and beta-agonists can partially block the response to SO_2 (15).

Carbon Monoxide

Carbon monoxide (CO) is derived from the burning of fossil fuel (coal, oil, gasoline) and wood as well as from cigarette smoke. CO can bind to hemoglobin (HbCO) and decrease the capacity for oxygen transport. The CO concentration in blood is generally less than 1% in nonsmokers but may be as high as 10% in smokers (49). As mentioned in chapter 4, beyond an HbCO concentration of 4.3%, there is a 1% reduction in $\dot{V}O_2$max for each 1% increase in the HbCO concentration. In contrast, when one exercises at about 40% $\dot{V}O_2$max, the HbCO concentration can be as high as 15% before endurance is affected. The cardiovascular system simply has a greater capacity to respond with a larger cardiac output when the oxygen concentration of the blood is reduced during submaximal work (30, 48, 49). This, of course, requires a higher HR for the same work rate, and participants need to reduce the intensity of exercise during exposure to CO to stay in the THR range. Because it takes about 2 to 4 hr to remove half the CO from the blood once the exposure has been removed, CO can have a lasting effect on performance (15). Unfortunately, it is difficult to predict what the actual CO concentration will be in any given environment. Because we must consider the previous exposure to the pollutant, as well as the length of time and rate of ventilation associated with the current exposure, the following guidelines are provided for exercising in an area with air pollution (49):

- Reduce exposure to the pollutant before exercise because the physiological effects are time and dose dependent.
- Stay away from areas where you might receive a high dose of CO: smoking areas, high-traffic areas, and urban environments.
- Do not schedule activities during the times when pollutants are at their highest levels because of traffic: 7 to 10 a.m. and 4 to 7 p.m.

Levels of health concern	Numerical value	Meaning
Good	0–50	Air quality is considered satisfactory, and air pollution poses little or no risk.
Moderate	51–100	Air quality is acceptable; however, for some pollutants there may be a moderate health concern for a very small number of people who are unusually sensitive to air pollution.
Unhealthy for sensitive groups	101–150	Members of sensitive groups may experience health effects. The general public is not likely to be affected.
Unhealthy	151–200	Everyone may begin to experience health effects; members of sensitive groups may experience more serious health effects.
Very unhealthy	201–300	Health alert: everyone may experience more serious health effects.
Hazardous	301–500	Health warnings of emergency conditions. The entire population is more likely to be affected.

FIGURE 11.13 Color-coded AQI chart.

Reprinted from AirNow, 2015, *Air quality index (AQI) basics*.

Air Quality Index

The air quality index (AQI) is a measure of air quality for five major air pollutants regulated by the U.S. Clean Air Act: ground-level ozone, particulate matter, carbon monoxide, sulfur dioxide, and nitrogen dioxide. The AQI is shown in figure 11.13 as a color-coded chart with interpretations of what the numerical values mean. This information is generally provided in a local community's weather forecast, can be found online at www.airnow.gov, and is available in smartphone apps, including a free version from the American Lung Association. The fitness professional should interpret the AQI information to suit the individual—some people experience symptoms at lower levels of pollution than others do (9).

Effect of Altitude

An increase in altitude decreases the partial pressure of oxygen and reduces the amount of oxygen bound to hemoglobin. As a result, the volume of oxygen carried in each liter of blood decreases. As mentioned in chapter 4, maximal aerobic power steadily decreases with increasing altitude, so by 2,300 m (7,500 ft) the value is only 88% of that measured at sea level. This means that an activity that demanded 88% of $\dot{V}O_2$max at sea level now requires 100% of the new $\dot{V}O_2$max.

More than maximal aerobic power is affected by altitude exposure; any submaximal work rate is going to demand a higher HR at altitude compared with sea level (shown in figure 11.14). This is because each liter of blood has less oxygen at altitude, and thus more blood is required to deliver the same quantity of oxygen to the tissues. Consequently, the HR response is elevated at any given submaximal work rate. To stay within the THR range, a person must decrease the intensity of the exercise when at altitude. As with exercising in high heat and humidity, monitoring the THR allows the exerciser to modify the intensity of the activity relative to any additional environmental demand (31).

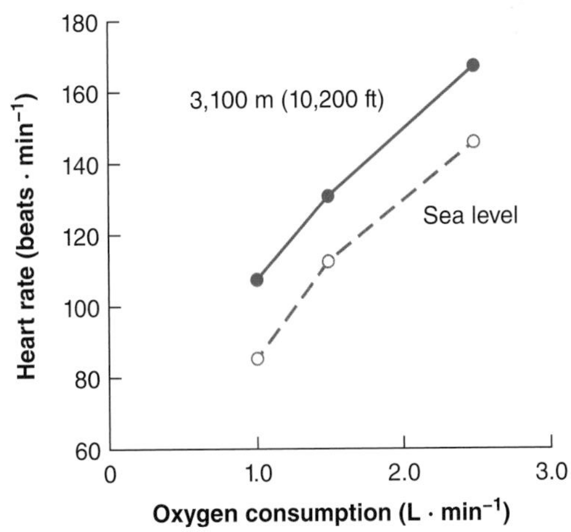

FIGURE 11.14 The effect of altitude on the HR response to submaximal exercise.

Based on Grover et al. 1967.

KEY POINT

In conditions of high heat and humidity, the exerciser should decrease the work rate to stay in the THR zone. Exercisers should acclimatize to heat over 7 to 14 days to reduce the risk of heat injury. Advise participants to drink water before, during, and after exercise and to exercise in the early morning to reduce environmental heat load. When exercising in cold weather, participants should wear clothing in layers and remove layers to minimize sweating and to stay dry. Participants should become aware of the AQI readings in their communities and avoid exercising at times and in places in which air pollution is a problem. When exercising at altitude, participants should decrease work intensity to stay in the THR zone.

LEARNING AIDS

REVIEW QUESTIONS

1. What do the terms *intensity*, *frequency*, and *duration* mean in describing the dose of physical activity?
2. How might you calulate the volume or amount of physical activity done in a week?
3. Explain the principle of overload.
4. What is the public health recommendation for physical activity for both moderate and vigorous intensities?
5. What is the range of exercise intensities, in %HRR, associated with increasing CRF? Where does moderate-intensity physical activity fit in that range?
6. What is the optimal range of exercise intensities associated with increasing CRF for most people who are cleared to participate in a structured exercise program?
7. What %HRmax values would you use to match the intensities in question 6?
8. What does *progression* mean when it comes to helping a person become physically active?
9. What should clients learn to check to help maintain the optimal relative intensity when the environmental temperature and relative humidity are elevated?
10. What is the air quality index (AQI), and how could you obtain information about air quality in your own community?

CASE STUDIES

In the first two case studies, you are given general information about a client, data on risk factors, and the results of an exercise test. Analyze each case, delineate the risk factors, and react to the person's responses to the test (whether normal or not). Then, on the basis of your analysis, make some recommendations for the client regarding an exercise program and risk-factor reduction program.

1. Paul, a Caucasian male, is 36 yr old, weighs 88 kg, is 178 cm tall, and has 28% body fat. Blood chemistry values indicate that his total cholesterol is 270 $mg \cdot dl^{-1}$ and HDL-C is 38 $mg \cdot dl^{-1}$. His mother died of a heart attack at the age of 63, and his father had a heart attack at the age of 68. He is sedentary and has engaged in no endurance training since college. The following are the results of a maximal GXT conducted by his physician.

Test: Balke, 3 mi · hr^{-1} (4.8 km · hr^{-1}); 2.5% Every 2 Min

% Grade	METs	SBP (mmHg)	DBP (mmHg)	HR (beats · min^{-1})	ECG	Symptoms
	Rest	126	88	70	Normal	—
2.5	4.3	142	86	142	Normal	—
5.0	5.4	184	88	150	Normal	—
7.5	6.4	162	86	160	Normal	—
10.0	7.4	174	84	168	Normal	—
12.5	8.5	186	84	176	Normal	—
15.0	9.5	194	84	190	Normal	Calf tight
17.5	10.5	198	84	198	Normal	Fatigue

2. Mary is a 38-yr-old Hispanic American female and is 170 cm tall, weighs 61.4 kg, and has 30% body fat. Blood chemistry values indicate a total cholesterol of 188 mg · dl^{-1} and an HDL-C of 59 mg · dl^{-1}. Her resting BP is 124/80 mmHg. Family history indicates that her father had a nonfatal heart attack at the age of 67. She has smoked one pack of cigarettes per day for the past 13 yr, and her lifestyle is sedentary. The table below is the result of her submaximal cycle ergometer test.

Test: YMCA Cycle Test

Work rate (kpm · min^{-1})	HR (min 2)	HR (min 3)
150	118	120
300	134	136

Pedal rate = 50 rev · min^{-1}; predicted HRmax = 182 beats · min^{-1}; seat height = 6; and 85% HRmax = 155 beats · min^{-1}.

3. You are asked to make a presentation to a group of sedentary faculty members at your school on how to begin a physical activity program to accrue the health-related benefits discussed in this chapter. What guidance would you provide to help them achieve their goals? Discuss the kind of general screening that you would recommend (that they could do at the meeting) and how you would instruct them to begin the program (specify the frequency, intensity, and time) that ultimately leads to the goal of 150 min of moderate-intensity physical activity per wk. You may assume that everyone can walk without pain.

Answers to Case Studies

1. If a person has a normal response to a GXT, HR and SBP increase with each stage of the test, whereas the DBP remains the same or decreases slightly. In addition, the ECG shows no significant ST segment depression or elevation and no significant arrhythmias. In these cases it can be assumed that the last load achieved on the test represents the true functional capacity (max METs). The GXT presented in this case study is representative of such a test.

   Paul has normal resting BP and a negative family history for CHD. Risk factors include a relatively high percentage of body fat, a sedentary lifestyle, and a poor blood lipid profile. Based on these findings, a THR range of 158 to 177 beats · min^{-1} was calculated (60%-80% $\dot{V}O_2$max as measured during the maximal GXT); this HR range corresponds to work rates equal to 6.3 to 8.4 METs. Initially, he will work below the lower end of the calculated THR range, with the emphasis on the duration of activity. As he becomes more active, he will be able to work within the THR range, depending, of course, on his interests. He was referred for nutritional counseling to improve his blood lipid profile. Paul has an estimated HRmax of 174 beats · min^{-1}; his measured HR was 24 beats · min^{-1} higher. Given the inherent biological variation in the estimated HRmax, use the measured values when they are available.

2. Mary's maximal work rate was estimated to be 750 kpm · min^{-1} by extrapolating the relationship between HR and work rate to the predicted maximal HR (see chapter 7). This is equivalent to a $\dot{V}O_2max$ of 29 ml · kg^{-1} · min^{-1}, or 8.3 METs.

   Her blood chemistry values and BP are normal. Her family history is negative for CHD. Her HR response to the test is normal and indicates poor CRF. Her maximal aerobic power is related to the sedentary lifestyle, the cigarette smoking (carbon monoxide), and the 30% body fat. She was encouraged to participate in a smoking-cessation program and was given the names of two local professional groups.

   The recommended exercise program emphasized beginning at or below the low end of the THR zone (70% HRmax: 127 beats · min^{-1}) with long duration. She preferred a walking program because of the freedom it gave her schedule; this is consistent with moderate-intensity physical activity. She was given the walking program in this chapter and was asked to record her HR response to each of the exercise sessions.

   A body-fat goal of 22% resulted in a target body weight of 121 lb (55 kg). She did not feel the need for dietary counseling at this time, but she agreed to record her food intake for 10 days to determine the patterns of eating behavior that would be beneficial to change (see chapters 5, 12, 18, and 23). She made an appointment with the fitness professional in 2 wk to discuss the progress with her program.

3. You might begin by talking about the importance of regular physical activity in reducing the risk of numerous chronic diseases. In addition, you could indicate that the risk associated with regular participation in moderate-intensity physical activity is very low. Have them complete one of the simple health screening questionnaires in chapter 2 to help them determine whether or not they should see their physician before beginning a physical activity program. Next, you might recommend a walking program that begins with short (e.g., 10 min) bouts of activity done at a comfortable pace each day. Encourage them to gradually increase the number of 10 min bouts per day until they can do a single 30 min walk each day. On the other hand, if some wanted to continue to do 10 min bouts because it fit their schedules, that would be fine. Finally, you might suggest that their weekly goal be at least 150 min of walking, but more is better relative to health benefits derived.

12

Exercise Prescription for Weight Management

Dixie L. Thompson

OBJECTIVES

The reader will be able to do the following:

1. Identify factors that contribute to obesity.
2. Describe the role that energy balance plays in weight loss and weight maintenance.
3. Provide guidelines for caloric intake to facilitate appropriate weight loss.
4. Discuss the role of exercise in weight loss and weight maintenance.
5. Prescribe safe and effective exercise programs for weight management.
6. Describe strategies for behavioral change for weight control.
7. List reasons to avoid quick-fix weight-loss techniques.
8. Recognize signs of eating disorders.
9. Provide healthy guidelines for gaining weight.

Americans spend billions of dollars each year on weight loss. The weight-loss industry provides a broad spectrum of goods and services, including over-the-counter and prescription drugs, motivational and educational books, weight-loss clinics, and online support for weight loss. Weight-loss support groups have sprung up in many environments, including schools, health clinics, and churches. Despite this multibillion-dollar industry, U.S. obesity prevalence is at an all-time high. Recent evidence shows that just over 68% of American adults are classified as either overweight or obese (35). Unfortunately, this same trend is found among U.S. children (38). Although many Americans lose the fight against obesity, many successfully lose excess weight, and some manage to maintain a healthy weight throughout their lives. The lessons from these people provide a road map for successful weight control (18, 47).

Increasing Prevalence of Obesity in the United States

In the early 1960s, 13.4% of American adults were obese (i.e., had a BMI $\geq$30 kg · m^{-2}) (10). Recent national statistics (from 2011-2012) revealed that obesity has soared to 34.9% (35). Figure 12.1 shows the increasing prevalence of obesity during the past five decades for both men and women. Some segments of the population have even more dramatic values. For example, obesity prevalence for non-Hispanic black women is currently 56.6%, and 16.4% of this group are classified with grade 3 obesity (35). Because of the rapid changes in obesity prevalence in the past few decades, this trend does not appear to be causally linked to genetics. As discussed later, lifestyle changes seem to be the major culprit.

Adults commonly accumulate additional adipose tissue as they age. This gradual accumulation of fat is sometimes called **creeping obesity**. Part of this change in body composition is attributable to a natural loss of muscle caused by aging. A decreasing metabolic rate, a more sedentary lifestyle, and unadjusted eating patterns, however, appear to be the most important factors in this increased body fat (8). Although some fat accumulation is acceptable (see chapter 8, table 8.1), when BMI climbs to obese levels, negative health consequences follow (33, 34).

KEY POINT

Although Americans spend billions of dollars each year on weight loss, the prevalence of obesity is high, with nearly 35% of adults classified as obese. Over two-thirds of adults are overweight or obese. People tend to accumulate fat as they age, but excessive fat accumulation is unhealthy.

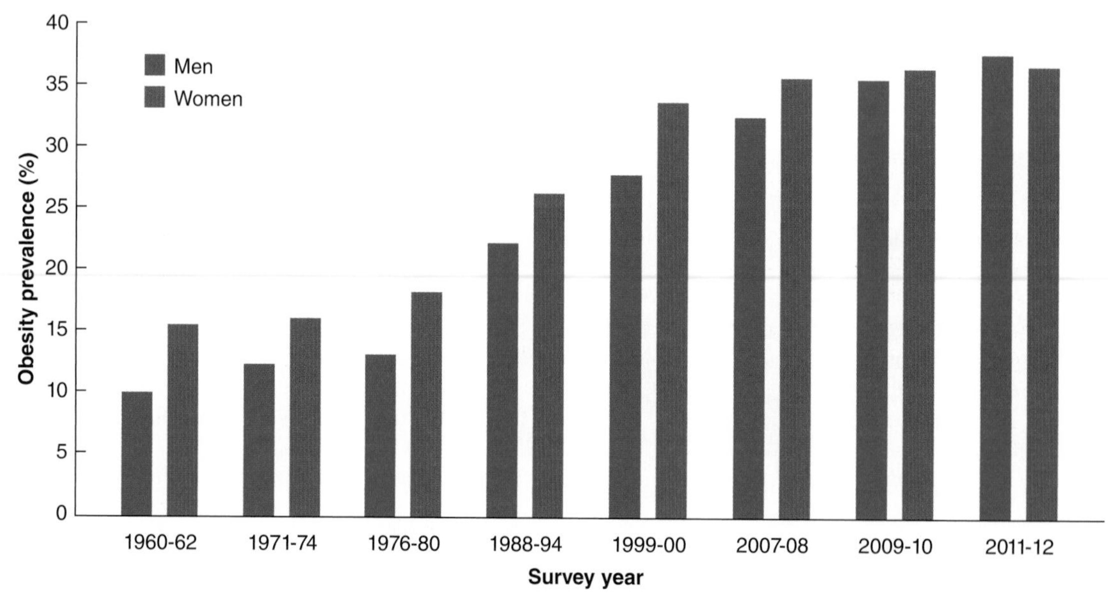

FIGURE 12.1 Prevalence of obesity among American adults.
Data from Flegal et al. 2012; Flegal et al. 2010; Flegal et al. 2002; Ogden et al. 2014

Etiology of Obesity

The cause of obesity cannot be described simply, because many factors contribute to its development. Ultimately, **positive caloric balance** (i.e., taking in more calories than are expended) leads to obesity. Factors contributing to obesity can be discussed under two broad categories: genetics and lifestyle.

Genetics

Although estimates vary based on study design, evidence generally suggests that inheritance contributes 30% to 70% of the interindividual variation in obesity (28). In evaluating the genetic influence on obesity, researchers have attempted to differentiate among factors that are genetic and sociocultural. Bouchard and colleagues (7) estimate that approximately 25% of the variance in percent body fat is attributable to genetics. Interestingly, these authors found that inheritance has a larger effect on total fat and deep deposits of adipose tissue than on subcutaneous fat. Additional evidence on the importance of genetics comes from data demonstrating that the BMI of adopted children is more similar to that of their biological parents than to that of their adoptive parents (39). The recent discoveries of genes linked with obesity provide additional evidence that genetic factors help determine the likelihood of being obese and developing diseases that accompany obesity (e.g., type 2 diabetes) (41). Research continues in an attempt to understand the link between genetics and obesity. See chapter 20 for more information.

Many genes are linked with obesity, and recently 97 new loci in the human genome were shown to be associated with BMI (29). The expression of each gene depends on environmental factors (e.g., availability of fatty foods, social influences); therefore, the genetics of obesity is complex and much is yet to be learned (6, 28). A negative consequence of our growing knowledge of the genetic link to obesity is that people with many overweight family members may become discouraged and believe that they can do nothing about their weight status. Although genetics can contribute to the development of obesity, a primary reason that people become obese is lifestyle. Loos and Bouchard (30) suggest that only a small percentage of individuals have true genetic obesity that would be present regardless of the environment. These authors suggest that the majority of people who develop obesity in modern Western societies (an environment where high-calorie food is abundant and physical activity is not a part of everyday life) might be normal weight or at worst overweight in a less obesogenic environment (28). Fitness professionals must emphasize to clients that genetics may predispose certain people to obesity, but those people still have a great capacity to affect their body weight.

Lifestyle

The choices people make about energy expenditure and caloric intake predominantly influence the development of obesity. The number of calories consumed, the types of foods eaten, and the amount of daily activity all affect body weight. If more calories are consumed than are expended, the positive caloric balance results in weight (fat) gain. To lose fat weight, a **negative caloric balance** must be established. This balance can be achieved by decreasing caloric intake, increasing caloric expenditure, or both. National data comparing 1971 with 2000 show that the American daily calorie intake increased by 168 kcal · day^{-1} for men and 335 kcal · day^{-1} for women (48), and daily physical activity rates during these same years did not increase to offset the change in energy intake. Thus the typical American today weighs just over 24 lb (18 kg) more than the typical American of 40 years ago (36). During the early part of the 21st century, caloric intake has remained steady (49). Likewise, obesity prevalence appears to have leveled off at around 34% (35). In recent examinations of national trends in caloric intake, it appears that there may be a slight decrease (<100 kcal · day^{-1}) in caloric intake (15).

Food Intake

When excess calories (particularly fat calories) are consumed, the energy is stored as fat. From an evolutionary standpoint, fat storage is a positive adaptation to variations in food availability. In other words, fat accumulation occurs during times of plenty, and this stored energy is used when food supplies are low. In populations that have a constant abundance of food with high caloric density, this mechanism often results in excessive fat accumulation.

Health professionals sometimes question whether individuals who are obese typically consume more calories than their counterparts who are average weight. Dietary-recall stud ies provide little clear information about this issue because people tend to underreport dietary intake and overestimate physical activity (27). Some research suggests that subjects who are obese particularly underreport consumption of high-fat and snack foods (45). Highly advanced research procedures in which people ingest isotopes of oxygen and hydrogen (doubly labeled water) indicate that individuals who are overweight expend and consume more calories than people of normal weight (44). The higher energy expenditure is caused by the metabolic cost of supporting excess body weight. The reason extra calories are consumed is not known and is likely related to a variety of complex factors.

Types of Food Eaten and Obesity

When fat is consumed, it is stored as adipose tissue more readily than is either protein or carbohydrate. From a theoretical perspective, the low thermic effect of fat (i.e., the energy needed to digest, absorb, transport, and store fat), the ease with which fat is stored as adipose tissue, and the high caloric density of high-fat foods make fat a likely culprit in the development of obesity. National data indicate that since the 1970s, the percentage of calories from fat in the typical American diet has gone down and the percentage of calories from carbohydrate has increased (15). However, since the total energy intake has increased, the actual number of calories from fat intake has changed very little.

Several studies indicate that people who are obese and overweight tend to consume a higher percentage of calories from fat than people of normal weight consume (45). However, it appears that the availability of foods high in fat and simple sugar puts people at higher risk for obesity. Recent evidence suggests that it might actually be the increase in carbohydrate, not fat, that is most closely associated with obesity (37).

Daily Energy Expenditure

Researchers have found a relationship between low physical activity and an increased likelihood of obesity (2, 25). Amish adults who live an active life that is similar to what was typical in the late 19th century have much lower rates of obesity compared with the average American (5). Additionally, women who walk more daily have a lower BMI, WC, and body-fat percentage compared with women who are less active (20, 24, 40). Because these are cross-sectional studies, it is impossible to say whether low physical activity leads to obesity or obesity causes people to reduce their activity levels. The longitudinal CARDIA study has shown that adults who maintain active lifestyles over a 20-yr period gain significantly less weight and add fewer inches to their waists (17).

The role of regular exercise in weight loss is complex and has been reviewed by several authors (2, 16, 34). Increased physical activity helps create a negative caloric balance, and in combination with dietary restriction, it can lead to weight loss (2). Although exercise without dietary restriction typically does not lead to major weight reduction, the long-term positive effects of physical activity on weight maintenance are clear (2). Exercise is a strong predictor of long-term weight maintenance (2, 26, 46, 47). Additionally, regular physical activity attenuates age-related weight gain (10, 17).

KEY POINT

Both genetics and lifestyle contribute to obesity. Caloric intake, food choices, and daily physical activity are all aspects of lifestyle that affect fat accumulation. A positive caloric balance results in weight gain; a negative caloric balance results in weight loss. Exercise is an important factor in prevention of weight gain and in weight management following weight loss.

Maintaining a Healthy Weight

Numerous methods can be used to maintain a healthy weight or to lose weight when necessary. Fitness professionals should encourage clients to choose weight maintenance or weight-loss techniques that are effective yet pose little threat to overall health. The following sections outline practices that most adults can implement safely.

Assessing Daily Caloric Need

Whether planning individualized programs for weight loss or weight maintenance, it is helpful to know the number of calories the client needs to sustain her current body weight. You can gain this knowledge by estimating daily caloric need. **Daily caloric need** is the number of calories a person needs to sustain current body weight, assuming that activity levels remain constant. The resting metabolic rate, **thermic effect of food**, and energy expended by daily activities determine the daily caloric need (figure 12.2).

Resting metabolic rate (RMR) is the number of calories expended to maintain the body during resting conditions. For most people, RMR is 60% to 70% of their daily caloric need. For people who engage in regular, vigorous exercise, the RMR may account for a smaller proportion of daily caloric need because the energy requirements of exercise account for a larger percentage. RMR can be measured in a laboratory using indirect calorimetry. To accurately measure RMR, assess the client when he has not eaten for several hours, has not exercised vigorously for the past 12 hr, and has been in a resting, reclined position for 30 min (31). Because of the cost of indirect calorimetry and the strict control needed to obtain accurate results, measuring RMR is not always practical; therefore, a number of equa-

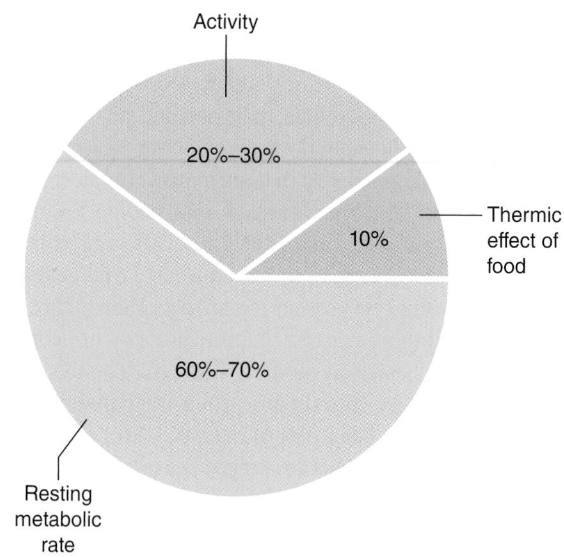

FIGURE 12.2 Contributors to daily caloric need.

tions have been developed to predict RMR. These RMR equations are based on the following principles:

- RMR is proportional to body size.
- RMR decreases with age.
- Muscle is more metabolically active than fat.

The larger the body, the more calories needed to sustain it. This relationship is reflected in all RMR equations. In addition to body size, age significantly affects RMR. As a person ages, RMR decreases, meaning that the daily caloric need decreases with age. Generally, RMR equations are sex-specific because males often have more fat-free mass than females have and fat-free mass requires more energy compared with fat tissue.

If a client's fat-free mass is known, the following equation can be used to predict RMR (9). There is no need for sex-specific equations when fat-free mass is known, because a gram of muscle has the same metabolic need whether it resides in a male or female body.

$$\text{RMR (kcal} \cdot \text{day}^{-1}) = 370 + (21.6 \cdot \text{fat-free mass in kg}).$$

When determining daily caloric need, an estimate of the calories burned in physical activity is needed. This assessment requires information about work and leisure activity. Although there are numerous ways to gather information about daily activity, one typical method is an activity log in which the client records work and leisure activity. Once the activity pattern is established, the caloric cost of various activities can be calculated (see chapter 6) and used to estimate the energy burned in activity. Estimating this energy is especially important if working with a client who trains extensively. Alternatively, you can estimate daily caloric need by using the methods outlined in *Calculating Daily Energy Needs*.

The smallest part of the daily caloric need comes from the thermic effect of food. This is the energy needed to digest, absorb, transport, and store the food that is eaten. Although this value may vary slightly depending on the food eaten, the thermic effect of food typically accounts for 10% of the daily caloric need (32).

Changing Lifestyle to Promote a Healthy Weight

Although each individual must assess which areas of her lifestyle contribute to excessive weight accumulation, common steps that benefit the majority of people who are attempting to lose weight include the following:

- Reduce total calories.
- Reduce fat and carbohydrate (particularly simple sugar) intake.
- Increase physical activity.
- Adopt healthy eating behaviors.

As previously mentioned, a negative caloric balance must be established for weight loss. The number of calories consumed while attempting to lose weight should be determined by the client's health, caloric need, and ultimate weight-loss goals. Most healthy adults who need to lose weight can institute a short-term low-calorie diet (LCD) consisting of 800 to 1,500 kcal $\cdot$ day^{-1} without major adverse consequences. Very-low-calorie diets (VLCDs)

Calculating Daily Energy Needs

The IOM (14) recommends the following equations for calculating a person's daily caloric need, or estimated energy requirement (EER). These formulas require the client's age in years, height in meters, weight in kilograms, and level of physical activity.

Adult Man

$$\text{EER} = 662 - 9.53(\text{age}) + \text{PA}\ [15.91(\text{weight}) + 539.6(\text{height})].$$

Adult Woman

$$\text{EER} = 354 - 6.91(\text{age}) + \text{PA}\ [9.36(\text{weight}) + 726(\text{height})].$$

PA reflects a person's level of daily physical activity. Use the following table to choose the appropriate PA value.

Activity Level	PA Value (Men)	PA Value (Women)
Sedentary—extremely limited activity	1.0	1.0
Low active—typical ADLs only	1.11	1.12
Active—regular moderate physical activity	1.25	1.27
Very active—regular vigorous exercise	1.45	1.45

consisting of <800 kcal · day^{-1} are sometimes used in specialized settings to treat individuals with extreme obesity (22). In these cases, physicians and dietitians provide patient oversight (22). VLCDs can lead to substantial weight loss, and years of study with this approach have yielded carefully monitored protocols with few negative side effects (42).

ACSM recommends that weekly weight-loss goals should target a loss of 1 to 2 lb or 0.5 to 0.9 kg (1). A general guideline is to establish a caloric deficit of 3,500 to 7,000 kcal · wk^{-1} (500-1,000 kcal · day^{-1}), which theoretically results in a 1 to 2 lb loss (0.5 to 0.9 kg) of fat each week (1 lb of fat = 3,500 kcal). ACSM also recommends that people restricting their caloric intake limit their fat intake to less than 30% of total calories (1). These are general recommendations, and people with special needs (e.g., athletes, older adults, people with metabolic disorders) may require a different approach to weight loss. Caloric restriction can lead to decreased RMR and fat-free mass. The decrease in RMR and loss of fat-free mass will be greater in dieters with large daily caloric deficits (34).

Exercise Prescription for Weight Management and Weight Loss

ACSM recommends a combined approach of exercise and moderate caloric restriction for people attempting weight loss (1, 2). Although debate continues over the precise contribution of exercise to weight management, a combination of exercise and moderate calorie restriction appears to be most effective in maintaining lean mass and avoiding excessive decreases in RMR. Existing data clearly demonstrate that people who are successful in maintaining weight loss engage in regular aerobic activity (47). Studies also show that regular exercise helps prevent weight gain (10, 17, 21). From a theoretical perspective, adding exercise to everyday life can significantly alter body weight. For example, expending just 100 kcal · day^{-1} beyond daily caloric need for a year creates a caloric deficit of 36,500 kcal. ACSM recommends that individuals engage in a minimum of 150 min of moderate-intensity exercise per wk and further states that additional exercise (200-300 min per wk) is more likely to be associated with successful weight control (1, 2). The following are specific recommendations for weight management and weight loss with exercise (1):

- Frequency: ≥5 days per wk.
- Intensity: Begin with moderate intensity (40%-60% HRR), eventually progressing to higher intensity (≥60% HRR).
- Time: Begin with short, easily tolerated bouts preferably totaling 30 min per day. Progress to 60 min per day. Multiple daily bouts can be used with bout duration of 10 min or longer.
- Type: Aerobic exercise targeting large muscle groups. Resistance and flexibility exercise is recommended as a supplement to aerobic activity.

In addition to the physical benefits, psychological variables improve with exercise. Improvements in self-esteem and self-efficacy are commonly reported outcomes of regular exercise. The empowerment that comes from becoming more fit can add to the resolve to live a healthy lifestyle and maintain a healthy weight.

KEY POINT

Daily caloric need is determined by RMR, the thermic effect of food, and activity levels. Reducing total calories, decreasing fat intake, increasing physical activity, and adopting healthy eating behaviors are some common steps that will benefit many people who are attempting to lose weight. The exercise prescription for weight management should involve weekly aerobic activity of at least 150 min. When weight reduction is needed, most healthy adults can safely initiate weight-loss goals of 1 to 2 lb (0.5 to 0.9 kg) per wk.

Behavior Modification for Weight Loss and Maintenance

The majority of attempts to lose weight and maintain long-term weight loss are unsuccessful. However, even a 3% to 5% sustained weight loss can provide important reductions in CVD risk factors (22). Behavior modification (changes in lifestyle habits) is an important component of successful weight-loss and maintenance programs (22, 34). A recent guideline issued by the AHA, the American College of Cardiology (ACC), and the Obesity Society emphasizes the importance of a comprehensive lifestyle intervention in the treatment of obesity (22). For additional information on behavior modification, see chapter 23.

When people are committed to changing eating and activity patterns, a number of strategies can improve the chances of long-term success. During the initial phase of weight loss (the action stage; see chapter 23), implementing these strategies requires a great deal of effort and there is a significant chance of failure (i.e., relapse). After 6 mo or more of using these strategies (the maintenance stage; see chapter 23), changes in diet and lifestyle become more natural. Some strategies effective for losing weight and maintaining weight loss are discussed next. Not every person responds well to the same techniques, so clients should be considered separately and an individualized plan developed for each.

Keeping Records

Before implementing a weight-loss or maintenance program, it is wise to examine current eating patterns. This is most easily done with an eating diary or food log. A sample food log is provided in chapter 5. Remember, it is important to gather information about the types and quantities of food eaten as well as the social and emotional circumstances surrounding eating.

Careful record keeping accomplishes several objectives. First, food logs document the problem areas of food intake. Many people are unaware of the total calories or the amount of fat they consume daily. Second, eating diaries document the social and emotional cues to eating. After keeping records for a while, individuals begin to recognize the factors other than hunger that lead to eating (e.g., socializing with friends, watching television, feeling stressed). To combat these cues to eating, the social and emotional situations that trigger overeating must be recognized and strategies developed to overcome them. Third, recording food intake makes eating a cognitive process. For many people, eating is a habit, and they automatically choose how much and what to eat without conscious consideration. As discussed next, planning appropriate meals and snacks is an important component of successful weight loss.

Planning Meals and Snacks

Weight loss does not occur by accident; it takes a concerted effort. Purchasing appropriate foods and planning meals are imperative for success. One of the most helpful practices in controlling food intake is not purchasing high-fat and calorie-dense food. Substituting low-calorie and low-fat foods for high-calorie and high-fat foods also can substantially affect weight loss. For example, substituting a cup (8 fl oz, or 237 ml) of 1% milk for a cup of whole milk decreases caloric intake by approximately 50 kcal. If a person drinks 2 cups of milk per day, this substitution will reduce caloric intake by 36,500 kcal in 1 yr!

Meal planning is also essential. In busy households, planning healthy meals often becomes a low priority, and this can lead to meals that are easy to prepare but do not promote health or weight control. One technique for overcoming time constraints is buying breakfast foods that are quick to prepare yet are nutritious and relatively low in calories (e.g., fresh fruit, low-fat yogurt, whole-grain cereals). These foods provide a morning meal that offsets hunger and includes important nutrients.

Because many Americans are not at home for the noon meal, they often eat at restaurants that are convenient, affordable, and quick, including fast-food restaurants. Although several fast-food chains have added healthier items to their menus, the majority of fast food is high in both fat and calories. Individuals who choose to eat fast food are less successful at maintaining weight loss compared with those who avoid these food choices (19). Planning ahead might allow some people to carry their lunch to work and ensure that they can choose from a variety of healthy foods for this important meal.

The evening meal contributes a significant percentage of the daily caloric intake of many Americans. It is not uncommon for people who have limited their food intake during the day to overindulge at night. Because of the effort required to cook a meal, many people eat at restaurants or purchase packaged meals that tend to be high in fat and calories. The effort necessary for cooking nutritious meals can be reduced by doing the following:

- Cook and store meals ahead of time.
- Find a variety of low-calorie meals that are quick and easy to prepare.
- Purchase food ahead of time to avoid unnecessary shopping.
- Keep a variety of fresh vegetables on hand.

It is also important to consider the foods available for snacks. Although avoiding food between meals may be ideal for some, there are times when snacks are necessary. Foods that are nutritious and also low in calories are the best choices (e.g., fresh fruit, raw vegetables, low-fat yogurt).

Establishing a Support System

Studies have shown the benefit of having a support system when trying to lose weight (34). The source of the support, however, will vary depending on the client. A support system may be a friend, significant other, parent, coworker, therapist, or support group. Fitness professionals should encourage clients in a weight-loss or maintenance program to seek out other people to encourage them in their efforts. For some people, the reasons for overeating are emotional and deeply rooted. In these cases, a trained therapist may be needed.

A lot of people are encouraged by supporting others who also are attempting to lose weight. Many commercial weight-loss centers provide support groups, which serve several functions: They provide a group to whom participants are accountable, a setting in which helpful hints and success stories can be shared, and a nonthreatening environment where all of the participants are pursuing the same objective. In addition, Internet support groups are gaining popularity. Some of these services are free and others charge a membership fee. Consumers should seek out Internet services that meet their needs.

Committing to Behavioral and Outcome-Oriented Goals

Clients must develop goals that encourage healthy eating. Goal setting is important to help individuals remain focused on weight loss or weight maintenance. It should be a mutual exchange between the fitness professional and the client. The fitness professional provides information about healthy weight-loss or management practices, and the client identifies the behavioral goals to which she is willing to commit.

Typically, weight loss is outcome oriented (i.e., the end result is the measure of success). Weight-loss goals should be reasonable for the client and should follow the guidelines listed previously in this chapter. In contrast to outcome goals, behavioral goals focus on the process of weight loss, not the final outcome. Behavioral goals can help the client make behavior and lifestyle changes that will affect weight loss or maintenance. These goals may target altering eating patterns, making wise food choices, and increasing daily energy expenditure. An example of a behavioral goal is, "I will walk the stairs to my office daily rather than riding the elevator." More specific information on goal setting can be found in chapter 23.

Designing a Reward System

Part of human nature is the desire to be rewarded for accomplishing goals. When designing a weight-loss or maintenance program, it is wise to provide motivation by rewarding success. As with goal setting, it is vital that the client be involved in developing the rewards that will be used. One rule that fitness professionals should encourage, however, is to avoid using food as a reward. The reward program should recognize the achievement of both outcome-oriented and behavioral goals. This is important because attaining an outcome goal may take much longer than it may take to change certain behaviors. Also, there will be times when a person's weight plateaus; behavioral goals should be rewarded during these times. Here are some examples of rewards:

- Purchasing new clothes
- Purchasing hobby items (e.g., books, music, tools)
- Taking a trip
- Attending special events (e.g., movies, concerts, lectures)

Avoiding Self-Defeating Behaviors

Certain situations increase the likelihood of overeating. A client trying to lose weight needs to acknowledge these situations and institute measures to minimize the chance of succumbing to self-defeating behaviors. For example, a person who snacks on high-calorie foods late at night might avoid purchasing such foods and also implement a behavioral objective of not eating after 7:00 p.m. A person who loves pizza but tends to overindulge when going out to a restaurant might make pizza at home using low-fat ingredients and vegetables as toppings.

There are special times (e.g., birthdays, holiday dinners) when people will want to eat foods that are not a part of their weight management plan. Fitness professionals should emphasize to clients that a lapse in eating (or activity) should not mean an end to the weight management plan. Clients should be encouraged to immediately return to their healthy eating and exercise plan after the lapse. Fitness professionals might help clients who feel guilty by suggesting they view the lapse not as a failure but as an opportunity for renewing the commitment to weight loss or maintenance.

Combining Moderate Caloric Restriction and Aerobic Exercise

Regular exercise is an important facet of successful weight loss and weight maintenance. As mentioned, ACSM (1, 2) and the National Institutes of Health (NIH) (34) support the use of exercise for weight loss and maintenance. The majority of weight-loss studies that compare diet with diet plus exercise show that the combined approach leads to greater weight loss (34). The standard aerobic activity recommendation of at least 150 min per wk should be considered a minimum for people attempting to lose or maintain weight (1, 2). Progressing to 200 to 300 min per wk is likely to provide additional assistance with weight control. See previous comments in this chapter and also chapter 20 for more information on exercise prescription for weight loss or weight maintenance.

Changing Unhealthy Eating Patterns

Specific eating patterns have been linked with excessive weight gain (8). Being aware of these behaviors and implementing plans to avoid them increases the likelihood of successful weight management. The following changes in eating patterns are recommended:

- Slow down.
- Make wise substitutions.
- Consume a variety of nutritious foods.
- Eat smaller and fewer portions.

People often eat rapidly and then feel uncomfortably full for several minutes after they finish eating. When food is eaten rapidly, inadequate time is allowed for the satiety mechanisms to help curb hunger. This results in people overeating before they realize that they are no longer hungry. To help slow their eating, people can put down eating utensils between bites, pause at least 30 sec between bites, and chew food completely and swallow before taking another bite (8).

Substituting foods that contain less fat and calories for foods that are high in fat and calories can significantly reduce caloric intake. For example, a person who eats a roasted chicken breast without the skin instead of a fried chicken breast with the skin will save approximately 160 kcal. The wise consumer looks closely at the total calories in a food as well as the calories that are contributed by fat. Reducing fat intake not only helps with weight control but also may help improve the blood lipid profile.

One problem that people face when trying to manage weight is diet burnout. It is not uncommon to find dieters who consume only certain foods. To avoid becoming bored and frustrated with a diet, it is important to consume a variety of healthy, low-calorie, and tasty foods. This objective is linked to the planning process. Maintaining variety in the diet not only helps avoid boredom but also provides nutritional balance.

When attempting to lose weight, one of the most helpful changes is to decrease the portion size as well as the number of portions consumed. Many people habitually fill their plates and eat everything on the plate. Also, social norms can contribute to the struggle to control weight. For example, Americans may demonstrate to their hosts that they enjoy the provided food by eating extra portions. Taking smaller portions of foods as well as avoiding second helpings can contribute significantly to caloric restriction.

Committing to Lifelong Maintenance

Weight loss is only temporary unless a plan is in place to maintain the loss. In examining the variables that predict success in maintaining weight loss, Lavery and Loewy (26) concluded, "There are no quick-fix, easy solutions to obesity. The solution is the harsh realization of the need for permanent lifestyle changes to maintain a desired weight status." Fitness professionals should help clients understand the need to commit to long-term lifestyle changes rather than focus solely on short-term weight-loss goals. It is encouraging, however, to learn that long-term maintenance of weight loss is much more likely once people have kept the weight off for 2 to 5 yr (47).

KEY POINT

Some strategies for successful weight management are keeping records, planning meals and snacks, developing a support system, designing a reward system, committing to both outcome-oriented and behavioral goals, avoiding self-defeating behaviors, combining moderate caloric restriction with aerobic exercise, changing unhealthy eating patterns, and committing to lifelong weight maintenance.

Gimmicks and Gadgets for Weight Loss

Over the years numerous devices have been marketed for weight loss. The majority of these devices are ineffective, and, unfortunately, some are potentially harmful.

Saunas and sweat suits have sometimes been recommended to help weight loss by burning off or melting away fat, but this is a false claim. These devices may induce short-term (i.e., a few hours) loss of weight by dehydration. They do not burn fat but can cause people to sweat profusely. Overusing saunas and sweat suits can lead to severe dehydration. Further, the warmer core temperature that is caused by these devices could harm fetuses during the first trimester of pregnancy.

Other devices such as vibrating belts, body wraps, and electrical stimulators have been used in attempted weight loss. Although these devices may not be harmful, the scientific evidence does not support their weight-loss claims. The money spent on these devices would be better spent on proven techniques. Additionally, people who put faith and effort into these unproven techniques may delay making lifestyle changes that lead to long-term weight loss and maintenance.

A widely held myth is that exercise emphasizing a particular body part will cause that area to lose fat faster than the rest of the body uses it. This false theory is called **spot reduction**. People commonly perform sit-ups or curl-ups in an attempt to decrease their waistlines. Although these are terrific exercises for increasing the strength and endurance of the abdominal muscles, they are not very effective for burning fat. As a person establishes a caloric deficit through regular aerobic exercise, fat loss occurs all over the body, not just at the parts he would like to see decrease.

Programs that advertise rapid, large weight losses are typically deceptive. The rapid weight losses at the beginning of such programs primarily result from lost water weight. Also, dietary plans that establish extremely large caloric deficits substantially reduce RMR and lean body mass and do not establish healthy, lifelong eating habits. As stated earlier, diets consisting of fewer than 800 kcal · day^{-1} are not generally recommended (22, 34). Information about fad diets is highlighted in the sidebar *Focus on Fad Diets*.

Disordered Eating Patterns

Certain conditions exist in which an eating pattern can have a serious negative effect on health. **Eating disorders** are clinically diagnosed conditions in which the unhealthy eating patterns may lead to severe declines in health and even to death. **Anorexia nervosa**, **bulimia nervosa**, and **binge-eating disorder** are three of the eating disorders recognized by the American Psychiatric Association (APA)

Focus on Fad Diets

Diet plans that promise incredible results can be found easily on bookshelves, in advertisements, and on the Internet. Many people are looking for quick, easy ways to lose weight, and entrepreneurs are eager to supply them. No one description summarizes all fad diets. Many focus on eating one food or food group, whereas others emphasize avoiding certain foods. Most of these plans are low in calories and may result in weight loss. However, these diets often do not emphasize a balanced diet with an adequate supply of essential nutrients. Over time, these nutritional deficiencies have the potential to lead to serious health consequences. Because of this potential for negative health consequences, the AHA has declared war on fad diets.

Another problem with these diets is that they do not lead to lifestyle changes that result in permanent weight loss. Many people follow these diets for a brief time and then regain their excess weight when they return to their previous pattern of overconsuming calories. These diets typically focus on food rather than on behavior change (e.g., increasing physical activity, using food substitution). For more information on making healthy diet choices, see the websites of the Academy of Nutrition and Dietetics (www.eatright.org), USDA (www.choosemyplate.gov), and National Institute of Diabetes and Digestive and Kidney Diseases (NIDDK; www.niddk.nih.gov).

(4). **Disordered eating** refers to subclinical, unhealthy eating patterns that are often the precursors of eating disorders.

In the United States, anorexia nervosa occurs at a rate of 0.5% to 1%, and bulimia nervosa occurs at a rate of 2% to 4% (22). No single mechanism has been identified as the primary cause of disordered eating or eating disorders. It appears that genetic, psychological, and sociocultural factors may predispose a person to these conditions. In the United States, these conditions are most common in young women from middle and high socioeconomic environments and in female athletes in sports that emphasize extreme leanness. It is hypothesized that the social pressure to be thin as well as discomfort with sexual development contribute to unhealthy eating patterns in young women. For female athletes, the pressure to perform in some sports is linked with extremely low body weights. For example, it has been reported that more than 60% of female gymnasts exhibit disordered eating patterns (23).

In anorexia nervosa, a preoccupation with body weight leads to self-starvation. People with anorexia nervosa typically view themselves as overweight even when their weight is substantially below normal. The APA lists the following criteria for diagnosis of anorexia nervosa (4):

- Purposefully maintaining weight at less than 85% of expected weight for age and height
- Extreme fear of gaining weight or fat
- Unhealthy body image in which the person feels overweight even when underweight; often associated with a severe intertwining of body image and self-esteem and a disregard for the seriousness of maintaining an extremely low body weight
- Absence of at least three consecutive menstrual cycles in postmenarchal women

Bulimia nervosa is characterized by consuming large amounts of food followed by food purging (4). Misuse of laxatives, self-induced vomiting, and excessive exercise are among the methods that may be used to purge. To meet the diagnostic criteria established by the APA, a person must engage in this behavior at least twice a week for 3 mo. Patients with bulimia nervosa, similar to those with anorexia nervosa, have an impaired body image and fear losing control over their body weight. Both anorexia nervosa and bulimia nervosa should be considered life-threatening disorders.

Binge-eating disorder is characterized by consuming large amounts of food in a short time (4). Unlike bulimia nervosa, binge eating is not associated with purging. Binge episodes are often initiated by emotional or psychological cues (e.g., loneliness, anxiety) rather than by physical hunger. These binges typically occur when the person is alone and may be followed by shame, guilt, and depression. To be clinically diagnosed with binge-eating disorder, a person must engage in at least two binges per wk for 6 mo (4). The prevalence of binge-eating disorder in the general population has been estimated at 2%. In contrast, 25% to 70% of obese individuals seeking treatment for weight loss may have this disorder (43).

Recognizing the signs of disordered eating is necessary for successful intervention. Some common signs of disordered eating are listed in the sidebar *Signs of Disordered Eating*. Fitness professionals who observe these signs should discuss the issue in a nonconfrontational manner with the client. However, when approached, many people will deny the existence of a problem. Asking gentle questions about the client's health (e.g., "How are you feeling?" or "Are you a little tired?") is one way to attempt to break the ice on this delicate subject. Successful intervention for eating disorders requires a multidisciplinary approach combining medical, nutritional, and psychological professionals (3). Knowledge of local support groups or professionals who work with patients who have eating disorders will allow fitness professionals to recommend places for clients to receive help. For additional information and support for dealing with eating disorders, refer to the National Eating Disorders Association (www.nationaleatingdisorders.org) and the National Institute of Mental Health (www.nimh.nih.gov).

KEY POINT

Eating disorders can significantly impair health and may even result in death. Anorexia nervosa, bulimia nervosa, and binge-eating disorder are three eating disorders recognized by the APA. Intervention for eating disorders should be multidisciplinary and should include psychological counseling.

Strategies for Gaining Weight

Before concluding this chapter, we must mention that some people struggle to increase their body weight. Fitness professionals should encourage these individuals to accumulate fat-free mass rather than all-fat weight. This will necessitate adding resistance training to the exercise routine. Various nutritional supplements are touted as supposedly guaranteed ways to increase muscle mass. However, as mentioned in chapter 5, even those who are training intensely need only about 1.5 g of protein per kilogram of body weight. Supplements such as creatine monohydrate may contribute somewhat to weight gain, but much of the change comes from greater water retention in the muscle.

The following are tips for increasing weight over time. When individuals continually lose weight or struggle to gain weight, a physician should be consulted about the possibility of underlying conditions.

- Increase caloric intake by 200 to 1,000 kcal $\cdot$ day^{-1} by increasing the meal size, number of meals, or number of between-meal snacks.

Signs of Disordered Eating

- A preoccupation with food, calories, and weight
- Repeatedly expressed concerns about being or feeling fat, even when weight is average or below average
- Increasing self-criticism about the body
- Secretly eating or stealing food
- Eating large meals and then disappearing or making trips to the bathroom
- Consuming large amounts of food not consistent with current body weight
- Bloodshot eyes, especially after trips to the bathroom
- Swollen parotid glands at the angle of the jaw, giving a chipmunk-like appearance
- Vomitus or odor of vomitus in the bathroom
- Wide fluctuations in weight over a short time
- Bouts of severe caloric restriction
- Excessive laxative use
- Compulsive, excessive exercise that is not part of the planned training regimen
- Unwillingness to eat in front of others
- Expression of self-deprecating thoughts after eating
- Wearing baggy or layered clothing
- Mood swings
- Appearing preoccupied with the eating behavior of others
- Continual drinking of diet soda or water

Based on Johnson 1994.

- Increase the number of healthy snacks consumed. Choose bread, fruit, granola, and other nutritious foods.
- Consume complex carbohydrate (e.g., whole-wheat pasta, whole-grain bread, brown rice, potatoes) to get the majority of additional calories.
- Add resistance training to the daily routine. Weight training is an effective means for increasing fat-free mass.
- When training intensely, make sure each day to consume 1.5 g of protein for each kilogram of body weight.
- Increase consumption of milk and fruit juices. These excellent choices not only provide additional calories but also essential nutrients.

KEY POINT

The additional calories needed to increase weight should come from increasing the number of healthy snacks or the size of meals. Adding resistance training to the exercise routine may help increase muscle mass.

12

LEARNING AIDS

REVIEW QUESTIONS

1. What is the current obesity prevalence for U.S. adults?
2. Define *positive caloric balance*. Does it lead to weight loss or weight gain?
3. What roles do genetic factors play in the development of obesity?
4. What three factors contribute to the daily caloric need?
5. What is the standard recommendation for daily caloric deficit when attempting weight loss?
6. Why is exercise important for those who are attempting weight loss or maintenance?
7. What are some behavioral strategies that can be useful for weight loss and maintenance?
8. List the signs of disordered eating.

CASE STUDIES

Ms. Kim is a 55-yr-old female who comes to your facility for an initial evaluation. She complains that she has gained 20 lb (9 kg) in the last 5 yr, and she wants to lose that extra weight. She is 5 ft 5 in. (165 cm) and weighs 160 lb (72.6 kg). She currently does not exercise and has a sedentary job.

1. Calculate her estimated daily energy requirements.
2. In order for her to lose approximately 1 lb (0.5 kg) a week, what calorie intake would you recommend?
3. Assume Ms. Kim begins a weekly exercise program in which she will walk (3.5 mph or 5.6 kph) for 30 min on 5 days per wk. How many additional calories will this expend each day? (Hint: See chapter 6.) Describe the effect this will have on weight loss.

Answers to Case Studies

1. Ms. Kim's estimated daily energy requirements are as follows:

$$\text{EER} = 354 - 6.91(\text{age}) + \text{PA}[9.36(\text{weight}) + 726(\text{height})]$$
$$= 354 - 6.91(55) + 1.12[9.36(72.7) + 726(1.65)]$$
$$= 2{,}078 \text{ kcal} \cdot \text{day}^{-1}.$$

2. Recommend 1,578 kcal · day^{-1} (deficit of 500 kcal · day^{-1}).
3. Approximately 4.5 kcal · min^{-1} × 30 · min per day = 135 kcal · day^{-1}.

   If Ms. Kim engages in this activity 5 days per wk, that will add up to 675 kcal · wk^{-1}, which will add an extra pound (0.5 kg) of weight loss every 5 wk.

13

Exercise Prescription for Muscular Fitness

Avery Faigenbaum

OBJECTIVES

The reader will be able to do the following:

1. Explain the physiological principles of overload, specificity, and progressive resistance and how they relate to exercise programming for developing muscular fitness.
2. Describe the following methods of resistance training: isometrics, dynamic constant external resistance training (DCER), variable resistance training, isokinetics, and plyometrics.
3. Describe the modes of resistance training.
4. Discuss the health and fitness benefits of resistance training, and understand precautions that enhance participant safety.
5. Describe the variables that are used to design resistance training programs, and discuss the relationship among the amount of resistance used, the training volume, the repetition velocity, and the rest intervals between sets and exercises.
6. Understand periodization and its application in the design of exercise programs, and differentiate between overreaching and overtraining.
7. Describe the following systems of resistance training: single set, multiple set, circuit training, preexhaustion, and assisted training.
8. Discuss the safety, benefits, and recommendations of resistance training for youth, older adults, pregnant women, and people considered to be at elevated cardiovascular or musculoskeletal risk.

Traditionally, resistance training was used primarily by adult athletes to enhance sport performance and increase muscle size. Today, resistance training is recognized as a method of enhancing the health and fitness of men and women of all ages and abilities (6, 32, 44, 108). Resistance training has become a popular method of conditioning in commercial, community, clinical, and corporate health and fitness facilities (78, 101, 102). Current public health guidelines aim to increase participation in resistance training to improve overall health and fitness (37, 103, 110).

Regular resistance training provides a variety of health and fitness benefits that may enhance quality of life while reducing the risk of several chronic diseases (see table 13.1). In addition to improving musculoskeletal strength, participation in a resistance training program is inversely associated with age-related weight and adiposity gains, risk of hypertension, and the prevalence and incidence of metabolic syndrome (7, 85, 105). Adequate levels of muscular strength and local muscular endurance enable people to perform ADLs and participate in other physical activities with energy and vigor. Resistance training is recommended by professional health, fitness, and medical organizations such as the AHA, ACSM, and National Strength and Conditioning Association (NSCA), and it is performed by everyone from children to older adults, pregnant women, and patients with chronic disease (6, 33, 44). For fitness professionals, the ability to design safe and effective resistance training programs for people of all ages, fitness levels, and health conditions is a valuable asset. This chapter focuses on principles of resistance training that can be used in designing exercise programs for enhancing muscular fitness in untrained and trained people. Photos and instructions for exercises that target major muscle groups are included in the appendix of this chapter. Advanced resistance training programs for developing speed, strength, and power for elite athletes are available elsewhere (18, 32, 44).

In this chapter, the term *resistance training* refers to a method of conditioning designed to increase a person's ability to exert or resist force. This term encompasses a wide range of resistive loads (from light manual resistance to plyometric jumps) and a variety of training modalities, including free weights (barbells and dumbbells), weight machines, elastic tubing, medicine balls, stability balls, and body weight. Resistance training should be distinguished from the competitive sports of **weightlifting**, **powerlifting**, and **bodybuilding**. Weightlifting and powerlifting are sports in which athletes attempt to lift maximal amounts of weight, and bodybuilding is a sport in which the goal is to enhance muscle size and symmetry. Although fitness enthusiasts may perform some of the same exercises used by weightlifters, powerlifters, and bodybuilders, the program goals and training regimens are different.

Local muscular endurance refers to the ability of a muscle or muscle group to perform repeated contractions against a submaximal resistance. **Strength** is defined as the maximal force that a muscle or muscle group can generate at a specified velocity, and **power** refers to the rate of performing work and is the product of strength and speed of movement. *Muscular fitness* is a general term that includes local muscular endurance, strength, and power and is related to promoting and maintaining good health and

Table 13.1 Effects of Aerobic Training and Resistance Training on Health and Fitness Variables

Variable	Aerobic training	Resistance training
Body composition	• Decrease in fat mass • Decrease in intra-abdominal fat • Little impact on lean mass or bone mass	• Increase in muscle mass • Increase in bone mass • Little impact on fat mass or intra-abdominal fat
Aerobic power and endurance	• Large increase in $\dot{V}O_2max$ • Large improvement in submaximal and maximal endurance times	• Little impact on $\dot{V}O_2max$ • Improvement in submaximal and maximal endurance times
Muscular factors	• Large increase in capillary and mitochondrial density • Little or no change in muscle mass or strength	• Large increase in muscular power and strength • Increase in number of actin and myosin filaments (hypertrophy)
Cardiovascular factors	• Decrease in RHR and submaximal exercise HR • Decrease in resting BP (in those with hypertension) • Decrease in submaximal exercise BP	• Little to no impact on resting or exercise BP or HR
Glucose control	• Improvement in insulin sensitivity	• Improvement in insulin sensitivity

fitness. For ease of discussion, the terms *youth* and *young athletes* are broadly defined in this chapter to include the preadolescent and adolescent years, and the terms *older* and *senior* refer to adults aged 65 and older.

Principles of Training

A key factor in any resistance training program is appropriate program design. Because the act of resistance training itself does not ensure gains in muscular fitness, the resistance training program needs to be based on sound training principles and must be carefully prescribed in order to maximize training outcomes. Although factors such as initial fitness level, heredity, nutritional status (e.g., diet composition and hydration), health habits (e.g., sleep), and motivation influence the rate and magnitude of the adaptation that occurs, there are four principles that determine the effectiveness of all resistance training programs: progression, regularity, overload, and specificity. These principles of resistance training can be remembered as the PROS.

Principle of Progression

According to the principle of progression, the demands placed on the body must continually and progressively increase over time in order to result in long-term fitness gains. Although it is impossible to improve at the same rate throughout long-term training programs, the systematic manipulation of training variables (e.g., intensity, repetitions) during the program can limit training plateaus and optimize training adaptations (5). This does not mean that heavier weights should be used in every workout but rather that over time exercise sessions should become more challenging in order to create a more effective exercise stimulus. Without a more challenging stimulus that is consistent with individual needs, goals, and abilities, the human body has no reason to adapt any further. This principle is particularly important after the first 2 or 3 mo of resistance training, when the threshold for training-induced adaptations in conditioned people is higher (5).

The importance of recovery between resistance training workouts should not be underestimated, but the training stimulus should increase at a rate that is compatible with the training-induced adaptations. Beginners can progress relatively fast whereas slower rates of improvement are appropriate for people with experience in resistance training. A reasonable guideline for a beginner is to increase the training weight about 5% to 10% and decrease the **repetitions** (the number of times a movement is completed) by 2 to 4 once a given load can be performed for the desired number of repetitions with proper exercise technique. For example, if an adult female can easily perform 12 repetitions of the chest press using 100 lb (45 kg), she should increase the weight to 110 lb (50 kg) and decrease the repetitions to 8 if she wants to continue to gain muscular strength. Alternatively, she could increase the number of **sets** (groups of repetitions), increase the number of repetitions, or add another chest exercise (e.g., dumbbell fly) to her routine. The decision on how to progress should be based on the person's training experience and personal goals.

Principle of Regularity

In order to make continual gains in muscular fitness, resistance training must be performed regularly several times per week. Inconsistent training will result in only modest training adaptations, and prolonged inactivity will result in a loss of muscular strength and size. The adage "Use it or lose it" is appropriate for exercise programming because training-induced adaptations cannot be stored. Although adequate recovery is needed between training sessions, the principle of regularity states that long-term gains in muscle strength and performance will be realized only if the program is performed on a regular basis.

Principle of Overload

For more than a century, the **overload** principle has been a tenet of resistance training. The overload principle states that to enhance muscular fitness, the body must exercise at a level beyond that at which it is normally stressed. For example, an adult male who can easily complete 10 repetitions with 20 lb (9 kg) while performing a barbell curl must increase the weight, the repetitions, or the number of sets if he wants to increase his arm strength. If the training stimulus is not increased beyond the level to which the muscles are accustomed, training adaptations will not occur. Overload is typically manipulated by changing the exercise intensity, total repetitions, repetition speed, rest periods, type of exercise, and training volume (5). This process is often referred to as *progressive overload* and is the basis for maximizing long-term training adaptations.

Principle of Specificity

The principle of **specificity** refers to the adaptations that take place as a result of a training program. The adaptations to resistance training are specific to the muscle actions, velocity of movement, exercise ROM, muscle groups, energy systems, and intensity and volume involved in training (5, 78). Specificity is often referred to as the *SAID principle*, which stands for **s**pecific **a**daptations to **i**mposed **d**emands. In essence, every muscle or muscle group must be trained to make gains in strength and local muscular endurance. For instance, exercises such as the squat and leg press can enhance lower-body strength, but they will not affect upper-body strength.

The adaptations that take place in a muscle or muscle group will be as simple or as complex as the stress placed on them. For example, because basketball requires multijoint and multiplanar movements (i.e., in the frontal, sagittal, and transverse planes), basketball players should perform complex exercises that closely mimic the movements and energy demands of their sport. The specificity principle also can be applied to designing resistance training programs for people who want to enhance their ability to perform ADLs such as stair-climbing and house cleaning, which also require multijoint and multiplanar movements. The most effective resistance training programs target specific muscle groups and energy systems.

KEY POINT

Gains in strength and local muscular endurance will occur only if the overload is greater than that to which the muscle or muscle group is normally accustomed. To make continual gains, training must progress gradually and be performed regularly. The program design will influence the training-induced adaptations that occur. The most beneficial resistance training programs are designed to meet individual needs, goals, and abilities.

RESEARCH INSIGHT

Reported Engagement in Resistance Training

Although regular participation in a resistance training program offers observable health and fitness benefits, the number of adults in the United States who are meeting muscle-strengthening guidelines is below expectations. Public health researchers performed a random-digit-dialed telephone survey of nearly 500,000 noninstitutionalized U.S. adults aged 18 yr or older (47). The median survey response rate for all states was 50%. The researchers reported that 51.6% of U.S. adults met the aerobic activity guideline, and only 29.3% met the muscle-strengthening guidelines. These findings highlight the importance of educating adults about the benefits associated with resistance training and of designing fitness programs that are consistent with each individual's needs, goals, and abilities.

Program Design Considerations

As with exercise programs that enhance CRF, resistance training programs should be based on the participant's interests, current fitness level, health needs, clinical status, and personal goals as well as on the principles of resistance training. By assessing the individual needs of each participant and applying principles of training to the program design, safe and effective resistance training programs can be developed for each person. However, because the magnitude of adaptation to a given exercise stimulus varies from person to person, fitness professionals must be aware of interindividual differences and be prepared to alter the program to reduce the risk of injury and to maximize training adaptations.

Health Status

The health status of each person should be assessed before the resistance training begins. As discussed in chapter 2, each participant should complete a health and medical questionnaire, and the fitness professional should review it to make decisions about further medical evaluation. Additional questions on the HRA regarding past resistance training experiences, previous musculoskeletal injuries, presence of known cardiovascular conditions, and personal goals can also help with designing the resistance training program.

Fitness Level

An important factor to consider when designing resistance training programs is the participant's previous experience with resistance training, or training age. Those who are the least experienced in resistance training tend to have a greater capacity for improvement compared with those who have been resistance training for several years. Although any reasonable program can increase the strength of untrained people, more comprehensive programs are often needed to produce desirable adaptations in trained people (5, 78). Thus, resistance training programs designed for beginners may not be effective for participants who have at least 3 mo of experience with resistance training. For example, a 32-yr-old person with 5 yr of resistance training experience (i.e., a training age of 5 yr) may not achieve the same strength gains in a given time as a 25-yr-old person who has no experience with resistance training (i.e., a training age of 0 yr). The potential for adaptation gradually decreases as training age increases. As people gain experience with resistance training, they need more advanced programs so that they may continue to enhance their muscular fitness (5, 14). Clearly, there is no single model of resistance exercise that will optimize training-induced adaptations in both untrained and trained people.

Therefore, it is reasonable for beginners to start with a general resistance training program and gradually progress to more advanced programs as performance and self-confidence in their ability to perform resistance exercise improve. However, as more advanced training programs are designed, fitness professionals must consider the additional time and effort that are required to make additional gains. For example, people with several years of training experience may need to devote a larger amount of time to training in order to make relatively small gains. Although athletes may be willing to make this type of commitment for small changes in performance, others may be less willing to devote a large amount of time to resistance training.

Because long-term progression in resistance exercise requires a systematic manipulation of the program variables, fitness professionals need to make critical decisions regarding the exercise prescription. These decisions require a solid understanding of training-induced adaptations that take place in both beginners and nonbeginners. Beginners need less variation, but as the program progresses, more variation and more complex training regimens are needed. More advanced training programs are available elsewhere (14, 18, 78).

Training Goals

After the preexercise screening, participants should establish realistic short- and long-term goals. The results of a muscular fitness evaluation (see chapter 9) along with the participant's interests can be used to help set realistic and measurable goals. To improve compliance, these goals ideally are set by the participant with guidance from a knowledgeable fitness professional. Typical goals are to increase muscle strength, decrease body fat, and improve overall health. An effort to establish realistic goals and increase confidence to achieve those goals is important because it may help people avoid unrealistic expectations that ultimately can lead to discouragement and poor adherence. Testing fitness periodically and reviewing individualized workout logs can help the fitness professional assess training progress and modify the program. Understanding that resistance training programs designed to improve health and fitness are quite different from training programs designed to enhance sport performance will further promote the development of and adherence to programs suited to a participant's needs.

Types of Resistance Training

Several types of resistance training can be used to enhance muscular fitness. Although each method has advantages and disadvantages, there are several factors to consider when selecting one type of training over another or including multiple types of training within a given program. The most common types of resistance training include isometrics, dynamic constant external resistance training, variable resistance training, isokinetics, and plyometrics.

Isometrics

Isometric training, or static resistance training, refers to muscle actions in which muscle length does not change. This type of training is usually performed against an immovable object such as a wall or a weight machine loaded with a heavy weight. The concept of isometric training was popularized in the 1950s when Hettinger and Muller reported remarkable gains in muscle strength resulting from one daily 6 sec isometric contraction at two-thirds of maximal force (49). Although subsequent studies also reported gains in strength resulting from isometric training, the reported gains were substantially less than those reported earlier (32).

An advantage of isometric training is that specialized equipment is not required and the cost is minimal. Increases in strength and muscle **hypertrophy** (an increase in size or mass) can occur from this type of training; however, a major limitation is that the strength gains are specific to the joint angle at which the training occurred. For example, if isometric training of the elbow flexors is performed at a joint angle of 90°, muscle strength will increase at this joint angle but not necessarily at other angles. Even though there seems to be about 20° of carryover on either side of the joint angle, the same isometric exercise must be performed at varying joint angles in order to increase strength throughout the full ROM. Isometric training may help to maintain muscle strength and prevent muscle **atrophy** (a decrease in size or mass) when a limb is immobilized in a cast, but gains in functional strength (e.g., stair-climbing) and motor performance (e.g., sprinting and jumping) as a result of isometric training are unlikely to occur if isometric training takes place only at one joint angle.

Factors such as the number of repetitions performed, duration of contractions, intensity of contractions, and frequency of training can influence the strength gains resulting from isometric training. In general, isometric training characterized by maximal voluntary muscle actions performed for 3 to 5 sec for 15 to 20 repetitions at least 3 times per wk tends to optimize strength gains (35). Because of the nature of isometric training, it is particularly important to avoid the breath-holding Valsalva maneuver, which reduces venous return to the heart and increases SBP and DBP. During all types of resistance training, regular breathing patterns (i.e., exhalation while lifting and inhalation while lowering) should be encouraged.

Dynamic Constant External Resistance (DCER) Training

Resistance training that involves a lifting and lowering phase is called *dynamic*. Exercises using free weights (e.g., barbells and dumbbells) and weight machines are dynamic because the weight is lifted and lowered through a predetermined ROM. Although the term *isotonic* traditionally was used to describe this type of training, it literally means "constant (*iso*) tension (*tonic*)." Because tension exerted by a muscle as it shortens varies with the mechanical advantage of the joint and the length of the muscle fibers at a particular joint angle, the term *isotonic* does not accurately describe this training method. As shown in figure 13.1, during a barbell curl, the elbow flexors are strongest at approximately 100° and weakest at 60° (elbows fully flexed) and at 180° (elbows fully extended). The same principle applies to other muscle groups. DCER better describes resistance training in which the weight does not change during the lifting, or **concentric** (muscle-shortening) **action**, and lowering, or **eccentric** (muscle-lengthening) **action**.

DCER training is the most common method of resistance training for enhancing health and fitness. Endless combinations of sets and repetitions and a variety of training equipment can be used for DCER training. Untrained people should perform each repetition deliberately at a slow to moderate velocity, whereas the performance of various training velocities from unintentionally slow (using heavy loads) to intentionally fast (using power training) will provide the most effective training stimulus for people with resistance training experience (78). Weight machines generally limit the user to fixed planes of motion. However, they are easy to use and are ideal for isolating muscle groups. Free weights are less expensive and can be used for a wide variety of exercises that require greater proprioception, balance, and coordination. Several free-weight exercises (e.g., barbell squat, bench press) require the use of a spotter who can assist the lifter in case of a failed repetition. In addition to improving health and fitness, DCER training is also used to enhance motor performance skills and sport performance.

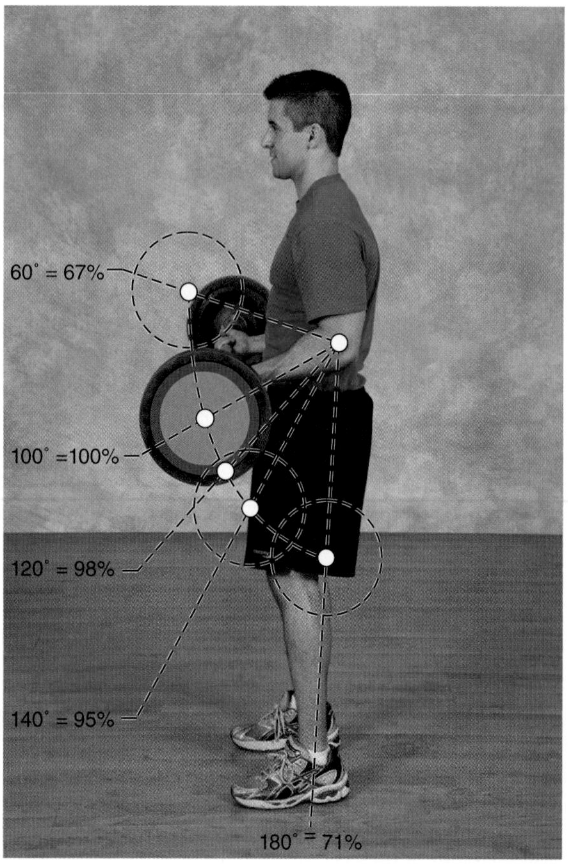

FIGURE 13.1 Variation in strength relative to the angle of the elbow flexors during the biceps curl.

During DCER training, the weight lifted does not change throughout the ROM. Because muscle tension can vary significantly during a DCER exercise, the heaviest weight that can be lifted throughout a full ROM is limited by the strength of a muscle at the weakest joint angle. As a result, DCER exercise provides adequate resistance to stimulate training adaptions in some parts of the movement range but not enough resistance in others. For example, during the barbell bench press, more weight can be lifted during the last part of the exercise than in the first part of the movement when the barbell is being pressed off the chest. This is a limitation of DCER training that should be recognized when choosing starting weights for beginners.

In an attempt to overcome the variation in strength across the ROM, mechanical devices that operate through a lever arm or cam have been designed to vary the resistance throughout the ROM of an exercise (see figure 13.2). These devices, called *variable resistance machines*, theoretically force the muscle to contract maximally throughout the ROM by varying the resistance to match the exercise strength curve. These machines can be used to train all the major muscle groups, and by automatically changing the resistive force throughout the movement range, they provide proportionally less resistance in weaker segments of the movement and more resistance in stronger segments of the movement. As with all weight machines, variable resistance machines provide a specific movement path. This makes the exercise easier to perform compared with free-weight exercises, which require balance, coordination, and the involvement of stabilizing muscle groups. These features make variable resistance machines a popular mode of resistance training for people who desire safe and simple exercise sessions.

Isokinetics

The term *isokinetics* refers to muscular actions performed at a constant angular limb velocity. Isokinetic training involves specialized and expensive equipment, and most isokinetic devices are designed to train only single-joint movements. Isokinetic machines generally are not used in fitness centers, but they are used by physical therapists and certified athletic trainers for injury rehabilitation. Unlike other types of resistance training, in isokinetics,

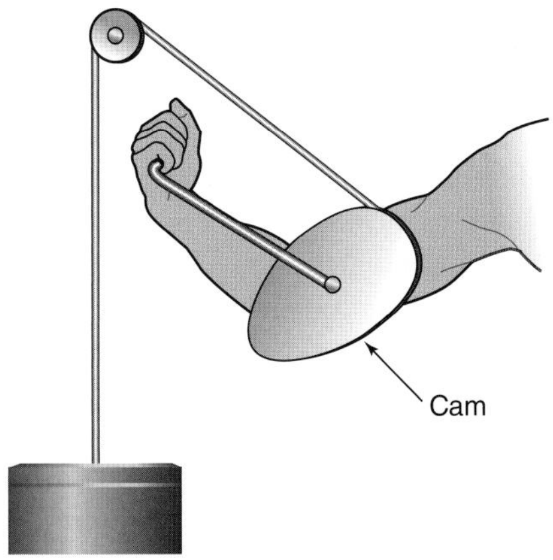

FIGURE 13.2 Variable resistance device for the biceps muscle in which a cam alters the resistance throughout the ROM.

Adapted, by permission, from D. Wathen and F. Roll, 1994, Training methods and modes. In *Essentials of strength training and conditioning,* edited by T.R. Baechle (Champaign, IL: Human Kinetics), 408.

the speed of movement rather than the resistance is controlled. During isokinetic training, any force applied to the isokinetic machine is met with an equal reaction force. Although it is theoretically possible for a muscle to contract maximally through the full ROM of an exercise, this seems unlikely during isokinetic training because of the acceleration at the beginning and deceleration at the end of the ROM.

Isokinetic training studies have generally found that strength gains are specific to the training velocity (15). Isokinetic training at a slow movement velocity (e.g., $60^\circ \cdot sec^{-1}$) will increase strength at that velocity, but strength gains at faster velocities are unlikely to occur. If the purpose of the training program is to increase strength at higher velocities (e.g., for enhanced sport performance), high-speed isokinetic training appears prudent. The best approach may be to perform isokinetic training at slow, intermediate, and fast velocities to develop strength and power at a variety of movement speeds.

Plyometrics

Plyometric training, first known simply as *jump training*, refers to a specialized method of conditioning designed to enable a muscle to reach maximal force in the shortest possible time (18). Unlike an exercise such as the bench press, plyometric training is characterized by quick, powerful movements that involve rapid stretching of a muscle (eccentric muscle action) immediately followed by rapid shortening (concentric muscle action). This type of muscle action, sometimes called *stretch–shortening cycle exercise*, provides a physiological advantage because the muscle force generated during the concentric muscle action is potentiated by the preceding eccentric muscle action (18). Although both muscle actions are important, the amount of time it takes to change direction from the eccentric to the concentric muscle action is a critical factor in plyometric training. This amount of time is the **amortization phase** and should be as short as possible (<0.1 sec) in order to maximize training adaptations. Both mechanical factors (i.e., increased stored elastic energy) and neurophysiological factors (i.e., change in the force–velocity relationship of the muscle) contribute to the increased force production resulting from plyometric training (18, 87).

Exercises that involve explosive jumping, skipping, hopping, and throwing can be considered plyometric. Although plyometric exercises often are associated with high-intensity drills such as depth jumps (i.e., jumping from a box to the ground and then immediately jumping up), common activities such as jumping jacks and hopscotch are also plyometric exercises because every time the feet hit the ground, the quadriceps go through a stretch–shortening cycle. Strength and power athletes in sports such as American football, volleyball, and track and field regularly perform plyometric exercises as part of their conditioning program. More recently, this type of training has become popular in group exercise classes and fitness programs.

VIDEO Watch **video 13.1**, which demonstrates plyometrics.

Because plyometric exercises can greatly stress muscles, connective tissues, and joints, they need to be carefully prescribed to reduce the likelihood of musculoskeletal injury. In some cases, the risks of performing plyometric exercises may outweigh the potential benefits for untrained or overweight people who may lack the strength and coordination to perform the exercises properly. In other cases, plyometrics may be a worthwhile addition to the exercise program of a trained individual who wants to join a recreational basketball league. Clearly, the prescription of plyometric exercises needs to be individualized and based on a person's health history, training experience, and personal goals. Although participants with different levels of physical fitness can benefit from plyometric training (87), it seems prudent to restrict plyometric training to people who have developed a foundation of muscular fitness by first participating in a general resistance training program.

It is also reasonable to begin plyometric training with lower-intensity drills and gradually progress to higher-intensity drills as technique and performance improve. In one case report, a 12-yr-old boy developed exertional rhabdomyolysis after he was instructed to perform excessive repetitive squat jumps (>250) in a physical education class (19). Exertional rhabdomyolysis is a serious medical condition that can result in severe muscle soreness and renal failure. Clearly, there is the potential for injury or illness to occur if the intensity, volume, or frequency of resistance training exceeds the ability of the participant.

Other considerations for plyometric training include proper footwear, adequate space, shock-absorbing landing surfaces (e.g., suspended floor or grass playing field), and training frequency (18). Also, plyometric training should not be considered a standalone training method but rather should be used in combination with other types of conditioning. Although research indicates that plyometric protocols with more than 40 jumps per session appear to maximize training adaptations (87), it is always better to undertrain than overtrain and risk an injury. It seems reasonable to begin plyometric training with 1 to 3 sets of 6 to 10 repetitions of several low-intensity exercises for the upper and lower body twice a week on nonconsecutive days. Fitness professionals who have experience with plyometric training should provide demonstrations and coaching cues in order to enhance learning, improve technique, and reduce the likelihood of injury. Additional training guidelines and examples of plyometric drills are available elsewhere (18).

KEY POINT

Various types of resistance training can increase muscular strength, local muscular endurance, and muscular power. The effects of isometric training are generally limited to the joint angle at which the training occurs. DCER training refers to exercises performed throughout a ROM with free weights and weight machines. Isokinetic training occurs at a constant limb velocity with maximal force exerted throughout the ROM of the joint. Plyometric training exploits the muscle cycle of lengthening and shortening to increase speed of movement and muscular power.

Modes of Resistance Training

Various modes of resistance training can be used to accommodate the needs of young people, adults, and seniors. Provided that the principles of training are adhered to, almost any mode of resistance training can be used to enhance muscular fitness. Some types of equipment are relatively easy to use, while others require balance, coordination, and high levels of skill. The decision to use a certain mode of resistance training should be based on each client's needs, goals, and abilities. The major modes of resistance training are weight machines, free weights (barbells and dumbbells), body-weight exercises, and a broadly defined category of balls, bands, and elastic tubing.

Single-joint exercises such as the biceps curl target a specific muscle group and require less skill. Multijoint exercises such as the bench press involve more than one joint or major muscle group and require more balance and coordination. Although both single-joint and multijoint exercises enhance muscular fitness, multijoint exercises are considered to be more effective for increasing muscle strength because they involve a greater amount of muscle mass and therefore enable a heavier weight to be lifted (5, 78). Multijoint exercises have also been shown to have the greatest acute metabolic and anabolic hormonal (e.g., testosterone and growth hormone) response, which could favorably influence resistance training that targets improvements in muscle size and body composition (32). The appendix of this chapter provides examples of resistance training exercises for the major muscle groups. Table 13.2 summarizes the advantages and disadvantages of weight machines, free weights (barbells and dumbbells), body-weight exercises, and balls, bands, and elastic tubing.

Weight machines are designed to train all the major muscle groups and can be found in most fitness centers. Both single-joint (e.g., leg extension) and multijoint (e.g., leg press) exercises can be performed on weight machines, which are relatively easy to use because the exercise motion is controlled by the machine and typically occurs in only one anatomical plane. This may be particularly important when designing resistance training programs for sedentary or inexperienced participants. Also, several weight-machine exercises such as the lat pull-down and leg curl are difficult to mimic with free weights. Weight machines are designed to fit the average male or female, so smaller people may not be able to properly position themselves on the equipment. A seat pad or back pad can be used to adjust body position to allow for a better fit. Some companies now manufacture weight machines specifically for children. These machines are smaller versions of adult-sized machines and have weight increments that are appropriate for younger populations.

Free weights are also popular in fitness centers and come in a variety of shapes and sizes. Although it may take longer to master proper exercise technique when using free weights compared with weight machines, free weights have several advantages. For example, proper fit is not an issue with adjustable barbells and dumbbells because one size fits all. Free weights also offer a greater variety of exercises than weight machines because they can be moved in many directions. Another benefit of free weights is that they require the use of stabilizing and assisting muscles to hold the correct body position during an exercise. As such, free-weight training can occur in different planes. This is particularly true with dumbbells because they train each side of the body independently.

Table 13.2 Comparison of Resistance Training Modes

	Weight machines	Free weights	Body weight	Balls and cords[a]
Cost	High	Low	None	Very low
Portability	Limited	Variable	Excellent	Excellent
Ease of use	Excellent	Variable	Variable	Variable
Muscle isolation	Excellent	Variable	Variable	Variable
Functionality	Limited	Excellent	Excellent	Excellent
Exercise variety	Limited	Excellent	Excellent	Excellent
Space requirements	High	Variable	Low	Low

[a]Medicine balls, stability balls, and elastic cords.

In general, free weights allow the participant to train functionally by encouraging different muscle groups to work together while performing exercises that are similar to the participant's chosen sport or activity. However, unlike weight machines, several free-weight exercises require the aid of a spotter who can assist the lifter in case of a failed repetition. Using a spotter is particularly important when performing the bench press. In an epidemiological evaluation of injuries related to resistance training, a large number of injuries occurred with free weights, and the most common mechanism of injury was weights dropping on the person (54). Accidents such as these underscore the importance of close supervision and an appropriate progression of training loads when training with free weights.

Body-weight exercises such as push-ups, pull-ups, and curl-ups are some of the oldest modes of resistance training. An example of using body weight as a form of resistance is Pilates exercise and to some extent certain forms of yoga that particularly target stability and core strength (i.e., abdominal muscles, lower back, hips). Obviously, a major advantage of body-weight training is that equipment is not needed and a variety of exercises can be performed. Conversely, a limitation of body-weight training is the difficulty in adjusting the body weight to the individual's strength level. Sedentary or overweight participants may not be strong enough to perform even one push-up or pull-up. In such cases, body-weight exercises not only may be ineffective, they may have a negative effect on program compliance. Exercise machines that allow people to perform movements that mimic body-weight exercises, such as pull-ups and dips, by using a predetermined percentage of their body weight are available. These machines provide an opportunity for participants of all abilities to incorporate movements similar to body-weight exercises into their resistance training program.

Stability balls, medicine balls, and elastic tubing are safe and effective alternatives to weight machines and free weights, provided qualified supervision and instruction are available. The first use of medicine balls dates back almost 3,000 years, and stability balls and elastic tubing have been used by therapists for decades. Now fitness professionals are using balls and bands for resistance training and conditioning. Not only are stability balls, medicine balls, and elastic tubing relatively inexpensive, they can also be used to enhance strength, local muscular endurance, and power. In addition, exercises performed with balls and tubing can challenge proprioception, which carries added benefits, including gains in agility, balance, and coordination.

Stability balls are lightweight, inflatable balls about 45 to 75 cm in diameter that add the elements of balance and coordination to any exercise while targeting selected muscle groups. Although many exercises can be performed with stability balls, they are often used to develop core (i.e., abdominal, hip, and low back) strength and improve posture. When participants sit on a stability ball, their feet should be at a 90° angle. The firmer the ball, the more difficult the exercise will be. Because proper body alignment is crucial when performing an exercise on a stability ball, fitness professionals should know how to perform each exercise correctly and when to modify an exercise to meet individual needs and abilities. Many types of exercise programs using stability balls can be created to enhance strength, local muscular endurance, and flexibility (42, 97). Figure 13.3 illustrates the performance of abdominal curls on a stability ball.

Medicine balls come in a variety of shapes and sizes (about 1 kg to more than 10 kg) and are a safe and effective alternative to free weights and weight machines. In addition to performing squats or chest presses with a medicine ball, participants can use the ball in throwing drills—such as throwing from participant to instructor or against the wall—to enhance upper-body explosive power. High-speed training with medicine balls adds a new dimension to resistance training that can benefit men and women of all ages. Further, because medicine balls typically require the body to function as a unit instead of as separate parts, they are particularly effective for mimicking natural body positions and movement speeds that occur in daily life and game situations. Progressive medicine-ball training that can be used in one-on-one settings or group fitness classes is available (42, 63). Figure 13.4 illustrates the medicine-ball squat.

Resistance training with an elastic band involves performing an exercise against the force required to stretch the band and then return it to its unstretched state. A variety of exercises can be performed by holding the ends of the cord with both hands or attaching one end of the cord to a fixed object. For safety reasons, fitness professionals should ensure that the cord is secured under both feet or to a fixed object before performing any exercise. Incorporating exercises with stability balls, medicine balls, and elastic tubing into a workout session can be challenging, motivating, beneficial, and fun. Figure 13.5 illustrates a chest press with an elastic band.

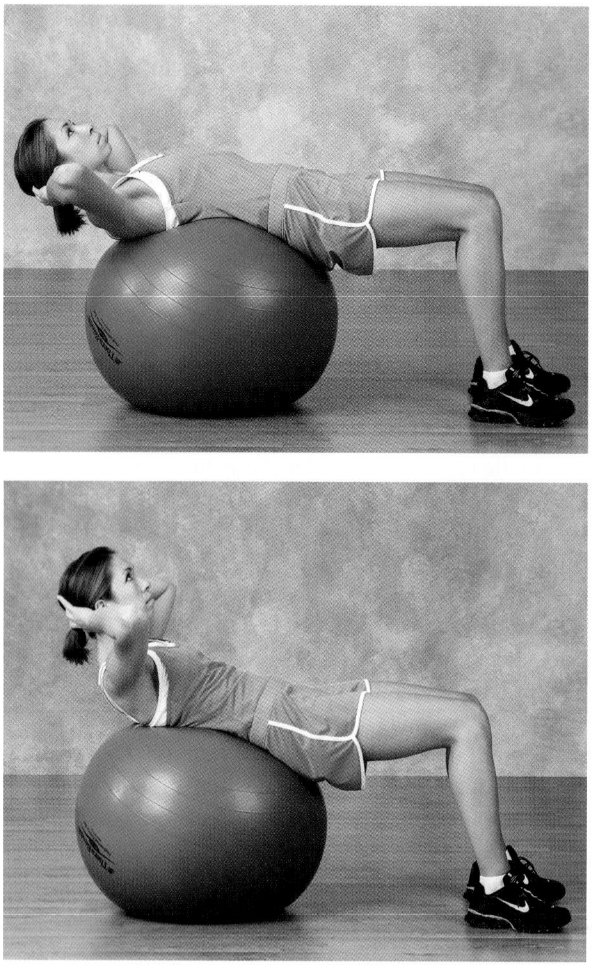

FIGURE 13.3 Abdominal curl on a stability ball.

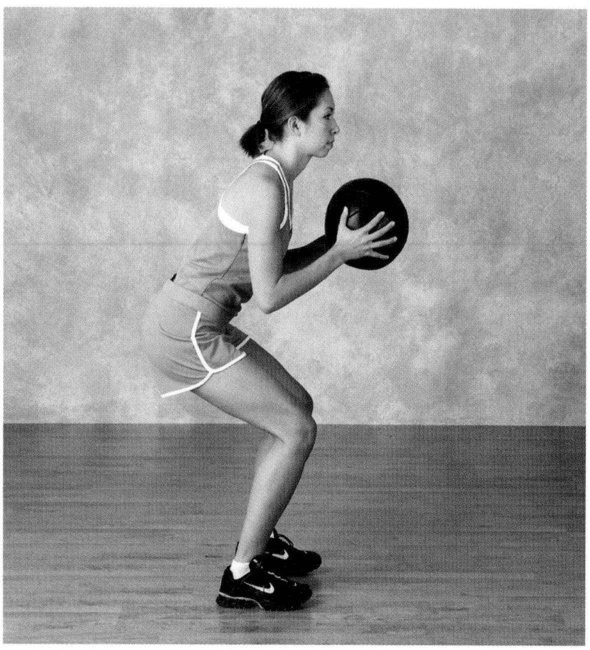

FIGURE 13.4 Medicine-ball squat.

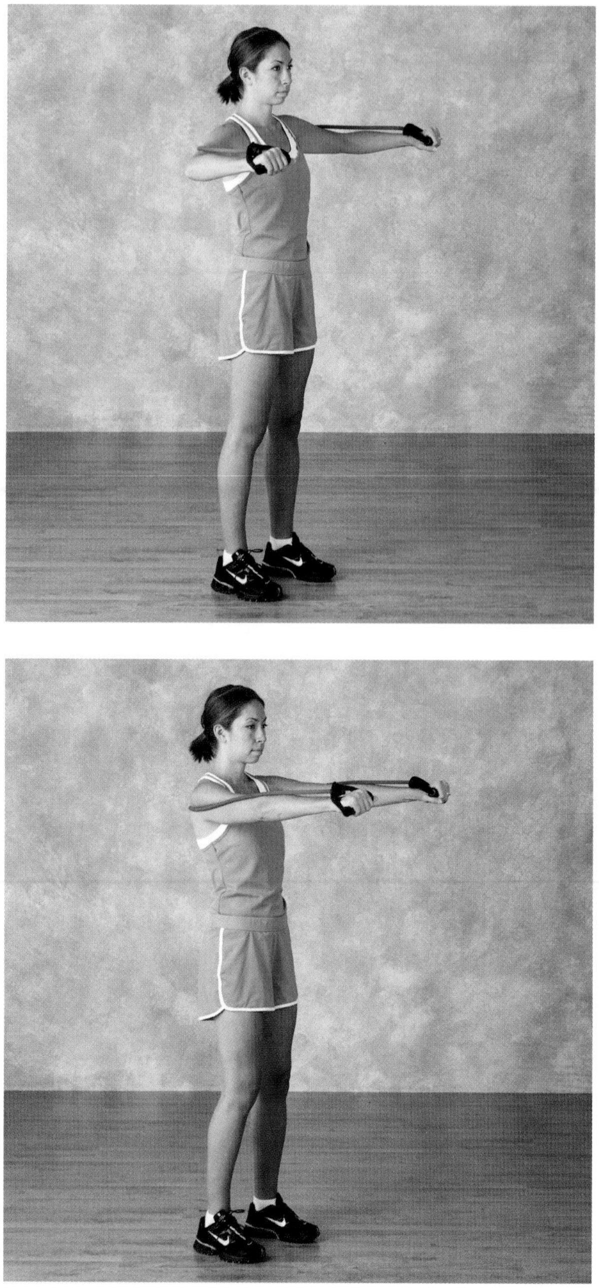

FIGURE 13.5 Chest press with elastic band.

KEY POINT

Weight machines, free weights, bodyweight exercises, medicine balls, stability balls, and elastic bands can be used to enhance muscular fitness. When designing resistance training programs, fitness professionals should evaluate the advantages and disadvantages of each training mode to meet individual needs, goals, and abilities while maximizing participant safety.

Safety Issues

Resistance training programs should be designed by fitness professionals who are knowledgeable about safe and effective training methods. Although all types of exercise have some degree of risk, the chance of injury during resistance training can be reduced by following established training guidelines and safety procedures. Without proper supervision and instruction, injuries that require medical attention may occur. An evaluation of resistance-training-related injuries presenting to U.S. emergency rooms revealed that 27% of all reported injuries in adults were considered accidental (e.g., dropped weights, improper use of equipment, tripping over equipment) and could have been prevented with strict adherence to safety guidelines (68). A majority of the reported injuries were considered nonaccidental because they resulted from exertion (sprain or strain), overuse, or equipment malfunction (68). Further, these researchers reported that men suffered more trunk injuries than women, whereas women had more foot and leg injuries than men (77), Figure 13.6 illustrates the percentage of resistance-training-related injuries at each body part for men and women who presented to U.S. emergency rooms (77). Clearly, people who resistance train should receive instruction on appropriate training guidelines and equipment use from qualified fitness professionals. General safety recommendations for designing and instructing resistance training programs are given next.

Supervision and Instruction

People who want to participate in resistance training should first receive guidance and instruction from qualified fitness professionals who understand principles of resistance training and appreciate individual differences. Fitness professionals should be able to correctly perform the exercises they prescribe and should be able to modify exercise form and technique if necessary. They should know which exercises require spotters and should be prepared to offer assistance in case of a failed repetition. When working in a health or fitness facility, the staff should be attentive and should try to position themselves with a clear view of the training center so that they can quickly access people who need assistance. In addition, the fitness staff is responsible

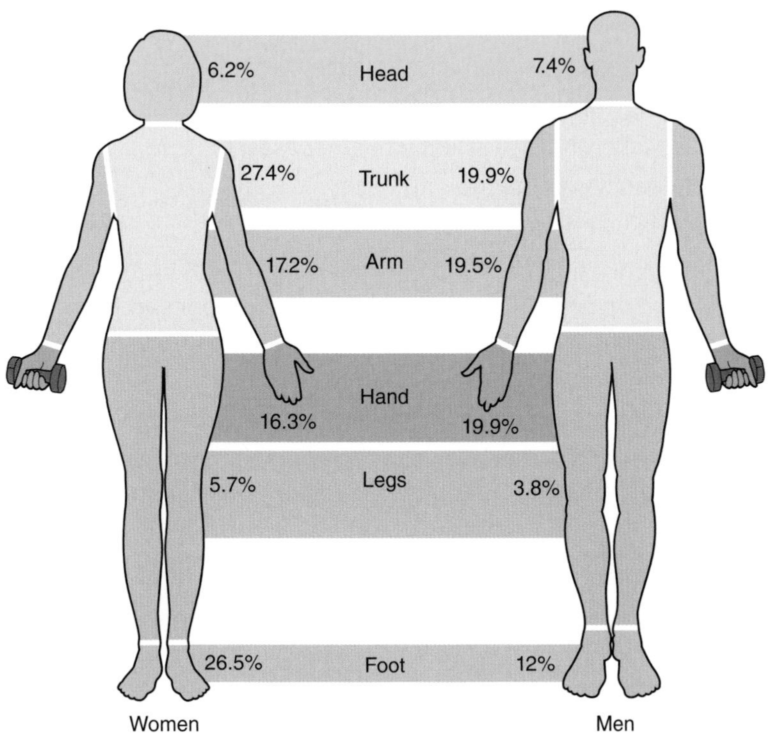

FIGURE 13.6 Percentage of injuries at each body location for men and women.

Based on from Quatman 2009.

for enforcing safety rules (e.g., wear proper footwear, store weights safely, no foolish play in the fitness center) and safe training procedures (e.g., emphasizing proper exercise technique rather than the amount of weight lifted). Not only can fitness professionals enhance the safety of resistance training, but they can help clients maximize strength gains when they develop and supervise personalized programs (40, 61, 79).

Training Environment

If exercise is to take place in a public, community, worksite, or school-based fitness center, the training area should be well lit and large enough to handle the number of people exercising in the facility at any given time. The facility should be clean and the equipment should be well maintained. Equipment pads that come in contact with the skin should be cleaned daily, and cables, guide rods, and chains on machines should be checked weekly. Equipment should be spaced to allow easy access to each resistance training exercise, and equipment such as free weights and collars should be returned to the proper storage area after each use. Recommended temperature (68-72 °F, or 20.0-22.2 °C), humidity (60% or less), and air circulation (at least 8 air exchanges every hr) should be maintained in the resistance training area (3). Additional recommendations for fitness facility maintenance and risk management are available elsewhere (3).

Warm-Up and Cool-Down

Resistance training should be preceded by warm-up activities. A general warm-up increases body and muscle temperature, increases blood flow, and may enhance performance (6). This type of warm-up typically includes 5 to 10 min of moderate- to high-intensity aerobic exercise such as slow jogging or stationary cycling. More recently, the benefits of static stretching as the sole activity during the warm-up have been questioned (95). However, dynamic warm-up protocols that include moderate- to high-intensity hops, skips, and jumps and various movement-based exercises for the upper and lower body have proven to be effective (10, 78). Although a general warm-up can elevate muscle temperature, a well-designed dynamic warm-up can also enhance motor unit excitability, improve kinesthetic awareness, and increase strength and power (10, 35). Although the combination of factors that are responsible for enhancing muscle performance after a dynamic warm-up might be unclear, most factors relate to a neuromuscular phenomenon known as *postactivation potentiation*, or PAP (84, 107). In this phenomenon, muscular performance is acutely enhanced as a result of prior activity performed at a relatively high intensity.

A specific warm-up involves movements that are similar to the resistance training exercises that are about to be performed. For example, after a general or dynamic

Safety Recommendations for Resistance Training

- Review participants' HRA before they begin resistance training.
- Select appropriate starting weights and exercises.
- Provide adequate supervision and instruction when necessary.
- Regularly practice emergency procedures.
- Encourage participation in warm-up and cool-down activities.
- Move carefully around the resistance training area, and don't back up without looking first.
- Place an out-of-order sign on broken or malfunctioning equipment and take the necessary steps to ensure that this equipment is not used by any client until it is completely repaired.
- Use collars on all plate-loaded barbells and dumbbells.
- Be aware of proper spotting procedures and offer assistance when needed.
- Model appropriate behavior and do not allow horseplay in the fitness center.
- Demonstrate correct exercise technique and do not allow participants to train improperly.
- Periodically check all resistance training equipment.
- Ensure the training environment is free of clutter and appropriately maintained.
- Stay up to date with current resistance training guidelines and safety procedures for special populations.

warm-up, a lifter could perform a light set of 10 repetitions on the bench press before performing the training set with a heavier weight. It makes sense to physically and mentally prepare for the demands of resistance training by spending a few minutes warming up. After a resistance workout, it's a good idea to cool down with general calisthenics and static stretching exercises. A cool-down may reduce the risk of cardiovascular issues (e.g., low BP).

KEY POINT

Qualified supervision and instruction, a safe training environment, sensible training loads, and adherence to established training guidelines will help minimize the risk of injury during resistance training. Fitness professionals should educate participants about safe training procedures and design programs that are consistent with each person's needs and abilities. Warm-up and cool-down activities can enhance performance and reduce the likelihood of muscle stiffness and injury.

Resistance Training Guidelines

Although fitness and sports medicine organizations recognize the importance of resistance training for health and fitness, there has been debate regarding training variables (e.g., sets, repetitions, weight lifted) and program design. Yet, despite various claims about the best training approach, there does not appear to be one optimal combination of sets, repetitions, and exercises that promotes long-term adaptations in muscular fitness for all people. Rather, many program variables may be altered to achieve desirable outcomes provided that the tenets of resistance exercise are followed. Clearly, resistance training programs need to be individualized and based on a person's training history and personal goals.

There are many factors to consider when designing a resistance training program, including the following (32, 78):

- Choice of exercise
- Order of exercise
- Resistance used
- Training volume (total number of sets and repetitions)
- Rest intervals between sets and exercises
- Repetition velocity
- Training frequency

Summary of ACSM's Resistance Training Guidelines for Healthy Adults

- Perform multijoint or compound exercises that involve more than one muscle group.
- Train each muscle group for 2 to 4 sets.
- Choose a resistance that allows 8 to 12 repetitions per set (60%-80% 1RM).
- A reasonable rest interval between sets is 2 to 3 min.
- Perform each exercise in a controlled manner with proper technique during the concentric and eccentric phases of the repetition.
- Perform each set to the point of muscle fatigue but not failure.
- Maintain a regular breathing pattern that typically involves exhaling during the lifting phase and inhaling during the lowering phase.
- Train each major muscle group 2 or 3 nonconsecutive days per wk.
- Periodically assess muscular strength so that a proper resistance is selected for each set.
- Progressively overload the muscles to create a greater training stimulus if continued gains in muscular fitness are desired.
- Seek instruction from a qualified fitness professional on proper exercise technique and program design.

Adapted from American College of Sports Medicine 2014, *ACSM's guidelines for exercise testing and prescription*, 9th ed. (Philadelphia: PA: Lippincott, Williams, & Wilkins).

By varying one or more of these variables, endless resistance training programs can be designed. But because different people will respond differently to the same resistance training program, decisions must be based on an understanding of exercise science, individual needs, and personal goals. The ACSM's guidelines are summarized in the sidebar *Summary of ACSM's Resistance Training Guidelines for Healthy Adults*.

Choice of Exercise

A limitless number of exercises can be used to enhance muscular strength, power, and local muscular endurance (78, 101). Selected exercises should be appropriate for a participant's exercise experience and training goals. Also, the choice of exercises should promote muscle balance across joints and between opposing muscle groups (e.g., quadriceps and hamstrings). Selected weight-machine and free-weight exercises and the primary muscle groups strengthened are listed in table 13.3.

Exercises generally can be classified as single joint (i.e., body-part specific) or multijoint (i.e., structural). Dumbbell biceps curls and leg extensions are examples of single-joint exercises that isolate a specific body part (biceps and quadriceps, respectively), whereas squats and deadlifts are multijoint exercises that involve two or more primary joints. Exercises also can be classified as closed kinetic chain or open kinetic chain. Closed-chain exercises are those in which the distal joint segment is stationary (e.g., squats), whereas open-chain exercises are those in which the terminal joint is free to move (e.g., leg extensions). Closed-chain exercises more closely mimic everyday activities and include more functional movement patterns (52).

Single-joint exercises and many machine exercises are often used by people who have limited experience resistance training or who simply enjoy this mode of training. This mode is also beneficial in activating specific muscles (e.g., during injury rehabilitation). With most machines, the path of movement is fixed and therefore the movement is stabilized. Conversely, exercises with free weights require additional muscles to stabilize the movement and are therefore more challenging. Also, dual-limb exercises with free weights (e.g., dumbbell lateral raises) may be particularly beneficial for people who need to strengthen a weaker limb. It is important to incorporate multijoint or compound exercises (e.g., leg press, squat, chest press) into a resistance training program to promote the coordinated use of multijoint movements.

The performance of single- and multijoint exercises on unstable surfaces (e.g., stability balls and wobble boards) has become popular in fitness centers. This type of training has been found to increase core activation and improve balance as well functional performance in recreationally active people (12). Although a multitude of exercises can be performed under a variety of conditions, when participants learn a new exercise they should start with a light weight so that they can master the technique before adding weight. Regardless of the exercise type, the concentric and eccentric phases of each lift should be performed in a controlled manner with proper technique.

Another issue concerning choice of exercise is including exercises for abdominal and low-back musculature. It is not uncommon for beginners to focus on strengthening the chest and biceps and not spend enough time strengthening their abdominal muscles and low back. Strengthening the midsection not only may improve force output and enhance body control during free-weight exercises such as the squat, it also may decrease the incidence of LBP (50, 105). Thus, prehabilitation exercises for the low-back and abdominal muscles should be included in all resistance training programs. In other words, as a preventive health

Table 13.3 Selected Weight-Machine and Free-Weight Exercises and the Primary Muscle Groups Strengthened

Weight-machine exercise	Free-weight exercise	Primary muscle groups strengthened
Leg press	Barbell squat	Quadriceps, gluteus maximus
Leg extension	Dumbbell lunge	Quadriceps
Leg curl	Barbell standing hip extension	Hamstrings
Chest press	Barbell bench press	Pectoralis major
Pec deck	Dumbbell fly	Pectoralis major
Front pull-down	Dumbbell pullover	Latissimus dorsi
Seated rows	Dumbbell one-arm row	Latissimus dorsi
Overhead press	Dumbbell press	Deltoids
Biceps curl	Barbell curl	Biceps
Triceps extension	Lying triceps extension	Triceps

A description of the proper exercise technique for each exercise is available in the appendix of this chapter.

measure, exercises that may be prescribed for the rehabilitation of an injury should be performed even though no injury is present. Exercises such as abdominal curl-ups and back extensions are useful, but they only train the muscles that control trunk flexion and extension. Multidirectional exercises that involve rotational movements and diagonal patterns performed with body weight or a medicine ball on a stable or unstable surface can strengthen the abdominal muscles and lower back. Depending on the needs and goals of the person, other prehabilitation exercises (e.g., internal and external rotation for the rotator cuff) can be incorporated into the exercise session.

Order of Exercise

The order of resistance exercises within a training session may influence the safety and effectiveness of the exercise program (94). Traditionally, exercises for large muscle groups are performed before exercises for smaller muscle groups, and multijoint exercises are performed before single-joint exercises. Following this order will allow participants to use heavier weights on the multijoint exercises because fatigue will be less of a factor. It is also helpful to perform more challenging exercises earlier in the workout when the neuromuscular system is less fatigued. However, in some cases (e.g., injury prevention or rehabilitation), it may be appropriate to reverse this order so that the smaller muscle groups are trained first. In general, it seems reasonable to follow the priority system of training in which the exercise order is dictated by the goals of the training program. Also, participants should perform power exercises such as plyometrics before strength exercises so that they can train for maximal power without undue fatigue. A sample resistance training program is illustrated in the Weekly Resistance Training Log (form 13.1).

Resistance Used

One of the most important variables in designing a resistance training program is the amount of weight used for an exercise (5, 32,). Gains in muscular fitness and performance are influenced by the amount of weight lifted, which is highly dependent upon program variables such as exercise order, training volume, repetition velocity, and rest-interval length (5, 32). By definition, the amount of weight that can be lifted with proper technique for only 1 repetition is the 1-repetition maximum (1RM). Similarly, the amount of weight that can be lifted with proper technique for 10 but not 11 repetitions is the 10RM. To maximize gains in muscular fitness while minimizing the risk of injury or residual muscle soreness, training sets should be performed with proper exercise technique to the point of muscular fatigue but not failure (6).

The use of RM loads is a relatively simple method to prescribe resistance training intensity. Research studies suggest that RM loads of 6 or fewer have the greatest effect on developing muscle strength, whereas RM loads of 15 to 20 or more have the greatest effect on developing local muscular endurance (16, 32). Although untrained people can make significant gains in muscle strength with lighter loads, people with resistance training experience need to train with a heavier resistance to optimize training adaptations (5, 82). ACSM recommends a repetition range between 8 and 12 to enhance muscle strength and local muscular endurance (see figure 13.7) (6). This repetition range translates to a training intensity of approximately

FORM 13.1 Weekly Resistance Training Log

Date	10/23			10/25			10/27			
Name ________________	Wt (lb)	Rep	Set	Wt (lb)	Rep	Set	Wt (lb)	Rep	Set	Comments
Leg press	150	10	2	150	11	2	150	12	2	
Leg curl	55	10	2	55	11	2	55	12	2	
Chest press	80	10	2	80	11	2	80	12	2	
Lat pull-down	80	10	2	80	11	2	80	12	2	
Biceps curl	30	10	2	30	11	2	30	11	2	
Triceps extension	40	10	2	40	11	2	40	12	2	Slight soreness in triceps
Kneeling trunk extension	No wt	10	2	No wt	11	2	No wt	12	2	
Abdominal curl	No wt	10	2	No wt	11	2	No wt	11	2	

From E.T. Howley and D.L. Thompson, 2017, *Fitness professional's handbook*, 7th ed. (Champaign, IL: Human Kinetics).

60% to 80% 1RM. However, deconditioned exercisers should start at a lower intensity with more repetitions (i.e., 10 to 15) to reduce the risk of a musculotendinous injury. Using weights that exceed a person's 6RM capacity minimally affects local muscular endurance, whereas training with very light weights (e.g., above 20RM) results in only small gains in maximal muscle strength. Each repetition zone (i.e., 3 to 6, 8 to 12, 15 to 20) has advantages, so the best approach for people with resistance training experience is to systematically vary the resistance used in order to avoid training plateaus and to optimize training adaptations (5, 14).

A percentage of a person's 1RM also can be used to determine the resistance training intensity. If the 1RM on the chest press is 100 lb (45 kg), a training intensity of 70% would be 70 lb (32 kg). It is reasonable for beginners to use a training resistance of approximately 60% to 70% 1RM because they are mostly improving motor performance at this stage (5). As participants get stronger and gain training experience, heavier resistances (~80% 1RM) will be needed to optimize gains in muscular strength and local muscular endurance (5, 76). Obviously, this method of prescribing resistance exercise requires testing the 1RM on all exercises in the training program. In many cases this is not realistic because of the time required to correctly perform 1RM testing on 8 to 10 exercises. Furthermore, maximal resistance testing for small-muscle-group exercises (e.g., biceps curls and lying triceps extensions) typically is not performed.

Fitness professionals should also be knowledgeable about the relationship between the percentage of 1RM and the number of repetitions that can be performed. In general, most people can perform about 10 repetitions using 75% of their 1RM. However, the number of repetitions that can be performed at a given percentage of the 1RM varies with the amount of muscle mass required to perform the exercise. For example, studies have shown that at a given percentage of the 1RM (e.g., 60%), adults can perform more repetitions of an exercise for large muscle groups such as the squat or leg press compared with an exercise for smaller muscle groups such as the arm curl or leg curl (51, 91). Therefore, prescribing a resistance training intensity of 70% of 1RM on all exercises warrants additional consideration because at 70% of the 1RM, a person may be able to perform 20 or more repetitions on a large-muscle-group exercise, which may not be ideal for enhancing muscle strength. If a percentage of the 1RM is used for prescribing resistance training, the prescribed percentage of the 1RM for each exercise may need to vary to maintain a desired training range (e.g., 8RM-10RM). Further, because self-

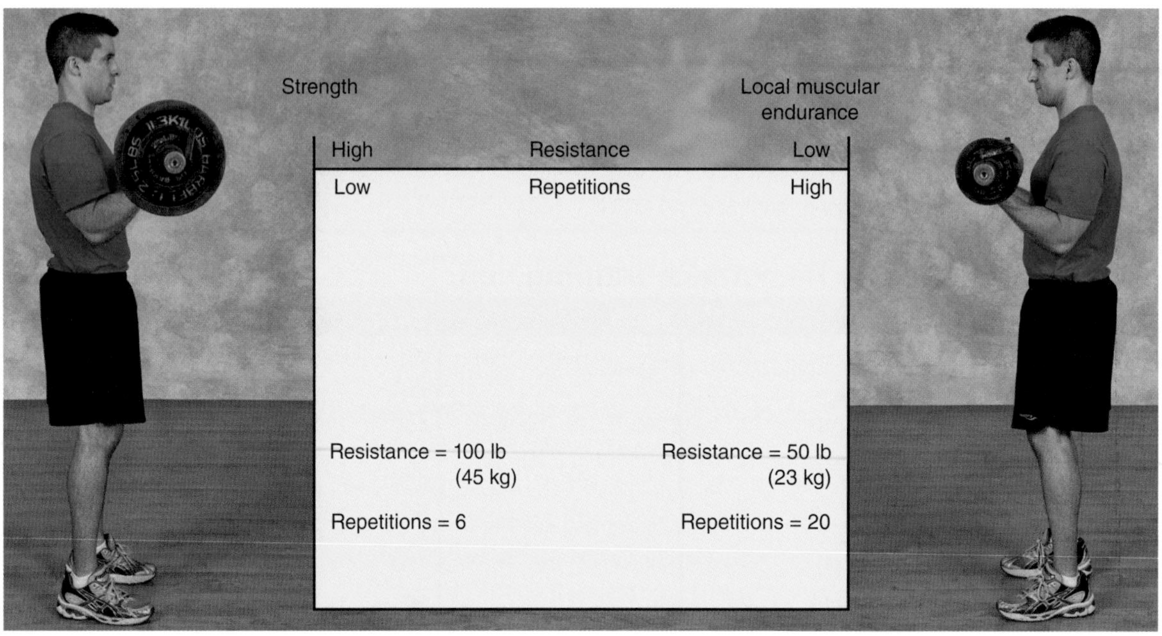

FIGURE 13.7 The strength–endurance continuum. The use of heavy weights and low repetitions has the greatest effect on strength and power, whereas the use of light weights and high repetitions has the greatest effect on local muscular endurance.

selected resistance exercise intensities tend to be lower than what is recommended (41, 79, 100), fitness professionals need to carefully prescribe the amount of weight used for each exercise to maximize training adaptations.

Training Volume

The number of exercises performed per session, the repetitions performed per set with a given weight, and the number of sets performed per exercise all influence the training volume (5). For example, if a participant performs 3 sets of 10 repetitions with 100 lb (45 kg) on the bench press, the training volume for this exercise is 3,000 lb ($3 \cdot 10 \cdot 100 = 3{,}000$), or 1,361 kg. Altering the training volume can influence neural, hypertrophic, metabolic, and hormonal responses and adaptations to resistance training (5, 69). Although there has been much discussion regarding training volume, it is important to remember that every training session does not need to be characterized by the same number of sets, repetitions, weights, and exercises.

ACSM recommends that apparently healthy adults train each major muscle group with 2 to 4 sets to improve muscular strength and power (6). These sets may be for the same exercise or for different exercises affecting the same muscle group. Although training programs with 1 set per exercise may be appropriate for beginners, the results of meta-analytical studies have found that multiple-set resistance training protocols are superior to single-set protocols for strength and power enhancement in untrained and trained populations (36, 56, 72, 82).

When fitness professionals design a resistance training program, they need to consider the person's training status and goals because of the numerous possibilities for program design. It seems reasonable for beginners and very deconditioned people to start with a single-set program of 10 to 15 repetitions of moderate intensity and gradually increase the number of sets depending on personal goals and time available for training. A single-set protocol reduces training time and may therefore increase the likelihood for exercise compliance in people who do not train regularly. However, it is also possible that a multiple-set protocol can be a time-efficient method of training. For example, instead of performing 1 set for each of 12 exercises during every workout, participants can perform 2 sets for each of 6 exercises or 3 sets for each of 4 exercises. With a careful selection of multijoint exercises, all muscle groups can be trained each exercise session regardless of the number of sets or exercises performed.

Nonetheless, it is important to point out that a dramatic increase in training intensity or volume may increase the risk of overtraining. By gradually varying the sets, repetitions, and number of exercises, the training stimulus will remain effective and therefore the adaptations to the training program will be maximized. Periods of low-volume or single-set training can provide a needed variation for people who have been participating in a high-volume or multiple-set conditioning program for a prolonged time.

Rests Between Sets and Exercises

The rest interval between sets and exercises is an important training variable that affects the acute responses and chronic adaptations to resistance training (21). In general, the length of the rest influences energy recovery and the training adaptations that take place. For example, if the primary goal of the program is to increase muscular strength, heavier weights and longer rests (e.g., 2-3 min) are needed, whereas if the goal is local muscular endurance, lighter weights and shorter rests (e.g., <1 min) are required. Obviously, training intensity, training goals, and fitness level will influence the length of the rest interval. For example, it has been shown that the number of repetitions performed is compromised with short rest intervals (<1 min), whereas performance can be maintained during a multiset protocol when 3 and 5 min rest intervals are used (80). As previously noted for the other program variables, the same rest interval does not need to be used between all sets and exercises. In addition, fatigue resulting from a previous exercise should be considered when prescribing the rest interval. In general, resting 2 to 3 min between sets is recommended for exercises with heavier loads, although for assistance exercises a shorter rest interval of 1 to 2 min may suffice (5). Short rests (<30 sec between sets and exercises) are not recommended for beginners because of the discomfort and high blood lactate concentrations (10-14 $\text{mmol} \cdot \text{L}^{-1}$) associated with this type of training (55). However, the rests can be shortened gradually over time to provide ample opportunity for the body to tolerate increased muscle and blood acid levels. For example, circuit training is a type of conditioning that is characterized by relatively short rest intervals between exercise stations.

Repetition Velocity

The velocity or cadence at which a resistance exercise is performed can affect the neural, hypertrophic, and metabolic adaptations to a training program (5, 78). According to the principle of training specificity, gains in muscle strength and performance are specific to the training velocity (32). For example, fast-velocity plyometric training is more likely to enhance speed and power than are slow-velocity exercises on weight machines. However, it is useful to recognize two types of slow-velocity training. *Unintentional* slow velocities are used when a heavy resistance is lifted and the velocity is slow despite the attempt to exert maximal force. On the other hand, *intentional* slow velocities are used when a person trains with a submaximal load and purposefully performs the exercise at a slow velocity. Increasing time under tension with intentionally slow velocities results in greater fatigue and less muscle fiber activation (48). Given that concentric force production is lower for an intentionally slower velocity compared with a moderate velocity, lighter loads performed at an intentionally slow velocity may not be optimal for maximizing strength development (53).

Because beginners need to learn how to perform each exercise correctly with a light resistance, it is generally recommended that untrained people perform exercises in a deliberately controlled manner (6). As they gain experience, they may use unintentional slow velocities with a heavier resistance to optimize strength gains. Of interest, the intent to maximally accelerate the weight during training is essential for maximizing strength gains in trained people (78). This concept has been termed *compensatory acceleration* and requires the trained person to accelerate the weight maximally throughout the concentric phase of the lift (78). Therefore, participants with resistance training experience can perform a continuum of velocities, from unintentionally slow to fast, in order to maximize performance adaptations.

Training Frequency

Training frequency typically refers to the number of training sessions per week. In general, a training frequency of 2 to 3 sessions per wk on nonconsecutive days is recommended (6). This training frequency allows for adequate recovery between sessions (48-72 hr between sessions) and has proven to be effective for enhancing muscle strength and local muscular endurance (32). However, trained people who perform more advanced programs may need more time between sessions (82, 83). Factors such as training volume, training intensity, exercise selection, sleep habits, and nutritional intake may influence the ability to recover from and adapt to the training program. For example, trained people who perform a split routine may resistance train 4 times per wk, but they only train each muscle group 2 times per wk; they might train muscles of the lower body on Monday and Thursday and muscles of the upper body on Tuesday and Friday. Although an increase in training experience does not necessitate an increase in training frequency, a higher frequency does allow for greater specialization characterized by more exercises and a higher weekly training volume.

Periodization

Periodization refers to systematic variation in a resistance training program. It is impossible to continually improve at the same rate over long-term training, but properly varying the training variables can limit training plateaus, maximize performance gains, manage fatigue, and reduce the likelihood of overtraining. Periodization is a process whereby fitness professionals regularly change the training stimulus in order to keep it effective. Although periodization has been part of program design for many years, the benefits of periodized programs compared with nonperiodized programs for long-term progression continue to be explored in the literature (5, 14, 45).

The concept of periodization, or program variation, is not just for athletes but for people with all levels of training experience who want to enhance their health and fitness. By periodically varying program variables such as choice of exercise, training weight (resistance), number of sets, rest intervals between sets, or any combination of these, long-term performance gains will be optimized and the risk of overuse injuries may be reduced (5, 14). Moreover, it is reasonable to suggest that people who participate in well-designed periodized programs and continue to improve their health and fitness may be more likely to adhere to an exercise program over the long term.

For example, if a person's lower-body routine typically consists of leg presses, leg extensions, and leg curls, performing step-ups and dumbbell lunges on alternate workout days will likely add to the effectiveness and enjoyment of the resistance training program. Further, varying the volume and intensity of training can help to prevent training plateaus, which are common after the first 2 mo of training. Many times participants can avoid a strength plateau by varying the training intensity and volume to allow for ample recovery. In the long term, program variation with adequate recovery will result in even greater gains because the body will be challenged to adapt to even greater demands. The underlying concept of periodization is based on the theory that, after a certain time, adaptations to a stimulus will no longer take place unless the stimulus is altered. Periodized resistance training has been shown to be superior to nonperiodized resistance training for promoting long-term training adaptations in strength and power (45, 83), and therefore fitness professionals should not underestimate the importance of training variety to keep the stimulus challenging and effective.

Although there are many models of periodization, the general concept is to prioritize training goals and then develop a long-term plan that varies throughout the year. In general, the overall training plan is divided into time periods called **macrocycles** (about 1 yr), **mesocycles** (3-4 mo), and **microcycles** (1-4 wk), with each cycle having a specific goal (e.g., hypertrophy, strength, or power). The classic periodization model is referred to as a *linear model* because the volume and intensity of training gradually change over time (99). For example, at the start of a macrocycle, the training volume may be high and the training intensity may be low. As the year progresses, the volume decreases as the intensity increases.

Although the linear training model was originally designed for weightlifters and track and field athletes who wanted to peak for a specific competition, it can be modified by fitness professionals in order to enhance health and fitness. For example, people who routinely perform the same combination of sets and repetitions may benefit from gradually increasing the weight and decreasing the number of repetitions as strength improves. The classic periodized model is outlined in table 13.4. After the four-phase program is complete, people should be encouraged to participate in recreational activities or low-intensity resistance training to reduce the likelihood of overtraining. This period of restoration is called *active rest* and typically lasts for 1 to 3 wk. After active rest, participants can then return to the first phase of their training program with more energy and vigor.

A second model of periodization is referred to as an *undulating (nonlinear) model* because of the daily fluctuations in training volume and intensity. For example, a person may perform 2 sets of 10 repetitions with a moderate load on Monday, 3 sets of 6 repetitions with a heavy load on Wednesday, and 1 set of 15 repetitions with a light load on Friday. The heavy training days will maximally activate the trained musculature, and selected muscle fibers will not be maximally taxed on light and moderate training days. By alternating training intensities, the participant can minimize the risk of overtraining and maximize the potential for maintaining training-induced strength gains. A sample nonlinear periodized workout plan for a trained adult is presented in table 13.5. In addition, fitness professionals should consider a participant's vacation schedule or travel plans when incorporating active rest into the year-long training schedule. Periods of restoration lasting from 1 to 3 wk will allow for physical and psychological recovery from the resistance training. A detailed review of periodization and specific examples of periodized programs are available elsewhere (5, 14).

KEY POINT

Designing a safe and effective resistance training program involves an understanding of exercise science along with an appreciation of the art of prescribing exercise. The specific exercises, the order of exercises, the resistance used, the number of sets, the rest intervals between sets and exercises, the training velocity, and the training frequency are variables that contribute to the design of a resistance training program. Periodization is the systematic variation of program variables to optimize long-term training adaptations.

Table 13.4 Sample Linear Periodized Workout for Maximizing Strength Gains in Healthy Adults

	Phase 1 General preparation	Phase 2 Hypertrophy	Phase 3 Strength	Phase 4 Peaking
Intensity	12RM-15RM	8RM-12RM	6RM-8RM	4RM-6RM
Sets	1-2	2	2-3	3
Rest between sets	60-120 sec	60 sec	60-120 sec	120-180 sec

The workout is for major-muscle-group exercises performed each phase; each phase lasts about 6 to 8 wk. RM = repetition maximum.

Table 13.5 Sample Nonlinear Periodized Workout for a Trained Adult

	Monday	Wednesday	Friday
Intensity	8RM-10RM	4RM-6RM	13RM-15RM
Sets	2	3	3
Rest between sets and exercises	2 min	3 min	1 min

This plan is for the major-muscle-group exercises performed each day.

RESEARCH INSIGHT

Effectiveness of Periodization Models

Although participation in a periodized resistance training program can enhance training adaptations, it is unclear which approach to muscular strength development is the most effective. Harries and colleagues (45) used meta-analytical techniques to combine and evaluate the treatment effects from 17 studies that directly compared linear and undulating periodized resistance training programs. The analyses determined there were no differences in the effectiveness of linear versus undulating periodization on upper- or lower-body strength, although the short-term nature of most training studies should be considered when evaluating these data. These findings indicate that program variation and novelty are important for optimizing resistance training adaptations, but there does not appear to be one optimal combination of program variables for all clients.

Resistance Training Systems

Many resistance training systems can be used to enhance muscular fitness. Some systems have been scientifically proven to be effective, whereas others are based on anecdotal evidence. The wide variety of systems illustrates the types of programs that can be developed by manipulating program variables. Five of the most common resistance training systems are the single-set system, multiple-set system, circuit training system, preexhaustion system, and assisted training system.

Single-Set System

This system of resistance training is one of the oldest and consists of performing a single set of a predetermined number of repetitions (e.g., 8 to 12) until volitional fatigue. This time-efficient method of resistance training can be an effective method for people who have no resistance training experience or who have not trained for several years. Because the acute adaptations to resistance training (i.e., 6 to 12 wk) are primarily due to neuromuscular adaptations (32), a single-set system can be an appropriate method of training for beginners or very deconditioned people.

Multiple-Set System

The multiple-set system is an effective training method for enhancing strength and power. This system of training became popular in the 1940s and originally consisted of 3 sets of 10 repetitions with increasing weights. For example, the classic multiple-set protocol used by DeLorme in his pioneering rehabilitation work involved performing the first set of 10 repetitions at 50% of 10RM, the second set of 10 repetitions at 75% of 10RM, and the third set of 10 repetitions at 100% of 10RM (22). Over the years, many multiple-set programs using various combinations of sets and repetitions have been shown to be effective. For example, the pyramid system is a multiple-set system in which the weight increases progressively over several sets so that fewer and fewer repetitions can be performed (see table 13.6). For continued progression in a resistance training program, multiple sets should be used. However, in order to reduce the risk of overtraining, the total number of sets performed per training session should gradually increase. In addition, not all exercises need to be performed for the same number of sets.

Table 13.6 Sample Light-to-Heavy Pyramid Training System

Set number	Repetitions	Intensity (%1RM)
1	10	75
2	8	80
3	6	85

Circuit Training System

This system of training involves performing a series of resistance exercises in a circuit with minimal rest (about 30 sec) between exercises (see figure 13.8). Generally, moderate weights are used (about 60% of 1RM), and 10 to 15 repetitions are performed at each exercise station. In addition to increasing muscular strength and local muscular endurance, circuit training also can improve CRF. However, gains in maximal oxygen consumption resulting from aerobic training are greater than those resulting from circuit training. Starting with a 1 min rest between exercises and gradually reducing the rest to the desired range as the body adapts is recommended when a person is beginning circuit training. A sample circuit training program is illustrated in figure 13.8

Preexhaustion System

This training method consists of performing successive sets of two exercises for the same target muscle or muscle group. For example, after performing a set to volitional fatigue on the bench press, the participant immediately performs a set of dumbbell flys to facilitate chest development. This type of training forces the target muscle group (e.g., pectoralis major) to work longer and harder and is often used to increase muscle hypertrophy.

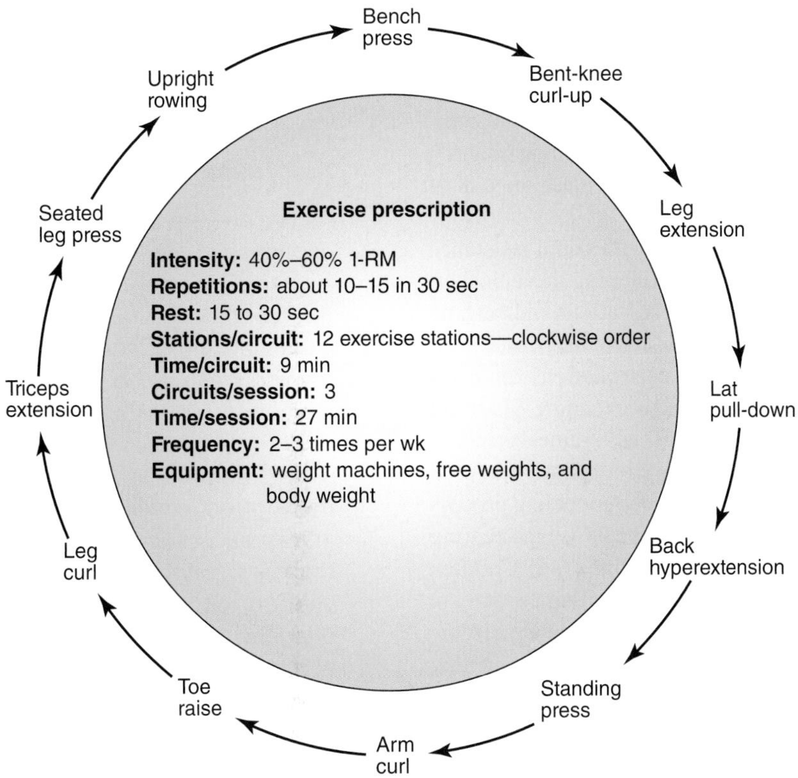

FIGURE 13.8 Sample program for circuit resistance training.

Adapted, by permission, from V.H. Heyward, 2014, *Advanced fitness assessment and exercise prescription*, 7th ed. (Champaign, IL: Human Kinetics), 189.

Assisted Training System

As the name implies, this method of training requires the assistance of another person who, after several repetitions of an exercise are performed to volitional fatigue, can provide just enough assistance to allow the lifter to complete 2 to 3 additional repetitions. Because muscles are stronger eccentrically than concentrically, assistance may not be needed during the eccentric phase of the forced repetitions. Although this advanced training system will enhance muscular fitness, it is not recommended for beginners because it typically results in muscle soreness attributable to the reliance on heavy eccentric muscle actions. Other training systems also may result in some muscle soreness, but assisted training increases the likelihood that soreness will result.

KEY POINT

A variety of resistance training systems can be used to enhance strength, power, and local muscular endurance. Although all training systems can be effective, the key is to match the system with the needs, goals, and abilities of each participant for long-term success. The resistance training system will influence the training-induced adaptations that take place.

Resistance Training for Special Populations

Resistance training can be a safe, effective, and beneficial method of conditioning for men and women of all ages and physical abilities. Although research on resistance training has focused predominantly on healthy adults, a growing body of evidence indicates that children, seniors, pregnant women, and people with certain chronic but stable conditions (e.g., high BP, diabetes, CHD) can participate safely in resistance training provided that appropriate training guidelines are followed.

Children

Despite previous concerns that children would not benefit from resistance training because of inadequate levels of circulating androgens, studies clearly demonstrate that boys and girls can benefit from resistance training (13, 28, 58). ACSM (6), CSEP (11), and the NSCA (29) support children's participation in resistance training provided that the program is appropriately designed and supervised. Furthermore, public health recommendations support regular participation in muscle-strengthening activities for children (103, 110). In addition to increasing muscular strength and power, regular participation in a resistance training program may favorably influence several measurable indexes of health, including body composition, BMD, and metabolic risk factors (29, 96). Further, because many aspiring young athletes who enter sport programs may not be prepared for the demands of training and competition, participation in a preseason conditioning program that includes resistance training may decrease the risk of sport-related injuries (67, 86).

A traditional concern associated with youth resistance training is that it may harm the developing musculoskeletal system. However, current observations indicate no evidence of a decrease in stature in young people who participate in resistance training in controlled environments (28, 60). In fact, the belief that resistance training is harmful to the immature skeleton of young weight trainers is inconsistent with current findings suggesting that childhood may be the time during which the bone-modeling process responds best to the mechanical loading of weight-bearing physical activities such as resistance training (43). Children and adolescents are now encouraged to participate daily in 60 min or more of physical activity that includes aerobic activities as well as age-appropriate muscle-strengthening and bone-strengthening activities (103, 110). Because a certain level of muscular strength is needed to perform fundamental movement skills such as jumping and throwing, the importance of resistance training during childhood should not be overlooked when designing youth fitness programs (27, 67).

Another corollary of youth resistance training is its influence on body composition. As the number of overweight young people in the United States and other countries continues to increase (20, 70), the effect of resistance training on body composition has received increased attention (88). Although aerobic exercise is typically prescribed for decreasing body fatness, researchers have reported that resistance training may be beneficial for treating children who are overweight (62, 89, 92). Of interest is the finding that progressive resistance training has been found to significantly increase insulin sensitivity in overweight youth (90, 104) and positively influence the self-concept of overweight and obese adolescent boys (89). It appears that young people who are overweight enjoy resistance training because it is not aerobically taxing and it gives all participants a chance to experience success and feel good about their performance. Further study is warranted, but the first step in encouraging these youth to exercise may be to increase their confidence in their ability to be physically active, which in turn may lead to an increase in physical activity and a decrease in body fat.

Although there is no minimum age requirement for participating in a youth resistance training program, all children who participate should have the emotional maturity to accept and follow directions and understand the benefits and risks associated with this type of training. In general, if children are ready for organized sport, then they are ready for some type of resistance training. As a point of reference, many 7- and 8-yr-old boys and girls have participated in closely supervised resistance training programs. Although some observers may be concerned about the stress that resistance training places on the developing musculoskeletal system, the sport-specific forces placed on the joints of children may be greater in both duration and magnitude than those resulting from moderate-intensity resistance training. Further, injury to the epiphyseal plate or growth cartilage has not been reported in any prospective study on youth resistance training (28). Nevertheless, fitness professionals should follow age-related training guidelines to decrease the likelihood of an accident or injury when young people perform resistance exercises (30).

Children should begin resistance training at a level that is commensurate with their physical abilities. No matter how big or strong a child is, adult training programs and philosophies (e.g., "No pain, no gain") should not be imposed on children. The focus of youth resistance training should be on learning proper technique for a variety of exercises. During each session, fitness professionals should listen to each child's concerns and closely monitor each child's ability to handle the prescribed training weight. Various combinations of sets and repetitions and a variety of training modes from child-sized weight machines to body-weight exercises have proven to be effective (30, 58). Although several combinations of exercises, sets, and repetitions have proven to be effective (58), ACSM recommends that children perform 8 to 15 repetitions of a variety of exercises that use all the major muscle groups (6).

RESEARCH INSIGHT

Benefits of Aerobic and Resistance Training in Obese Adolescents

As the prevalence of obesity among youth continues to increase worldwide, effective strategies are needed to treat and manage this condition. Sigal and colleagues (92) examined the effects of 22 wk of aerobic training, resistance training, or combined training in previously inactive adolescents who were obese. Following the training period, aerobic, resistance, and combined training reduced total body fat and WC in obese adolescents. In participants with the best adherence to the exercise intervention, combined training appeared to offer the greatest benefit. These findings demonstrate that interventions that include resistance training may be most beneficial for youth who are sedentary and obese.

When working with children, remember that the goal of the program should not be limited to increasing muscle strength. Teaching children about their bodies and promoting a lifelong interest in physical activity are equally important. Consider the following guidelines for program design when developing resistance training programs for children:

- Parents or legal guardians should complete an HRA for each child.
- Children with diseases or disabilities should have their exercise program tailored to their condition, symptoms, and functional capacity.
- Qualified instructors should supervise youth fitness activities.
- The exercise area should be free of clutter and adequately ventilated.
- Children should use a light weight or a wooden dowel when learning a new exercise.
- Resistance should be increased only when the child can perform the desired number of repetitions with proper exercise technique.
- Two or three nonconsecutive training sessions per wk are recommended.
- Include a range of exercises that are designed to enhance muscular strength and motor skill competency.

Seniors

The number of men and women over the age of 65 in the United States is increasing (see chapter 17), and research studies and clinical observations indicate that seniors can benefit from exercise programs that include resistance training (4, 8, 93). Even people over the age of 90 can enhance their muscular fitness through resistance training (31). Regular participation in a resistance training program can help offset the age-related declines in bone, muscle mass, and strength that often make ADLs—such as climbing stairs—more difficult.

Further, structured physical activity programs that include resistance training may help reduce the risk of major mobility disability in seniors (71, 109). Bones become more fragile with age because of a decrease in bone mineral content that results in an increase in bone porosity (69). Advancing age also is associated with a loss of muscle mass, or sarcopenia, which generally includes a loss of both Type I (slow-twitch) and Type II (fast-twitch) fibers (4, 76). Evidence indicates that seniors who resistance train can improve muscle strength, muscle power, gait speed, and balance, which in turn can enhance overall function and reduce the potential for injuries caused by falls (33, 81, 98). Moreover, there is emerging evidence for significant psychological and cognitive benefits from regular exercise participation by older adults (4, 17, 57). Fitness professionals should educate seniors on the benefits of resistance training because a majority of adults do not participate regularly in strength-building activities (47, 59).

Seniors can adapt readily to resistance training exercises. If the training intensity is adequate, they can make relative gains in strength that are equal to or greater than those of younger people. Of interest is the observation that resistance training trials comparing training intensities show strong resistance training effects in a dose–response manner, with high-intensity training being more effective than moderate- and low-intensity training in seniors (98). Research studies using CT and muscle-biopsy analysis have also reported evidence of muscle hypertrophy in seniors who resistance train, and others have reported that resistance training can increase the RMR and BMD of older adults who resistance train (4, 31). Although both aerobic and resistance exercise are important for seniors, only resistance training can increase muscle strength and muscle mass. These potential benefits may be particularly important for seniors who are at increased risk for falls and osteoporotic fractures. However, adults will retain the beneficial effects of resistance training only as long as they continue their exercise program. During prolonged inactivity, adaptive changes in skeletal muscle strength and bone regress toward preexercise levels (25, 46). This is sometimes referred to as the **principle of reversibility**.

Before starting a resistance training program, seniors should undergo preparticipation health screening because many have a variety of known, coexisting medical conditions. In addition, at least during the initial phase of training, fitness professionals should provide instruction and offer assistance as needed. Older adults should begin resistance training at a light intensity (i.e., 40%-50% 1RM) during the first few weeks to allow time for musculoskeletal adaptation and to practice exercise technique (6). Over time, the intensity can gradually increase to 60% to 80% 1RM (6). People who are very frail may need to perform muscle-strengthening activities before aerobic training because of their physical limitations (6). Although there are no specific recommendations for neuromuscular training, exercises that combine balance, agility, and proprioceptive training can be effective in reducing and preventing falls in older adults (6). Over time, exercises that gradually reduce the base of support (e.g., tandem stand and one-legged stand), stress postural muscle groups (e.g., heel stands and toe stands), and reduce sensory input (standing with eyes closed) can be sensibly incorporated into senior training programs provided that qualified supervision and instruction are available (6). ACSM recommends the following program design considerations for seniors who want to resistance train (6):

- Perform ≥1 to 3 sets of 8 to 12 repetitions for each of 8 to 10 exercises involving the major muscle groups.
- Use a rating between moderate (5-6) and vigorous (7-8) on a scale of 0 to 10 for level of physical exertion.
- Maintain proper breathing patterns while exercising.
- Perform all exercises within a pain-free ROM.
- Individualize progression of all resistance training activities.
- Gradually incorporate balance, agility, and proprioceptive training into the exercise program.
- Resistance train at least 2 days per wk.
- Use behavioral strategies such as social support to enhance adherence.

RESEARCH INSIGHT

Qualified Supervision Enhances Fitness Gains in Seniors

Although many people resistance train at home, the extent to which home-based resistance exercise can improve muscular strength is unclear. Thiebaud and colleagues (100) systematically reviewed the literature to examine the effects of home-based resistance training on strength and functional ability in older adults (average age 76 yr). The researchers reported that home-based resistance training can improve muscular strength and functional ability, but the observed gains were generally small. Also, they noted that the more supervised research studies reported greater gains. The intensity of home-based resistance training programs may be below levels needed to optimize adaptations in older adults. Qualified supervision and instruction are needed to sensibly progress and properly modify resistance training programs.

Pregnant Women

Research evidence suggests that regular exercise during a low-risk pregnancy poses little risk to either the mother or the fetus and improves overall maternal fitness and well-being (2, 26, 66). Indeed, regular exercise may reduce the risk of developing conditions associated with pregnancy, including pregnancy-induced hypertension and gestational diabetes mellitus (23, 66, 75). Furthermore, regular exercise during pregnancy may influence psychological health, reducing feelings of depression, fatigue, and anxiety (39). Participation in a wide range of physical activities appears safe during and after pregnancy, but resistance training may be particularly beneficial because it enhances muscular fitness, which allows expectant mothers to perform ADLs with greater ease and possibly minimizes LBP, which is common during pregnancy (2, 38, 106). Along with moderate-intensity aerobic exercise, resistance training at an appropriate intensity, duration, and frequency may offer significant health value to women with an uncomplicated pregnancy.

Exercise is not advised for all women who are pregnant, especially those who have medical complications. Thus, pregnant women should undergo a medical evaluation with their personal physician or qualified medical care provider and ask about activities that may or may not be appropriate during pregnancy. The American College of Obstetricians and Gynecologists (ACOG) established the following absolute contraindications for exercise during pregnancy: hemodynamically significant heart disease, restrictive lung disease, incompetent cervix or cervical cerclage, multiple gestation at risk for premature labor, persistent second- to third-trimester bleeding, placenta previa after 26 wk of gestation, premature labor during the current pregnancy, ruptured membranes, and preeclampsia or pregnancy-induced hypertension (2).

Limited data are available regarding resistance training for pregnant women (9, 73, 74, 106). General guidelines for resistance training are outlined in this chapter, and recommendations for exercising while pregnant are discussed in chapter 18. General exercise recommendations include maintaining adequate hydration, wearing appropriate clothing, and exercising at a comfortable intensity. Also, because pregnancy requires an additional 300 kcal · day^{-1}, pregnant women who exercise should be particularly careful to maintain adequate calories and a well-balanced diet (2, 6).

The following ACSM program design considerations are appropriate for pregnant women who perform resistance training (6):

- Resistance train 2 to 3 nonconsecutive days a week.
- Perform multiple repetitions (i.e., 8 to 10 or 12 to 15) to the point of moderate fatigue.
- Perform 1 to 3 sets on exercises that target the major muscle groups.
- Gradually increase the weight as strength improves.
- Practice proper breathing patterns while resistance training.
- Perform Kegel exercises and others that strengthen the pelvic floor.
- Avoid isometric muscle actions and the Valsalva maneuver.

- Avoid exercise in the supine position after 16 wk of pregnancy.
- Avoid sports and activities that may cause a loss of balance or trauma to the mother or fetus.
- Exercise in a thermoneutral environment and stay hydrated.
- Stop exercise in the event of any discomfort or complications such as vaginal bleeding, dyspnea before exertion, dizziness, headache, chest pain, muscle weakness, calf pain or swelling, preterm labor, decreased fetal movement, or amniotic fluid leakage.
- Exercise in the postpartum period may begin about 4 to 6 wk after a normal vaginal delivery or about 8 to 10 wk (with medical clearance) after a cesarean section.

Adults With Heart Disease

CHD is a leading cause of morbidity and mortality, and patients with CHD typically have multiple risk factors. Secondary prevention programs are designed to not only control these risk factors but to improve exercise capacity, psychosocial well-being, and quality of life (65). Also, by preventing or delaying the progression of this disease, longevity is likely to increase and yearly health care costs are likely to decrease (33). Cardiac rehabilitation programs traditionally have emphasized aerobic exercise to maintain and improve CRF. However, muscular strength and local muscular endurance are also important to prepare the patient for return to work and leisure activities (33, 34, 108). Many ADLs, as well as most occupational tasks, place demands on the cardiovascular system that closely resemble resistance exercise. Because many cardiac patients are deconditioned and lack the strength and confidence to perform common activities involving muscular effort, adding resistance training to an overall physical activity program provides patients with an opportunity to restore or gain optimal physiologic, vocational, and psychosocial status. The AHA (108), ACSM (6), and AACVPR (1) recommend resistance training as part of a comprehensive cardiac rehabilitation program.

Research indicates that medically stable cardiac patients can safely engage in resistance training provided that the program is appropriately designed and carried out within the prescribed guidelines (1, 6, 108). Regular participation in a resistance training program may favorably affect muscular strength, local muscular endurance, cardiorespiratory endurance, cardiac risk factors, and psychosocial well-being. Training-induced gains in muscular strength also can decrease the rate–pressure product (and associated myocardial demands) during daily activities such as carrying groceries and gardening (7, 108). In general, improving physical fitness can improve a patient's quality of life and help older patients live independently.

Before patients begin a resistance training program, a qualified health care provider should review their health and medical history to identify any condition that may exclude participation. Although most low- to moderate-risk patients can safely participate in resistance training, programs for patients with low fitness levels or severe left ventricular dysfunction may be safer in a medically supervised environment. According to ACSM (6), contraindications for inpatient and outpatient cardiac rehabilitations include the following: unstable angina, resting SBP >180 mmHg or resting DBP >110 mmHg, orthostatic BP drop of 20 mmHg with symptoms, significant aortic stenosis, acute systemic illness or fever, uncontrolled atrial or ventricular arrhythmias, uncontrolled sinus tachycardia (>120 beats $\cdot$ min^{-1}), uncompensated CHF, third-degree AV block (without pacemaker), active pericarditis or myocarditis, recent embolism, acute thrombophlebitis, uncontrolled diabetes mellitus, severe orthopedic conditions, and other metabolic conditions such as thyroiditis or hypokalemia.

KEY POINT

Resistance training can be a safe and beneficial component of a comprehensive fitness program for people of all ages and those with medical conditions provided that appropriate guidelines are followed and qualified instruction is available. Despite previous concerns, children, seniors, pregnant women, and patients with heart disease can benefit from participation in a well-designed resistance training program. Participants should first be screened to identify those who may be contraindicated for resistance training, as determined by a qualified health care provider.

All patients entering cardiac rehabilitation should be considered for resistance training, particularly those who jobs involve manual labor (6). Although patients can use elastic bands and light weights (1-5 lb, or 0.5-2 kg) in a progressive fashion immediately upon entry into an outpatient program, consistent participation in a cardiac rehabilitation program should precede a traditional resistance training program in which patients lift weights corresponding to 40% to 60% 1RM for 10 to 15 repetitions for each exercise (6). ACSM recommends that patients perform 1 to 3 sets of 8 to 10 exercises that focus on the major muscle groups (6). Further, patients should maintain a regular breathing pattern and avoid sustained, tight gripping, which may evoke an excessive BP response. The decision to begin a resistance training program should be based on current health status as determined by a qualified health care provider. The guidelines for designing a resistance training program for cardiac patients are the same as those for older adults—namely, patients should start with a light weight and gradually progress as they adapt to the training program. For patients returning to work, exercise training should be specific to the muscle groups and energy systems used for occupational tasks in order to increase physical work capacity, improve safety, and enhance self-efficacy (6).

Overreaching and Overtraining

Fitness professionals need to balance the demands of training with adequate recovery between workouts in order to optimize training adaptations. A resistance training program characterized by an excessive frequency, volume, or intensity of training, combined with inadequate rest and recovery, eventually results in overtraining syndrome. In essence, overtraining syndrome may occur when the training stimulus exceeds the rate of adaptation. Overtraining syndrome typically includes a plateau or decrease in performance. Other observable manifestations of overtraining include decreased body weight, decreased appetite, sleep disturbances, decreased desire to train, muscle tenderness, and increased risk of infection (24, 64).

Overtraining on a short-term basis has become known as *overreaching* (64). Unlike overtraining syndrome, which can last for months, recovery from overreaching can occur within a few days. In fact, overreaching is sometimes a planned part of conditioning programs as participants train at higher volumes and intensities. Nevertheless, overreaching should be considered the first stage of overtraining and therefore warrants attention because not all people recover quickly from overreaching. Participants may need to decrease the intensity and volume of their training program to recover from overreaching.

A downfall of many fitness programs is not allowing adequate recovery between workouts. For example, if a person resistance trains on Monday, Wednesday, and Friday and jogs on Tuesday and Thursday, the repetitive forces placed on the lower body can injure muscles and connective tissue and decrease performance in the weight room and on the track. Overtraining can result from poor programming characterized by frequent training sessions without adequate rest and recovery between workouts. From a practical perspective, it is important to consider a person's training experience as well as all fitness activities regularly performed. Periodized resistance training, which should include periods of less intense training and active rest, can help to avoid overtraining and promote long-term gains in muscular fitness (14). In addition, lifestyle factors such as sensible nutrition, proper hydration, and adequate sleep can influence how people adapt to resistance training.

KEY POINT

Resistance training programs should be characterized by an appropriate overload and progression combined with planned periods of rest and recovery. Overreaching is often the first stage of the overtraining syndrome, which is characterized by a decrease in performance and other physical and psychological effects. Adequate rest and recovery between workouts can help to avoid overtraining syndrome.

Program Design for People With Heart Disease

- A physician or other qualified health care provider should review the health and medical history.
- Begin with a light weight and focus on controlled movements for 10 to 15 repetitions.
- Following initial adaptations, gradually increase the load to 40 to 60% 1 RM.
- Perform each exercise initially for 1 set and progress to 2 or 3 sets as tolerated.
- A perceived exertion rating of 11 to 13 on a scale of 6 to 20 may be used to guide effort.
- Include multijoint exercises that involve more than one muscle group.
- Progress slowly as the individual adapts to the training program.
- Train 2 to 3 times per wk on nonconsecutive days.
- Maintain regular breathing and avoid straining.
- Stop exercise in the event of any warning signs or symptoms such as dizziness, dysrhythmias, unusual shortness of breath, or anginal discomfort.

LEARNING AIDS

REVIEW QUESTIONS

1. What four training principles determine the effectiveness of resistance exercise programs?
2. Distinguish between isometric, concentric, eccentric, and isokinetic muscle actions.
3. What musculoskeletal, cardiorespiratory, and metabolic adaptations may result from resistance training in healthy adults?
4. List four resistance training systems that can enhance muscular fitness, and provide an example of each method.
5. What are the advantages and disadvantages of resistance training with weight machines, free weights, medicine balls, and body-weight exercises?
6. Discuss the benefits and concerns associated with youth resistance training.
7. What resistance exercises should pregnant women avoid after the first 16 wk?
8. What resistance training guidelines are appropriate for low-risk patients with CHD?
9. What resistance training system would be most appropriate for a deconditioned client, for a healthy adult who wants to enhance general fitness, and for a trained person who wants to increase muscle hypertrophy?

CASE STUDIES

1. A 25-yr-old member of your fitness center has been resistance training for 4 mo and claims to have made significant gains in strength. He performs 1 set of 12 to 15 repetitions on eight weight machines 2 days per wk. However, over the past 6 wk he's noticed that he isn't making the strength gains that he used to. His goal is to get stronger and increase his muscle mass. How would you modify his training program to optimize his desired gains in muscular fitness over the long term?
2. A 48-yr-old female currently swims for 45 to 60 min, 3 to 4 days per wk, at the local recreation center. Although she has been a swimmer for years, she was recently advised by her doctor to participate in weight-bearing physical activities to increase her musculoskeletal strength. She has no previous experience resistance training and is excited about incorporating this type of exercise into her training program. However, she is somewhat concerned about lifting heavy weights and doesn't want to get hurt. Address her concerns regarding resistance training and modify her current exercise program to optimize gains in musculoskeletal strength.
3. The director of a local assisted living center for seniors wants to offer a new activity class at the facility, and she asks you for guidance and recommendations. In addition to a walking program that is already established, she wants you to develop a proposal for a senior resistance training program that not only enhances muscular fitness, but is safe and enjoyable for men and women over 65 yr old who have no resistance training experience. The facility does not have weight machines, but it does have several pairs of lightweight (1-5 lb, or 0.5-2 kg) dumbbells and a variety of elastic bands. Comment on program design considerations for seniors that will enhance muscular fitness and reduce the risk of falling.

Answers to Case Studies

1. Because it is not possible to improve at the same rate over long-term training, it is important to vary the resistance training program over time to limit training plateaus and optimize adaptations. By periodically varying the program variables (e.g., choice

of exercise, sets, and repetitions), long-term performance gains will be optimized and exercise adherence will be improved. One option for this member is to follow an undulating or nonlinear training program, which is characterized by daily fluctuations in volume and intensity. For example, over time he could progress to 2 or 3 sets of 8 to 10 repetitions with a moderate load on Monday, 3 or 4 sets of 6 repetitions with a heavy load on Wednesday, and 1 or 2 sets of 12 to 15 repetitions with a light load on Friday. In addition, he should seek advice from a fitness professional and learn how to safely incorporate free-weight exercises and other training systems (e.g., preexhaustion and assisted training) into his program.

2. Although this client should be encouraged to continue swimming, resistance training can offer additional benefits in terms of musculoskeletal strength. A fitness professional should review the potential health and fitness benefits of regular weight-bearing physical activity with the client and should discuss the importance of proper exercise technique and a gradual progression of training weights to avoid injury. This client does not have any resistance training experience, so she should begin with a single set of 8 to 12 repetitions on a variety of single-joint and multijoint exercises to improve her confidence and exercise compliance. Over time, she should progress to a multiple-set system at a higher training intensity to optimize gains in musculoskeletal strength.
3. Regular resistance training can offer observable health and fitness benefits to older adults; however, the health status of seniors should be assessed before resistance training begins in order to identify any preexisting medical conditions. Also, fitness professionals who have experience working with older populations should be available to provide instruction and assistance as needed. General program design considerations to discuss with the director of this assisted living center include the following: (1) Resistance training should begin with minimal resistance during the first few weeks so participants can learn proper exercise technique and have time for musculoskeletal adaptation; (2) the resistance, repetitions, or number of sets should be gradually increased to maximize gains in muscular fitness; and (3) over time, exercises that reduce the base of support, stress postural muscle groups, and reduce sensory input should be sensibly incorporated into the program to enhance balance, agility, and proprioception. Further, the importance of exercising in a group setting should be emphasized because social support can enhance exercise adherence in older populations.

APPENDIX 13.1: SELECTED RESISTANCE TRAINING EXERCISES FOR THE MAJOR MUSCLE GROUPS

Leg Press

Prime muscle movers: Quadriceps, gluteus maximus

Exercise technique: The exerciser starts in a sitting position with the knees bent at 90° and the feet placed about shoulder-width apart on the foot pad. The torso should be erect and the back should be pressed against the back of the seat. The participant extends the legs almost completely (without locking the knees) and then slowly returns to the starting position.

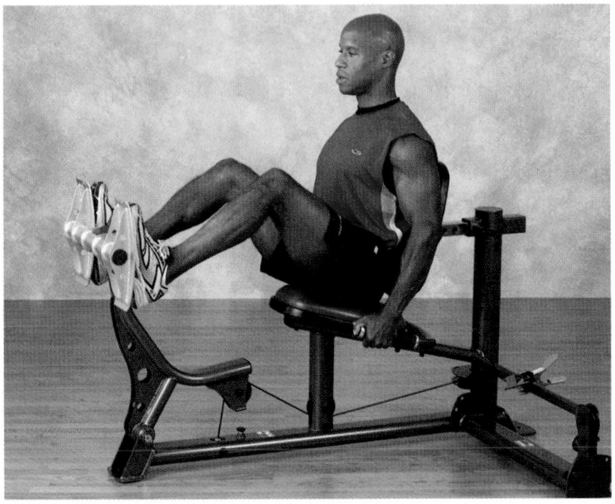

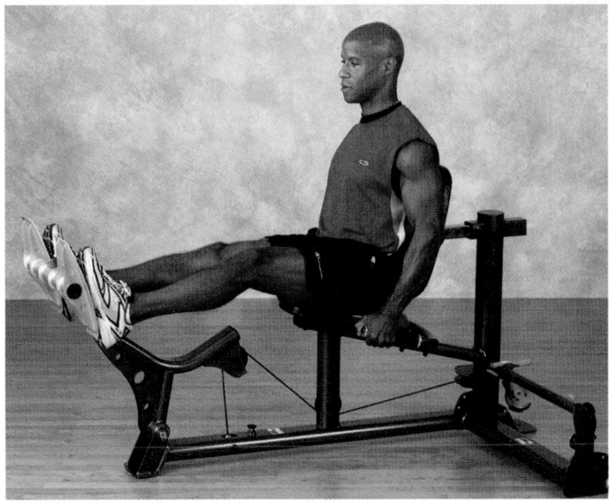

Leg Curl

Prime muscle movers: Hamstrings

Exercise technique: The participant faces the machine with one ankle in front of the pad. After grasping the handles and stabilizing the body, the participant bends the knee to lift the weight. Slowly return to the starting position and repeat the movement. Do not use momentum to complete the lift. After the desired number of repetitions, switch legs.

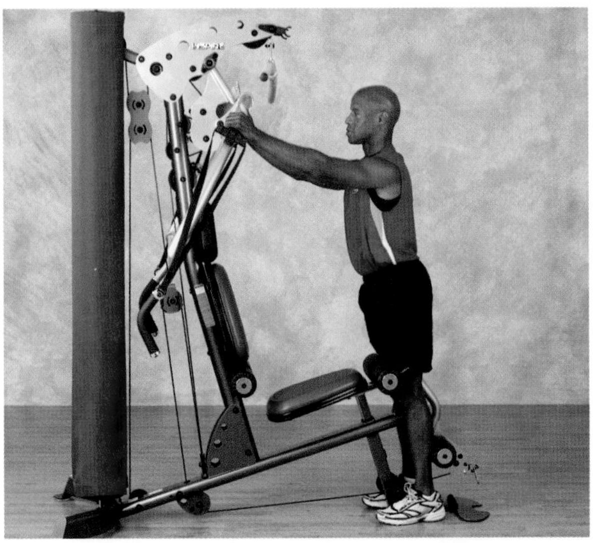

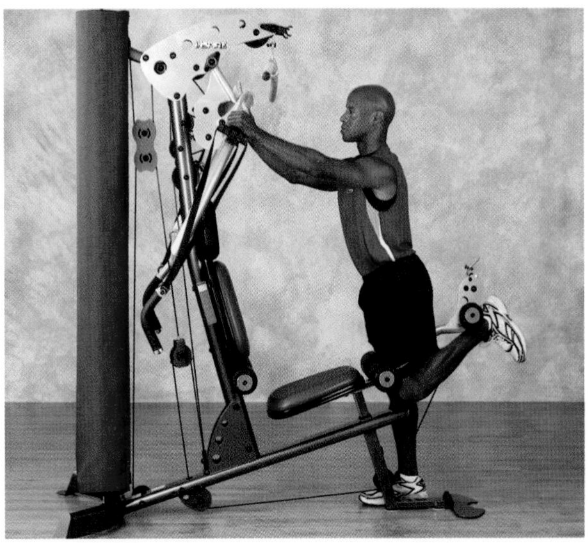

Dumbbell Heel Raise

Prime muscle movers: Gastrocnemius, soleus

Exercise technique: The participant stands, holding a dumbbell in the right hand and placing the left hand on a wall for support. The left foot is lifted off the floor. The participant raises the heel of the right foot as high as possible and then slowly lowers it to the starting position. This exercise should be performed on both sides of the body. The participant should concentrate on keeping the torso and knees straight to avoid upper-leg involvement. To increase the ROM, a 1 to 2 in. (2.5-5.0 cm) board or weight plate can be placed under the ball of the exercising foot. If this is too difficult, the exercise can be performed with both feet on the floor or board.

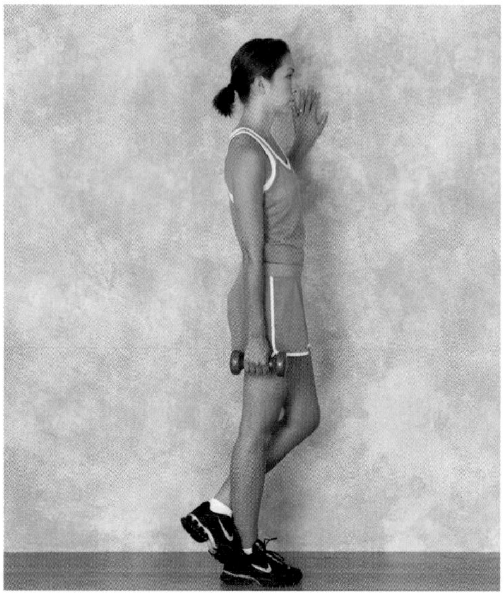

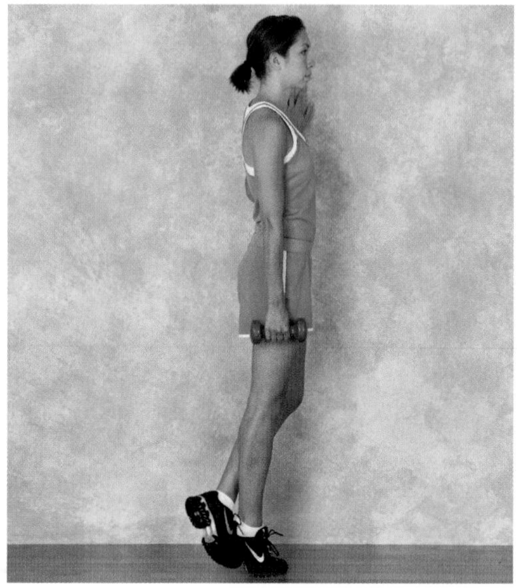

Bench Press

Prime muscle movers: Pectoralis major, anterior deltoid, triceps

Exercise technique: The participant lies flat on the bench and holds the barbell with a wider-than-shoulder-width grip directly above the chest, with arms straight and feet flat on the floor. The participant slowly lowers the barbell to the chest and then presses the barbell back up to the starting position. The barbell should not be bounced on the chest, and a spotter should stand by in case of a failed repetition.

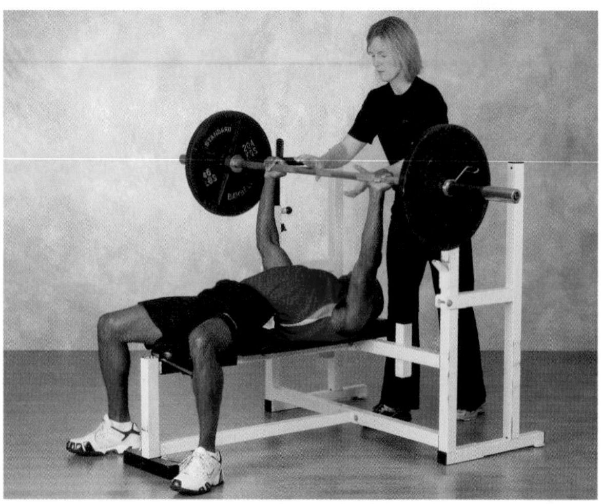

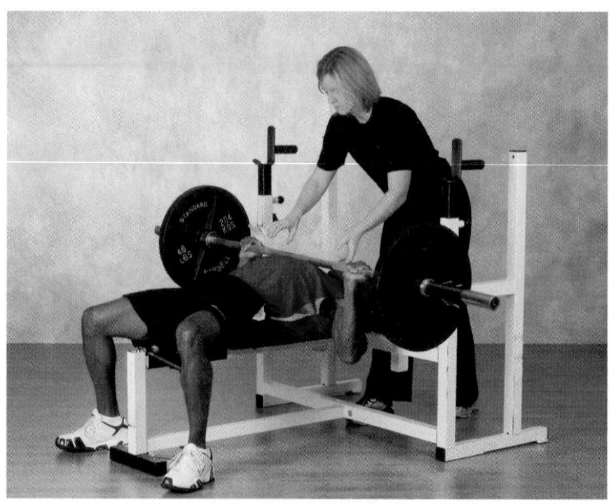

Front Pull-Down

Prime muscle movers: Latissimus dorsi, biceps

Exercise technique: The participant sits on the seat with the arms fully extended, places both knees under the exercise pad, and grips the bar underhand (palms toward the face) using a shoulder-width grip. The participant should lean slightly backward from the waist and maintain this position throughout the duration of the exercise to avoid getting hit by the bar. The bar is pulled down just under the chin and then returned slowly until the arms are fully extended.

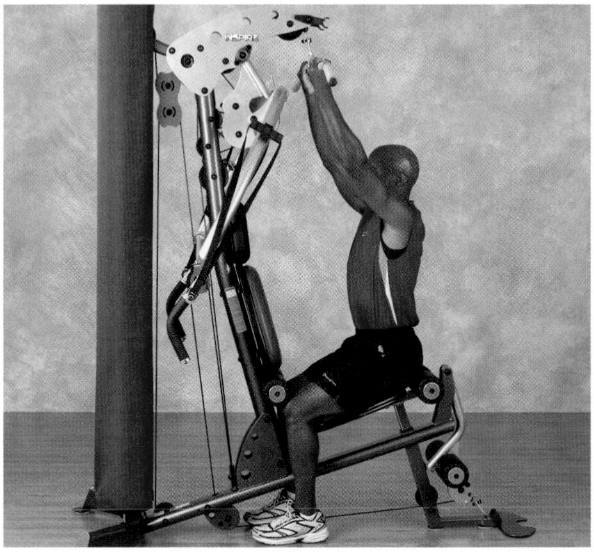

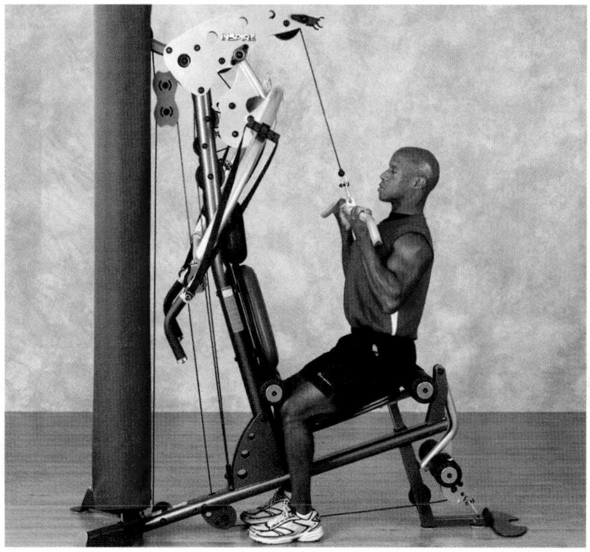

Dumbbell Overhead Press

Prime muscle movers: Deltoids, triceps

Exercise technique: In the standing position, the participant holds a dumbbell in each hand at shoulder level with palms facing forward. The participant presses the weights overhead to a straight-arm position and then slowly returns to the starting position. The participant should not bend or sway the back to complete a repetition.

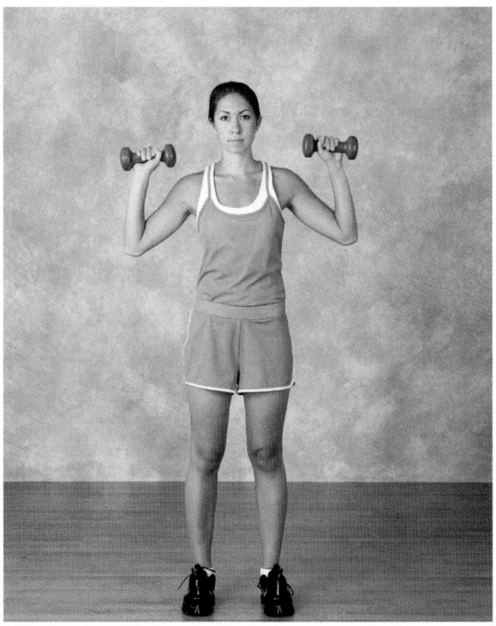

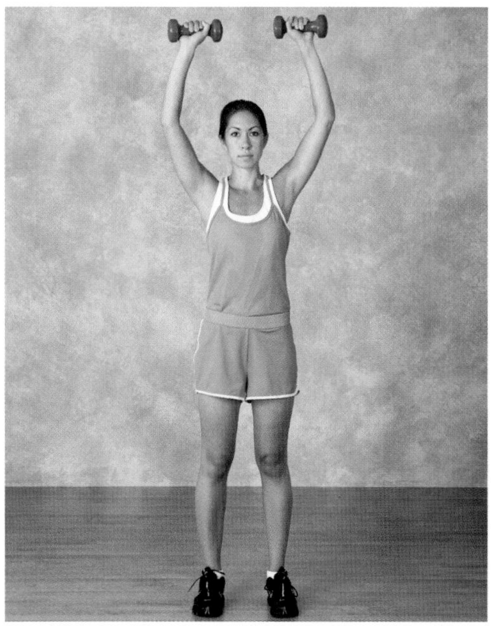

Dumbbell Curl

Prime muscle movers: Biceps
Exercise technique: The participant stands with a dumbbell in each hand (palms facing forward) and the arms at the sides of the body. The participant bends the elbows to bring the weights toward the shoulders and then slowly returns to the starting position. The back should not be bent or swayed to complete a repetition.

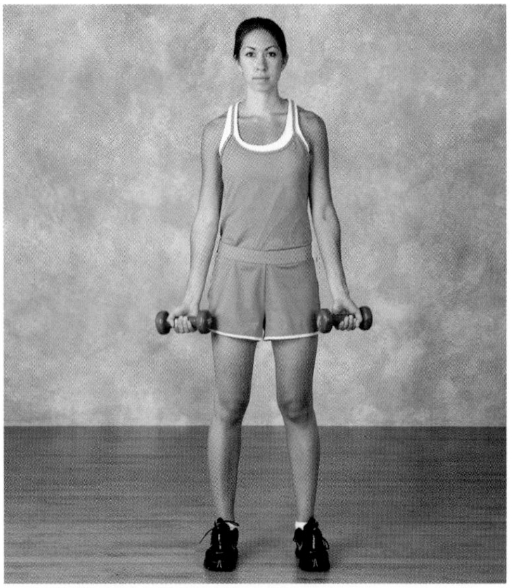

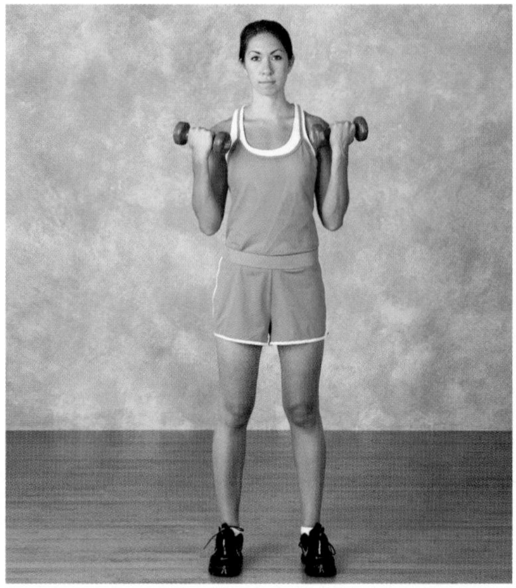

Lying Triceps Extension

Prime muscle movers: Triceps
Exercise technique: The participant lies flat on the back on an exercise bench and holds a dumbbell in each hand with arms straight over shoulders and palms facing each other. The participant lowers both dumbbells to the side of the head by bending only at the elbows and then slowly returns to the starting position. The upper arm should not be swayed to complete a repetition.

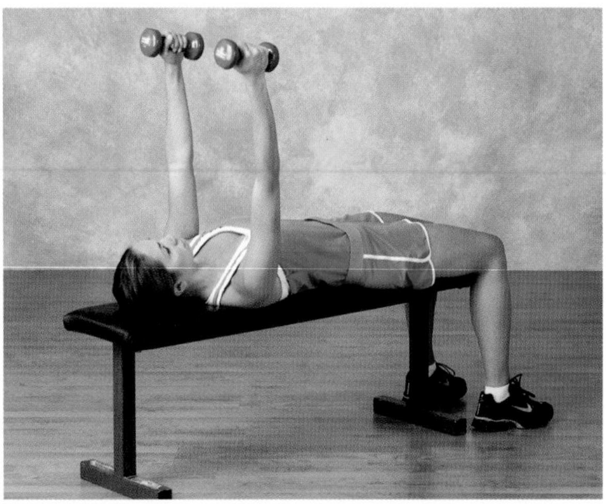

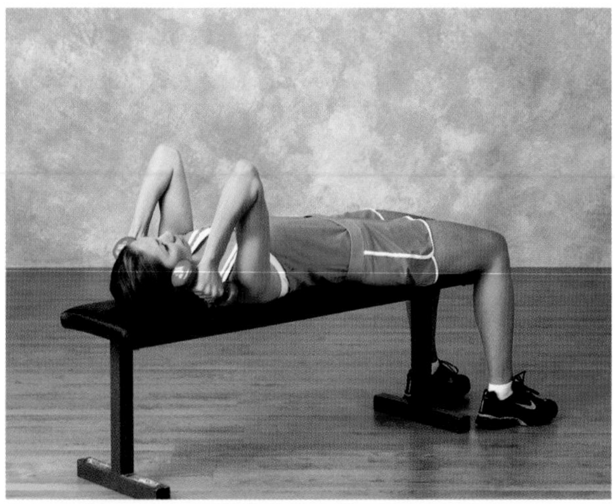

Kneeling Trunk Extension

Prime muscle mover: Erector spinae

Exercise technique: The participant kneels on the floor and supports the body on both hands and knees. The participant extends the right leg backward until it is parallel to the floor, pauses briefly, returns to the starting position, and then extends the left leg backward. To make this exercise more challenging, the participant can raise the left arm parallel to the floor while extending the right leg (and vice versa).

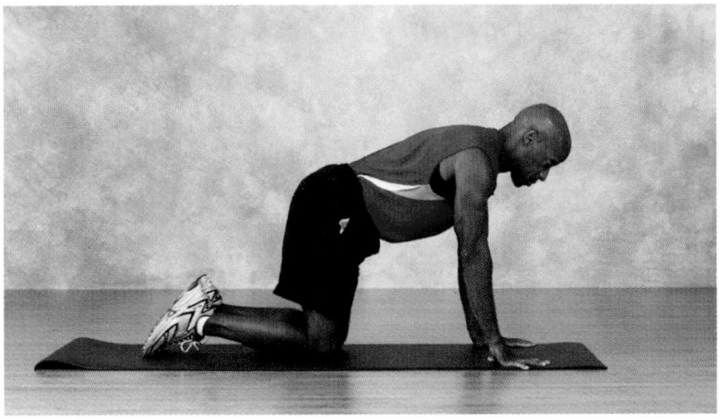

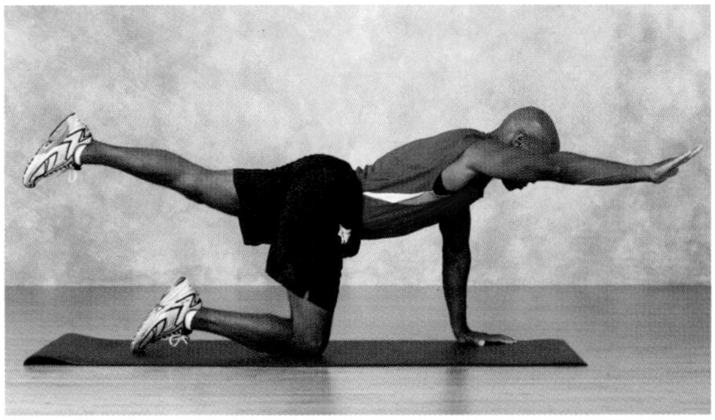

Abdominal Curl

Prime muscle mover: Rectus abdominis

Exercise technique: The participant lies flat on the back with the knees bent, feet about 12 to 15 in. (30.5-38.0 cm) from the buttocks, and hands placed on the thighs (or across the chest). Leading with the chin, the participant lifts the shoulders and upper back off the mat (about 30°-45°) while moving the hands toward the knees, pauses briefly, and then returns to starting position. If the hands are placed behind the head, the participant must not pull the head forward with the hands.

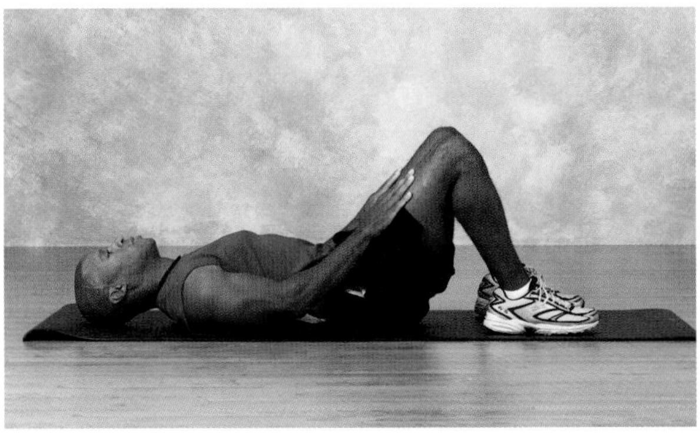

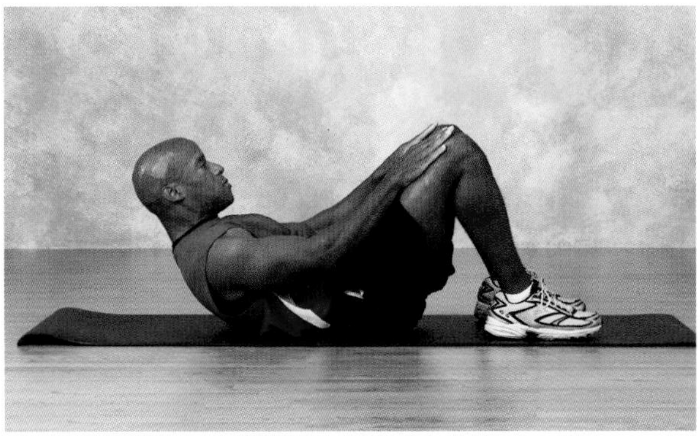

14

Exercise Prescription for Flexibility and Low-Back Function

Laura Horvath Gagnon

I am pleased to have been able to build on the work of Dr. Wendell Liemohn.

OBJECTIVES

The reader will be able to do the following:

1. Describe a motion segment and explain the role of the facet joints.
2. Differentiate between functional and structural spinal curves.
3. Describe flexibility exercises for the spine.
4. Describe flexibility exercises for the upper and lower extremities.
5. Explain why it is important for the trunk muscles to be able to control pelvic positioning.
6. Identify the musculature of the local and global stabilizing systems.
7. Describe the ideal ways to activate the deep abdominal layers.
8. Describe exercises that increase the strength and endurance of muscles that are fundamental to the development of core stability.
9. Describe the current recommendations for stretching exercises.

ADLs and recreational activities can be significantly affected by flexibility. The capacity to move a joint smoothly through its full ROM allows for more efficient and comfortable movement. The exte nsibility of the major muscles crossing the lumbosacral region can have a significant impact on low-back function. ACSM's current recommendations include flexibility training at least 2 days per wk to increase or maintain the normal ROM at joints (26).

Exercises directed at improving flexibility and low-back function are both diverse and common in the fitness setting. Many are aimed at promoting and maintaining a healthy spine, and others are meant to address deficits from low-back dysfunction and pain. Given that LBP (low-back pain) is so common in the adult population (45, 83), with about one-fourth of American adults experiencing LBP in the past 3 mo (34), fitness professionals need to be able to design an appropriate individualized program for clients that strengthens the lumbopelvic region and protects it from injury. Many clients who sign up for fitness training will have either a history of or current low-back dysfunction. The ability to create and refine a program that addresses low-back function and flexibility requires an understanding of basic spine anatomy and biomechanics.

This chapter presents spinal anatomy and biomechanics relevant to core stability and reviews spinal movement. Core stability principles and exercises are presented, including some popular alternatives such as Pilates. In addition, flexibility exercises addressing the major joints and muscles are presented with the current recommendations for stretching. The chapter closes with a discussion concerning the potential need to refer a client for a medical consult.

Anatomy of the Spine

Figure 14.1 depicts the lumbar spine. Appreciating the anatomy of the spine allows for an understanding of LBP. The fundamental unit of the lumbar spine is the motion segment, which consists of two vertebrae and their intervening **disc**. The bodies of the vertebrae and their intervening disc are sometimes referred to as the *anterior aspect* of the motion segment. The posterior aspect of the motion segment is attached to the anterior aspect by the pedicles, which provide the lateral boundary of the foramen (vertical passageway) for the spinal cord and its nerves. In addition to the transverse and spinous processes, the posterior elements of the vertebrae include the superior and inferior articular processes, and each of their junctions is referred to as a *zygapophyseal joint*, or **facet joint**. In addition to supporting loads on the spine, the facet joints control the amount and direction of vertebral movement based on their joint surface orientation (64).

A series of ligaments reinforces the vertebrae of the spine. The anterior and posterior longitudinal ligaments provide stability for the anterior portion of the motion segments; they run the length of the spine on the anterior and posterior surfaces of the vertebrae bodies as well as the intervertebral discs. The ligaments that support the posterior aspect of the motion segment include the ligamentum flavum, which is located immediately behind the spinal cord and serves as its posterior boundary. Also reinforcing the posterior aspect of the motion segments are the facet joint capsular ligaments that span the synovial joints formed by the superior and inferior articular processes between each vertebral pair. The posterior aspects of each motion segment are reinforced further by

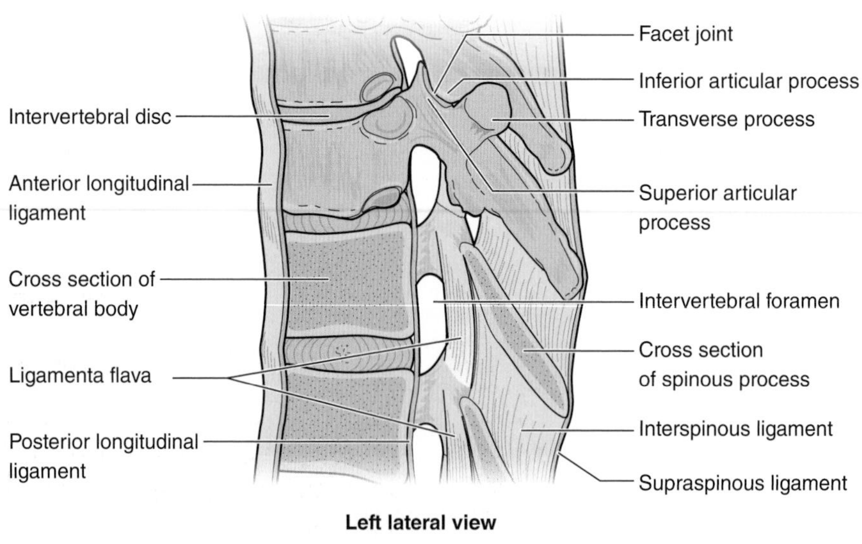

FIGURE 14.1 The lumbar spine. Note the vertebral bodies, facet joints, intervertebral discs, pedicles, and lordotic curve. The facet joints (i.e., the junction of the superior and inferior articular processes) are positioned to provide stability and control the amount and direction of movement.

the interspinous and supraspinous ligaments, which are attached to the spinous processes. All of these ligaments have pain receptors, and therefore a sprain to any of them can signal a back problem.

The discs enable each vertebra to be more mobile and distribute forces (figure 14.2). Each intervertebral disc consists of a centrally placed nucleus, which is a gelatinous mass (nucleus pulposus). This nucleus is surrounded by a ligamentous sheath of connective-tissue fibers (annulus fibrosis peripherally and vertebral end plates superiorly and inferiorly). This structure is somewhat analogous to a jelly donut (the central nucleus is the jelly and the peripheral annulus fibrosis and vertebral end plates are the surrounding donut). The annulus has fibers that run parallel in concentric layers at an angle 45° to 65° (32) to the vertebral body. Each layer runs perpendicular to the previous layer. When rotation is applied to the disc, half the fibers tighten and the other half loosen. This is particularly important when a flexion and rotation force is applied, as in bending forward with a twist. In this position the posterior annulus has a tension force with only half the fibers taut and ready to respond and is therefore more vulnerable. Intervertebral discs act as spacers and shock absorbers, and when compressive forces are placed on the spine (e.g., when a person carries a load), the nucleus of the disc exerts pressure in all directions to help absorb the force. The nucleus bears the compressive force, and the annulus, a tensile force (64); the position of the nucleus changes based on the direction of spine motion (see figure 14.2*c*). Force can also be transferred from the nucleus pulposus through the vertebral end plates into the trabeculae of adjacent vertebrae (64).

Disc injuries are common in the low back, and an area that is particularly vulnerable is between the fifth lumbar vertebra and the sacrum (the L5-S1 disc). Its load is greater than that of any other disc due, in part, to the angle at which it sits. In a standing position with the sacrum at a 30° angle to the vertical, the shear force across the lumbosacral joint is 50% of body weight, and this increases if the angle increases (32), such as in an anterior tilt of the pelvis. When a person bends forward so that the sacral angle is approximately 50°, the shear force can increase to 75% of body weight. It makes sense, then, that an increase in body weight has a significant impact on the load on the L5-S1 disc both as a shear force and compression (30, 32). Another disc that is often injured in the low back is the one between L4 and L5, which is the only disc in the lumbar spine that has a vertical compressive force (in contrast to shear force) in upright standing (32).

Except for their periphery, the discs do not have pain receptors; however, if the nucleus of a disc breaks through its normal boundaries (e.g., distends or ruptures its annulus), the peripheral pain receptors of the disc respond. (The pain receptors in the ligaments of the spine can also quickly communicate when something is wrong in a ligament or in an adjacent damaged disc that exceeds its normal confines.)

Why is it important to appreciate the loads on the lower spine? It is essential to understand and educate clients in the ideal alignment of the spine during exercises to promote the best transfer of forces across the spinal components to avoid injury. The fitness professional needs to be aware of positions that may compromise the spinal structures. If a disc is diseased or injured, its ability to withstand stress is adversely affected and the motion segment to which it belongs may become unstable.

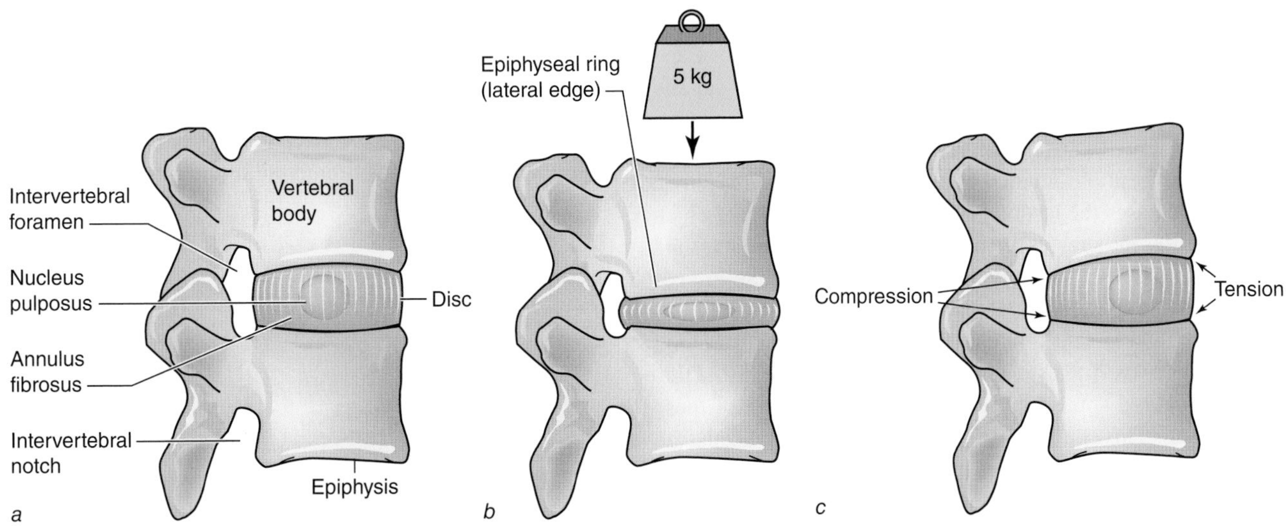

FIGURE 14.2 *(a)* Discs allow flexibility and act as shock absorbers. *(b)* When weight is added (in this case perpendicular to the disc), the force is absorbed in all directions; however, if the external force is applied obliquely, the pressure within the disc is away from the direction of the applied force. *(c)* Compression force is on the side of the bend, tension on the opposite side. Spine extension brings compression on the posterior disc and tension on the anterior annulus.

Figures 14.2*a* and 14.2*b* adapted from Liemohn 2001.

The disc is avascular (i.e., without a blood supply), and motion in the spine enhances its nutrition (i.e., motion enables the disc to absorb nutrients through the vertebral end plates). It is wise to frequently change positions, altering the loads on the discs and promoting the flow of fluid and nutrition to the disc (84). When we sleep, discs imbibe fluid and become tighter than they were at the end of the day. During the day we lose about 15 to 25 mm of height due to water loss in the discs (32). For this reason back injuries often occur in the morning, when these fuller discs permit less movement. Thus, slow warm-ups before strenuous exercise or work are especially important in the morning or following sleep.

KEY POINT

The fundamental unit of the spine is the motion segment, which consists of two vertebrae and their intervening disc. The spinal discs absorb shock to the vertebral column by exerting pressure in all directions. Although the facet joints help support loads, one of their primary responsibilities is controlling the amount and direction of spinal movement, such as that seen in rotation. A lack of proper mechanics can compromise the discs, ligaments, facets, and musculature of the spine, causing injury.

Spinal Curves

The curvatures of the spine as viewed from the side are described as a **lordotic curve** when they are concave and as a **kyphotic curve** when they are convex. Cervical and lumbar curves are normally lordotic and the thoracic curve is kyphotic. Exaggerations of these curves are not desirable; for example, an increased anterior (or forward) pelvic tilt increases the lordotic curve in the lumbar area, which increases the stresses on the ligaments, discs, vertebrae, and musculature of the spine (especially L5). A small lumbar lordotic curve is natural and, along with the cervical lordosis and thoracic kyphosis, assists the discs in cushioning compressive forces occurring in the spine during ADLs. The neutral spine concept is based on a balance of these curves. (This concept will be revisited later in a discussion of core exercises.) Factors such as being overweight, wearing high heels, and lacking appropriate muscle length or strength can affect the degree of lordosis. Tightness in the hip flexors (i.e., the psoas) can increase the lordotic curve by causing an anterior pelvic tilt; conversely, tightness in the hamstrings can reduce the lordosis (see figure 14.3).

When the spine is viewed from the back, ideally a straight vertical line is seen. As noted in chapter 10, if a lateral curve is seen (see figure 14.3), the fitness professional should refer the client to a medical doctor or physical therapist for evaluation and clearance for a fitness program that includes spinal flexibility and core strengthening.

Functional and Structural Curves

Spinal curves may be either functional or structural. Spinal curves are functional if the curve can be removed by assuming a posture that takes away the force responsible for the curve. A **functional curve** may be present due to a spasm or tightness of a particular muscle group and will disappear when the client is lying down or bending or when the spasm has dissipated. In contrast, a **structural curve** is always present independent of the person's position; it is fixed and not flexible. However, a functional curve may eventually become structural if one assumes an unhealthy posture over several years. For example, a person sitting at a desk for many hours each day often assumes a slumping posture during this time, which may result in an increase in thoracic kyphosis and rounded shoulders, a forward head position, and a decrease in the lumbar curve. If this person does not extend the spine or retract the shoulders periodically, the ability to perform these movements may decrease and the poor posture may become structural. A structural curve is not easy to straighten and is associated with a loss of spinal flexibility.

Why does this matter when working with a client? If a client has a structural lumbar lordosis or thoracic kyphosis, obtaining an ideal spine position from which to perform both stretching and core exercises may be difficult or painful. The fitness professional can teach the client to obtain the most comfortable position midway between flexion and extension where there is no pain, or the client may need supportive props such as yoga blocks or pillows to support the structural curve. Gentle stretching exercises to facilitate movement in the restricted direction may help the client to obtain a more ideal position in the future.

KEY POINT

Functional curves can be removed by assuming a posture that reduces the force that caused the curve. Structural curves can develop over several years and are not easily removed. Structural curves increase the difficulty of obtaining the ideal spine position needed for flexibility and core exercises. Helping the client find a comfortable position midway between flexion and extension or providing props such as yoga blocks or pillows to support the structural curve can help.

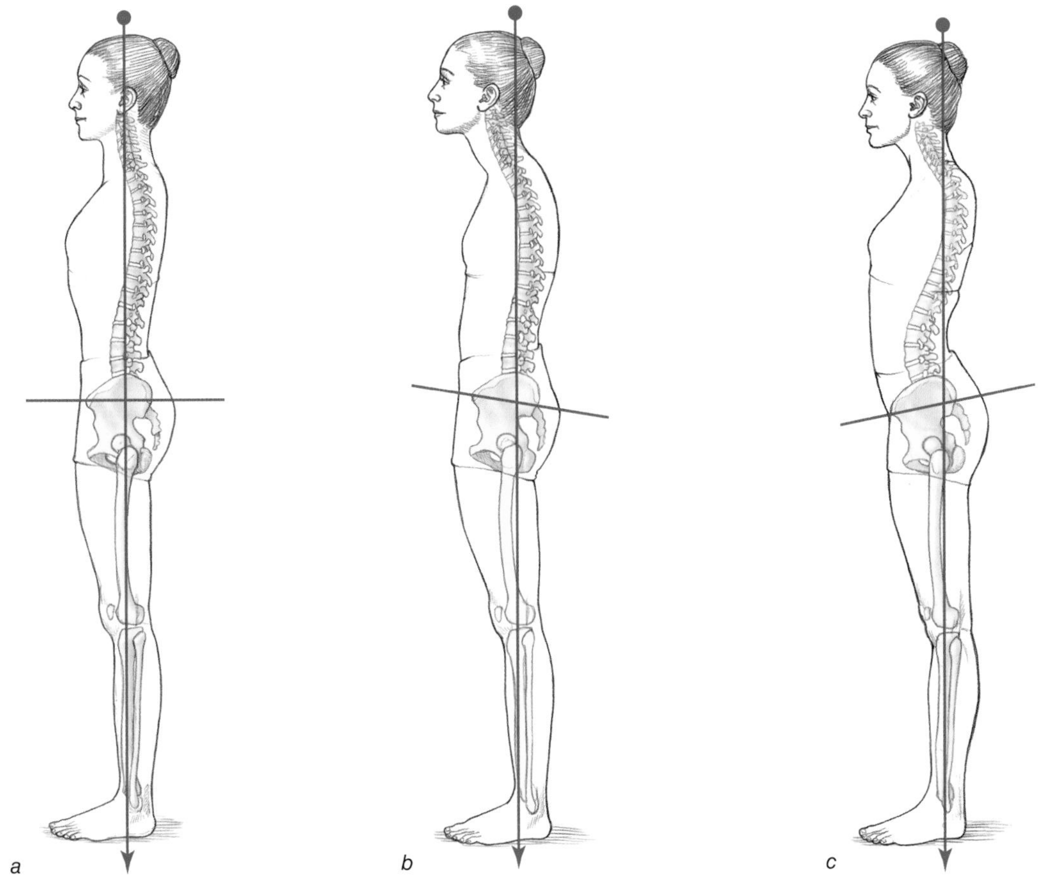

FIGURE 14.3 *(a)* Ideal spinal alignment, *(b)* posterior pelvic tilt with decreased lordosis and forward placement of the head, and *(c)* anterior pelvic tilt with increased lordosis.

Spinal Movement

When the whole spine moves in any direction, each vertebra contributes motion in a complex pattern of simultaneous rotation and translation (64). With injury, such as degenerative disc disease, the vertebral motion pattern changes (64) and influences the motion of the whole spine, potentially causing pain and hypermobility (28). There is a region of intervertebral motion around a neutral position that has little restraint from the passive spinal components, similar to the wiggle room between two vertebrae without passive restraint (i.e., ligaments). The spine is like the mast of a sailboat. If the mast has too much movement, or wiggle room, it cannot provide a stable base for the sail, or the attaching muscles. Panjabi (69) termed this region of intervertebral motion that has little resistance from the passive spinal components the *neutral zone*, and it is used to quantify the amount of segmental instability that is present (67, 75, 85). It is thought that the neutral zone is a better measurement of instability than spine ROM is (66, 70). If the neutral zone grows larger as disc degeneration or ligamentous injury occurs, there is more laxity or instability in the spine to control and more demands are placed on the stabilizing systems.

Therefore, an important question to ask is, what are the stabilizing systems? How can one improve the stability of the spine? Panjabi (68) defined the stabilizing system as an interconnected set of three subsystems:

1. Passive
2. Active
3. Neural control

The passive system consists of the bony structures, ligaments, joint capsules, discs, and passive portion of the musculotendinous units (68). This system is thought to send feedback to the neural subsystem about joint positions and challenges to stability at the passive level (68). The active system is composed of the muscles and tendons and is the subject of the core exercises later in this chapter. The neural subsystem receives and transmits information from and to the other two systems to manage spinal stability. Neuromuscular control can be compromised in patients with LBP and must be considered in a core stabilization program (41, 44).

Most spinal motions in functional activities and some exercises use some combination of the three planes of motion: sagittal (flexion and extension), frontal or coronal (lateral flexion or side bending), and transverse (rotation). Because some of the most forceful stresses on the discs occur during movements that combine bending and rotation, exercises involving these movements should always be done under muscle control. In other words, exercises involving intervertebral movement should not be ballistic (e.g., movements in which momentum plays a major role). If the movement results from momentum rather than muscle control, normal end ROM may be exceeded and connective-tissue structures such as spinal ligaments or discs may be damaged. As mentioned, the spine is particularly vulnerable at the beginning of the day because the discs imbibe tissue fluid while recumbent in sleeping postures, resulting in tighter discs that are more vulnerable to sprain or other injury.

Mechanics of the Spine and the Hip Joint

The muscles crossing the hip joint (hip flexors, hamstrings, ITB) can be viewed as guy-wires bracing the pelvis. If any of these guy-wires are too tight, the abdominal musculature has difficulty controlling pelvic positioning. Because the sacrum (in the pelvis) is the foundation for the 24 vertebrae stacked on it, pelvic positioning is important to the integrity of the spine. Tightness in the hamstrings can severely affect the ability of the pelvis to tilt anteriorly and thus can diminish pelvic ROM. Tightness of the hip flexors (iliopsoas and rectus femoris) can also be detrimental to low-back function because the pelvic girdle may rest in an anterior tilt, causing increased load to L5-S1 (64). If there is an asymmetry in the length of the iliopsoas from one side to the other, a pelvic girdle asymmetry may occur, creating a sacroiliac joint dysfunction. A shortened ITB may restrict lower-extremity adduction, and a tightened piriformis also might restrict hip rotatory motion. When healthy subjects were compared with LBP patients in terms of their hip ROM (21), there was an association between hip rotation imbalance (internal and external rotation) and the presence of LBP.

A neutral position of the pelvic girdle and spine is one in which the joints are in an optimal position for performing daily activities and exercise. The person in figure 14.3*a* is displaying a good neutral spine posture in which the convex curves in the thoracic and sacral areas are balanced by the concave curves in the cervical and lumbar areas. Energy expenditure is minimal because body segments are in balance and forces on the discs are minimized. The people in figures 14.3*b* and 14.3*c* demonstrate altered pelvic positions that change the rest of the spinal curves, placing additional strain on the spinal components. An anteriorly tilted pelvis may be from tight hip flexors or trunk extensors, whereas a posteriorly tilted pelvis may result from tight hamstrings. Both flexibility and core exercises need a neutral spine alignment as a starting point. As mentioned previously, a structural spinal curve may prevent a person from obtaining the ideal neutral spine position; finding a position that is pain free and as close to neutral as possible is usually the best solution. A person who is unable to obtain a neutral position while standing due to tight hamstrings or hip flexors may be able to reach a neutral position in a supine position because the tight hip muscles are in a slack position. Frequently the first goal of flexibility and spine exercises is to teach clients how to obtain a neutral spine position. It is common for this position to feel foreign to them if they have had poor posture for some time. Consequently, for effective stretching and core strengthening programs, it is important that they learn what a neutral spine position.

KEY POINT

The pelvis serves as the foundation for the spine, so the ability of the trunk muscles to control pelvic positioning is essential for maintaining a neutral spine and a healthy back. If either the hip flexors or hip extensors are too tight, posture may be compromised.

Exercise Considerations: Preventive and Therapeutic

ACSM recommends both flexibility and core strengthening exercises (1). Although core stability training is often used to train athletes to perform better in their particular sports, it is also emphasized in LBP prevention and in therapeutic programs. Good isometric endurance of the trunk musculature may prevent a first occurrence of LBP (10, 29), and deconditioning of the lumbar extensor musculature is a risk factor for low-back injury and pain (29, 38, 78). The core exercise of drawing in the abdominal muscles, which activates the transversus abdominis (TrA) and multifidus (MF), has been shown to reduce the 3 yr recurrence rate of LBP from 75% to 35% (37). The rationale behind flexibility and strength training for the core will be noted and suggestions for specific exercise programs will be presented.

Core Stability

Core stability is the ability to control the forces across the spine and pelvic girdle while protecting the integrity of the spinal structures. It is the ability to achieve and sustain control of the trunk region at rest and during precise movements (55). The objective of core stability training is to challenge the muscular systems enough to achieve functional stability without excessive load to the spine (59). Two components of core stability are the muscles themselves and neuromuscular control. Core stability results when the passive structures of the spinal column (i.e., the vertebrae, discs, rib cage, pelvis, and all associated connective tissue) are stabilized by the active component (i.e., the neuromuscular component).

Stability can be viewed both from a larger perspective of trunk stability during ADLs (55) and from the stability present at the vertebral segments in the neutral zone (66, 75). Can a client keep the spine stable while performing a squat, chest press, or plank, or are extra motions occurring at the spine to compensate for the arm and leg muscular contractions that pull on the spine? Table 14.1 presents a model of spine stability that divides the muscles into local and global musculature; the local muscles are recruited in a coordinated fashion to keep the segments stable, while the global muscles generate **torque (*T*)** and control spinal motion during trunk or extremity movement (9). Figure 14.4 presents a cross-section of these muscles.

There are some extremely small muscles that are close to the spinal column, including the intertransversarii mediales, interspinales, and rotatores. These muscles have a high density of muscle spindles (63) and are thought to act as vertebral position sensors and maintain core stability

Table 14.1 Local and Global Core Muscle Divisions

LOCAL MUSCLES (STABILIZATION SYSTEM)		GLOBAL MUSCLES (MOVEMENT SYSTEM)
Primary	**Secondary**	
Transversus abdominis (TrA)	Internal oblique (IO)	Rectus abdominis (RA)
Multifidus (MF)	Medial fibers of external oblique (EO)	Lateral fibers of external oblique (RA)
	Quadratus lumborum (QL)	Psoas major
	Diaphragm	Erector spinae (ES)
	Pelvic floor muscles	Quadratus lumborum (QL)
	Iliocostalis and longissimus (lumbar portion)	

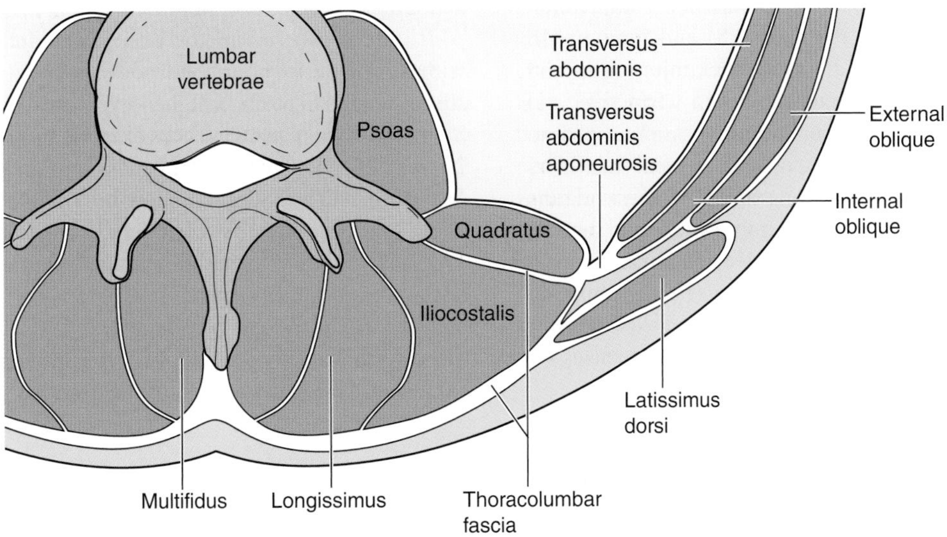

FIGURE 14.4 Cross section of the major trunk muscles that contribute to core stability. Note how the TrA attaches to the connective-tissue sheath that houses the ES (iliocostalis and longissimus) and MF; with the obliques, the TrA envelops the RA anteriorly as its sides meet at the linea alba. Although the IO also attaches to this sheath, its attachment is narrow and hence it cannot exert as much of a lateral stabilizing force (hoop tension) as the TrA exerts.

by providing feedback on the amount of contraction needed by other muscles (11, 56).

The coordination or neural control of the local and global musculature is important to core stability (3, 12, 39, 41-44). As noted in table 14.1, the local system includes the deeper core muscles of the TrA, MF, and IO, which provide support to the individual segments of the spinal column (66). The global system, including the superficial trunk muscles RA and ES, responds to the loads on the spine, maintaining equilibrium (9). If the local musculature is not performing well, the contraction of the global muscles may add loads to the local segments that may cause injury. For example, when a person performs an exercise engaging the latissimus dorsi, such as a pull-down or row, the latissimus dorsi (originates at the spinous processes of T7-L5) pulls on the spine, creating a load that must be managed with the local musculature. A person performing any leg lift during a core routine uses the psoas, which originates from and thus pulls on the spine, again creating a load that must be managed by the local system of muscles. These systems need to work in a coordinated fashion to simultaneously perform the movement needed (e.g., bench press, lunge) and protect the spine (12).

When healthy people lift an arm or leg, the TrA and IO contract before the limb moves (41, 42, 44). TrA and IO recruitment is significantly delayed or nonexistent (41) in those with back pain (41). This means there is a good chance that the person with a history of LBP, who is in the fitness setting performing various arm and leg movements during weightlifting or core work, may have a delayed response in the deep stabilizing abdominal muscles. In addition, the psoas (8) and lumbar MF atrophy (8, 34, 35, 38) after low-back injury (29), and MF recovery is not spontaneous even when pain and disability improve (38). The fitness professional needs to teach the client how to activate the deep local stabilizers (TrA and MF) before suggesting strengthening workouts using the upper and lower extremities. It would then be wise to incorporate cuing of the deep stabilizers during any other fitness exercise to restore this trunk stabilizing component. Healthy subjects can change muscle recruitment patterns with a training program that focuses on this neuromuscular control (79).

Assessment of Core Stability

Because the deep local system of abdominal muscles, the TrA and MF, consists of spine stabilizers, the fitness professional needs to be adept at teaching the use of these muscles and recognizing when they are engaged. The most commonly used tool is the hollowing maneuver or drawing in, which is taught at the beginning of the core exercise program. This is simply drawing in the abdomen or belly button toward the spine. During the drawing-in motion, the TrA contracts bilaterally to form a musculofascial band that appears to tighten like a corset (36). The TrA increases the stiffness of the lumbar intervertebral joints (39) and significantly decreases the laxity of the sacroiliac joint (71). The ability to contract the MF is related to the ability to contract the TrA (35). It has been shown that an inward movement (drawing in or hollowing) of the lower abdominal wall when the client is in a supine position produces the most independent activity of the TrA compared with the other abdominal musculature and may be an ideal position to teach TrA recruitment (81).

The IO and TrA can also be activated with minimal activity from the RA and EO in other exercise positions, such as hook lying, bridging, prone lying, four-point kneeling, and wall-support standing with a squat (14-16). The drawing in or hollowing is effective in engaging the TrA and MF and can be performed in a variety of positions. This exercise should be included even as the program progresses to more advanced levels such as doing exercises on unstable surfaces.

When the drawing-in motion is done correctly, the abdominal region has a scooped or flat appearance. If the client is bracing and recruiting the most superficial muscle, the RA, the abdominal region will have a tentlike appearance rather than a scooped-out appearance. The RA will need to be recruited for certain core exercises, but with proper involvement of the TrA and MF, the abdominal muscles will not tent.

If clients can recruit the deep abdominal muscles with a drawing-in motion, how do you know if they are strong enough to perform higher-level core exercise? The Sahrmann assessment and core exercise progression (4, 23) is an excellent tool for the fitness setting. It is simple to perform and provides important information about the client's core stability. As the client learns to recruit the TrA, it is important to pay attention to breathing patterns during these stability exercises. There is an interaction between the diaphragm, breathing, and TrA in the control of postural stability (39, 40, 53). It is usually ideal to exhale on the leg lift portion of the exercise.

VIDEO Watch **video 14.1**, which demonstrates the Sahrmann assessment.

Procedures for Level 1 Sahrmann Assessment

1. The client begins on her back with both legs bent and feet on the floor. The spine should be in a neutral position with a normal lordosis. This is the base position from which to progress to all other levels.
2. If the client has difficulty controlling the pelvic girdle and tends to go into an anterior tilt during the first couple of exercises, a slight posterior tilt will help protect the spine. This pelvic tilt creates slight flexion of the lumbar spine, with the spine gently pressing into the mat or floor surface. This position is sometimes called *imprint*.
3. A cue is provided to draw in the navel toward the spine in order to activate the deep abdominal musculature.
4. While the navel is maintained in an inward position, the client slowly lifts one foot off the surface without moving the spine.
5. If the deep core musculature cannot control the force of the leg's motion on the spine, the pelvis will shift anteriorly and possibly laterally. The goal of this exercise is to lift and lower one leg and have no motion in the spine.
6. The exercise progresses by alternating lifting and lowering one leg and then the other.

Once the client can maintain a stable pelvic girdle during the one-leg lift and lower, the next level may be attempted. This second level may be the most revealing of core weakness.

Procedures for Level 2 Sahrmann Assessment

1. The client performs the first level while in an imprint position, holds the first leg in the air, and slowly lifts the second leg off the ground.
2. If the deep core musculature is not able to stabilize the spine, the pelvis will tilt as the psoas contracts to lift the second leg.
3. If the client cannot lift the second leg without the pelvis tilting, she needs to remain at this level of core strengthening and recruitment, practicing this exercise until she can lift the second leg with ease and control.
4. The second leg can be lifted partially or the foot slid along the ground until lifted to make a safer progression to the full lift.
5. When the second leg can be lifted while the spine and pelvic position is maintained, the upper body may be lifted in a curl or the legs can progress to an alternating toe touch on the floor.
6. This exercise can also be performed on a foam roller for a greater challenge as shown in figure 14.5.

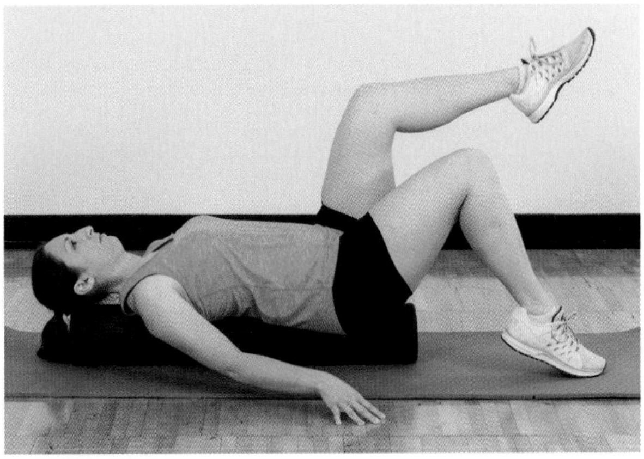

FIGURE 14.5 Sahrmann assessment and core exercise program variation on the foam roller for an additional challenge.

Once clients can control the movement of the spine and pelvic girdle when lifting one leg and then the other, they can challenge themselves by lifting the upper body, extending the arms or legs, holding a weighted ball, or placing the body on a moving object (such as a ball or roller), with confidence that the spine will be protected. If the spine and pelvic girdle move out of a neutral spine or imprint position during any of these core exercises, clients should stop the exercise and rest until they're able to control the motion again. They can learn to obtain this neutral spine control in an upright posture for weightlifting and other exercises to provide ideal support to the spine.

Three other exercises that are easily performed in a fitness setting can be used as tests for core stability (80). Figure 14.6 illustrates these tests: the single-leg stance, march on a ball and hold for 20 sec, and side plank on the knees. A negative (meaning no problem) response is the maintenance of a neutral spine without upper- or lower-extremity compensations for the standing and march tests. In the side plank, the QL is tested on the side that is toward the floor. A positive test for weakness is the inability to lift the hips (28). These tests can also be used as strengthening tools.

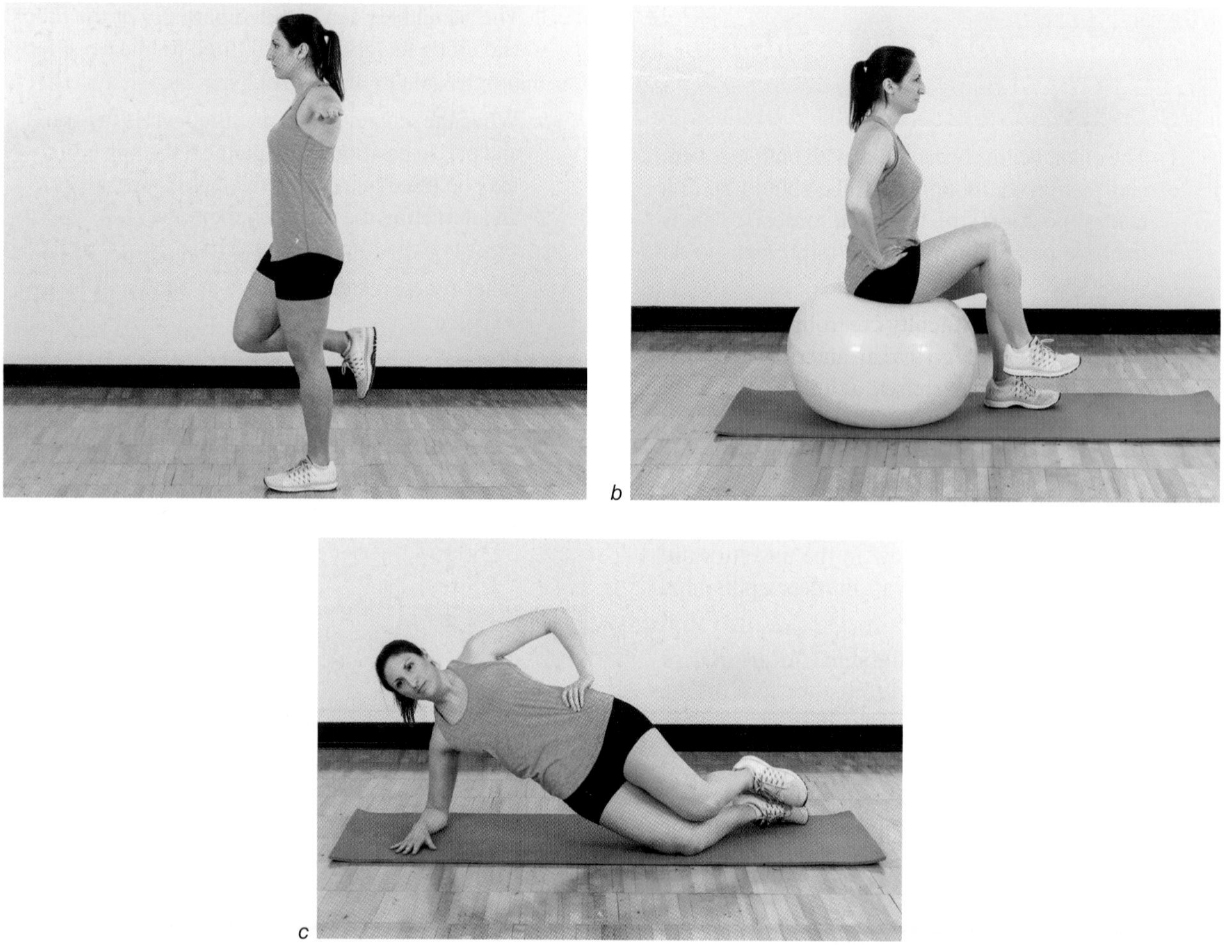

FIGURE 14.6 Supplemental tests for core stability include the *(a)* single-leg stance; *(b)* march on the ball (hold for 20 sec and watch for maintenance of neutral spine) (80); and *(c)* side plank (lift the hips off the floor to test for same-side QL strength) (28).

KEY POINT

The TrA is controlled independently of the other trunk musculature and should be trained separately from other trunk muscles with hollowing or drawing in. Its function needs to be assessed when beginning a core strengthening program. The TrA and MF are the principal deep core muscles affected by LBP; when atrophied, they predict a high rate of recurrence of LBP and dysfunction. Cueing for use of the deep abdominal muscles with the drawing-in or hollowing motion can be included with any strengthening or flexibility exercise to promote protection of the spine.

Core Muscle Exercises

Table 14.2 presents exercises aimed at recruiting and improving neuromuscular control of the deep spine stabilizers, the TrA and MF, and stabilization exercises aimed at recruiting both the local stabilizers and the global musculature. Address the deep abdominal recruitment exercise progression first (23, 73), and then add the more global exercises.

A variety of abdominal exercises are required to sufficiently challenge all of the abdominal muscles (see table 14.2) with minimal stress to the spine (5). Four exercises in particular are appropriate for enhancing spine stability with low loads to the spine (60):

1. Trunk curl—progressing with variations noted in table (exercise focus 4)
2. Dead bug—increasing range of extremities during motion (exercise focus 2)

Table 14.2 Common Core Exercises and Their Progressions

Exercise focus	Level 1	Level 2	Level 3
1. Basic stability progression to recruit TrA	Drawing in with one leg lifted 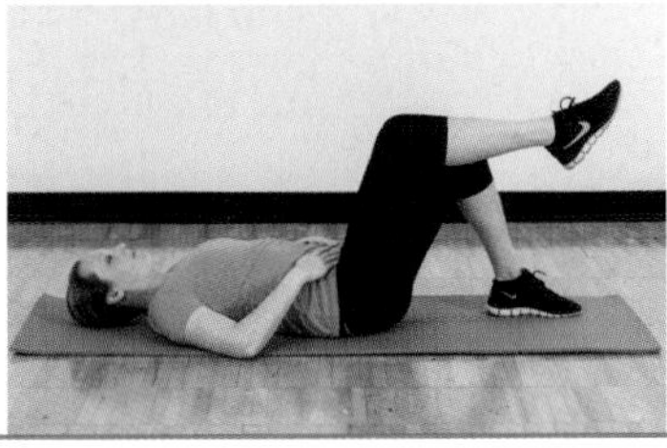	Addition of second leg 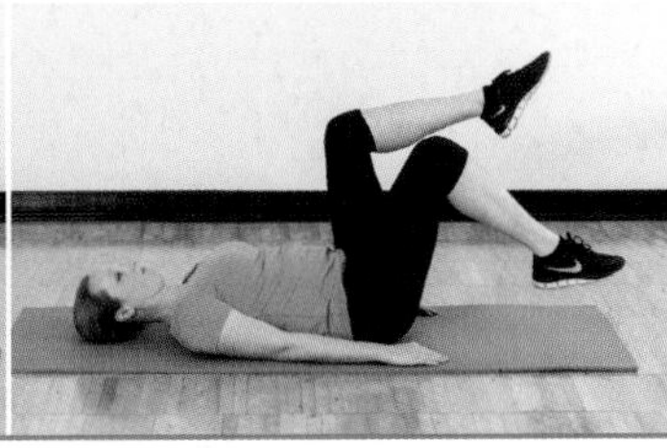	Addition of a trunk curl 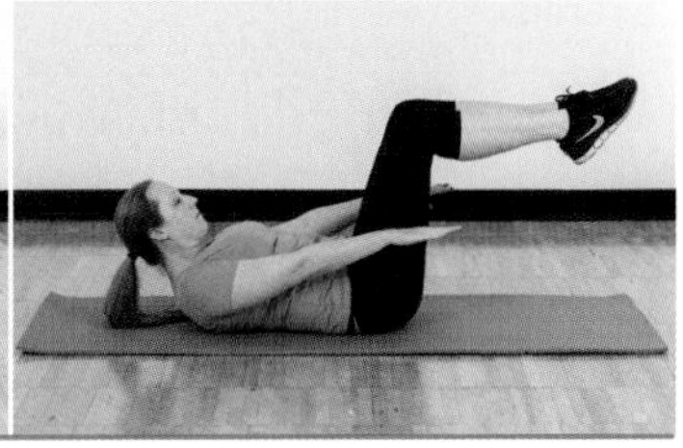
2. Focus 1 with addition of arm and leg motion (dead bug variations)	Toe tapping with the spine held in neutral or imprint position 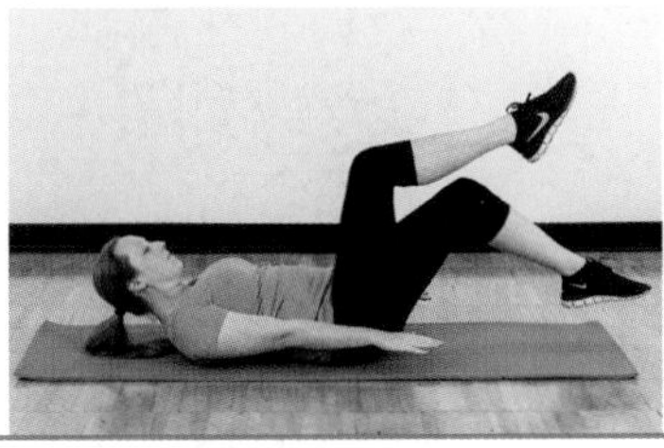	Arms and legs added as neutral spine maintained 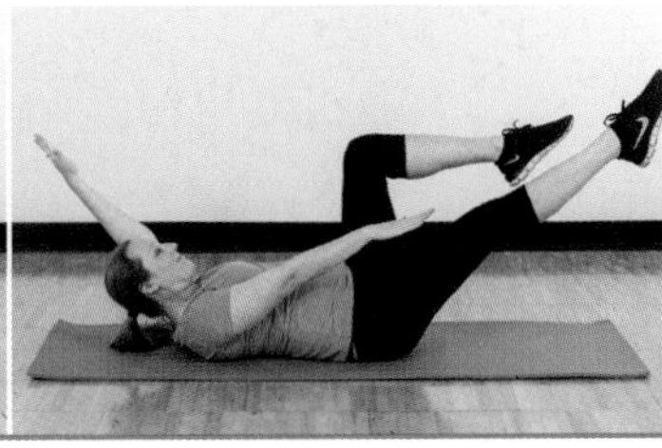	Addition of a twist 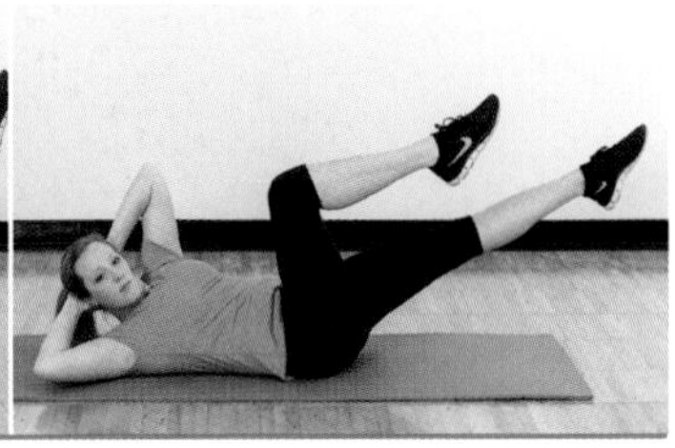
3. Bridge series	Basic bridge 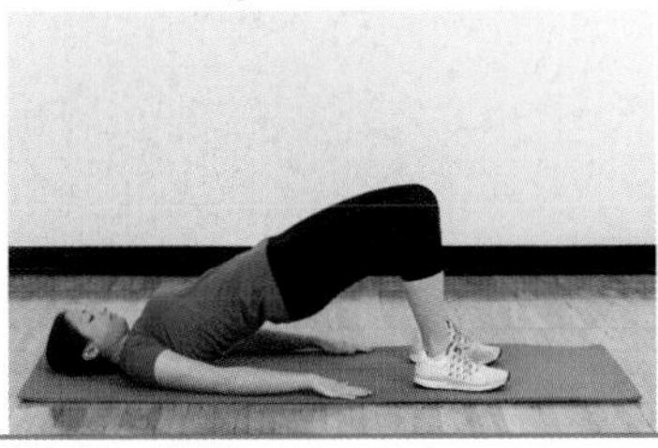	Bridge with leg extension 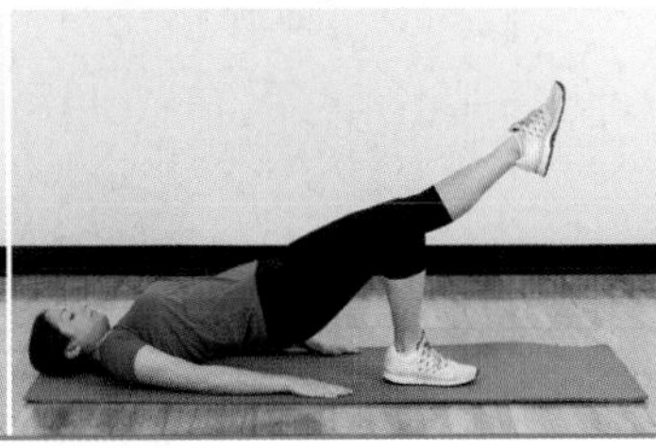	Bridge with a march 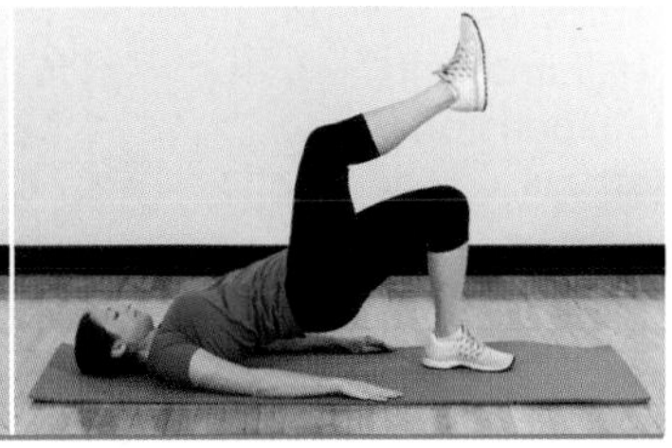
4. Basic trunk curl	Basic trunk curl (twist may be added while keeping the TrA drawn in) 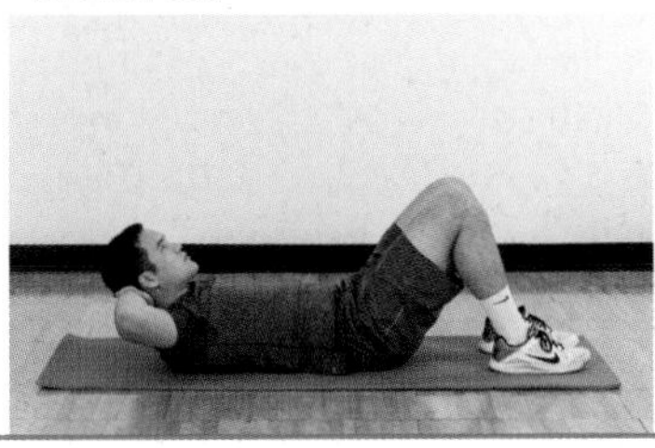	Supine trunk curl with a ball 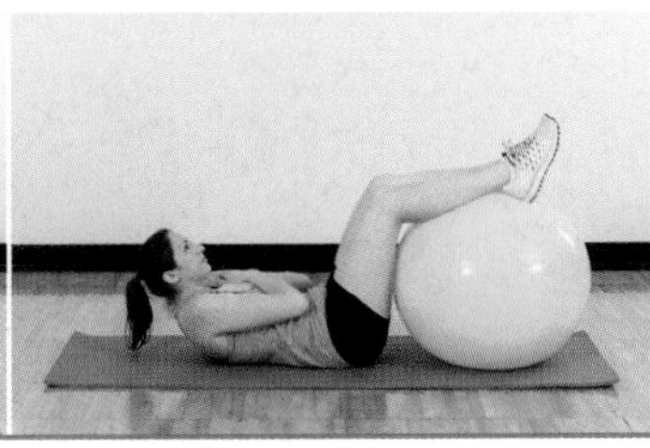	Seated ball trunk curl 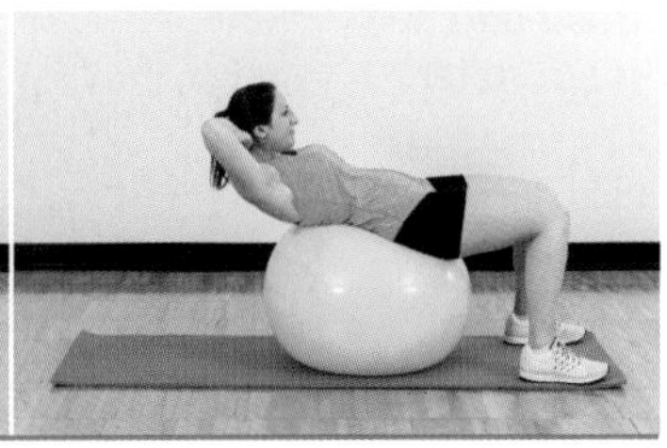
5. Swimmer exercise and bird dog to recruit MF and TrA	Performed with alternating just the arms or just the legs before adding them together Opposite arm and leg are lifted Pillow may be needed under the abdomen 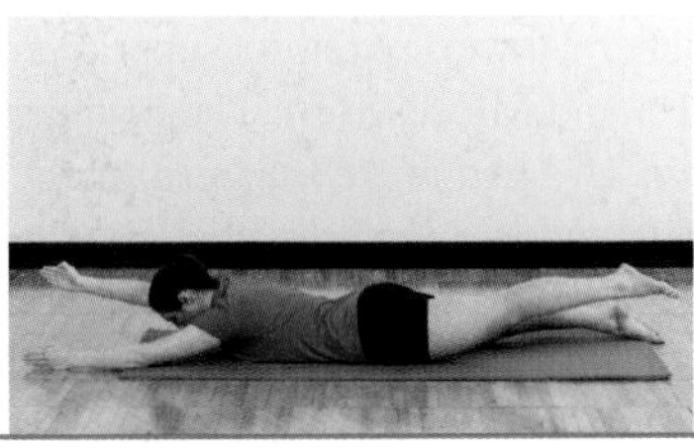	Progression to quadruped and the ball 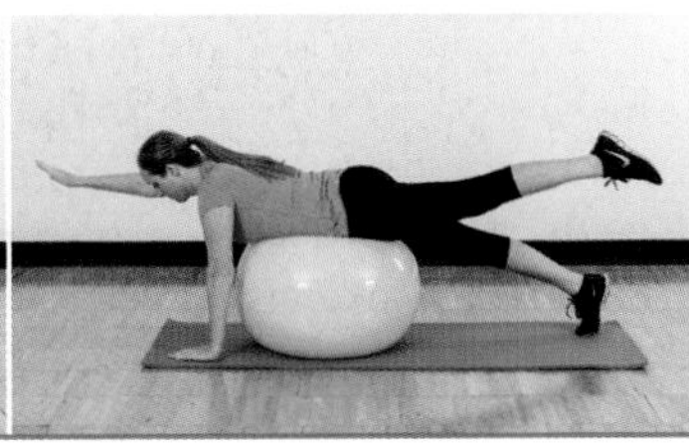	Trunk extension on ball Trunk may be lowered and lifted or held Legs may be separated to increase support 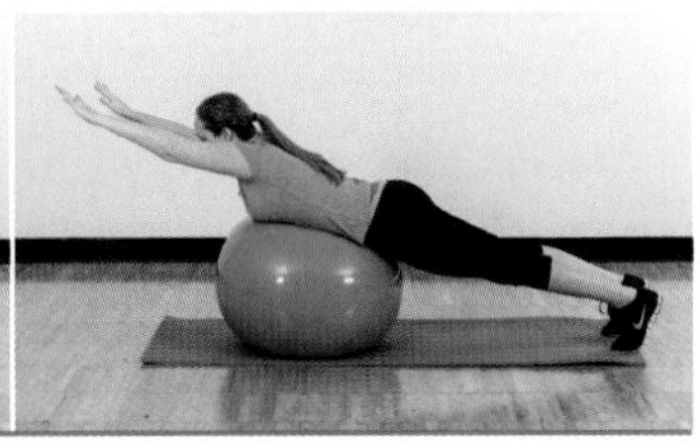

(continued)

Table 14.2 *(continued)*

Exercise focus	Level 1	Level 2	Level 3
6. Plank exercises	Plank on the elbows 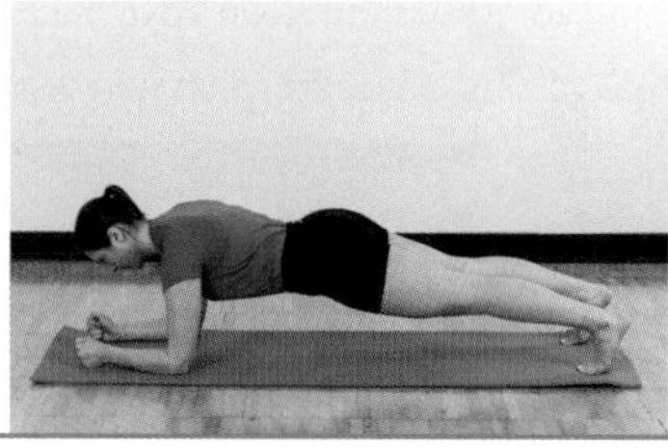	Plank with full arm extension 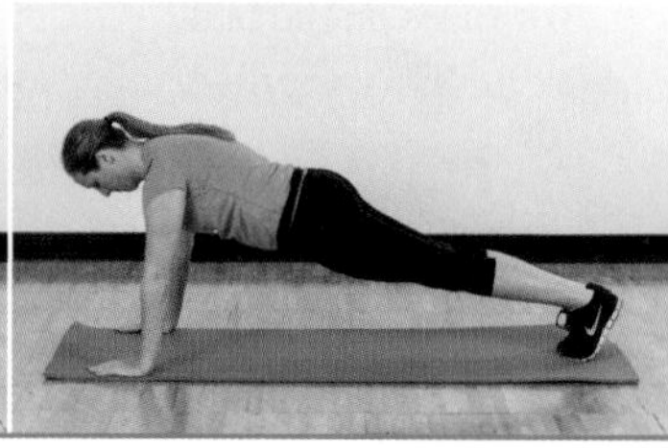	Plank with alternating arms and legs 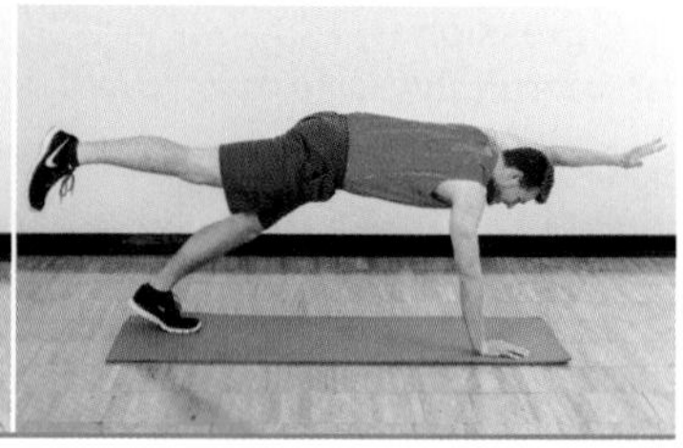
7. Side plank variations	Progressing from knees to feet 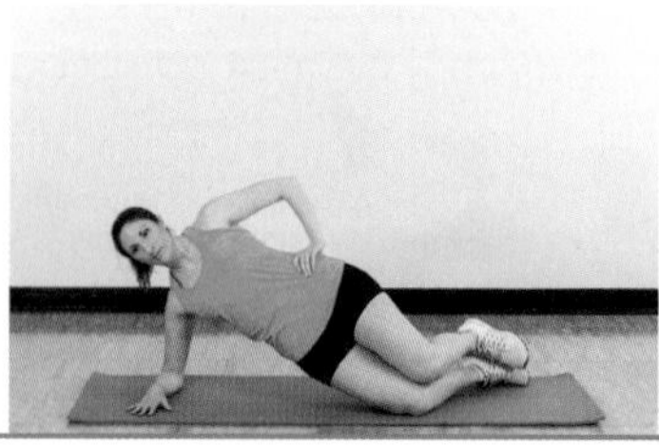	Full leg extension in a side plank 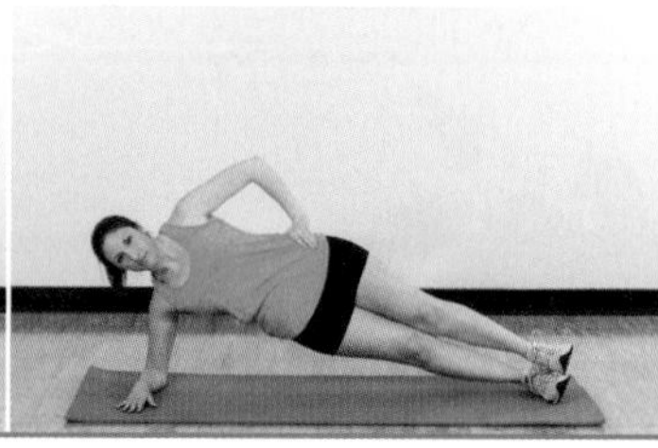	Focus change and rotation 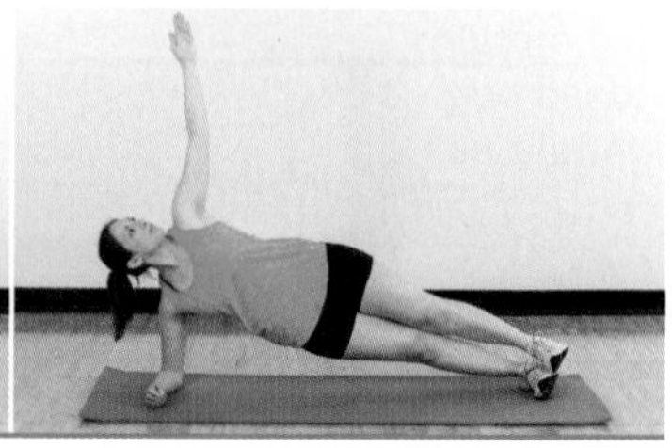
8. Unstable surfaces: ball and suspension straps	Dynamic variations of planks 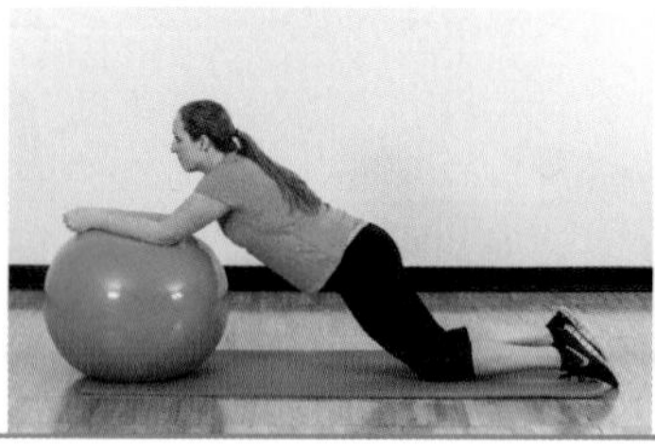	Plank into lower-extremity curl 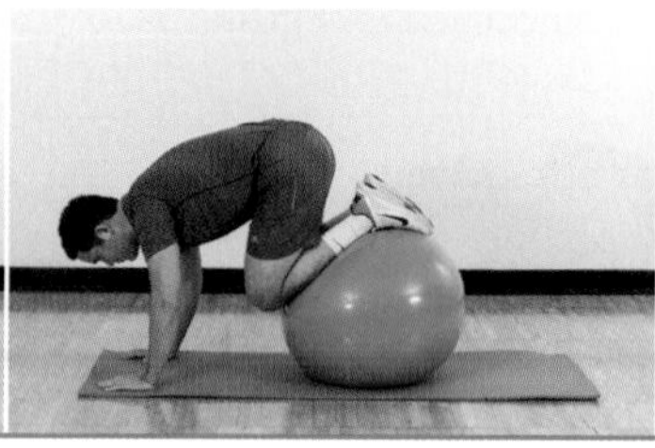	Suspension exercises 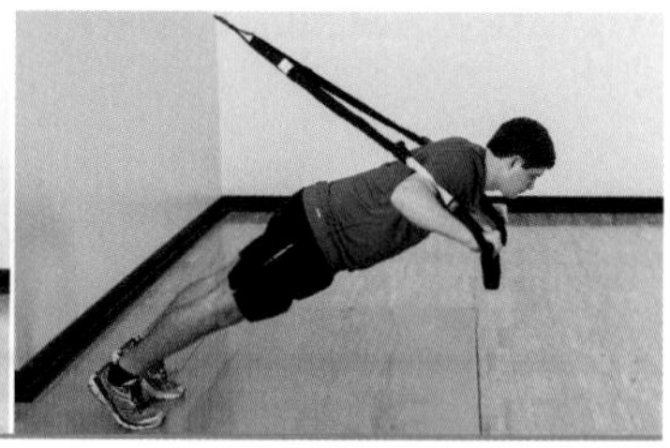
9. Unstable surfaces: Bosu and foam roller	Bridge on Bosu 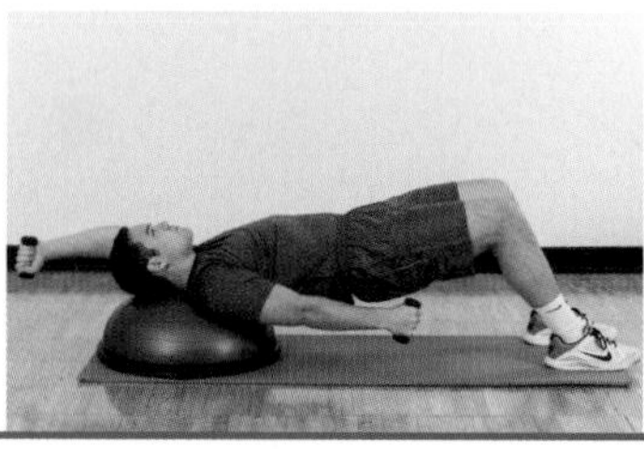	Side plank on Bosu 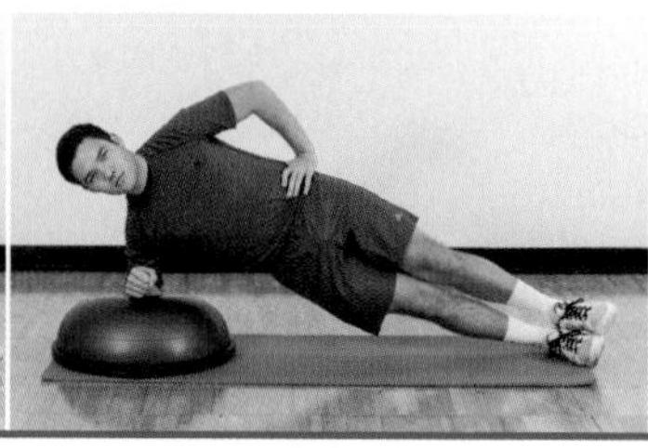	Foam roller with one leg lifted at a time into a balance 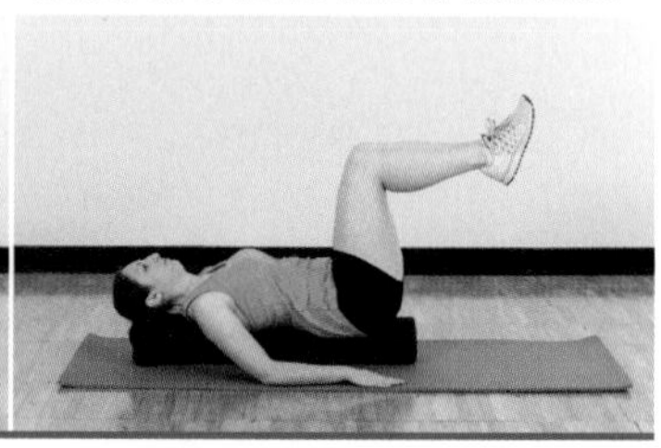

3. Side bridge (plank)—knee support progressing to foot support; addition of rotation to a prone plank; and transition to the other side bridge (exercise focus 6 and 7)
4. Bird dog—beginning with one extremity and then alternating both an arm and opposite leg (33, 60) (exercise focus 5)

McGill et al. suggest using the side bridge because it produces high activation levels in the QL, which is a significant stabilizer of the spine (58). Because this exercise involves only nominal contraction of the psoas, it does not place much compressive pressure on the intervertebral discs of the lumbar vertebrae; moreover, it emphasizes both strength and endurance (57). Bridging exercises are commonly prescribed for core strengthening. A study investigating trunk muscle activity during the front bridge (plank), supine bridge, and side bridge (plank), all with unilateral and bilateral support, showed that the exercises with bilateral lower-extremity support provided a challenge to the ES and MF (27, 65). The bridging exercises with a leg lifted revealed more IO recruitment on the side of the raised leg and an increased challenge to all musculature.

Core stability exercises can be performed on stable (floor) or unstable surfaces (exercise ball, foam roll, Bosu) (table 14.2). In general, exercises performed on an unstable base provide a greater challenge based on core muscle activity (46, 74, 82). A trunk curl on a ball increases RA recruitment (82), performing a bridge on an exercise ball increases both IO and MF activity, and integrating arm movements increases IO activity (49). Exercises on the ball have been shown to be effective in a core stability training program (77), and foam roller exercises induce greater abdominal recruitment compared with the same exercises done on the floor (50).

Suspension exercises have become a popular core training approach that is in the unstable category. One or both limbs are supported on handle straps at the end of a suspension cable with an overhead anchor point. One study showed that the hip abduction in plank most effectively activated the EO, IO, and TrA (table 14.2) and the hamstring curl most effectively activated the lumbar MF (61) while performing these exercises using suspension straps. The authors concluded that this approach is appropriate for healthy young adults.

Exercises to Enhance Flexibility

What amount of stretching results in improved flexibility? ACSM guidelines (2) suggest the following:

- Stretches should be done at a frequency of 2 to 3 days per wk with daily stretching producing the best results.
- Each stretch should be performed for a total of 60 sec (10 to 30 sec per repetition can be effective), repeated 2 to 4 times. Older adults may benefit from 30 to 60 sec duration with each stretch.
- Stretches can be passive, static (muscle fully relaxed), dynamic (as in actively straightening the leg in a hamstring stretch), ballistic, or contract-relax style as in proprioceptive neuromuscular facilitation (PNF).
- The stretch position should not cause pain or take the joint past the normal ROM; it can be to the point of tightness or slight discomfort.
- It is most effective to perform the flexibility exercises when the muscle temperature has increased through warmup exercise. It is suggested that flexibility exercises follow cardiorespiratory exercise, resistive exercise or sports (especially when power and strength are important), or be used as a standalone program. Static stretching exercises may acutely reduce power and strength.
- Suggestions for PNF include a 3 to 6 sec light-to-moderate (20% to 75% maximum) volitional muscle contraction with a 10 to 30 sec assisted stretch.

There have been many approaches to stretching various muscle groups, and a discussion of some recent approaches for the hamstrings is presented next.

Precautions for Core Stability Exercises

According to Axler and McGill (5), four exercises are not recommended: the supine bilateral straight-leg raise, bent-leg raise, hanging bent-leg raise, and static cross-knee curl-up. Unfortunately, these are common exercises in the fitness setting. The supine straight-leg raise appears to be challenging, but the load and shear to the spine can be dangerous and most people cannot stabilize their spine sufficiently to perform the exercise safely. When performing flexion trunk curls, it is only necessary to lift the shoulder girdle off the exercise surface. It is critical to minimize the role of the hip flexors (i.e., the paired psoas) in any trunk flexion exercise, particularly for people who are less fit. Many people believe that bending the knees reduces the role of the psoas muscles, but this is not so, particularly if the feet are supported (e.g., held by another person). Moreover, the psoas muscles place extreme compressive forces on the discs of the lumbar-motion segments of the vertebral column in activities such as sit-ups or bilateral leg lifts (5, 47). Posterior rotation of the pelvis is often incorporated into abdominal strengthening exercises, but for someone with disc disease, it is not always appropriate. Posterior rotation of the pelvis typically removes the lumbar lordosis, and such movement can prompt the nucleus of the intervertebral disc to migrate posteriorly. If the disc is damaged, pressure can be placed on the damaged tissue and its pain receptors or even on spinal nerves. Exercisers can place the palm of one hand on the exercise surface under the lumbar lordotic curve (i.e., the small of the back) to provide feedback to maintain the lumbar lordosis.

Many variations have been suggested as the most efficient way to create more flexible hamstrings. The variables that may be altered are the type of stretch, the duration of the stretch, the repetitions performed in one session, and the number of days per week the stretches are done. Many combinations have been successful in increasing hamstring flexibility:

- 3 days per wk, 6 repetitions of 30 sec, active stretching (6)
- 5 days per wk, 6 repetitions of 5 sec, active stretching (7)
- 5 days per wk, 1 repetition of 30 sec, passive stretching (7) (with more than two times the improvement than the active stretch of 5 sec previously noted)
- 7 days per wk, 2 times a day, 2 repetitions of 30 sec (17)
- 7 days per wk, 2 times a day, 6 repetitions of 10 sec (17)
- 3 days per wk, 15 to 45 sec per repetition totaling 120 sec per day, active or passive (20)

These studies show that some variation is allowed for individual prescription of stretching, ranging from 3 to 5 days per wk of active or passive stretching, a stretch duration of 5 to 45 sec, and a daily duration of 30 to 180 sec.

How does age affect these observations? Subjects who were 65 or older with tight hamstrings stretched 5 days per wk for 6 wk with a 15, 30, or 60 sec stretch (24). The group that performed the 60 sec stretch had a better outcome at the end of the 6 wk, an improvement that persisted longer than the gains of the other groups. Therefore, one might recommend that adults over the age of 65 stretch for 60 sec 5 days per wk.

Stretches to avoid include the standing toe touch, hurdler stretch, and full-circle neck stretch (figure 14.7). Unfortunately, these are commonly seen in fitness settings.

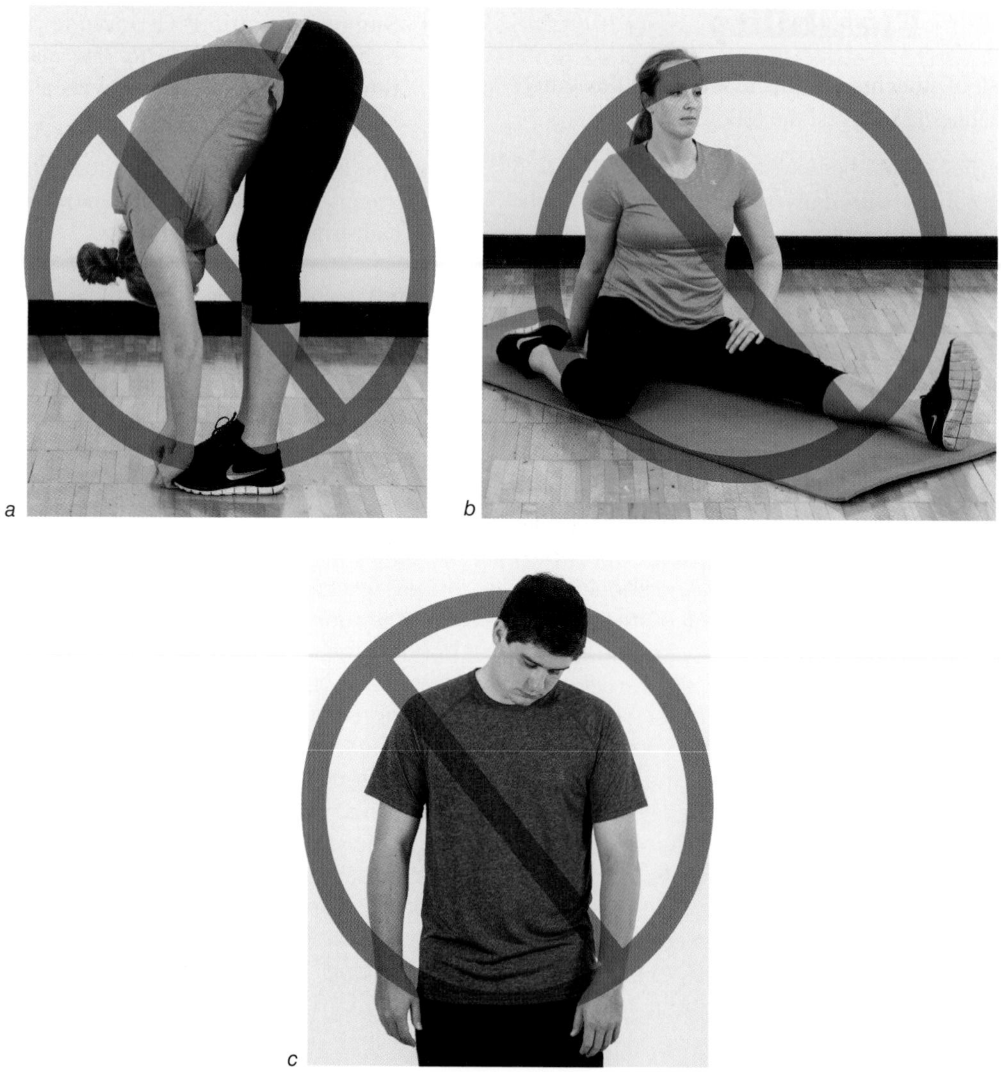

FIGURE 14.7 Stretches to avoid are the *(a)* standing toe touch, *(b)* hurdler stretch, and *(c)* full-circle neck stretch.

Stretching Techniques

- Static stretching: In static stretching, the muscle is slowly lengthened to a point where further movement is limited, and the stretch is held for a period of time (e.g., 10-60 sec).
- Active stretching: In active stretching, you assume a position with a muscle in a lengthened position and hold it there with no assistance other than the strength of the agonist muscles (the muscles that produce the main action). For example, the quadriceps (agonist) holds the leg straight in the active hamstring (antagonist) stretch. The tension of the agonists in an active stretch helps to relax the muscles being stretched (the antagonists) by reciprocal inhibition.
- Passive: A passive stretch is one in which there is no active muscular contraction in the stretched muscle. An example of this is where a fitness professional holds the leg of a client in a hamstring stretch and gently presses the leg into a stretch as the client is totally relaxed.
- Ballistic: This type of stretching uses velocity and a fast, bouncy movement to stretch a muscle or body region. It may be considered, when properly performed, for adults who participate in sports that involve ballistic movements (e.g., basketball) (2). For most it may not be safe because the forces involved with bouncing may push tissues past a safe length (the end point of normal ROM) where the client can control the movement and prevent injury from occurring.
- Dynamic: This type of stretching involves moving while stretching, but it does not include bounding or pushing muscles past their normal ROM. An example of dynamic stretching would be arm circles, progressing from smaller to larger as the shoulders warm up.
- Proprioceptive neuromuscular facilitation (PNF): PNF includes stretching techniques that are commonly used in the clinical setting. They are aimed at improving active and passive ROM as well as optimizing motor performance and neuromuscular performance. The active PNF stretches common in a fitness setting combine stretching with alternating contraction and relaxation of muscles to improve flexibility.

Stretching Program

When designing a fitness program for a client, it is important to include a general stretching program addressing flexibility of all the major muscle groups. Following are some suggested stretches for most major muscle groups and body regions. It is wise to address all areas of the body in flexibility training. Remember to not take the joint past the normal ROM and to avoid ballistic stretching. The stretch position should not elicit pain. If clients experience pain, refer them to the appropriate medical provider for further evaluation.

Neck Stretches

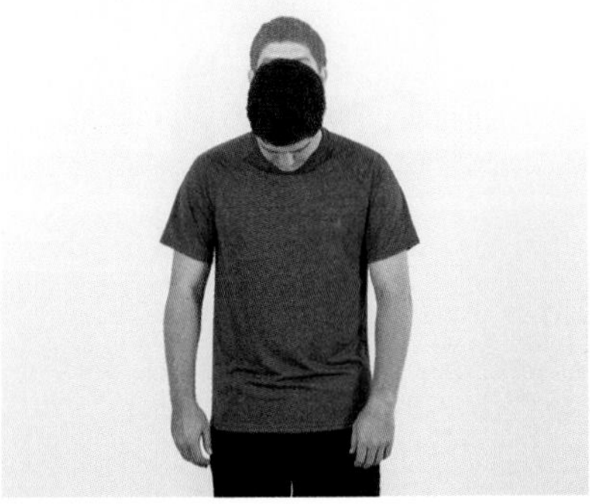

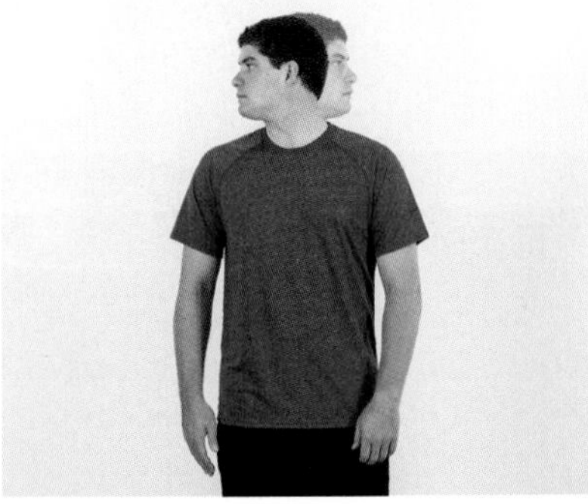

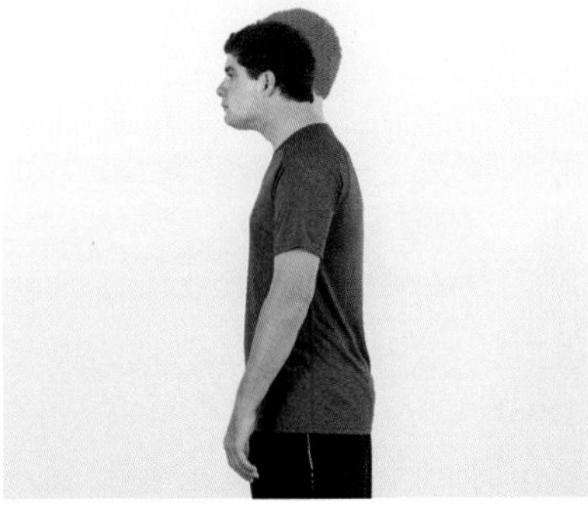

(continued)

Stretching Program *(continued)*

Upper-Back and Chest Stretches

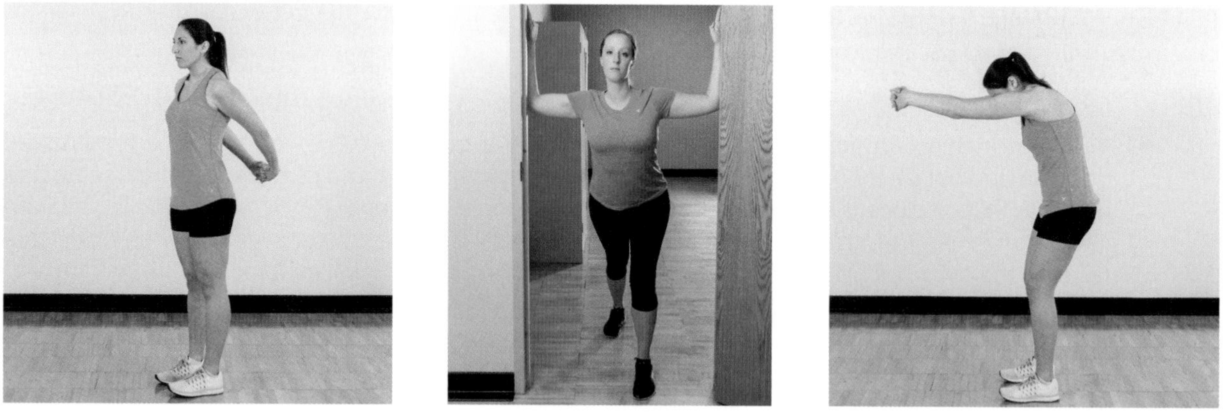

Spine Stretches

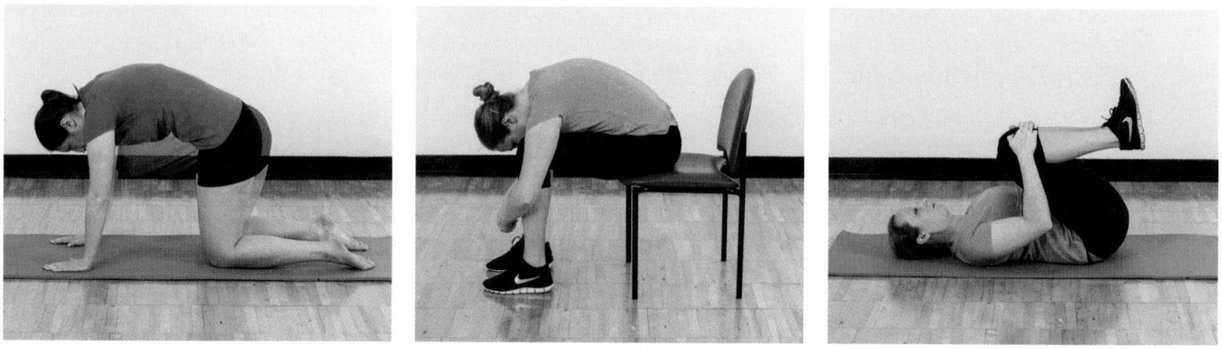

Spine Stretches

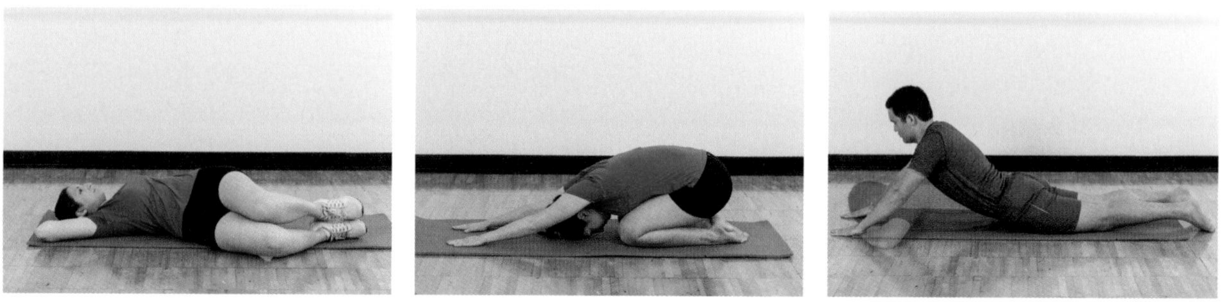

Back and Hip Stretches (Piriformis)

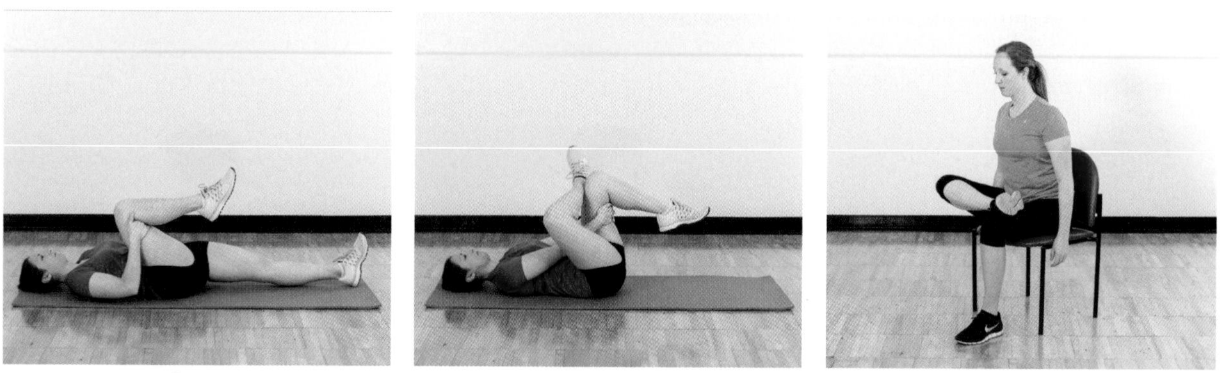

Hamstring Stretches

It is best if the natural lumbar lordosis is maintained to protect the disc from added stress (52). This can be performed with a strap passively or actively extending the leg.

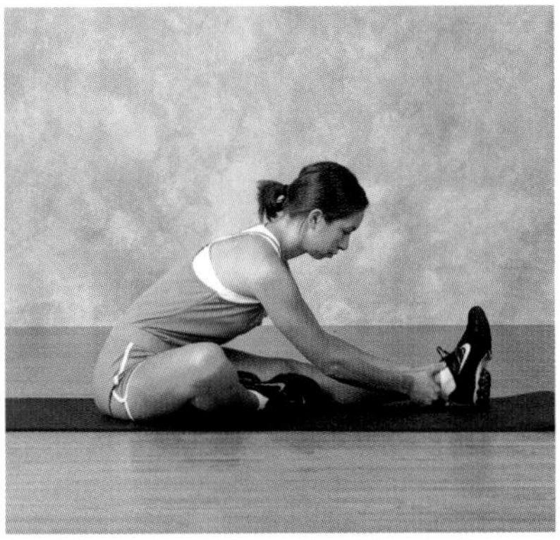
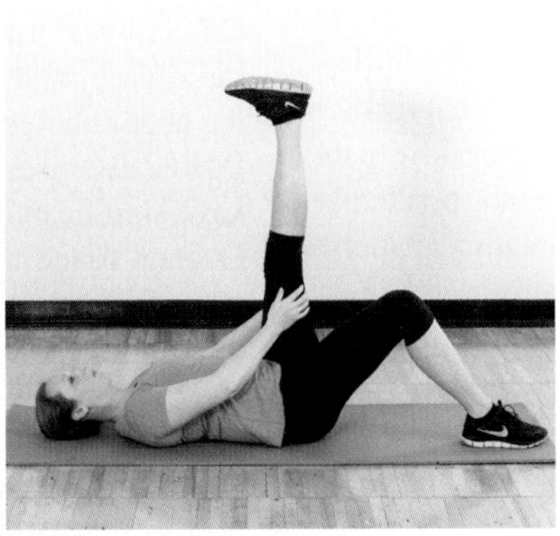
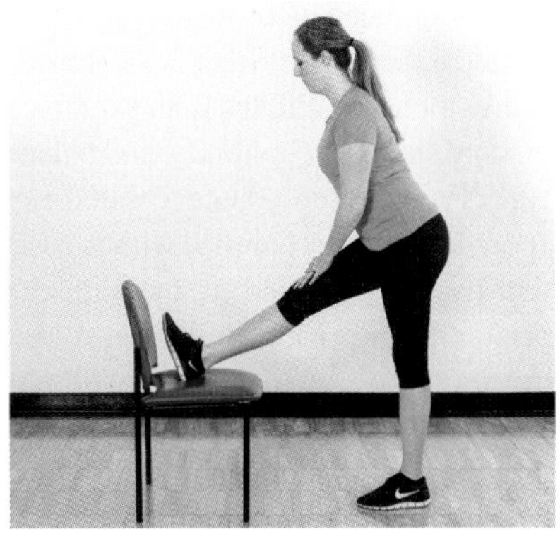

ITB Stretches

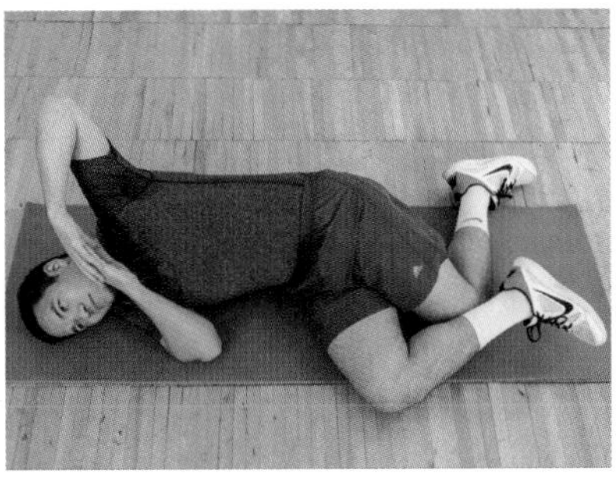
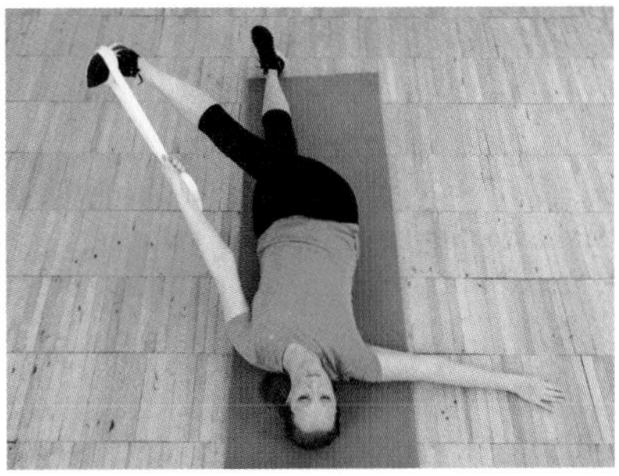
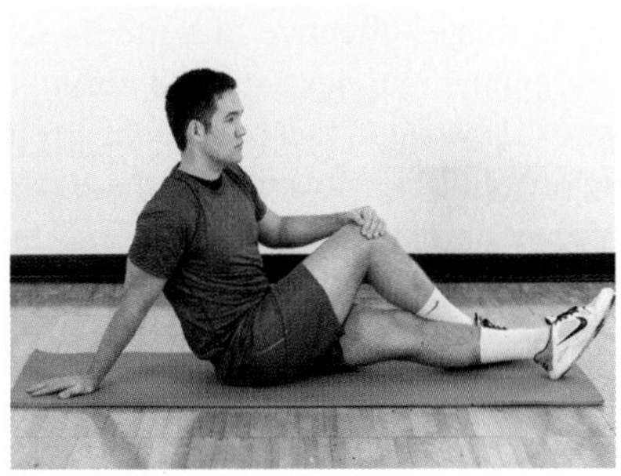

Hip, Thigh (Quadriceps), and Inner Thigh Stretches

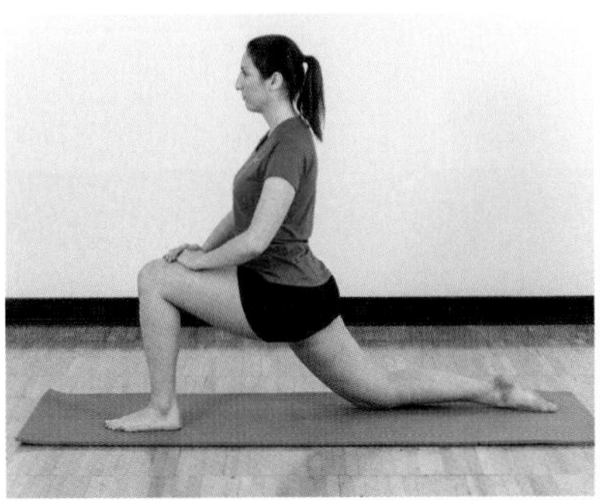
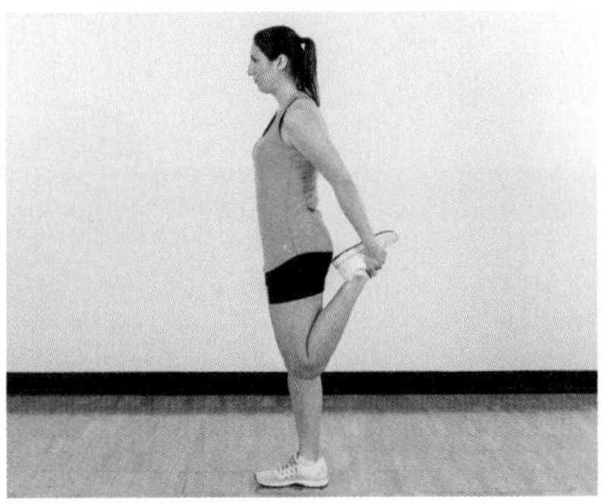
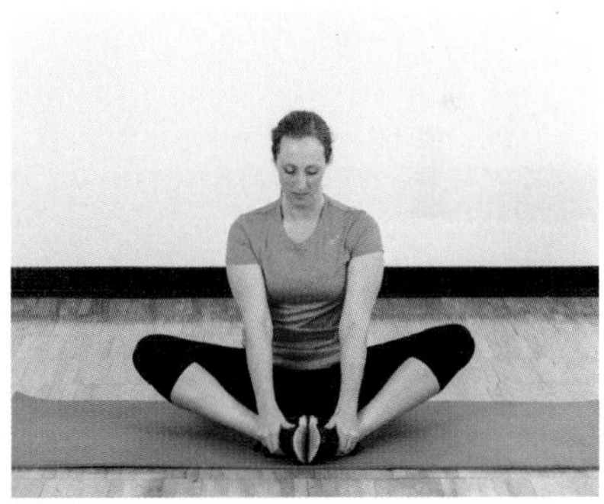

Calf Stretches (Soleus and Gastrocnemius)

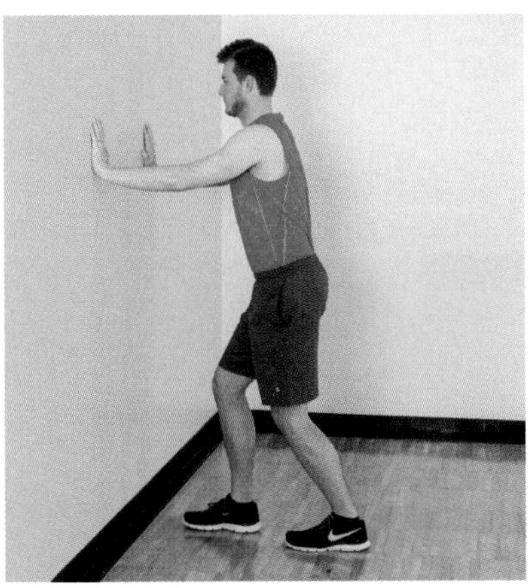
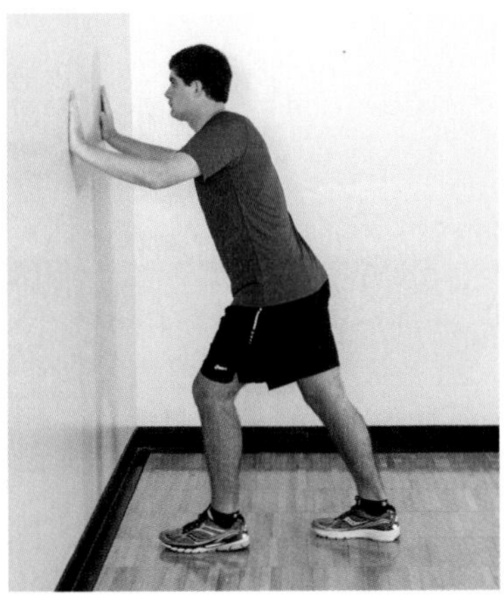
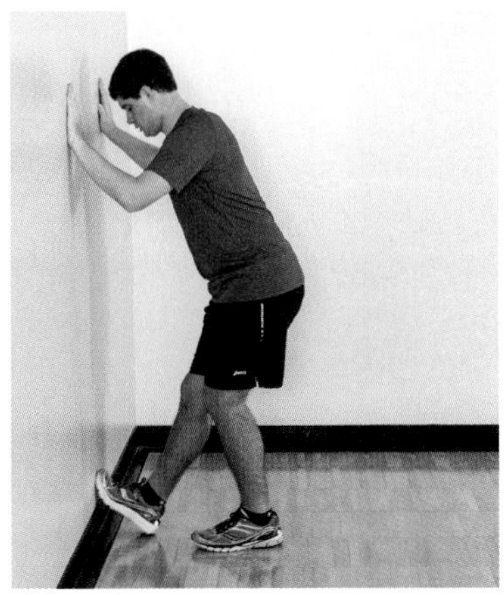

Pilates, Yoga, Tai Chi, and Aquatic Approaches

Pilates has been incorporated into both fitness settings and physical therapy settings as a core strengthening and flexibility tool (76). Pilates is an exercise method that focuses on core strength, flexibility, and balance in the body. In the early 1900s, Joseph Pilates created a systematic practice of specific exercises coupled with focused breathing patterns that has been refined to integrate current biomechanical principles to protect the spine. A variety of certification programs are available. The Pilates Method Alliance (PMA) is a professional association with a certification program for Pilates teachers. Its goal is to establish the teaching of Pilates as a profession by validating that a PMA-certified Pilates instructor meets entry-level standards for safety and competency.

Is Pilates effective in a fitness setting? Are the deep abdominal muscles activated during typical Pilates exercises? How important is it to correctly perform the drawing-in or hollowing movement in these exercises? Studies have shown an increase in the use and thickness of the TrA following performance of the hundred (a common Pilates exercise; see figure 14.8) 2 days per wk for 8 wk (19). The TrA recruitment (drawing-in action) also has been shown to be increased and thicker (improved contraction) during the correctly performed mat imprint, two styles of the hundred, the roll-up, and the leg circle as compared with resting the abdominal muscles (22) (see figure 14.9). Two prone Pilates exercises, swimming and leg beat (figure 14.10), have significantly high activation levels of the MF (48). Gagnon found that a Pilates program with LBP patients was as effective as the traditional lumbar stabilization program in lowering pain, improving functional reports, and improving balance stability testing (25). Measures of pain were lower and function was significantly higher in experimental groups of subjects with LBP who participated in a Pilates program compared with subjects who had medication only (62) and other medical consultations (72). It appears that, with the appropriate application of the hollowing deep abdominal activation, Pilates is a good method of core stability training. It is important to note that one needs proper training to teach Pilates. The PMA website is a good place to begin for people who are interested in this training (www.pilatesmethodalliance.org).

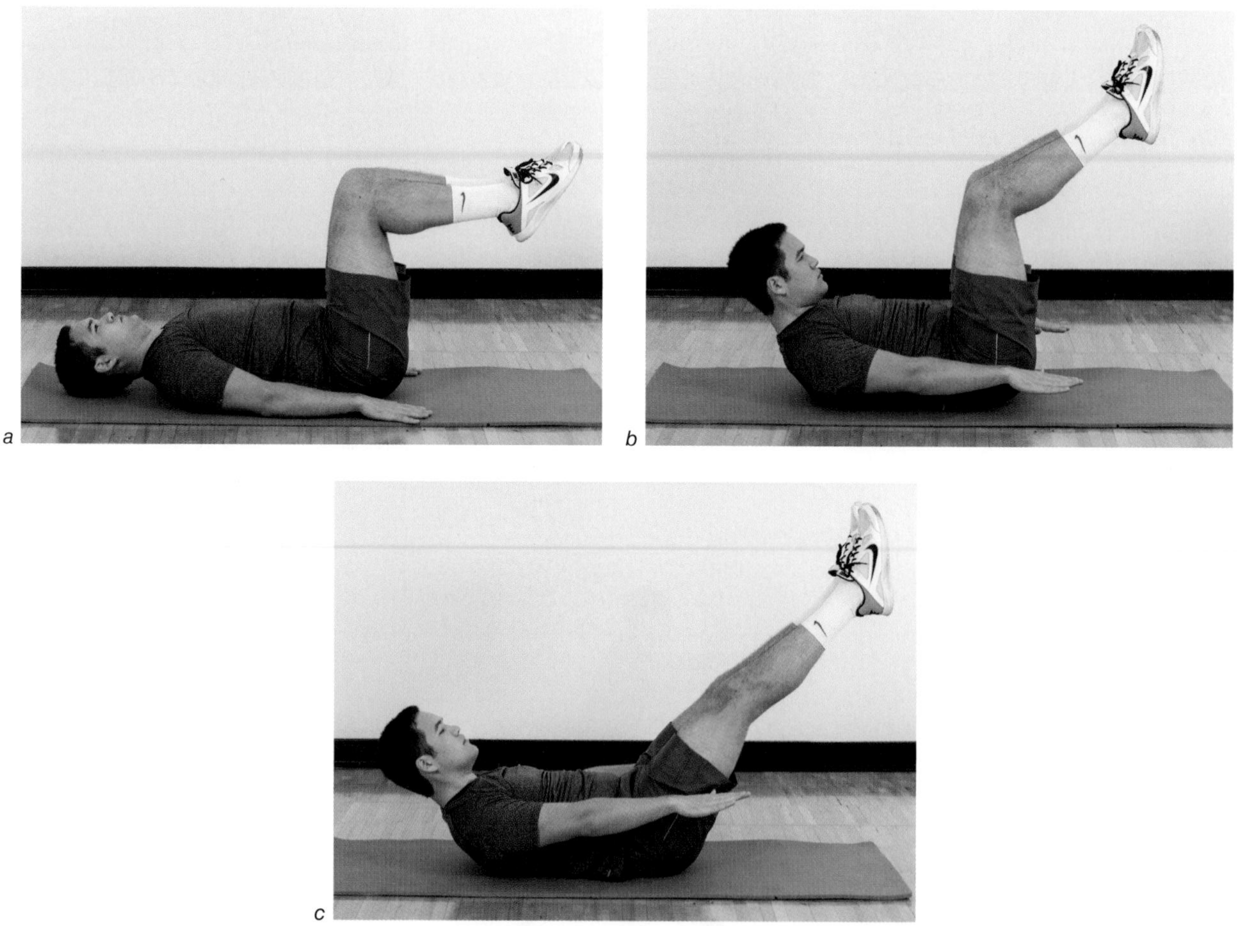

FIGURE 14.8 Pilates hundred exercise. Note the scooped shape of the abdomen with the drawing in of the TrA and the lumbar spine in contact with the mat to safely perform this exercise.

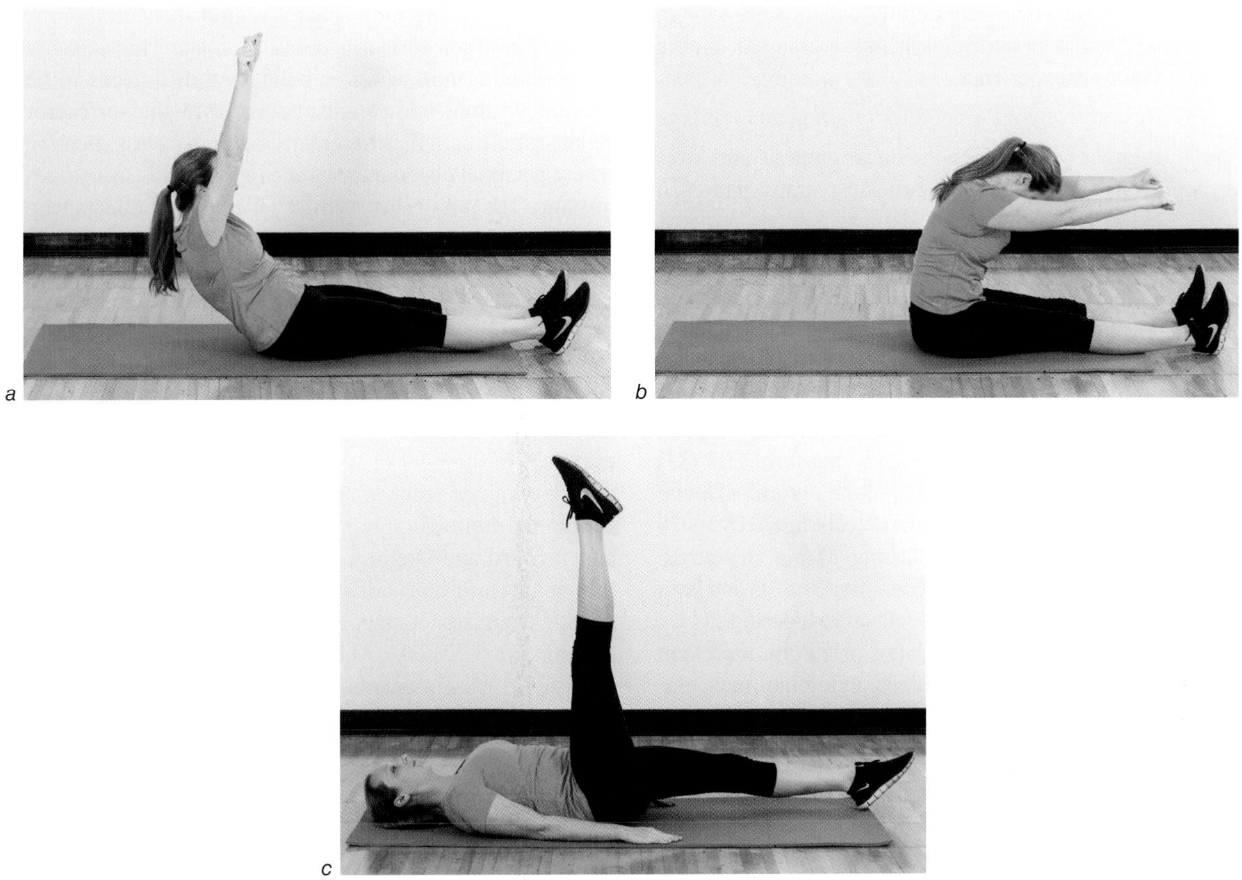

FIGURE 14.9 Pilates exercises for TrA recruitment: *(a)* roll-up midpoint, *(b)* roll-up end position, and *(c)* leg circle.

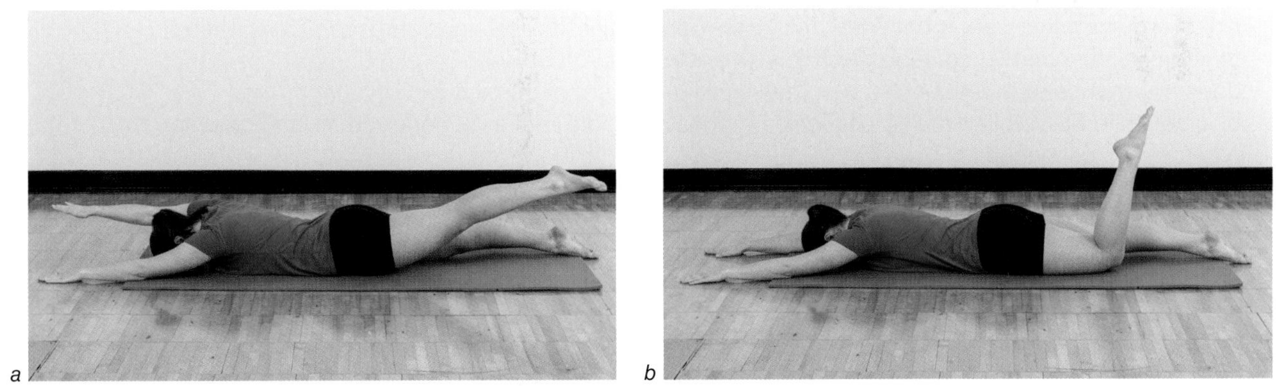

FIGURE 14.10 Pilates exercises to activate the MF: *(a)* swimming and *(b)* leg beat.

Yoga has been recommended for many reasons, including improving flexibility, reducing stress, and reducing pain (76). Some fitness settings offer yoga classes, and the fitness professional may need to determine whether yoga is appropriate for a particular client. Some research points to yoga being a supportive adjunct to other fitness activities. For example, Cramer et al. found strong evidence for short-term effectiveness and moderate evidence for long-term effectiveness of yoga for chronic LBP (18). There are many forms of yoga:

- Hot yoga—performed in 105 °F (40 °C) heat and 40% humidity
- Hatha yoga—focuses on slow, gentle movements using a repertoire of poses, or asanas; common in fitness settings
- Vinyasa yoga—flows from one pose to the next; the most popular style of yoga in the United States

- Ashtanga yoga—commonly called *power yoga*; best suited for athletes or people looking for a more vigorous experience
- Restorative yoga—good for quieting and relaxing
- Iyengar yoga—focuses on alignment and uses props such as blocks, harnesses, straps, and even cushions

As with Pilates, fitness professionals interested in teaching yoga should seek certification in this area. Yoga Alliance is a nonprofit organization that credentials yoga teachers and may be found at www.yogaalliance.org.

Another popular group exercise aimed at flexibility, balance, and control of the spine is tai chi. Tai chi is a good alternative for those aged 18 to 70 with long-term LBP (31) and those with chronic conditions of the musculoskeletal system (54). A 2011 study had subjects aged 18 to 70 participate in 18 sessions, each lasting 40 min, in a group setting for 10 wk. Overall functional fitness tests and pain improved for these subjects over the 10 wk period (51).

Before performing yoga, Pilates, or tai chi, the client needs to be able to recruit the deep abdominal musculature stabilizing the lumbosacral region in neutral spine position or slight flexion for any exercise. This capacity for abdominal hollowing or pelvic stability needs to be present without additional cueing from the instructor because these activities frequently occur in a class situation where personal observation of the individual is sometimes missing. The possibility of injury increases if clients who cannot stabilize the lumbosacral region are asked to perform larger movements. The neutral zone needs to be stabilized by the local system before adding a larger challenge from the global muscular system.

Aquatic exercise can be extremely beneficial for clients needing flexibility and core stability training. Some researchers recently investigated spine stabilization exercises in the pool (13). They found that the exercises that maximized trunk muscle activity in the pool were abdominal hollowing and resistance against an exercise ball forward and laterally (holding the ball and pressing into it forward and sideways). For more details about aquatic exercises, contact the United States Water Fitness Association (USWFA), which offers national certifications for water fitness instructors (www.uswfa.com).

A Note About Medical Intervention

When might the fitness professional need to refer a client to a medical professional? A fitness professional spends a lot of time with a client and may have the opportunity to hear concerns that the client has not shared with others. The discussion here is not about emergency situations that occur in a fitness setting but rather when there is slow or no progression or when unusual signs and symptoms are mentioned. If clients report any of these signs and symptoms related to low-back function, encourage them to visit a medical professional: unrelenting pain, pain that does not change with rest or change of position, persistent night pain when younger than 20 yr or older than 55 yr, bilateral leg pain or paresthesia, saddle region (where you sit on a saddle) paresthesia, or changes in bowel or bladder control (28). If these are reported, the client should see a doctor before continuing.

Clients might also comply with a program that has been well designed for them but make slow or nonexistent progress. This may be evident in a lack of progression in specific exercises, no change or an increase in pain, or no change in flexibility. Such cases might be an opportunity to refer the client to a physical therapist to address potential biomechanical and alignment needs. Ahmed et al. (2) found that patients with mechanical LBP showed more improvement with lumbar mobilization (manual therapy) and core strengthening combined than with core strengthening alone. The client may need manual therapy or orthotic assessment to support the fitness program. Referral to a physical therapist does not mean the client needs to stop attending the fitness sessions but that the addition of another tool may help the client progress faster and further. The fitness professional should communicate with the medical professional to create a cohesive approach for the client.

LEARNING AIDS

REVIEW QUESTIONS

1. What constitutes a motion segment? What is a function of the facet joints?
2. Describe the difference between a structural and a functional spinal curve.
3. Which muscles are important in controlling pelvic position (guy-wires)?
4. Explain the roles of the local and global trunk musculature.
5. Explain why knowing a client's back history is important.
6. Describe the hollowing or drawing-in abdominal exercise and its purpose.
7. Describe the progression from the basic drawing-in abdominal motion to a trunk curl with the feet off the floor, and explain when to take the precaution of stopping the progression.
8. Describe a good exercise for developing each of the following muscles: quadratus lumborum (QL), rectus abdominis (RA), transversus abdominis (TrA), and erector spinae (ES).
9. Why is good flexibility important to spinal health?
10. Describe flexibility exercises for the major areas of the body and the ACSM guidelines for performing them.

CASE STUDIES

1. A fitness professional is using a double-leg-lowering task with a group of relatively fit adults, ostensibly to improve the strength of the abdominal muscles. Discuss the appropriateness or inappropriateness of the exercise.
2. A client shares that his favorite hamstring stretches are the hurdler stretch and toe touch, which he has performed since high school. Should he change this stretching routine?
3. A fitness professional reads a book on Pilates exercises and feels successful in performing them. She decides to teach them to a training client at the next session. Discuss the appropriateness of this decision.
4. A fitness professional is progressing a client through the beginning-level hollowing abdominal exercises and sees a tentlike appearance of the abdominal region. What is occurring, and is this person ready to add global musculature strengthening?

Answers to Case Studies

1. The double-leg-lowering task is not an appropriate core exercise if the legs are taken to the floor. According to Axler and McGill (5), four exercises are not recommended, including the supine bilateral straight-leg raise. Some exercises, such as the Pilates hundred (figure 14.8), may be appropriate for people who can stabilize the spine and pelvic girdle with both legs extended out at an angle; however, the legs should never be lowered to the floor and lifted again.
2. The hurdler and toe touch are not safe, effective stretches. The fitness professional can instruct this client in alternative hamstring stretches, explaining that research has revealed more effective ways to address hamstring tightness.
3. A fitness professional should have significant training in an area such as Pilates, yoga, or tai chi before accepting the responsibility of teaching these specialized exercise techniques to clients.
4. The tentlike appearance is most likely the RA (the most superficial abdominal muscle, which runs superior to inferior on the abdomen) contracting as the hollowing exercise is performed. This client is not ready to progress to the next level because the tenting reveals that the TrA is not yet activated as the primary abdominal stabilizer. The client should continue to work on recruiting the TrA in a variety of positions and activities.

15

Training for Performance

Scott A. Conger

OBJECTIVES

The reader will be able to do the following:

1. Describe the elements of an aerobic training program.
2. Understand the importance of establishing a training base before prescribing more advanced training methods.
3. Design an aerobic interval workout for athletes who compete in endurance events.
4. Understand the benefits of cross-training and tapering for athletes.
5. Understand the benefits and risks of ballistic resistance training.
6. Describe the various methods used to improve running speed.
7. Describe the benefits of high-intensity interval training.

Numerous health benefits of physical activity and exercise have been discussed throughout this text. For example, aerobic exercise improves cardiovascular function and reduces the risk of heart disease and type 2 diabetes. Resistance training is important throughout the life span and helps maintain bone health and functional independence later in life. However, when performance enhancement is the goal, the application of training principles is considerably different. Every athlete, whether competing at a world-class level or in a recreational setting, needs a specific training program to realize performance goals.

To train safely for performance, a baseline level of fitness (e.g., healthy body composition, cardiorespiratory endurance, muscular strength) is needed. In that regard, all athletes should perform some training in areas not central to their primary focus. For example, endurance athletes should spend a majority of their training time completing endurance exercise, but resistance and flexibility training should also be part of the overall training program.

This chapter provides a brief overview of training strategies for achieving performance goals. The focus of the chapter is the recreational athlete rather than the elite athlete competing at the collegiate or national level. Also, we direct the interested reader to the Human Kinetics website (www.humankinetics.com) for resources that contain more detailed treatments of how to train for competitions. After briefly reviewing the need for a warm-up, we begin with training programs for endurance events.

Warm-Up and Cool-Down

There is no question that a warm-up and cool-down are essential parts of every workout, especially when the focus is on performance. (Please see chapters 11 and 13 for more details.) The warm-up before a training session or a competition allows an athlete to physically and mentally prepare for the activity. It increases muscle and core temperature, circulation to the active muscles, and neuromuscular activity.

A warm-up should include a general warm-up and an activity-specific warm-up. The general warm-up consists of 5 to 10 min of moderate-intensity activity, such as walking, light running, or stationary cycling. During this period, the HR and respiratory rate increase to modest levels. The general warm-up should be followed by an activity-specific warm-up that incorporates movements that are specific to the sport. Traditionally, static stretching was included in the warm-up, but research suggests that static stretching before exercise provides no performance benefits (35) and may even hinder performance (24, 54). A better option is to complete dynamic warm-up exercises through the complete ROM of the joints. The dynamic exercises should mimic the movements used in the training session and can include some prescribed movements that address any injuries or deficiencies. For example, a warm-up routine for a runner may include dynamic movements such as walking lunges and butt kicks. To address problems related to ITB syndrome, the athlete would also incorporate dynamic lateral leg swings to loosen the hip and ITB. Additional activity-specific movements at progressively greater intensities can also be included. The total duration of the activity-specific warm-up should be between 5 and 15 min.

Immediately after completing the workout, the athlete should perform a 5 to 15 min cool-down that includes light aerobic activity and static or PNF stretching (see chapter 14). If the athlete has any lingering soft-tissue issues, foam rollers or trigger-point therapy may be included during this time. During or immediately after completing the cool-down, the athlete should begin to rehydrate and consume a small amount of carbohydrate and protein. See chapter 5 for more information on postexercise nutrition.

Training for Aerobic Events

What kind of workouts can you design for clients who are interested in competing in local road races, such as a 5K or 10K, or in triathlons that involve a combination of swimming, biking, and running? The common variables for success in these races include maximal aerobic power ($\dot{V}O_2$max), the muscle's ability to use fuel aerobically, the LT (lactate threshold), and training to perform at race pace. Although the principles outlined in this section can apply to many kinds of competitions, we focus on these events for the following reasons:

- 5K and 10K runs are popular distances in community charitable races (e.g., Susan G. Komen Race for the Cure). The world record for the 10K (6.2 mi) is about 27 min for men and 30 min for women, but many adult recreational runners might be happy with those times for a 5K (3.1 mi). These distances are well within the abilities of many adult fitness participants who are interested in performance.
- Sprint triathlons typically require a .75K (.5 mi) swim, 20K (12.4 mi) bike ride, and 5K (3.1 mi) run, and Olympic triathlons require a 1.5K (.93 mi) swim, 40K (24.8 mi) bike ride, and 10K (6.2 mi) run. In addition to the overall performance in the triathlon, each element has an endurance component. Triathlons are popular with many recreational athletes who enjoy finding challenges beyond a single sport.

As with any new training program, progression is key when moving clients from where they are (in terms of aerobic fitness, volume and intensity of exercise, and experience) to where they need to be to compete in the events like those just described. One size does not fit all. So, where does one begin? How do we systematically challenge the various systems and tissues to improve endurance performance?

Training Base

To engage in and benefit from the various training programs described later, an athlete needs to have already established a routine exercise program—a **training base**—on which to improve. Before initiating a strenuous exercise program, the athlete typically should already be working out 3 or 4 days per wk with a rest day between each. In establishing a training base, the focus is on exercise volume, generally done at an intensity below that of race pace. For running performance, a classic approach has been long, slow distance (LSD) training involving continuous exercise at an intensity less than 70% of $\dot{V}O_2max$ (<80% of HRmax) for a distance or duration approaching what is required for competition in shorter road races. To ensure the training runs are performed at the appropriate intensity, a heart watch would be helpful for providing feedback about HR. When the athlete is ready to increase the volume of activity, a change of no more than 10% per wk is recommended. For example, if the athlete is completing 30 min workouts 3 days per wk, an increase to 33 min per workout would meet that recommendation.

Establishing a training base using an existing skill is recommended, and for many people that means a focus on running. That may not be so for swimming, where skill is quite varied and can have a significant impact on the ability to compete. That said, adults do learn to swim better with training. For swimming, developing a training base requires enhancing skill as well as building endurance in muscle groups that are not typically used. For that reason, in addition to choosing a speed that can be comfortably tolerated, the workout includes brief (10 sec) rest periods between elements of the workout. The times for each element are not recorded; the focus is on completing the workout and building the base. The following would help accomplish that goal for a person working toward completing a triathlon:

- Ten 50 m swims with 10 sec between each; repeat after 2 min recovery
- Pyramid workout (e.g., 50, 100, 150, 100, and 50 m swims) with 10 sec between each; repeat after 2 min recovery

As the person's fitness improves, the distance of each swim interval (e.g., 50 m) increases while the rest interval remains the same. This progression continues until the athlete can swim continuously for the desired distance (e.g., .75K).

Cyclists with a goal of completing a half-century ride (50 mi, or 80 km) can build the training base using stationary bikes at the gym, spin classes, their own bikes on a trainer, or their own bikes on the road. Cyclists are not just increasing their fitness; they are also building up seat time that allows adaptation to the focused pressure on the sitting area and crotch for long periods of time. In that regard, ensuring that the bicycle is properly fitted and wearing padded cycling shorts are recommended. The base is built over many weeks, beginning with two to three short rides per wk of 30 min or less. The frequency and duration of rides should increase each week, but keep in mind that the weekly volume of exercise should increase by no more than 10% per wk.

Aerobic Training Methods

Once a training base has been established, the focus can shift to specific aspects of performance during each training session. A variety of aerobic training methods can be used to achieve performance goals, and each method is unique in how it adjusts training intensity and duration to achieve a particular outcome. The major methods of aerobic training are tempo training, aerobic interval training, fartlek training, and anaerobic interval training (discussed later in the chapter).

Tempo Training

Tempo training uses an intensity that is at or slightly below that used in the competition (14). For improvements in $\dot{V}O_2max$, this type of training is superior to LSD training (33). The purpose of these training sessions is to develop a sense of an appropriate pace for competitions, and the duration of each session is usually 20 to 40 min. Hanc (29) suggests four methods to choose the appropriate intensity for these runs:

1. Recent race: Add 30 to 40 sec to the current 5K pace or 15 to 20 sec to the 10K pace.
2. HR: Should be 85% to 90% of maximum HR.
3. Perceived exertion: Should be an 8 on a scale of 1 to 10 (a comfortable effort would be 5; racing would be close to 10).
4. Talk test: A question like "Pace okay?" should be possible, but conversation won't be.

Jack Daniels has written extensively about this topic in his book *Daniels' Running Formula* (14). In addition, a website with a calculator based on Daniels' principles is available to determine the pace for a tempo training session (www.runsmartproject.com/calculator). This calculator was used to determine the pace for the following two runners: Anna, who is currently able to run a 10K at a race pace of 10 min · mi^{-1} (62:10 finishing time), and Rodney, who is able to run a 10K at a race pace of 7 min · mi^{-1} (43:30 finishing time). The pace during their tempo training session will vary slightly depending on the total duration of the session. For a 20 min tempo run, each should be able to maintain an intensity similar to their LT pace but below race pace. For each additional 5 min of exercise duration, the pace should slow by about 1% (14). Table 15.1 shows the tempo training pace for each runner based on the exercise duration and the runner's personal performance in the 10K using Daniels' calculator.

Interval Training

Interval training consists of alternating periods of exercise with periods of recovery. It is also referred to as *intermittent* or *repetition training*. Though there is some debate about the appropriate use of these terms, they all refer to the same general concept (15). The duration and intensity of the exercise period (known as the *work interval*) varies based on the goals of the workout. As the duration of the work interval increases, the relative intensity is reduced. Longer work intervals emphasize the aerobic system to a greater extent. In contrast, as the intensity of the work interval increases and the duration decreases, the anaerobic pathways supply more energy to the muscles. The time between work intervals is termed the *recovery interval*. In most cases, the recovery interval should be active rather than passive, meaning that the body stays in motion at a low intensity. Low-intensity activity, such as walking or slow running, helps to prevent some of the negative repercussions associated with stopping an exercise session suddenly.

The work and recovery intervals are expressed as a ratio. For example, a 60 sec work interval followed by a 30 sec recovery interval would result in a 2:1 work-to-recovery ratio. Interval training can be subdivided into two categories based on the duration of the intervals: aerobic interval training and anaerobic interval training (discussed later in this chapter).

Aerobic intervals are characterized by work intervals of between 1 and 5 min, with brief recovery intervals that may be as short as 10 sec (3, 13). The goal of aerobic interval training is to spend as much time during the workout as possible at 95% to 100% of $\dot{V}O_2$max. For our clients Anna and Rodney, this speed would be faster than they could maintain for a mile. Based on their 10K performances mentioned earlier, we can use Daniels' calculator (www.runsmartproject.com/calculator) to determine the pace to maintain in an aerobic interval workout:

Anna: 9:15 min · mi^{-1} pace(2:18 per .25 mi [.4 km] and 4:36 per .5 mi [.8 km])

Rodney: 6:37 min · mi^{-1} pace (1:39 per .25 mi [.4 km] and 3:18 per .5 mi [.8 km])

In general, the work-to-recovery ratio during aerobic interval training is around 1:1 but can be up to 8:1. A short recovery interval does not allow the cardiovascular system to completely recover, but it does allow a brief break from the stress associated with the strenuous exercise (13). During 2 min intervals at 100% of the velocity of $\dot{V}O_2$max (running speed estimated from the runner's $\dot{V}O_2$max and running economy that was obtained during a separate testing session [47]), Demarie et al. (17) found that the time spent at 100% of $\dot{V}O_2$max during interval training was twice as long when the recovery interval was shortened from 2 min to 1 min. Because the recovery interval (i.e., 1 min) was not long enough to allow the cardiovascular system to recover completely, the time that it took for oxygen consumption to return to $\dot{V}O_2$max was shorter during the next work interval (17).

The design of an aerobic interval program should incorporate many of the same elements that are used in designing a CRF program (see chapter 11). Elements to consider in the aerobic interval program include: (1) duration or distance of work intervals, (2) intensity of work intervals, (3) number of work intervals, (4) duration of recovery intervals, and (5) frequency of workouts (37, 40, 43).

1. The interval duration will vary based on the workout, but in general the duration should be 2 to 3 min. An alternative would be to select a distance that requires the athlete to complete it within the selected duration at the appropriate intensity.
2. The intensity of the work interval will vary based on the duration, but it will typically be between 90% and 100% of $\dot{V}O_2$max. Due to the relatively short duration of the intervals, using percentage of HRmax or HRR may not be appropriate because of the time needed for the HR to plateau.
3. Determining the number of work intervals will also depend on the length of the intervals. A good working rule is to limit the total duration of the work intervals to between 10 and 20 min. For example, if a workout has the athlete completing 2 min work intervals at a 2:1 work-to-recovery ratio, the total number of work intervals should be between 5 and 10. The entire workout (including warm-up, cool-down, and work and recovery intervals) may be 60 min in duration, but only 10 to 20 min will be at the prescribed work-interval intensity.
4. For aerobic interval workouts, the recovery duration should be equal to or less than the work duration. The recovery intervals should be active at a low intensity (20%-30% of $\dot{V}O_2$max).
5. Due to the intensity of these workouts, the typical athlete should only complete one or two aerobic interval workouts per wk. For most training programs, one interval workout per wk is sufficient. If multiple aerobic interval workouts are completed during a week, at least 2 full days of recovery should be allowed between workouts (e.g., workout 1 on Monday and workout 2 on Thursday).

These same principles can be applied to all endurance exercise modes. For example, a 1,000 yd (914 m) swim interval workout could consist of 20 intervals of 50 yd (46 m) with a 1:1 work-to-rest interval. For cycling, find a relatively flat route and select a comfortable, moderate to high pedaling cadence during the warm-up. Shift to a higher gear and try to maintain the same cadence for 3 min. After 3 min, shift to the lowest gear for the 3 min recovery interval.

Table 15.1 Average Running Pace ($min \cdot mi^{-1}$) for Tempo Training Sessions for Two Clients With Different Race Paces

	20 min	25 min	30 min	35 min	40 min
Anna (10 $min \cdot mi^{-1}$ race pace)	10:04	10:11	10:17	10:20	10:24
Rodney (7 $min \cdot mi^{-1}$ race pace)	7:11	7:17	7:21	7:23	7:26

Table 15.2 Sample Interval Workout for Two Athletes at Different Fitness Levels

	Distance	Intensity	Repetitions	Recovery
Anna (10 $min \cdot mi^{-1}$ 10K race pace)	.25 mi (.4 km) .50 mi (.8 km)	.25 mi: 2:18 .50 mi: 4:36	Repeat three times	2 min rest between work intervals
Rodney (7 $min \cdot mi^{-1}$ 10K race pace)	.25 mi (.4 km) .50 mi (.8 km)	.25 mi: 1:39 .50 mi: 3:18	Repeat three times	1.5 min rest between work intervals

Repeat this pattern for 4 to 6 intervals. An interval workout for any endurance activity can be designed in a number of formats, such as alternating durations (e.g., 1.5 min and 3 min repeated four times), pyramid distance (e.g., 400 m, 800 m, 1,200 m, 800 m, 400 m), or using a hill for running or cycling that takes 2 to 3 min to ascend. Hill workouts also allow a built-in recovery interval by having the athlete run or cycle up the hill and walk or coast down the hill during the recovery interval. Table 15.2 provides an example of an interval running workout for our clients Anna and Rodney (www.runsmartproject.com/calculator).

Fartlek Training

A form of endurance training that combines LSD training with aerobic interval training is **fartlek training** (from the Swedish word meaning "speed play"). The distinction between fartlek training and interval training is that, in fartlek training, the exercise is continuous with intensity alternating between moderate and high levels (in contrast to low and high levels during interval training). Two examples of fartlek workouts for runners would be to break a continuous 45 min run into several short intervals as follows:

1. Run 4 min at a normal LSD pace followed by 1 min at a pace that is 20 to 30 sec faster than the LSD pace (e.g., a 7:30 $min \cdot mi^{-1}$ pace compared with an LSD pace of 8:00 $min \cdot mi^{-1}$); repeat this pattern for the duration of the workout.
2. Run at LSD pace for 20 steps and then slightly increase the pace for 20 steps, run at a LSD for 40 steps and then slightly increase the pace for 40 steps, run at LSD pace for 60 steps and then slightly increase the pace for 60 steps, and so on (14).

Interval Training History

Interval training has a rich history. In 1912, interval training was a cornerstone of Finnish 10,000 m Olympic champion Hannes Kolehmainen's training plan (6). Following World War II, interval training became common among elite distance runners. Emil Zatopek is commonly considered the father of interval training, although some of his training is better characterized as fartlek training (42). Zatopek's training usually consisted of two training sessions per day. One training session consisted of a fartlek-style training run of 1 to 2 hr through the forest, frequently running 50 repetitions of 200 to 400 m, alternating between high and moderate intensity (42). The second session consisted of 50 × 200 m runs at race pace or 40 × 200 m runs at 100% of maximal velocity and 6 × 400 m at 90% of maximal velocity (6). Using these training methods, Zatopek won the 10,000 m in the 1948 Olympics. At the following Olympic Games, he won the gold medal in the 5,000 m and the 10,000 m. He capped off the 1952 Olympics by winning a gold medal in the marathon in his first race ever at that distance (52). Two years later, Roger Bannister broke the 4 $min \cdot mi^{-1}$ barrier by employing a training plan that consisted primarily of repeated 400 m intervals at near-maximal effort (5). With the success of these athletes, interval training became an important component of endurance athletes' training programs. It is clear that endurance athletes' training programs should include some type of interval training to realize their performance goals.

This type of training can be used as an alternative to interval training for athletes who do not enjoy repeating laps around a track. It also helps reduce boredom during a daily workout. The benefits of fartlek training are similar to those of aerobic interval training and tempo training: improvements in $\dot{V}O_2max$ and LT.

Cross-Training

The repetitive nature of some sports can lead to staleness and increase the chance for overuse injuries. Lap after lap in the pool or on a track can cause training at the appropriate intensity to become boring and the athlete to lose motivation. To break up the monotony, it can be beneficial to build cross-training into a program. **Cross-training** refers to an alternative training mode that is outside the athlete's competition sport. For example, a runner may include a cycling workout in his training program once per wk to break up the routine of a typical running workout. Beyond overcoming boredom, there are a number of reasons why cross-training may be beneficial to performance. One of the biggest benefits is that the risk of overtraining injuries may be reduced (7, 41). Cross-training can train the same energy system without the repetitive stress to muscles and joints that accompanies sport-specific training. Cross-training is also a useful way to maintain aerobic fitness when an athlete is injured or is on a reduced training volume while recovering from an injury. Further, as mentioned previously, it can help maintain an athlete's motivation by breaking up the monotony of a training program. There is perhaps a greater need to break up the repetitive nature of workouts during the off-season when competitions are infrequent.

Although cross-training has benefits, the principle of specificity reinforces the importance of sport-specific training. In most cases, cross-training for the healthy athlete should be no more than 20% to 30% of the total training volume during the off-season. Unless there is an injury, cross-training will be more infrequent during the competitive season (1 cross-training session every other wk).

Cross-training options vary depending on the competitive sport. An ideal cross-training exercise would be an activity that uses many of the same muscle groups used during the athlete's sport but gives the body a break from the repetitive nature of the sport. A runner may select cycling or elliptical exercise during her cross-training days. For non-weight-bearing sports such as swimming and cycling, athletes may choose weight-bearing cross-training activities to mitigate the potential negative effects of non-weight-bearing activities on bone health (53). Swimmers may also choose endurance activities that incorporate the upper body, such as arm or rowing ergometry.

Tapering

Tapering is a purposeful decrease in training frequency and duration (i.e., total volume) or intensity leading up to a competition in order to attain peak performance at the time of competition. An effective taper allows for a break from the cumulative physiological and psychological fatigue that occurs during training, without compromising the physiological adaptations leading up to a competition. Finding the appropriate reductions in exercise frequency, intensity, and duration, along with the appropriate duration of the taper, can be complicated. Mujika and Padilla (48) provided a list of practical suggestions for tapering:

1. The goal of the taper is to reduce cumulative fatigue of training rather than to continue to improve fitness.
2. Maintaining training intensity and frequency while reducing volume is important to minimize the effects of detraining. Many athletes are noncompliant during the taper and do not reduce the training volume enough for fear of losing fitness gains. Maintaining exercise intensity and frequency is effective in reducing the mental stress of the approaching race and fear of losing the training effect.
3. Reductions in training volume as high as 90% may be effective for highly trained athletes. During a taper for a 10K, the training volume would typically be reduced by about 50%.
4. Physiological and performance adaptations may be seen in tapers lasting 4 to 28 days. However, 2 wk may be the maximal taper length for most athletes (39). In general, the longer the race distance, the longer the taper. For a 10K, a taper will begin 6 or 7 days before the race. For a marathon, the taper is usually about 3 wk.
5. The goal of a taper is to increase performance during the competition. But, a realistic improvement in performance following a taper is only about 3%.

For sports with few competitions during a calendar year, the taper may be much longer than for sports with competitions on a weekly schedule. Completing a marathon is a common goal for recreational runners. A marathon can take anywhere from slightly over 2 hr for elite runners to 5 or more hr for recreational runners. For this 26.2 mi (42.2 km) race, it is common to begin tapering about 3 wk before race day. Table 15.3 gives an example of a 3 wk taper for a marathon runner.

KEY POINT

Once a training base is established, training for aerobic events focuses on progression in volume and intensity. The major methods of aerobic training are tempo training, aerobic interval training, fartlek training, and anaerobic interval training.

Table 15.3 Sample Taper Leading Up to a Marathon

	Monday	Tuesday	Wednesday	Thursday	Friday	Saturday	Sunday
Last normal training wk	5 mi (8 km) easy pace	Interval workout	5 mi (8 km) LSD pace	40 min tempo pace	Rest	10 mi (16 km) race pace	20 mi (32 km) LSD
Taper wk 1	5 mi (8 km) easy pace	Interval workout	5 mi (8 km) LSD pace	30 min tempo pace	Rest	4 mi (6 km) race pace	12 mi (19 km) LSD
Taper wk 2	4 mi (6 km) easy pace	Interval workout	4 mi (6 km) LSD pace	30 min tempo pace	Rest	4 mi (6 km) LSD pace	8 mi (13 km) LSD
Taper wk 3	3 mi (5 km) easy pace	Interval workout	3 mi (5 km) LSD pace	Rest	Rest	2 mi (3 km) LSD pace	Marathon race day

Training for Sprint Events

The 100 m sprint uses the same muscles and movement patterns as a 10K, but because of the short duration, training to improve performance is very different. Although there is benefit from some of the same training methods used for an event lasting 30 min or more, those methods are not training at the event-specific movement speed. In contrast, although many of the methods used to train athletes for explosive events are also beneficial for sprinters, the specificity of the sport is missing. The following section discusses specific training strategies for an athlete training for sprint events lasting less than 20 sec.

Speed Training

Running speed is achieved through the interaction between stride frequency and stride length. The goal of a **speed training** program for running is to achieve high stride frequency while maintaining optimal stride length. At lower running velocities, both stride length and stride frequency increase linearly as velocity increases (18). At higher velocities, stride length begins to plateau, and any further increases in running velocity are due to increases in stride frequency (18). Thus, peak running velocity depends on peak stride velocity (18). The optimal stride length varies from person to person and is primarily related to body height and leg length (46). Hence, stride frequency is more trainable than stride length. Once optimal stride length has been reached, the time that the foot is in contact with the ground must decrease to increase running velocity (16). This depends on the ability to generate explosive ground reaction forces, often approaching a force that is four times the athlete's body weight (46). For improvements in peak running velocity, training methods should focus on improving explosive strength and power. A number of training methods can improve speed, and the key to success is to incorporate a combination of these methods.

Sprint Training

Based on the principle of specificity, athletes must regularly practice an activity in order to increase performance during that activity. Sprint training initially should focus on mastery of the movement techniques and mechanics at submaximal intensities. Sprint distance should also start with short distances (20 m) with a rolling or falling start and progress to starting from a down or starting-block position. This progression allows the intensity to increase gradually so that the athlete can focus on the mechanics at a submaximal intensity. The sprint distance can gradually increase up to the race distance and the intensity can increase up to maximal effort as the athlete progresses in the training (36).

Overspeed Training

Overspeed training helps increase speed by helping athletes achieve velocities greater than they can attain on their own. The principle behind this training method is related to the shorter ground-contact times demonstrated by elite sprinters (30). By specifically addressing this variable, maximal velocity may be enhanced. Methods to increase velocity include high-speed towing, gravity-assisted (downhill) running, and unloading body weight on a treadmill with a harness (figure 15.1) or altered lower-body pressure (figure 15.2). These methods have demonstrated improvements in peak running velocity (38). However, during downhill running or high-speed towing, athletes may overstride or brake in an attempt to protect themselves from falling. A conservative downhill grade and towing speed should be used to reduce the risk of injury.

Sprint-Resistance Training

Sprint-resistance training includes gravity-resisted (uphill) running or running against an added resistance (e.g., parachute, sled, harness, stretch cord, weighted vest). This principle is based on increasing resistance without directly affecting the athlete's running mechanics (2). Sprint-resistance training should be used conservatively; large increases in resistance can have negative effects on form and technique by causing the athlete to change running mechanics to maintain velocity.

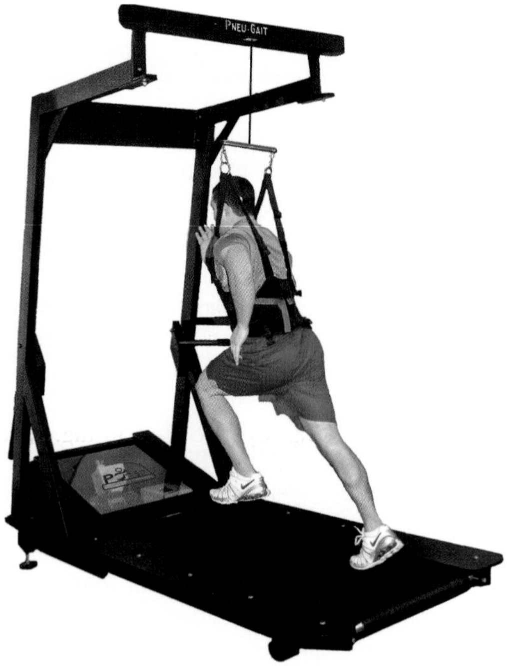

FIGURE 15.1 Harness-supported treadmill sprinting.
Photo courtesy of Pneumex (www.pneumex.com).

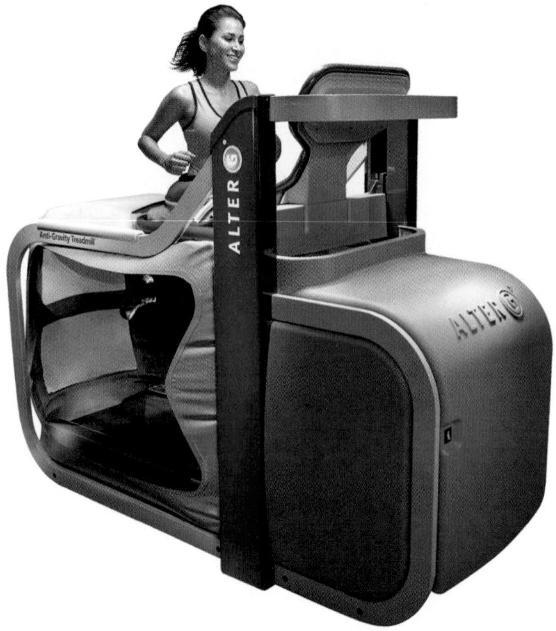

FIGURE 15.2 AlterG air-pressure-supported treadmill running.
Courtesy AlterG, Inc.

Strength Training for Sprinters

Strength training has been used to improve running speed by targeting the primary muscles that are involved in sprinting. The training program should include as much of the force–velocity spectrum as possible. There should be some high-resistance, low-speed movements as well as training at low resistance and high velocity. Most of the resistance training exercises should use multijoint movements (such as squats or dumbbell step-ups). The program should also include explosive, dynamic movements (such as squat jumps while holding dumbbells) and plyometric exercises (such as depth jumps and bounds) that test the stretch–shortening cycle used during sprinting (see chapter 13).

KEY POINT

The goal of a training program for running speed is to achieve peak stride frequency while maintaining optimal stride length. Training methods should focus on improving explosive strength and power.

Training for Explosive Power Events

Many aspects of sport performance require high explosive power output. Sports such as the high jump or the shot put rely almost entirely on the ability to generate force quickly. High power output is also needed for specific aspects of other sports, such as during a tennis serve or a volleyball spike. Although a considerable amount of training for these sports requires focused attention on technique, training to improve the ability to generate force quickly is also important for performance. Therefore, training to improve both force and power is the cornerstone for athletes competing in these sports. As mentioned in chapter 13, strength represents the maximal force that can be generated, and power is the product of strength and speed of movement. There is a fundamental relationship between muscular strength and power: For an athlete to be able to generate a high power output, there must be a relatively high amount of strength. Thus, both strength and power are important for athletes to improve their performance. For a more thorough treatment of this topic, see Cormie, McGuigan, and Newton (12).

Resistance Training

Every athlete's training program should include resistance training (see chapter 13). Resistance training programs are primarily designed to increase strength, but maximal muscular power may also increase during this type of training. Increasing movement velocity during traditional resistance training has been investigated as a possible method of increasing muscular power (28, 61). However, using light loads (<60% 1RM) during traditional resistance exercises has been shown to be less effective for improving strength or power because it does not provide an adequate stimulus for adaptations to occur (51). Therefore, the traditional resistance training methods discussed in chapter 13 should be used primarily to increase muscular strength. Dynamic, multijoint power movements may be a more effective approach to increase muscular power.

Olympic Power Lifts

Olympic power lifts are explosive lifts that move a barbell from the floor to a position over the head. The Olympic lifts are the clean and press (also known as the clean and jerk) and the snatch. Both lifts require complex multijoint movements, and they are often broken into smaller segments. For example, an athlete may focus on the deadlift, hang clean (figure 15.3), and push press (figure 15.4) portions of the clean and press separately during a training session. These movements require the athlete to rapidly accelerate and decelerate body mass and the barbell. Because the movements are so complex and involve large amounts of neuromuscular activity, these exercises are often considered to be similar to sport-specific movements such as sprinting and jumping (58). Olympic power lifts are frequently included in training programs for athletes in all types of sports (20, 21, 55). Many strength and conditioning coaches believe that Olympic power lifts improve the athlete's maximal power output, but evidence to support this is limited (51).

Although athletes of any age can learn these exercises, due to the high risk of injury they should be limited to athletes with a considerable background in resistance training. Teaching these movements should start with no resistance on a bar or a lightweight alternative to a bar (such as a PVC pipe) until the movements are mastered. The athlete needs to understand techniques related to the hand grip, body position, and breathing before using resistance. It is also important to have appropriate powerlifting equipment, including a platform, rubber-coated bumper plates, and enough dedicated space to prevent equipment damage or injuries to others who may be working in the area.

Unlike other resistance training movements, a spotter should not be used during Olympic powerlifting. Spotting these exercises can be dangerous for both the athlete and the spotter. The athlete should be trained to push the bar away or drop the bar if he or she fails during a lift attempt (19).

Ballistic Resistance Training

Chapter 13 described the importance of plyometric exercises to increase muscular strength and power. In contrast to plyometric training, in which body weight is the resistance, **ballistic resistance training** uses external resistance.

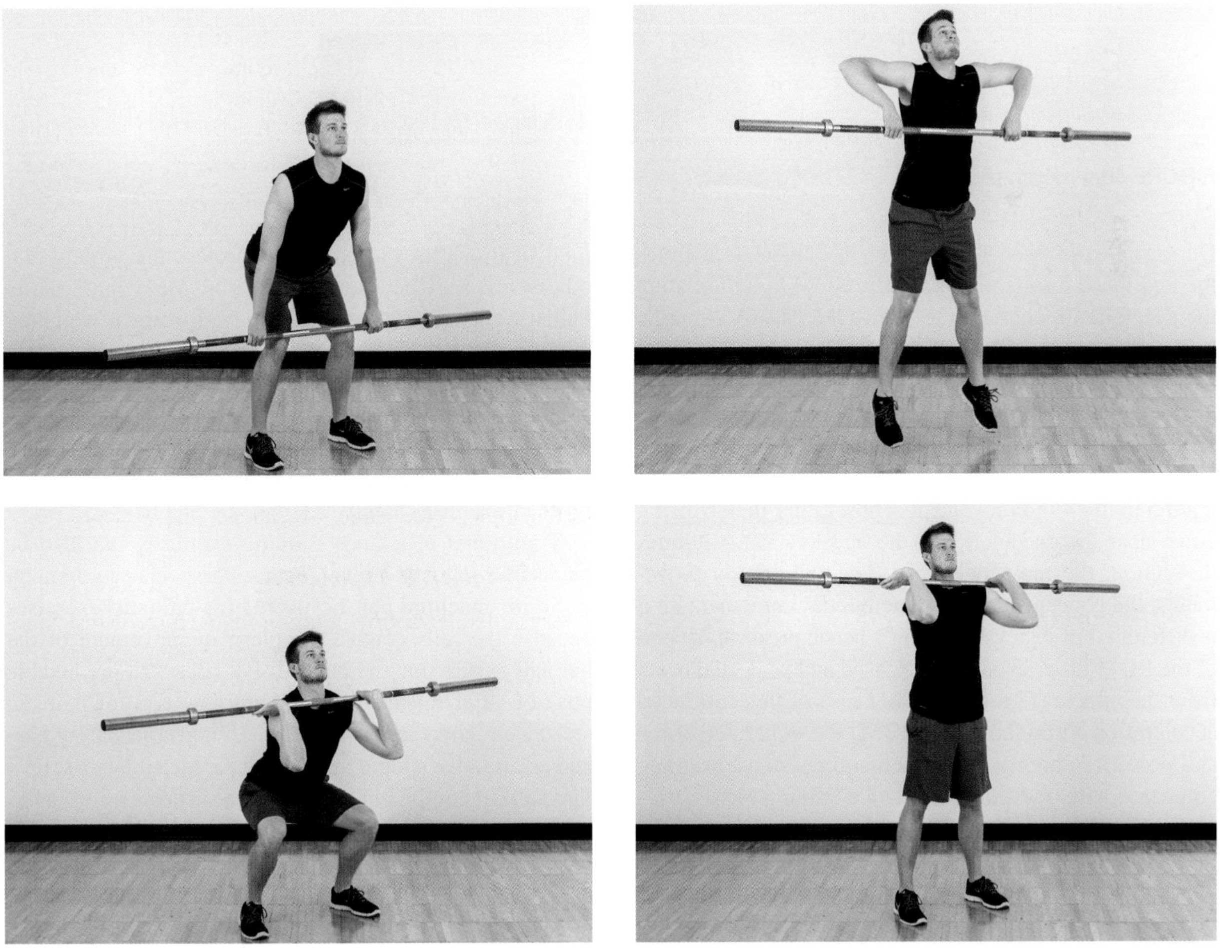

FIGURE 15.3 Hang clean.

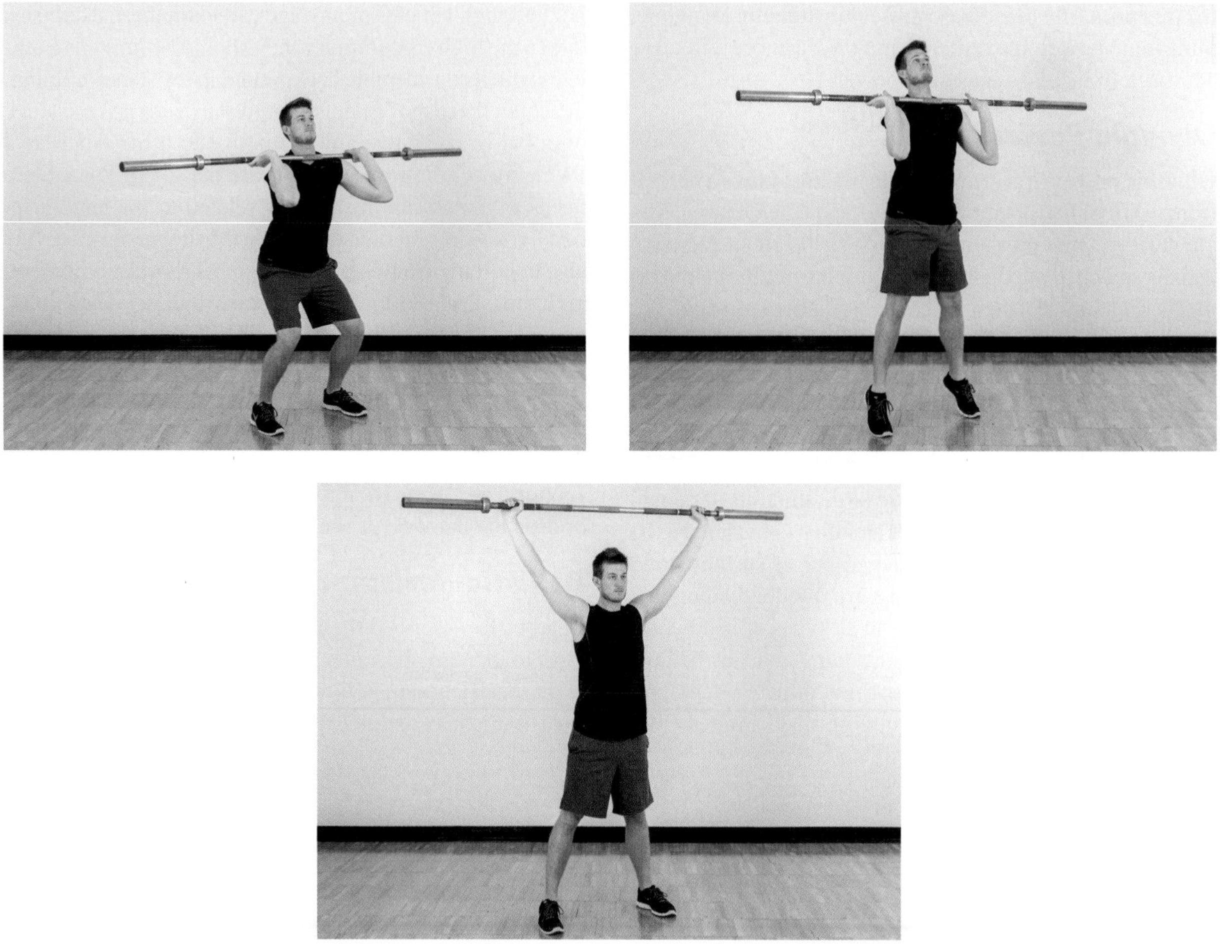

FIGURE 15.4 Push press.

During ballistic resistance training, the athlete accelerates the resistance throughout the entire ROM by eliminating the deceleration phase at the end ROM (50). A common ballistic resistance exercise is the dumbbell squat jump (34, 45). While holding the dumbbells at the side in a low-carry position, the athlete completes a squat through the normal ROM. But, rather than stopping when the back, legs, and hips are in the extended position, the athlete continues to a jump in one fluid movement. Thus, rather than slowing down near the end of ROM, the acceleration continues throughout the movement (50). For upper-body movements, the concepts are the same but the implementation is different. For example, during a bench press, at the end of the ROM the resistance is released and projected away from the athlete (figure 15.5). Because of this continued acceleration throughout the ROM, the generated force and power are higher during ballistic resistance training compared with traditional resistance training (45).

During a ballistic bench press, once the athlete releases the barbell and projects it away from his body, gravity dictates that the barbell must come back down. Because of safety concerns during these types of advanced upper-body ballistic exercises, special equipment or exercise modifications are necessary to protect the athlete and others who may be exercising nearby. Many upper-body ballistic movements can be achieved using a weighted medicine ball. A ballistic medicine ball chest-press throw requires activation of the chest, shoulders, and arms. To create a more sport-specific movement and activate the lower body as well, add a jump squat (figure 15.6). Space and flooring must be adequate to be able to complete these types of exercises safely.

Traditional resistance training exercises can also be made into ballistic movements with special equipment. A Smith machine can be useful for ballistic exercises because the rails control the plane of movement of the bar and ensure that the bar will fall back to a predictable position after release. When doing any type of ballistic resistance movement using a Smith machine, safety bars and an attentive spotter are critical for the athlete's safety. Specialized equipment for ballistic resistance training has been developed to reduce the risk of injury and eliminate the need for a spotter. A plyometric leg press can turn a leg press into a ballistic movement. This can also be achieved to some extent using light weight on a leg press machine or using a standard free weight leg press sled. Other

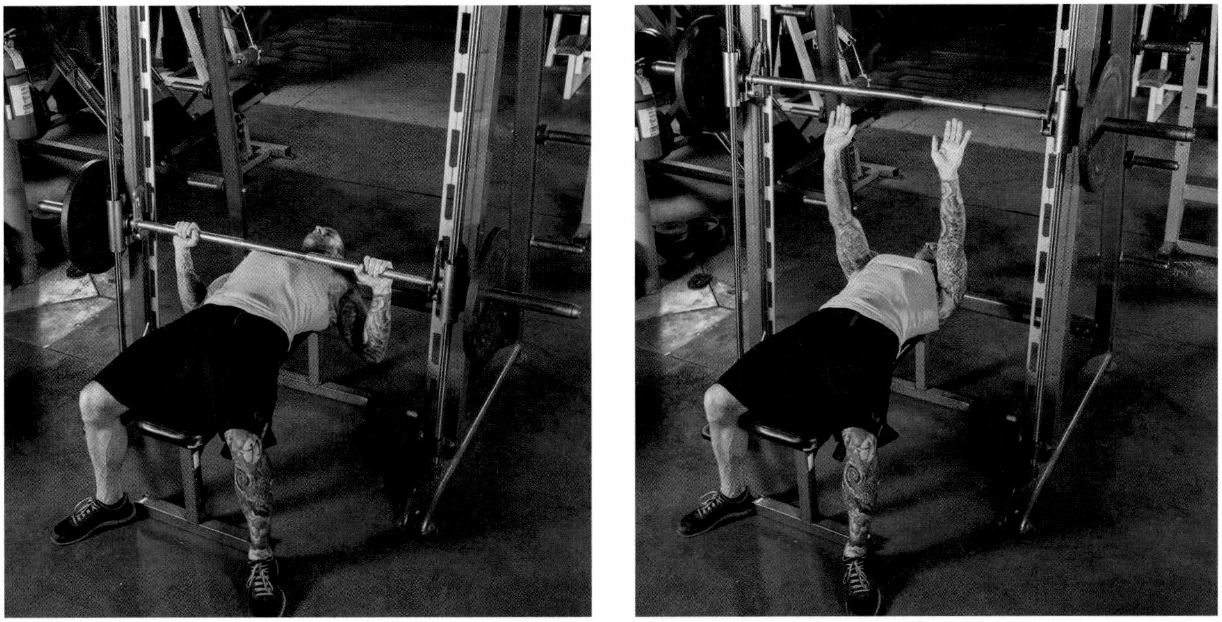

FIGURE 15.5 Ballistic bench press on a Smith machine. (Note that the bar hooks are in place in the second panel for purposes of capturing the photo. They would normally remain released throughout the movement).

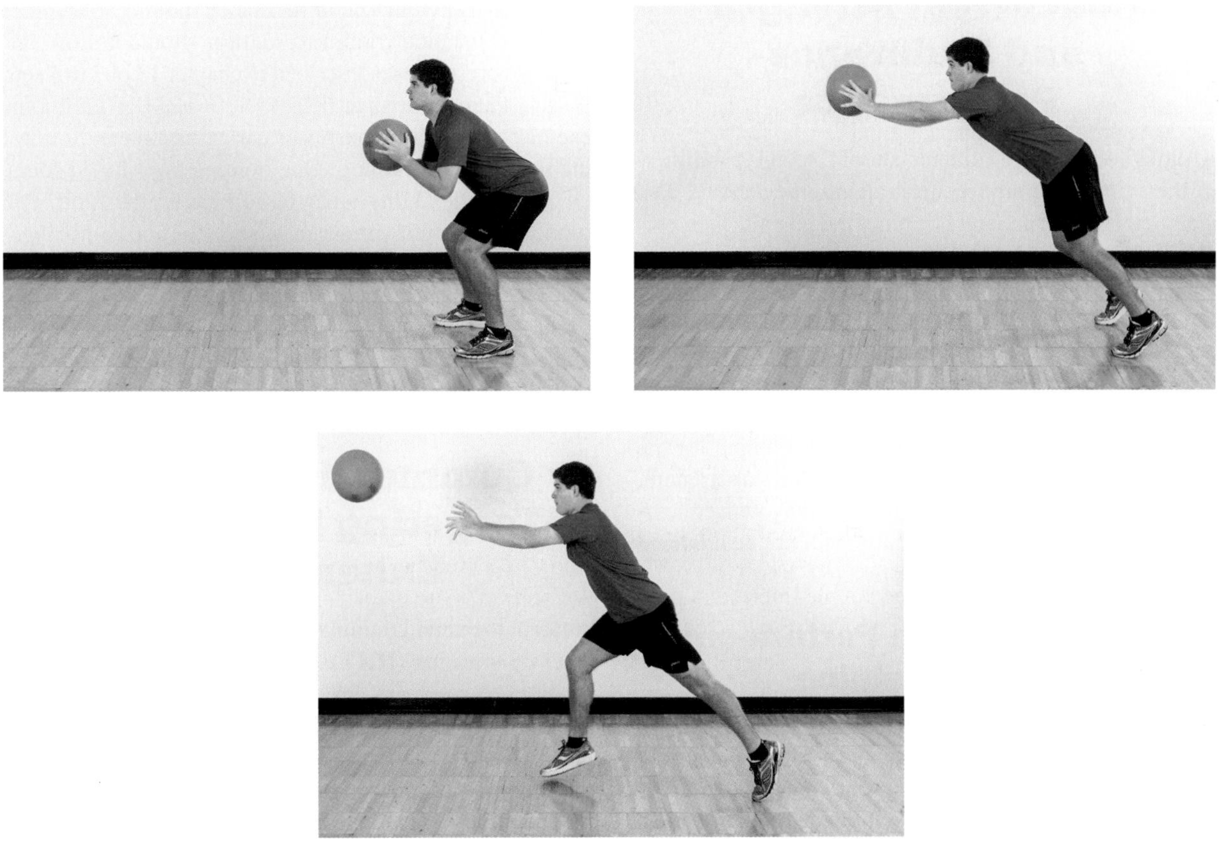

FIGURE 15.6 Ballistic medicine ball toss.

companies have developed a hydraulic cylinder system that controls the fall rate of the resistance back to the starting position after it is released at the end of the ROM. For example, Cormax (www.trainingsafely.com) has developed several machines specifically designed for ballistic resistance training. With this equipment, the speed of the fall can be adjusted, allowing many traditional resistance exercises to be adapted into ballistic movements.

KEY POINT

Resistance training programs can be tailored to increase strength and muscular power. Complex Olympic powerlifting focuses on maximal power output, and ballistic resistance training uses continued acceleration throughout the ROM, generating higher force and power than traditional lifts.

Concurrent Strength and Endurance Performance

Although endurance athletes should spend a majority of their time in sport-specific training, they should also incorporate resistance and flexibility training into their programs. Some endurance athletes worry that their endurance performance may be impaired if they include resistance training in their program. They neglect resistance training because of the fear that adding body weight (even if it is muscle) will hinder their development or performance in their endurance event. Athletes whose sport relies on anaerobic power may neglect endurance training for the opposite reason: fear of losing muscle mass or strength. Research indicates that success in an activity with concurrent strength and endurance training will not be hindered if the endurance training occurs first (62, 63).

Improved Strength Performance With Endurance Training

In 1980, Hickson (32) demonstrated that muscular strength was lower in subjects who completed a 10 wk concurrent strength and endurance training program when compared with a group that completed only strength training. Subsequent studies have found mixed results. There do seem to be competing intracellular signaling cascades that decrease the capacity to gain strength with concurrent endurance training (25, 31, 49). One fact that should be pointed out about the Hickson study is that a third group that completed endurance training improved aerobic power but had no change in muscular strength. The group that completed strength training improved muscular strength but had no change in aerobic power. But, the group that completed concurrent strength and endurance training increased *both* aerobic power and muscular strength (32). This demonstrates that athletes who compete in sports requiring high levels of aerobic power and muscular strength can improve both with concurrent training.

Improved Endurance Performance With Strength Training

For endurance athletes, strength training appears to enhance performance in endurance events (1, 59, 62, 63). The improvements seem to be due to enhanced mitochondrial biogenesis (59) and increased Type IIa muscle fibers (1). The research indicates that the combination and order of exercises may be important (11). Based on this research, a general recommendation for athletes is to complete sport-specific training first, followed by supporting exercises such as plyometric or resistance training.

The resistance training program should follow the standard prescription described in chapter 13 of 2 to 4 sets of 8 to 12 repetitions at 60% to 80% 1RM of multijoint exercises. Flexibility exercises can be completed following each day of training. One training day should focus on specific flexibility areas of concern in the sport. For runners, a flexibility program should focus on hamstrings, hips, and calves. For cyclists, extra attention should be given to the quadriceps, calves, and lower back. Swimmers should include stretches for the shoulders, chest, and back. Table 15.4 provides an example of a training program that includes resistance training and flexibility.

Commercial Programs Targeting Performance Enhancement

Anaerobic interval training, also known as **high-intensity interval training (HIIT)**, has become a popular training mode in recent years. Programs such as CrossFit, P90X, and Insanity have introduced a training method to the public that is rooted in a solid body of evidence. Much of the research supporting HIIT is related to enhancing CRF; however, there is no question that these programs are also effective at increasing muscular strength and power as well as decreasing body fat.

Table 15.4 Training Week With Resistance and Flexibility Training for an Endurance Runner

Monday	Tuesday	Wednesday	Thursday	Friday	Saturday	Sunday
Resistance and flexibility training	Interval workout or 40 min tempo	5 mi (8.0 km) LSD pace or cross-training	3 mi (4.8 km) LSD pace and resistance training	Rest	4 mi (6.4 km) race pace	9 mi (14.5 km) LSD pace

Anaerobic Interval Training and Endurance Enhancement

Anaerobic interval training consists of work intervals greater than $\dot{V}O_2max$ followed by longer recovery intervals. This type of speed training provides tremendous neuromuscular stress. The work-to-recovery ratio is generally 1:4 or higher. The goal of these training sessions is to improve speed and increase anaerobic capacity. HIIT has a demonstrated ability to improve not only anaerobic capacity but also aerobic capacity. During a 7 wk training protocol that consisted of 4 to 10 intervals of 30 sec each with 2 to 4 min of active recovery between each, peak power output and $\dot{V}O_2max$ increased along with anaerobic and aerobic enzyme activity (44). Even with no changes in $\dot{V}O_2max$, exercise time until fatigue at a submaximal intensity has been shown to increase by 100% (10) and time-trial performance by almost 10% (8). When compared with LSD training (40-60 min at 65% $\dot{V}O_2peak$, 3 days per wk), anaerobic interval training (4-6 intervals, 1:9 work-to-recovery ratio, 3 days per wk) produced similar increases in pyruvate oxidation enzyme activity and lipid oxidation with one-third of the weekly time commitment (9). Many people also find anaerobic interval training more enjoyable than moderate-intensity continuous endurance training despite higher perceived exertion (4).

HIIT Training Programs

Popular exercise programs such as CrossFit use various combinations of the anaerobic power training methods described in the previous sections. A HIIT workout in these programs typically consists of Olympic lifts, plyometric exercises, sprint training, body-weight exercises (e.g., push-ups, pull-ups, squats), and traditional resistance training exercises. These exercises are often completed in rapid succession with little or no rest between sets. There is usually a time component to the workout: either time intervals for each exercise or total time to complete the workout. The workouts have gained popularity in part due to the fitness gains and weight loss experienced through regular participation (56). The results of these studies are similar to those that have been demonstrated when performing anaerobic interval training on a cycle ergometer (57).

However, some concerns have been raised about safety when doing these types of training programs, including reports of injuries that have led to lawsuits (22). Although it is not clear that injury rates during anaerobic interval training are higher than during other exercise programs (23, 26, 27, 60), the fitness professional needs to be aware of the potential risks associated with these types of programs. Professionals should use caution when prescribing these programs to people who are sedentary or detrained, obese, previously injured, or elderly or who have known cardiovascular or metabolic conditions. People in these categories who are interested in anaerobic interval training should first establish a baseline level of muscular strength

RESEARCH INSIGHT

HIIT and Markers of Aerobic Performance

The purpose of a study by Burgomaster et al. (10) was to examine the effects of six HIIT sessions on muscle biochemistry, $\dot{V}O_2max$, and submaximal exercise capacity. Sixteen healthy, college-aged men and women were assigned to either an exercise training group or a control group. The exercise group completed six HIIT sessions over the course of 2 wk. Each session was separated by 1 to 2 days to allow for recovery. The exercise sessions consisted of 4 (progressing up to 7) all-out 30 sec sprints on a stationary cycle ergometer followed by 4 min of active recovery. Pre- and posttesting included $\dot{V}O_2max$, endurance capacity at 80% of $\dot{V}O_2max$, and muscle biopsies to examine changes in muscle biochemistry. The results of the study found that HIIT increased Krebs cycle enzyme activity and oxidative potential in the muscles. Submaximal exercise capacity increased from 26±5 min to 51±1 min. There were no significant changes in $\dot{V}O_2max$. Even though the training consisted of anaerobic intervals, this study demonstrated that HIIT can increase the capacity for aerobic exercise.

and endurance and CRF. Given the vigorous intensity of the exercise, the client's HRA should be evaluated to determine if this exercise is appropriate (see chapter 2). When appropriate, medical clearance should also be obtained before beginning anaerobic interval training.

Professionals should be sure to emphasize proper form and technique throughout the training session. Because there is a time component to many of the exercises, once athletes become fatigued, their form or technique may begin to break down, making them more susceptible to injury. It is the responsibility of the fitness professional to recognize these signs and help protect the athlete from a preventable injury. Once the athlete reaches this point of fatigue, an alternative movement (such as marching in place) should be used for the duration of the interval. It should also be emphasized that these programs should not be an athlete's only form of exercise; rather, they should be part of a larger program that includes other performance training methods described in this chapter.

15

LEARNING AIDS

REVIEW QUESTIONS

1. What are the four major training methods used by endurance athletes?
2. Compare and contrast an interval training session and a fartlek workout.
3. Name two benefits of cross-training for athletes.
4. Describe one upper-body and one lower-body plyometric exercise.
5. How does the work-to-recovery ratio differ between HIIT and aerobic interval training?
6. What two variables of running can be altered to increase running speed?
7. Describe the precautions to take before recommending a HIIT program to a new client.

CASE STUDIES

1. A recreational marathon runner mentions that she has a goal of qualifying for the Boston Marathon next year. She asks for your advice on modifying her training program. What recommendations would you give her?
2. A junior college baseball coach approaches you for advice on how to improve the speed of his outfielders. What types of training activities could he add to his program to improve his outfielders' speed?
3. A recreationally competitive 10K runner tells you that he doesn't do any resistance training because he is afraid that the extra muscle will impair his performance. What advice would you give him about the benefits of resistance training for his running performance and the types of exercises he should incorporate?

Answers to Case Studies

1. In addition to her LSD workouts, she should incorporate one interval training or fartlek session into her weekly workouts and one or two tempo runs. She can also include one cross-training session in her workout to reduce the risk of overtraining injuries. She should begin to taper about 3 wk before the race by reducing her training volume but maintaining the high-intensity workouts.
2. Several methods could improve his athletes' speed, including sprint training, overspeed training using a treadmill with harness system, and resistive sprint training using a parachute or sled as resistance. The athletes should also include resistance training focusing on lower-body multijoint movements such as squats and step-ups.
3. Resistance training can enhance an endurance athlete's performance if the resistance training follows the endurance training. If completing multiple types of training in the same day, endurance runners should complete endurance training first, followed by resistance training.

Special Populations

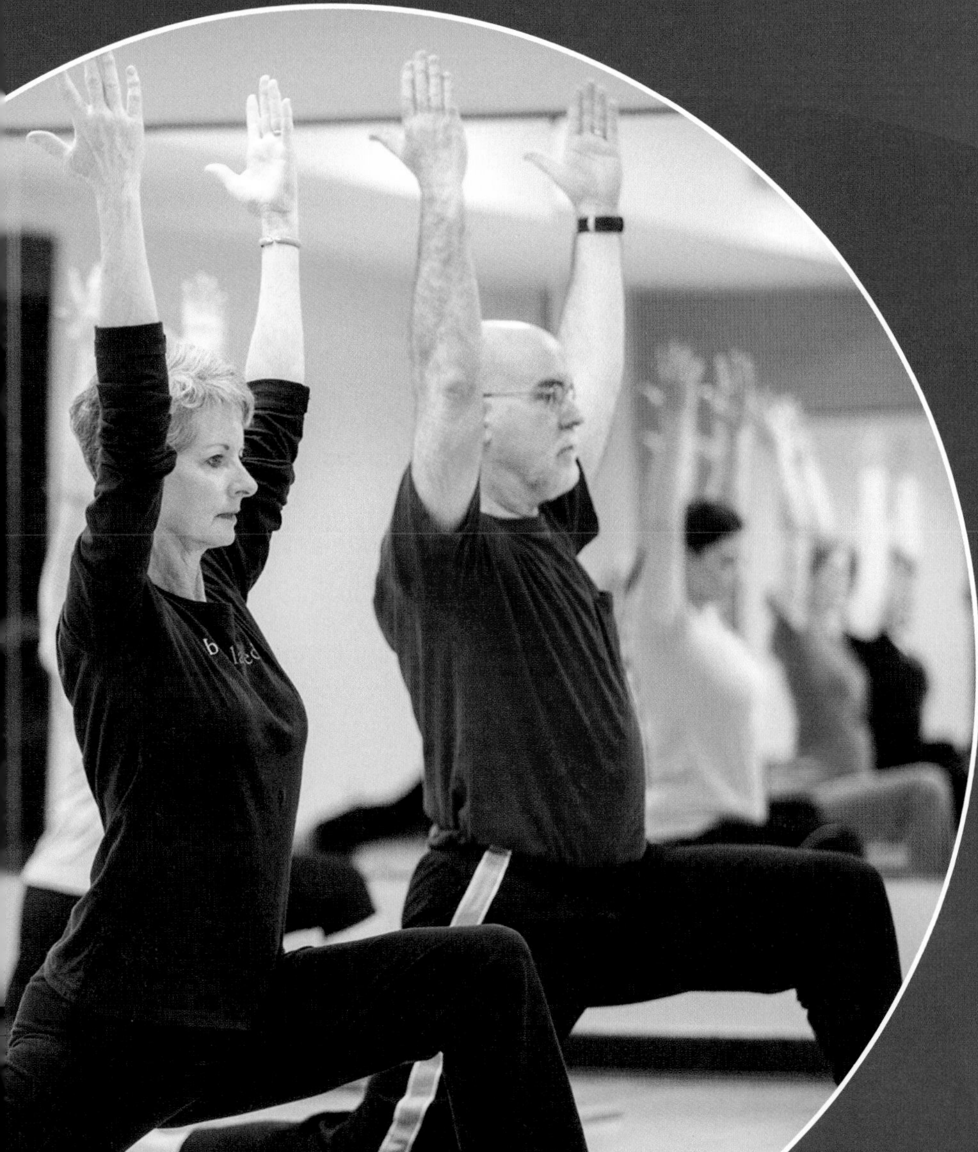

PART V

This section is based on several interrelated factors:

- Physical activity benefits people of both sexes, of all ages, and with a variety of medical conditions.
- Recommendations for physical activity need to address unique factors that can have a bearing on the exercises selected for the individual (age, medical condition, and so on).
- Fitness professionals are increasingly expected to work with people with a variety of clinical conditions.

In chapters 16, 17, and 18, we explain special characteristics and health challenges for children, older adults, and women. In chapters 19, 20, 21, and 22, we provide recommendations to promote safe and effective physical activity for people experiencing some of the major health problems of today, including

- heart disease (chapter 19),
- obesity (chapter 20),
- diabetes (chapter 21), and
- pulmonary disease (chapter 22).

Any one of these topics could make a complete book in and of itself. Our purpose is to help fitness professionals understand the role of physical activity in the quality of life for all people and to provide practical guidelines for special screening, testing, supervision, and activity modifications for each population.

16

Exercise for Children and Youth

Edward T. Howley

OBJECTIVES

The reader will be able to do the following:

1. Compare the physiological responses of children and youth with those of adults for both acute and chronic exercise.
2. Describe health-related physical fitness testing for children and youth.
3. List the health-related benefits realized by children and adolescents who participate in physical activity.
4. Describe special precautions for exercise participation and testing of children and youth.
5. Describe the public health physical activity guidelines for children and youth.
6. Contrast the public health physical activity guidelines for children and youth with those for children and youth with disabilities.
7. Describe the physical activity guidelines for children from birth to 5 yr of age.
8. Describe the characteristics of structured exercise programs consistent with achieving CRF, strength, body composition, and bone health goals in children and youth.
9. Identify social and psychological benefits derived from participation in physical activity.

Evidence shows that physical activity is essential for attaining the highest quality of life throughout the life span; however, most of the experimental research on how exercise affects fitness has been conducted on young adults, and most of the epidemiological research on how physical activity improves health outcomes has emphasized older adults. One of the common conclusions drawn from the research is that regular physical activity needs to be integrated with one's lifestyle, and it is recommended that this active lifestyle be established early in life. Although the correlations for tracking physical activity across various ages are not high, Malina (17) concludes, "Allowing for the different methods for estimating habitual physical activity, change associated with normal growth and maturation, and lack of control for important covariates in studies of tracking, physical activity tracks reasonably well from childhood into young adulthood" (p. 7). Further, there is evidence that both cardiovascular risk factors and obesity track across age, emphasizing the need to address these issues as early as possible. The good news is that increasing evidence shows that physical activity enhances the health and fitness of children and youth. This evidence serves as the basis for the U.S. Physical Activity Guidelines for Children and Adolescents (44), which are addressed later in this chapter.

In the United States, there is increasing emphasis on motivating people of all ages to begin and continue regular physical activity (43). In addition, physical fitness testing for children and youth is part of many physical education programs. This chapter deals with physical activity programs for children and youth, the role of fitness testing, and activity guidelines for health and fitness. We focus on school-aged children and youth. Although only briefly covered in this chapter, motor skill development is vital in preschoolers (11, 20, 22). The emphases of activity during the first years of life are primarily on motor development and healthy growth and are very individualized.

Response to Exercise

This section reviews the immediate (acute) and long-term (chronic) effects of physical activity on children and youth. It also compares the physiological responses of children and youth with those of adults (see chapter 4).

Acute Effects

There are a variety of similarities and differences between children and adults in how they respond to acute and chronic (e.g., endurance training) exercise (2, 10, 15, 33, 49).

Children are similar to adults in

- $\dot{V}O_2$max in ml · kg^{-1} · min^{-1} (endurance tasks can be performed well),
- phosphocreatine and ATP (children can deal well with brief, intense exercise), and
- ventilatory threshold (VT).

Children are higher than adults in

- maximal HR and
- HR and ventilation responses at a given absolute $\dot{V}O_2$.

Children are lower than adults in their

- capacity to generate ATP via glycolysis (children have a lower capacity to do intense activity lasting 10-90 sec),
- absolute energy production (kcal · min^{-1}; this is due to differences in body size),
- ability to dissipate heat via evaporation and acclimatize to heat (children have an increased potential for heat-related illness),
- ability to deal with cold (due to a higher ratio of surface area to mass and less subcutaneous fat),
- economy of walking and running (children require more oxygen to walk or run at the same speed; standard equations listed in chapter 6 for estimating energy expenditure of walking and running cannot be used for children),
- BP response to exercise (in general, BP is lower in children),
- RPE (for most children, RPE is lower at the same HR or %HRmax), and
- oxygen deficit (children achieve the steady state faster than adults).

Chronic Effects

Children and youth experience many of the same health and fitness benefits from regular physical activity and structured exercise programs that adults experience.

- Gains in $\dot{V}O_2$max due to endurance training are slightly lower (5%-15%) in children compared with adults.
- Strength gains occur across age in children, youth, and adults.
- In prepubertal children, most strength gains are due to neural adaptations.
- In older adolescents and adults, strength gains are due to both hypertrophy and neural adaptations (see chapter 13 for more on this).

An active lifestyle seems to be natural for most children, and activity is a normal and essential part of the growth and development that take place during these years (11, 21). This chapter emphasizes the fitness and health aspects of activity for children and youth, but achieving fundamental motor skills (e.g., moving, throwing, catching) is also an important aspect of the active lifestyle for this age group (49). See the sidebar for a brief summary of the benefits of physical activity in children and youth.

KEY POINT

Children are well suited for endurance and intermittent activities, but caution should be used in extreme environmental conditions. Regularly active youth not only prepare for maintaining active lifestyles as adults but also derive health and fitness benefits during childhood and adolescence.

Special Considerations

Children and youth with various medical problems need special attention (5). Young children need to be protected from overemphasizing a specific sport or activity and the intense training that often accompanies it, which can lead to physical or emotional problems. Children and youth should be encouraged to choose a variety of activities in an enjoyable and fun atmosphere. Young children do not adapt well to extreme environmental conditions; thus, more precautions need to be taken when exercising in very hot or cold conditions (1, 2, 3, 49).

Although exercise-related deaths are rare in children, when they do occur, they are most often linked to congenital heart defects (i.e., abnormalities of the heart resulting in imperfect oxygenation of the blood as manifested by cyanosis and breathlessness) or acquired myocarditis (i.e., inflammation of the myocardium). Children with these conditions should avoid intense activities. Children (as well as adolescents and adults) with other medical conditions (see chapters 19-22) need to modify their activities, but in almost all cases activity can still be healthful. These children, and their parents, should work with health care professionals to modify activities (e.g., longer warm-up and cool-down, lower intensity) to facilitate an active lifestyle.

KEY POINT

Children and young people should be screened for cardiovascular problems that might cause exercise-related deaths. Other medical problems can be addressed by modifying activities. The fitness professional should encourage children to enjoy a variety of activities with less emphasis on intense training for competition in one specific sport.

Fitness Measurements

Concern for the fitness of children and youth goes back over a century. Park's (26) historical review of the topic of fitness and fitness testing indicates that leaders of physical education from the latter part of the 19th century were convinced of the connections among exercise, fitness,

Benefits of Regular Physical Activity in Children and Youth

Strong Evidence

- Improved cardiorespiratory and muscular fitness for boys and girls
- Improved bone health
- Improved cardiovascular and metabolic biomarkers (impact is greater in those at higher risk)
  - Insulin sensitivity (increased)
  - HDL-C (increased)
  - Type 2 diabetes (lower risk)
- Favorable body composition

Moderate Evidence

Reduced symptoms of anxiety and depression

Reprinted from U.S. Department of Health and Human Services, 2008, *Physical activity guidelines advisory report.*

and health. Not surprisingly, fitness testing was part of physical education. Initially, testing in the United States was concerned more with anthropometry and strength, and it sometimes included a medical exam. Tests of motor ability also were developed, but it was a long time before a national battery of fitness tests for young people became a reality.

The driving force for promoting fitness in the United States in the first half of the 20th century was war or the threat of war, attributable to the concern raised when a large number of young men could not pass a fitness exam for induction into the armed forces. In the early 1950s, a new alarm was sounded when a study showed that a large percentage of American children could not pass basic flexibility and power tests. In response to this concern, President Eisenhower established the President's Council on Youth Fitness. Soon after that, the American Association for Health, Physical Education and Recreation (AAHPER) published its Youth Fitness Test, with fitness items such as the pull-up, sit-up, shuttle run, standing broad jump, 50 yd (45.7 m) dash, softball throw for distance, and 600 yd (548.6 m) run-walk. This test battery focused on skill-related fitness with an emphasis on muscular power (26).

In the early 1980s, two U.S. government publications, *Healthy People* and *Promoting Health/Preventing Disease: Objectives for the Nation*, shifted the focus to health-related fitness. Major organizations such as the American Alliance of Health, Physical Education, Recreation and Dance (AAHPERD), Cooper Institute, and President's Council on Fitness, Sports and Nutrition developed and promoted the use of fitness tests with test items related to health. These included tests such as the 1 mi (1.6 km) run for CRF, skinfold measurements to evaluate body composition, and the sit-and-reach and the sit-up test to evaluate low-back function.

Field Tests

The President's Council on Fitness, Sports and Nutrition now recommends Fitnessgram as the field test to evaluate fitness in children. Table 16.1 lists the Fitnessgram items for evaluating the components of fitness. In contrast to tests that use percentile values to categorize a child's performance, these tests use criterion-referenced standards to focus on health-related goals (26). See the Research Insight for more on criterion-referenced standards.

VIDEO Watch **video 16.1**, which demonstrates the PACER test.

RESEARCH INSIGHT

Cardiorespiratory Fitness Standards for Children

Determining the best way to evaluate fitness in children has been a concern for educators and scientists for the past century (26). One of the most important questions related to fitness tests is the type of standards to use in making judgments about a child's level of fitness. Normative standards such as percentile scores have traditionally been used to describe children's fitness values relative to their peers (e.g., 75th percentile—see chapter 7). The current thinking, especially for health-related fitness tests in Fitnessgram (e.g., 1 mi [1.6 km] walk or run test, skinfold test), is that criterion-referenced standards might be more appropriate. Criterion-referenced standards attempt to describe the minimum level of fitness consistent with good health, regardless of what percentile that might be in a normative data set.

For example, Blair et al. (7) showed that in adults, $\dot{V}O_2max$ values associated with a low risk of disease were not that high (i.e., 35 ml · kg^{-1} · min^{-1} for men and 30 ml · kg^{-1} · min^{-1} for women 20 to 39 yr of age). This information was used in setting the criterion-referenced standards for Fitnessgram, the fitness evaluation program developed by the Cooper Institute. $\dot{V}O_2max$ standards were set at 42 ml · kg^{-1} · min^{-1} for boys aged 5 to 17 yr. For girls, the values were set at 40 ml · kg^{-1} min^{-1} for ages 5 to 9 yr, with a decrease of 1 ml · kg^{-1} · min^{-1} per year until age 14, where the 35 ml · kg^{-1} · min^{-1} value held until age 17. Once these standards were set, the investigators had to translate the ml · kg^{-1} · min^{-1} values into equivalent 1 mi (1.6 km) run times, one of the tests children could take to evaluate aerobic fitness. The investigators had to consider the percent of maximal aerobic power the children would perform at during the run and the fact that economy of running improves with age. The result is that we now have nationwide standards to classify whether children's CRF is consistent with a low risk of disease (12). See the following for more details on this topic:

- www.cooperinstitute.org/youth/fitnessgram
- www.pyfp.org/doc/teacher-guide.pdf

Table 16.1 Physical Fitness Tests in Fitnessgram*

Fitness component	Recommended	Alternative 1	Alternative 2
Cardiorespiratory	PACER	1 mi (1.6 km) run	1 mi (1.6 km) walk test
Muscular strength and endurance	Curl-up; trunk lift; 90° push-up	Modified pull-up	Pull-up or flex-arm hang
Flexibility	Back-saver sit-and-reach	Shoulder stretch	
Body composition	Skinfold measurements	BMI	BIA

*Fitnessgram is a trademarked product of The Cooper Institute.

BMI = body mass index; BIA = bioelectrical impedance analysis; PACER = Progressive Aerobic Cardiovascular Endurance Run (see chapter 7).

Clinical Tests

Although fitness professionals are rarely involved in the diagnostic testing of children, a brief overview is appropriate given that fitness professionals may be directly involved in the delivery of exercise programs resulting from such tests (see Exercise is Medicine at www.exerciseismedicine.org/support_page.php?p=12). In addition to the contraindications to exercise testing listed for adults in chapter 7, Zwiren (49) provided the following contraindications for performing exercise testing in children:

- Dyspnea at rest (or forced expiratory volume <60% of predicted value)
- Acute renal disease or hepatitis
- Insulin-dependent diabetes (in subjects who do not take insulin as prescribed) or ketoacidosis
- Acute rheumatic fever with carditis
- Severe pulmonary vascular disease
- Poorly compensated heart failure
- Severe aortic or mitral stenosis
- Hypertrophic cardiomyopathy with syncope

Measuring $\dot{V}O_2$max in children using the cycle ergometer or the treadmill has a sound historical foundation (4, 30). The GXT format is used for children, and the test (initial grade and speed on the treadmill, increments per stage) must match the child in the same way as tests are matched to adults (see chapter 7). Treadmill testing may be easier because the child's shorter attention span can interfere with a cycle protocol. In addition, local muscle fatigue may shorten a cycle ergometer test before the child reaches maximum aerobic power. If a cycle is used for young children, the handlebars, seat height, crank length, and resistance scale must be adjusted (49). Many laboratories use the Bruce protocol, with 2 min stages, or a Balke protocol in which a speed of 3 to 3.5 mi · hr^{-1} (4.8-5.6 km · hr^{-1}) for walking or 5 mi · hr^{-1} (8.1 km · hr^{-1}) for running is constant and the grade increases 2% per stage (1).

A variety of cycle ergometer protocols exist to test children, with the initial work rate and the work rate increment per stage based on characteristics of the child (1, 47). To set the values,

- the James protocol uses body surface area,
- the Strong protocol uses weight, and
- the McMaster protocol uses height.

In all cases, shorter, lighter children begin at a lower work rate with smaller increments per stage compared with taller, heavier children. This is similar to the YMCA cycle ergometer protocol for adults described in chapter 7 in that a smaller person would have a higher HR response to the first fixed work rate and would progress through the test with smaller increments per stage. Karila et al. (16) recommended an individual approach based on the child's predicted max, from which a maximal power output can be calculated. Then these procedures are followed:

- The child maintains a cadence of 60 rpm, and the test typically lasts 11 min.
    - It begins with a 3 min warm-up at 20% of the calculated maximal power output.
    - The remaining 80% of the calculated power output is divided by 8 to obtain 1 min increments.
- A 2 min recovery follows the test at the warm-up intensity, plus 3 min of passive recovery.

These investigators also have a treadmill protocol that follows a similar pattern once the initial speed is selected.

What is important to remember is that there is no one best test for everyone in all circumstances. Depending on the clinical issue that the child brings to the table (e.g., asthma, cystic fibrosis, obesity, congenital heart disease), one test format will be preferred over another (1, 29).

KEY POINT

Fitness testing of children and adolescents is part of many school and youth agency programs. The field tests focus on health-related components of physical fitness. Children and youth with various diseases can be tested with a GXT, with the protocol selected based on their clinical condition.

Recommendations for Physical Activity

Children and youth enhance their health and well-being through regular physical activity. At a time when many adult diseases are increasingly diagnosed in young people, we must be concerned with health throughout the life span. Risk factors for heart disease are increasingly appearing in young people, including obesity, hypertension, and type 2 diabetes (43). The recent increase in childhood obesity is considered a public health epidemic (38, 41). Both healthy and unhealthy behaviors often begin early in life and are more difficult to acquire or change as age progresses. Thus, encouraging children and youth to incorporate physical activity into daily life may provide the basis for a lifetime of this healthy habit (17). It is now well established that regular physical activity can reduce the risk of developing a wide variety of health problems at all ages (42-44). Currently, the trend is to emphasize the physical activity behavior more than the fitness test scores. The major question is, what kinds of physical activities should children do?

Most motor skills (e.g., throwing, jumping, running, riding bikes, swimming) develop during childhood. Children are inherently active, and one of the most important elements adults must provide for them is an opportunity to play (11, 21). The need for children to develop motor skills must be kept in mind when attending to fitness goals (49).

Fitnessgram and the President's Council (27, 28) recognize the behavior of physical activity through the Activitygram (https://www.cooperinstitute.org/vault/2440/web/files/662.pdf) and the Presidential Active Lifestyle Award (PALA+; see the Participate in Programs tab at www.fitness.gov). These allow teachers and youth leaders to reward both the behavior of regular physical activity and the physical fitness outcomes. There are three major reasons for emphasizing an active lifestyle for children and youth:

1. Enhancing health and fitness
2. Beginning an active lifestyle that can be continued throughout life
3. Reducing risks for health problems throughout life

In 2012, a midcourse report for the Physical Activity Guidelines for Americans was published (46), with a focus on how to improve physical activity among youth. Following are the key findings and the level of research support (sufficient, emerging, suggestive, or insufficient) for each:

- With almost all youth enrolled in schools 6 to 7 hr per day, 5 days per wk, for most of the year, school is an ideal place in which to increase the physical activity of this population. The evidence is sufficient that structured physical education programs accomplish that goal. There is emerging evidence that taking activity breaks throughout the day increases physical activity, and the evidence is suggestive that active transport (walking or biking to school) is also effective.
- More than 4.2 million children aged 3 to 5 are enrolled in preschool, and the evidence is suggestive that well-designed interventions increase the physical activity level in these children.
- The evidence is suggestive that changes to the built environment (e.g., parks, walking and biking trails, wider sidewalks) increase activity in all youth.
- The report also provides clear directions for future research in which the evidence is currently insufficient. These include camps and organizations, family and the home setting, and the primary care setting.

In 2014, the National Physical Activity Plan Alliance published a report card on how well the United States is providing physical activity for children and youth (24). Although the authors gave a grade of C^- to the school setting, they felt that the built environment deserved a B^-. Active transportation did not fare so well (grade of F). Clearly we have much to do to improve the physical activity and fitness of youth. By becoming a fitness professional who is an advocate for community-wide physical activity initiatives, you can have an impact in your community well beyond what you accomplish in your job.

In the past, physical activity recommendations were separated for children and adolescents (9), but in the *2008 U.S. Physical Activity Guidelines*, they were combined (see the sidebar *U.S. Physical Activity Guidelines for Children and Adolescents*) (44). What follows is a brief description of each guideline related to fitness goals.

Cardiorespiratory Fitness

In general, the same exercise prescription for CRF for adults (see chapter 11) can be used for children. For example, in the *Physical Activity Guidelines Advisory Committee Report* (45), the review of the literature used to write the *2008 U.S. Physical Activity Guidelines*, gains in $\dot{V}O_2max$ were achieved in structured exercise programs in which the intensity was ≥80% HRmax, done 3 to 4 days per wk,

U.S. Physical Activity Guidelines for Children and Adolescents

1. Children and adolescents (6-17 yr old) should do 60 min (1 hr) or more of physical activity daily:
   - *Aerobic:* Most of the 60 min per day should be either moderate- or vigorous-intensity aerobic physical activity, and it should include vigorous-intensity physical activity at least 3 days per wk.
   - *Muscle strengthening:* As part of their 60 min of daily physical activity, children and adolescents should include muscle-strengthening physical activity on at least 3 days per wk.
   - *Bone strengthening:* As part of their 60 min of daily physical activity, children and adolescents should include bone-strengthening physical activity on at least 3 days per wk.
   - It is important to encourage young people to participate in physical activities that are appropriate for their age, that are enjoyable, and that offer variety.
2. Children and adolescents with disabilities
   - are more likely to be inactive than those without disabilities,
   - should work with their health care provider to understand the appropriate types and amounts of physical activity,
   - should meet the guidelines (see number 1) when possible, and
   - should be as active as possible and avoid being inactive when the guidelines cannot be met.

Adapted from Office of Disease Prevention and Health Promotion 2008.

for 30 to 60 min per day over the course of 1 to 3 mo (45). However, the actual gains in $\dot{V}O_2$max in children are typically less than those seen in adults. This suggests that the focus should be on health-related benefits of aerobic exercise rather than simply $\dot{V}O_2$max. When the focus is on health-related benefits, using a variety of continuous physical activities (e.g., cycling, running, in-line skating), team sports (e.g., basketball, soccer), individual and dual sports (e.g., tennis, racquetball), and recreational activities (e.g., hiking) can contribute to energy expenditure and its associated benefits. Parents, schools, and communities must provide opportunities for children to have safe places to walk, run, and cycle; provide organized programs for children to learn and play sports; and focus on personal achievement rather than winning at all costs. Lastly, parents should limit the time youth spend using computers, mobile devices, and gaming systems and watching TV. Based on the report card mentioned earlier, we are not doing well in that department (grade of D) (24).

KEY POINT

Children should focus on health-related physical activity with a variety of endurance activities appropriate for their age. Prolonged inactivity should be avoided.

Strength

Both boys and girls can improve muscular strength and endurance by participating in formal resistance training programs. In the *Physical Activity Guidelines Advisory Committee Report* (45), the typical program associated with strength gains included the following characteristics: intensity of 75% 1RM, 2 to 3 days per wk with a day of rest between sessions, done over 8 to 12 wk. Safety precautions must be taken, however, because children are anatomically, physiologically, and psychologically immature (6, 32, 49). Chapter 13 discusses resistance training programs, including those for children. Here we highlight some of the more important considerations for children:

- Have the parent or legal guardian complete a health history for each child.
- Children with diseases or disabilities should have their exercise program tailored to their condition, symptoms, and functional capacity.
- Ensure that trained personnel supervise each session.
- Adapt equipment to children.
- Teach proper lifting techniques, beginning with a light weight or wooden dowel.
- Have children perform 1 or 2 sets of 8 to 10 exercises (8 to 15 repetitions per set) and include major muscle groups.

- Increase resistance only when the child can perform the desired number of repetitions in good form.
- Individualize progression of all resistance activities.
- Do 2 or 3 nonconsecutive sessions each week.
- Perform a range of exercises that are designed to enhance strength and motor skill.

KEY POINT

Children can benefit from resistance training. Such training should emphasize safety, supervision for proper form, and muscular endurance (i.e., less resistance and more repetitions).

Body Composition

Obesity continues to be a major public health problem, affecting about 17% of children and about 35% of adults (25). In the *Physical Activity Guidelines Advisory Committee Report* (45), physical activity programs that included 30 to 60 min of moderate- to vigorous-intensity activity done 3 to 5 days per wk were effective in reducing adiposity and visceral obesity in those who were overweight or obese. Keep in mind that when working with overweight or obese children who are sedentary, it is necessary to use a progression model to introduce the physical activity, just as you would do for a sedentary adult (see chapter 11 for more on progression) (44).

Bone Health

In the *Physical Activity Guidelines Advisory Committee Report* (45), studies that demonstrated gains in BMD in children included the following types of activities: jumping, weight-bearing activities (e.g., running), games, and resistance exercises. These were better than weight-supported activities such as swimming and cycling (45). The evidence suggests that one of the best times to influence bone health is during puberty and the premenarchal years. The effect of such exercises on bone health is realized over many months of training, in contrast to the gains in CRF and strength that can be realized in a shorter period of time.

Developmental Concerns

All of the fitness component can be positively affected by following the recommendations of the U.S. Physical Activity Guidelines (44). Doing more vigorous activity would have a greater effect on these fitness outcomes. In addition, children and adolescents who do at least 360 min $\cdot$ wk^{-1} of physical activity have good health risk profiles.

Infants and Young Children

All of the previously described guidelines are for children and adolescents aged 6 to 17 yr. What about the younger crowd? An overriding recommendation is that adults responsible for the well-being of infants and young children should be aware of the importance of physical activity and facilitate the development of the child's movement skills. The National Association of Sport and Physical Education (NASPE) (2009) outlined the following recommendations for children from birth to age 5.

Infants (birth-12 mo) should

- interact with parents and caregivers in daily physical activities dedicated to exploring their environment and promoting the development of movement skills, and
- be active in a safe environment.

Toddlers (12-36 mo) should

- accumulate at least 30 min of structured physical activity per day,
- engage in at least 60 min and up to several hr of unstructured physical activity per day,
- not be sedentary for more than 60 min at a time,
- develop movement skills, and
- be active in safe indoor and outdoor areas.

Preschoolers (3-5 yr) should

- accumulate at least 60 min of structured physical activity per day,
- engage in at least 60 min and up to several hr per day of unstructured physical activity,
- not be sedentary for more than 60 min at a time,
- develop competence in fundamental movement skills, and
- be active in safe indoor and outdoor areas.

School-Aged Children and Teens

Rowland (31) pointed out that the motivation for activity shifts from a biological one in children to a more psychosocial one in adolescence. Many of the adolescent psychosocial factors negatively influence physical activity, resulting in the well-known decline in physical activity, especially among females. Although the recommendations for physical activity are essentially the same as those for adults (37), the strategy for enhancing motivation must target these adolescent psychosocial factors (34). Youth sport provides an excellent opportunity and motivation for millions of young people to be active (39). In 2012 and 2013, 3,267,664 girls and 4,527,994 boys participated in high school sports (23). Such participation is an important part of overall physical activity for this age group, but because of disparities in participation rates between boys and girls and across ethnic groups, the National Physical Activity Plan Alliance gave it a grade of C^- (24). Physical activity programs that promote mastery of motor and sport-specific skills contribute to a wide variety of psychological and social assets (8, 48) (see the sidebar *Developmental Assets Attained Through Sport-Specific Activity Programs*).

The best way to attain these outcomes is through the involvement of physical activity leaders (e.g., coaches, fitness professionals), family members, health care providers, fellow participants and friends, and community leaders (48). Children are dependent on adults for a physically active lifestyle, be it though safe parks and playgrounds, bike trails, sidewalks, or, of course, physical education programs.

Increasing the percentage of children involved in school-based physical education is a major goal of *Healthy People 2020* (43). As Morrow and Jackson (19) have indicated, physical education helps promote physical activity for children and adolescents. A number of programs, such as Coordinated School Health (18), SPARK (31), and PATH (13), have shown that physical education programs can have a positive effect on both children (35) and youth (13). In addition, the increased time spent on physical education does not diminish achievement in other subject areas (36); in fact, higher levels of aerobic fitness, as measured by the PACER test, tracked with academic performance (14). Finally, a principal recommendation from the evidence-based review of physical activity and youth was to restore daily physical education programs and after-school intramural programs to address the lack of physical activity in adolescents (40). In the United States, we must invest in our children when we can influence their physical activity—when they are at school. If we don't invest the money now, we will pay a penalty in the form of higher disease-related costs in the years ahead.

KEY POINT

Young people gain physical, social, and psychological benefits through participation in physical activity, especially when it includes mastery of motor and sport-specific skills. Adults play a major role in providing opportunities for children to be physically active.

Developmental Assets Attained Through Sport-Specific Activity Programs

Psychological Assets

- Self-determined motivation toward physical activity
- Positive values toward physical activity
- Feelings of self-determination, autonomy, and choice
- Positive identity, body image, and self-esteem
- Perceived physical competence and self-efficacy
- Positive affect and stress relief
- Moral identity, empathy, and social perspective-taking
- Cognitive functioning and intellectual health
- Hope and optimism about the future

Social Assets

- Support from significant adults and peers
- Feelings of social acceptance
- Close friendship and friendship quality
- Leadership, teamwork, and cooperation
- Respect, responsibility, courtesy, and integrity
- Sense of civic engagement and contribution to community
- Resistance to peer pressure to engage in risky behavior

16

LEARNING AIDS

REVIEW QUESTIONS

1. How do children compare with adults in terms of $\dot{V}O_2$max (per kg body weight), maximal HR, ability to produce ATP through glycolysis, and absolute energy production during exercise?
2. Describe some of the health-related benefits derived when children and adolescents participate in physical activity.
3. What common field test is used to assess CRF in children and youth?
4. What are criterion-referenced fitness standards?
5. Describe the 2008 U.S. Physical Activity Guidelines for children and adolescents aged 6 to 17 yr. How do they compare with the adult standards?
6. What are the physical activity guidelines for children and adolescents with disabilities?
7. How much physical activity is recommended for infants and toddlers?
8. List some of the social and psychological benefits children and adolescents experience as a result of participation in physical activity.

CASE STUDIES

1. A parent has read that for major strength gains, weightlifters should use a resistance that can be lifted for only 3 to 6 repetitions. He knows that strength is important for some of the sports his 9-yr-old son wants to play, so he asks for your advice. What do you tell him?
2. A parent's group is recommending that additional reading and math be included in the schools by reducing time for physical education and recess. The school board has asked you to respond to this recommendation. How do you respond?
3. A friend is considering not allowing her daughter to participate in sports in school because of the risk of injury. Although that risk is real, what information could you provide to indicate the benefits of participation in school sports?

Answers to Case Studies

1. Refer the parent to the recommendations for resistance training in children, explaining that the emphasis should be on proper form, supervision, and endurance at this age. After puberty, he can include resistance training with fewer repetitions.
2. Acknowledge that reading and math are important. The school needs to provide a good foundation in these areas, but it cannot possibly do it all—some reading and math work will need to be done at home. Including physical activity (through physical education and recess) is essential for the health of the children. Basic health is a prerequisite for other learning. In the same way that the school cannot provide all the necessary math and reading, the school cannot provide all the recommended physical activity, but it can provide a foundation that can be supplemented in the home and community.
3. You might provide a summary of the psychological and social benefits that can be realized through participation in sport. These benefits are considerable and include the following:

   Psychological assets

   - Self-determined motivation toward physical activity
   - Positive values toward physical activity

- Feelings of self-determination, autonomy, and choice
- Positive identity, body image, and self-esteem
- Perceived physical competence and self-efficacy
- Positive affect and stress relief
- Moral identity, empathy, and social perspective-taking
- Cognitive functioning and intellectual health
- Hope and optimism about the future

Social assets

- Support from significant adults and peers
- Feelings of social acceptance
- Close friendship and friendship quality
- Leadership, teamwork, and cooperation
- Respect, responsibility, courtesy, and integrity
- Sense of civic engagement and contribution to community
- Resistance to peer pressure to engage in risky behaviors

17

Exercise and Older Adults

Edward T. Howley

OBJECTIVES

The reader will be able to do the following:

1. Describe the changes in the number of people older than 65 yr that will take place during the first six decades of the 21st century, and provide a brief profile of older adults, indicating factors that affect the delivery of fitness-related programs.
2. Describe the typical changes in $\dot{V}O_2$max, strength, body composition, and flexibility that occur with age and the effect of exercise training on each.
3. Describe modifications to exercise tests to accommodate typical limitations seen in older adults.
4. Describe functional tests used to evaluate the components of fitness.
5. Explain why it is necessary to address individual differences in older adults regarding exercise prescription.
6. Provide current physical activity guidelines for CRF, muscular fitness, bone health, and flexibility for older adults.

A constant theme throughout this text is the importance of physical activity and exercise in leading a healthy life. This message is especially important for older people, the fastest growing segment of the U.S. population. The baby boom generation (those born between 1946 and 1960) was a spike in the birth rate in the United States after World War II, and these individuals are now coming to full maturity. Figure 17.1 shows the changes in the number of people over age 65, projected to the year 2060 (32). The number more than doubles between 2000 and 2040 because of the baby boomers. In addition, because of advances in hygiene and medicine over the past century, life expectancy has increased in general and with it the number of people living to advanced ages. Shephard (25) described the following age classifications and characteristics of those aged 40 and older:

- Middle age—40 to 65 yr; 10% to 30% loss of biological functions
- Old age—also called *young old age*; 65 to 75 yr; further loss of function
- Very old age—75 to 85 yr; substantial impairment in function but can still lead an independent life
- Oldest old age—over 85 yr; institutional or nursing care typically needed

Currently, there are 17 times more people in the 75-to-84 age group and 48 times more people in the 85+ age group than there were in 1900 (32). These latter age groups already have had a major effect on health delivery systems, financing of health care, family issues in caring for parents and grandparents, and general concerns about quality of life for those contemplating retirement. These changes also affect the role of the fitness professional in providing appropriate physical activity and exercise programs to increase and maintain health and fitness in older adults. Are fitness clubs ready to welcome older participants when the focus has been on younger, healthier age groups? Are personnel trained to serve the special needs of older adults? This chapter summarizes important health and fitness information related to this age group.

Demographic Profile

A variety of demographic and physiological characteristics of the older population (>65 yr of age) affect the planning of fitness facilities, the programming options available, and the kinds of emergencies to anticipate. The following information, from *A Profile of Older Americans: 2013* (32), provides some insights into the population as a whole:

- There are almost four times as many widows (8.7 million) as widowers (2.3 million) in this age group.
- The majority live in a family setting; however, as the population ages, the number living alone or in an institution increases.
- In 2010 to 2012, 46% of older white Americans rated their health as excellent or very good, versus 26% of African Americans and 31% of Hispanics.
- Physical activity limitations increase with age, with 36% reporting a severe disability. There is a strong link between disability and reported health status. Disabilities interfere with the capacity to carry out ADLs (activities of daily living), such as bathing,

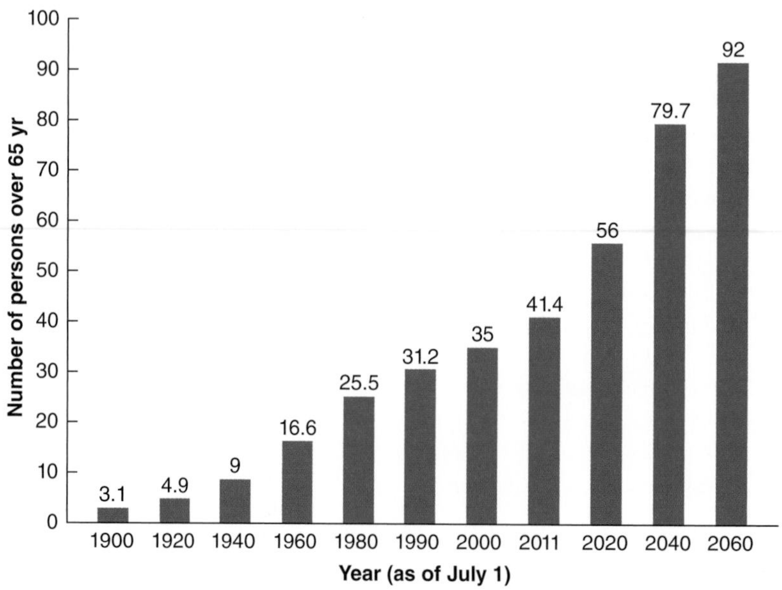

FIGURE 17.1 Number of people (in millions) aged 65 yr and older from 1900 to 2060. Increments in years are uneven.
From U.S. Department of Health and Human Services 2013.

dressing, and feeding, and instrumental activities of daily living (IADLs), such as preparing meals, shopping, and doing housework.

- Most older adults have at least one chronic condition and many have several. These include hypertension (72%), arthritis (50%), heart disease (30%), cancer (24%), and diabetes (20%).

This brief demographic profile indicates that fitness programs must address health-screening issues, the need for socialization, joint-protective activities, prevention and treatment of chronic diseases, and pragmatic goals to maintain independent living (7, 25). However, these characteristics (i.e., type and severity of disease, physical limitations, fitness) are not uniformly distributed across the older population, and fitness professionals must attend to individual differences. We address this issue in the sections dealing with exercise prescription.

KEY POINT

The number of older adults in the United States is increasing as the baby boom generation enters retirement age. Older participants present special challenges to fitness professionals because of chronic disease conditions and physical activity limitations. Programs must focus on preventing and reducing the progression of chronic diseases as well as increasing or maintaining fitness to allow for independent living.

Effects of Aging on Fitness

There is no question that physiological function decreases with age; however, some functions decrease faster than others. Further compounding the problem, each person displays a unique rate of aging that is influenced by genetic and environmental factors (e.g., education, health care, economic status, nutrition, exercise) (27). Consequently, it is not uncommon to find a person who is intellectually young but physically old, or an active 70-yr-old who has the physiological capacity of a sedentary 40-yr-old.

In general, the common chronic diseases that contribute to mortality in older adults respond to exercise interventions in a manner similar to that of younger adults. Endurance training

- improves blood lipids (linked more to a reduction in body fatness than an increase in exercise),
- lowers BP to the same degree as shown for younger individuals with hypertension, and
- improves glucose tolerance and insulin sensitivity (1).

As described earlier in the text, the primary fitness components (CRF, muscular fitness, body composition, and flexibility) affect our ability to perform work and engage in recreational pursuits at any age. Although natural changes in these fitness components occur with age, the evidence is overwhelming that regular physical activity and exercise maintain fitness at considerably better levels than does a sedentary lifestyle. The following sections address each fitness component.

Cardiorespiratory Fitness

Figure 17.2 shows that maximal aerobic power ($\dot{V}O_2max$) decreases at the rate of about 1% per year in healthy men and women after the age of 20 (15, 29). This decrease is due to both inactivity and weight gain as well as to the physiological effects of aging (1). Some studies show that this rate of decline is reduced by half in men who maintain a vigorous exercise program (2, 15). The most notable example of this effect of chronic training is from a study that tracked a world-class rower who won a medal in five consecutive Olympics. $\dot{V}CO_2max$ was unchanged (~5.9 $L \cdot min^{-1}$) over that 20 yr period when measured in the year leading up to the Olympics when training was most intense (19). In addition, figure 17.2 shows that the $\dot{V}O_2max$ values of 80-yr-old athletes were much higher (average: 38 $ml \cdot kg^{-1} \cdot min^{-1}$) compared with age-matched untrained subjects (average: 21 $ml \cdot kg^{-1} \cdot min^{-1}$). In fact, the $\dot{V}O_2max$ values of the trained subjects were similar to those of typical untrained subjects several decades younger (29).

In contrast to men, women show a 10% decline per decade independent of activity status (8). However, trained women, as expected, have a higher $\dot{V}O_2max$ at any age compared with their sedentary counterparts (10).

It should be no surprise that the decrease in $\dot{V}O_2max$ affects endurance performance. Average running speed in distance races decreases about 1% per year, suggesting a link between the decrease in $\dot{V}O_2max$ and performance in distance running. However, a variety of other factors (e.g., running economy, LT, joint trauma) also might affect running performance (15).

The fact that most people experience a decline in $\dot{V}O_2max$ with age means that by the time of retirement, the ability to engage in routine physical activities has been compromised. This reduced capacity for work can further reduce physical activity, setting up a vicious cycle leading to lower and lower levels of CRF. This may result in the inability to perform ADLs, which affects quality of life and the ability to live independently (27). Figure 17.2 clearly shows the impact of this decline in $\dot{V}O_2max$. The dashed line (at a $\dot{V}O_2max$ of 17.5 $ml^{-1} \cdot kg^{-1} \cdot min^{-1}$) represents a threshold for independent living, and all of the untrained octogenarians are just above that value. Also, remember that a $\dot{V}O_2max$ value of 17.5 $ml^{-1} \cdot kg^{-1} \cdot min^{-1}$

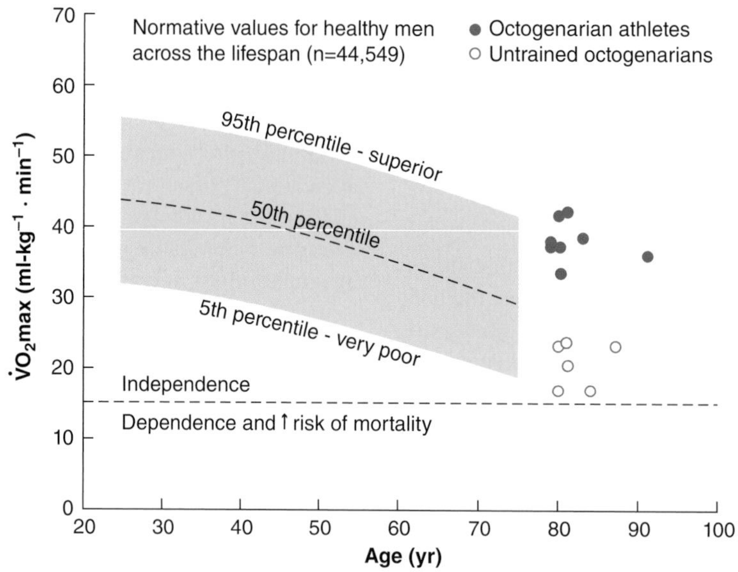

FIGURE 17.2 Change in $\dot{V}O_2$max with age in men. Data points represent octogenarian lifelong endurance athletes (filled circles) and healthy untrained octogenarians (open circles).

Reprinted, by permission, from S. Trappe et al., 2013, "New records in aerobic power among octogenarian lifelong endurance athletes," *Journal of Applied Physiology* 114: 3-10.

is associated with a much higher risk of death—a risk that is reduced 12% for every 3.5 ml^{-1} · kg^{-1} · min^{-1} increase in $\dot{V}O_2$max (29).

Maximal oxygen uptake (see chapter 4) equals the product of maximal cardiac output (maximal HR · maximal SV) and maximal oxygen extraction (systemic arteriovenous oxygen difference). There is no question that maximal HR decreases with age (e.g., 220 – age) and is the major contributor to the age-related decrease in maximal cardiac output. The Frank–Starling mechanism (greater stretch of the ventricle due to higher venous return) appears to compensate for the lower maximal HR in middle age and so reduces the magnitude of change in maximal cardiac output, but this mechanism is less effective in old age (1, 15). Maximal oxygen extraction is also lower in the elderly compared with younger sedentary adults, but this decrease is probably attributable more to their level of inactivity and its impact on mitochondrial number than to a true aging effect.

The good news is that endurance training increases $\dot{V}O_2$max about 10% to 30% in previously sedentary older adults, an increase similar to that of younger adults (1, 15). The increase in $\dot{V}O_2$max is due to an increase in both maximal cardiac output and oxygen extraction in older men, but it is due almost entirely to an increase in oxygen extraction in older women. This may be related to the observation that older women show little or no increase in left ventricle mass, end-diastolic volume, or maximal SV after endurance training. The increase in oxygen extraction is due to increases in capillary number and mitochondrial enzymes, the same as in younger adults (1, 15).

KEY POINT

$\dot{V}O_2$max decreases about 1% per year in sedentary men and women because of a decrease in both maximal cardiac output and maximal oxygen extraction. Endurance training increases $\dot{V}O_2$max in older adults just as it does in younger adults. The greater $\dot{V}O_2$max results from gains in both maximal cardiac output and oxygen extraction in men but is due solely to an increase in oxygen extraction in women.

Muscular Strength and Endurance

Figure 17.3 shows that muscular strength in untrained men begins to decline at about age 30, but the majority of the decrease occurs after age 60, when it falls at a faster rate (17, 24). The loss of strength relates directly to a loss of muscle mass, or **sarcopenia**, which is attributable primarily to a loss of muscle fibers (motor units) and secondarily to an atrophy of those muscle fibers (primarily Type II) that remain. However, the distribution of fiber types is maintained across age, as is strength per cross-sectional area of muscle (1, 15, 17, 24). The pattern is very different in strength-trained men, in that strength was maintained until after age 60.

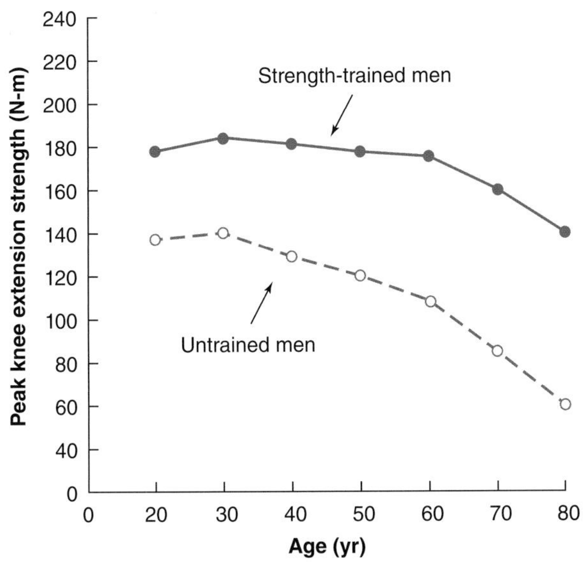

FIGURE 17.3 Changes in peak knee extension strength in trained and untrained men at various ages.

Adapted by permission, from W.L. Kenney, J.H. Wilmore, and D.L Costill, 2015, *Physiology of sport and exercise,* 6th ed. (Champaign, IL: Human Kinetics), 462.

This loss of strength and muscle mass is not due to aging alone. Figure 17.4 shows computed tomography scans of the upper arm of three 57-year-old men of similar body weights. Please note the large differences in the muscle cross-sectional area and subcutaneous fat as you go from strength trained (on the right) to swim trained to untrained. Similar observations were made in a 70-year-old triathlete, in which a MRI scan of his thigh showed little difference in muscle mass compared to a 40-year-old triathlete. In contrast, a 70-year-old sedentary man showed dramatically reduced muscle mass and a much more fat (34).

Clearly, it is important to maintain muscle mass as we age. Muscle mass is necessary not only for preserving the ability to carry out daily activities but also for its link to RMR (see chapter 12) and the risks of type 2 diabetes and hypertension (2, 24). Considerable evidence shows that an intense (80% 1RM) resistance training program increases both muscle mass and strength in 60- to 96-yr-old individuals (1, 9, 13). These training programs result in modest increases in muscle fiber area (10%-30%) but large increases (>100%) in 1RM strength. The disproportionate increase in strength is similar to what is observed when young adults participate in intense resistance training programs (see chapter 13) and is ascribed to neural adaptations. There is also evidence that resistance training can increase $\dot{V}O_2$max in this population (12). For some frail elderly, resistance training should precede aerobic conditioning because exercisers must be able to rise from a chair and maintain balance and posture in order to walk (1).

KEY POINT

Muscular strength decreases with age because of a loss of motor units (muscle mass) as well as a reduction in the size of the remaining muscle fibers. Intense resistance training (80% 1RM) can cause large (>100%) increases in strength; this is attributable primarily to neural factors because fiber size increases only 10% to 30%.

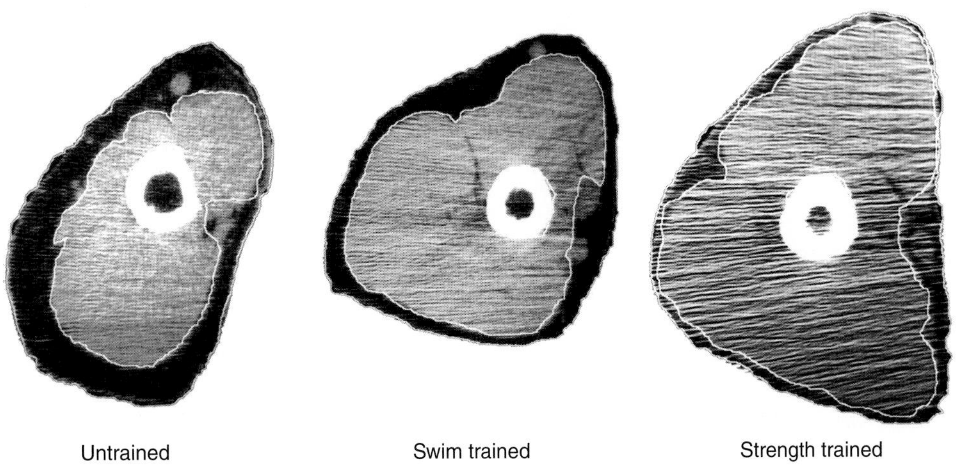

FIGURE 17.4 These scans show bone (dark center surrounded by white ring), muscle (striated gray area), and subcutaneous fat (dark perimeter).

Reprinted, by permission, from L.W. Kenney, J. Wilmore, D.L. Costill, 2015, *Physiology of sport and exercise*, 6th ed., (Champaign, IL: Human Kinetics), 463.

Body Composition

Chapters 8 and 12 provided details about health risks, measurement issues, and recommendations for achieving body composition goals. In general, body fatness increases from about 16% (males) and 25% (females) in 25-yr-olds to 28% (males) and 41% (females) in 75-yr-olds. This amounts to a gain of about 10 kg of fat for both groups during that time. Fat-free mass is stable until about age 40 but decreases 3% (males) and 4% (females) per decade between age 40 and 60 and 6% (males) and 10% (females) per decade from age 60 to 80 (15). As mentioned, exercise can play an important role in battling sarcopenia.

Evidence indicates that the increase in body fat relates to a sedentary lifestyle rather than to an increase in food intake or an aging effect. Cross-sectional and longitudinal studies on older male and female athletes suggest that regular vigorous exercise is associated with maintaining a stable weight during aging (15). However, observations of highly trained athletes indicate that body fatness still increases about 2% per decade. Consequently, vigorous exercise attenuates, but does not prevent, the increase in body fatness that accompanies age. Importantly, when body composition in older adults changes due to exercise, most of the body fat is lost from central stores, which reduces the risk of metabolic and cardiovascular diseases (15). Exercise is also important in dealing with the loss of bone mineral density (BMD) with age, but there is more to that story (see the sidebar).

KEY POINT

An increase in body fat with age is attributed more to a decrease in physical activity than to an increase in caloric intake. Vigorous exercise is associated with maintaining a stable body weight with increasing age, and exercise intervention results in the loss of body fat from central stores, which is associated with reduced risk of cardiovascular and metabolic diseases.

Flexibility

The ability to move a joint through its normal ROM is an important factor related to the ability to carry out daily activities and to the risk of low-back problems (see chapter 10). Joint motion is influenced by the condition of the

Bone Mineral Density

Bone mineral density (BMD), a measure of bone mass, decreases with age at about the same rate as the fat-free mass; however, in women bone loss accelerates after menopause (15). Accelerated bone loss is a major concern because the risk of fractures increases as BMD decreases. A general recommendation is to maximize BMD through adequate calcium intake and physical activity before age 30 and then reduce the rate of loss from that point in time (3, 5). Hormone levels (estrogen and testosterone), calcium intake, and physical activity affect the rate of loss of BMD. The higher rate of loss after menopause can be prevented by hormone-replacement therapy, but some women may choose not to use this therapy because of an increased risk of CHD and cancer (1, 21). In addition, there are certain drugs (e.g., bisphosphonates) that can prevent bone loss. Vigorous exercise, calcium intake, and vitamin D are important in maintaining BMD. Older adults need additional calcium (see chapter 5) to help maintain BMD and possibly to realize the full benefits of increased physical activity. The most effective exercise programs for bone health in older women include activities that

- involve a wide variety of muscle groups and movement directions,
- are weight-bearing activities (e.g., walking, jogging; higher-impact activities are more effective),
- strengthen most muscle groups, and
- generally exceed 75% of maximal capacity for both strength and endurance.

Regarding the last point, the fitness professional needs to introduce activity (aerobic and strengthening) in an appropriate and progressive manner to help the client make a smooth and safe transition to higher-intensity activities (1, 5, 7). Further, in older adults with severe osteoporosis, impact-producing exercises and those that involve forward spinal flexion should be avoided (1, 5). Please see chapter 18 for more on women's health.

muscle, connective tissues, and cartilage associated with the joint. In general, the increase in collagen cross-links in tendons and ligaments and a degradation of articular cartilage contribute to decreased joint ROM with age (1). However, in evaluating the health of a joint, it is difficult to separate aging effects from those associated with chronic inactivity.

It is difficult to provide a general profile of the effect of training on flexibility as was done for $\dot{V}O_2$max and strength due to the variability in the number of subjects, the types of research design, and the methods used to assess flexibility (1, 22, 27). However, general physical activity programs that incorporate stretching exercises, as well as special ROM exercise programs, have been shown to improve flexibility in older adults (1, 25). See the later section on exercise prescription for improving flexibility for more details.

KEY POINT

Possessing adequate flexibility throughout old age contributes to the ability to perform ADLs and maintain independence. Flexibility can be improved through general programs of physical activity that incorporate stretching exercises, as well as through programs using special ROM exercises.

Special Considerations Regarding Exercise Testing

Age is a risk factor because the likelihood of developing serious conditions increases with age. The passage of time allows the consequences of poor health behaviors (e.g., smoking, high-fat diet, inactivity) to add up and manifest themselves as major medical problems (e.g., lung cancer, atherosclerosis, glucose intolerance). Consequently, fitness professionals should closely follow the ACSM guidelines for risk classification (3) when working with the elderly (1).

Risk classification provides guidance for test selection and personnel requirements (see chapter 2). Clearly, with the higher incidence of CVD in older age groups, diagnostic exercise testing may be used as part of a medical exam. However, standard submaximal CRF tests (see chapter 7) may be used as part of a fitness assessment. Independent of the reason for testing, modifications may be necessary to address certain limitations (3, 7, 8, 26):

INSTRUMENTATION

- A cycle ergometer may be a better choice for those with arthritis of the knee or hip or those with balance problems.
- Tracking cadence may be a problem unless an electronic cycle ergometer is available.
- If a treadmill is used, additional practice may be needed, with emphasis on slow walking speeds.

INTENSITY AND PROGRESSION

As mentioned in chapter 7, for deconditioned people with low $\dot{V}O_2$max values, the initial intensity of a GXT should be low, increments per stage should be small, and perhaps the time (3 versus 2 min) per stage should be longer so the person can achieve a steady state. See the sidebar *Functional Testing* for alternatives to traditional exercise testing for older adults.

Exercise Prescription

Only half as many American adults aged 65 yr or older (15.9%) meet both the aerobic and muscle-strengthening guidelines compared with younger adults 18 to 24 yr of age (30.7%) (14). Consequently, the general recommendation that adults should participate in moderate-intensity physical activity for at least 150 min per wk and do muscle strengthening activity at least 2 days per wk is essential for all ages, but especially for older people, who are positioned to benefit substantially from an increase in physical activity (1, 3, 20, 30). When working with this age group, the fitness professional needs to keep in mind that an activity that is moderate work for a younger adult may be classified as very hard for an older adult (see figure 11.8) (16).

Older adults are not all the same, and fitness professionals must treat them as unique individuals. The only thing two 65-yr-old men in the same fitness class may have in common is their age! They may differ substantially in their health risk (chronic diseases), CRF ($\dot{V}O_2$max), and experience with exercise. Scientists and clinicians (11, 23, 27) have developed a variety of classification schemes to deal with this reality; Rimmer's (23) classification scheme is representative of these:

- Level I *Healthy:* No major medical problems; in relatively good condition for age; has exercised the past 5 yr.
- Level II *Ambulatory, nonactive:* No major medical problems; has never participated in a structured exercise program.
- Level III *Ambulatory, disease failure:* Diagnosed as having severe CAD, arthritis, diabetes, or COPD.
- Level IV *Frail elderly:* Relies on partial assistance from professional staff for ADLs; can stand or walk short distances, usually less than 100 ft (30.5 m) with an assistive device; spends most of the day sitting.
- Level V *Wheelchair dependent:* Relies on total assistance from professional staff for ADLs; cannot stand or walk.

Functional Testing

A common method used to evaluate the capabilities of older adults involves a series of performance tests that are linked to underlying fitness components. The Senior Fitness Test (SFT), developed by Rikli and Jones (22), uses the following tests to evaluate the various fitness components:

- Chair stand—number of times within 30 sec a person can stand from a seated position with arms folded across the chest (assesses lower-body strength).
- Arm curl—number of curls that can be completed in 30 sec with a 5 lb (2.3 kg) dumbbell (women) or 8 lb (3.6 kg) dumbbell (men) while the participant is seated (assesses upper-body strength).
- 6 min walk—number of yards the participant can walk in 6 min around a 50 yd (46 m) course (assesses aerobic endurance).
- 2 min step—number of full steps the participant can complete in 2 min, raising knee to midway between knee and hip while standing in place. This is an alternative to the 6 min walk.
- Chair sit-and-reach—number of inches between extended fingertips and tips of toes when the participant is sitting in a chair with legs extended and hands reaching toward toes (assesses lower-body flexibility).
- Back scratch—number of inches between the extended middle fingers when the participant reaches with one hand over the shoulder and the other hand up the back (assesses upper-body flexibility).
- 8 ft up-and-go—number of seconds required to get up from a seated position, walk 8 ft (2.4 m), turn, and return to the seated position (assesses agility and dynamic balance).
- Height and weight—used to calculate BMI.

These tests have been shown to be valid and reliable, and normative data are provided for men and women aged 60 to 94 yr (22). These practical and easy tests can be used to track progress over the course of a training program or to document loss of function that might necessitate additional medical attention.

These classifications of abilities and problems should be viewed as a continuum rather than discrete categories. As a person moves across the continuum, the following occurs:

RISK OF DISEASE INCREASES

- Need for supervision by medical personnel is greater.
- Use of medication increases.
- Testing moves from fitness to diagnostic to functional (see the sidebar *Functional Testing*).

FITNESS LEVEL DECREASES

- Range of suitable fitness activities decreases.
- Fitness professionals must be creative and adapt conventional activities to the limitations of the participant.
- Fitness professionals must incorporate socialization as part of the activity.

PERSONNEL NEEDS CHANGE

- Personnel need more education in gerontology, pathophysiology, and pharmacology.
- Staff mix may include fitness, nursing, physical therapy, and therapeutic recreation personnel.

Given the variation that exists among people in this age group, it should be no surprise that physical activity recommendations are equally diverse. These recommendations are discussed in the next sections of the chapter.

Aerobic Activity for Health and Cardiorespiratory Fitness

Physical activity recommendations for older adults were addressed in both the *2008 U.S. Physical Activity Guidelines* (30) and in the 2009 update of the ACSM position stand, "Exercise and Physical Activity for Older Adults" (1). What follows is a summary of those recommendations

Osteoarthritis

Osteoarthritis (OA), a common problem in many older adults, is a degenerative joint disease associated with damage to the articular cartilage that lines joint structures. The swelling and pain associated with OA affect joint ROM and may prevent some individuals from participating in physical activity. A variety of over-the-counter and prescription medications can reduce pain and inflammation and allow participation in physical activity. Activity programs should not excessively load the involved joint (e.g., participants with a knee or hip problem should perform stationary cycling or pool work instead of jogging or stair-climbing). Select the modes that provide the least discomfort; poor choices may cause pain and lead to noncompliance. Gradual warm-up and flexibility exercises should be included, and the intensity and duration of the endurance exercise program should be at the low end of the spectrum. For example, moderate-intensity aerobic activity (40%-59% HRR) is appropriate for most people with OA, but 30% to 39% HRR might be better for those who are extremely deconditioned. A frequency of 3 to 5 days per wk is recommended, with a goal of 150 min per wk of moderate-intensity activity. However, a series of short (e.g., 10 min) bouts may be better tolerated than one longer bout. Resistance training should begin with an intensity of 50% to 60% 1RM (goal is 60% to 80% 1RM) using only a few repetitions and gradually progress to 8 to 12 repetitions using pain threshold as a guide (3, 18).

for health and fitness outcomes from the U.S. Physical Activity Guidelines (30).

The following physical activity guidelines are the same for adults and older adults:

- All older adults should avoid inactivity, some activity is better than none, and older adults who participate in any amount of physical activity gain some health benefits.
- For substantial health benefits, older adults should do at least 150 min per wk of moderate-intensity physical activity, 75 min per wk of vigorous-intensity aerobic activity, or an appropriate combination of both. The physical activity should be done in bouts of at least 10 min, and the total amount should be spread throughout the week.
- On a scale of 0 to 10 for level of physical exertion, use 5 to 6 for moderate-intensity activity and 7 to 8 for vigorous-intensity activity.
- For additional and more extensive health benefits, older adults should increase their aerobic physical activity to 300 min per wk of moderate-intensity activity or 150 min per wk of vigorous-intensity activity. Additional health benefits can be gained by going beyond this amount.

The following guidelines are just for older adults:

- If older adults cannot do 150 min of moderate-intensity activity because of chronic conditions, they should be as active as their abilities and conditions allow.
- Older adults should determine their level of effort for physical activity relative to their level of fitness.
- Older adults with chronic conditions should understand how their conditions affect their ability to do regular physical activity safely.

Consistent with the breadth of these guidelines and the diversity of the older adult population, special attention must be given to progression. The physical activity must be suited to each individual, with an emphasis on a conservative approach for the most deconditioned older adults. Although a formal program of activities aimed at improving CRF should be built on a base of regular moderate-intensity activities, some older individuals may need to begin with light-intensity activities (1). As with any workout, it should begin with a formal warm-up and end with a cool-down during which flexibility exercises can be done.

It is crucial to adapt the activities to the abilities of the group. Those at the high end of the fitness continuum can participate in a wide variety of activities similar to those used for younger adults. Those who have the $\dot{V}O_2$max of cardiac patients (5-7 METs) can follow exercise routines that would not be too different from those used in a cardiac rehabilitation program (see chapter 19). However, prescribing activities for those at the low end of the functional continuum, in whom $\dot{V}O_2$max may be only 2 to 4 METs, demands special creativity and attention to safety. Exercises can be done standing with support, seated on a chair, or in the water (4, 22). Because of the prevalence of joint-related problems, exercise modes should be chosen that do not aggravate the problem. The need for additional assistance with balance and attention to safety regarding the risk of a fall should be incorporated into the routine (see the sidebar *Balance and Falls*).

The general exercise prescription for older adults is similar to what was described in chapter 11 for the typically sedentary person (2, 3):

- **Frequency:** Even though the recommendation is given in minutes per week, there is no question that the total volume of activity should be spread over the course of the week, and as mentioned previously, over the course of a day if the person cannot do a single 30 min bout of moderate-intensity physical activity. Formal vigorous-intensity exercise sessions should be done 3 to 4 times each week, with a rest day between exercise days.
- **Intensity:** THR can be used to set the exercise intensity, but measured maximal HR is preferred to predicted maximal HR. Intensity guidelines are similar to those for younger adults, but the low end of the THR zone should be emphasized at the beginning of the program, and RPE or an equivalent relative intensity scale should be used to determine whether the intensity is suitable.
- **Time (duration):** If the client is extremely deconditioned, the exercise sessions should be divided into segments (5-10 min) that can be done throughout the day (or within the context of a single class). Some participants may not be able to exercise continuously for 30 min.

The National Institute on Aging (NIA) provides information and examples of exercises that address all of the fitness components for this population. You can browse publications by topic under the Health and Aging tab at www.nia.nih.gov.

Muscular Strength and Endurance

Again, we emphasize the need for progression. The goal is to slowly and safely help the client progress to strength training exercises at a vigorous level. The exercise prescription for increasing strength in older adults was described in chapter 13 and is highlighted here (1, 3, 30):

- Instruct participants on safety, proper lifting technique, and breathing.
- Individualize progression of all resistance training activities.
- Begin with light intensity (40%-50% 1RM) for the first few weeks to allow for adaptation to the activity.
- Participants should perform at least 1 set of 10 to 15 repetitions of 8 to 10 exercises that use the major muscle groups.

Balance and Falls

Loss of balance can lead to a fall, with dire consequences. The lower bone density in elderly people predisposes them to fractures, and about half are unable to return to regular walking after a fracture (27). The ability to maintain balance is influenced by a variety of factors, such as strength, vision, proprioception, medications, illnesses, flexibility, and environmental hazards (27). Considerable information shows that exercise programs improve balance and reduce falls, but not without exception (1, 25). In older adults at greater risk for falling, the research shows that regular physical activity is safe and reduces the risk of falls. However, due to inadequate research there is no firm recommendation regarding intensity, frequency, and type of balance exercises (1). That said, successful programs include balance training, moderate-intensity strength training, and moderate-intensity aerobic training. Balance exercises may include backward walking, sideways walking, heel walking, toe walking, and standing from a seated position. Following is a progression of difficulty in balance exercises for each of three ways to stress balance (7):

1. *Narrow the base of support:* Stand with feet apart with assistive device; with feet apart without assistive device; with feet together; heel to toe; one-legged stand.
2. *Displace the center of mass:* Turn in a circle; shift weight side to side; step over obstacles; do crossover or sideways walking; move weighted arms to front and side.
3. *Minimize contributions of visual and proprioceptive pathways:* Close eyes with movements mentioned previously; stand on foam, pillow, or mattress.

Needless to say, these exercises should be done under supervision until the individual has demonstrated enough control to work independently. The frequency of balance exercises will vary considerably from several times a day for someone in a rehabilitation setting to 1 day per wk for someone who is simply maintaining gains in balance (7). Tai chi exercises may be useful in this regard (30, 31). However, medications, environmental hazards, and vision also must be addressed to reduce the risk of falls (27).

- For intensity, use a rating between moderate (5-6) and vigorous (7-8) on a 10-point scale.
- Participants should exercise at least twice a week on nonconsecutive days.
- Participants should stay within the pain-free ROM.
- Participants should not exercise if an arthritic joint is painful or inflamed (see the sidebar *Osteoarthritis*).

Flexibility

A flexibility program should involve all joints with the goal of maintaining their normal ROM. However, there are few studies that compare or contrast various ROM exercises and their flexibility outcomes, and as a result there is little consensus on the frequency, duration, or type of exercise (static versus dynamic) to use (1). That said, the results do suggest that flexibility can be increased in major joints by doing ROM exercises specific to the joint (see chapter 14 for more information). Tai chi and yoga programs can be used to achieve and maintain flexibility goals. However, for most people, flexibility goals can be achieved within the context of a regular exercise class. Elements of a flexibility program include the following (3):

- Movements should be performed as a regular part of the warm-up and cool-down, the same as for younger participants.
- Doing stretching exercises after a workout when the muscles are warm is more effective.
- Static stretches are preferred, although others can be done (1).
- For static stretches, use slow movements through pain-free ROM, with stretches held for 15 to 60 sec; do at least 4 repetitions per muscle group.
- Stretching should be performed at least 2 days per wk.

Psychological Health and Well-Being

This chapter has focused on the fact that regular participation in physical activity is associated with better health (lower risk of chronic diseases) and fitness (cardiovascular function, strength, body composition, and flexibility) during aging. However, regular participation in physical activity also has been shown to improve psychological health and well-being (1, 6, 28, 33). Short-term benefits due to a single exercise session include enhanced relaxation and mood state, enhanced social and cultural integration, and empowerment to be more independent (31). A review of the long-term benefits shows that physical activity (1)

- improves overall psychological well-being (mediated through effects on self-concept and self-esteem),
- decreases risk of clinical depression and anxiety,
- decreases risk of cognitive decline and dementia,
- improves cognitive performance in previously sedentary adults, and
- has a positive impact on quality of life.

This is a good example of how regular physical activity affects the whole person, leading to a more active and fulfilling life.

17

LEARNING AIDS

REVIEW QUESTIONS

1. By the year 2040, how many people in the United States will be over the age of 65 yr compared with the year 2000?
2. Briefly describe the kinds of chronic conditions that exist in older adults that are less common in younger adults.
3. What happens to $\dot{V}O_2$max, muscular strength, and body fatness with age?
4. How might you have to modify a fitness test for CRF to accommodate the problems present in older adults?
5. What are some functional tests to evaluate flexibility, muscular endurance, and CRF?
6. Would you implement the same exercise program for all 65-yr-old adults? Why or why not?
7. Present the newest physical activity guidelines for older adults that address health and CRF, muscular strength, and flexibility.

8. If older adults cannot meet the activity guidelines you just stated, they should do nothing. Do you agree? Why or why not?
9. Discuss the role that progression plays in implementing physical activity programs for older adults, with specific emphasis on how to deal with duration and intensity in deconditioned individuals.
10. What are some psychological benefits that older adults experience as a result of regular participation in physical activity?

CASE STUDIES

1. A 67-yr-old male who has been actively involved in jogging and tennis most of his life has developed arthritis in his left knee. The problem has caused him to reduce his jogging, and his lack of fitness, as he calls it, is affecting his tennis game, which he is determined to continue. He comes to your health club for testing and advice about what he can do to increase and maintain his fitness. How do you address his concerns?
2. A 55-yr-old woman does three workouts every week, with an emphasis on vigorous aerobic exercise in a competitive masters swim class. Her doctor is concerned that her bone density is decreasing in spite of the exercise, and she comes to you for help. What do you recommend to address this concern?
3. A 70-yr-old woman has been referred to you for advice. She indicates that she has not been able to comfortably do her ordinary activities, and she would like your help. What tests do you perform, and what physical activities do you recommend to improve her CRF and muscle endurance to help her regain her confidence in doing routine activities?

Answers to Case Studies

1. You should begin by finding out when he had his last physical and what his physician told him about his arthritis. After appropriate screening (see chapter 2), a submaximal cycle ergometer test should be carried out to obtain some baseline measures (HR, RPE) to use as reference points for subsequent follow-ups. Establish a THR zone for him (e.g., 50%-70% of HRR), and verify that this elicits an RPE of about 10 to 13 on a 20-point scale. Have him begin his exercise program at 50% HRR, performing work–relief intervals (5 min on, 1 min off) to determine if he can do a series of these intervals with little or no joint discomfort. The goal is 30 min of continuous activity as long as the discomfort is little or nothing. Increase the work interval to 10 min in the second week. If joint discomfort is a problem, stay with intervals within his tolerance. Intensity can be increased after he has achieved 30 min of total exercise time. Introduce him to a variety of weight-supported exercise modes (cycling, rowing, water aerobics) that he should be able to use with less joint discomfort than what he experienced with jogging. Workouts should be done 3 to 4 days per wk and include regular warm-up and flexibility activities.
2. This 55-yr-old woman is clearly fit, but she needs to add other types of activities to her regular routine to improve bone health. You might recommend that she add a resistance training program that will not only improve bone strength but also her swimming performance. In addition, you might suggest that she add regular walking to her weekly activities to provide some downward loading to the bone that she is not experiencing in her swim workouts.
3. You might begin by using the Senior Fitness Test to obtain some baseline values for the various fitness components. Based on those test results, you should develop a program of activities that include walking (graduated in a manner that encourages multiple short walks with plenty of rest) and muscle strengthening activities using either very light dumbbells or low-tension elastic bands (again, with only a few repetitions in the beginning).

18

Exercise and Women's Health

Dixie L. Thompson

OBJECTIVES

The reader will be able to do the following:

1. Describe the risks and benefits of exercise during pregnancy, and suggest ways to alter exercise to make it more comfortable and safe for pregnant women.
2. Describe osteoporosis and its risk factors, and prescribe exercise to promote bone health.
3. Define the female athlete triad, and describe how a fitness professional might assist someone exhibiting signs of the triad.

Women and men share many of the same obstacles to good health (e.g., CVD, type 2 diabetes, obesity). Likewise, the benefits of exercise that combat these diseases are similar for men and women, as are exercise guidelines. However, some conditions are faced exclusively or primarily by women. In this chapter, we examine three of these: pregnancy, osteoporosis, and the female athlete triad.

Pregnancy and Exercise

Pregnancy places enormous demands on a woman's body. Concern about the safety of the fetus and the mother leads to questions about whether exercise is wise during pregnancy. Fortunately, there is substantial evidence that for healthy pregnant women, exercise is safe and beneficial during this critical time (4). Although difficult to document, proposed benefits of exercise during pregnancy include greater psychological well-being, less fatigue, and shorter and easier delivery (6, 24). Exercise during pregnancy can be helpful in avoiding excessive gestational weight gain (21), and leading an active life before and during early pregnancy is associated with a lower risk of developing gestational diabetes mellitus (22).

However, some conditions require a cautious approach to exercise. Pregnant women with cardiovascular, pulmonary, or metabolic disease, as well as those with severe obesity or who are considerably underweight, should seek physician guidance concerning exercise (11). The contraindications for exercise during pregnancy as determined by ACOG (5) are listed later in the chapter. In addition, CSEP has created the Physical Activity Readiness Medical Examination for Pregnancy (PARmed-X for Pregnancy). This tool screens for potential medical problems and assists with exercise prescription, and it can be found on the CSEP website (csep .ca/home). ACSM recommends that fitness professionals use the PARmed-X for Pregnancy when working with pregnant clients (4).

Potential Problems of Exercising During Pregnancy

Concerns about exercise during pregnancy target four crucial areas: heat dissipation, oxygen delivery, nutrition supply, and premature delivery. During the first trimester, the fetus is particularly vulnerable to developmental defects caused by excessive heat. Although the body's core temperature can increase with exercise, there are no known links between exercise and a greater prevalence of birth defects. An increase in the woman's blood volume provides adequate blood for heat dissipation, exercise demands, and nourishment of the fetus. Increases in skin blood flow also help protect against excessive changes in body temperature (24). Additionally, the temperature at which sweating begins decreases as pregnancy progresses, providing another protective mechanism against higher core temperatures (11).

Concern that vigorous exercise could compromise uterine blood flow is also unsubstantiated. The increase in maternal blood volume, coupled with a decrease in systemic vascular resistance, results in an increase in cardiac output that provides adequate blood flow, and therefore oxygen, to the fetus (6, 24). The fact that fetal HR is only modestly, if at all, affected by exercise provides evidence that this type of physical activity does not significantly distress the fetus (6, 24). Because of the nutritional demands of pregnancy, greater caloric consumption is needed. The nutritional demands of exercise and fetal development must be adequately met by the exercising woman. For most women, the energy demands of pregnancy are approximately 300 kcal · day^{-1} (4). Evidence that exercise does not compromise the nutritional needs of the developing fetus comes from studies showing little difference between the weights of newborns from exercising and nonexercising mothers (6, 24).

Another major concern is that exercise may cause premature delivery. For normal pregnancies, there is no evidence that the length of the pregnancy is affected by exercise (6, 24). Care should be taken, however, to avoid activities (e.g., contact sports) in which injury could lead to fetal injury or premature delivery (4, 5).

Exercise Testing and Prescription During Pregnancy

Maximal exercise testing should be avoided unless it is medically necessary and under the direction of a physician (4, 9). Submaximal exercise testing, with termination <75% HRR, can be used if specific information is required for exercise prescription.

Moderate and even vigorous exercise can be performed safely by previously active pregnant women. The type, intensity, frequency, and duration of activity should conform to the woman's health and comfort. The U.S. Physical Activity Guidelines (23) and ACSM (4) suggest that healthy pregnant women should accumulate at least 150 min per wk of moderate-intensity activity. Encourage regular (at least 3 days per wk) rather than periodic exercise (4). Intensity can be gauged with RPE, with a recommended range of 12 to 14 (9). THR ranges for moderate-intensity exercise based on age and fitness can also be used in exercise prescription (see table 18.1). For women who were overweight or obese prior to pregnancy, light-intensity exercise is recommended (see table 18.1).

Following are general recommendations for healthy women during pregnancy:

- Frequency:≥3 to 5 days per wk
- Intensity: moderate intensity (see table 18.1 for HR ranges; RPE 12-13); light intensity for overweight and obese women. For women who were highly active before pregnancy, vigorous intensity (≥6 METS, RPE 14-17) is acceptable.

Table 18.1 Heart Rates Corresponding to Moderate-Intensity Exercise in Pregnant Women Based on Age and Fitness Level*

BMI (kg · m^{-2})	Age (yr)	Fitness level	HR range (bpm)
<25	<20	Any fitness level	140-155
	20-29	Unfit	129-144
		Active	135-150
		Fit	145-160
	30-39	Unfit	128-144
		Active	130-145
		Fit	140-156
≥25	20-29	Any fitness level	102-124
	30-39	Any fitness level	101-120

*The recommended HR ranges for women who were overweight or obese prior to pregnancy correspond to light-intensity exercise.

Adapted, by permission, from American College of Sports Medicine, 2014, *ACSM guidelines for exercise testing and prescription,* 9th ed. (Philadelphia, PA: Lippincott, Williams, and Wilkins), 198

- Time: approximately 30 min per day of accumulated moderate-intensity exercise for 150 min per wk of accumulated moderate-intensity exercise (or 75 min of accumulated vigorous exercise for those engaging in high-intensity exercise prior to pregnancy)
- Type: rhythmic, dynamic activities that use large muscle groups

Although the physiological response patterns described in chapter 4 generally hold true for pregnant women, the variables themselves (e.g., HR, oxygen consumption) are changed due to the increased metabolic demands (9, 15). For example, HR, SV, and minute ventilation at rest and during exercise are higher than they were before pregnancy. These variables change throughout the pregnancy to meet the needs of the mother and the growing fetus (15).

Return to exercise in the postpartum period should be gradual and based on the woman's health (4, 5, 9). Because it is common that women's level of physical activity is less following childbirth, it provides an opportunity to encourage a healthy lifestyle (5). Often women can return to light- to moderate-intensity exercise 4 to 6 wk following vaginal delivery. Following a cesarean delivery, return to exercise requires medical clearance, which typically happens 8 to 10 wk following the birth. Deconditioning occurs in the period leading up to and following delivery, so women need to gradually regain their endurance when returning to exercise.

Because of the demands of pregnancy, the exercise mode should be based on comfort and convenience. Some women find that non-weight-bearing exercises such as swimming and stationary cycling are more comfortable, especially as pregnancy advances. During the postpartum stage, the return to activity should be gradual and based on individual response. A pregnant client should take the following precautions when exercising (4, 5, 23).

- Avoid exercise in a supine position after the first trimester. The enlarged uterus can apply pressure to the surrounding blood vessels and limit venous return.
- Take steps to avoid heat injury. To prevent hyperthermia, avoid exercising in hot and humid environments, ensure adequate hydration (before, during, and after exercise), and dress appropriately for the heat. It is prudent to avoid exercise classes that are held in a heated space.
- Limit exposure to falling and impact injury. Although completely eliminating risk is impossible, it is prudent to avoid competitive contact sports (e.g., soccer, boxing) and activities where trauma risk is great (e.g., skydiving, waterskiing). As pregnancy advances, center of gravity and balance change; therefore, exercise that requires rapid changes in direction may be more problematic than it was before pregnancy.
- Be aware that joint laxity increases during pregnancy. The release of relaxin allows the pelvis to undergo the changes needed during pregnancy and delivery. However, this hormone also leads to greater laxity in other joints. Follow the precautions in the previous point to help prevent joint injury.
- Resistance training can be used during pregnancy, but observe the following precautions: Avoid the Valsalva maneuver during lifting, keep the program at low to moderate intensity (resistance should be low enough that at least 12 repetitions can be completed without fatigue), and use slow and steady rather than ballistic movements. For more information on resistance training during pregnancy, see chapter 13.

Contraindications for Exercise During Pregnancy

Absolute Contraindications

- Hemodynamically significant heart disease
- Restrictive lung disease
- Incompetent cervix or cerclage
- Multiple gestation at risk for premature labor
- Persistent second- or third-trimester bleeding
- Placenta previa after 26 wk of gestation
- Premature labor during current pregnancy
- Ruptured membranes
- Preeclampsia or pregnancy-induced hypertension
- Severe anemia

Relative Contraindications

- Anemia
- Unevaluated maternal cardiac arrhythmia
- Chronic bronchitis
- Poorly controlled type 1 diabetes
- Extreme morbid obesity
- Extreme underweight (BMI <12 $kg \cdot m^{-2}$)
- History of extremely sedentary lifestyle
- Intrauterine growth restriction in current pregnancy
- Poorly controlled hypertension
- Orthopedic limitations
- Poorly controlled seizure disorder
- Poorly controlled hyperthyroidism
- Heavy smoker

Adapted, by permission, from American College of Obstetricians and Gynecologists, 2015, "Exercise during pregnancy and the postpartum period. Committee Opinion No. 650," *Obstetrics and Gynecology* 126: e135-142.

- Exercises that strengthen the pelvic floor (Kegel exercises) are recommended to decrease the risk of incontinence.
- Avoid exercise in which extremes in air pressure occur. Scuba diving should be avoided because it puts the fetus at risk for decompression sickness. Exercise at altitudes over 6,000 ft (1,829 m) could be potentially dangerous for unacclimatized women and should be performed with caution.
- Be aware of the body's warning signs (5). Each woman should closely monitor her body for signs or symptoms that something may be wrong. If any of the following occur, stop exercise and consult a physician:
  - Vaginal bleeding
  - Regular, painful contractions
  - Dyspnea before exertion
  - Dizziness
  - Headache
  - Chest pain
  - Muscle weakness affecting balance
  - Calf pain or swelling
  - Amniotic fluid leakage

KEY POINT

Exercising during pregnancy is safe and beneficial for most women. Light- and moderate-intensity aerobic exercise is recommended for women who are pregnant. Protecting against traumatic impact, heat injury, musculoskeletal injury, and overexertion is the key to planning safe exercise programs for pregnant women.

Osteoporosis

Osteoporosis is a disease characterized by fragile bones. Approximately 10.2 million Americans over age 50 have osteoporosis, and another 43.4 million have low bone mass, or **osteopenia**, and are at risk for developing osteoporosis (25). Osteoporotic fractures account for $22 billion in medical expenses each year (7). The most common sites for osteoporotic fractures are the hip, vertebrae, and wrist. Bone strength is determined by **bone mineral density (BMD)** and the structural integrity of the bone. BMD is measured by dual-energy X-ray absorptiometry (DXA; see chapter 8) and reflects the amount of bone mineral per unit area ($g \cdot cm^{-2}$). BMD accounts for about 70% of bone strength and is highly correlated with resistance to fractures (17). Structural integrity is determined by the microarchitecture of the bone, which is much more difficult to assess, requiring invasive testing of bone (1). Because of the low risk, the ease, and the availability of DXA, it has become the preferred method for diagnosing osteoporosis.

According to WHO guidelines, *osteoporosis* is defined as a BMD that is 2.5 SDs below the mean for young white women. When BMD is in the osteoporotic range, fracture risk is high. Common pharmaceutical treatments for osteoporosis are selective estrogen receptor modulators, hormone-replacement therapy (for women), and bisphosphonates. These drug interventions slow bone loss, and some even increase BMD. Recently developed drugs such as RANKL (receptor activator of nuclear factor kappa-B ligand) inhibitors show promising results. More information about osteoporosis and its treatment can be found at the website of the National Institute of Arthritis and Musculoskeletal and Skin Diseases (www.niams.nih.gov).

Risk Factors for Osteoporosis

Osteoporosis can affect both males and females across all ages and ethnicities. However, older women, particularly of Caucasian and Asian descent, are especially at risk. One in three women and one in five men aged 50 or older will experience an osteoporotic fracture in their lifetime (18). Bone accumulates during childhood and generally peaks in early adult life (14). Although BMD declines somewhat during the middle adult years, the most rapid loss in women occurs in the years surrounding menopause (14). The decline in estrogen levels around the time of menopause is the reason for the rapid bone loss, which can be as great as 3% to 5% of bone mass each year. In men, bone loss is typically slow but steady from the time of peak accumulation until death. In general, men are somewhat less likely than women to experience osteoporotic fractures because their peak BMD is higher than women's. In addition to sex, race is a factor in determining peak bone mass. Peak BMD is generally higher in individuals of African descent compared with those of European and Asian ancestry (17).

Risk factors for osteoporosis include the following:

- Female
- Older age
- Estrogen deficiency
- Caucasian or Asian race
- Low weight or BMI
- Diet low in calcium
- Alcohol abuse
- Inactivity
- Muscle weakness
- Family history of osteoporosis
- Smoking
- History of fracture

Sometimes osteoporosis results from other medical conditions or is related to use of prescription medications; examples include endocrine disorders, gastrointestinal diseases, nutritional deficiencies, and the long-term use of glucocorticoid medications. Because many factors lead to low bone density, people of all ages, including children, can develop osteoporosis. Low intake of calcium and vitamin D can limit the accumulation of bone during childhood, and it is estimated that only 25% of boys and 10% of girls achieve the recommended levels for calcium intake (17). Attaining a peak bone density that is lower than expected increases the risk of osteoporosis in later life. The International Osteoporosis Foundation (IOF) has developed a screening tool to assess risk for osteoporosis. This simple online test, designed to help identify people at particularly high risk for osteoporosis, is found in the sidebar *IOF One-Minute Osteoporosis Risk Test.* When BMD is known, an estimate of one's 10 yr fracture risk can be calculated using the Fracture Risk Assessment Tool (FRAX), an assessment measure published by WHO. In addition to BMD, the FRAX algorithm includes biological factors (e.g., age, sex), family history, and lifestyle factors (e.g., alcohol use). Information on the screening tool and FRAX can be found at the IOF website (www.iofbonehealth.org).

IOF One-Minute Osteoporosis Risk Test

Your Family History

- Has either of your parents been diagnosed with osteoporosis or broken a bone after a minor fall (a fall from standing height or less)? ❍Yes ❍No
- Did either of your parents have a dowager's hump? ❍Yes ❍No

Your Personal Clinical Factors

- Are you 40 years old or older? ❍Yes ❍No
- Have you ever broken a bone after a minor fall, as an adult? ❍Yes ❍No
- Do you fall frequently (more than once in the last year) or do you have a fear of falling because you are frail? ❍Yes ❍No
- After the age of 40, have you lost more than 3 cm in height (just over an inch)? ❍Yes ❍No
- Are you underweight (is your BMI less than 19 $kg \cdot m^{-2}$)? ❍Yes ❍No
- Have you ever taken corticosteroid tablets (cortisone, prednisone, etc.) for more than 3 consecutive months (corticosteroids are often prescribed for conditions like asthma, rheumatoid arthritis, and some inflammatory diseases)? ❍Yes ❍No
- Have you ever been diagnosed with rheumatoid arthritis? ❍Yes ❍No
- Have you been diagnosed with an over-reactive thyroid or over-reactive parathyroid glands? ❍Yes ❍No

For Women

- For women over 45, did your menopause occur before the age of 45? ❍Yes ❍No
- Have your periods ever stopped for 12 consecutive months or more (other than because of pregnancy, menopause, or hysterectomy)? ❍Yes ❍No
- Were your ovaries removed before age 50, without you taking hormonal replacement therapy? ❍Yes ❍No

For Men

- Have you ever suffered from impotence, lack of libido, or other symptoms related to low testosterone levels? ❍Yes ❍No

Your Lifestyle Factors

- Do you regularly drink alcohol in excess of safe drinking limits (more than 2 units per day)? ❍Yes ❍No
- Do you currently, or have you ever, smoked cigarettes? ❍Yes ❍No
- Is your level of physical activity less than 30 minutes per day (housework, gardening, walking, running, etc.)? ❍Yes ❍No
- Do you avoid, or are you allergic to, milk or dairy products, without taking any calcium supplements? ❍Yes ❍No
- Do you spend less than 10 minutes per day outdoors (with part of your body exposed to sunlight), without taking vitamin D supplements? ❍Yes ❍No

If you answered *yes* to one or more of these questions, it is possible that you are at increased risk for osteoporosis, and consultation with your physician is recommended.

Exercise Testing and Prescription for Individuals With Osteoporosis

For individuals with osteoporosis, particularly severe osteoporosis, precautions should be taken with both exercise testing and prescription. There are no specific special considerations for exercise testing of clients with osteoporosis beyond those for the general population. The benefits versus the risks of exercise testing must be weighed (4, 18). For individuals with severe kyphosis that limits forward vision or balance, modifications to testing protocols include using handrail support during treadmill walking and using stationary cycling (4). Those with compression fractures may find cycle ergometry less painful than walking. Testing muscular strength can be important in designing programs for osteoporotic clients; however, maximal exertion and exercises that involve significant spinal flexion should be avoided because of the risk of compression fractures. Tests of balance and functionality can be useful in designing programs to reduce the risk of falling. Improving functional muscle strength and balance is important in reducing the risk of falls (see chapters 13 and 17 for more on this topic).

Exercise prescription for the osteoporotic client must be individualized and based on the severity of disease and the presence of other conditions. In general, exercise prescription should include aerobic activity, exercises that strengthen muscle, and activities that improve balance. This combination incorporates three major components: cardiovascular health, bone health, and reduced risk of falling. It is common for individuals with osteoporosis to be deconditioned, so initial exercise prescription may involve low-intensity activity and slow progression. Ultimately, clients should attempt to reach the following exercise levels (4):

- Frequency: weight-bearing endurance exercise 4 to 5 days per wk; resistance exercise of 8 to 10 repetitions performed on 1 or 2 days per wk (may progress to 2 to 3 days per wk of resistance exercise)
- Intensity: moderate-intensity aerobic exercise (40%-59% HRR); moderate loading force for resistance exercise (60%-80% 1RM for 8 to 12 repetitions)
- Time: Begin with 20 min per day of aerobic exercise (progress to 30 to 60 min per day); for resistance exercise, begin with 1 set of 8 to 12 repetitions (may increase to 2 sets)
- Type: weight-bearing aerobic exercise (walking, stair-climbing) and resistance exercise

Explosive, high-impact activities generally should be avoided by people with osteoporosis. Clients should be counseled to note any new pain, and this information should be carefully considered in modifying exercise. Exercises that improve balance should also be incorporated into the overall exercise program. Tai chi is an example of activity that can be used to improve balance and functional ability. For more details on exercise testing and prescription for osteoporotic clients, see Smith, Wang, and Bloomfield (19).

Exercise in Prevention and Treatment of Osteoporosis

One of the primary means for preventing osteoporosis is maximizing bone accumulation during childhood and adolescence. In addition to adequate calcium and vitamin D intake, physical activity is important for developing strong bones. Studies demonstrate that children who exercise regularly have higher bone mineral levels than their sedentary peers, and this increase in bone carries over into adulthood (3). The primary goal for children is to participate in activities that maximize bone accrual.

The research examining exercise as a tool to increase bone density among adults has produced mixed results. Although some studies have demonstrated gains in bone density with exercise, others have shown that exercise has little effect. The wide variety among research protocols is one reason for the mixed results. Some common elements among studies that yielded the most profound effect on adult bone health are moderate to vigorous activity, adequate calcium intake (1,000-1,500 mg · day^{-1}) in conjunction with exercise, and movements that involve either impact loading or resistance training. For older adults, exercise alone may not be adequate to prevent age-related bone loss; however, exercise is essential in slowing this potentially devastating condition. Older adults with osteoporosis should be encouraged to engage in exercises designed to lower the risk of falling (e.g., balance and resistance training) in order to help protect against osteoporotic fractures.

Exercise for children and adolescents helps maximize bone density. Regular participation in high-intensity loading activities should be encouraged. ACSM recommends the following (3):

- Frequency: at least 3 days per wk
- Intensity: high-loading forces in jumping; moderate (<60% 1RM) resistance training
- Time: 10 to 20 min (multiple bouts per day if possible)
- Type: activities and sports that involve weight bearing and jumping (e.g., volleyball, gymnastics) and moderate resistance training

For nonosteoporotic adults, loading exercises and muscle-building activities promote bone health. An excellent example of this type of program is described by Metcalfe and colleagues (16). Using the evidence available, ACSM recommends the following approach to preserve bone during adulthood (3):

- Frequency: weight-bearing endurance exercise 3 or 4 times per wk; resistance exercise 2 or 3 times per wk
- Intensity: moderate to high loading forces
- Time: 30 to 60 min, combining weight-bearing and resistance exercise
- Type: weight-bearing aerobic exercise, jumping activities (e.g., basketball), and resistance exercise

KEY POINT

Osteoporosis, a disease characterized by fragile bones, affects millions of Americans. Although males and females of all ages can develop osteoporosis, it is most commonly seen in postmenopausal women. Healthy eating practices and an active lifestyle are keys to promoting bone health. Exercises that involve impact loading or resistance training appear most beneficial for promoting bone development. Special care should be taken when testing and prescribing exercise for osteoporotic clients. Building strength, endurance, and balance should be special considerations when planning exercise for those with osteoporosis.

Female Athlete Triad

The female athlete triad includes three interrelated components: energy availability, bone health, and menstrual status (2). As shown in figure 18.1, athletes at the healthy end of the continuum eat healthy diets with an adequate number of calories to meet energy needs; have normal menstrual cycles; and have healthy, strong bones. Unfortunately, athletes who continually underconsume calories may have irregular or absent menses (amenorrhea) and compromised BMD (osteoporosis). If left untreated, this condition can produce significant health consequences, including glycogen depletion, anemia, and electrolyte imbalances (2).

The precipitating factor in the female athlete triad is low energy availability (with or without disordered eating). Anorexia nervosa and bulimia nervosa are two eating disorders commonly associated with the female athlete triad. However, among athletes who develop the triad, there is a wide range of unhealthy eating practices. Some athletes clearly present with eating disorders, whereas others limit calories without meeting the strict clinical definitions of an eating disorder (2, 12). The unhealthy eating pattern with insufficient calories and nutritional density leads to amenorrhea. The estrogen deficiency seen in amenorrhea leads to osteopenia and potentially even osteoporosis. This loss of bone puts the athlete at great risk for stress fractures and for osteoporotic compression fractures.

In the general adult population, anorexia nervosa occurs at a rate of 0.5% to 1% and bulimia nervosa occurs at a rate of 2% to 4% (13). Although it is difficult to determine the percentage of athletes struggling with unhealthy eating practices, the prevalence of these eating disorders among athletes seems to be at least as high as that for the general population and is often found to be higher, particularly in sports with an emphasis on thinness (2). A meta-analysis found that some athletes are at particular risk for eating disorders (elite athletes, dancers, athletes in sports that emphasize thinness), whereas others (nonelite status, athletes in sports that do not emphasize thinness) may actually have some protection from unhealthy eating (20). Several studies have reported that one-third to one-half of elite female athletes report habits indicative of disordered eating (2). When left untreated, eating disorders can lead to seriously deteriorating health and potentially even death (see chapter 12).

Amenorrhea, or lack of menses, is clinically divided into two categories. **Primary amenorrhea** is characterized by the absence of menarche (i.e., first menses) in girls

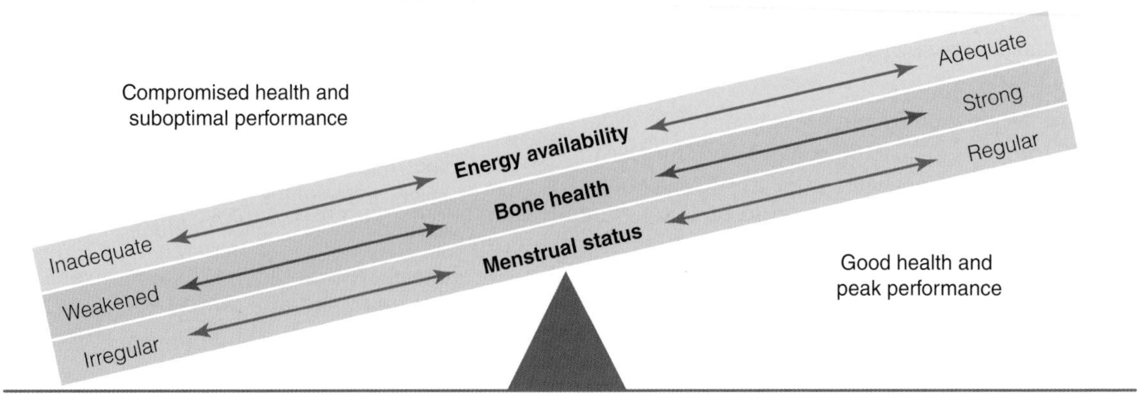

FIGURE 18.1 Female athlete triad.

aged 16 or older. When there is a lack of menses for 3 or more consecutive months in females after menarche, it is classified as **secondary amenorrhea**. The cause of amenorrhea can be difficult to establish and involves a complex interaction among the hypothalamus, pituitary gland, and ovaries. Because of inadequate stimulation, the ovaries do not function normally, resulting in lower-than-normal estrogen and progesterone levels. The high prevalence of irregular menstruation has been observed in athletic women for a number of years, but the consequences on bone largely were ignored until Drinkwater and colleagues' landmark study (10) in which the bones of young amenorrheic athletes were found to be comparable in density to those of postmenopausal women. To help protect against bone loss, physicians sometimes treat amenorrheic athletes by replacing the missing endogenous estrogen with oral contraceptives, but the results of this treatment are minimal at best (2). Restoring a healthy eating pattern and achieving a normal weight are keys to assisting bone health (2).

Recognizing the signs of disordered eating (see chapter 12) is necessary before successful intervention. Often coaches and athletes are ill informed about the female athlete triad. Therefore, education is an important first step in battling this condition. Successful intervention for the female athlete triad requires a multidisciplinary approach that includes input from medical, nutritional, and psychological professionals (2, 12). Screening and diagnosis of the female athlete triad falls under the scope of practice for physicians and mental health professionals (2). The preparticipation physical or annual exam is an opportune time to screen for the triad.

Prevention of the female athlete triad takes effort on the part of many individuals: coaches, parents, nutritionists, health care providers, and officials providing oversight for sport governing bodies. Creating an environment that values optimal health as well as athletic performance is key. To create a healthy environment for female athletes, the National Athletic Trainers' Association (NATA) makes several recommendations, including that ideal weight and body-fat percentage be deemphasized and that public discussion of results from body composition testing be avoided (8). For more information on eating disorders, refer to chapter 12.

KEY POINT

The female athlete triad is characterized by low energy availability, amenorrhea, and osteoporosis. Anorexia nervosa and bulimia nervosa are eating disorders frequently seen in the female athlete triad and can lead to significant health impairment and even death if left untreated. Intervention for the female athlete triad should be multidisciplinary and should include psychological counseling.

18

LEARNING AIDS

REVIEW QUESTIONS

1. What are the benefits of exercising during pregnancy?
2. What special precautions should a pregnant woman take when exercising?
3. What are the relative and absolute contraindications to exercise for pregnant women?
4. What is the standard exercise recommendation for pregnant women?
5. What is osteoporosis?
6. What are risk factors for osteoporosis?
7. What exercise recommendations for children will help promote good bone development?
8. What precautions should be taken when testing clients with osteoporosis?
9. What is the standard exercise prescription for a person with osteoporosis?
10. Describe the female athlete triad.
11. What steps might help prevent the female athlete triad?

CASE STUDIES

1. A sedentary 52-yr-old woman with a family history of osteoporosis comes to your facility for information on exercise to promote bone health. Her doctor says she is in generally good health and does not have osteoporosis, but there are signs that her bones are weaker than when she was younger (i.e., osteopenia). What type of exercise do you recommend?
2. Janice is an active, healthy, 32-yr-old woman who is pregnant for the first time. She is in her first trimester. Although she has been a runner for years, she has been told by her mother-in-law that she should give up running while pregnant. Her doctor told her that it is perfectly healthy to continue running. What is your advice?
3. Samantha is a 17-yr-old runner who has dreams of someday competing in an Olympic marathon. You have been helping to plan her workouts for the past year, and you notice some disturbing signs: Her weight has decreased dramatically, she is constantly battling stress fractures, her mood is negative and characterized by self-criticism, and her performance times are worse than a few months earlier. What do you do?

Answers to Case Studies

1. This client will benefit from both weight-bearing aerobic activity and resistance training. To increase her aerobic fitness, protect her against chronic disease, and load her bones, a walking program is appropriate. She should gradually progress to a 30 min brisk walk on most, preferably all, days of the week. Additionally, she should engage in resistance training 2 to 3 days per wk. The program should include upper- and lower-body exercises and focus on areas at high risk for osteoporotic fractures (hip, spine, wrist). Three sets of approximately 70% of 1RM (8-12 repetitions) are appropriate. Suggested exercises include the standing toe raise, leg press, leg extension, leg curl, back extension (use care to avoid hyperextension), bench press, shoulder press, biceps curl, triceps extension, and wrist curl. Additionally, the client should consume adequate amounts of calcium and vitamin D (see chapter 5).
2. Given that Janice's physician cleared her to continue running, there is no medical reason to stop running at this point in her pregnancy. However, it is understandable that both Janice and her mother-in-law have concerns. The first step is to alleviate fears through education. Give Janice background information on the health benefits of remaining active during pregnancy. Also, provide her with the warning signs that she should seek medical help (e.g., vaginal bleeding, dyspnea before exertion). Then encourage her to remain as active as she feels comfortable with during her pregnancy. Talk with her about using HR and RPE as a guide to her exercise intensity. Also, acknowledge that the types and intensity of exercise will likely need to change as she gets closer to term. Discuss with her the types of exercise that should be avoided (e.g., supine exercise).
3. This is a potentially difficult and dangerous situation. At the very least, Samantha is exhibiting signs of poor physical and emotional health. Begin a dialogue with Samantha addressing your concerns. Gently ask questions about her weight and eating habits (e.g., "Have you been doing anything different with your eating or exercise?"). Encourage her to take her health seriously. Explain to her how important it is to eat a healthy diet in order to optimize performance as well as remain healthy. Encourage her to discuss with her health care providers the recurrent stress fractures that she is experiencing. She is still a minor, so if you have a relationship with her parents, you may also want to engage them in a conversation. But before you engage either Samantha or her parents in conversation about your concerns, you need to seek out a support system for assistance. Find out the names of nutritionists, physicians, and mental health professionals in your area who specialize in eating disorders, particularly with athletes. Given that Samantha is already exhibiting diminished health and signs associated with disordered eating, she is likely going to require the assistance of a multidisciplinary team.

19

Exercise and Heart Disease

David R. Bassett, Jr.

Dr. Glenn Farr, PharmD (University of Tennessee College of Pharmacy), provided expert assistance in revising and updating the medications section of this chapter.

OBJECTIVES

The reader will be able to do the following:

1. Describe the atherosclerotic process and the resulting outcome if blood flow becomes obstructed in the arteries of the heart, brain, or periphery.
2. Quantify the magnitude of CVD as a health problem in the United States and list the various subcategories of CVD.
3. Identify the various patient populations found in cardiac rehabilitation programs.
4. Describe the physiological and mental health benefits of exercise for individuals with CVD.
5. Explain what is meant by secondary prevention of CHD.
6. Describe tests that can help diagnose the presence or absence of CHD, including those that use exercise and nonexercise challenges to stress the heart.
7. Describe how to prescribe aerobic exercise (frequency, intensity, and duration) in cardiac rehabilitation programs.
8. Discuss special considerations in prescribing exercise intensity for individuals who are taking beta-blocker medications.
9. List the common categories of prescription medications used to treat CVD, some examples of each category, and the probable effect of these medications on exercise performance.

Coronary heart disease (CHD) is a major problem in the United States and other industrialized nations. This chapter provides the fitness professional with a basic understanding of the development of CHD, the types of patients found in cardiac rehabilitation programs, the benefits of exercise for a cardiac population, and the special considerations for exercise prescription in this group. It is not a comprehensive guide to exercise in cardiac rehabilitation; a number of excellent texts provide more complete information on the topic (2, 8, 18).

Atherosclerosis

Atherosclerosis refers to a thickening of the artery wall that blocks blood flow to a certain region of the body (figure 19.1). It occurs because of genetic predisposition, high-fat diets, physical inactivity, and other CVD (cardiovascular disease) risk factors. The atherosclerotic process begins early in life, as evidenced by studies of soldiers killed in the Korean War. Approximately three-fourths of the 300 soldiers examined (mean age 22.1 yr) had some degree of blockage in their coronary arteries (11). The theory at that time was that cholesterol builds up inside the arteries, much like rust building up inside a pipe. However, it is now believed that the atherosclerotic process begins when the **endothelial cells** lining the artery become damaged because of smoking, toxic agents, or high BP (see *Hypertension* sidebar). Subsequently, the white blood cells invade the artery wall and cause chronic inflammation. LDLs that contain cholesterol and triglycerides pass through the endothelial cells and are deposited at the site of inflammation, and plaque formation (or atherosclerosis) occurs (23). Over time, these atherosclerotic plaques may gradually build up to the point where they impede blood flow in the affected arteries, sometimes to the point of complete occlusion (30, 17). But more often than not, the thin, fibrous cap that covers a plaque ruptures, causing a blood clot to suddenly form. This is known as a **plaque hemorrhage**, and it results in a sudden blockage of blood flow (23).

Atherosclerosis can occur in various arteries throughout the body and have various results. Blockages in the coronary arteries lead to **myocardial ischemia** (reduced blood flow, and thus inadequate oxygen, to the heart) and in severe cases to **myocardial infarction (MI)**. If arteries in the brain become occluded, a **stroke** will result. **Peripheral artery disease (PAD)** is characterized by blockages in the peripheral arteries. PAD can result in **claudication**, or intermittent muscle pain that occurs with exertion

Cardiovascular Disease

In the United States, CVD is the leading cause of death, with nearly 787,000 people dying from CVD (including congenital cardiovascular defects) in 2011. CHD accounts for 51% of these deaths, with stroke (17%), hypertensive disease (7%), and congestive heart failure (CHF) (7%) making up most of the other leading causes (5). (CVD is any disease of the heart and the blood vessels or circulation; CHD is a more specific condition resulting from reduced blood flow in the coronary arteries.) The death rate attributable to coronary artery disease (CAD) has declined in recent decades, but it remains a problem of huge proportions. According to the AHA, approximately 735,000 Americans have heart attacks each year. About 635,000 of these are first heart attacks, and the rest are recurrent attacks. Of those experiencing a heart attack, 80% will survive, and some of the survivors will be referred to cardiac rehabilitation programs (5). Although CVD is often thought of as a man's disease, it is the leading cause of death in women as well as men.

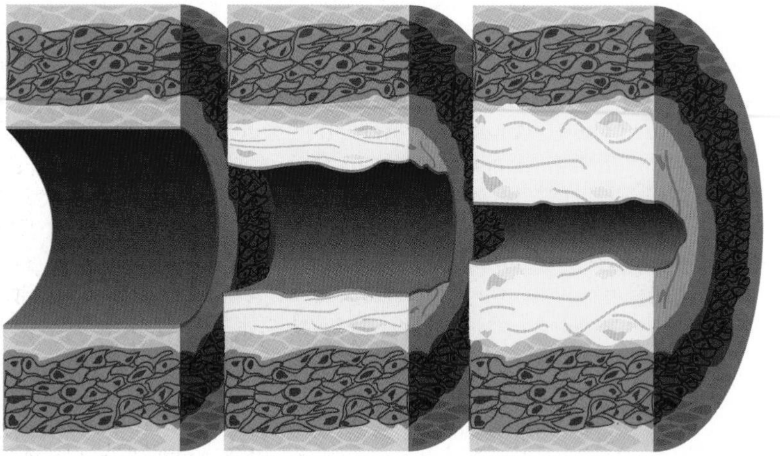

FIGURE 19.1 Stages of atherosclerosis: *(a)* normal artery, *(b)* partially blocked artery, and *(c)* significantly blocked artery.

KEY POINT

Atherosclerosis is a disease that starts early in life and leads to blockages in the arteries of the heart, brain, or peripheral muscles. If a blockage occurs in a coronary artery, myocardial ischemia or infarction results. There is a high prevalence of such health problems in the United States.

Populations in Cardiac Rehabilitation Programs

Cardiac rehabilitation programs include people who have experienced angina pectoris, MI, **coronary artery bypass graft (CABG)**, and angioplasty (12, 13). **Angina pectoris** refers to the chest pain attributable to ischemia of the ventricle resulting from an occlusion of one or more of the coronary arteries. The pain appears when the oxygen requirement of the heart (estimated by the double product SBP · HR) exceeds a value that coronary blood flow can meet. The ischemia can be transient and may subside once the oxygen demand of the heart returns to normal.

MI patients have heart damage (death of ventricular muscle fibers) caused by the occlusion of one or more of the coronary arteries. The degree to which ventricular function is affected depends on the mass of the ventricle permanently damaged. Individuals who have experienced an MI usually take medications (beta-blockers) to reduce the work of the heart and control the irritability of the heart tissue so that dangerous arrhythmias (irregular heartbeats) do not occur. Generally, when these individuals engage in regular exercise, they experience a training effect similar to that of people who have not had an MI.

CABG patients have had surgery to bypass one or more blocked coronary arteries. In this procedure, a blood vessel is sewn into existing coronary arteries above and below the blockage in order to reroute the blood flow (see figure 19.2). People with chronic angina pectoris before CABG find a relief of symptoms, with 50% to 70% experiencing no more pain. Generally, with an increased blood flow to the ventricle, left ventricular function and the capacity for work improve (31). These patients benefit from systematic exercise training because most are deconditioned before surgery as a result of activity restrictions related to chest pain.

Hypertension

Hypertension, or high BP, greatly increases the risk of developing CVD. It is estimated that 80 million people in the United States have hypertension (5), defined as a BP of 140/90 or higher. **Stage 1 hypertension** is defined as an SBP of 140 to 159 mmHg or a DBP of 90 to 99 mmHg. For those who have this type of hypertension, a variety of nonpharmacological approaches to reducing BP are often recommended at first; however, if BP is not normalized with lifestyle changes, medications may be prescribed. Dietary change includes reducing sodium intake, which has been shown to independently lower SBP and DBP by 5 and 3 mmHg, respectively (16, 20). Obesity is linked to hypertension, and research shows that a loss of 1 kg of body weight decreases SBP and DBP by 1.6 and 1.3 mmHg, respectively (16, 20). Also, participating in an endurance exercise program has been shown to decrease SBP and DBP by 7 and 6 mmHg, respectively, in hypertensive individuals (3).

Stage 2 hypertension (SBP of 160-179 mmHg or DBP of 100-109 mmHg) is more serious, and it is typically controlled through medication (see chapter 24). **Stage 3 hypertension** refers to a persistent elevation in BP (SBP >180 mmHg or DBP >110 mmHg) with target-organ damage. This may include damage to the heart (such as enlargement of the left ventricle); damage to the kidneys, leading to renal insufficiency; and damage to the eyes caused by small hemorrhages in the blood vessels.

The standard ACSM exercise prescription for improving $\dot{V}O_2$max (see chapter 11) also reduces BP in previously hypertensive individuals (3, 16). In addition, endurance exercise at moderate intensities (40%-60% $\dot{V}O_2$max) has been shown to reduce BP. Moderate-intensity exercise should be done frequently and for durations long enough to expend a large number of calories. Furthermore, for people with higher BPs who are taking medication, this type of exercise program along with changes in diet, smoking, and body weight can lower BP. In these cases, BP should be checked frequently so medications can be reduced as needed. Gradually establishing appropriate diet and exercise habits improves the chance that a person will maintain an appropriate BP once it has been normalized.

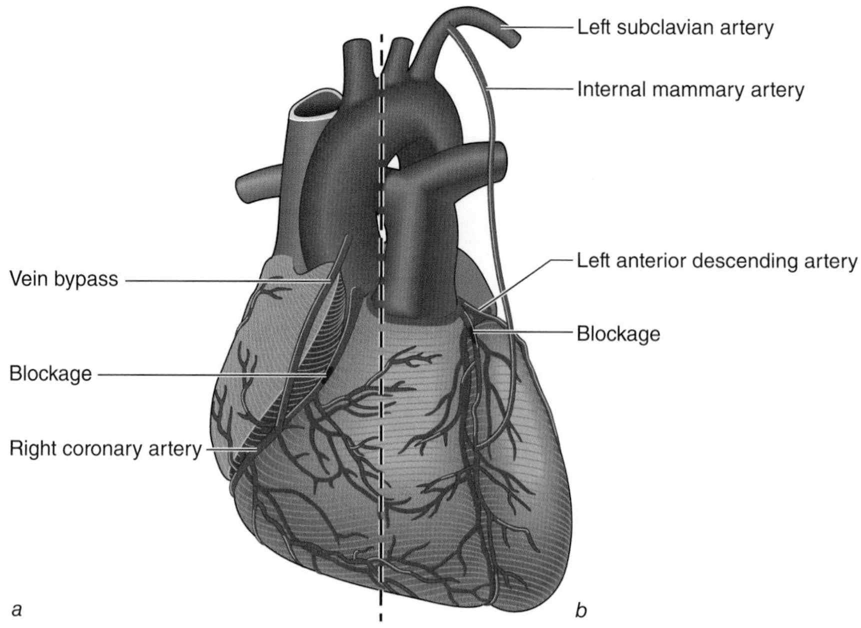

FIGURE 19.2 Coronary artery bypass surgery. *(a)* CABG using saphenous vein and *(b)* CABG using mammary artery. Blood flow is rerouted around the site of obstruction by taking a blood vessel from another part of the body and sewing it to the affected coronary artery, distal to the site of the obstruction. Blood vessels typically used in the procedure are the saphenous (leg) vein and the mammary artery.

Some CHD patients undergo a special procedure, **percutaneous transluminal coronary angioplasty (PTCA)**, to open occluded arteries. In this procedure, the chest is not opened; instead, a balloon-tipped catheter (a long, slender tube) is inserted into the coronary artery, where the balloon is inflated to push the plaque back toward the arterial wall (see figure 19.3). These patients tend not to have as severe CHD as those who undergo CABG. For these patients, PTCA has some advantages, including being less invasive, requiring a shorter hospital stay (1-2 days instead of 6-9 days), and costing less (13). However, with PTCA the coronary artery becomes reoccluded in approximately one-third to one-half of patients within 6 mo of the procedure (15).

To help prevent reocclusion, **intracoronary stents** are often used to help keep the **lumen** of the coronary artery open. A stent is composed of a metal mesh that is inserted into the artery on a balloon catheter and positioned in the area of obstruction. Some stents slowly release a drug that helps to prevent restenosis; these are known as drug-eluting stents. The balloon is first inflated to increase the lumen size, and then it is deflated and pulled back while the stent remains embedded in the artery. The main disadvantage of metal stents is that they increase the risk of blood clots; hence, anticoagulation therapy is needed to reduce this risk (7).

KEY POINT

CHD is treated by CABG, angioplasty, or intracoronary stent. Patients who have undergone these procedures are candidates for a hospital-based cardiac rehabilitation program.

Evidence for Exercise Training

Sixty years ago, the most common advice given to patients who had experienced an MI was to take several weeks of complete bed rest (2). Today, however, exercise training is an ordinary part of treatment for people with CHD. Cardiac rehabilitation programs use a multidisciplinary approach of education and exercise to help clients with heart disease return to normal function within the limits of their disease (18).

There is no question that patients with CHD have improved cardiovascular function as a result of exercising. This is evidenced by higher $\dot{V}O_2max$ values, higher work rates achieved without ischemia (as shown by angina pec-

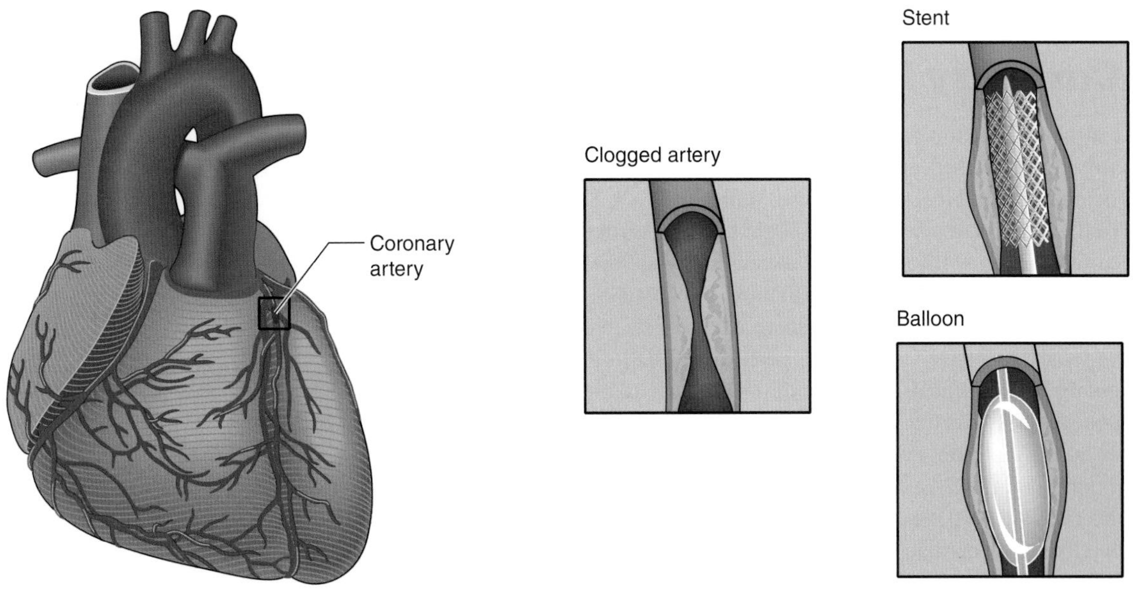

FIGURE 19.3 Percutaneous transluminal coronary angioplasty (PTCA). The cardiologist locates a clogged section of a coronary artery by injecting a contrast dye into the artery, allowing it to be seen on an X-ray machine. A guide wire is inserted into a femoral artery and is pushed up to the heart, where it is used to position the balloon catheter at the site of obstruction inside the coronary artery. The balloon is temporarily inflated, increasing the lumen size and capacity for blood flow. The balloon catheter is then deflated and removed. In some cases, a metal stent is placed inside the coronary artery to help keep it open. The stent is expanded by inflation pressure, and it remains inside the patient.

toris or ST segment changes), and an increased capacity for prolonged submaximal work (9, 27, 29). Moderate reductions in body fat, BP, total cholesterol, serum triglycerides, and LDL-C have been shown to occur with regular exercise, along with increases in HDL-C. The improved lipid profile is a function of more than the exercise alone, given that weight loss and the saturated-fat content of the diet can modify these variables.

A major focus of cardiac rehabilitation programs is to reduce the occurrence of subsequent MIs (2). This is referred to as **secondary prevention** of CHD. The Framingham Heart Study has shown that people who have experienced one heart attack are at increased risk of a second heart attack. Further, the likelihood of recurrence clearly is associated with many of the same risk factors that caused atherosclerosis in the first place. Thus, cardiac rehabilitation personnel must monitor BP, blood cholesterol levels, and smoking in their patients. In general, research has shown that a cardiac rehabilitation program involving exercise results in a 20% to 25% reduction in all-cause and cardiovascular mortality after an MI. This is good news, because it indicates that such patients derive a substantial benefit from participating in cardiac rehabilitation. In addition, patients gain an improved sense of well-being (18).

One of the most exciting developments in cardiac rehabilitation is the demonstration that lifestyle modification can reverse CAD. Ornish and colleagues (25) conducted a series of studies in which they showed that a program consisting of a strict vegetarian diet, yoga, meditation, smoking cessation, and physical activity reversed the atherosclerotic process. Patients in this study showed actual reversal of blockages in their coronary arteries, lending credibility to the idea that this condition can, in some cases, be treated with nonsurgical interventions. The lifestyle intervention group had more regression of CHD after 5 yr than after 1 yr, while the control group (which made more modest changes in lifestyle) showed continued progression of atherosclerosis and more than twice as many cardiac events.

KEY POINT

Cardiac rehabilitation programs help people with heart disease regain their fitness and return to normal, everyday activities. The benefits of such programs include increased work capacity and reduced cardiovascular risk factors. Cardiac rehabilitation programs generally lower the risk of a second heart attack.

Diagnostic Tests to Detect Coronary Heart Disease

Tests of heart function include radionuclide procedures, typically administered in conjunction with either exercise or pharmacological (nonexercise) stress tests (7, 8, 22). In the latter case, the pharmacologic agents provoke myocardial ischemia through either increased myocardial oxygen demand or peripheral vasodilation. For instance, **thallium-201** (a radioactive substance) can be injected intravenously to assess myocardial perfusion. Thallium is taken up by well-perfused myocardium similarly to the way potassium is taken up. Ischemic myocardium tends not to take up the thallium, thus identifying areas of the heart with poor blood flow. Another technique involves a radioisotope that binds to the red blood cells, **technetium-99m**, which is useful for cardiac blood pool imaging. This allows the end-systolic volume (ESV) and end-diastolic volume (EDV) to be measured, and the ejection fraction then can be computed as follows: Ejection fraction = (EDV – ESV) ÷ EDV. A normal ejection fraction is 55% to 70%, but a person with a severely damaged myocardium may have an ejection fraction of only 30%. This technique can identify ventricular wall motion abnormalities that occur with a ventricular **aneurysm** (7).

The most definitive tests for CHD are **coronary angiography** and **positron emission tomography (PET)** scans. In angiography, a cardiac catheter is inserted into the femoral artery and pushed all the way up the aorta until it reaches the entrance to a coronary artery, where the curved tip of the catheter guide allows it to be inserted into the artery. A contrast dye is injected through the catheter into the coronary artery. By viewing an image of the coronary arteries on a screen, the cardiologist can measure the degree of occlusion (narrowing) that exists (see figure 19.4). PET scans use [^{18}F]deoxyglucose or [^{13}N]ammonia. These substances allow the level of myocardial cell metabolism to be assessed. Metabolically active areas, indicative of good perfusion, can be distinguished from underperfused areas by color.

KEY POINT

Special types of diagnostic tests can determine whether a patient has CHD. Using GXTs on the treadmill (with close monitoring of the ECG and BP) is a common method of detecting signs and symptoms of heart disease. Radionuclide tests can more definitively confirm the presence or absence of heart disease.

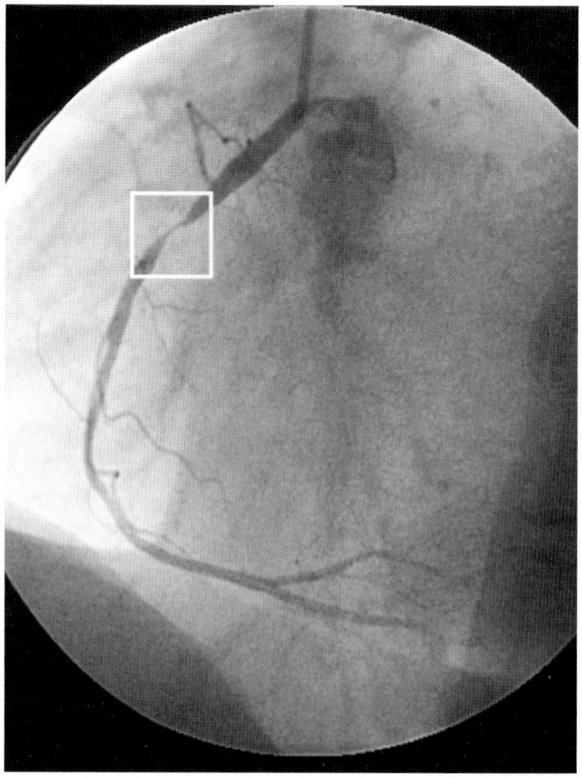

FIGURE 19.4 Coronary angiogram showing occlusion (narrowing) of a coronary artery. A catheter has been inserted into a coronary artery and radiographic contrast dye injected to allow the artery to be seen.
Courtesy of David R. Bassett Jr.

Exercise Testing in Patients With Coronary Heart Disease

Testing a patient with CHD is much more involved than testing the apparently healthy person. There are some classes of patients with CHD for whom exercise or exercise testing is inappropriate and dangerous (4). (See chapter 7 for absolute and relative contraindications to exercise.) In others, however, the benefits of a graded exercise test (GXT) outweigh the risks. Diagnostic exercise testing is nearly always performed in a hospital environment with a physician present. A 12-lead ECG is monitored at discrete intervals during the GXT, and three leads are displayed continuously on an oscilloscope. BP, RPE, and various signs and symptoms also are noted. Emergency equipment includes a defibrillator, supplemental oxygen, and emergency medications. Personnel trained and certified in advanced cardiac life support (ACLS) are on hand to provide assistance if needed.

Treadmill tests commonly used in diagnostic exercise testing are the Naughton, Balke, Bruce, and Ellestad protocols, named after their developers (4). These protocols are all GXTs that increase speed or grade at regular intervals to increase the exercise intensity. For those who are unable to perform treadmill exercise, a cycle test or arm ergometer test may be used. The criteria for terminating the GXT focus on various pathological signs (e.g., ST segment depression on the ECG) or symptoms (e.g., angina pectoris) rather than on achieving some percentage of age-adjusted maximal HR (4). A subjective angina scale may be used to assess the severity of the symptoms (see table 19.1).

Table 19.1 Angina Rating Scale

1	Mild, barely noticeable
2	Moderate, bothersome
3	Moderately severe, very uncomfortable
4	Most severe or most intense pain ever experienced

This scale is used in rating the subjective pain associated with myocardial insufficiency.

Adapted from American College of Sports Medicine 2006.

Typical Exercise Prescription

Fitness professionals who work in health clubs and other fitness settings often encounter clients who have gone through a cardiac rehabilitation program. Thus, it is important to have an understanding and appreciation of what these clients have experienced during their recovery process. In addition, many individuals with a master's degree in exercise physiology can, with the proper training, find jobs in cardiac rehabilitation. As part of a team of medical professionals that includes physicians, nurses, dietitians, physical therapists, and clinical psychologists, the fitness professional can play an important role in helping patients to resume a healthy life after a heart event (28). A fitness professional working in cardiac rehabilitation must be vigilant about monitoring the signs and symptoms of heart disease. This involves knowing how to read an ECG, take BP readings, and administer the angina rating scale (refer back to table 19.1). Fitness professionals should be trained in emergency procedures and preferably should achieve certification in ACLS.

The details of how to design and implement cardiac rehabilitation programs, from the first steps taken after patients are confined to bed to the time that they return to work and beyond, are provided in the AACVPR guidelines (2). This section briefly introduces these programs.

Cardiac rehabilitation programs are organized in progressive phases of programming to meet the needs of clients and their families. Phase I (the acute phase) begins when a patient arrives in the hospital step-down unit after leaving the intensive or coronary care unit (18). Within 1 to 3 days of the MI or revascularization procedure, the patient has already been taught the risk factors for atherosclerotic disease and has begun the rehabilitation process. Patients are exposed to orthostatic or gravitation stress by intermittently sitting and standing. Later, bedside activities and slow ambulation (i.e., walking) in the hallways are recommended (2).

Phases II and III refer to outpatient exercise programs conducted in a hospital environment. Rhythmic activities using large muscle groups are recommended for physical conditioning; these activities include treadmill exercise, cycle ergometry, combined arm and leg exercise, rowing, and stair-climbing. Light to moderate resistance training is accomplished with free weights (dumbbells) and elastic tubing. Special care must be taken when prescribing upper-body exercises to clients who have undergone CABG procedures because of limitations related to the chest incision. See chapter 13 for more details on resistance training in cardiac populations.

Recommendations for aerobic exercise programming in outpatient cardiac rehabilitation (phases II and III) are as follows, with patients progressing on an individual basis (4, 12-14):

- Frequency: 3 to 5 days per wk
- Intensity: moderate intensity equivalent to 40% to 80% of $\dot{V}O_{22}$max or HRR; or RPE 12-16 (on a 20-point scale)
- Duration: 20 to 60 min per day of continuous or accumulated exercise; if patient is unable to exercise continuously for 30 min, use intermittent exercise bouts of 10 min, interspersed with rest or light intensity
- Type: prolonged, rhythmic, dynamic exercises using large muscle groups (e.g., treadmill, cycle ergometer, rower, elliptical, stair climber, arm ergometer, or combined arm-and-leg ergometer)
- 5 to 10 min of warm-up and cool-down exercises

Fitness professionals who work in cardiac rehabilitation must have knowledge of cardiovascular medications (for a description of these, see chapter 24). Patients who are on beta-blockers require special consideration, because the Karvonen formula for computing THR range is invalid if the client was not on beta-blockers at the time of testing. For these patients, a THR is sometimes computed by adding 20 to 30 beats · min^{-1} to the client's standing, resting HR. However, in view of the wide differences in physiological responses to beta-blockade, another approach is to use RPE ratings around *somewhat hard*, which correspond to 11 to 14 on the original Borg RPE scale (2).

In phase II, clients are monitored carefully for vital signs (HR, BP, ventilation), and the ECG is monitored at a central observation station via telemetry (radio signals). A single-channel recording of 6 to 10 patients can be monitored simultaneously on a computer screen, and in the event of arrhythmias or ST segment changes, a rhythm strip is printed out. The rate–pressure product (SBP · HR) is sometimes used as an indicator of myocardial oxygen demand. After training, the rate–pressure product at a fixed work rate is reduced, allowing the cardiac patient to exercise at higher work rates before the onset of angina (28). In addition to exercise classes, patient education classes are offered, and they cover topics such as healthy eating, stress management, cardiovascular medications, and principles of behavior modification. Phase II programs typically last about 12 wk and are covered by health insurance.

Phase III programs are hospital-based programs in which outpatients are encouraged to continue their exercise regimens and are provided access to continuing health care and patient education. In these cases, the client's ECG usually is not monitored by telemetry, but clients continue to follow an individualized exercise prescription and attend patient education classes. Eventually, clients may enter the maintenance phase and move to a phase IV program in a nonhospital setting (e.g., sports medicine clinic).

For heart patients who are unable to attend a traditional cardiac rehabilitation outpatient program due to geography or finances, there are other options. Many hospitals offer rehabilitation programs following a distance-education model and can even monitor a client's ECG over the Internet. In addition, a group called *Mended Hearts* (http://mendedhearts.org) offers support-group meetings and online resources to help clients with heart disease and their families deal with the physical and emotional effects of heart disease.

KEY POINT

Cardiac rehabilitation programs are divided into four phases. Phase I is the acute phase, performed while the patient is still in the hospital. Phases II and III are conducted on an outpatient basis, and phase IV is the maintenance phase. Cardiac patients can benefit from aerobic and resistance training, but working with this population requires special knowledge of their medical conditions.

Medications

A variety of medications are used to treat people with heart disease. Some control BP, others control HR or rhythm, and still others affect the force of contraction of the ventricles. Other drugs the fitness professional will likely encounter include medications to control blood glucose concentrations, medications for patients with hyperlipidemia to control abnormal blood lipid levels, and bronchodilators for individuals with asthma. Fitness professionals do not prescribe medications or deal on a day-to-day basis with patients taking these medications, but they do encounter participants taking some of them. This section summarizes the major classes of drugs, describes how they affect the exercise HR response, and indicates possible side effects.

Beta-Adrenergic Blockers

Beta-adrenergic blocking medications (beta-blockers) are commonly prescribed for patients with CAD, CHF, or hypertension and occasionally for patients with migraine headaches. They compete with epinephrine and norepinephrine for the limited number of **beta-adrenergic receptors** located in various target organs. Beta-blockers are generally used to reduce the HR and the vigor of myocardial contraction, thus lowering the oxygen requirement of the heart. Because these medications influence submaximal and maximal HR, they have a profound effect on exercise prescription. Subjects should be tested while on beta-blockers if they will be training while taking them. All beta-blockers lower HR at rest and particularly during exercise, as seen in figure 19.5.

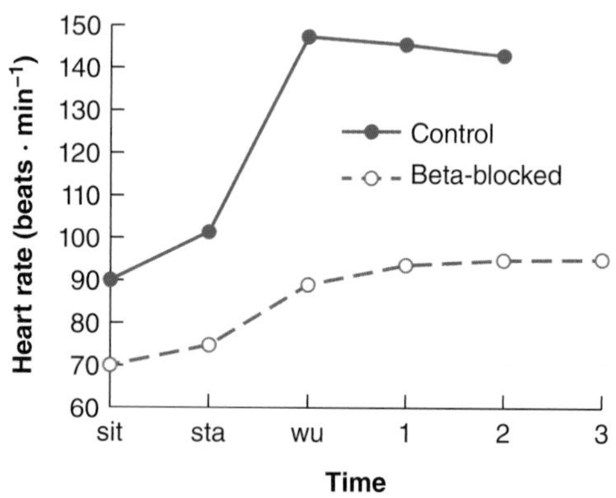

FIGURE 19.5 HR before and after beta-blockade (2 days of 40 mg of Inderal per day) in an apprehensive patient undergoing treadmill testing. Sit = sitting; sta = standing; wu = warming up at 1.0 mi · hr^{-1} (1.6 km · hr^{-1}), 0% grade. Min 1 and 2 are 2.0 mi · hr^{-1} (3.2 km · hr^{-1}), 0% grade. Min 3 is 2.0 mi · hr^{-1} (3.2 km · hr^{-1}) and 3.5% grade.

The generic names of all beta-blockers end in *–lol*. Two types of beta-adrenergic receptors are recognized: β_1 and β_2. The β_1 receptors are found mainly in the heart, and the β_2 receptors are located primarily in the smooth muscle in the lungs, arterioles, intestine, uterus, and bladder. Some beta-blockers selectively block the β_1 receptors in the heart. (Here's a tip for remembering this: You have one heart and two lungs.) The $\beta\beta_1$-selective (cardioselective) blockers include metoprolol (Lopressor, Toprol XL), atenolol (Tenormin), nebivolol (Bystolic), and acebutolol (Sectral). Other beta-blockers are less selective and act on both the β_1 and β_2 receptors. These nonselective beta-blockers include propranolol (Inderal), nadolol (Corgard), labetalol (Trandate, Normodyne), and carvedilol (Coreg). An undesirable side effect of the nonselective beta-blockers is contraction of the smooth muscle surrounding the airways in the lungs and reduction of the airway lumens, which increases the work of breathing. This side effect can result in labored breathing, shortness of breath, and other asthma-like symptoms.

Indications for using beta-blockers include treatment of hypertension, angina pectoris, and supraventricular arrhythmias. In addition, as previously mentioned, some beta-blockers are used to prevent migraine headaches. Nonselective beta-blocking medications are not recommended for patients with asthma, COPD, bronchitis, or similar lung problems. Beta-blocking medications may also blunt some symptoms of hypoglycemia in people with insulin-dependent diabetes, an undesirable side effect (6), although this is less likely with the selective agents and with Coreg (because it has some alpha-blocking activity as well as beta-blocking). The alpha receptors are located on vascular smooth muscle cells, and norepinephrine stimulates them to cause vasoconstriction of the blood vessels.

Using Inderal and presumably other beta-blocking medications does not invalidate the THR (target HR) method of prescribing exercise intensity. Hossack, Bruce, and Clark (19) showed that the regression equations relating %HRmax to %$\dot{V}O_2$max are similar in beta-adrenergic-blocked and nonblocked patients with CAD. Thus, the THR method of exercise prescription is assumed valid if the measured HRmax is determined *while the patient is on beta-blocking medications*.

Because beta-blockers lower HRmax, their use invalidates estimating THR by taking 70% to 85% of age-adjusted, predicted HRmax (predicted HRmax = 220 − age). For example, a 40-yr-old individual has a predicted HRmax of about 180, with an estimated 70% to 85% THR of 126 to 153 beats · min^{-1}. If this individual takes a beta-blocker, HRmax could easily drop to 150 beats · min^{-1}. If the estimated THR of 126 to 153 beats · min^{-1} is used for training, this participant may be training at HRmax. HRmax must be measured to calculate an appropriate THR for anyone taking beta-blockers, and this measurement should be repeated after any change in beta-blocking medicines.

There has been some question as to whether beta-blocking medicines reduce or block the effectiveness of endurance training. In general, work capacity and endurance training are impaired more after nonselective beta-blockade than after β_1-blockade (29). Ades and coworkers (1) examined the effects of endurance training in 30 adults with hypertension taking a placebo, metoprolol (a β_1-selective blocker), or propranolol (a nonselective beta-blocker). $\dot{V}O_2$max increased 24% in the placebo group and 8% in the metoprolol group but did not increase in the propranolol group. Pavia and colleagues (26) found that chronic use of a β_1-selective blocker (metoprolol) in post-myocardial patients did not interfere with the typical effects of endurance training. They observed similar increases in $\dot{V}O_2$peak in patients taking metoprolol and in those who were not on beta-blockers.

Nitrates

The **nitrates** exist in several forms, including patches, ointments, long-acting tablets, and sublingual tablets, and they are used to prevent or stop attacks of angina pectoris. Nitrates are produced from amyl nitrate (a volatile agent), which is rendered nonexplosive by adding an inert chemical such as lactose. Nitrate preparations relax venous smooth muscle, which reduces venous return and the quantity of blood the heart has to pump. Arterial smooth muscle is also relaxed, although to a lesser degree than venous smooth muscle, thus lowering the peripheral vascular resistance against which the heart has to pump. Both actions help reduce the work and oxygen requirement of the heart. Many patients use NTG (nitroglycerin) on a 24 hr basis with ointment or patches. Patients may take longer-acting tablet forms of NTG such as isosorbide dinitrate (Isordil) and isosorbide mononitrate (ISMO, Monoket, Imdur) before beginning activities that are likely to provoke anginal attacks, whereas sublingual NTG tablets (Nitrostat) are used to treat acute anginal episodes. Headaches, dizziness, and **hypotension** are the main side effects of NTG (6). Beta-adrenergic-blocking medications may potentiate the hypotensive actions of NTG.

Calcium Channel Blockers (Calcium Antagonists)

The **calcium channel blockers (CCBs)** currently include nifedipine (Procardia), felodipine (Plendil), amlodipine (Norvasc), verapamil (Calan, Isoptin) and diltiazem (Cardizem). These drugs interfere with the slow calcium currents that occur during depolarization in cardiac and vascular smooth muscle. Verapamil is used primarily to treat atrial and ventricular arrhythmias, whereas nifedipine and diltiazem are used to treat exertional angina and variant angina pectoris, or angina pectoris attacks that occur at rest (6).

The effects of CCBs on exercise prescription and training have been studied. Chang and Hossack (6) showed that the regression equations relating %HRmax and %$\dot{V}O_2$max are the same in patients taking diltiazem and in unmedicated patients. Verapamil and nifedipine (Procardia) are assumed not to alter the relationship between %HRmax and %$\dot{V}O_2$max. CCBs are not thought to adversely affect endurance training in healthy subjects or in patients with CAD (22). MacGowan and colleagues (24) showed that verapamil does not diminish training responses in healthy, young subjects. The public perception of a calcium blocker may be that it blocks the absorption of dietary and supplemental calcium, thus leading to increased risk of osteoporosis. This is not true because the CCBs work at the cellular level.

Antiarrhythmic Medications

Common **antiarrhythmics** include quinidine (Quinaglute), procainamide (Pronestyl), disopyramide (Norpace), lidocaine (Xylocaine), fosphenytoin (Cerebyx), mexiletine (Mexitil), flecainide (Tambocor), propafenone (Rythmol), many beta-blockers, and the CCBs verapamil and diltiazem. In recent years, however, amiodarone (Cordarone, Pacerone) has become the most widely used antiarrhythmic agent. With the exception of the beta-blockers, these medications have little influence on the HR response to exercise; in fact, the reduction in arrhythmias may improve work capacity.

Digitalis Preparations

The primary **digitalis** medication is digoxin (Lanoxin, Digitek) and is used to increase the vigor of myocardial contractions (contractility or inotropic effect) and treat atrial flutter and fibrillation. However, recent evidence has questioned the efficacy and safety of digoxin, especially in the treatment of CHF (6). In individuals with poor ventricular function, the increased contractility resulting from digitalis preparations may increase work capacity. Digitalis medications are marketed under several trade names, including Lanoxin, Lanoxicaps, and Digitek. Cardiac side effects of the digitalis group include **premature ventricular contractions** (PVCs), Wenckebach AV block, and atrial tachycardia. Digitalis drugs can cause false-positive tests for CHD due to ST segment depression during exercise testing (10).

Antihypertensives

Antihypertensives can be divided into five groups according to the mechanism of action. Drugs in the first group, *diuretics*, work by increasing the excretion of electrolytes and water. These drugs include hydrochlorothiazide (HCTZ), chlorthalidone (Hygroton), and furosemide (Lasix). This group is often used as the first treatment for hypertension. Side effects include hypokalemia, or low blood levels of potassium. Hypokalemia can induce arrhythmias and is a potentially serious problem. Diuretic-induced hypokalemia often can be prevented by consuming more citrus fruits, which are high in potassium. If dietary sources of potassium prove to be ineffective, a prescription potassium supplement (K-Tab, Kay Ciel) can be used (6). Alternatively, a potassium-sparing diuretic such as spironolactone (Aldactone) or triamterene (Dyrenium or Dyazide and Maxzide when combined with HCTZ) can be prescribed.

The second group of antihypertensive medications comprises the *antiadrenergic agents*. These include drugs that act at the level of the central nervous system, such as clonidine (Catapres), to reduce sympathetic outflow from the brain. In addition, this group includes drugs that block beta-adrenergic receptors (see previous section) to decrease cardiac output, renin release, and sympathetic outflow from the brain.

In an important side effect, the diuretics and beta-blockers elevate triglyceride and cholesterol levels and impair glucose and insulin metabolism. Thus, although they effectively lower BP and reduce the incidence of stroke and severe kidney disease, they have a less-than-predicted effect on preventing heart attacks.

Vasodilators make up the third group of antihypertensive medications. These medications decrease BP by relaxing vascular smooth muscle. The primary drug in this category is hydralazine (Apresoline). Its side effects include hypotension, dizziness, and tachycardia. The active chemical in Loniten is also marketed under the name *Rogaine* as a topical solution for stimulating hair growth in male-pattern baldness. Rogaine has little or no antihypertensive effect.

Antihypertensive medications in the fourth group work through the renin–angiotensin system. These drugs lower BP by inhibiting angiotensin-converting enzyme (ACE), which converts angiotensin I to angiotensin II, a powerful vasoconstrictor. They are called *ACE inhibitors* for that reason. Some of the drugs in this category are captopril (Capoten), lisinopril (Prinivil, Zestril), and perindopril (Aceon). The ACE inhibitors are expensive and may produce a dry cough in a fairly large percentage of patients. They decrease left ventricular hypertrophy, reduce proteinuria in diabetic patients with macroalbuminuria, and maintain blood lipid levels. In addition to the ACE inhibitors, the angiotensin receptor blockers also work through the renin-angiotensin system. These agents block the effects of angiotensin II without affecting ACE. Thus, they do not produce a cough and have a lower risk of causing angioedema than do the ACE inhibitors. The angiotensin receptor blockers include losartan (Cozaar), valsartan (Diovan), irbesartan (Avapro), telmisartan (Micardis), and olmesartan (Benicar). One hint for identifying drugs that act on the renin–angiotensin system is that all generic names of ACE inhibitors end in *–pril* and angiotensin receptor blockers end in *–sartan*.

The fifth group of antihypertensive medications includes the *calcium antagonists* (CCBs; see the section on calcium channel blockers). As with the ACE inhibitors, drugs in this class do not adversely affect lipid, glucose, and insulin metabolism.

Lipid-Lowering Medications

Several types of medications are used by people who are unable to adequately control lipids through diet and exercise. The first group is the sequestering agents, which include cholestyramine (Questran) and colesevelam (Welchol), as well as ezetimibe (Zetia), which prevents intestinal absorption of lipids. Niacin (Niaspan) is also used for lipid disorders and can cause significant flushing, which could interfere with exercise. Fibrates are used primarily for elevated triglycerides and include gemfibrozil (Lopid), fenofibrate (Tricor), and fenofibric acid (Trilipix). The primary class of lipid-lowering medications is the statins; these drugs block an enzyme necessary to synthesize cholesterol. These are some of the best-selling drugs in the world and include simvastatin (Zocor), pravastatin (Pravachol), atorvastatin (Lipitor), rosuvastatin (Crestor), and pitavastatin (Livalo). The statins can cause a significant degree of muscle problems (myalgia, myositis, and even rhabdomyolysis) that could negatively affect exercise.

Anticoagulants and Antiplatelets

The **anticoagulants** delay blood clotting and are used to prevent strokes and heart attacks in those who are at risk for those conditions. The antiplatelet drugs block platelet activation and decrease the potential of clotting. Oral agents in this category include aspirin, warfarin (Coumadin), clopidogrel (Plavix), prasugrel (Effient), ticagrelor (Brilinta), dabigatran (Pradaxa), rivaroxaban (Xarelto), and apixaban (Eliquis). Cilostazol (Pletal) is a platelet inhibitor and vasodilator used for the treatment of intermittent claudication (IC). It seems to improve the maximum walking distance (MWD) or absolute claudication distance (ACD) on a treadmill or the time to initial pain, known as the pain-free walking distance (PFWD). These medications are unlikely to directly affect exercise testing or training, but they do increase the risk of bruising. Aspirin and some other medications (e.g., nonsteroidal anti-inflammatory drugs [NSAIDS] such as Motrin, Advil, and Aleve) can potentiate anticoagulants and increase the risk of bruising with minimal trauma.

LEARNING AIDS

REVIEW QUESTIONS

1. Define *atherosclerosis*, and list three alterable cardiovascular risk factors that promote the atherosclerotic process.
2. Describe what will happen if an atherosclerotic plaque leads to a blockage of blood flow within a coronary artery, cerebral artery, or femoral artery.
3. Where does CVD rank among causes of death in the United States today? What are four subcategories of CVD?
4. Describe the effects of aerobic exercise on people with hypertension. What are some other recommended treatments for hypertension?
5. List four specific patient populations who are commonly referred to cardiac rehabilitation programs.
6. What evidence is there that exercise training can be beneficial for individuals with CHD?
7. One of the goals of any cardiac rehabilitation program is secondary prevention of CHD. Explain what this means.
8. Identify diagnostic tests that can be used to detect the presence of CHD.
9. Outline the recommendations for aerobic exercise programming in phase II and phase III cardiac rehabilitation in terms of frequency, intensity, duration, and mode. Is weight training recommended? Why is the Karvonen formula often not very useful in establishing a THR for a cardiac patient?
10. List the general categories of cardiovascular medicines and describe their physiological effects on the body.

CASE STUDIES

1. John is a 46-yr-old male. He is an insurance executive who is married with two children. John is active in his church and plays golf on the weekends. He went to see his cardiologist because he experienced recent fatigue with chest pain on exertion. He has never smoked but he consumes one to two alcoholic drinks a day. His medical history reveals a blood cholesterol level of 263 $mg \cdot dl^{-1}$, a triglyceride level of 195 $mg \cdot dl^{-1}$, and an HDL-C value of 45 $mg \cdot dl^{-1}$. Considering his sex, age, symptoms, and risk factors, what do you think is the likelihood he has CHD? What would be a reasonable next step to diagnose the presence or absence of CHD?
2. Jane is a 61-yr-old retired female. She recently underwent a left heart catheterization, which revealed significant occlusion in the left anterior descending artery and the circumflex artery. Therefore, a balloon angioplasty procedure was performed. Approximately 2 wk later, she performed a GXT with the following results:

   - Protocol: Balke (3.3 $mi \cdot hr^{-1}$, or 5.3 $km \cdot hr^{-1}$)
   - Resting: HR = 72 $beats \cdot min^{-1}$, BP = 130/72 mmHg
   - End point: stage 3 for 1 min (approximately 7 METs)
   - HR = 126 $beats \cdot min^{-1}$, BP = 160/90 mmHg
   - Reason for termination: Fatigue
   - No ST segment depression, no reported symptoms

   Jane was taking atenolol (a beta-blocker) at the time of her test, and her physician instructed her to continue taking this medication. She was referred to the cardiac rehabilitation center for supervised exercise and risk-factor modification. List some types of exercise that would be appropriate for her. In addition to the mode, be sure to recommend an appropriate frequency, intensity, and duration of exercise.
3. Ralph is a 65-yr-old male who had CABGs on two coronary arteries (left anterior descending and circumflex). Both arteries were 75% occluded at the time of his surgery, which involved a sternectomy. His sternum was cut and separated, and the saphenous vein in his leg was harvested to obtain the grafting material; the sternum was then closed and fastened with stainless steel wires that are still in his chest. Ralph has completed phase I cardiac rehabilitation and has now been referred to an outpatient cardiac rehabilitation program 3 wk postoperative. He has inquired about a weight training program as part of his 12 wk phase II cardiac rehabilitation. What type of resistance training program would you design for this cardiac patient?
4. A participant in your exercise program has been taking a beta-blocking medication for several years without experiencing any significant side effects. He was recently given a prescription for Isordil and now reports that he often becomes dizzy upon standing suddenly. Could this be related to his medication? If so, why?

Answers to Case Studies

1. Because John is a 46-yr-old male with typical effort-induced angina and an elevated total cholesterol–HDL ratio over 5.0 (signifying increased risk), he has a high likelihood of CHD. A reasonable next step would be to refer him for a GXT in the presence of a physician to see if signs or symptoms of CHD occur. If they do, a more definitive diagnostic test such as coronary angiography might be recommended.
2. Jane's GXT results indicated that her maximal aerobic capacity was 7 METs; therefore, prescribing exercise at about 60% of this value, or around 4 METs, would be appropriate. Suitable exercises would include treadmill walking, stationary cycling, and arm cranking. Realize that her maximal HR is low because she is taking a beta-blocker. Thus, exercise could be prescribed on the basis of RPE (e.g., a target rating of *somewhat hard* on the Borg RPE scale). Light resistance exercises using dumbbells and elastic bands, as tolerated, would also be acceptable. The resistance should be selected so as to allow her to perform 12 to 15 repetitions with good form.
3. Because Ralph has had a chest incision and heart surgery, he must proceed cautiously. A resistance training program consisting of light, seated exercises using 1 to 2 lb (.5-.9 kg) dumbbells and lightweight elastic bands is appropriate in the beginning. He could perform 12 to 15 repetitions of several exercises while maintaining good form and proper breathing. The goal should be to slightly overload the muscles and maintain ROM. He should stop if he feels pain or movement in the area of the incision. Also, he should be instructed to avoid holding his breath or straining while lifting. Over time, the weights can be gradually increased.
4. Isordil contains a nitrate, similar to NTG, and is used to reduce the chance of having an angina attack. The drug relaxes vascular smooth muscle and might cause pooling of blood in the extremities. This pooling could decrease blood pressure and result in symptoms of dizziness.

20

Exercise and Obesity

Dixie L. Thompson

OBJECTIVES

The reader will be able to do the following:

1. Define *obesity* and describe its health risks.
2. Describe the role that exercise plays in preventing and treating obesity.
3. Explain the modifications to standard testing procedures necessary for clients who are obese.
4. Write an exercise prescription for someone who is obese.

20

Obesity is characterized by excessive adiposity. It can be documented by examining the relationship between height and weight (e.g., BMI) or by evaluating percent body fat (%BF). Because BMI requires simple measurements and, for the majority of adults, closely relates to body fatness, it has become the clinically preferred method of assessing obesity (see chapter 8). Generally accepted guidelines classify a BMI of 30 kg · m^{-2} or higher as obese (8). The following are subclasses of obesity:

- Grade 1 obesity—30.0 to 34.9 kg · m^{-2}
- Grade 2 obesity—35.0 to 39.9 kg · m^{-2}
- Grade 3 (extreme) obesity—40 kg · m^{-2} or higher

Although there are no universally agreed-upon standards for classifying obesity from %BF, a %BF of >38% for females and >25% for males generally is considered to be obese (26). Another tool used to screen for obesity is WC (waist circumference; see chapter 8 for more details). Adiposity located in the abdominal region is strongly linked with chronic disease risk; therefore, a WC of ≥102 cm (40 in.) in men or ≥88 cm (35 in.) in women is used to classify individuals with abdominal obesity (8).

Potential Causes of Obesity

Although consuming calories in excess of daily caloric need is an easily identified culprit in the etiology of obesity, this condition is much more complex than suggested by that simple explanation. Both biological (e.g., genetic predisposition attributable to lower-than-normal metabolic rate) and psychological (e.g., poor body image) factors can contribute to obesity and can pose significant obstacles when a person attempts to lose weight (8, 9). Some studies show that genetics contribute around 25% to 40% of the variation in body composition (6), but others argue that genetics are responsible for 50% to 70% of this variation (5).

Many biological factors have been identified as possible mechanisms that predispose a person to obesity. These factors include leptin (a protein), activity of the sympathetic nervous system, several neuropeptides, and some hormones (5). Suggested pathways through which these factors work include lowering RMR, influencing eating behaviors, and slowing the rate of fat oxidation. Recent genome-wide association studies (GWAS) are providing new insight into the role of genetics in obesity. One study identified 97 BMI-associated loci in the human genome, and the loci were associated with important physiological processes including synaptic function, glutamate signaling, insulin secretion and action, and adipogenesis (21). In another study of the human genome, 49 loci were associated with WHR, even after adjustment for BMI (30). GWAS are helping to uncover the links among obesity, body-fat distribution patterns, and disease. Because of the attention recently focused on the genetic roots of obesity, individuals who are obese can become discouraged from attempting to lose weight. Although biological factors clearly contribute to obesity, the imbalance between energy intake and expenditure ultimately leads to fat accumulation. Educating clients on the role of appropriate nutrition and exercise in maintaining a healthy weight is an important aspect of the fitness professional's responsibilities.

Prevalence of Obesity

The prevalence of obesity in the United States and in many countries around the world increased dramatically during the last part of the 20th and the first part of the 21st century (24). Between 1980 and 2013, the worldwide prevalence for overweight and obesity combined rose 27.5% in adults and 47.1% in children (24). The U.S. prevalence of obesity rose from less than 15% in the early 1960s to 34.9% in 2011 and 2012 (25). Recent surveys reveal that 68.5% of American adults now have a BMI of 25 kg · m^{-2} or higher and thus are classified as overweight or obese (25). Certain minority groups appear particularly at risk for overweight and obesity, with non-Hispanic blacks and Hispanics having prevalence rates of 76.2% and 77.9%, respectively, for BMI ≥25 kg · m^{-2} (25). Currently, over half (56.6%) of non-Hispanic black women are classified as obese using BMI criteria (25). Also, abdominal obesity has increased for women and men in the last decades (see figure 20.1). Based on waist circumference, 43.5% of men and 64.7% of women have abdominal obesity (15).

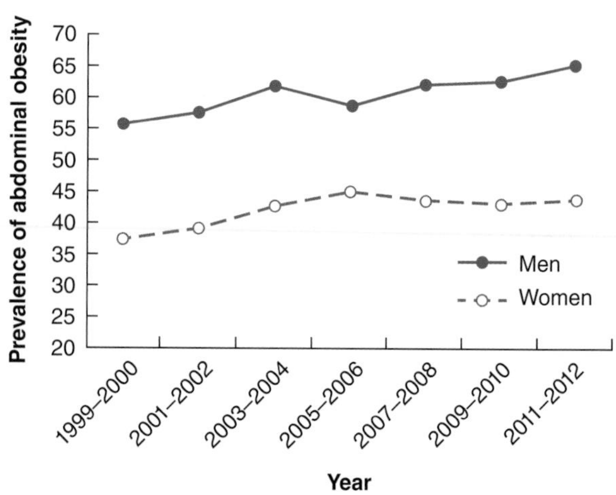

FIGURE 20.1 Recent changes in the prevalence of abdominal obesity.

Data from Ford, Maynard, and Li 2014.

KEY POINT

Obesity is a complex condition with biological and lifestyle links. Over one-third of U.S. adults and over 17% of U.S. children are classified as obese, and the prevalence has risen dramatically in recent decades. Comorbidities of obesity include type 2 diabetes, CHD, stroke, and some cancers. In the United States the economic cost of obesity is nearly $150 billion per year.

Another disturbing trend is the increasing rate of obesity among children. Recent national surveys (2011-2012) reveal that 32.2% of American children are overweight (at or above the 85th percentile for BMI) and 17.3% are obese (at or above the 95th percentile for BMI) (31). Of greatest concern is that 5.9% are classified with grade 2 obesity and 2.1% with grade 3 obesity (31). Some researchers have linked the rising prevalence of childhood obesity to an increase in inactive leisure pursuits such as television viewing (16, 27). The rapid increase in obesity in the United States over the last four decades supports the contention that lifestyle choices (i.e., diet and physical activity), not genetics, are primarily responsible for the increasing prevalence of obesity.

The increasing prevalence of obesity is important because of the negative health complications that accompany it. Obesity, particularly grades 2 and 3, is linked with increased mortality and morbidity rates (13). Diseases and conditions associated with obesity include CHD, CHF, stroke, type 2 diabetes, hypertension, dyslipidemia, gallbladder disease, OA, some cancers (e.g., breast, colon), sleep apnea, and respiratory problems. Women who are obese are more likely to experience menstrual irregularities and complications with pregnancy. Estimates of annual U.S. deaths attributable to obesity range from 112,000 (11) to 300,000 (3). Deaths due to CVD, diabetes, and kidney disease are particularly related to obesity (12). Recent studies of the costs related to obesity reveal the toll this condition takes on the economy (10, 34, 43). It is estimated that the medical costs of an obese person are 30% higher than those of a person of normal weight (43). In 2008, nearly 10% of health care spending in the United States, approximately $147 billion, was attributed to overweight and obesity (10).

Clearly, obesity results in major personal as well as financial strains. The serious effects of overweight and obesity are reflected by the issuance of *The Surgeon General's Call to Action to Prevent and Decrease Overweight and Obesity* (35) and *The Surgeon General's Vision for a Healthy and Fit Nation* (37). These reports outline the problem of overweight and obesity and call for both public and private commitments to address this health concern.

Physical Activity in Prevention and Treatment of Obesity

The rapid increase in obesity prevalence appears linked to both low physical activity and excessive energy intake (33). This suggests that increasing physical activity and reducing caloric intake will lower rates of obesity. Although the evidence is indirect, an overview of cross-sectional and prospective studies suggests that active people are less likely to be obese, and those who maintain an active lifestyle are least likely to become obese over time (2, 7, 20). Research shows that both leisure and workplace physical activity are inversely associated with obesity (29). An international consensus meeting concluded that 45 to 60 min of daily moderate activity are needed to prevent obesity (28). However, estimating energy intake and expenditure on a population level is crude, the studies do not always agree, and much additional research is needed to clarify these issues. Despite the need for more research, there is general agreement in the medical (32) and public health (35) communities that both exercise and dietary modification should be used in treating patients who are obese.

A number of studies have used exercise as a means for treating obesity. Most of these trials were short term, and many had design flaws that limit the conclusions that can be drawn. In general, well-controlled, randomized control trials typically have found modest weight reduction when exercise is used to treat obesity (2, 12, 36). Slightly greater weight loss typically is seen when caloric restriction is combined with exercise. There is also evidence that a combination of dietary restriction and exercise is better at helping maintain weight loss than is either method alone (17, 40). The data from the National Weight Control Registry (NWCR) suggest that regular aerobic exercise is common among those who successfully maintain significant weight loss (41, 42). See the Research Insight for more information on the characteristics of people who are successful at maintaining weight loss.

Screening and Testing Clients With Obesity

Several conditions frequently coexist with obesity (e.g., type 2 diabetes, hypertension) (8). The high prevalence of

KEY POINT

Active people are less likely to be overweight or obese. Exercise can be an important part of a weight-loss program and is a key to maintaining weight loss.

RESEARCH INSIGHT

Data From the National Weight Control Registry

The NWCR was established in 1994 to provide insight into ways that people successfully lose weight and then maintain weight loss (41, 42). Approximately 5,000 people participate in the NWCR, with an average weight loss of 30 kg maintained for 5.5 yr. About half of these participants used commercial weight-loss programs, whereas the others lost weight without formal guidance. Several interesting facts have been gathered from these successful losers: (1) The vast majority (over 85%) used exercise in their weight-loss programs, (2) the most common dietary approach involved choosing a diet low in total calories and low in fat (<25% of calories from fat), (3) most participants weighed themselves frequently to provide feedback on the success of their behaviors, (4) a typical exercise routine was 1 hr per day of moderate physical activity, and (5) walking was the most frequently reported exercise (80% of participants), while about 29% used resistance training. An overwhelming majority (>90%) of NCWR participants report that their weight loss has been associated with higher energy levels, better mobility, improved mood, higher self-confidence, and overall better quality of life. For more information on the NWCR, visit its website (www.nwcr.ws).

these comorbidities requires that fitness professionals carefully screen participants who are obese before performing exercise testing. Health histories and pretesting screenings should be designed to identify any comorbidities (see chapter 2). These comorbidities, as well as the person's overall physical condition, will determine the types of exercise testing needed before exercise programming. Once the initial health history screening is completed, the ACSM risk classification (1) can be used to determine the need for medical clearance and physician supervision of exercise tests.

Medications

As with all clients, a person who is obese should provide documentation of medications. Because of the wide-ranging comorbidities that can exist with obesity, a variety of medications may be prescribed. It is common to find clients who are obese and who take several medications, including those for hypertension and glucose control. Before exercise testing and prescription, fitness professionals should consider the possible effect of these medications.

Prescription medications for weight loss or weight control are available for individuals under a physician's care. Several medications have been approved by the FDA for weight loss. One of the FDA-approved drugs, orlistat, can be obtained with a physician's prescription (Xenical) or over the counter (Alli). Orlistat interferes with the absorption of fat in the digestive system and commonly results in weight loss and improved blood lipid profile. There is a slight chance of liver injury from using orlistat, but more common side effects are oily discharge and fecal urgency. Phentermine, diethylpropion, and phendimetrazine are appetite suppressants and are approved for short-term use (up to 12 wk) with a prescription. Sleeplessness, nervousness, and increased BP are sometimes reported while using these medications. Recently, the FDA approved two new drugs, Belviq and Qsymia, for long-term weight management.

Over-the-counter weight-loss aids and herbal supplements are also taken frequently by people desiring weight loss. In 2004, the FDA banned ephedrine alkaloids (ephedra) in over-the-counter products because of the reported occurrence of tachycardia, hypertension, strokes, and heart attacks. It is beyond the scope of this chapter to review all products used to promote weight loss. Fitness professionals should encourage clients to be wise consumers of such products by learning about the potential side effects and discussing these substances with their physicians.

Exercise Testing

Typically, standard testing modes and protocols can be used when testing people who are obese; however, the initial intensity as well as the incremental increases should reflect the individual's fitness and activity level (see chapter 7). This is particularly important because of the severe deconditioning that often exists with obesity. With severe obesity or when ambulation is problematic, it may be preferable to use cycle or arm ergometry for testing. However, when walking is the exercise of choice for programming, treadmill testing provides useful insight into the velocity that the client can maintain during walking. This can be helpful information when designing a workout with a targeted caloric expenditure.

The physiological response to exercise typically is similar in people who are obese and people who are normal weight, except that excessive weight often reduces cardiorespiratory function. However, comorbidities, especially hypertension and type 2 diabetes, can alter the exercise or postexercise response. For more information on testing clients who are obese, refer to the review by Wallace and Ray (38).

KEY POINT

The large number of comorbidities that accompany obesity necessitates careful screening of clients who are obese. Exercise testing of these clients should be individualized, taking into account any special needs.

Exercise Prescription

Weight loss, greater fitness, and improved chronic disease risk factors are the focus of exercise programs for individuals who are obese. ACSM guidelines state that all adults, including those who are obese, should exercise on most, if not all, days of the week for a minimum of 150 min per wk in order to protect against chronic disease (1). However, evidence indicates that an even greater caloric expenditure (i.e., 200-300 min per wk) may be most beneficial for long-term weight control (1, 2). Some groups advocate 45 to 60 min of daily moderate activity to prevent weight gain and 60 to 90 min for individuals who were previously obese in order to prevent weight regain (14, 28). The Physical Activity Guidelines for Americans encourage people who are using exercise for weight loss or weight control to accumulate 300 min per wk of moderate-intensity exercise, or 150 min per wk of vigorous-intensity activity (36). When first beginning an exercise program, participants may be unable to exercise this long, so an initial focus of programming is to build enough endurance to sustain aerobic activity to reach these duration goals. Accumulating activity in shorter bouts throughout the day is also an option.

ACSM recommends the following approach to exercise for weight loss (1):

- Frequency: 5 or more days per wk
- Intensity: initially moderate (40%-60% HRR), with progression to higher intensity (≥60% HRR)
- Time: begin with short, easily tolerated bouts totaling 30 min per day, progressing to 60 min per day; multiple daily bouts can be used with bout duration of 10 min or longer
- Type: aerobic exercise targeting large muscle groups, with resistance (2 to 3 days per wk) and flexibility (2 to 3 days per wk) exercise recommended as supplements to aerobic activity

Designing exercise programs for clients who are obese requires some special considerations. One of the primary aims of any exercise program should be safety. For participants who are obese, avoiding orthopedic injuries is a particular concern because of the additional loading to joints. Therefore, low-impact activities (water exercise, cycling, and walking) are preferable when individuals who are obese begin to exercise regularly. After some weight loss and conditioning occur, they may participate in higher impact sports and activities. Another safety concern is thermoregulation (38). Because of excessive body fatness and the increased energy demands of activity, keeping the body cool during exercise can be problematic for people with a lot of body fat. They should be encouraged to exercise at cool times of the day or in temperature-controlled environments. They should also maintain hydration by drinking adequate amounts of water.

Resistance training is an important component of the overall exercise program. Although resistance training typically does not burn a large number of calories, it can serve important functions in weight loss (2). Maintaining muscle mass benefits both functional capacity and metabolic rate. Compared with fat, muscle is a metabolically active tissue, so maintaining lean mass helps minimize decreases in metabolic rate and thus promotes weight loss. A growing body of evidence suggests that resistance training can be an important tool in preventing chronic diseases such as diabetes and is essential in maintaining function as we age.

Individuals who are obese rarely begin exercising without also setting goals related to weight loss (although exercise provides benefits even in the absence of weight

Surgical Procedures for Weight Loss

For individuals with extreme obesity (BMI >40 $kg \cdot m^{-2}$) who have been unsuccessful in previous weight-loss attempts and who have serious comorbid conditions, **bariatric surgery** may be an option (22, 23, 32). There are a variety of surgical options (23), but all modify the gastrointestinal system so that food intake is restricted and nutrient uptake is diminished. These procedures often lead to significant weight loss, but they also have a number of serious side effects (22, 23). The cost of these procedures is in excess of $20,000 but may be supported by health insurance. These surgeries require major modifications in eating patterns. Once patients recover from surgery, exercise programming is recommended. The dietary planning and exercise programming for these patients should be overseen by medical professionals.

loss; see *Exercise Without Weight Loss*). Fitness professionals should assist the client in developing healthy weight-loss goals. An appropriate goal is 0.5 to 1 kg · wk^{-1}. For example, reducing caloric intake by 500 kcal · day^{-1} and expending an additional 300 kcal · day^{-1} creates a caloric deficit that approximates a 0.7 kg loss in 1 wk: 7(500 + 300) = 5,600 kcal · wk^{-1}. A well-planned, low-fat diet with a caloric deficit of 500 to 1,000 kcal · day^{-1} gradually reduces weight without sacrificing nutritional needs (2). An appropriate distribution of macronutrients along with the necessary amounts of vitamins and minerals should be included in the dietary planning (see chapter 5). Diets that are low in fat, particularly saturated fat, not only are effective for weight loss but also are associated with long-term weight maintenance. See chapter 12 for additional information on weight-loss and management strategies. Individuals who are overweight and obese should reduce body weight by at least 5% to gain health benefits such as lower BP and a more favorable blood lipid profile. For some individuals, an even greater reduction in body weight may optimize health improvement (2).

Long-term adherence to exercise is problematic for people who have been sedentary and are obese. Fitness professionals should help clients overcome perceived barriers to living an active lifestyle. Commonly reported barriers are feeling too fat to exercise, believing that their health is too poor for exercise, and believing that an injury or disability precludes participation in exercise (4). Fitness professionals should provide education about the risks of leading an inactive life, the health benefits of regular exercise (which occur independent of body weight), and the variety of exercise options available. A dialogue between the fitness professional and client determines program needs, client likes and dislikes, and level of support needed to increase adherence. These discussions can lead to decisions about the specific nature of the exercise routine (e.g., structured versus lifestyle, intermittent versus continuous) (18, 19). Look for opportunities to increase energy expenditure through structured exercise (e.g., taking brisk 30 min walks) and lifestyle activity (e.g., substituting active for sedentary leisure pursuits). When it comes to long-term adherence, finding an approach that fits the needs of the client is critical.

KEY POINT

Prudent weight-loss goals for clients who are overweight and obese range from 0.5 to 1.0 kg · wk^{-1}. Daily or near-daily moderate aerobic activity is suggested. Although 30 min per day of moderate-intensity exercise is a minimum goal, better success is seen with 45 to 90 min. People who are obese can use both aerobic exercise and resistance training. For weight loss, exercise programs should be combined with a low-fat, reduced-calorie diet. When prescribing exercise, emphasize avoiding musculoskeletal injuries and heat injury as well as finding ways to improve adherence.

Exercise Without Weight Loss

Even without weight loss, exercise benefits people who are overweight. These benefits (e.g., improved blood lipid profile, lower BP, better stress management) are much the same as those seen in people who are normal weight. Although both reducing weight and improving fitness optimize health benefits, participation in regular exercise significantly protects against disease even when the person remains overweight. Data from the Cooper Clinic in Dallas have demonstrated that fitness protects against early death in people who are overweight (39). Because of these findings, it is important to emphasize an active lifestyle even if weight loss is not an outcome.

LEARNING AIDS

REVIEW QUESTIONS

1. What are potential causes of obesity?
2. Describe how the prevalence of obesity has changed over the past 50 years.
3. Describe the costs associated with obesity, both in terms of dollars and excess deaths.
4. Compare the exercise recommendation for health benefits with the exercise recommendation for weight control.
5. What is the National Weight Control Registry (NWCR)? What useful information has been obtained from this resource?
6. What special considerations should be applied when screening obese patients prior to exercise testing?
7. What special considerations should be applied to administering exercise tests to obese clients?
8. What medications have FDA approval for use in weight loss?

CASE STUDIES

1. Marsha is a 51-yr-old female who comes to your fitness facility and expresses interest in purchasing a membership. She is responding to a series of advertisements that your facility is using to attract people interested in weight loss. Your screening reveals the following:

   - Her height is 5 ft 5 in. (165 cm) and her weight is 240 lb (109 kg).
   - Her blood pressure is 152/88 mmHg.
   - She has never exercised regularly, has a desk job, and has no active leisure pursuits.
   - It has been more than 3 yr since she had a medical examination.
   - There is a history of heart disease on her father's side of the family, and her mother developed type 2 diabetes after menopause.

   a. What, if any, medical screening do you recommend before this client enrolls in your facility's programs?
   b. What fitness testing do you suggest for her?
   c. Assuming that no medical conditions are revealed with the screening and initial testing, describe a diet and exercise program that Marsha could use to achieve her weight-loss and fitness goals.

2. You have a new client, Kevin. He is a healthy, somewhat active 38-yr-old man who is coming to you for advice on exercise and maintaining a healthy weight. Kevin's BMI is 25.5. He reports that over the past 2 yr he has lost more than 75 lb (34 kg) using a commercial weight-loss plan. He is beginning to feel diet burnout and his weight has crept up 5 lb (2.3 kg) over the past month. What exercise and other lifestyle advice would you provide?
3. Shala comes to you for help in becoming more active. She is a 32-yr-old woman who underwent bariatric surgery 6 mo earlier. Her doctor has cleared her for moderate-intensity activity and has encouraged her to become more active. Shala has never been active. Her BMI is still in the extreme obesity range, and you noticed that she was breathless from just walking in from her car. What are the initial steps to take in helping Shala?

Answers to Case Studies

1. For the case study of Marsha, consider the following:

    a. Because Marsha is hypertensive, has extreme (grade 3) obesity, is inactive, has a strong family history of CVD and diabetes, and has not undergone a medical examination in several years, medical clearance before beginning an exercise program is recommended. The medical examination should reveal any underlying medical conditions that would make it unsafe for Marsha to engage in moderate or vigorous exercise.

    b. In addition to height and weight, measurement of waist and hip circumference is recommended. In addition to BMI calculations and examination of abdominal adiposity, an estimate of body-fat percentage could be useful, but only if methods are chosen that are both reliable and accurate for obese individuals (see chapter 8). CRF could be assessed with either a treadmill or a cycle ergometer protocol. Standard flexibility and strength tests could be used.

    c. A conversation with Marsha is crucial to determine her goals and interests. To increase adherence, close attention should be paid to her willingness to engage in various activities. Attempts should be made to increase lifestyle activity and structured exercise. Assuming that Marsha is willing to invest 1 hr a day, 3 days per wk, in structured exercise and is willing to exercise on her own on other days, the following program would target a weight loss of 2 lb per wk (0.9 kg per wk).

    Exercise 6 days per wk and try to expend 300 kcal of energy on each of these days. The structured exercise should focus on improving CRF, strength, and flexibility. On 3 days per wk, Marsha could walk on her own or preferably with an exercise partner for 1 hr (could be divided into shorter sessions). This increase in activity will increase her caloric expenditure by approximately 1,800 kcal · wk^{-1}. Given that Marsha is inactive now, a progressive program must be included in order to build up to this level of exercise.

    She should target an energy intake that is approximately 745 kcal below her estimated calorie need. Using the formula in chapter 12, Marsha's daily energy need is approximately 2,480 kcal. Targeting a daily caloric intake of approximately 1,735 kcal · day^{-1} will result in a caloric deficit of 5,200 kcal · wk^{-1} from caloric restriction.

    The combination of caloric restriction (5,200 kcal · wk^{-1}) and energy expenditure (1,800 kcal · wk^{-1}) will result in a weight loss of approximately 2 lb (0.9 kg) each week. Weekly weigh-ins and consultation with the fitness professional are recommended in order to adjust the program as needed.

2. For Kevin's exercise goals, develop a plan that will allow Kevin to accumulate 300 min per wk in moderate-intensity exercise. Better yet, given that Kevin is healthy and young, encourage him to spend at least some of his exercise time in vigorous exercise. Determine Kevin's exercise preferences and develop a program that meets aerobic recommendations and also addresses muscular fitness needs (resistance training 2 days per wk and flexibility training during cool-downs from all workouts).

    For lifestyle goals, encourage Kevin to eat a well-rounded diet as described in chapter 5. He is at a fairly healthy BMI, so making weight loss a major consideration is unnecessary. However, for a person like Kevin, weight-loss maintenance can be a struggle. Therefore the following can be useful: (1) Encourage him to weigh himself each morning, (2) encourage him to keep a journal of his food intake and exercise, and (3) encourage him to seek out a support system. As his fitness trainer, you will be a primary part of his support system, but encourage him to seek out friends who can provide additional support and encouragement for his healthy eating and exercise habits.

3. Shala has a long way to go to become an active person, but the fact that she has undergone bariatric surgery and is following her doctor's advice to become more active suggests that she is serious about improving her health. It is imperative that you begin the process of encouraging her to take small steps toward fitness. Given that she has never been active, it is unlikely that she has ever found enjoyment with exercise. Additionally, ADLs (e.g., walking in from her car) leave her breathless. This means you must start with small steps and build up.

   During the first week, encourage her to walk at a pace that feels comfortable for 10 min each day. Also, encourage her to decrease her TV viewing time. Ask her to keep a journal of her daily exercise and how she feels during and following the exercise bouts. Reassess and modify goals the following week based on any symptoms or difficulties she experiences. Use this process to gradually build up her exercise time. Encourage her to try a variety of exercise modes. In addition to aerobic activity, devise a resistance training and flexibility program, again with a focus on slow progression. Encourage her to get additional support through either personal training or a facility with a focus on helping people with extreme obesity. She will need to develop a supportive network if she is to evolve into an active person. Because she has undergone bariatric surgery, she should follow her doctor's orders regarding her nutritional needs.

21

Exercise and Diabetes

Dixie L. Thompson

OBJECTIVES

The reader will be able to do the following:

1. Define *diabetes mellitus* and describe the characteristics of type 1 and type 2 diabetes.
2. Describe the role that exercise plays in the prevention and treatment of type 2 diabetes.
3. Describe special considerations in exercise testing for clients with diabetes.
4. Describe special considerations in exercise prescription for clients with diabetes.

Diabetes mellitus refers to metabolic diseases characterized by **hyperglycemia** (i.e., elevated plasma glucose). The criteria used to diagnose diabetes are fasting blood glucose levels, the blood glucose response to ingesting carbohydrate, and the hemoglobin A1c level (see table 21.1). **Hemoglobin A1c** (i.e., glycosylated hemoglobin) is a form of hemoglobin that is typically found in low concentrations but exists in higher concentrations when blood glucose is constantly higher than normal. Thus, hemoglobin A1c reflects overall blood glucose control during the past 2 to 3 mo.

Comparison of Type 1 and Type 2 Diabetes

The cause of hyperglycemia varies depending on the form of diabetes present, with the most common forms being type 1 and type 2 diabetes. **Type 1 diabetes**, accounting for about 5% of diabetes cases, is characterized by a deficiency of insulin often attributable to an autoimmune destruction of the insulin-producing beta cells of the pancreas. Without insulin, the cells are unable to take in glucose. In **type 2 diabetes**, the insulin receptors in the cells become insensitive or resistant to insulin. Although there are other forms of diabetes mellitus (e.g., gestational diabetes), type 1 and type 2 account for the vast majority of cases. Regardless of the type, a number of complications may result from diabetes. These complications typically affect the blood vessels and nerves and include vision impairment, kidney disease, peripheral vascular disease, atherosclerosis, and hypertension (8). The economic burden (direct and indirect costs) of diabetes in the United States in 2012 was estimated at $245 billion (3).

In the United States, 29.1 million people have diabetes, and 8.1 million of them are unaware that they are diabetic (8). Between 90% and 95% of the cases are type 2 diabetes (8). This form of diabetes has both lifestyle and genetic roots. Many people with type 2 diabetes are relatively inactive and overweight or obese, particularly with excessive abdominal fat. Other risk factors include a family history of type 2 diabetes, older age, and belonging to an ethnic minority (prevalence is higher among Hispanics, Native Americans, and African Americans compared with Caucasians). Type 2 diabetes frequently coexists with other conditions such as hypertension and dyslipidemia. Although type 2 diabetes can appear at any age, the highest rates are seen among people aged 60 yr and older (8, 15). However, there is an increasing prevalence of type 2 diabetes among children, and this trend seems to be linked to increasing obesity rates (8, 15).

Approximately 1.25 million Americans have type 1 diabetes (8). Unlike type 2 diabetes, type 1 diabetes often appears early in life and is more closely linked to genetic than lifestyle factors. People with type 1 diabetes require insulin injections. There are many types of insulin, and they vary by how rapidly they begin working, their peak time of action, and how long they continue to work. Types of insulin used to treat diabetes are listed in table 21.2. Some people with type 2 diabetes also require insulin injections. More often, however, they take other types of prescription medications to lower blood glucose. Many types of medications are used for this purpose (see table 21.3). For more information on medications used to treat diabetes mellitus, see the websites of the American Diabetes Association (ADA) (www.diabetes.org) and the National Institute of Diabetes and Digestive and Kidney Diseases (NIDDK) (www.niddk.nih.gov).

Table 21.1 Criteria for Diagnosis of Prediabetes, Diabetes, and Gestational Diabetes

Prediabetes	FPG: 100 mg · dl^{-1} (5.6 mmol · L^{-1}) to 125 mg · dl^{-1} (6.9 mmol · L^{-1})
	PG 2 hr after OGTT: 140 mg · dl^{-1} (7.8 mmol · L^{-1}) to 199 mg · dl^{-1} (11 mmol · L^{-1})
	A1c: 5.7-6.4%
Diabetes	FPG: ≥126 mg · dl^{-1} (7.0 mmol · L^{-1})
	PG 2 hr after OGTT: ≥200 mg · dl^{-1} (11.1 mmol · L^{-1})
	Random PG: ≥200 mg · dl^{-1} (11.1 mmol · L^{-1}) (in patient with diabetic symptoms)
	A1c: ≥6.5%
Gestational diabetes	FPG: ≥92 mg · dl^{-1} (5.1 mmol · L^{-1})
	PG 1 hr after OGTT: ≥180 mg · dl^{-1} (10.0 mmol · L^{-1})
	PG 2 hr after OGTT: ≥153 mg · dl^{-1} (8.5 mmol · L^{-1})

FPG = fasting plasma glucose (no caloric intake for at least 8 hr); PG = plasma glucose; OGTT = oral glucose tolerance test using 75 g glucose load; A1c = hemoglobin A1c.

Data from American Diabetes Association 2011.

Table 21.2 Forms of Insulin Used to Control Diabetes Mellitus

Type of insulin	Onset of action	Peak	Duration
Rapid acting	15 min	30-90 min	3-5 hr
Short acting	30-60 min	2-4 hr	5-8 hr
Intermediate acting	1-3 hr	8 hr	12-16 hr
Long acting	1 hr	Lowers evenly for 24 hr	20-26 hr
Premixed (intermediate + short acting)	5-15 min	Varies	10-16 hr
Premixed (intermediate + rapid acting)	5-15 min	Varies	10-16 hr

Table 21.3 Examples of Medications Used to Control Type 2 Diabetes

Class of medication	Example	Mode of action
Sulfonylureas	Glyburide (DiaBeta)	Stimulates insulin production and release
Biguanides	Metformin (Glucophage)	Reduces glucose release from liver
Alpha-glucosidase inhibitors	Acarbose (Precose)	Slows absorption of carbohydrate
Thiazolidinediones	Rosiglitazone (Avandia)	Increases insulin sensitivity
Meglitinides	Repaglinide (Prandin)	Stimulates insulin production and release
Dipeptidyl peptidase-4 inhibitor	Sitagliptin (Januvia)	Increases insulin release and inhibits glucagon release (helpful in managing hemoglobin A1c levels)

Type 2 diabetes is characterized by **insulin resistance**, a condition in which the body's insulin receptors no longer respond normally to insulin. Thus glucose entry into cells is impaired and hyperglycemia results. Plasma insulin levels of people with type 2 diabetes may be normal, suppressed, or elevated depending on the individual. Regardless, type 2 diabetes is considered a disease of relative insulin deficiency because the insulin available is inadequate to maintain normal glucose concentrations. Although some people with type 2 diabetes can control their disease through exercise and weight loss, others require medications such as oral hypoglycemic agents and possibly even insulin injections (see table 21.3).

Type 2 diabetes usually develops over time, first appearing as **impaired fasting glucose** (100-125 mg · dl^{-1}) or **impaired glucose tolerance (IGT)**. IGT is a condition in which the increase in blood glucose after ingestion of carbohydrate is higher than normal and remains elevated longer than normal. A glucose level of 140 to 199 mg · dl^{-1} 2 hr after an oral glucose tolerance test (OGTT) indicates IGT. Examples of normal and abnormal blood glucose responses are shown in figure 21.1. A person with either impaired fasting glucose or IGT is classified as having **prediabetes**. Without intervention, prediabetes generally evolves into type 2 diabetes. It is estimated that at least 86 million Americans have prediabetes (8).

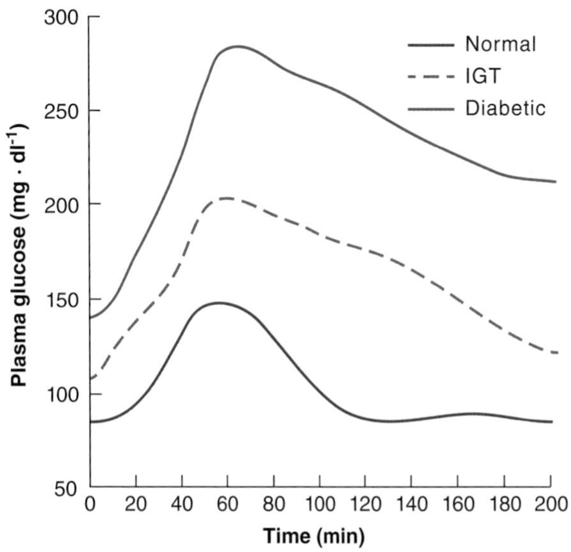

FIGURE 21.1 Comparison of glucose response with carbohydrate ingestion.

KEY POINT

Diabetes mellitus is characterized by hyperglycemia. Approximately 29 million Americans have diabetes mellitus, and the economic cost is approximately $245 billion each year. Type 1 diabetes results from a lack of insulin production. Type 2 diabetes, the most common form of diabetes, is characterized by the cells becoming insensitive to insulin. Risk factors for type 2 diabetes include older age, a family history of type 2 diabetes, excess weight, and inactivity.

Exercise for Clients With Diabetes

Exercise can provide many benefits to individuals with type 1 or type 2 diabetes. This is particularly true because of the strong link between diabetes and CVD and the role that exercise plays in reducing CVD risk. Unfortunately, people with diabetes are much less likely to exercise than their nondiabetic peers (16). Although exercise will not prevent or cure type 1 diabetes, exercise should be encouraged in this population for a number of reasons (4). Exercise improves insulin sensitivity and reduces disease risk for people with diabetes, much like in those without diabetes. Because of the high rate of CVD among people with diabetes, exercise can promote overall well-being. Exercise protects against CAD, dyslipidemia, hypertension, and obesity. Increased physical activity and improved physical fitness also promote psychological health and quality of life.

Exercise has been shown to be effective in preventing and treating type 2 diabetes. Inactivity and obesity are common characteristics of people with type 2 diabetes. Research has shown that individuals who are regularly active are 30% to 50% less likely to develop type 2 diabetes compared with their inactive counterparts (7). Additionally, people who have IGT are less likely to develop type 2 diabetes if they begin to exercise regularly (2, 13). Evidence is mounting that people with type 2 diabetes experience better glucose tolerance and improved insulin sensitivity through regular exercise (2, 10). There are a number of reasons why exercise can benefit the treatment of type 2 diabetes (1, 2, 9), including the following:

- Lower fasting blood glucose concentrations
- Better glucose tolerance (less of a spike in glucose after eating)
- Improved insulin sensitivity (more glucose uptake with a given amount of insulin)
- Weight control (increased lean mass and reduced fat mass)
- Improved lipid profiles
- Reduction in BP for those with hypertension
- Lower risk of CVD
- Stress management (stress can affect glucose control via increased levels of catecholamines)

KEY POINT

Exercise has been shown to be effective in preventing and treating type 2 diabetes. Regardless of the type of diabetes, exercise benefits people with diabetes by improving blood glucose and weight control and by lowering the risk of CVD.

Screening and Testing Clients With Diabetes

Clients with diabetes are at high risk for CVD; thus, screening prior to exercise participation is critical (1, 14). Medical clearance is recommended for all previously sedentary clients with diabetes mellitus to ensure that they can safely perform exercise; however, if the client is asymptomatic and is already engaging in regular physical activity, medical clearance is not needed prior to light- or moderate-intensity exercise (1). Individuals should discuss with their physicians how to modify their insulin dosage and other diabetes medications with exercise. Because exercise increases glucose uptake from peripheral tissues regardless of insulin levels, hypoglycemia may result if insulin intake is not adjusted (see the next section for tips on avoiding hypoglycemia). Diabetes is a primary risk factor for the development of CVD, so clients with diabetes should be screened carefully for signs and symptoms of disease (chapter 2).

People with type 2 diabetes frequently are overweight and hypertensive and have a poor blood lipid profile; therefore, they may be taking a number of medications that can influence the exercise response. For people who have had diabetes for a number of years, peripheral neuropathy may be a problem. Damage to the sensory nerves in the feet can lead to ulcerations, and if there is damage to blood vessels, healing can be slow. Because of these and other issues, conducting a thorough medical history is particularly important with these clients.

The need for medical clearance prior to exercise participation depends on the client's current level of physical activity and the intensity of the exercise program. For currently active clients with diabetes who are asymptomatic, they may continue with light-intensity (< 40% HRR) or moderate-intensity (40-60% HRR) exercise without medical clearance. For these clients, medical clearance is recommended prior to beginning a vigorous-intensity (≥ 60%) exercise program. For any diabetic client who is currently inactive, medical clearance is recommended prior to beginning an exercise program. Typically, exercise testing (or other ECG stress testing) may not be necessary for these individuals unless they intend to undertake vigorous-intensity exercise. The need for exercise testing before exercise programming depends on the person's risk factors and the intensity of the exercise program (1, 2, 14). Diagnostic exercise stress testing under the supervision of a physician may be necessary for people with numerous risk factors. The decision of whether to perform exercise testing should be made in consultation with the client's physician. Generally, before any diabetic client begins a vigorous exercise program, exercise testing with CAD screening is recommended (14). For additional information on testing clients who have diabetes, see *ACSM's Resource Manual for Guidelines for Exercise Testing and Prescription* (9, 14) and *ACSM's Exercise Management for Persons With Chronic Diseases and Disabilities* (12).

When performing exercise testing on diabetic clients, the protocol will depend on the client's age and functional ability. Submaximal exercise testing can be used to estimate aerobic power (see chapter 7). However, autonomic neuropathy can cause unusual HR and BP responses during exercise. In a medically supervised setting, diagnostic techniques such as echocardiography or radionuclide imaging may be used during the exercise test (14).

KEY POINT

Screening clients with diabetes mellitus is important prior to performing any exercise testing. Medical clearance is needed for clients who have been sedentary. If exercise testing is needed, the type of tests will depend on the client's needs and the intensity of the exercise program.

Exercise Prescription

The goals of exercise programming for clients with diabetes (e.g., increasing aerobic power, reducing disease risk, increasing flexibility, increasing muscular strength and endurance, limiting sedentary time) are similar to those for clients who do not have diabetes, with the exception of increased attention to improving glucose control. The basic elements of exercise prescription should be applied for clients with diabetes but with special considerations, as outlined in the following sections.

Type 1 Diabetes

A person with type 1 diabetes must carefully consider modifying insulin dosage and carbohydrate ingestion before beginning an exercise program. Increasing the intake of carbohydrate or reducing insulin dosage is often necessary to maintain glucose control and to avoid hypoglycemia that can result from exercise. The adjustment in carbohydrate intake and insulin dosage depends on the intensity and duration of activity. Glucose should be measured before initiating an exercise session. If glucose is <100 mg · dl^{-1}, carbohydrate (20-30 g) should be ingested before beginning exercise (9). If glucose is >250 mg · dl^{-1} but without ketosis, participants can undertake moderate-intensity exercise only if they are feeling well and are well hydrated; otherwise exercise should be delayed (9).

For the client with type 1 diabetes who was previously inactive, progression should be slow, with careful monitoring of blood glucose and symptoms of cardiovascular and metabolic distress. Initially, supervised exercise is recommended. After the person is able to maintain glucose control with exercise, unsupervised exercise is acceptable. However, it is always preferable that clients with diabetes do not exercise alone because of the need to have someone nearby in case of a hypoglycemic event. Symptoms of hypoglycemia include dizziness, nausea, headache, confusion, and irritability. The following precautions should be observed for avoiding exercise-induced hypoglycemia:

- Measure blood glucose immediately before and 15 min after exercise (also during exercise if the exercise lasts longer than 30 min).
- Consume carbohydrate if glucose is <100 mg · dl^{-1}.
- Avoid exercising during times of peak insulin action.
- Reduce insulin dose (and inject into inactive areas) on days of planned exercise.
- Consume carbohydrate (5-30 g) after exercise, particularly after high-intensity, glycogen-depleting exercise. Hypoglycemia can appear several hours after exercise, so monitoring after exercise is crucial.
- Avoid exercise late at night, because hypoglycemia could occur while sleeping.
- Extend the warm-up and cool-down if needed.

Regular (3 or more days per wk) aerobic exercise is recommended to maximize blood glucose control. The intensity of the exercise should match the characteristics of the client. Although moderate-intensity resistance exercise is safe for most people with diabetes, those with advanced complications (e.g., kidney disease, vision impairment) should avoid heavy lifting, where extreme BP elevation is possible. The ADA provides specific examples of recommended and discouraged exercises depending on the severity of the disease (4).

Dehydration due to polyuria can be problematic for diabetic clients. Dehydration can lead to a number of complications, including poor thermoregulatory control. Diabetic clients should be encouraged to maintain adequate hydration and watch for signs of heat or cold illness (see chapters 4, 7, and 25).

Because peripheral neuropathy can lead to ulcerations of the feet, good foot care is essential. Properly fitting and supportive shoes are particularly important for clients with diabetes who are engaging in weight-bearing exercise. For those with advanced peripheral neuropathy, low-impact and potentially non-weight-bearing exercises are more appropriate (4). Clients may find ACSM's exercise guide for people with diabetes helpful (6).

General recommendations for aerobic exercise by diabetic patients are as follows (1, 9):

- Frequency: 3 to 7 days per wk
- Intensity: 40% to 89% $\dot{V}O_2R$ or HRR; RPE 11-17
- Type: rhythmic, large-muscle-group activities dependent on personal preferences and needs
- Time: 20 to 30 min in bouts of at least 10 min for a total of at least 150 min per wk of moderate-intensity exercise, at least 75 min per wk of vigorous-intensity exercise, or a combination

In the absence of retinopathy, recent laser treatments, or other contraindications (1, 9), resistance exercise is also recommended for diabetic patients. General guidelines are as follows (9):

- Frequency: 2 to 3 days per wk
- Intensity: 50% to 85% of 1RM (lower initially)
- Time: 1 to 3 sets of 8 to 10 repetitions (10 to 15 repetitions initially)
- Type: all major muscle groups, with four to five upper-body and four to five lower-body or core exercises (avoid static contractions and sustained gripping; avoid Valsalva maneuver)

Type 2 Diabetes

The ADA and ACSM recommend that people with type 2 diabetes engage in both endurance and resistance training, unless significant complications or limitations exist (1, 2, 9). Individuals should accumulate at least 150 min per wk in moderate-intensity exercise (1, 2). When possible, additional minutes (e.g., 150-300 min per wk) should be encouraged in order to achieve additional benefits. For those who are overweight or obese, aerobic activity should focus on caloric expenditure and weight control. Although at least 3 nonconsecutive days of exercise per week are recommended, individuals may choose to engage in daily physical activity to maximize glucose control and caloric expenditure.

Moderate-intensity exercise is generally recommended (1, 2), although the participant's characteristics should be considered when determining intensity. Activity at higher intensities is acceptable for those who are conditioned and choose more vigorous exercise. Because of the possibility of autonomic neuropathy, using HR to monitor exercise intensity may be problematic. Therefore, RPE may be a better choice for self-monitoring exercise intensity (see chapter 7). Exercise intensity and duration should be balanced to achieve goals for caloric expenditure. Typically, exercise sessions lasting at least 10 min are suggested, with physical activity accumulating to 30 to 60 min each day. The mode of aerobic exercise should fit the client's needs and abilities. Walking is the mode of choice for many, but for those with peripheral nerve damage, other modes (e.g., swimming, nonimpact exercise equipment) may be preferable.

General recommendations for aerobic exercise by type 2 diabetic patients are as follows (9):

- Frequency: 3 to 7 days per wk (no more than 2 consecutive inactive days)
- Intensity: 40% to 89% $\dot{V}O_2R$ or HRR; RPE 11-17
- Time: 30 to 60 min in bouts of at least 10 min
- Type: rhythmic, large-muscle-group activities dependent on personal preferences and needs

Resistance training also is suggested for many people with type 2 diabetes (1, 2, 9). Resistance training maintains or even increases muscle mass and improves glucose tolerance and insulin sensitivity. The program should focus on major muscle groups (8-10 exercises) and should be performed regularly (see the following guidelines). People without advanced complications can follow more aggressive programs. However, for those with eye or kidney damage resulting from diabetes, particular caution should be taken to avoid extreme BP elevations (4). In the absence of retinopathy, recent laser treatments, or other contraindications (1, 9), resistance exercise is recommended for diabetic patients. General guidelines are as follows (9):

- Frequency: 2 to 3 days per wk
- Intensity: 50% to 85% of 1RM (lower initially)
- Time: 1 to 3 sets of 8 to 10 repetitions (10 to 15 repetitions initially)

- Type: all major muscle groups, with four to five upper-body and four to five lower-body or core exercises (avoid static contractions and sustained gripping; avoid Valsalva maneuver)

Because many clients with type 2 diabetes have a history of being relatively inactive and are often overweight, beginning and then maintaining an active lifestyle presents particular challenges. Creating a supportive environment is critical to the success of these clients. Early in the exercise program, it is especially important to provide information on the benefits of a lifetime commitment to exercise. The program should progress slowly, be based on realistic goals, and incorporate the client's needs and desires. Additional information on increasing adherence to exercise can be found in chapter 23 and in the ACSM and ADA position statement on exercise and type 2 diabetes (2).

KEY POINT

Exercise prescription for the client with diabetes must take into account special needs caused by the disease. Careful monitoring of blood glucose levels is needed to help avoid hypoglycemic events. For people who have diabetes without complications, the exercise recommendation is a minimum of 150 min per wk of moderate-intensity aerobic exercise. Resistance training can be used with clients who have diabetes as long as the client avoids damage to already weakened blood vessels.

Metabolic Syndrome

Metabolic syndrome (also called *syndrome X*) is a condition in which a number of CAD risk factors exist together. People with metabolic syndrome have a much higher risk for atherosclerotic CVD. In order to be diagnosed with metabolic syndrome, a person must have at least three of the following (11):

- Abdominal obesity: WC ≥102 cm (men) or ≥88 cm (women)
- High triglycerides: ≥150 mg · dl^{-1}, or drug treatment
- Low HDL-C: <40 mg · dl^{-1} (men) or <50 mg · dl^{-1} (women), or drug treatment
- Elevated BP: ≥130/85 mmHg, or drug treatment
- Elevated fasting glucose: ≥100 mg · dl^{-1}, or drug treatment

It is estimated that over 30% of American adults have metabolic syndrome. Without intervention, chronic disease risk (e.g., CVD, diabetes) is much higher for these individuals. The approach to control metabolic syndrome depends on the symptoms that are present. Because abdominal obesity is common, weight loss is frequently suggested (7%-10% weight loss the first year and then continued reduction to reach a BMI of <25 kg · m^{-2}) (10). Physical activity is also commonly recommended because of the positive effect of regular exercise on all characteristics of metabolic syndrome.

Exercise testing for individuals with metabolic syndrome should follow the screening guidelines outlined in chapter 2. It is critical to screen for signs and symptoms of CVD and make decisions based on findings. See chapter 20 for more information about testing clients who are obese.

Exercise prescription for people with metabolic syndrome should include aerobic, resistance, and flexibility components as outlined in chapters 11, 13, and 14. Information on exercise prescription for obese clients is included in chapter 20. Achieving a healthy body weight and managing CVD risk factors are vital for clients with metabolic syndrome.

LEARNING AIDS

REVIEW QUESTIONS

1. List the two major types of diabetes.
2. What are the similarities and differences between type 1 and type 2 diabetes?
3. What is prediabetes?
4. What are the diagnostic criteria for diabetes?
5. What characteristics in a diabetic client will lead you to recommend ECG stress testing prior to exercise prescription?
6. What are general aerobic exercise recommendations for diabetic clients?
7. What are general resistance training recommendations for diabetic clients?
8. What precautions should be taken to avoid hypoglycemia?
9. What is metabolic syndrome?

CASE STUDIES

Mr. Conner is a 40-yr-old man who, in response to doctor's orders, appears at your medical wellness facility for exercise programming. He recently sought the care of his physician after experiencing fatigue and headaches. Mr. Conner's physician ordered a series of tests, including a diagnostic exercise stress test. Here are Mr. Conner's test results:

Weight = 265 lb (120 kg)

Cholesterol = 270 mg · dl^{-1}

Fasting glucose = 132 mg · dl^{-1}

Height = 5 ft 9.5 in. (177 cm)

LDL-C = 190 mg · dl^{-1}

BP = 148/94 mmHg

Nonsmoker

HDL-C = 32 mg · dl^{-1}

$\dot{V}O_2max$ = 22 ml · kg^{-1} · min^{-1}

High stress

Previously inactive

No ischemia with GXT

Mr. Conner was diagnosed with type 2 diabetes, placed on medication to lower his cholesterol, and placed on a diuretic to lower his BP. He was told to begin to exercise and lose weight in an attempt to lower his blood glucose.

1. Design a 3 mo supervised exercise program for Mr. Conner.
2. What are reasonable weight-loss goals for Mr. Conner? What recommendations will you make to help him achieve these goals?
3. What additional support systems will you recommend to help Mr. Conner achieve success with his exercise and weight-loss goals?

Answers to Case Studies

1. Recommend aerobic and resistance training for Mr. Conner.

   Month 1: Begin with 5 days per wk of supervised sessions (3 days of aerobic exercise and 2 days of aerobic exercise and resistance training). Although this may seem like a lot of supervised sessions, it is designed to assist with compliance and to help him make the significant lifestyle adjustment. His history indicates he is not likely to exercise without support. Additionally, because he is new to the medication regiment, he needs supervision in case of a hypoglycemic event.

   - Aerobic component—begin with 2 bouts of walking, 10 min each in duration, separated by 5 min of stretching. Use RPE (target 12 on 2-20 scale). If joint pain is an issue, use walking for one bout and select another mode of aerobic activity for the other bout. After the second week, move to 12 min bouts.
   - Resistance component—select 8 multijoint exercises with upper- and lower-body exercises as a part of the workout. Have Mr. Conner complete 1 set of 8 to 12 repetitions during the first month. Do these exercises following his walking bouts on 2 days per wk.

   Month 2: Continue with 5 days of supervised exercise, but also encourage him to build activity into his daily life and on his unsupervised days. Focus on building activity into his routine (e.g., parking farther from his office door, taking stairs). Encourage him to buy a pedometer and track his steps during the day. On his unsupervised days, encourage him to engage in active leisure activities (e.g., trips to the park, walking at the mall, visiting local outdoor markets).

   - Aerobic component—gradually build up to 2 bouts of 20 min each, separated by 5 min of stretching. Use RPE (target 13-14 on the 6-20 scale).
   - Resistance component—continue with same exercises, but add a second set.

   Month 3: Continue with 5 supervised sessions per week. If Mr. Conner is doing well (no hypoglycemic events and he appears motivated), you might consider dropping off to 3 supervised sessions per week. On his days off, set specific exercise goals and have him report his activity.

   - Aerobic component—gradually convert his walking to a 30 min bout followed by a 15 min bout, separated by 5 min of stretching. Use RPE (target 12-16 on the 6-20 scale).
   - Resistance component—same as month 2.

2. Weight-loss goals: Mr. Conner should restrict calories and increase exercise to achieve a weekly weight loss of 1 to 2 lb (0.5-0.9 kg). Use strategies outlined in chapter 12 to calculate caloric intake goals at approximately 500 kcal $\cdot$ day^{-1} below energy needs. Focus on low-fat food options. He has likely been given eating recommendations by his physician; incorporate those recommendations into his plan.
3. Mr. Conner will benefit from building a supportive network. Help him identify friends, family members, coworkers, and so on who will encourage his healthy lifestyle. Encourage him to keep a journal of his eating and exercise. Help him develop strategies to deal with challenges (e.g., travel, time management). Encourage him to monitor his weight and check in with his physician regularly. It will be important to monitor his CVD risk factors. If he makes the changes you suggest and he follows the medication regiment prescribed by his physician, his risk-factor profile should improve.

22

Exercise and Pulmonary Disease

David R. Bassett, Jr.

Dr. Glenn Farr, PharmD (University of Tennessee College of Pharmacy), provided expert assistance in revising and updating the medications section of this chapter.

OBJECTIVES

The reader will be able to do the following:

1. Describe the differences between chronic obstructive lung diseases and restrictive lung diseases.
2. Define the underlying physiological problems associated with asthma, emphysema, bronchitis, and cystic fibrosis.
3. List physiological and mental health benefits of exercise for individuals with pulmonary disease.
4. Describe how pulmonary function testing can be used to diagnose chronic obstructive lung diseases versus restrictive lung diseases.
5. Describe how signs (e.g., dyspnea) and symptoms (e.g., hypoxemia) of pulmonary disease are monitored during a GXT.
6. Describe how to prescribe aerobic exercise (frequency, intensity, and duration) in pulmonary rehabilitation programs.
7. Identify the benefits of upper-body training in pulmonary rehabilitation.
8. Discuss the use of supplemental oxygen therapy and pursed-lip breathing for individuals with COPD.
9. List the common categories of medications used to treat pulmonary disease as well as examples of each category, and discuss the probable effect of these medications on exercise performance.

Pulmonary diseases can be subdivided into two major categories. In **chronic obstructive pulmonary disease (COPD)**, the airflow into and out of the lungs is impeded. In **restrictive lung diseases**, the expansion of the lungs is reduced because of conditions involving the chest cavity or parenchyma (lung tissue). Some pulmonary diseases are genetically inherited (e.g., cystic fibrosis), but in other cases a history of cigarette smoking, environmental pollutants, or occupational exposure to silica, coal dust, or asbestos is the primary contributing factor. All pulmonary diseases show a disruption in the exchange of gases between the ambient air and the pulmonary capillary blood. As a result, $\dot{V}O_2$max is reduced, the work of breathing is increased, and the ability to perform exercise is limited.

Chronic Obstructive Pulmonary Disease

COPD causes a reduction in airflow that can dramatically affect a person's ability to perform daily activities. Characteristics of COPD include expiratory flow obstruction and shortness of breath on exertion. Types of COPD include chronic bronchitis, emphysema, and bronchial asthma. All of these diseases obstruct airflow, but the underlying reason for obstruction differs for each (7):

- Bronchial asthma is caused by bronchial smooth muscle contraction and increased airway reactivity.
- Chronic bronchitis results from persistent production of sputum attributable to a thickened bronchial wall with excess secretions.
- Emphysema is caused by loss of elastic recoil of alveoli and bronchioles and enlargement of those pulmonary structures.
- Cystic fibrosis is a genetic disorder that results in excessive mucous production in the airways, which hinders ventilation of the lungs.

In 2011, 14.7 million American adults were estimated to have COPD, not including asthma (5). Unfortunately, the mortality rates associated with COPD have increased over the past two decades. Chronic bronchitis and emphysema are not reversible. The patient with COPD perceives an inability to perform normal activities without dyspnea, but, tragically, by the time this occurs the disease is well advanced (7). COPD is the fourth leading cause of death in the United States (17), accounting for 133,965 deaths in 2009 (5).

Asthma

An estimated 25.9 million people in the United States have asthma; 27% of those are children under the age of 18 (4). It is a condition that can reverse itself, and it varies from wheezing and slight breathlessness to severe attacks that may result in suffocation. Causes of asthma include allergic reactions to antigens such as dust, pollen, smoke, and air pollution. Nonspecific factors such as emotional stress and exercise as well as viral infections of the bronchi, sinuses, or tonsils can also result in asthma. People with exercise-induced asthma may have normal resting pulmonary function but experience bronchospasms during exercise. In some cases, no specific cause of the asthma can be identified. Treatment involves bronchodilators (often administered by inhalers) and other drugs that thin the mucous secretions and help eject them (expectorants) (10).

Exercise-induced asthma is a reactive airway disease affecting between 4% and 20% of the U.S. population (22). With this condition, exercise tends to cause the bronchioles to constrict. One method of diagnosing exercise-induced asthma is to have a patient run for 6 to 8 min on the treadmill at 85% to 90% of maximal HR (2). The forced expiratory volume in 1 sec (FEV_1) is measured before exercise and 3 to 9 min after exercise. A positive test occurs when the postexercise FEV_1 is 15% below the pretest value (2).

People with exercise-induced asthma can usually engage in exercise training (20). In fact, some notable Olympians such as Jackie Joyner-Kersee (gold medalist in heptathlon, 1988 and 1992) and Amy Van Dyken (gold medalist in four swimming events, 1996) have had this condition. Oral inhalers, such as Ventolin and Flovent, are helpful for managing exercise-induced asthma. Other strategies to improve exercise tolerance include exercising in warm, moist environments rather than in cold, dry ones. Many people with asthma tolerate swimming better than running. In addition, a long warm-up can lessen the airway constriction that is more likely to occur with sudden, strenuous exercise (2, 22).

Chronic Bronchitis

According to data from the U.S. National Center for Health Statistics, 10 million American adults were diagnosed with chronic bronchitis in 2011 (5). Bronchitis is characterized by inflammation of the bronchi, anatomical structures that carry air from the trachea to the lungs. Symptoms of chronic bronchitis include a cough, often with the production of sputum (i.e., mucous that is coughed up from the respiratory tract). Airflow into the lungs is restricted due to inflammation of the airways and excess mucous production. Upon exertion, a patient with chronic bronchitis may experience wheezing and **dyspnea** (shortness of breath) (18).

The most common risk factor for chronic bronchitis is cigarette smoking. Chronic bronchitis can also be caused by air pollution, secondhand smoke, occupational exposure to airborne irritants, and genetic factors (17). Chronic bronchitis is much more serious than acute bronchitis. About 90% of the time, acute bronchitis results from an acute virus such as the common cold or flu. Over time, acute bronchitis goes away and normally does not pose a problem for long-term health.

If the patient is a smoker, the most important treatment for bronchitis is to stop smoking. This helps relieve symptoms and halt progression of the disease. Treatment for chronic bronchitis often involves the administration of a bronchodilator (e.g., albuterol), typically through the use of an inhaler. Short-term steroid therapy can reduce inflammation of the bronchial tubes. Good hydration is essential to help remove bronchial secretions, and over-the-counter medicines such as Mucinex and Robitussin may also help in that regard. If the patient suffers from hypoxemia, supplemental oxygen can help to increase arterial oxygenation and relieve symptoms of dyspnea (6).

Emphysema

In 2011, an estimated 4.7 million American adults reported ever being diagnosed with emphysema (5). Emphysema is characterized by destruction of the alveolar walls and enlargement of air spaces distal to the terminal bronchioles. As a result, the lung loses its elasticity and the airways tend to collapse on exhalation. Symptoms include coughing and severe shortness of breath upon exertion. The inability of the lungs to saturate the arterial blood with oxygen leads to hypoxemia (13).

As with chronic bronchitis, cigarette smoking is the most common cause of emphysema. Other causes of emphysema include environmental air pollutants and, in rare cases, a hereditary deficiency of alpha-1 antitrypsin. (Alpha-1 antitrypsin inhibits neutrophil elastase, a compound that breaks down the fibroelastic network of the lungs.) Patients with emphysema may have a barrel-shaped chest due to hyperinflation of the lungs. Breathing rate is often rapid and tidal volume is smaller than normal (18).

Treatment for emphysema cannot cure or reverse the lung damage. Smoking cessation and prevention of respiratory infections with antibiotics are important in medical management of emphysema. Supplemental oxygen is often needed, and this can be administered for 18 to 24 hr per day. Bronchodilators are sometimes given to relax and open the airways, and corticosteroids are used to reduce inflammation of the respiratory tract. Expectorants can help loosen the mucous secretions, enabling the patient to cough them up.

Cystic Fibrosis

Cystic fibrosis, another type of COPD, is a recessively inherited genetic disorder. Three decades ago, most cystic fibrosis patients died in childhood, but better treatments have prolonged life expectancy by 20 yr (16). In Caucasian children, 1 in 2,500 is born with the condition, although the disease is rare in Asians and African Americans (16). Thick mucous secretions by the exocrine glands affect many systems in the body. In fact, clinical diagnosis is based on excessive chloride concentration in the sweat. In the lungs, the mucous secretions plug the airways, causing inflammation and chronic bacterial infections. Treatment for cystic fibrosis consists of having patients lie with the head facing downhill while percussion is used to enhance mucous drainage. In addition, aerobic exercise has been shown to help clear the lungs and prevent bacterial infections. The increased use of antibiotics is yet another reason that survival of cystic fibrosis patients has increased dramatically in recent years (18).

KEY POINT

COPD reduces the capacity for airflow during respiration. Bronchitis and emphysema are irreversible. Bronchial asthma is an intermittent condition caused by restriction of airways; it can be relieved with bronchodilator medications. Cystic fibrosis is a fatal disease that results from a genetic defect.

Restrictive Lung Diseases

Restrictive lung diseases have many causes, including diseases of the rib cage and spine such as kyphoscoliosis and pectus excavatum (sunken chest). Other causes include pulmonary edema, pulmonary **embolism**, exposure to toxic substances (coal workers' pneumoconiosis, silicosis, asbestosis), chemotherapy, and radiation therapy. Often, these inflame the interstitium and fibrotic tissue develops. Various types of neuromuscular diseases (spinal cord injury, amyotrophic lateral sclerosis or Lou Gehrig's disease, Guillain-Barré syndrome, tetanus, myasthenia gravis) can also cause restrictive lung disease. Obesity and pregnancy can restrict lung expansion because of the abdomen pushing up into the thoracic cavity. In general, people with restrictive lung diseases have reduced residual volume (RV), inspiratory reserve volume (IRV), expiratory reserve volume (ERV), forced vital capacity (FVC), and maximal tidal volume (TV) (see figure 22.1). Breathing is more difficult because the respiratory muscles must work harder to inflate the lungs (11).

KEY POINT

Restrictive lung diseases have numerous causes, but all are characterized by the reduced capacity to expand the lungs. Thus, smaller lung volumes, assessed through pulmonary function testing, typically are seen in people with these diseases.

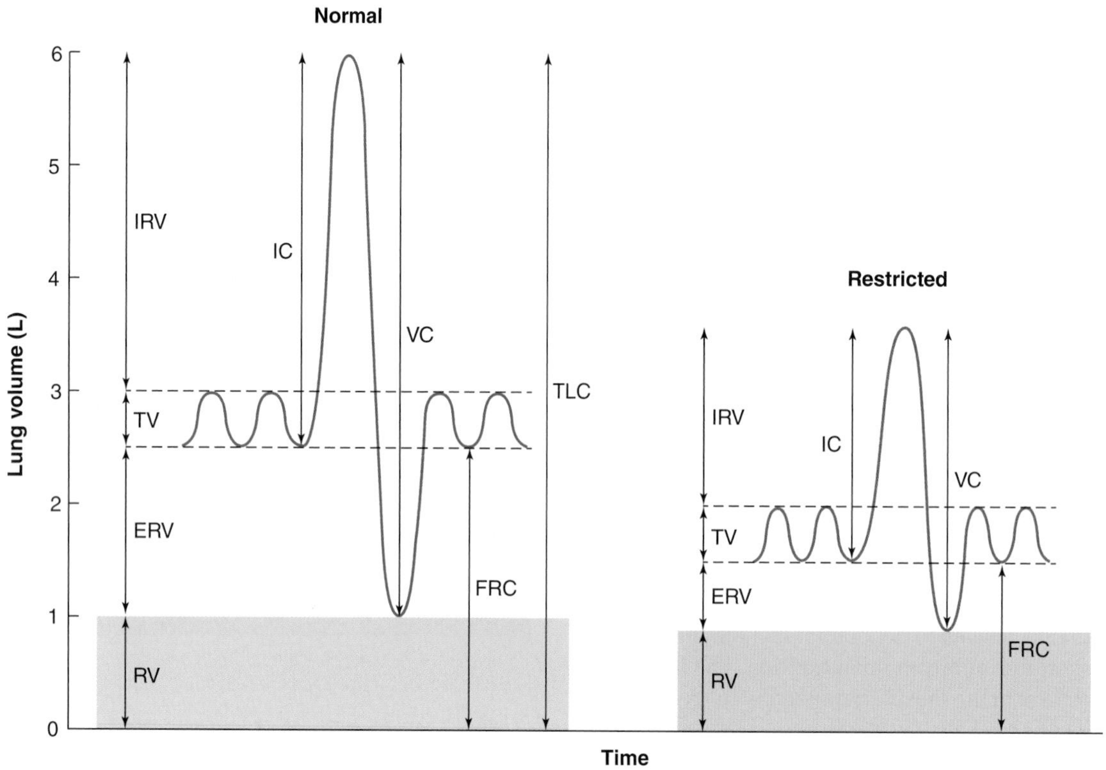

FIGURE 22.1 Lung volumes in a person with restrictive lung disease versus a person with normal pulmonary function. Lung volumes are total lung capacity (TLC), vital capacity (VC), inspiratory capacity (IC), inspiratory reserve volume (IRV), tidal volume (TV), functional residual capacity (FRC), expiratory reserve volume (ERV), and residual volume (RV).

Evidence for Exercise Training

Pulmonary rehabilitation programs are often found alongside cardiac rehabilitation programs in many hospitals. Most pulmonary rehabilitation programs focus on people with COPD, although people with other types of pulmonary disease may also benefit from exercise (6). Support for pulmonary rehabilitation programs is limited by the fact that patients typically show little or no improvement in $\dot{V}O_2$max, tests of lung function, and mortality rates. As a result, many insurance providers are reluctant to pay for pulmonary rehabilitation because they view it as medical management rather than a way to restore the patient to normal function (as much as possible).

However, most pulmonary rehabilitation patients do improve in functional outcomes, including symptom-limited GXT, symptoms of dyspnea, quality of life, and frequency of hospitalization (6). Thus, pulmonary rehabilitation should be viewed as a desirable part of the patient's medical treatment (13, 14). The overall goals are to improve the patient's general health, to optimize oxygen saturation, to make ADLs more easily accomplished, and to improve self-efficacy (6).

KEY POINT

Patients with lung diseases can benefit from a pulmonary rehabilitation program. Although patients usually demonstrate little improvement in $\dot{V}O_2$max and pulmonary function tests, they do improve in their ability to carry out tasks and in other measures of quality of life.

Diagnostic Tests to Detect COPD

In most instances, **pulmonary function testing** is carried out for diagnostic purposes and to assess the severity of the disease (19). Computerized spirometry systems measure lung volumes and flow parameters (see figure 22.2). In COPD, the principal measure is **forced expiratory volume (FEV_1)**, which reflects the maximum volume of air that can be moved in 1 sec (see figure 22.3). Sometimes forced expiratory volume is expressed as FEV_1/VC, where **vital**

capacity (VC) is the volume of air that can be breathed out when going from maximal inhalation to maximal exhalation. Because of airway obstruction, individuals with COPD have a decreased ability to exhale quickly; if the FEV_1 is below 80% of the expected value, the test is considered abnormal (9). In addition, if the value of FEV_1/VC is below 0.70, it is considered indicative of COPD. In restrictive lung disease, the lung volumes (i.e., RV, IRV, ERV, FVC, and maximal TV) are smaller than normal because lung expansion is limited. People with restrictive lung disease compensate by taking faster, smaller breaths, which reduces the work that the respiratory muscles must perform to inflate the lung.

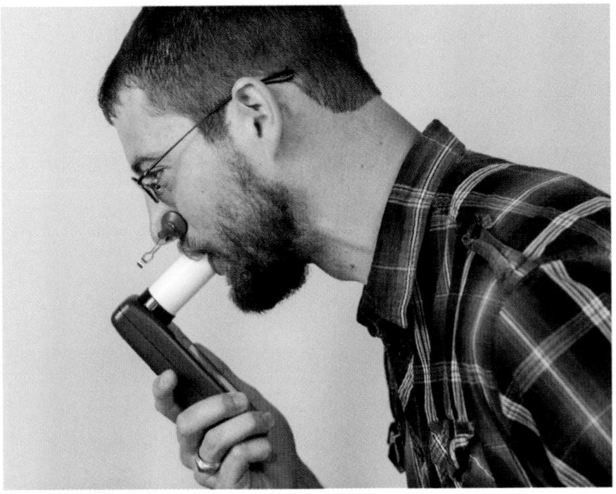

FIGURE 22.2 Pulmonary function testing is used to examine lung volumes and flow parameters.

Exercise tests are often administered to assess the patient's ability to exercise. The test may be a standard GXT on a treadmill or cycle ergometer or a simple 6 or 12 min walk test on a flat surface. In a pulmonary patient, exercise capacity is limited more by the lungs than the cardiovascular system. As a result, these patients typically experience **hypoxemia** (low arterial oxygen content) and dyspnea. Measurements of maximal ventilation rates ($\dot{V}O_2$max), obtained during the final minute of an exercise test, are also clinically useful. $\dot{V}O_2$max is typically 60% to 70% of the maximal voluntary ventilation (MVV), although in COPD patients it may approach 80% to 100%. MVV can be measured via a special spirometry test, or it can be predicted from the following formula: MVV = $FEV_1 \cdot 40$.

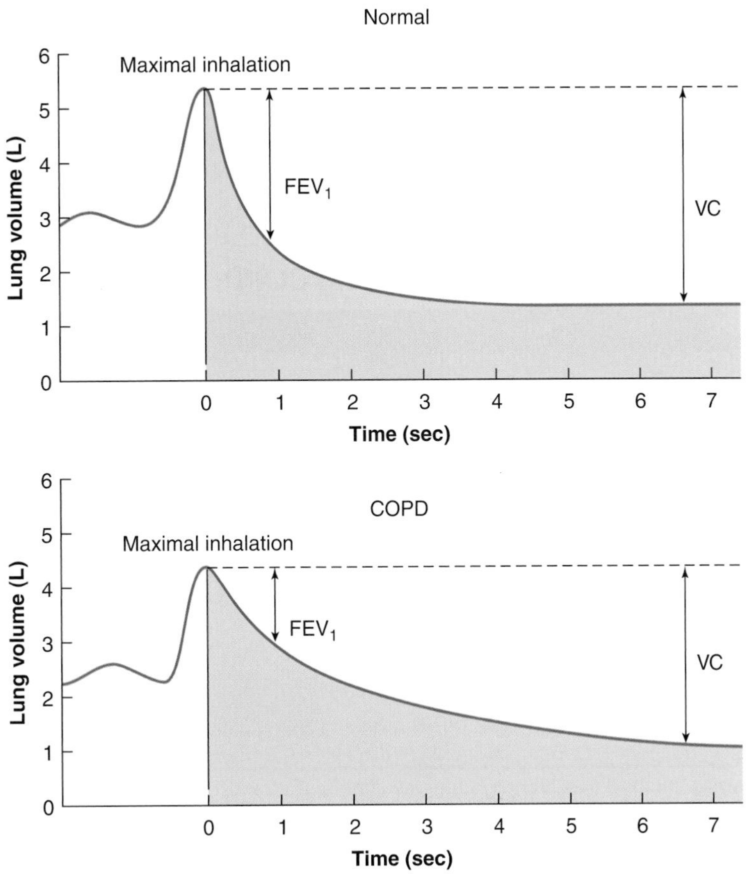

FIGURE 22.3 Pulmonary function test showing the volume versus time curves in a normal person and a person with obstructive lung disease. FEV_1 = forced expiratory volume in the first second of exhalation; VC = vital capacity.

A **pulse oximeter** is used to assess the percent saturation of hemoglobin in the arterial blood (S_aO_2) of pulmonary patients (figure 22.4). This noninvasive device shines a light beam through the finger or earlobe. The absorption characteristics of oxygenated and deoxygenated hemoglobin in the red or infrared region are used to assess the arterial oxygen saturation. Values for S_aO_2 below 90% indicate that the client needs supplemental oxygen to increase the driving force for diffusion of oxygen into the lungs. Frequently, a dyspnea rating scale is used to evaluate symptoms during exercise testing (8, 21). Cardiovascular, pulmonary, metabolic, and power output measurements are obtained and used to evaluate the severity of disability (see table 22.1).

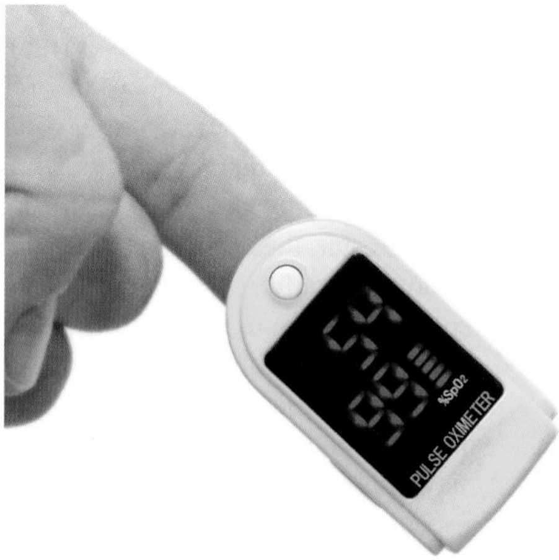

FIGURE 22.4 Portable pulse oximeter used to assess a person's arterial O_2 saturation. The finger probe shines a light through the fingertip, and the absorption of light due to the pulsing arterial blood is measured. The number on the bottom of the display shows the percent saturation of hemoglobin in arterial blood (S_aO_2), and the number on the top shows the HR.

VIDEO Watch **video 22.1**, which demonstrates arterial oxygen saturation measurement.

KEY POINT

One of the main pulmonary function tests for COPD is the FEV_1. COPD patients demonstrate a reduced ability to exhale quickly because of obstructed airways. In restrictive lung diseases, lung volumes are often reduced because the ability to expand the lungs is compromised. Exercise testing of patients with lung diseases, with appropriate monitoring of signs (hypoxemia) and symptoms (dyspnea) to assess the severity of the patient's condition, is beneficial.

Table 22.1 GOLD Classifications for Grading COPD

Grade	COPD description	Cause of dyspnea	FEV_1 (predicted)*	$\dot{V}O_2max$ (ml · kg^{-1} · min^{-1})	S_aO_2
GOLD 1	Mild COPD	Fast walking and stair-climbing	≥80	>25	Normal
GOLD 2	Moderate	Walking at normal pace	≤50 to <79	>20 or >75% predicted	Above 90% at rest and with exercise
GOLD 3	Severe	Slow walking	≤30 to <49	10-20 or >30%-75% predicted	Below 90% with exercise
GOLD 4	Very severe	Walking less than one block	<30	>10 or >30% predicted	Below 90% at rest and with exercise

*Spirometric classification using the fixed post bronchodilator ratio of $FEV_1/FVC < 0.70$.

Data from the Global Initiative for Chronic Obstructive Lung Disease, a collaboration between the National Institutes of Health and the World Health Organization; www.goldcopd.org; accessed November 4, 2015.

Typical Exercise Prescription

Given the high prevalence of pulmonary diseases, especially among older adults, fitness professionals can expect to encounter clients who have these conditions in health clubs and other fitness settings. If a client has severe symptoms of pulmonary disease, the fitness professional should refer the individual to a hospital-based pulmonary rehabilitation program. With a master's degree in exercise physiology, it is possible to get a job in pulmonary rehabilitation, which requires knowledge of the various types of pulmonary diseases, their pathology, and their treatment. Because exercise is recommended for increasing the health and life quality of pulmonary patients, the fitness professional should know how to prescribe exercise for this population.

The goal of a typical pulmonary rehabilitation program is the client's self-care, and to achieve that goal, physicians, nurses, respiratory therapists, exercise specialists, nutritionists, and psychologists are recruited to deal with the various manifestations of the disease (3). The pulmonary patient receives education about ways to deal with the disease, including breathing exercises, ways to approach ADLs at home, and ways to handle work-related problems. The emphasis in most pulmonary rehabilitation programs is on the COPD patient, although patients with restrictive lung disease often participate as well (6, 22). The AACVPR published a detailed description of exercise testing and prescription in its *Guidelines for Pulmonary Rehabilitation Programs* (1).

Aerobic training is usually accomplished with rhythmic, dynamic exercise that uses large muscle groups. Recommended modes are walking, cycling, and swimming (table 22.2). The exercise modes should be enjoyable and improve the ability to perform normal daily activities (13). As with healthy individuals and other clinical populations, the frequency for aerobic activity is typically 3 to 5 days per wk, with each session lasting 20 to 60 min (2). For muscular strength activity, the session duration recommended is 2 to 4 sets of 10 repetitions for strength training, and 1 to 2 sets of 15 to 20 repetitions for endurance training (2). For flexibility activity, the session duration recommended is to spend 10 to 30 sec on each static stretch, and 2 to 4 repetitions per exercise (2). However, assigning appropriate exercise intensities poses a particular problem. Pulmonary patients usually cannot achieve the same peak HRs as healthy individuals of the same age. Thus, computing a THR from a typical percentage of age-predicted HRmax often results in target intensities that are too high. On the other hand, using THR values computed from a typical percentage of measured HRmax underestimates the appropriate training intensity (1, 9).

Various methods can be used to estimate the appropriate exercise intensity for pulmonary patients. Generally, the method of assigning exercise intensity varies with the level of the disability. In patients with mild or moderate impairment, setting the intensity just below the VT (ventilatory threshold) or the point where the person became noticeably dyspneic is appropriate. A **dyspnea rating scale** (table 22.3) should

Table 22.2 COPD Exercise Prescription

Modes	Goals	Frequency	Time to goal
Aerobic Large-muscle activities (walking, swimming, cycling)	• Increase $\dot{V}O_2$max. • Increase LT and VT. • Become less sensitive to dyspnea. • Develop more efficient breathing patterns. • Facilitate improvements in ADLs.	3-5 days per wk	2-3 mo to ensure completion
Strength Weight machines, free weights, or body weight exercises	• Increase maximal number of reps. • Increase isokinetic torque and work. • Increase lean body mass.	2-3 days per wk	2-3 mo
Flexibility Static, dynamic, or PNF stretching Tai chi	• Increase ROM.	2-3 days per wk	Ongoing
Neuromuscular Walking Balance exercises Breathing exercises	• Improve gait and posture. • Improve breathing efficiency.		

PNF = proprioceptive neuromuscular facilitation

Reprinted, by permission, from C.B. Cooper, 2009, Chronic obstructive pulmonary disease. In *ACSM's exercise management for persons with chronic diseases and disabilities*, 3rd ed. (Champaign, IL: Human Kinetics), 134.

Table 22.3 Dyspnea Rating Scale

1	Light, barely noticeable
2	Moderate, bothersome
3	Moderately severe, very uncomfortable
4	Most severe or intense dyspnea ever experienced

Adapted from American College of Sports Medicine 2014, *ACSM's guidelines for exercise testing and prescription*, 9th ed. (Philadelphia: PA: Lippincott, Williams, & Wilkins).

be used to determine the patient's symptoms of shortness of breath. In clients with more severe disability, it is often necessary to let symptoms of dyspnea be the guiding factors (9). Intermittent exercise, interspersed with rest, may be all that the client can tolerate. If the impairment is severe, supplemental oxygen will be needed to maintain S_aO_2 above 90% (15).

Individuals with emphysema should be instructed in pursed-lip breathing, which involves pressing the lips together and exhaling through a small opening in the center of the mouth. This slows the rate of respiration and prevents collapse of small airways, resulting in better oxygenation (6, 14). In some instances, a resistive breathing device may be recommended to train the respiratory muscles at rest.

Upper-body exercise is recommended for pulmonary patients. This exercise can be achieved using modalities that require both arm and leg muscles, such as the Schwinn Airdyne or the rowing ergometer. Additionally, resistance training can be accomplished with dumbbells, machines, or elastic bands. Increasing arm strength and endurance improves the client's ability to perform functional activities and decreases local muscle fatigue (6, 9). Flexibility training (e.g., stretching, tai chi) and balance training may also be incorporated to improve the patient's functional ability (13).

KEY POINT

Pulmonary rehabilitation programs involve many types of health professionals. The primary goals are to educate patients about dealing with their disease and to help them improve their exercise capacity. A health professional in pulmonary rehabilitation must understand the client's medical conditions and physiological limitations. Sensations of dyspnea and pulse oximeter readings are frequently used to determine the appropriate exercise intensity.

Medications

Guidelines for the diagnosis and management of asthma from the National Heart, Lung, and Blood Institute (NHLBI; www.nhlbi.nih.gov) recommend a stepwise approach to asthma in which medication doses or types are stepped up as needed and stepped down when possible. Treatment is based on the level of asthma control.

Drugs for asthma are classified as the following:

1. Quick-relief or rescue bronchodilators for *treatment* (e.g., inhaled β_2 agonists). Oral steroids can be used for exacerbations but do not act quickly enough for rescue.
2. Long-term control or anti-inflammatories for *prevention* (e.g., inhaled steroids, mast cell stabilizers, leukotriene inhibitors, theophylline). Oral steroids can be used for exacerbations or chronically for severe persistent asthma, but they cause several systemic side effects when used chronically.

Corticosteroids act as anti-inflammatory agents and thus have a major role in the treatment and prevention of asthma as controllers given by inhalation (inhaled corticosteroids, or ICS). Examples of corticosteroids include the following:

- Prednisone—only given orally for severe asthma
- Flunisolide (AeroBid)
- Triamcinolone (Azmacort)
- Beclomethasone (Vanceril, Qvar)
- Fluticasone propionate (Flovent, Flonase)
- Fluticasone furoate (Veramyst, Arnuity Ellipta)
- Budesonide (Pulmicort, in Symbicort)
- Mometasone (Asmanex, in Nasonex)
- Ciclesonide (Omnaris, Alvesco, Zetonna)

Bronchodilators are classed as short-acting and long-acting. They stimulate the β_2 receptors that relax smooth muscle surrounding airways in the lungs and relieve the symptoms of asthma, bronchitis, and related lung disorders (10, 13). These medications can be taken orally or from an inhaler. Because of their beta-adrenergic stimulating effect, these medications can increase HR and BP, although they mostly focus on the smooth muscle found in airways. Some inhaler brand names include the following.

SHORT-ACTING BRONCHODILATORS

- Bitolterol (Tornalate)
- Pirbuterol (Maxair)
- Terbutaline (Bricanyl)
- Albuterol (Ventolin, Proventil)
- Levalbuterol (Xopenex)

LONG-ACTING BRONCHODILATORS

- Salmeterol (Serevent, in Advair)
- Formoterol (Foradil, in Symbicort, in Dulera, Perforomist)
- Arformoterol (Brovana)

The methylxanthines, which include aminophylline and theophylline, are another class of drugs. These cause bronchodilation via a different mechanism from the $ß_2$ agonist and are not as effective as a $ß_2$ agonist. Side effects of this class are similar to caffeine and include tachycardia, arrhythmias, central nervous system (CNS) stimulation, and risk of seizures.

Anticholinergic bronchodilators are also used. Short-acting agents include ipratropium (Atrovent), which can be combined with albuterol as Combivent Respimat. Long-acting anticholinergics include muscarinic tiotropium (Spiriva, Spiriva Respimat).

Another class of drugs, called *mast cell stabilizers*, is used for preventive therapy. These agents reduce the release of histamine, serotonin, leukotrienes, and other things that precipitate asthmatic attacks. The primary agent in this class is cromolyn (Intal).

Also used for preventive therapy are the leukotriene inhibitors. These drugs reverse the primary biological effects of the cysteinyl leukotrienes in relation to the pathogenesis of asthma, including bronchoconstriction, mucus hypersecretion, and airway inflammation. The primary agent is this class is montelukast (Singulair), which is also FDA approved for seasonal allergies and exercise-induced asthma.

The most recent introduction is Xolair (omalizumab), the first biotechnology product indicated for asthma caused by allergies. It works by disabling a naturally occurring antibody called *IgE* that triggers the release of chemicals that cause inflammation, asthma, and allergies (e.g., peanut allergies). Due to its expense and side effects, a patient must qualify to receive injections of this agent.

Additional medicines are used to treat common respiratory disorders. These include **decongestants** (phenylephrine, pseudoephedrine) to dry out the mucous membranes; traditional **antihistamines** such as diphenhydramine (Benadryl), brompheniramine (Dimetane), and chlorpheniramine (Chlor-Trimeton, Teldrin); and low-sedating antihistamines such as loratadine (Claritin), desloratadine (Clarinex), cetirizine (Zyrtec), fexofenadine (Allegra), and levocetirizine (Xyzal). These agents are given to relieve symptoms of seasonal allergies (e.g., hay fever): anti-inflammatory agents (ibuprofen, naproxen), expectorants (guaifenesin), and cough medications (dextromethorphan, codeine, hydrocodone). Antibiotics such as amoxicillin, azithromycin (Z-Pak), doxycycline, levofloxacin (Levaquin), and moxifloxacin (Avelox) are often given to fight off infections (8), which tend to occur if mucous secretions block the airways.

Diuretics such as hydrochlorothiazide (HCTZ) and furosemide (Lasix) are important in treating cor pulmonale, a condition that occurs in about half of pulmonary patients with severe disease. *Cor pulmonale* is defined as pulmonary hypertension with right ventricular hypertrophy. Because failure of the right ventricle often follows, diuretics may be needed to enhance fluid excretion (10, 12).

KEY POINT

Inhaled corticosteroids are the primary controller medication, and short-acting $ß_2$ agonists are bronchodilators used for rescue therapy for asthma. The same types of drugs or combinations are also used for patients with COPD. Decongestants, antihistamines, anti-inflammatory agents, and antibiotics are often prescribed to treat respiratory disorders. Diuretics are sometimes needed for patients with severe pulmonary disease who also develop heart failure.

LEARNING AIDS

REVIEW QUESTIONS

1. What is the major problem in COPD, and what are the physiological consequences of severe COPD?
2. What is the major problem in restrictive lung disease, and what are the physiological consequences of severe restrictive lung disease?
3. Define the underlying problems associated with the following subcategories of COPD: asthma, emphysema, bronchitis, and cystic fibrosis.
4. Identify which of the static lung volumes are decreased in people with restrictive lung disease.

5. Describe how the FEV_1 and VC are affected in people with COPD (e.g., asthma).
6. What two physiological variables can be monitored noninvasively via a pulse oximeter?
7. Describe a therapeutic treatment that is available in case a client's SaO_2 falls below 90%.
8. Outline the recommendations for aerobic exercise programming for people with COPD in terms of frequency, intensity, duration, and mode. What are the recommendations for strength training?
9. List the types of medicines used to treat pulmonary disease as well as their physiological effects on the body.
10. Why is upper-body training often recommended for people with pulmonary disease?

CASE STUDIES

1. A 38-yr-old woman with asthma would like to enter your fitness program. What kinds of questions do you ask her during your screening interview?
2. A 50-yr-old man with a history of smoking a pack of cigarettes a day for the past 25 yr enters a hospital complaining of dyspnea. A chest X-ray shows that his lungs are hyperinflated, and spirometry tests show that his FEV_1 is only half the normal value. What type of pulmonary disease does he have, and what is the logical course of treatment?
3. A middle-aged patient with severe kyphoscoliosis is referred to a pulmonary rehabilitation program. He has restrictive pulmonary disease, demonstrating a vital capacity of only 1.5 L (compared with the normal value of 5.0 L). During a 6 min walk test, he manages to cover 865 ft (264 m), stopping once because of shortness of breath. His S_aO_2 at the end of the test has fallen to 87%. What type of exercise training would you recommend? What other therapies might assist him in completing his exercise sessions?

Answers to Case Studies

1. Find out if she has worked with her physician and is currently experiencing any problems with her medication. In addition, ask if she carries a bronchodilator with her to class, and determine that she knows how to use it when she has shortness of breath. Lastly, pay special attention to her during the early phases of the class.
2. The patient likely has emphysema and possibly bronchitis, two forms of COPD that commonly result from cigarette smoking. This is shown by his reduced ability to exhale air quickly (decreased FEV_1). The logical course of treatment is a program to help him stop smoking, followed by a pulmonary rehabilitation program to help him regain his ability to exercise so that he can carry out ADLs.
3. The patient has a limited ability to exercise, but intermittent treadmill walking (with treadmill level), cycle ergometry, and rowing would be suitable. Arm exercises with very light weights or stretch cords for upper-body conditioning are also appropriate. During physical training, his oxygen saturation, ECG, and symptoms of dyspnea should be closely monitored. Supplemental oxygen will help increase his oxygen saturation, maintaining it above 90%.

Comprehensive Exercise Program Considerations

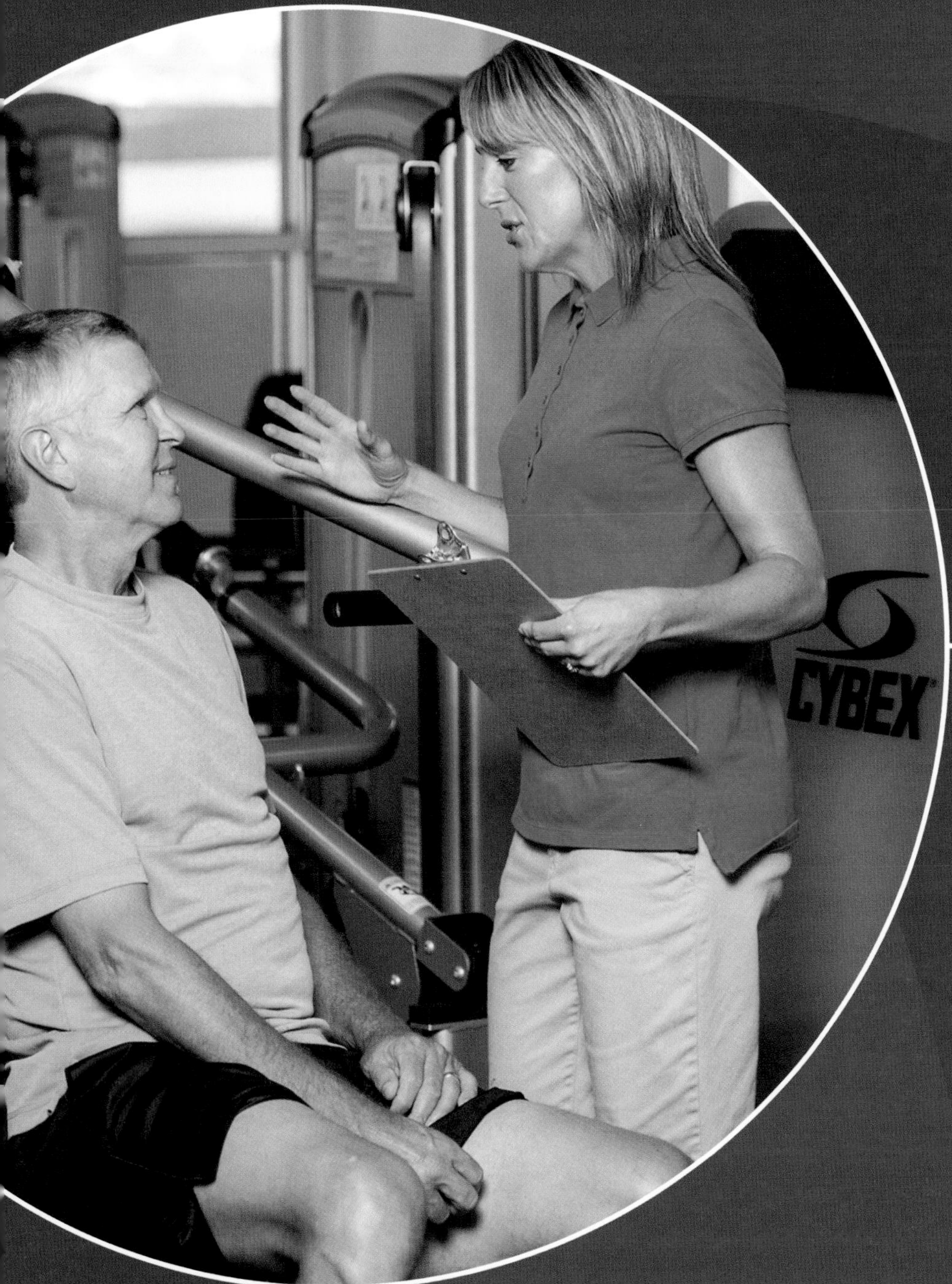

PART VI

The previous parts of this textbook covered assessment and exercise prescription for components of physical fitness for people with a variety of characteristics and health conditions. This section includes other elements needed for a comprehensive and effective fitness program. In chapter 23, we go over ways to help motivate people to adopt and maintain a healthy lifestyle. In chapter 24, we review analysis of the electrocardiogram (ECG) at rest and during exercise. Chapter 25 provides information on the prevention and treatment of injuries. Finally, in chapter 26 we describe important legal considerations for fitness professionals.

23

Behavior Change

Janet Buckworth

OBJECTIVES

The reader will be able to do the following:

1. Describe theories involved in healthy behavior change.
2. Discuss the role of motivation in exercise adoption and adherence, and identify behavioral strategies for enhancing motivation.
3. Describe six strategies that fitness professionals can use to monitor and support behavior change.
4. Describe ways to apply relapse prevention to exercise behavior.
5. Identify effective communication skills useful in motivating and fostering healthy behavior change.
6. Explain the effects of weight bias on the quality and effectiveness of individual interventions.

Translating the desire to change a health-related behavior into action is a challenge for most people. They may wish to be more active or to eat a healthier diet but may not have the knowledge, skills, or motivation to make the necessary behavior modifications and stick to them. To help people adopt and maintain a healthier lifestyle, the fitness professional should understand basic principles of behavior change and develop the skills to put those principles into practice.

This chapter begins with a brief description of theoretical models for explaining and predicting human behavior, in particular the transtheoretical model of behavior change (also known as the *stages of change model*) and self-determination theory (SDT). Methods and strategies are presented in the context of behavior change as a process, with suggestions for use based on readiness to change and the promotion of intrinsic motivation. For an excellent review of the transtheoretical model applied to exercise, refer to Prochaska and Marcus (17), and for SDT, see Teixeira and colleagues (23). Factors for fitness professionals to consider as they help participants move through each stage of the model are discussed along with strategies for enhancing intrinsic motivation to adopt and maintain healthy behaviors. Additional strategies and suggestions for interventions can be found in *ACSM's Behavioral Aspects of Physical Activity and Exercise* (16) and in *Motivating People to Be Physically Active* by Marcus and Forsyth (11). The last section in this chapter examines communication skills that fitness professionals should possess in order to motivate participants and foster healthy behavior change.

Theories of Behavior Change

Several theories guide strategies for changing exercise behavior, such as behavior modification, social cognitive theory, SDT, and the transtheoretical model of behavior change (1). Behavior modification theory is based on the assumption that behavior is learned and can be changed by modifying the antecedents (stimuli, cues) and consequences (rewards, punishments). A cue could be a flier listing the benefits of walking during lunch, and a reward could be a certificate presented to the aerobics participant with the best attendance. Social cognitive theory offers the view that behavior is influenced by the dynamic relationships among the person's characteristics, the environment, and the behavior itself. Someone training for a marathon would be more motivated than a novice fitness walker to exercise outside in the rain, but even the most dedicated marathoner would not run in a lightning storm. Finally, SDT is a theory of motivation that explains human behavior in respect to one's motivation for meeting basic needs (competency, autonomy, and relatedness). People may start exercising to lose weight but later train for a road race because they enjoy a sense of accomplishment from running. Although effective strategies for behavior change have been developed with these and other theories, most theories of behavior treat change as an all-or-none event. In other words, participants go from being sedentary to being regularly active in response to an intervention.

The transtheoretical model presents change as a dynamic process whereby attitudes, decisions, and actions evolve through stages over time. This model has been applied with some success to promoting exercise (26). The transtheoretical, or stages of change, model can help people think about, decide to begin, and continue an active lifestyle. SDT has gained popularity as a basis for understanding and promoting healthy behaviors by addressing the continuum of rewarding contingencies from external reinforcement to engagement simply for enjoyment and pleasure.

Transtheoretical Model

The **transtheoretical model** is a model of intentional behavior modification. Behavior change is a dynamic process that occurs through a series of interrelated stages that are mostly stable but open to change (18). This model emphasizes the individual's motivation, readiness to change, and personal history regarding the target behavior. For example, people who exercised successfully in the past would have more confidence in their ability to exercise again than would people who have been sedentary most of their lives. The problem with most interventions is that they are for people who are prepared to take action (17). According to the transtheoretical model, traditional strategies for participant recruitment will not affect people who are not ready to change. Different strategies must be used to persuade people to consider change and then motivate them to take action. Other approaches will be more effective in supporting adherence to the new behavior.

The transtheoretical model has two key components: stages of change (see *Transtheoretical Model Stages of Change*) and attitudes, beliefs, and skills for change (18). By evaluating the participant in respect to these factors, the fitness professional can design individually tailored and stage-specific interventions.

The *how* of behavior change in the transtheoretical model includes attitudes, beliefs, and behavioral skills that change as someone progresses through the stages. These change elements are self-efficacy, decisional balance, and processes of change.

- *Self-efficacy* is confidence in one's ability to engage in a positive behavior or abstain from an undesired behavior. Expectation of success is important in making the decision to change and in maintaining the new behavior. Types of self-efficacy include confidence to accomplish the elements of a task, which is important when beginning a new behavior, and confidence to overcome personal and environmental barriers (coping, barrier self-efficacy), which is important for adhering to the behavior.

- *Decisional balance* refers to evaluating and monitoring potential gains (pros, benefits) and losses (cons) arising from any decision. Perceived gains increase and perceived losses decrease in respect to the target behavior as the person moves through the stages of change.
- *Processes of change* are strategies used to change behavior. Experiential or cognitive processes are strategies that involve thoughts, attitudes, and awareness. Behavioral processes involve taking specific actions directed toward yourself or the environment. For example, seeking out information about the best exercise for losing weight is a cognitive process, and creating reminders to register for a water aerobics class is a behavioral process.

Self-Determination Theory

Self-determination theory (SDT) is a theory of human motivation developed by Deci and Ryan in the 1980s that has been applied to promoting exercise (3). According to this theory, humans are naturally inclined toward growth and development and have a set of universal psychological needs. Motivation to engage in activities results from the fundamental needs for competency, autonomy, and relatedness. Satisfying these three psychological needs will foster intrinsic motivation and therefore enhance positive behaviors and mental health as well as the persistence of healthy behaviors. SDT is based on the assumption that motivation to engage in a behavior falls on a continuum from extrinsic (avoiding negative consequences or gaining rewards outside of the particular behavior) to intrinsic (engaging in the behavior for enjoyment of the act itself). Behaviors that are more intrinsically motivated have a greater chance of persisting.

For example, two clients may both want to join a HIIT class, but one wants to lose weight and the other wants to spend time with friends in the class. The *what* is the same, but the *why* is the key to how long each will stick with the class. Losing weight is more extrinsic, and once the weight is lost, so is the reason for participating in the exercise class. Spending time with friends is associated with meeting the basic need for relatedness.

SDT is based on the assumptions that human beings are active in controlling their lives and naturally inclined toward growth and development (3). *Self-determination* describes the motivation for intentional behavior that comes from the person. Motivation stems from efforts to meet the basic psychological needs of autonomy, competence, and relatedness. Deci and Ryan (3) proposed that these needs are universal and vary in terms of self-determination from intrinsic, in which motive for a task is determined (regulated) by the person, to extrinsic, in which the motive is determined (regulated) by others or outside influences. Thus, behavioral regulation is the degree to which behavior is perceived to be regulated or controlled by oneself. Regulation can be more external, such as joining a swimming class because a physical therapist recommended non-weight-bearing exercise, or more internally regulated, such as when someone runs faster simply because it feels good. The more internal the regulation is, the greater sense of personal choice, or autonomy.

BASIC NEEDS ACCORDING TO SELF-DETERMINATION THEORY

- Autonomy—to be the causal agent of one's own life
- Competence—to experience mastery
- Relatedness—to interact, be connected to, and experience caring for others

Transtheoretical Model Stages of Change

1. *Precontemplation:* In this stage, the individual is not seriously thinking about changing an unhealthy behavior in the next 6 mo or is denying the need to change.
2. *Contemplation:* The individual is seriously thinking about changing an unhealthy behavior within the next 6 mo.
3. *Preparation:* This is a transitional stage in which the individual intends to take action within the next month. Some plans have been made, and the individual tries to determine what to do next.
4. *Action:* This stage is the 6 mo following the overt modification of an unhealthy behavior. Motivation and investment in behavior change are sufficient in this stage, but it is the busiest and least stable stage and has the highest risk of relapse.
5. *Maintenance:* Maintenance begins after the individual has successfully adhered to the healthy behavior for 6 mo. The longer someone stays in maintenance, the lower the risk of relapse.

Applying Theories to Promote Healthy Behaviors

The transtheoretical model is applied to exercise by matching or targeting the appropriate intervention strategy to the person's physical activity history and readiness for change (18) (see table 23.1). For example, the goal in working with people in the precontemplation stage is to get them to begin thinking about changing their level of physical activity. Discussing information from a fitness test or HRA followed by education about personal benefits of physical activity is an appropriate strategy for participants in the precontemplation stage. The goal with people in the contemplation stage is to motivate them and help them prepare to take action. They would benefit from learning about the pros of exercise coupled with accurate, easy-to-understand information about how they can start an exercise program or begin to be more active. Someone in the preparation stage is doing some exercise but realizes that it is not enough and needs help setting up a personalized exercise program. There is awareness of the benefits of exercise, but there are still barriers that must be resolved. Whereas participants in the contemplation stage may not be ready to set goals, those in the preparation stage are ready to set goals and get a personalized exercise prescription.

Participants in the action stage are participating in regular activity, but exercise is not a habit. They are at a high risk of relapsing into a more familiar, inactive lifestyle. Relapse prevention, which is discussed later, can help keep them on track to the maintenance stage. Movement from the action stage to the maintenance stage follows a decrease in the risk of relapse and an increase in self-efficacy. Helpful strategies include periodic reevaluations of goals and updates of plans for coping with life events such as travel, inclement weather, or medical events that can disrupt regular exercise.

KEY POINT

The transtheoretical model addresses the dynamic nature of behavior change. Practitioners apply this model by selecting interventions based on characteristics of the participant, environment, and stage of change. Interventions should match the stage the individual is in and address self-efficacy and perceptions of benefits and costs of exercise (see table 23.1). Understanding motivation and using concepts from SDT involves distinguishing between what clients want (i.e., the content of goals or aspirations) and why they want this (i.e., the regulatory reasons). According to SDT, behaviors that meet basic needs are more likely to be sustained. Behaviors that people engage in for less intrinsic reasons are less stable.

Promoting Exercise in Sedentary and Low-Active Individuals

A variety of strategies and programs can be used to motivate people to consider becoming more active and adopt regular exercise. These approaches are based on understanding the knowledge, attitudes, beliefs, and behavioral skills that foster adoption of a regular exercise program and understanding the person's motivational orientation to exercise. Specific factors related to promoting the adoption

Table 23.1 Intervention Strategies for the Stages of Change

Stage of change	Intervention strategies
Precontemplation	Implement a media campaign promoting exercise, educate about personal benefits of exercise, foster values clarification, conduct HRAs and fitness testing
Contemplation	Market benefits of exercise, foster self- and environmental reevaluation, provide clear and specific guidelines for starting an exercise program, be a positive role model, identify social support for exercise
Preparation	Conduct psychosocial and fitness assessments, evaluate supports/benefits and barriers/costs, design personalized exercise prescription, set goals, develop behavioral contracts, teach time management skills
Action	Identify social support for maintaining exercise, set up stimulus control, teach self-reinforcement, implement self-efficacy enhancement strategies, set goals, teach self-monitoring, employ relapse prevention
Maintenance	Encourage new activities with others, reinforce self-regulatory skills, review and revise goals, introduce cross-training, conduct periodic fitness testing

of regular exercise are presented next, followed by a review of strategies to market exercise and increase motivation.

Encouraging the Inactive and Unmotivated

People in precontemplation are sedentary and have no plans to start exercising. They may be in this stage because they lack information about the long-term personal consequences of physical inactivity. They also may be demoralized from previous unsuccessful attempts to stick with an exercise program and may have low self-efficacy for exercise. People in the precontemplation stage may feel defensive about their lifestyle because of social pressures to be physically active. They have no personally compelling reasons to change, and the costs of exercising seem to outweigh the benefits. Given these attitudes and beliefs, the clients' perceptions about the benefits of exercise should be strengthened and the costs reduced. Activities to help people develop a personal value for exercise and information about the role of exercise in a healthy lifestyle are useful in moving people to the next stage (11).

Sedentary individuals move to the contemplation stage because of information that is convincing, personal, and timely (12). Contemplators are planning to become more physically active, but they are still ambivalent about changing. For them, the costs of starting to exercise outweigh the perceived benefits. Experiences and information that support the contemplator's desire and motivation to exercise and counter perceived costs and barriers can initiate the move to preparation. Exposure to physically active role models, enhancement of perceived benefits, and strengthening of psychosocial variables such as self-efficacy for exercise are other factors that influence exercise adoption. The cognitive processes of change, such as increasing knowledge about the health benefits of regular exercise and being aware of how one's inactivity affects others, are critical in these early stages of change.

Although initial motivation for starting exercise is often tied to achieving goals that are a consequence of the behavior, such as weight loss or rehabilitation from an injury, many novices exercise primarily because they know they should. Being physically active keeps them from feeling guilty. Behavior that is regulated to avoid guilt through self-imposed pressure can be the spark that gets someone active, but to sustain the behavior, motivation needs to be more self-determined. Linking exercise with improved health or with other highly valued behaviors, such as playing with grandchildren, can move the person to internal regulation.

Influencing Motivation and Action for Exercise Adoption

People in the preparation stage may be doing some exercise, but not enough to meet health and fitness guidelines. The fitness professional's goal is to help them become more intrinsically motivated and move to the action stage and regular exercise. The aim is to shift motivation from avoiding guilt at one end of the continuum to exercising because of consistency with personal values or for pleasure at the other end. A thorough assessment of personal, social, and environmental factors that support the person's current level of activity can be particularly useful. A comprehensive assessment can establish physical fitness, motivation, goals, supports, barriers, and other factors to consider when developing a specific plan for change and implementing strategies. Behavioral strategies come into play more as someone begins to move from the preparation stage. Goal setting, behavioral contracts, and time management

Motivational Principles From Self-Determination Theory

Fitness professionals can nurture participants' exercise motivation by setting up exercise tasks to develop a sense of mastery (competence), making sure they have a say in their exercise program (autonomy), and helping them feel connected to others in the exercise setting (relatedness). Teixeira and colleagues published a comprehensive review of SDT-based intervention strategies and concluded that fostering more autonomous forms of motivation can promote enduring exercise (23). Other examples of strategies to foster autonomy—that is, a greater sense of choice and control—include providing information for more informed choices, encouraging choice and self-initiation, and providing options. The fitness professional can make sure that clients on the fence about adopting an active lifestyle know about types of activities available to them, such as walking clubs, dance classes, and videos, and that they understand they are the ones who get to choose what they want to do. Behavior that is consistent with values, goals, and lifestyle is also more intrinsically motivated and likely to be sustained. For example, reframing exercise to be something that fits with a client's priorities, such as supporting the community, can put working on a community garden in a whole new light and shift meaningful physical activity into part of the client's identity.

training are practical strategies to use with participants in the preparation stage, and information from an assessment will help tailor an intervention to the person's needs and situation.

Personal Influences

Individual characteristics that influence the initiation of exercise include demographics, activity history, past experiences, perception of health status, perception of access to facilities, time, enjoyment of exercise, aptitudes, beliefs, self-motivation, and self-efficacy (24). Higher education, higher income, gender (male), and younger age are positively associated with level of physical activity (24). Exercise history is an important factor in current level of physical activity. Past participation is li nked with physical activity in supervised exercise programs and in treatment programs for patients with CHD and obesity (4). Past exercise experience also can influence expectations about exercise and self-efficacy, and high exercise self-efficacy is associated with increased exercise participation.

Motivation is another variable influencing exercise adoption. Motivation depends on expectations for future benefits or outcomes from exercise, such as good health, improved appearance, social outlets, stress management, enjoyment, and opportunities for competition (13). It also varies in degree of self-determination (e.g., autonomy, personal choice)—intrinsic motivation is the most self-determined, whereas extrinsic motivation is based on satisfying others or on the consequences of the behavior.

Self-motivation for exercise is the ability to continue an exercise program without the benefit of external reinforcement. Participants high in self-motivation are probably good at goal setting, monitoring exercise progress, and self-reinforcement (21) and are high in intrinsic motivation. People with little self-motivation may need more external reinforcement and encouragement (e.g., group activities and social support) to adopt and adhere to exercise, but even people with high intrinsic motivation can benefit from social support.

Perceived behavioral control is significantly correlated with the intention to exercise (5). If participants believe they have more control over the exercise and have choices about when and how to exercise, they are more likely to begin a program. It follows that participants who set their own goals will have a greater chance of success than if goals are assigned to them (10), and they will be more likely to meet the need for autonomy.

Social Influences

Social support involves comfort, assistance, and information provided by individuals or groups. Practical help, such as providing problem-solving tips or a ride to the fitness facility, can result in tangible benefits to the participant, but emotional support also plays a key role. For example, emotional support (encouragement and expressions of care, concern, and sympathy) could be helpful when a participant is emotionally stressed. Other types of emotional support include esteem support (reassurance of worth, expressions of liking or confidence in the other person), network support (expressions of connection and belonging), and even informational support (information and advice). Exercising with a group can also meet the need for relatedness described by SDT.

Social support for exercise from family, friends, and physicians is usually associated with physical activity (24). Spouses appear to provide a consistent, positive influence on exercise participation; in one study, people who joined a fitness center with their spouse had better adherence and lower dropout rates than married people who joined without a spouse (25). Group factors may be particularly important for older adults and people who are motivated to exercise primarily for social reinforcement.

Environmental Influences

Research has shown that social support, environmental prompts, and convenience are factors in exercise adoption (2). Environments that have easily accessible facilities with few real or perceived barriers make it easier to sustain an exercise program. Posters, e-mails, texts, self-sticking

RESEARCH INSIGHT

Social Support in Women's Exercise Adherence

Social support plays a big role in exercise adherence, especially for women. In a 12 mo social support intervention with sedentary postpartum Latinas, 139 women were randomized to an attention control group or an intervention of walking plus social support (6). Women in the intervention received various types of support, such as practical assistance (e.g., offering child care or strollers so they could walk with their babies) and emotional support (e.g., encouragement) (6). Women attended weekly sessions for 12 wk, and physical, psychological, and behavioral variables were measured at baseline, 6 mo, and 12 mo. The authors found that social support was effective at increasing physical activity during the intervention but not afterward. Beyond support, the environment (e.g., safety) was suggested as a factor in sustaining physical activity in these women.

notes, visibly located exercise equipment, and attractive bike and walking paths are environmental attributes that also serve as cues for exercise.

The convenience of exercise is influenced by the sequence, or chain, of behaviors that must be accomplished for the person to complete each exercise session. The longer and more complicated the behavior chain, the more barriers there are to exercise. For example, there is a greater potential for a break in the link if a person must leave work, drive home, gather exercise clothes, drive to a facility, park, sign in, and change clothes to walk on a treadmill than if the person walks around the neighborhood first thing in the morning. For many people, exercising in the morning may be easier to stick with than exercising during the day, when numerous demands compete for time.

Researchers and practitioners recognize that the physical environment powerfully influences the level of physical activity in communities. For example, accessible, attractive, and safe places to walk, bike, or run can make physical activity more appealing and convenient. Certainly, workout facilities that are clean, are well ventilated, and have a good selection of equipment and adequate parking will be more enticing to novice exercisers compared with poorly maintained or managed fitness centers.

RESEARCH INSIGHT

Location Effects on Physical Activity Behavior

The physical environment is the context in which many fitness professionals must provide guidance and support for regular physical activity. McCormack and Shiell (15) conducted a systematic review of the relationship between the built environment and physical activity. Factors commonly considered included street and pedestrian connectivity, land-use mix (i.e., are shops, housing, and workplaces close together?), recreation proximity, transit proximity and access, population density, employment density, aesthetics, parks, traffic, neighborhood type, pedestrian and cyclist amenities, and trails, pathways, bike paths, and sidewalks. They found that street and pedestrian connectivity, pedestrian density, mixed land use, walkability, and neighborhood type were associated with more activity, and generally, built environment was more supportive of walking and cycling than other types of activity. This is important for the fitness professional to keep in mind when recommending walking for fitness—location makes a difference!

Marketing and Motivational Strategies for Early Stages of Change

The goal of fitness professionals may be to help people maintain regular exercise, but they may also be called on to promote regular exercise to people who are inconsistently active (i.e., preparation stage) or have not yet considered starting a fitness program (i.e., precontemplation stage). For example, the primary goal of a media campaign may be to capture the attention of inactive people and motivate them to contemplate beginning an exercise program or another healthy behavior. This might involve putting informational prompts at the point of decision to act, such as hanging catchy posters next to elevators encouraging people to take the stairs (8) (see figure 23.1). Bulletin boards, pamphlets, fliers, handouts, websites, and other media with upbeat information about the benefits of exercise and practical suggestions for increasing physical activity can also catch the attention of potential exercisers. Handing out passes at local restaurants for an aerobics class is a proactive form of recruitment. Fun runs and walks supporting charities may motivate people who primarily want to help the organization to begin thinking about exercise for its own sake. Wellness fairs, HRAs, and fitness testing in communities and at work sites can also prompt contemplation and enhance motivation to become more active.

To increase participation in the early stages of behavior change, the fitness professional's role is to provide education about benefits of being physically active, to describe

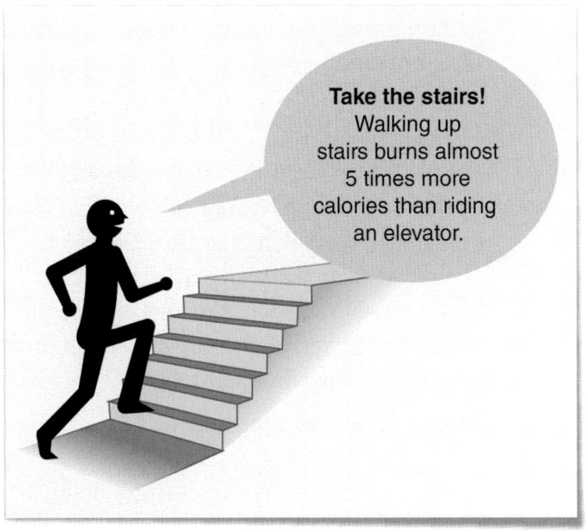
Take the stairs!
Walking up stairs burns almost 5 times more calories than riding an elevator.

FIGURE 23.1 This sign is an example of a point-of-decision prompt to take the stairs.

how to exercise sensibly, and to offer encouragement to follow through with a personal exercise program. Specific strategies to increase adoption and early adherence are recommended (2, 12, 17):

- Ask participants about their exercise history. They may need accurate information to dispel myths (e.g., the myth of no pain, no gain) and to develop positive attitudes about exercise.
- Explore ways exercise can benefit them personally. Find out what they think they will get out of being physically active and provide information and resources about additional benefits.
- Help participants develop knowledge, attitudes, beliefs, and skills to support the behavior change. In addition to providing information and training in self-management skills, the fitness professional may use cognitive restructuring to identify discouraging thoughts and replace them with positive statements (see *Cognitive Restructuring: Reframe Negative Statements Into Positive Statements*).
- Bolster the participant's exercise self-efficacy and sense of competency with success-producing learning experiences. There are four sources of information that contribute to self-efficacy beliefs and can be addressed by the fitness professional:

    1. *Mastery experiences.* These experiences include behavioral rehearsal with proper supervision and positive feedback. The fitness professional can make sure participants have chosen activities that are appropriate for their fitness and skill level so they can experience a sense of accomplishment when they exercise. Practical feedback will also help participants be successful and thus feel more confident. In addition, an increased sense of competency is motivating. We like to do things we are good at!
    2. *Verbal persuasion or self-persuasion.* Suggesting to people that they can succeed in behaviors they have not been successful in previously and giving specific feedback to help enhance their skills and foster success will promote self-efficacy. The fitness professional can provide verbal encouragement and teach participants positive self-talk.
    3. *Modeling.* Observing others can serve as a guide to performing a specific behavior. When people see someone successfully doing what they have little confidence to do, they start to expect that they, too, can succeed. The fitness professional can set up situations in which participants see someone like themselves succeed (e.g., post a newspaper story about seniors who now exercise regularly) or watch a peer who has trouble with the task succeed (e.g., point out to a new participant that "Lynette also had difficulty jogging three miles when she first started the program, but after months of hard work, she has now reached her goal!").
    4. *Interpretations of physiological and emotional responses.* Physiological arousal associated with a behavior can be stressful and contribute to lower self-efficacy for that behavior. The typical increased HR, respiration, and muscle tension that occur during exercise may make novices feel anxious or uncomfortable and less confident. The fitness professional can make sure that participants have information about the normal physiological responses to exercise and know how to interpret their physiological responses accurately.

- Clarify expectations and make sure they are reasonable and realistic. Use guidelines for goal setting to ensure initial successes.
- Identify potential barriers to behavior change and brainstorm with the participant about ways to overcome these barriers. Barriers can be personal (low exercise self-efficacy), physical (past injuries), interpersonal (peer pressure from sedentary friends to engage in sedentary behaviors instead of exercising), or environmental (inclement weather or lack of transportation to an exercise facility). For example, one person may want to exercise but does not have access to facilities and another person may think she does not have the willpower to stick with a program. The first person would be helped with a home exercise program, whereas the second would benefit from social support and reconsidering discouraging thoughts.
- Foster motivation to adopt and maintain an exercise program. Set up incentives to exercise. Incentives can be tangible (e.g., T-shirts, certificates, water bottles, recognition on a bulletin board) or intangible (e.g., sense of competence, enjoyment). Tangible incentives are useful early in a program, but intrinsic motivation is associated with better adherence (20). Offer a variety of incentives, but focus on fostering more intrinsic and self-regulated motivation, such as a sense of accomplishment or enjoyment. Strategies to increase motivation are listed in *Motivational Strategies*.

Cognitive Restructuring: Reframe Negative Statements Into Positive Statements

Negative Statements

- I'm never going to get in shape.
- I'm fatter than everyone else in the class.
- I've tried to stay with exercise and each time I fail.
- It's impossible to find time to exercise with my schedule.

Positive Statements

- Change takes time. I didn't get out of shape overnight, and I am making progress bit by bit.
- Everyone has to start somewhere. Other people have worked long and hard to get where they are.
- Every time I begin a new exercise program, I get closer to sticking with it for good.
- I can take a little time for myself to exercise every day because I deserve it. I'm the one in control.

Motivational Strategies

- Provide positive, practical behavioral feedback.
- Encourage group participation and group support to offer the opportunity for social reinforcement, camaraderie, and commitment and to meet the need for relatedness.
- Recruit partner and peers to support the behavioral change.
- Make the program enjoyable.
- When using music, make it upbeat, positive, and matched to the client's preferences.
- Provide a flexible routine to decrease boredom and increase interest and enjoyment. Consider activities such as games and backpacking as alternatives to traditional exercise modes to provide a variety of exercise options.
- Provide periodic exercise testing to show progress toward goals, increase a sense of competency, and offer an opportunity for positive reinforcement.
- Use strategies for behavioral change, such as personal goal setting, contracts, and self-management, to foster personal control and perceived competency, and emphasize goals that are meaningful to the participant.
- Chart progress using record cards, graphs, or software applications. Note and record progress daily to give immediate, positive feedback. Encourage self-monitoring.
- Recognize goal achievement in newsletters, websites, and bulletin boards. Individual effort increases when that effort is identifiable.
- Set up group or individual competitions.
- Offer lotteries based on individual or group accomplishment of a specific goal. Set a winning criterion (such as the first person to walk a certain distance each week for 5 wk wins) for which the winner is featured in a newsletter or gets money that each participant has contributed. An alternative is to set a criterion (e.g., attending 20 of 24 aerobic classes) for participation in a random drawing.
- Organize teams to train for a charity-sponsored fun run or road race.

KEY POINT

Individual, social, and environmental factors motivate people to move from not thinking about starting an exercise program to setting up a plan to begin. A variety of strategies can be used, from mass-media campaigns to fitness testing, to motivate people to move from contemplation into the preparation and action stages. Six strategies to facilitate adopting and maintaining exercise are to (1) ask participants about exercise history and use what you learn to set up a personalized plan; (2) help participants develop knowledge, attitudes, beliefs, and skills to support behavior change; (3) bolster self-efficacy; (4) involve participants in setting clear and realistic goals; (5) identify and resolve barriers to change; and (6) foster multiple motivators for exercise that have purpose and meaning for participants.

Enhancing Sustained Motivation and Behavioral Adherence

Various strategies have been discussed to illustrate principles of behavior change and to describe ways to market and motivate exercise. Once a participant has started an exercise program (action stage), the fitness professional plays an important role in monitoring and supporting the establishment and maintenance of regular exercise. For example, the fitness professional and the participant should work together to set goals that are consistent with capabilities, values, resources, and needs. Exercise self-efficacy predicts adoption and maintenance, and it can be increased with mastery experiences, which also help meet the need for competency. Thus, initial goals should be challenging but certain to be met, which will foster increased exercise self-efficacy. The fitness professional and participant also should evaluate environmental and social supports and barriers and use this information to determine ways to manage barriers in order to promote the new behavior, enhance coping strategies, and lessen the influence of perceived barriers.

Assessment

Regardless of the intervention, comprehensive fitness and psychosocial assessments are necessary to select and carry out the appropriate strategies of behavior change for participants in the preparation and early action stages. Reassessment should be conducted periodically to evaluate the effectiveness of the plan.

First, the problem must be identified and defined in behavioral terms. For example, the focus on being overweight is shifted to the behaviors—overeating and underexercising—that contributed to weight gain. The fitness professional can also help the participant decide what can be realistically changed and what cannot.

Next, examine past attempts at behavior change. Find out what worked, what did not, and why. This information will be useful in setting goals and identifying high-risk situations (see the section on relapse prevention later in this chapter).

Also, find out if initiation of the behavior change is voluntary or recommended by someone else. This will give a sense of the participant's motivation and commitment to change. Participants who are there because a doctor prescribed exercise may need help finding self-determined motives for exercising. There are many reasons for beginning an exercise program (e.g., health, weight loss, anxiety reduction), but the initial motivation may not be why someone continues to exercise. Most often, people start exercising to achieve an outcome of exercise or to avoid guilt (extrinsic motivation) rather than for personal enjoyment, expression of creativity, or demonstration of mastery (intrinsic motivation). Extrinsic motivation can be useful to get people started, but research has shown that developing intrinsic motivation for exercise is necessary for long-term maintenance. Ask participants what they expect to get out of exercise and be prepared to pique their interest by presenting additional short- and long-term benefits.

Another useful assessment tool is the decisional balance sheet. The participant lists all short- and long-term consequences, positive and negative, of both changing and not changing the behavior. The participant and the fitness professional then brainstorm ways to avoid or cope with the projected negative consequences of behavior change while also emphasizing and building upon perceived benefits.

Self-Monitoring

Part of the assessment process can be accomplished by self-monitoring, in which the participant records information about the target behavior and also indicates thoughts, feelings, and situations before, during, and after the behavior. The participant can identify the internal and external cues and behavioral consequences that inhibit and prompt exercise. Barriers and supports also become evident with self-monitoring. The fitness professional can help the participant develop strategies to cope with the barriers and use the supports. The chain of behaviors encompassing exercise can also be evaluated and weak links identified. For example, if the participant discovers she always skips her 5:30 a.m. aerobics class when she oversleeps and doesn't have time to pack her workout clothes before she leaves for work, you can suggest that she pack her workout bag the night before. Immediate benefits and reinforcements tailored to individual preferences can also be established at critical links in the chain (e.g., if she packs her workout bag the night before, she can push the snooze button for an extra 10 min of sleep the next morning). Tablets, computer programs, calendars, graphs, and charts can be used for self-monitoring as part of the initial assessment and as a way to record progress. Exercise tracking apps are also available for smartphones and other handheld devices, making self-monitoring more convenient than ever.

Time Management

The number one reason most people give for not exercising or for stopping a regular exercise program is lack of time (2). This is a reason we can all understand, but is the real reason that they don't have enough motivation or enough skills to manage the available time? Though fitness professionals want to be empathetic in response to life's demands, they need to help clients identify the underpinnings of their reason for not becoming or staying active. The fitness professional can help the client identify how time is a barrier and then choose appropriate interventions, such as modification of an exercise schedule or referral to a time management class.

Self-monitoring is an important strategy for getting at the root of the time problem, and there are a number of electronic tools that can relieve the burden of recording with paper and pencil. When people keep a diary of how they spend their time for at least a week, the payoffs are worth the effort. First, reviewing the diary with the client provides a sense of how much and when discretionary time is available. The goal is to free up blocks of time when the client can be physically active while at the same time accomplishing other necessary tasks. Flexibility in an exercise program (e.g., classes offered at many times, a lunchtime walking group) can also help with time problems. Accumulating several shorter bouts of exercise throughout the day may be another effective strategy. In addition, finding patterns in how tasks are organized can reveal ways to be more efficient. For example, fixing lunch during TV commercial breaks the night before can free up 15 to 20 min for a brisk walk before work in the morning. Task priorities can also be identified and time blocked out to protect that time from interruptions. For example, setting aside time for social media after studying for an exam can eliminate extra time spent repeatedly settling in where you left off.

Goal Setting

The purpose of **goal setting** is to accomplish a specific task in a specific time frame. Goals can be as simple and time limited as making a sandwich for lunch and as complicated and encompassing as earning an advanced degree. Goal setting provides a plan of action that focuses and directs activity and emphasizes a clear link between behavior and outcome.

Goals should be behavioral, specific, and measurable. Plans are easier to make if the goal is stated in behavioral terms. For example, a goal of walking 4 days per wk for 30 to 45 min is easier to implement than a goal to get in shape. Specific, measurable goals make it easier to monitor progress, make adjustments, and know when the goal has been accomplished.

Goals also must be reasonable and realistic. A goal might be achievable, but personal and situational constraints can make it unrealistic. Losing 2 lb · wk^{-1} (0.9 kg · wk^{-1}) through diet and exercise is reasonable for many people, but it may be almost impossible for the working parent of three who has minimal time for exercise and cooking. Unrealistic goals set the participant up to fail, which can damage self-efficacy and adherence to the program for behavior change. By using information from the assessment and self-monitoring, the fitness professional can help participants set positive, realistic behavioral goals based on their age, sex, fitness, health, interests, exercise history, skills, and schedule. Both short-term and long-term goals should be included. Short-term goals mobilize effort and direct present actions, but both short- and long-term goals lead to a more effective plan of action (10) (see *Characteristics of Effective Goals*).

CHARACTERISTICS OF EFFECTIVE GOALS

- Behavioral: Aim for actions, such as lifting weights, rather than outcomes, such as losing weight.
- Flexible: Absolute goals can set someone up for a sense of failure if the goal is not met, whereas planning to jog or cycle 4 to 5 days per wk, for instance, allows for options to work around the unexpected.
- Specific: Make the goal absolutely clear. For example, walking 3 mi (4.8 km) without stopping is much more specific than simply working out.
- Measurable: Be able to quantify the goal in miles, minutes, reps, and so on.
- Reasonable: Goals should be practical and achievable—in other words, are they possible?
- Realistic: The outcome should stand a good chance of happening based on the person's circumstances and the amount of effort required.
- Challenging: The goal should be difficult enough to be challenging but not overwhelming.
- Meaningful: The goals should be important to the participant.
- Reward for specific accomplishments: Set up benchmarks with rewards. For example, buy a new music album after completing a yoga course.

- Have a time frame: Establish a time frame for short- and long-term goals.
- Designate the situation: When, where, and under what conditions will the participant engage in the target behavior?

RESEARCH INSIGHT

Effects of Short-Term Process Goals

Goal setting is an essential strategy for exercise behavior change and adherence, and the importance of short-term process goals for fostering intrinsic motivation and adherence was demonstrated by Wilson and Brookfield (27). They conducted a 6 wk intervention based on SDT to examine the impact of goal setting and motivation on adherence. Sixty adult recreational exercisers were randomly assigned to one of three groups: process goal (weekly goals related to behavior, such as maintaining THR or pace), outcome goal (goal to achieve by the end of 6 wk), and no goal (control group). Intrinsic motivation (interest and enjoyment, perceived choice, and pressure and tension [negative indicator]) was measured at the beginning and end of the intervention and 3 mo and 6 mo later. The process-goal group had greater increases in interest, enjoyment, and perceived choice and better adherence than the other groups after the intervention and at each follow-up assessment. The outcome-goal group had lower perceived choice and higher pressure and tension than the control group, implying that using only an outcome goal may be detrimental to motivation and success.

Reinforcement

Social **reinforcement** and self-reinforcement are crucial in the action phase, especially because the longer someone has been inactive before starting to exercise, the longer it takes until exercise itself becomes reinforcing. Immediate consequences of exercise can be soreness and fatigue, so external, immediate, positive rewards are necessary for beginners. Monitoring progress is rewarding and can involve charting miles walked after each session or asking for feedback from instructors after a difficult exercise class. Positive reinforcement from others can enhance self-efficacy, especially when feedback comes from people who are important to the participant. Praise is more effective if it is immediate and behaviorally specific (7). "You worked hard in class last week" is not as effective as "You did a great job getting through all the leg lifts today," especially if the participant has been struggling with leg lifts.

Self-reinforcement should involve rewards that are important to the participant. Using special spa soaps and creams only after an aerobic workout and getting tickets to the big game after logging a certain number of miles are rewards that are personalized and self-administered.

Social support can be verbal or tangible, such as transportation to exercise class. It can come from the class instructor, exercise partners, family members, and so on. Significant others must be involved in the exercise plan and educated about the differences between support and nagging. Constructive verbal feedback, praise, encouragement, and positive attention will help a family member stick with exercise, whereas punishing comments, jokes about the person's efforts, and discouraging social comparisons can hinder adherence. Support focuses on what has been accomplished ("You're being consistent in your walking to lose weight. I'm proud of you."), whereas nagging harps on what has not been accomplished ("You should walk faster to lose weight. Why can't you pick up the pace?").

Friends in an exercise program can provide both social support and cues to exercise. They can be positive role models to enhance self-efficacy and part of a buddy system to support the exercise effort. Some participants are more likely to stick with a program if they know someone else is counting on them to be there to work out. Being part of an exercise group can also help participants feel connected to others and support the basic need for relatedness (from SDT).

Behavioral Contracts

Behavioral contracts are written, signed, public agreements to engage in specific goal-directed behaviors, and they have been used effectively to increase exercise adherence (2, 4). Contracts should include clear, realistic objectives and deadlines. Developing a contract engages the participant in a way that is motivating, challenging, and public. The public nature of contracts is especially important because public goals are more likely to be met compared with private or semiprivate goals (10). Having the participant make decisions about the nature of the contract fosters a sense of autonomy and can contribute to intrinsic motivation.

Contracts can be set by individuals or groups. The benefits of a group contract include the feeling it gives participants about not wanting to let others down and the desire to be part of a group. Individual contracts, however, can be tailored to the participant's specific situation and goals.

Consequences of meeting and not meeting the contracted goals should be clear and relevant to the participant. Contingency reinforcement can be set up so that the participant agrees to do a low-preference activity (e.g., squats) before a high-preference activity (e.g., sauna). Material and extrinsic reinforcers may be necessary initially but should become limited as natural reinforcers develop, such as social reinforcement. Inherent benefits of exercise, such as enjoyment and a sense of accomplishment, can foster more intrinsic motivation and better adherence, as can fostering a sense of autonomy, relatedness, and mastery through the goal-setting process. A sample behavioral contract for a middle-aged woman starting a walking program is shown in form 23.1.

FORM 23.1 Behavioral Contract

Goal: To walk 10,000 steps each day for a full week

Time frame: By the first week in June

Benefits of meeting the goal: Have more energy, lose weight, take my mind off stress at work, lower my risk for heart disease, and be a better role model for my children.

When I walk 10,000 steps a day for a full week (target behavior), I will go shopping at the outlet mall all day (reward).

THINGS I WILL DO TO REACH MY GOAL

1. Wear my pedometer every day and record daily steps in my diary.
2. Walk for at least 20 min during my lunch break and 20 min after supper.
3. Take the stairs at work instead of the elevator.
4. Walk around the field during my daughter's soccer practice.

GOAL-SUPPORTING ACTIVITIES

1. Keep a spare pair of walking shoes and exercise clothes at work.
2. Ask my husband to walk with me after dinner.
3. Tell my friends at work about my plan.
4. Create some upbeat playlists to listen to on my mobile device while I walk.
5. Use the list of step values for various exercises my fitness instructor gave me so I can add my water aerobics to my daily steps.

BARRIERS AND COUNTERMEASURES

1. Forget my pedometer: I will estimate my steps from other days with similar levels of walking and other activities.
2. Snow and ice: I will walk on the treadmill.
3. Fatigue: I will remind myself that a short, brisk walk is better than no walk.

MY FIRST SHORT-TERM GOAL

I will wear my pedometer for at least 5 days this week and record my steps each night before I go to sleep. This will help me see how many more steps I have to walk to achieve 10,000 each day.

Signed ________________________________ Date____________

Fitness professional ________________________________ Date____________

This contract will be evaluated every 2 weeks:

Date____________ Revisions________________________________

Date____________ Revisions________________________________

From E.T. Howley and D.L. Thompson, 2017, *Fitness professional's handbook*, 7th ed. (Champaign, IL: Human Kinetics).

Relapse Prevention

Over time, most people experience lapses in absolute adherence to an exercise program. The cyclical nature of long-term adherence to behavior change is addressed by the relapse prevention model (22). The relapse prevention model is based on relapses in alcohol abuse, smoking, and drug abuse; the goal is to decrease a high-frequency, undesired behavior. This model is best applied to voluntary behavior. Although exercise is voluntary, the goal is to increase and maintain a low-frequency, desired behavior. Even so, the concepts and techniques of relapse prevention can be used with exercise adherence (9, 23).

Relapse occurs when people who have been exercising regularly or engaging in other positive health behaviors stop the healthy behavior and go back to the old, unhealthy behavior. It is important to understand the concept of relapse as it applies to exercise because relapse is likely for many people, especially if they don't have many coping skills, such as positive self-talk or good time management. The fitness professional must help participants understand that relapse does not mean failure. Together, they can devise strategies to cope with temporary setbacks in the fitness program and foster an arsenal of coping strategies.

KEY POINT

Assessment is an important first step in the action stage of behavior change. Self-monitoring is useful in determining the antecedents and consequences of the target behavior as well as the potential costs of and barriers to behavior change. Strategies such as goal setting and behavioral contracts must be tailored to the individual and should be reevaluated regularly during the maintenance stage. Some of the variables that influence exercise maintenance are enjoyment, motivation, convenience, exercise intensity, program flexibility, social support, and skills such as self-regulation and self-reinforcement.

Defining High-Risk Situations

Relapse begins with a **high-risk situation** that challenges an individual's perceived ability to maintain the desired behavioral change. High-risk situations can be bad weather, stress at work, boredom, fatigue, and social situations. A wedding reception with all her favorite foods can be a high-risk situation for a dieter, and weekend guests can challenge a jogger's motivation to keep up with his afternoon runs. People are predisposed to high-risk situations if they have a lifestyle imbalance in which *shoulds* exceed *wants*. This imbalance leads to feelings of deprivation and desires for indulgence. Rationalization, denial, and apparently irrelevant decisions can then occur (9).

Successful coping in a high-risk situation leads to increased self-efficacy and decreased probability of relapse. Not coping or inadequate coping leads to decreased self-efficacy and positive expectations about not maintaining the behavior change (e.g., being able to eat like so-called normal people, having more time to spend with friends). If this leads to a slipup, the abstinence violation effect (or for exercise, the adherence violation effect) occurs in which participants perceive that they have failed. All-or-none thinking, such as the belief that you cannot skip a weekend of jogging and still be a jogger, makes the participant more susceptible to this effect. Feelings of failure lead to self-blame, lowered self-esteem, guilt, perceived loss of control, increased probability of relapse, and possibly giving up (9).

Fostering Coping Strategies for Exercise

Relapse prevention, as described by Marlatt and Gordon (14), is a method used to identify and deal with high-risk situations. The strategy begins by educating people about the relapse process and enlisting their help as active participants in preventing a relapse. The next step for the fitness professional is determining specific strategies to prevent exercise relapse:

- Identify situations with a high risk of relapse. High-risk situations are those that involve behaviors that are incompatible with exercise, such as eating, drinking, overworking, or smoking. High-risk situations can also involve relocation, medical events, travel, and inclement weather. Personal high-risk situations can be determined from information gathered during assessment and self-monitoring. The fitness professional should help the participant recognize aspects of the exercise behavior itself, such as intensity, time of day, place, people, moods, thoughts, and particular situations, that can threaten exercise adherence.
- Revise plans in order to avoid or cope with high-risk situations. Flexible, short-term goals can be adapted to uncontrollable situational demands. Temporarily resetting goals can decrease the sense of noncompliance and increase a sense of control (e.g., "While my weekend guests are here, I will jog one day in the morning before they get up instead of trying to jog on both Saturday and Sunday afternoons").

- Improve coping responses by referring participants to classes covering techniques related to time management, relaxation, assertiveness, stress management, confidence building, and so on.
- Provide realistic expectations of potential outcomes from not exercising so the behavioral consequences of relapse are placed in perspective.
- Encourage participants to expect and plan for potential lapses in an exercise routine. They should plan for some alternative modes of exercise, times of day, places, and so forth. If someone is likely to skip a day of exercise when all the treadmills are in use, suggest the cycle or stair-climber on those days.
- Minimize the tendency to interpret a lapse (e.g., missing one class, not exercising during a business trip) as inevitably leading to a relapse and then defining a relapse as a total failure. Use cognitive restructuring to change the definition of a missed exercise class from "the end of my exercise program" to "a temporary lapse that most exercisers experience."
- Correct a lifestyle imbalance in which *shoulds* outweigh *wants*. Make exercise something participants want to do instead of something they feel they should do. Help them find activities that have purpose and meaning for them. Use positive reinforcement and other strategies to make exercise fun.

KEY POINT

Because missing regular exercise is inevitable for many people, the fitness professional must be prepared to help participants prevent lapses in an exercise routine from ending the exercise program. Strategies such as being flexible in setting and revising goals, realizing that the occasional lapse is just temporary, and building self-confidence and coping skills can help participants deal successfully with a potential relapse.

Health and Fitness Counseling

The fitness professional is called on to provide counseling during assessment, exercise prescription, and ongoing monitoring of exercise programs. More and more professionals are implementing principles of motivational interviewing, such as expressing empathy and fostering self-efficacy in a client-centered, semidirective format (19). Regardless of the approach the fitness professional uses, communication skills are the foundation of effective counseling. Developing good communication skills takes time and focus, so patience is critical to listening and understanding. For additional information, see the excellent chapter on health behavior counseling skills by Whiteley et al. in the ACSM resource manual (26) and the Rollnick et al. text on motivational interviewing in health care (19).

Communication Skills

To be able to communicate well, the fitness professional must be able to listen effectively and respond empathetically. Listening involves being able to accurately discriminate the feeling and meaning of the speaker's message. It is more complicated than simply hearing words. **Communication** occurs at many levels, and thus we should not always assume that what people say is what they mean. The message includes the objective meaning of the words, or the content of the message; however, tone of voice, loudness or softness of speech, speed, and nonverbal behavior can change the meaning of a statement. A participant who smiles, looks you in the eyes, and says, "My program is going really well," is not saying the same thing as a person who mumbles the same words and looks away. To enhance our understanding of the message, we must be able to attend to the verbal and nonverbal as well as overt and covert messages. The fitness professional should pay attention to facial expressions, body language, and tone of voice in addition to listening to the actual words.

The context of the message, determined by the social and cultural implications of the situation, can create noise that will interfere with sending and receiving the message. Noise is also created by the ideas, experiences, expectations, and prejudices of the speaker and listener. Barriers to communication occur not only in the context of the message but also in the way a listener responds. Ordering, threatening, criticizing, interpreting, interrupting, interrogating, and diverting (often by humor) are responses that shut off understanding and make the speaker feel you do not care. Backing away, looking over your shoulder, and checking your watch are other obvious ways to shut down communication. If you don't have time to talk, be honest about it, but make sure you arrange another time when you won't be distracted and can give the participant the attention she needs and deserves.

Do not automatically assume you understand what a person is saying. We react to a communicated message according to our own perceptions of the nature of the message. Use responsive listening to clarify communication and confirm with the speaker that you comprehend his message. Reflect back what you have heard, and then ask questions and make statements that respond to the feeling and meaning of the message. Responsive listening lets people know you understand what they have expressed, helps build a relationship with them, encourages them to keep talking, and clarifies what they mean.

Characteristics of an Effective Helper

The role of the fitness professional as counselor is to help clients achieve their health-related goals. It is easier to provide this help when the fitness professional responds to the client with empathy, respect, concreteness, genuineness, and confrontation.

- Empathy is an expression of understanding the personal meaning of events and experiences to the participant. It is different from sympathy, which is an attempt to experience another person's feelings. Empathy is also not the same as knowing what the problem is. You may know that John has 28% body fat because he eats fast food every day and does not exercise, but empathy means you have a sense of what it must be like for him to be overweight and inactive, and you are able to communicate your understanding in a nonjudgmental manner. Even if you are not sure you are being empathetic, when the participant perceives that you are trying to understand, he will be encouraged to communicate more about the problem. The additional information will help you empathize more and give you clues to the underlying nature of the problem and how to come up with a more realistic intervention plan. Your effort to understand also communicates to the participant that you value him as an individual.
- Respect is a feeling of positive regard for the participant. You display warm acceptance of the participant's experiences and place no conditions on your acceptance and warmth. This means not making judgments. It is often hard for the fitness professional to respect a person whose behavior (e.g., smoking, sedentary lifestyle, high-fat diet) shows a lack of self-respect for his body. We must prize the person but not necessarily the behavior. When we respect another person, we help that person develop self-respect.
- Concreteness is the ability to help the participant be specific about feelings and goals she is trying to communicate. Reflective listening enables the participant to become more precise in communicating what she experiences and wants to accomplish, which aids in setting goals.
- Genuineness is being authentic and sincere in a relationship with another person. In a helpful relationship, the counselor is honest and open with the client. Some

Putting Responsive Listening Into Practice

Participant: I'm the only one in this class who can't get the new step routines. (The fitness professional should observe the tone of voice, eye contact, and posture.)

Fitness professional: You think the other members of the class catch on before you do. That must be really frustrating. (The fitness professional paraphrased the participant's statement and interpreted probable underlying feelings. Other feelings could be discouragement or a sense of futility or failure. Responding with an offer to teach the participant the steps might not have addressed an underlying lack of confidence. Responsive listening keeps the communications open so the participant can express what kind of help she wants.)

Participant: Yes, I wonder if I can even do aerobics. The steps change faster than I can follow them. (The participant has low self-efficacy for this step aerobics class. The fitness professional now has more information about the problem and can offer a better solution.)

Fitness professional: You doubt this is for you because it is so fast paced, but did you know that many of the people in this class started with Jenny's class? Jenny teaches all the basic routines at a slower pace and focuses on helping everyone learn the steps. (The fitness professional acknowledged the participant's beliefs and provided more information to put her perceptions into another context. She is not the only one who couldn't get the routine without some basic training. A beginners' class could provide mastery experiences to increase the participant's self-efficacy.)

Participant: I've always felt I didn't fit in, but I thought it was just me. Maybe I could try Jenny's step class. (The fitness professional should observe what the participant said and how she said it to see if the information met the underlying need.)

Fitness professional: This class was not the right one for you, but Jenny's class can be a good way for you to learn the steps. We can check the schedule and I can introduce you to Jenny. (The fitness professional paraphrased the participant's statement and offered help rather than telling her what to do. This acknowledges the participant's ability to make choices, promoting her autonomy.)

self-disclosure is appropriate and can help develop trust, but the goal of the relationship is to help the client, not deal with the fitness professional's personal issues.

- Confrontation involves telling the other person that you see things differently from how they are being presented to you. You point out incongruities that are observable facts about which the participant may not be consciously aware. Confrontation should be used only after you have an established relationship, and it should be directed toward the behavior, not the person.

Other qualities important in effective health counseling are listed in *Qualities of an Effective Healthy-Behavior Counselor*.

Weight Bias

What is weight bias? The tendency to stereotype and negatively judge an overweight or obese person based on preconceived or unreasoned assumptions and false character traits, such as being lazy, unintelligent, awkward, ugly, or unmotivated. In other words, it's general negativity toward people who are perceived as carrying excess weight.

Currently, more than two-thirds of American adults are overweight or obese. Disturbingly, studies have shown that a significant proportion of health care workers demonstrate bias toward their overweight patients. Given that many of the fitness professional's clients may be overweight or obese, attitudes and beliefs that can harm effective programming must be identified and addressed. Bias and stigma involve negative attitudes that affect our interpersonal interactions and activities in a detrimental way. This can include stereotypes, derogatory names, teasing, and ridicule, although much of bias against obesity can be implicit, or not within conscious awareness. Environmental barriers, such as examination gowns, tables, and BP cuffs that are too small, compound the difficulties associated with adequate health care for people who are obese.

Unfortunately, society promotes the idea that people are responsible for their life situation and get what they deserve, and that weight is a function of personal responsibility and under a person's control. The fitness professional can become sensitive to this bias by first recognizing the complex etiology of obesity, including not just individual behavior but also genetics, biology, the environment, and sociocultural influences. Challenge assumptions that obesity is only the result of eating too much and exercising too little and that the solution is greater motivation. Identify assumptions about someone based on weight regarding health, lifestyle, personality, professional success, character, intelligence, and abilities. Online resources for addressing personal assumptions and bias can be found at the Weight Bias and Stigma resource page of the Rudd Center for Food Policy and Obesity (www.uconnruddcenter.org/weight-bias-stigma).

Qualities of an Effective Healthy-Behavior Counselor

- Knowledgeable
- Supportive
- Model of healthy behavior
- Trustworthy
- Enthusiastic
- Innovative
- Patient
- Sensitive
- Flexible
- Self-aware
- Able to access material resources and services
- Able to generate expectations of success
- Committed to providing timely, specific feedback
- Capable of providing clear, reasonable instructions and plans
- Sensitive to physical barriers to communication while respectful of the physical limits of someone's personal space
- Aware of personal limitations

Ethical Considerations

There is an ethical dilemma in promoting healthy behavior change in people who don't want to change. The fitness professional must weigh the importance of persuading people to behave in ways conducive to good health versus the clients' right to do as they please with their own health as long as it does not impinge on the rights of others. Informed consent theoretically gives participants a free choice after they have been given all the information needed to make a decision. If an unhealthy lifestyle is based on ignorance or incorrect information, we should provide the information necessary for an informed choice, not aggravate feelings of guilt or failure. But if someone has chosen an unhealthy lifestyle as a matter of free will, we must accept this informed refusal, although fitness professionals often have difficulty doing so. Thus, an awareness of our own value preferences is essential in helping others set goals. We must consider whose values are to be served by the intervention, the clients' or ours, and we must respect their choices even if we disagree with them.

Confidentiality is another ethical concern for the fitness professional. In addition to client information that is clearly confidential, such as medical records, the fitness professional may become aware of other information the participant wants to keep private. Trustworthiness is an important characteristic of an effective helper and reflects an ethical stand. Participants will trust someone who keeps information confidential, treats them with respect, and keeps the relationship professional.

Also, recognize your limitations and know when to refer your client to a professional therapist. It is the role of the fitness professional to help people change unhealthy behavior, but marital problems, eating disorders, and affective disorders such as depression are a few of the areas that should be handled by someone trained to work with these issues. We must know our limits and help connect participants with the best resources for handling their unique problems.

KEY POINT

Listening to the actual words and the nonverbal message in context is the foundation of good communication skills. To communicate effectively, the fitness professional should practice reflective listening and empathetic responding. Characteristics of an effective helper include empathy, respect, concreteness, genuineness, and confrontation.

23

LEARNING AIDS

REVIEW QUESTIONS

1. What are the five stages of change as applied to exercise? Provide examples of factors fitness professionals must consider in working with clients in each stage.
2. What are the basic human needs according to SDT, and how can participation in a group exercise class help to meet each of these needs?
3. What are strategies fitness professionals can use to target sources of self-efficacy information and to help increase task *and* barrier self-efficacy in a novice exerciser?
4. List the personal, social, and environmental links in a behavioral chain for an overweight woman to participate in a walking program during her lunch hour. Explain how fitness professionals could target the weak links to increase the likelihood of long-term adherence.
5. Discuss and give examples of motivational strategies that could be used with participants who are just starting to exercise regularly and those who have been exercising for at least 6 mo.
6. Describe the elements of successful goal setting and write one long-term and one short-term goal for an older adult who wants to be fit enough to enjoy a vacation at the beach with his grandchildren 4 mo from now.
7. Explain the steps in relapse prevention and why each step is important in helping participants stick with an exercise program and resist relapse.

8. Describe the characteristics of an effective helper and explain how each characteristic is related to good communication skills.
9. Define *weight bias* and explain how bias toward people who are obese can affect fitness programming.

CASE STUDIES

1. Dana was given a 3 mo membership to your facility by her boyfriend, Mike, who attends aerobics classes regularly. They are going on a backpacking trip to Colorado this summer, and Mike thought you could help her get ready for the physical strain of the trip. She is a self-proclaimed couch potato. She started aerobics classes with Mike last year but got so sore that she stopped after 1 wk. Yesterday you completed her fitness assessment—Dana is in good health, has 20% body fat, and is slightly below average in aerobic fitness. She said her goal is to be prepared for the trip, and she wants to try aerobics again. However, she confides she is afraid she will disappoint Mike because she is out of shape and doesn't enjoy aerobics. What stage of behavior change is she in, and what strategies could you use to help her?
2. Jack is a middle-aged college English professor who joined the walking club in your facility after you conducted his fitness and psychosocial assessment 3 mo ago. His long-term goal was to walk around the world (in terms of total miles walked), and his progress has been marked on the walkers' promotional map at the front entrance. His office is two blocks from your facility, and he usually walks on your indoor track before he goes home for the day. You notice his mileage has decreased over the past 2 wk, and another walker tells you that Jack said, "I won't make it out of the state thanks to term papers and final exams." What stage of behavior change is he in, and what strategies could you use to help him?
3. Your club has sponsored a 10K race every Thanksgiving for the past 10 yr, and Marty has always placed in the top five of his age group. His brother Jim will be in town this Thanksgiving and they plan to run the 10K together. Marty is determined to beat Jim, so he has been coming into your club at least once a week for the past month to do speed work on the treadmill. However, he's discouraged by his minor increase in speed and the increased tightness in his legs. When you ask Marty about his training program, you discover that he does no resistance training and rarely stretches, but he has doubled his weekly mileage over the past 4 wk and plans to increase even more to be ready for the race and competition with Jim in 6 wk. What stage is Marty in, and what strategies could you use to help him?

Answers to Case Studies

1. Dana is in the preparation stage and has low exercise self-efficacy. She has had a bad experience with exercise in the past, so you want to educate her about what to expect at the beginning of an exercise program and make sure the prescription is appropriate for her fitness level. Use the fitness evaluation to give her a realistic idea of her current fitness level and how much progress she can expect based on a sensible prescription. In setting goals with her, find out what *she* wants to achieve and activities she might enjoy. Brainstorm about her barriers to exercise and how to counter them. Identify supports and ways she could reward herself during the program. Target her low exercise self-efficacy with a beginners' exercise class where she will have social support. Make sure she gets individual attention and encouragement, especially during the first few weeks. A behavioral contract with Mike doing something she wants him to do when she meets short-term goals could provide incentives and support that she needs to keep her program going.

2. Jack is in the action stage and is especially susceptible to relapse. You could make a point of walking with Jack the next time he comes in to provide support and education about relapse prevention. Extra work at the end of the term is a high-risk situation for him; he is discouraged and at risk of relapse. Talk with him about setting short-term goals that can be readjusted during exams. Help him to make the goals realistic and reachable. He might want to take walk breaks for 10 to 15 min during the days he can't get to the facility. Point out that these breaks will help him stay on track and give him a way to manage stress at work. Praise him for how far he has come and for continuing even though he is busy. Help him see that the high-risk situation is time limited, and brainstorm ways he can reward himself for the walking he can do. Recruit veteran walkers to provide support and encouragement.
3. Marty is in the maintenance stage, but his motivation has shifted from intrinsic to extrinsic by focusing on beating his brother Jim in the Thanksgiving race. His relationship with Jim is beyond your role, but you can help him train most effectively for this race. Ask if he has an exercise log you could review together to learn more about his training, or get him to log his miles, speed, and physical and psychological responses over the next week. Find out his experiences with resistance training and stretching to discover why he skips these activities. He might not know their benefits, or he might not enjoy lifting weights and stretching. Invite Marty to a resistance class that has several runners who have benefited from lifting weights. Introduce him to a fast runner who has a balanced training program and can show Marty stretching routines that have helped his running performance.

24

ECG and Exercise Performance

David R. Bassett, Jr.

OBJECTIVES

The reader will be able to do the following:

1. Describe the basic anatomy of the heart.
2. Describe the basic electrophysiology of the heart.
3. Define *electrocardiogram (ECG)* and identify the standard settings for paper speed and amplitude.
4. Identify the basic electrocardiographic complexes and calculate HR from ECG rhythm strips.
5. Describe the types of atrioventricular conduction defects and their probable effect on a subject's exercise response.
6. Identify the normal and abnormal cardiac rhythms, and predict the probable effect of the abnormal rhythms on exercise performance.
7. Describe electrocardiographic signs and biochemical markers of a heart attack.

This chapter provides background information on the heart, ECG analysis, and cardiovascular medications and how these factors affect exercise testing and prescription in the basically healthy population. This chapter is not intended to be a complete guide to ECG interpretation and cardiovascular medications; there are several excellent texts on these topics (3, 6, 8, 9).

Structure of the Heart

The heart is a muscular organ composed of four chambers: the right atrium, right ventricle, left atrium, and left ventricle (see figure 24.1). The flow of blood through the heart is directed by pressure differences and valves between the chambers. Venous blood from the body is returned to the heart by the inferior vena cava and superior vena cava, which empty into the right atrium. From the right atrium, blood passes through the **tricuspid valve** into the right ventricle. The right ventricle pumps blood through the **pulmonary valve** into the pulmonary arteries leading to the lungs. In the lungs, blood gives up carbon dioxide and picks up oxygen. The oxygen-rich blood is returned to the heart via the pulmonary veins emptying into the left atrium. From the left atrium, blood passes through the **mitral valve** into the left ventricle. The left ventricle pumps oxygenated blood past the **aortic valve** into the aorta and coronary arteries and to the rest of the body. The left ventricle, which generates more pressure than the right ventricle, is thicker.

Coronary Arteries

The heart muscle, or **myocardium**, does not receive a significant amount of oxygen directly from blood in the atria or ventricles. To meet the heart's need for oxygen, oxygenated blood is supplied to the myocardium via the **coronary arteries**, which lie on the surface of the heart. There are two coronary artery systems (the right and left coronary arteries), which branch off the aorta at the coronary sinus. The left main coronary artery follows a course between the left atria and the pulmonary artery and branches off into the left anterior descending and left circumflex arteries (figure 24.2). The left anterior descending artery follows a path along the anterior surface of the heart and lies over the interventricular septum, which separates the right and left ventricles. The left circumflex artery follows the groove between the left atrium and left ventricle on the anterior and lateral surface of the heart. The right coronary artery follows the groove that separates the atria and ventricles

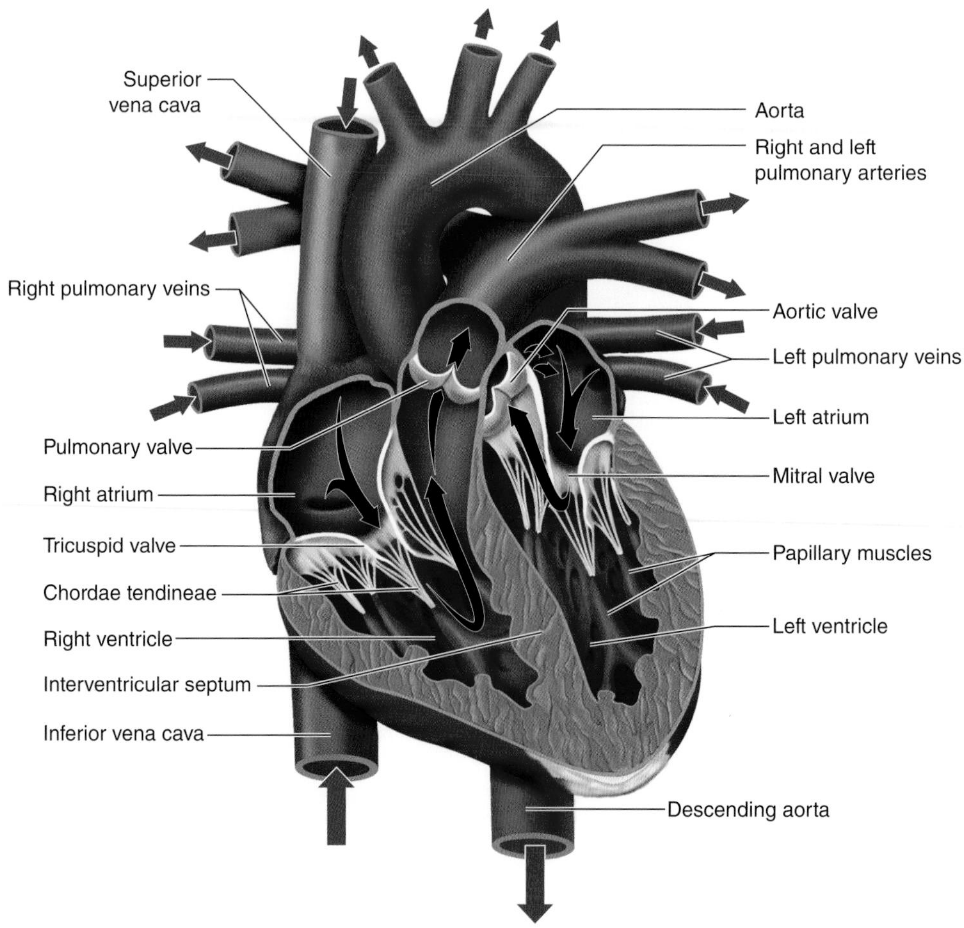

FIGURE 24.1 The chambers and valves of the heart.

around the posterior surface of the heart and forms the posterior descending artery. Numerous smaller arteries split off the major arteries, becoming smaller and smaller until finally they form the capillaries that transport oxygen to the muscle cells of the heart, where gas exchange occurs.

A major obstruction in any of these coronary arteries results in **myocardial ischemia**, or reduced blood flow to the myocardium and decreased ability of the heart to pump blood. If the coronary arteries become blocked and the heart muscle does not receive oxygen, then a portion of the heart muscle might die, which is known as a **myocardial infarction (MI)**, or heart attack. In contrast, if the ventricles cease to contract in a rhythmic fashion, blood stops circulating throughout the body, which is known as a **cardiac arrest**.

Coronary Veins

Venous drainage of the right ventricle occurs via the anterior cardiac vein, which normally has two or three major branches and eventually empties into the right atrium. The venous drainage of the left ventricle occurs primarily through the anterior interventricular vein, which roughly follows the same path as the left anterior descending artery, eventually forming the coronary sinus and emptying into the right atrium.

Oxygen Use by the Heart

The myocardium is well adapted to use oxygen to generate ATP. Approximately 40% of the volume of a myocardial cell is composed of mitochondria, the cellular organelle responsible for producing ATP with oxygen. The oxygen consumption of the heart in a resting person is about 8 to 10 ml · min^{-1} per 100 g of myocardium; in comparison, the total resting oxygen consumption for the body is about 0.35 ml · min^{-1} per 100 g of body mass (4). Myocardial oxygen consumption can increase six- to sevenfold during heavy exercise in young adults, whereas the total body oxygen consumption can easily increase 12 to 15 times. Heart muscle has a limited capacity to produce energy via anaerobic pathways and depends on the delivery of oxygen to the mitochondria to produce ATP. At rest, the whole body extracts only about 25% of the oxygen present in each 100 ml of arterial blood, and the body can meet an increased need for oxygen by simply extracting more from the blood. In contrast, the heart extracts about 75% of the oxygen available in the arterial blood. Consequently, an increase in the oxygen needs of the heart must be met by delivering more blood via the coronary arteries. An adequate oxygen supply to the heart is needed not only to allow the heart to pump blood but also to maintain normal electrical activity, which is covered in the next section.

KEY POINT

The heart is a muscular organ composed of four chambers: the right atrium, the right ventricle, the left atrium, and the left ventricle. The coronary arteries supply the heart muscle (myocardium) with blood, and the heart meets increasing oxygen demands by increasing blood flow.

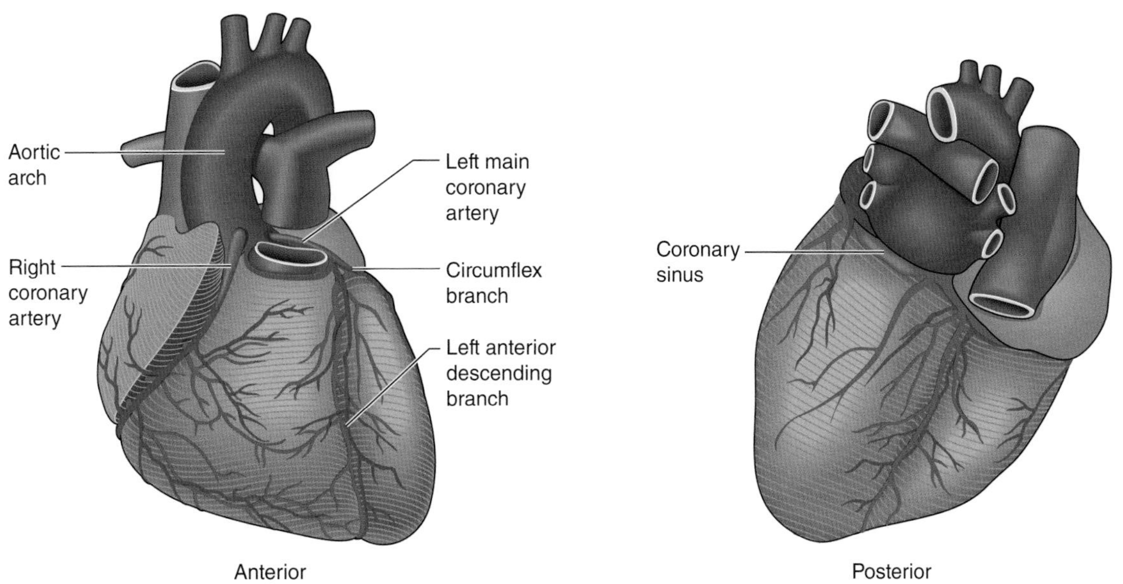

FIGURE 24.2 Coronary blood vessels.

Electrophysiology of the Heart

The electrical activity of the heart leads to mechanical activity (contraction), which pumps the blood. At rest, the insides of the myocardial cells are negatively charged and the exteriors are positively charged. This charge difference is due to the fact that the cell membrane is selectively permeable, and the concentrations of certain ions (Na^+, K^+, Ca^{++}, Cl^-) differ inside and outside of the cells (5). When the cells are depolarized (stimulated), the insides of the cells become positively charged and the exteriors become negatively charged. Depolarization occurs as positively charged Na^+ ions enter the cells. If a recording electrode is placed on the chest so that the wave of depolarization spreads toward the electrode, the ECG records a positive (upward) deflection. If the wave of depolarization spreads away from the recording electrode, a negative (downward) deflection occurs. When the myocardial cell is completely polarized or depolarized, the ECG does not record any electrical potential but shows a flat baseline, known as the *isoelectric line.* After depolarization, the myocardial cell undergoes repolarization to return to its resting electrical state. During repolarization, positively charged K^+ ions leave the cells. The steps leading from rest (complete polarization) to complete stimulation (complete depolarization) back to rest (repolarization) are shown in figure 24.3.

The **sinoatrial (SA) node** is the normal pacemaker of the heart and is located in the right atrium near the supe-

1 Completely polarized

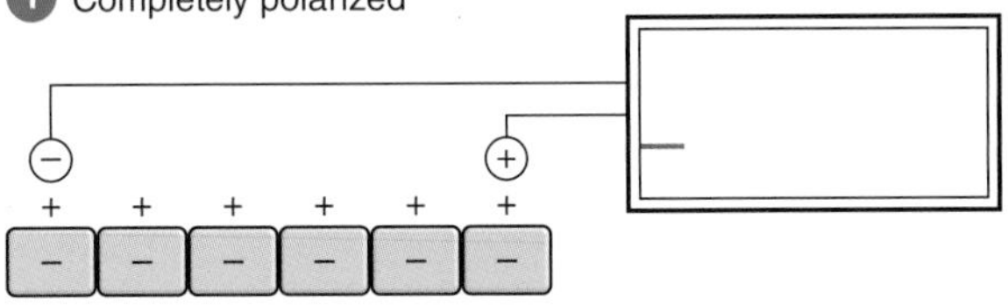

The myocardial cells shown on the left are at rest and are completely polarized. Because both of the recording electrodes are surrounded by positive charges, there is no voltage difference between them, and the electrocardiogram (ECG) shown on the right records the isoelectric line (0 mV).

2 Partially depolarized

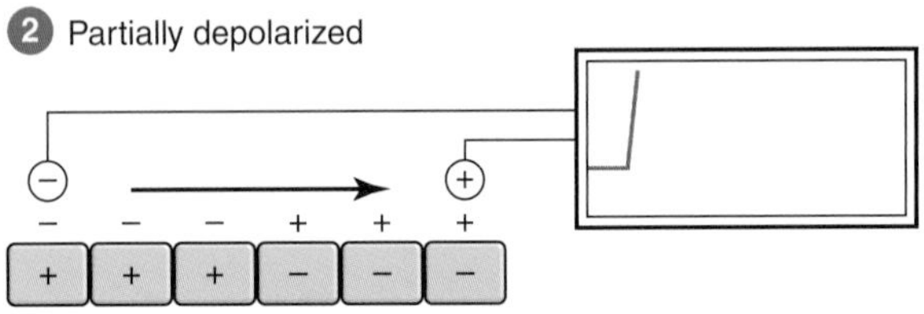

The process of depolarization (positive charges inside the cell and negative charges outside) is spreading from left to right. Because the electrode on the right is surrounded by positive charges, the ECG records a positive deflection. The amplitude of the deflection is proportional to the mass of the myocardium undergoing depolarization.

3 Completely depolarized

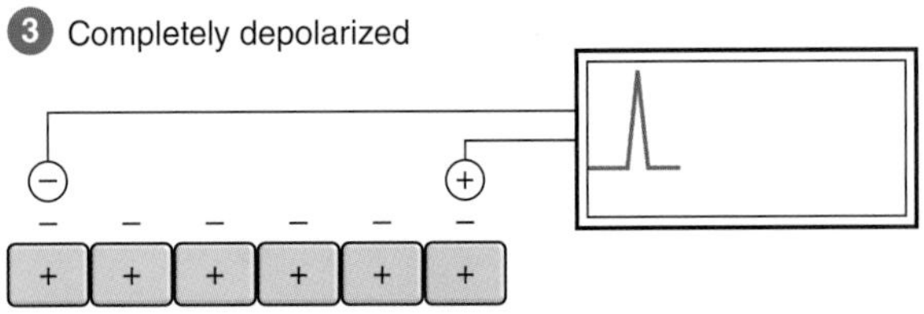

Depolarization is now complete, and both electrodes are surrounded by negative charges. Because there is no voltage difference between electrodes, the ECG is now recording 0 mV, or the isoelectric potential.

4 Partially repolarized

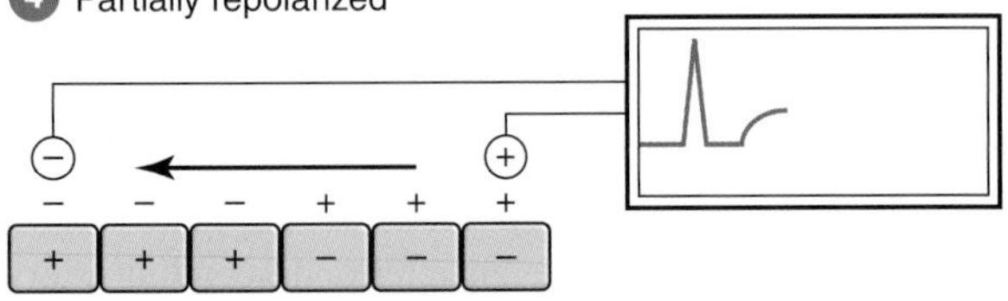

Repolarization has started from the right and is moving to the left. The ECG shows a positive (upward) deflection, because the right-hand electrode is surrounded by positive charges. Note that repolarization occurs in the opposite direction from depolarization in the human heart, and this is the reason the depolarization and repolarization complexes are both normally positive. If repolarization had started on the left and moved to the right, the ECG deflection would have been negative.

5 Completely repolarized

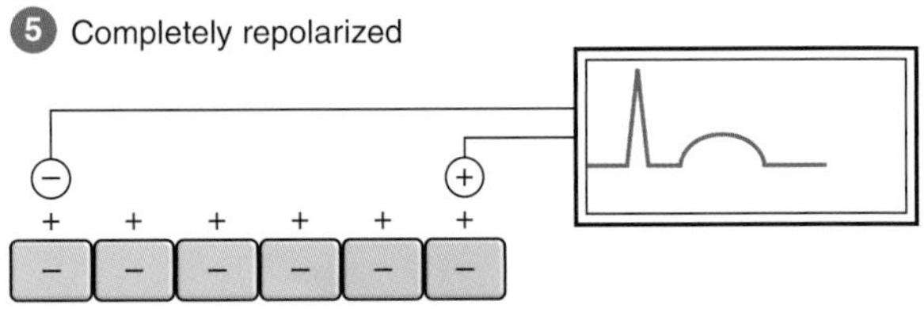

The muscle cells are now completely repolarized, or in the resting state, and the ECG records the isoelectric line. The myocardial cells are now ready to be depolarized again.

FIGURE 24.3 Steps in an electrocardiographic cycle.

rior vena cava (figure 24.4). The pacemaker cells in the SA node can depolarize on their own, without any input from the brain. This occurs because the slow movement of ions across the cell membrane causes the membrane potential to creep up to the threshold, and then an action potential occurs. Depolarization spreads from the SA node across the atria and results in the P wave (see the section Basic Electrocardiographic Complexes). There are three tracts within the atria that conduct depolarization to the **atrioventricular (AV) node**. Impulses travel from the SA node through the atrial muscle and conduction tracts and enter the AV node, where conduction slows to allow the atrial contraction to empty blood into the ventricles before the start of ventricular contraction. The **bundle of His** is the conduction pathway that connects the AV node with **bundle branches** in the ventricles. The right bundle branch splits off the bundle of His and forms ever-smaller branches that serve the right ventricle. The left bundle splits into two major branches that serve the thicker left ventricle. **Purkinje fibers** are the terminal branches of the bundle branches and form the link between the specialized conductive tissue and the muscle fibers. Small electrical junctions between adjacent cardiac muscle cells, known as **intercalated discs**, allow the electrical impulses to pass from cell to cell. The intercalated discs allow for coordinated contraction of the ventricular muscle fibers, which is needed for effective pumping of the heart. Because of the conduction pathways and the interconnected myocardial cells, a depolarization of the SA node results in a predictable electrical pattern, coordinated contraction of the heart's muscle cells, and effective pumping of the blood.

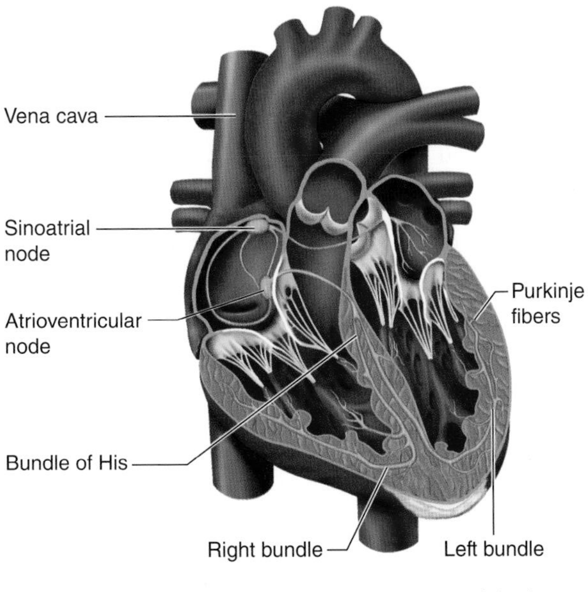

FIGURE 24.4 Electrical conduction system of the heart. These are the normal pathways used to ensure the rhythmic contraction and relaxation of the heart chambers.

KEY POINT

The electrical impulse originates in the SA node, located in the right atrium. From there the electrical impulse spreads to the AV node, the bundle of His, the left and right bundle branches, and the Purkinje fibers. Waves of depolarization then spread from cell to cell throughout the ventricular muscle by passing through the intercalated discs. Any restriction in blood flow to the myocardium could upset the electrical activity of the heart or damage the myocardium.

Interpreting the ECG

The **electrocardiogram (ECG)** is a graphic recording of the heart's electrical activity. As waves of depolarization travel through the heart, electrical currents spread to the tissues surrounding the heart and then travel throughout the body. If recording electrodes are placed on the skin, small voltage differences between various regions of the body can be detected. Thus, the electrocardiograph is a sensitive voltmeter that records the electrical activity of the heart.

This section on analyzing the ECG may appear to go beyond what a fitness professional needs to know about the topic; the physician is the person to judge whether an ECG response is normal. However, the fitness professional must be aware of the basic ECG interpretation in order to communicate effectively with the physician, program director, and clinical exercise specialist.

Systematically evaluating the ECG allows the examiner to determine the HR, rhythm, and conduction pathways and to search for signs of ischemia or infarction. Physicians normally evaluate a 12-lead ECG, but for our purposes a single ECG lead is adequate to describe the heart's electrical activity. A commonly used single ECG lead for exercise testing is the CM5, which looks similar to lead V5 on a 12-lead ECG. A 12-lead ECG (see figure 24.5) allows a cardiologist to look at the heart from 12 different views. (Six limb leads provide views of the heart from various angles in the frontal plane of the body, and six precordial leads provide views of the heart from various angles in the transverse plane of the body.) These 12 leads are made up of various combinations of 10 electrodes. The 12-lead ECG contains much more information than a single ECG lead, and it allows a more detailed picture of the heart's electrical activity. A detailed discussion of 12-lead ECG electrode placement and interpretation is beyond the scope of this chapter. For further information, consult the texts by Dubin (8) or Stein (13).

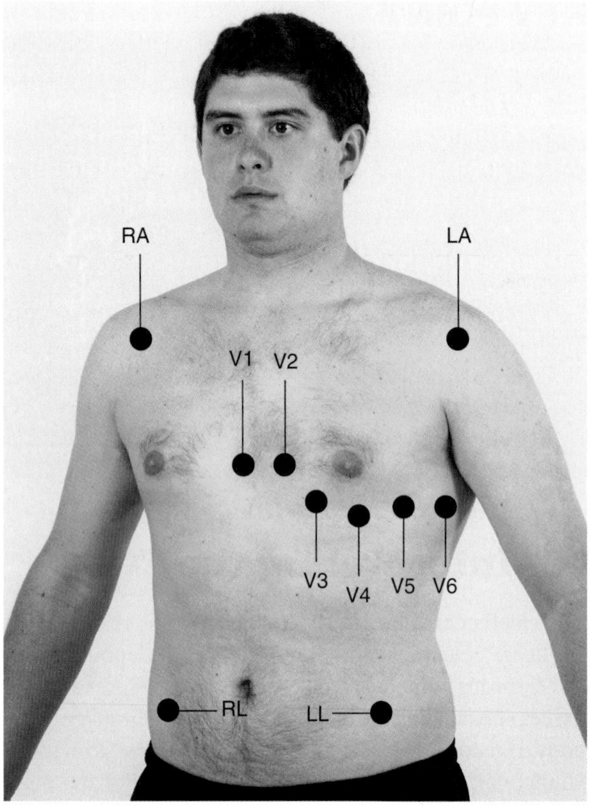

FIGURE 24.5 Electrode placements for a 12-lead ECG.

Watch **videos 24.1** and **24.2**, which demonstrate electrode placements for single- and 12-lead ECGs.

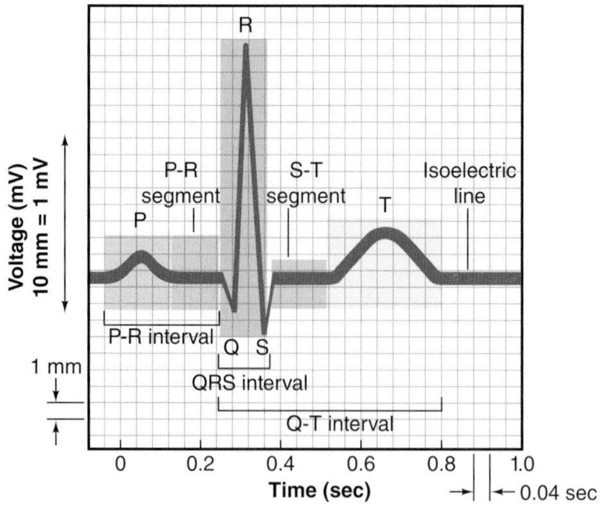

FIGURE 24.6 ECG complex with time and voltage scales.

KEY POINT

The pattern of electrical activity across the heart is called the *electrocardiogram (ECG).* The ECG is recorded with an electrocardiograph, and it provides information about the rhythm of the heart. The ECG paper speed is normally 25 mm · sec^{-1}, and at this speed each 1 mm mark represents 0.04 sec. The standard calibration factor is normally 0.1 mV per millimeter of deflection.

Time and Voltage

ECG paper markings are standardized to allow measurement of time intervals and voltages. Time is measured on the horizontal axis, and the paper normally moves at 25 mm · sec^{-1}. Most ECG machines can run at 50 or 25 mm · sec^{-1}, so one must know the paper speed when measuring the duration of ECG complexes (see the section Basic Electrocardiographic Complexes). ECG paper is marked with a repeating grid (see figure 24.6). Major grid lines are 5 mm apart, and at a paper speed of 25 mm · sec^{-1}, 5 mm correspond to 0.20 sec. Minor lines are 1 mm apart, and at a paper speed of 25 mm · sec^{-1}, 1 mm equals 0.04 sec. Voltage is measured on the vertical axis, and the standard calibration factor is normally 0.1 millivolt (mV) per mm of deflection. Most ECG machines can be adjusted to reduce this factor by 50% or to double it. You must know the voltage calibration before evaluating an ECG. All ECG measurements in this chapter refer to a paper speed of 25 mm · sec^{-1} and a voltage calibration of 0.1 mV · mm^{-1}.

Electrocardiographic Wave Forms

The **P wave** is the graphic representation of atrial depolarization. The normal P wave lasts less than 0.12 sec and has an amplitude of 0.25 mV or less. The T_a wave is the result of atrial repolarization. It is not normally seen because it occurs during ventricular depolarization and the larger electrical forces generated by the ventricles hide the T_a wave. The **Q wave** is the first downward deflection after the P wave, and it signals the start of ventricular depolarization. The **R wave** is a positive deflection following the Q wave; it results from ventricular depolarization. If there is more than one R wave in a single complex, the second occurrence is called *R'*. The **S wave** is a negative deflection preceded by Q or R waves, and it is also the result of ventricular depolarization. Collectively, the Q, R, and S waves are referred to as the **QRS complex.** The **T wave** follows this complex, and it results from ventricular repolarization.

Electrocardiograph Intervals

The **R-R interval** is the time between successive R waves. When the heart rhythm is regular, the duration of an R-R interval can be used to determine the HR (beats · min^{-1}). If the heart rhythm is irregular, the R-R interval varies and HR must be determined from the number of R waves in a 6 sec time interval (see figure 24.7).

The PP interval is the time between two successive atrial depolarizations. The **PR interval** is measured from the start

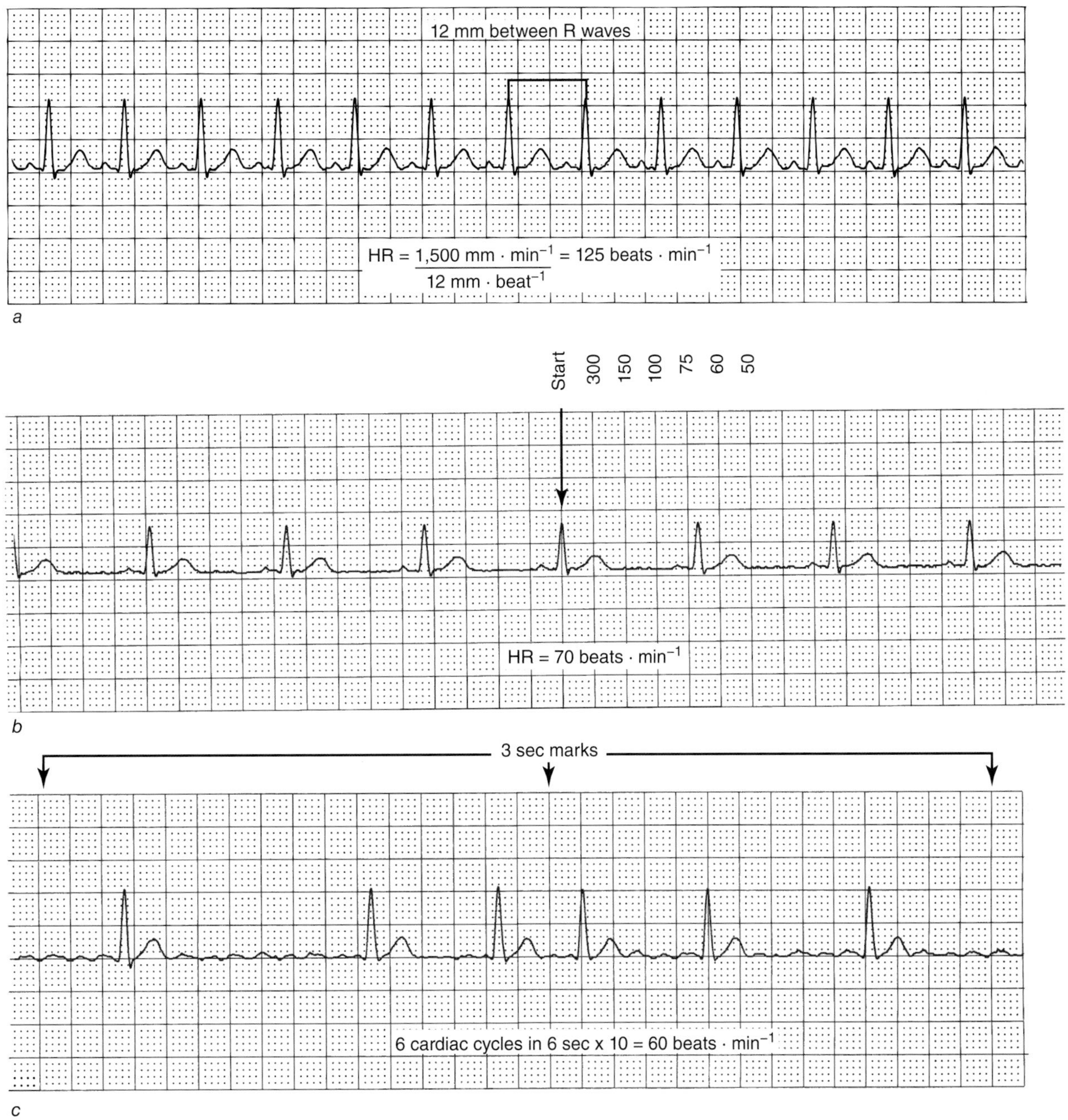

FIGURE 24.7 Three methods of determining HR from the ECG. *(a)* An approximate HR (beats · min^{-1}) can be determined by dividing 1,500 (60 sec at 25 mm · sec^{-1}) by the number of millimeters between adjacent R waves. *(b)* A second method is to begin with an R wave that falls on a thick black line. As you move to the right, count off the next six black lines as 300, 150, 100, 75, 60, and 50 (memorize these numbers). If the next R wave falls on one of these lines, the corresponding number indicates the HR. If the next R wave falls in between two thick black lines, you can estimate the HR by interpolation. *(c)* A third method is commonly used when the HR is irregular. With this method, you count the number of complete R-R intervals in a 6 sec ECG strip and multiply by 10.

of the P wave to the beginning of the QRS complex. The interval is called *PR* even if the first deflection after the P wave is a Q wave. Thus, the PR interval includes the time periods corresponding to atrial depolarization and the delay in the electrical impulse at the AV node. The upper limit for the normal PR interval is 0.20 sec, or 5 small blocks on the grid of the ECG paper.

The width of the QRS complex depends on the time for depolarization of the ventricles. A normal QRS complex lasts less than 0.10 sec, or 2.5 small blocks on the ECG paper. The **QT interval** is measured from the start of the QRS complex to the end of the T wave and corresponds to the duration of ventricular systole.

Segments and Junctions

The **PR segment** is measured from the end of the P wave to the beginning of the QRS complex. This segment forms the isoelectric line, or baseline, from which ST segment deviations are measured. The **J point** is the point at which the S wave ends and the ST segment begins. The **ST segment** is formed by the isoelectric line between the QRS complex and the T wave. During an exercise test this segment is examined closely for depression or elevation, which may indicate the development of myocardial ischemia or perhaps MI. A description of the process for determining MI and myocardial ischemia can be found later in this chapter. ST segment deviation usually is measured 60 or 80 ms after the J point.

Heart Rhythms

The ECG provides vital information about heart rhythms. Abnormalities in the electrical activity of the heart can be diagnosed from the ECG.

KEY POINT

The P wave signifies atrial depolarization, the QRS complex signifies ventricular depolarization, and the T wave signifies ventricular repolarization. If the rhythm is regular, HR can be determined by dividing 1,500 by the number of millimeters between successive R waves. HR also can be determined by starting with an R wave that falls on a thick black line and counting off the next six black lines as 300, 150, 100, 75, 60, and 50 and determining at which corresponding number the next R wave occurs. If the rhythm is irregular, HR can be determined by counting the number of R-R intervals in a 6 sec ECG strip and multiplying by 10.

Sinus Rhythm

Sinus rhythm is the normal rhythm of the heart (see figure 24.8). The HR is 60 to 100 beats · min^{-1} and the pacemaker is the SA node.

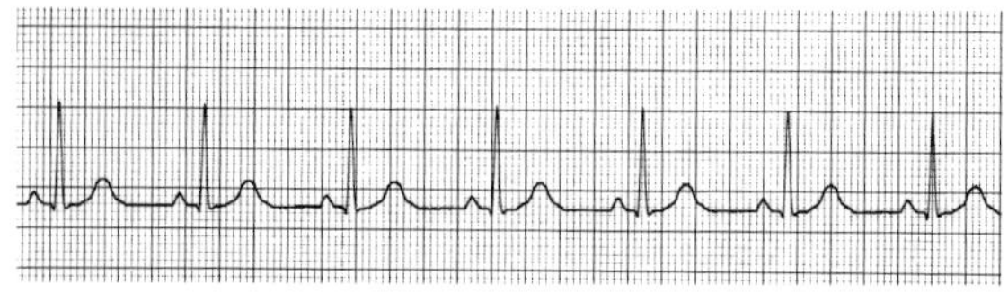

FIGURE 24.8 Normal sinus rhythm. In this example, the HR is 71 beats · min^{-1}.

Sinus Bradycardia

The HR in **sinus bradycardia** is less than 60 beats · min^{-1} (see figure 24.9). This is a normal rhythm, and it is often seen in conditioned subjects and patients taking beta-blockers.

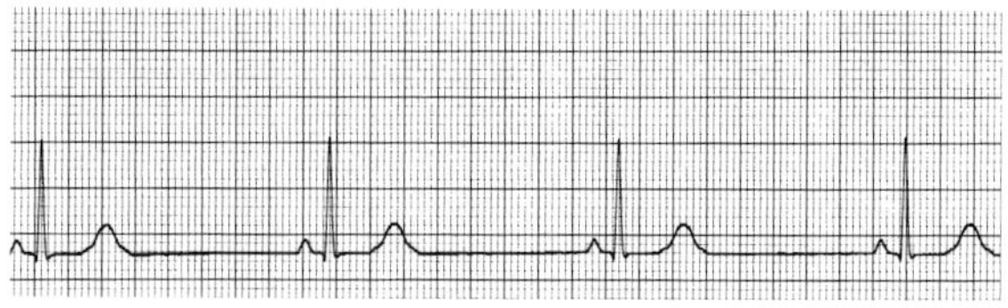

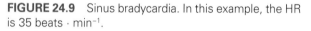

FIGURE 24.9 Sinus bradycardia. In this example, the HR is 35 beats · min^{-1}.

Sinus Tachycardia

Sinus tachycardia (HR >100 beats · min^{-1}) is normally seen during moderate and heavy exercise (see figure 24.10). Thus, exercise-induced sinus tachycardia is perfectly normal. Resting sinus tachycardia may be seen in deconditioned people or in patients who are apprehensive before exercise testing. In these heart rhythms, the SA node still functions as the pacemaker.

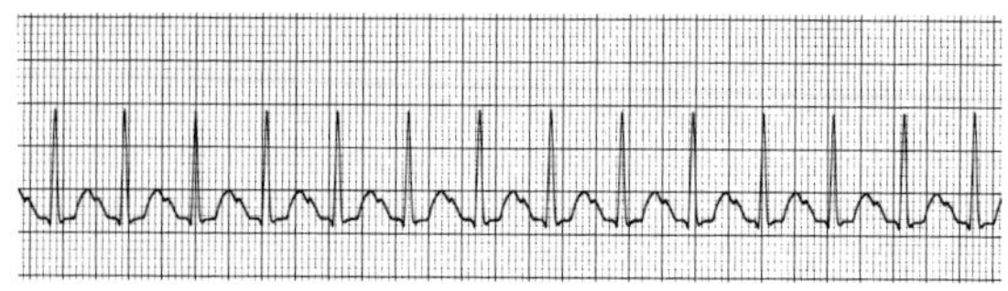

FIGURE 24.10 Sinus tachycardia. In this example, the HR is 143 beats · min^{-1}.

Atrioventricular Conduction Disturbances

Atrioventricular conduction disturbances are caused by a blockage of the electrical impulse at the AV node. The blockage may be either partial or complete.

KEY POINT

If the SA node is pacing the heart and the HR is between 60 and 100 beats · min^{-1}, the heart is in normal sinus rhythm. Bradycardia is an HR less than 60 beats · min^{-1}, and tachycardia is an HR greater than 100 beats · min^{-1} (normally seen during moderate and heavy exercise).

First-Degree AV Block

When the PR interval exceeds 0.20 sec and all P waves result in ventricular depolarization, a **first-degree AV block** exists (see figure 24.11). Causes of a first-degree AV block include medications such as digitalis and quinidine, infections, and vagal stimulation.

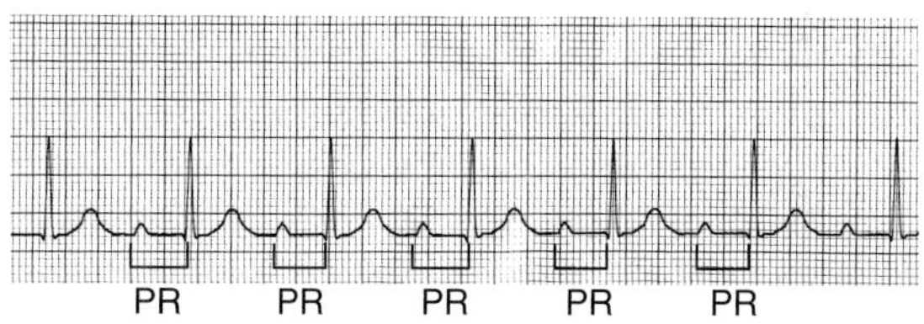

FIGURE 24.11 First-degree AV block. PR marks the prolonged PR interval (0.28 sec in this example).

Second-Degree AV Block

The distinguishing feature of **second-degree AV block** is that some, but not all, P waves result in ventricular depolarization. There are two types of second-degree AV blocks: Mobitz type I and Mobitz type II. **Mobitz type I AV block,** or Wenckebach AV block, is characterized by a PR interval that progressively lengthens until an atrial depolarization fails to initiate a ventricular depolarization and the QRS complex is skipped (see figure 24.12). This conduction disturbance is seen most commonly after an MI. The site of the block is within the AV node and is probably the result of reversible ischemia.

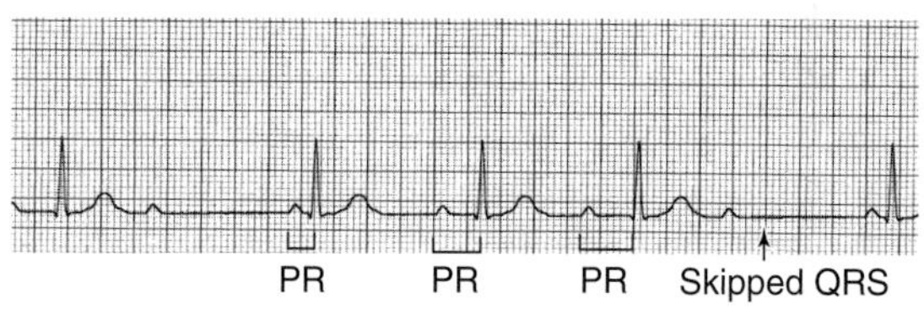

FIGURE 24.12 Mobitz type I (Wenckebach) AV block. The PR interval gradually lengthens until finally a QRS complex is skipped.

Mobitz type II AV block is the more serious of the second-degree AV blocks, and it is characterized by atrial depolarization occasionally not resulting in ventricular depolarization, even though PR intervals remain constant (i.e., do not lengthen; see figure 24.13). The site of the block is beyond the bundle of His, and it is usually the result of irreversible ischemia of the intraventricular conduction system.

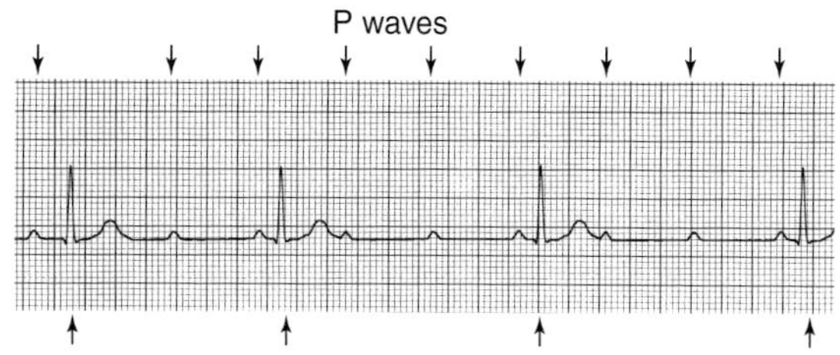

FIGURE 24.13 Mobitz type II AV block. Occasionally, and without lengthening of the PR interval, QRS complexes are skipped.

Third-Degree AV Block

Third-degree AV block is present when the ventricles contract independently of the atria (see figure 24.14). The PR interval varies and follows no regular pattern. The ventricular pacemaker may be the AV node, the bundle of His, Purkinje fibers, or the ventricular muscle, and it almost always results in a slow ventricular rate of fewer than 50 beats · min^{-1}.

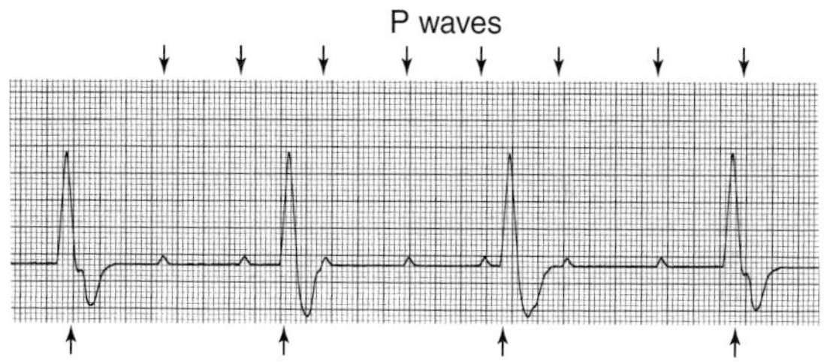

FIGURE 24.14 Third-degree AV block. There is no relationship between the atrial rate (e.g., 94 beats · min^{-1}) and the ventricular rate (e.g., 36 beats · min^{-1}), indicating complete blockage of the AV node.

Arrhythmia

An arrhythmia is an irregular heartbeat. Arrhythmias often arise when the myocardium becomes hyperexcitable due to a lack of blood flow or the use of stimulants.

Sinus Arrhythmia

Sinus arrhythmia is a sinus rhythm in which the R-R interval varies by more than 10% from beat to beat. In sinus arrhythmia, a P wave precedes each QRS complex, but the QRS complexes are unevenly spaced. Sinus arrhythmia is seen often in highly trained subjects and occasionally in patients taking beta-adrenergic blocking medications. The rhythm may be associated with respiration because HR increases with inspiration and decreases with expiration.

Premature Atrial Contraction

In **premature atrial contractions**, the rhythm is irregular and the R-R interval is short between a normal sinus beat and the premature beat (see figure 24.15). The premature beat originates somewhere other than the sinus node and is known as an **ectopic focus** (an irritable spot on the myocardium that depolarizes on its own). An ectopic focus often is caused by stimulants (e.g., caffeine), antihistamines, diet pills, cold medications (e.g., ephedrine), and nicotine. Premature atrial contractions may be seen before exercise testing in apprehensive subjects.

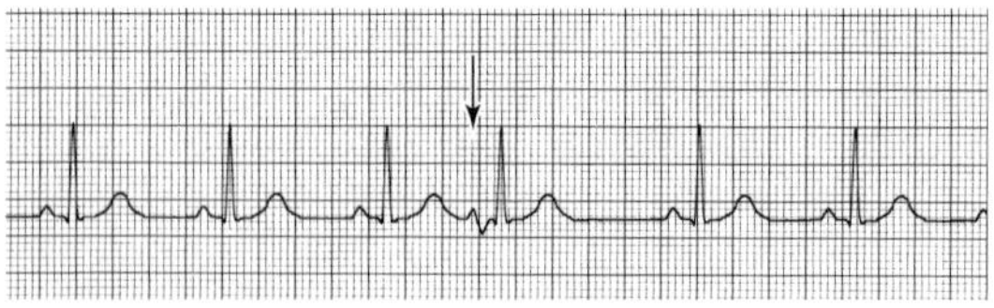

FIGURE 24.15 Premature atrial contraction. The arrow indicates a premature, diphasic P wave coming from an ectopic focus in the atria.

Atrial Flutter

During **atrial flutter**, the atrial rate is from 200 to 350 beats · min^{-1}, whereas the ventricular response is 60 to 160 beats · min^{-1}. The atrial rhythm is usually irregular, whereas the ventricular rhythm is either regular or irregular. The pacemaker site during atrial flutter is not the SA node but an ectopic focus, so normal P waves are not present. F waves, resembling a sawtooth pattern, may be seen (see figure 24.16). The causes of atrial flutter include increased sympathetic drive, hypoxia, and CHF (congestive heart failure).

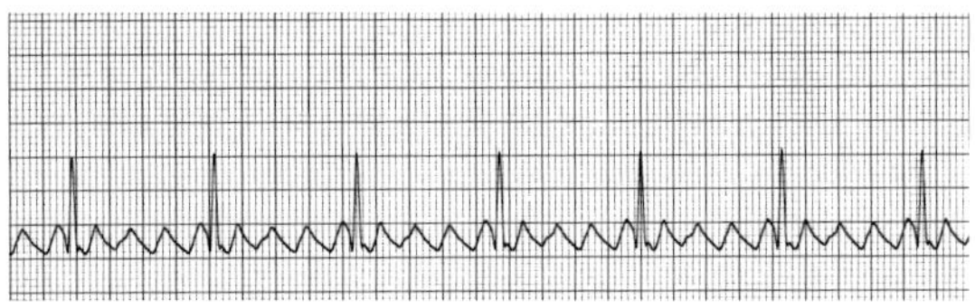

FIGURE 24.16 Atrial flutter. The atrial rate is 200 to 350 beats · min^{-1} (300 beats · min^{-1} in this example), but the ventricular rate is much slower.

Atrial Fibrillation

During **atrial fibrillation**, the atrial rate is 400 to 700 beats · min^{-1}, while the ventricular rate is usually 60 to 160 beats · min^{-1} and irregular. Multiple pacemaker sites are present in the atria, and P waves cannot be discerned (see figure 24.17). The significance of atrial fibrillation in exercise testing and training lies in its effect on ventricular function. During atrial fibrillation, the atria and ventricles are not coordinated, and the ability of the left ventricle to maintain an adequate cardiac output may be impaired. The causes of atrial fibrillation are essentially the same as those for atrial flutter. Recurrent atrial fibrillation may have little effect on the exercise response of a person with good left ventricular function, but it may cause significant symptoms in a person with poor ventricular function. Another problem with chronic atrial fibrillation is that the blood in the atria may clot and lead to a stroke because there is no concerted pumping action with atrial fibrillation.

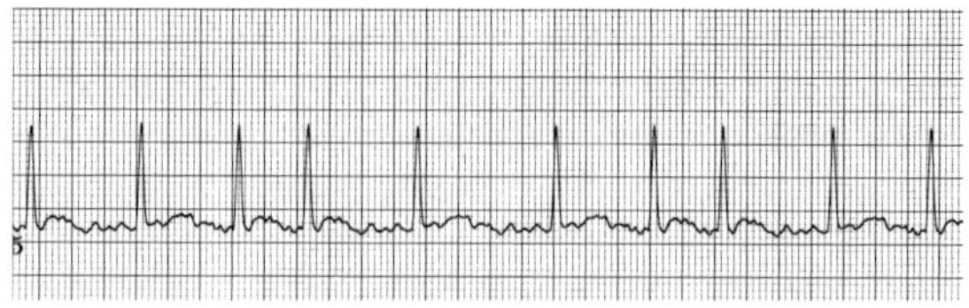

FIGURE 24.17 Atrial fibrillation. A jagged baseline and irregularly spaced QRS complexes are seen.

Premature Junctional Contractions

A **premature junctional contraction (PJC)** results when an ectopic pacemaker in the AV junctional area depolarizes the ventricles. Inverted P waves frequently accompany PJCs as the atrial depolarization proceeds in an abnormal direction (see figure 24.18). This characteristic of PJCs may distinguish them from premature atrial contractions, which frequently have notched or diphasic P waves. If these two conditions cannot be distinguished, the more general term *premature supraventricular contraction* may be used to indicate an ectopic focus above the ventricles.

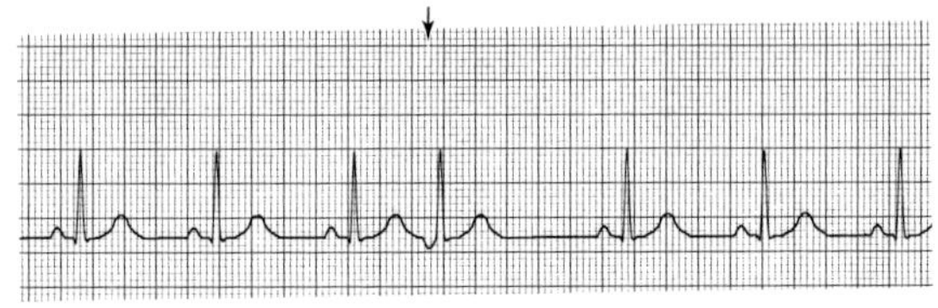

FIGURE 24.18 Premature junctional contraction (PJC). The arrow indicates a premature, inverted P wave coming from the AV node.

If the nodal tissue remains in the refractory phase after a PJC, then normally conducted waves of depolarization initiated from the sinus node will not pass into the ventricles and a compensatory pause will develop. PJCs usually result in a QRS complex of normal duration, or they may slightly prolong the QRS complex. They may be caused by catecholamine-type medications, increased parasympathetic tone on the AV node, or damage to the AV node. PJCs are of little consequence unless they occur frequently (more than 4-6 PJCs · min^{-1}) or compromise ventricular function (8).

Although supraventricular arrhythmias may concern fitness professionals and patients, Ellestad (9) found that exercise-induced supraventricular arrhythmias do not seem to compromise the long-term prognosis of patients with CAD (coronary artery disease). The significance of the supraventricular arrhythmias lies in the uncoupling of the atria and ventricles and in the resulting effect on the ability of the ventricles to maintain an adequate cardiac output.

Premature Ventricular Contractions

Premature ventricular contractions (PVCs) result from an ectopic focus in the His-Purkinje system, which initiates a ventricular contraction. PVCs have a QRS complex that is wide (>0.12 sec) and irregularly shaped (see figure 24.19). They often result in the ventricles being in the refractory phase of depolarization when the normal sinus depolarization wave reaches the ventricle, and a compensatory pause develops. PVCs are among the most common arrhythmias seen with exercise testing and training in patients with CAD. If PVCs have the same shape, they originate from the same site (ectopic focus) and are called *unifocal.* Multiple-shape PVCs that originate from multiple sites in the ventricles are called *multifocal* and are much more serious than unifocal PVCs. The rhythm of normal contractions alternating with PVCs is called *bigeminy*; if every third contraction is a PVC, the rhythm is called *trigeminy.* Three or more consecutive PVCs are known as **ventricular tachycardia**. If a single PVC falls on the descending portion of the T wave, the ventricles may be thrown into fibrillation. PVCs adversely affect the prognosis of patients with CAD; generally, the more complex the PVC, the more serious the problem. Ellestad (9) showed that the combination of ST segment depression and PVCs increases the incidence of future cardiac events.

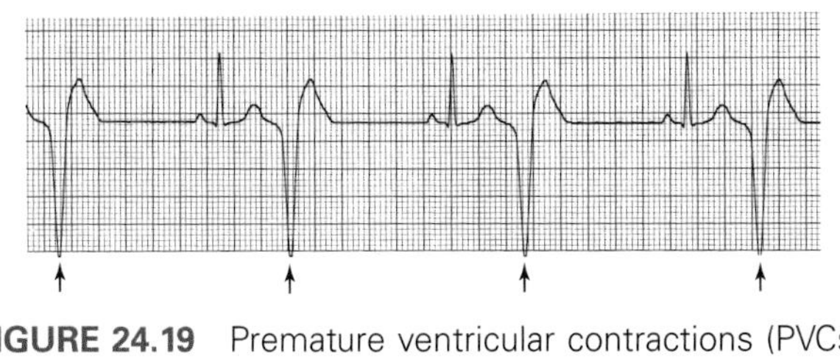

FIGURE 24.19 Premature ventricular contractions (PVCs). The arrows indicate PVCs coming from a single ectopic focus in the ventricles (unifocal PVCs).

If a PVC occurs during pulse counting, patients may report that the heart skipped a beat and may undercount their HR. They should be instructed to not increase the exercise intensity in an attempt to keep the HR in the target zone as a result of skipped beats. They should immediately reduce the exercise intensity and should report the appearance of (or increase in) skipped beats to the fitness professional and physician.

Ventricular Tachycardia

Ventricular tachycardia is present whenever three or more consecutive PVCs occur (see figure 24.20). This situation is an extremely dangerous arrhythmia that may lead to ventricular fibrillation. The HR is usually 100 to 220 beats $\cdot$ min^{-1}, and the heart may be unable to maintain adequate cardiac output during ventricular tachycardia. Ventricular tachycardia may be caused by the same factors that initiate PVCs, and it requires immediate medical attention.

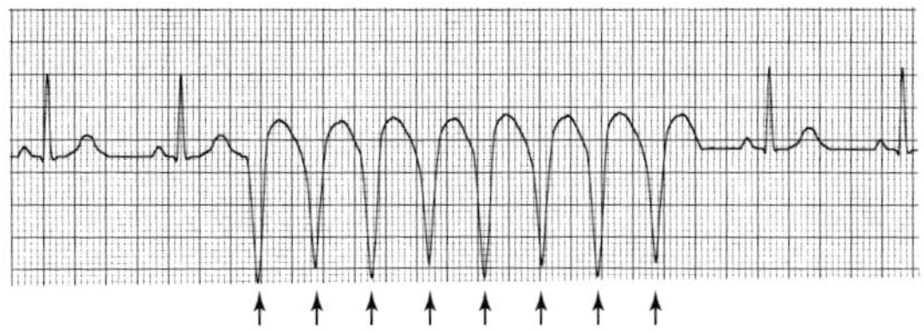

FIGURE 24.20 Ventricular tachycardia. A succession of three or more PVCs in a row is seen.

Ventricular Fibrillation

Ventricular fibrillation is a life-threatening rhythm. It requires immediate CPR until a defibrillator can be used to restore a coordinated ventricular contraction; otherwise, death will result. A fibrillating heart contracts in an unorganized, quivering manner, and the heart is unable to maintain significant cardiac output. P waves and QRS complexes are not discernible; instead the electrical pattern is a fibrillatory wave (see figure 24.21).

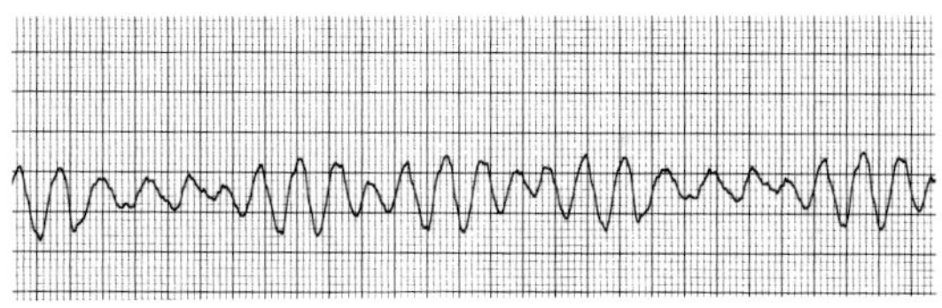

FIGURE 24.21 Ventricular fibrillation. When there are no discernible P waves or QRS complexes, the heart contracts in a disorganized, quivering manner.

KEY POINT

The ECG can be used to detect disturbances in the electrical conducting system of the heart, such as first-, second-, or third-degree AV block. The ECG can also indicate arrhythmias (abnormal heart rhythms), including sinus arrhythmia, premature beats, tachycardia, flutter, and fibrillation. Abnormal rhythms may limit exercise performance by decreasing cardiac output. In the case of severe arrhythmias, the fitness professional should terminate the exercise session and obtain immediate medical assistance.

Automated External Defibrillators

Defibrillators are devices used to treat ventricular fibrillation. They send a momentary electrical shock to the heart, often causing the heart to return to its normal rhythm. Recent technology has permitted the development of portable, battery-powered devices called *automated external defibrillators*, or AEDs. The operator applies two surface electrodes to the person's chest. These electrodes are connected to the AED, which has software that determines the person's heart rhythm. If ventricular fibrillation is detected, the AED gives a command to stand clear and then signals the operator to deliver a shock by pushing a button. Police, fitness professionals, and flight attendants should be certified in adult CPR (cardiopulmonary resuscitation) and AED training. This can be done through organizations such as the AHA and the American Red Cross. Research studies have shown that AEDs result in earlier treatment and greatly improve the chance of survival (2).

Myocardial Ischemia

Myocardial ischemia is a lack of oxygen in the myocardium attributable to inadequate blood flow. Obstruction of the coronary arteries is the most common cause of myocardial ischemia. A coronary artery is significantly obstructed if more than 50% of its diameter is occluded. A 50% reduction in diameter equals a loss of 75% of the arterial **lumen** (10). An obstructed coronary artery may supply an adequate blood flow at rest, but it will probably be unable to provide enough blood and oxygen during increased demand such as during exercise. Ischemia often, but not always, results in **angina pectoris**.

Angina pectoris is pain or discomfort caused by temporary, reversible ischemia of the myocardium that does not result in death or infarction of heart muscle. The pain often is located in the center of the chest, but it also may occur in the neck, jaw, or shoulders or may radiate into the arms and hands. Angina pectoris tends to be reproducible; patients often report anginal symptoms at roughly the same level of exertion. During exercise, patients experiencing anginal discomfort may deny pain, but on further questioning, they will admit to the sensation of burning, tightness, pressure, or heaviness in the chest or arms. Patients frequently confuse angina pectoris with musculoskeletal pain and with the discomfort resulting from the sternal incision of coronary artery bypass surgery. Anginal pain generally does not alter with movements of the trunk or arms, whereas such movement may decrease or increase musculoskeletal pain. Discomfort is probably not angina if the pain changes in quality or intensity when pressure is applied on the affected area (10).

Myocardial ischemia may cause **ST segment depression** on the ECG during an exercise test. ST segment depression usually occurs at a relatively constant rate–pressure product. The rate–pressure product equals HR · SBP, and it is a good estimate of the amount of work the heart is doing. Three types of ST segment depression are recognized: upsloping, horizontal, and downsloping (figure 24.22). Ellestad (9) has shown that the prognostic implications of upsloping and horizontal ST segment depression are roughly similar. Downsloping ST segment depression, however, affects survival more adversely.

ST segment elevation also may occur during exercise testing. ST segment elevation during an exercise test usually indicates an **aneurysm**, or a weakened area of noncontracting myocardium or scar tissue.

Myocardial Infarction

If the myocardium is deprived of oxygen for a sufficient length of time, a portion of the myocardium dies; this partial death is called a *myocardial infarction* (MI). Pain is the hallmark symptom of an MI. It is often very similar to anginal pain, only

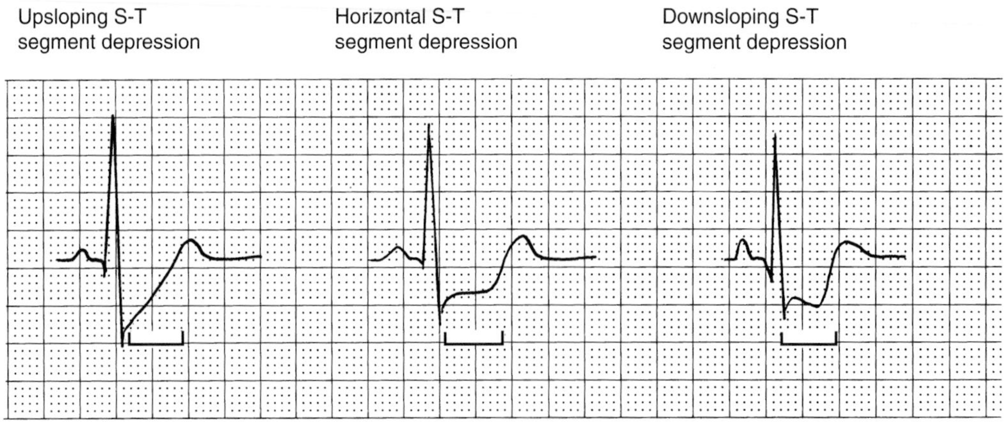

FIGURE 24.22 ST segment depression.

more severe, and may be described as a heavy feeling, a squeezing in the chest, or a burning sensation. Other symptoms that may accompany an MI are nausea, sweating, and shortness of breath.

ST segment elevation is often the first ECG sign of an acute MI. Later, pronounced Q waves and T wave inversion may appear in certain leads. Over time, the ST segment changes subside and the T wave returns to normal (see figure 24.23)

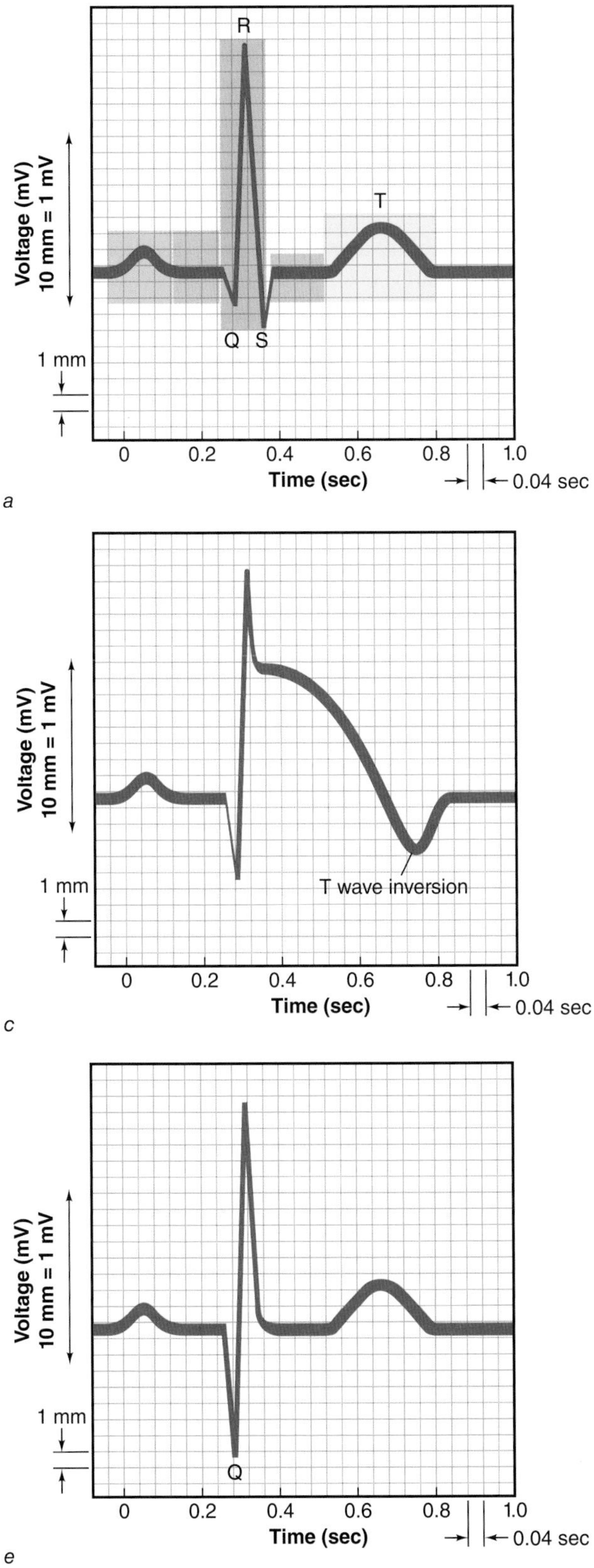

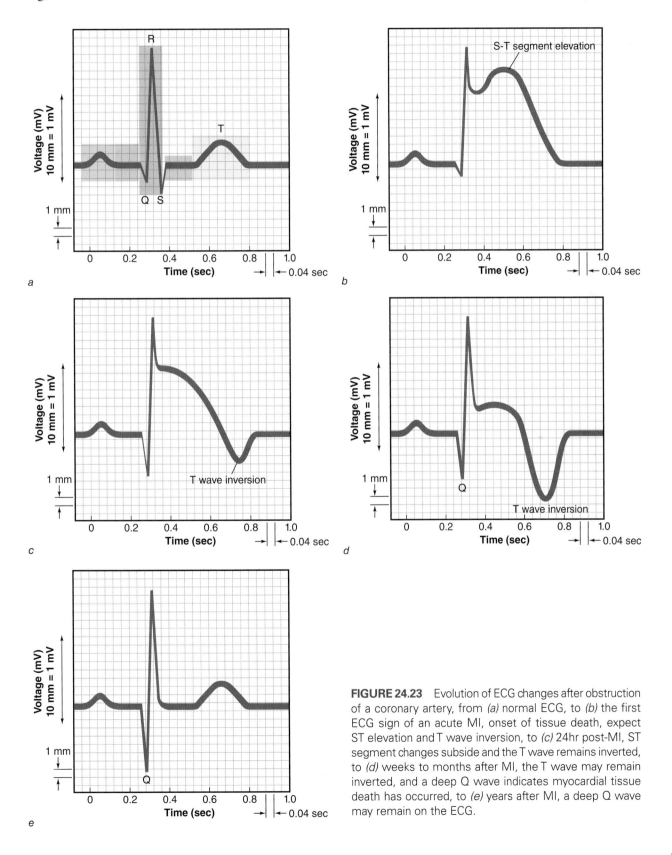

FIGURE 24.23 Evolution of ECG changes after obstruction of a coronary artery, from *(a)* normal ECG, to *(b)* the first ECG sign of an acute MI, onset of tissue death, expect ST elevation and T wave inversion, to *(c)* 24hr post-MI, ST segment changes subside and the T wave remains inverted, to *(d)* weeks to months after MI, the T wave may remain inverted, and a deep Q wave indicates myocardial tissue death has occurred, to *(e)* years after MI, a deep Q wave may remain on the ECG.

(13). Other clinical signs of an acute MI include elevations in cardiac muscle enzymes (serum lactate dehydrogenase and creatine phosphokinase), which leak into the blood after the myocardium is damaged (10).

The Framingham Heart Study demonstrated that up to 25% of MIs may be silent infarctions, meaning that the infarction does not cause sufficient symptoms for the person to seek medical attention (11). These silent infarctions may be recognized later during routine ECG examinations by the presence of significant Q waves in certain leads.

Patients with CAD should be instructed how to differentiate anginal attacks from possible MIs. If an anginal attack occurs, the patient should stop the activity, if any, that precipitated the discomfort and should take a nitroglycerin (NTG) tablet under the tongue. If the anginal discomfort persists after 5 min, the patient takes a second sublingual NTG tablet. This procedure is repeated, if needed, one more time. If the pain persists 5 min after the third NTG tablet, the patient should seek immediate medical attention (3).

KEY POINT

Inadequate blood flow to the myocardium often, but not always, results in symptoms of chest pain (angina pectoris). ST segment depression or elevation on the ECG can indicate inadequate blood flow (ischemia). Significant Q waves on the ECG can indicate that a portion of the heart muscle has died (MI).

Medications That Affect Heart Rate Response

Fitness professionals do not prescribe medications or deal on a day-to-day basis with people taking all of the following medications, but they do encounter participants taking some of them. Often drugs that don't specifically target cardiovascular function still affect the HR response to exercise, such as medications for smoking cessation, bronchodilators for asthma, medications to control blood glucose concentrations, and mood stabilizers such as antidepressants. This section summarizes how those drugs affect the exercise HR response and possible side effects.

Nicotine Gums, Nasal Sprays, and Patches

Nicotine gums, nasal sprays, and patches are used as smoking substitutes for people who are trying to stop smoking. With **nicotine gum**, the nicotine is absorbed through the oral mucosa, providing sufficient plasma nicotine concentrations to curb the craving to smoke. Nicotine gums are marketed under such names as Nicorette and Nicogum. Nicotine nasal sprays allow nicotine to be rapidly absorbed through blood vessels in the nose. With transdermal nicotine patches, the nicotine is slowly absorbed through the skin. Nicotine may affect the exercise response, particularly if a person chews nicotine gum but also continues to smoke. Nicotine may increase HR and BP as well as the incidence of cardiac arrhythmias (1).

Bronchodilators

The **bronchodilators** relax smooth muscle surrounding airways in the lungs and relieve the symptoms of asthma, bronchitis, and related lung disorders. These medications can be taken orally or from an inhaler. The inhalers are generally used for acute asthma episodes, whereas long-term bronchodilation is usually obtained with oral preparations. Most of these drugs stimulate the β_2 receptors that relax bronchial smooth muscle and increase the airway lumen. Because of their beta-adrenergic stimulating effect, they can increase HR and BP, although most of their effect is on the smooth muscle found in airways. Some of the inhaler brand names include Advair, Ventolin, Alupent, and Maxair. The oral bronchodilators include Theobid, Aminophylline, Theo-Dur, and many others (3).

Oral Antiglycemic Agents

A substantial number of obese participants in fitness programs have hyperglycemia, or elevated levels of blood glucose. In this condition the pancreas is able to produce insulin, but it is unable to produce sufficient quantities to maintain normal blood glucose control or the body has become resistant to the insulin that is produced. This condition is called *type 2 diabetes mellitus* or *non-insulin-dependent diabetes mellitus*, and it often can be controlled with **oral antiglycemic agents**. The oral antiglycemic medications that stimulate the pancreas to secrete more insulin include the sulfonylureas glyburide (Glynase, DiaBeta, Micronase), glipizide (Glucotrol), and glimepiride (Amaryl). These agents often cause hypoglycemia, or low blood sugar. Hypoglycemia is potentially dangerous, and the fitness professional should be cognizant of any changes in alertness and orientation in clients taking any medication that can lower plasma glucose concentrations.

Metformin (Glucophage), the most used oral antiglycemic agent, is classed as a biguanide. This agent reduces insulin resistance, thereby lowering blood sugar.

Several new classifications of drugs to treat type 2 diabetes have recently been introduced. These include the GLP-1 agonists such as exenatide (Byetta, Bydureon), liraglutide (Victoza), and albiglutide (Tanzeum). A similar class called the *DPP-4 inhibitors*, or gliptins, includes sitagliptin (Januvia), saxagliptin (Onglyza), linagliptin (Tradjenta), and alogliptin (Nesina). The most recent class of drugs introduced is the sodium glucose cotransporter 2 (SGLT2) inhibitors (flozins). These agents reduce resorption of glucose in the kidney, resulting in increased urinary glucose excretion and a consequent lowering of plasma glucose levels. The SGLT2 inhibitors include canagliflozin (Invokana), dapagliflozin (Farxiga), and empagliflozin (Jardiance). These newer agents also result in weight loss in some patients, but none are FDA approved for weight loss.

Type 1 or insulin-dependent diabetes mellitus is a more serious disorder of carbohydrate metabolism. It is characterized by an absence of insulin and requires frequent insulin injections. Insulin cannot be taken orally because it is a protein and would be inactivated by the digestive process. However, in 2014 the FDA approved an insulin nasal spray called *Afrezza*. When working with an insulin-dependent diabetic, the fitness professional should be aware of the possibility of hypoglycemia. Signs of hypoglycemia include bizarre behavior and slurred speech. When people with insulin-dependent diabetes mellitus are exercising, it is a good idea to have a source of sugar or quickly absorbed carbohydrate readily available in the event of a hypoglycemic episode. An injectable drug called *glucagon*, or a concentrated dextrose solution (D50W), can be administered in an emergency. See chapter 21 for additional details on diabetes.

Depressants

Tranquilizers, or anxiolytics, reduce anxiety. Antianxiety medications, such as alprazolam (Xanax), may lower HR and BP by controlling anxiety, but otherwise the exercise response is not affected. With some of the neuroleptic agents (previously called *major tranquilizers*), HR may increase while BP either drops or remains unchanged (1). **Alcohol** is a depressant that can affect the exercise test by impairing motor coordination, balance, and reaction times. Chronic alcohol consumption tends to elevate resting and exercise BP. The acute effects of alcohol ingestion on the exercise response have been examined. During brief maximal exercise, small to moderate doses of alcohol do not affect oxygen uptake, SV, ejection fraction, cardiac output, arteriovenous oxygen difference, and peak lactate concentration (14). However, higher doses (blood alcohol content = 0.20 mg · dl^{-1}) may impair myocardial function, as shown by a 6% decrease in ejection fraction (12). Alcohol intake can provoke arrhythmias at rest and during exercise.

KEY POINT

Medications are prescribed for a variety of reasons, including high BP, abnormal heart rhythms, elevated blood lipids, asthma, and other medical concerns.

24

LEARNING AIDS

REVIEW QUESTIONS

1. Draw a picture of the heart, and label the four heart chambers, the four heart valves, the pulmonary artery, and the aorta.
2. Name the coronary arteries, and identify what region of the myocardium they supply blood to.
3. Draw the major components of the heart's electrical conducting system, and label the SA node, AV node, bundle of His, left and right bundle branches, and Purkinje fibers.
4. Define the term *electrocardiogram (ECG)* and give the standard settings for paper speed and amplitude.
5. Identify the electrical event in the heart that corresponds to the P wave, PR segment, QRS complex, and T wave of the ECG.
6. If an individual in normal sinus rhythm has 20 mm between two adjacent R waves, what is the HR? If an individual in atrial fibrillation has 11 complete cardiac cycles in a 6 sec strip, what is the HR?
7. Describe the following conduction abnormalities: first-degree AV block, second-degree AV block (Mobitz type I and type II), and third-degree AV block.
8. Examine the ECGs in this chapter and point out abnormalities of HR, conduction defects, and arrhythmias.
9. What are the clinical signs (both electrocardiographic signs and plasma markers) associated with an MI (i.e., heart attack)? What are the symptoms of a heart attack?

CASE STUDIES

1. The following ECG tracing was obtained on a 38-yr-old female before she took a GXT on the treadmill.

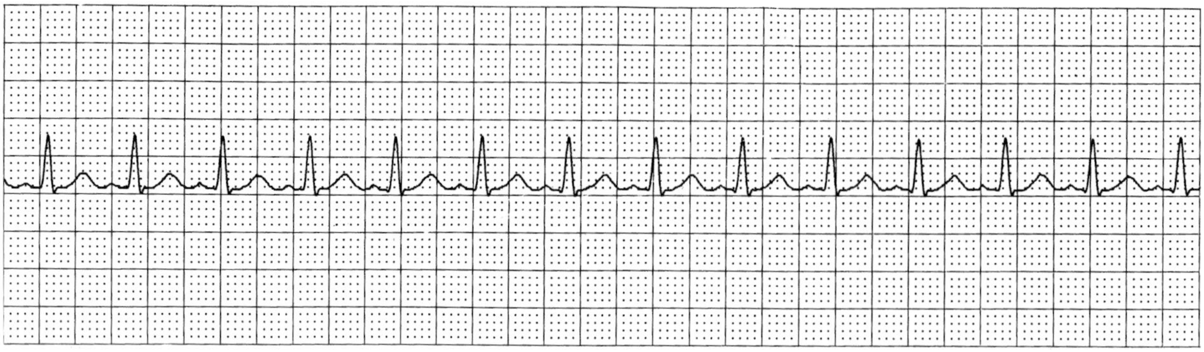

   a. Determine the HR (beats · min^{-1}) and the durations of the PR interval, QRS complex, and QT interval (in seconds).
   b. What condition does she have?
   c. What factors might cause this condition?

2. A 21-yr-old male college student who was taking a cold medication containing ephedrine showed the following ECG tracing at rest.

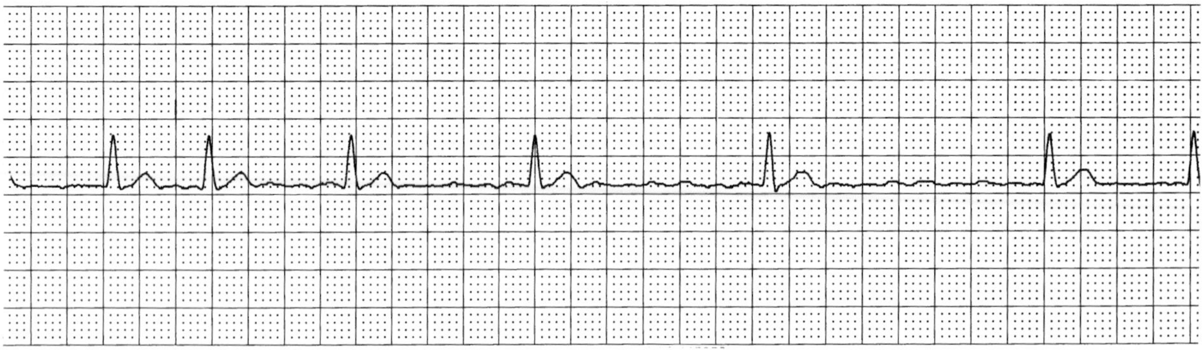

   a. What type of arrhythmia does he have?
   b. What is the ventricular rate?

3. A 57-yr-old participant in your exercise program showed the following ECG tracing while she was exercising at 3.5 mi · hr^{-1} on a 6% grade on the treadmill.

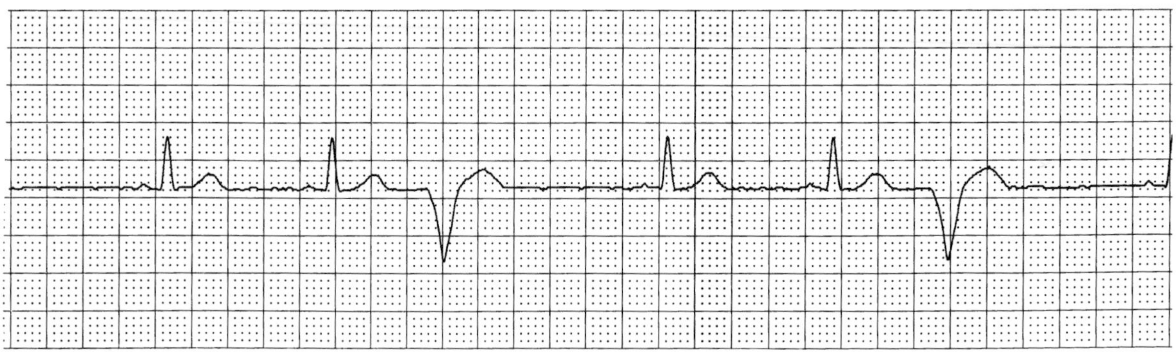

   a. What ECG abnormality is shown?
   b. What action should be taken?

Answers to Case Studies

1. For case study 1:
   a. HR = 1500 / 12 = 125 beats · min^{-1}.
      PR interval duration = 0.12 sec
      QRS complex duration = 0.08 sec
      QT interval duration = 0.32 sec
   b. Sinus tachycardia is a fast HR (over 100 beats · min^{-1}).
   c. Common causes of sinus tachycardia are anxiety, nervousness, caffeine, and low fitness.
2. For case study 2:
   a. He has atrial fibrillation (jagged baseline with irregularly spaced PVCs).
   b. Ventricular rate = 6 cardiac cycles in a 6 sec strip × 10 = 60 beats · min^{-1}.
3. For case study 3:
   a. He has trigeminy—every third heartbeat is a PVC.
   b. Gradually decrease treadmill speed and grade, and notify the physician.

25

Injury Prevention and Treatment

Jenny Moshak

OBJECTIVES

The reader will be able to do the following:

1. Design and implement an emergency action plan (EAP).
2. Describe the signs and symptoms of soft-tissue injuries (sprains, strains, contusions, tendinitis, tendinosis, dislocations, and subluxations), and describe how to provide acute care for injuries.
3. Define *delayed-onset muscle soreness (DOMS)* and *exertional rhabdomyolysis*, and explain how to prevent, identify signs and symptoms of, and provide care for these conditions.
4. Identify signs, symptoms, and initial proper treatment for bone injuries, wounds, and associated bleeding.
5. Provide prevention strategies to deter the occurrence and spread of community-associated methicillin-resistant *Staphylococcus aureus* (CA-MRSA).
6. Describe the causes, prevention, and treatment of heat-related disorders and emergencies, and provide guidelines for fluid replacement before and after exercise.
7. Explain the causes, prevention, and treatment of cold-related disorders and emergencies, including superficial and deep frostbite and hypothermia.
8. Provide direction using the 30–30 rule when lightning poses a threat during outdoor activities.
9. Identify and manage diabetic reactions, seizures, and respiratory disorders that occur during exercise participation.
10. Identify complications associated with conditioning and the environment related to sickle cell trait (SCT) and exertional sickling, including prevention, recognition of signs and symptoms, and care during an emergent situation.
11. Identify the signs and symptoms of a concussion, and determine when to remove a participant from activity.
12. Describe the appropriate action and techniques needed in emergency situations, including treating shock, monitoring vital signs, performing cardiopulmonary resuscitation (CPR), and using an automated external defibrillator (AED) for adults.

The fitness professional must be prepared to respond in an emergency medical situation and recognize signs and symptoms in order to manage common injuries and conditions to protect the safety, health, and well-being of fitness participants. This chapter discusses injury prevention, injury recognition, and common treatment approaches as well as planning for and handling medical emergencies.

Fitness enhances performance and aids in injury prevention. Improper conditioning is often a cause of sport- and activity-related injuries. Fitness professionals who appropriately develop and implement programs designed to improve flexibility; muscular strength, endurance, and power; balance and proprioception; and cardiorespiratory endurance can help increase performance and decrease the risk of injury.

There are inherent injury risks associated with sport and physical activity. The signs and symptoms of injury often include the following:

- Exquisite point tenderness
- Pain that persists even when the body part is at rest
- Joint pain
- Pain that does not go away after a warm-up
- Swelling or discoloration
- Increased pain with weight-bearing activities or with active movement
- Changes in normal bodily functions

Injury risk in exercise programs may be reduced by assessing the fitness level of the participant, designing a program that gradually increases in intensity and duration while meeting the participant's goals, and monitoring progress in order to modify the workouts if necessary. Safety regarding external factors such as equipment, facilities, and weather should also be considered. Advanced planning, emergency preparedness, adequate equipment and facilities, and counseling in activity selection can mitigate injury.

Emergency Action Plan

Emergency situations may arise at any time. An **emergency action plan (EAP)** is a written document used to facilitate and organize employee actions during workplace emergencies (see chapter 26 for more details on the legal aspects of EAPs). A professional staff member should be designated as the EAP coordinator to supervise and document the plan. The development and implementation of an EAP, along with personnel training so that employees understand their roles and responsibilities within the plan, will result in the best possible care during an emergency or life-threatening conditions (14, 23, 31). The importance of being prepared when emergencies arise cannot be overemphasized: A client's survival may hinge on the training and preparedness of emergency team members. ACSM recommends that staff emergency training be conducted at least four times a year (34). The EAP should be reviewed at least once a year with all staff, along with CPR and first aid recertification training. It is also critical that staff have clear documentation of the EAP, maintain records of staff training, and keep detailed records of any injuries that occur on-site (see form 25.1 for a sample EAP). The responsibility of maintaining these records often falls to the EAP coordinator. Following are considerations related to documenting the EAP:

- The EAP should be posted in a public area and kept on file.
- The EAP should be reviewed annually by the staff. Documentation of annual AED and CPR training by personnel, as well as documentation of all fitness professional staff present at the annual review of the EAP, should be recorded and filed.
- Documentation of regular emergency equipment checks and maintenance should be kept on file.

An EAP consists of three components:

1. Trained EAP personnel
2. Communication plan
3. Access to emergency equipment

Trained Personnel

Fitness professionals who are trained to react to emergency situations are essential in a workplace EAP. Fitness professionals should hold certification in **cardiopulmonary resuscitation (CPR)** with automated external defibrillators (AEDs), have knowledge of basic first aid and prevention of disease transmission, and be able to implement the EAP.

When forming the emergency team, it is important to develop team members' skills so that they can respond to a variety of situations. If each member is able to act in a wide range of capacities, the team will be better able to respond to situations that arise. This allows the emergency team to function even though certain members may not be present.

ROLES WITHIN THE EMERGENCY TEAM

1. Immediate care of the injured participant
2. Emergency equipment retrieval (e.g., first aid supplies, AED)
3. Activation of **emergency medical services (EMS)**
4. Direction of EMS to scene
5. Documentation

Communication Plan

Rapid and effective communication is a key to quick delivery of care in emergency situations. Access to a working telephone or other telecommunications device, whether fixed or mobile, should be ensured. The communications

FORM 25.1 Sample Emergency Action Plan

Effective November 2016

Emergency communication: Fixed telephone lines are located in the main office (555-555-1212) and at the front desk (555-555-1234). Supervisors on staff carry cellular telephones.

ROLES OF EMERGENCY TEAM PERSONNEL (FITNESS STAFF TRAINED AND CERTIFIED IN EMERGENCY CARE)

1. Immediate care to the injured participant
2. Activation of emergency medical services (EMS)
   - Call 911 (provide name, location, telephone number; number of people injured; condition of injured; first aid treatment; specific directions; other information as requested).
   - Provide venue directions: Our facility is located at 2000 N. Main Street on the corner of Main Street and Central Ave. The main entrance doors are on the north side of the building off of Main Street. Notify supervisor and other personnel needed to respond to the emergency.
3. Direction of EMS to scene
   - Open appropriate doors.
   - Designate a person to make initial contact with EMS and direct them to the scene.
   - Scene control: Limit scene to first aid providers and move bystanders away from area.
4. Emergency equipment retrieval
   - Centrally located AED is on the wall next to the main reception desk.
   - A second AED is located on the second floor on the wall between the weight room and multipurpose gymnasium.
   - First aid kits are located at the main reception desk and in the storage closet on the second floor.
5. Following the event: Staff present at the event shall document the incident by completing an injury or accident report of the emergency situation.

From E.T. Howley and D.L. Thompson, 2017, *Fitness professional's handbook*, 7th ed. (Champaign, IL: Human Kinetics).

system should be checked on a regular basis to guarantee working order. A backup communication plan should be in effect in case the primary communication system fails. The most common method of communication today is a cellular phone; however, it is important to know the location of all workable telephones. Prearranged access to the phones should be established. An example of a facility plan for activating EMS is provided.

Access to Emergency Equipment

All emergency equipment should be quickly accessible at the facility and stored in a clean, environmentally controlled area. Emergency equipment should be checked and calibrated on a regular basis. Personnel should be familiar with the function and operation of each type of emergency equipment and rehearse their use regularly. The emergency equipment should be appropriate for the emergency team personnel's training level and certification.

KEY POINT

The development and implementation of an EAP helps ensure the safety and well-being of fitness participants when an emergency situation arises. Key components of an EAP are a trained staff, a communication plan, and access to emergency equipment.

Activating Emergency Medical Services

Making the Call

- 911 (or local emergency number)
- Additional contacts required by the center (e.g., college campus fitness center may require communication with campus safety unit)

Providing Information

- Name, address, and telephone number of caller
- Number of injured people
- Condition of injured people
- First aid treatment initiated by first responder
- Specific directions to the emergency scene (e.g., "Come to the south entrance of the facility on Main Street")
- Other information as requested by dispatcher

Injury Management

The fitness professional should be knowledgeable about common activity-related injuries and may be called upon to give initial care. Actual diagnosis and long-term care of injuries is the responsibility of medical professionals. This section provides information to assist in identifying common injuries, administering appropriate acute care, and making referrals to medical personnel.

Managing an injury requires an understanding of the structures involved and the severity of trauma. An acute injury occurs when a force acts on tissue and produces a macrotrauma. A chronic injury occurs over a period of time when repetitive forces produce a microtrauma. Forces involved in the injury process consist of compressive, tensile, and shear. For example, a contusion, or bruise, is caused by a compressive direct force acting on the involved tissue. Damage to a ligament involves a tensile force that pulls the tissue apart, causing a stretch or tear. A **blister** occurs when a shear force acts in opposite directions on layers of the skin. Some traumatic injuries involve multiple forces and structures. For example, a knee injury that results in tears of the anterior cruciate ligament (ACL), medial collateral ligament (MCL), and meniscus and a bony contusion on the joint surface is an all-too-common complex injury involving multiple structures.

Signs and symptoms associated with an injury often include one or more of the following: swelling, discoloration, pain, instability, muscle spasms, point tenderness, decreased range of motion (ROM), decreased strength, and dysfunction. Some signs and symptoms may manifest immediately, whereas others may take several hours or days to present.

Soft-Tissue Injuries

Common activity-related injuries include the following:

- Contusion: caused by single or multiple forces over time, resulting in bleeding and tissue damage of the skin or muscle (e.g., deep thigh bruise)
- Acute sprain: caused by a single tensile force that produces a stretch or tear (partial or complete) of a ligament (e.g., lateral ankle sprain)
- Chronic sprain: occurs from repetitive forces acting on a ligament (e.g., Little League elbow)
- Muscle or tendon strain: involves a tensile force causing an overstretching or partial or complete tear (e.g., hamstring strain)
- Tendinitis: inflammation of a tendon caused by single or repetitive tensile forces (e.g., Achilles tendinitis)
- Tendinosis: degeneration of collagen in a tendon over time (e.g., tennis elbow)
- Bursitis: inflammation caused by compression or friction to a bursa sac (e.g., olecranon bursitis)
- Dislocation: when bone is forced out of its normal joint position and remains there until manually or surgically replaced (e.g., shoulder dislocation)
- Subluxation: when bone is partially forced out of the joint and spontaneously returns (e.g., patella subluxation)
- Nerve damage: occurs from a compressive or tensile force (e.g., sciatica); signs and symptoms include change in sensation, decrease in strength, numbness, and pain (nerve pain is often described as shooting, aching, sharp, dull, throbbing, tingling, or burning)

Soft-tissue injuries are classified by their severity and dysfunction:

- Mild or first degree: microtearing or stretching of the tissue involving minor tissue damage, mild to moderate pain, minimal swelling, full to limited ROM, and little to no dysfunction.
- Moderate or second degree: partial tearing of the tissue resulting in moderate tissue damage, moderate to severe pain, moderate swelling, limited ROM, and limited function. Muscle spasms may occur around the injury.
- Severe or third degree: major disruption to tissue, often resulting in a complete tear with moderate to severe pain, moderate to severe swelling, and loss of function. Palpable deformity may be present along with muscle spasms in the area.

Fitness professionals are not expected to diagnose the degree of injury, but they should have a basic understanding of the continuum of injuries and be able to provide first aid, including applying common elements of care for injuries.

Protection, rest, ice, compression, and elevation (PRICE principle) is the basis for providing injury care.

PRICE

P—Protection is necessary to avoid further tissue damage when a severe injury occurs. This requires complete immobilization (stabilizing the injury and the areas above and below) until further evaluation by medical personnel. Items that offer protection include crutches, splints, braces, and arm slings.

R—Rest is necessary to allow damaged tissue to begin the healing process and depends on the severity of injury. It can range from modifying activity, to not using the injured body part, to stopping activity all together.

I—Ice (cold application) results in an immediate decrease in pain and spasm around the injury. Vasoconstriction of local blood vessels occurs, which may help minimize swelling. Cold applications including ice bags and gel and chemical packs are applied for 20 to 30 min. Some individuals cannot tolerate ice directly on the skin due to tissue sensitivity or circulatory impairment. This typically occurs in older adults, young children, or people with systemic disease. In these cases, or when using a cold gel or chemical pack, a barrier such as a towel should be placed between the pack and the skin. Depending on the severity of the injury, ice can be reapplied several times during the first 24 to 72 hr.

C—Compression is applied using an elastic wrap or sleeve to help prevent swelling. The elastic wrap should be applied beginning distal to the injury, completely covering the body part, and extending proximal to the injury site. Compression should be applied firmly but not so tightly that circulation is impaired.

E—Elevation of the injured body part above the heart will maximize the effect of gravity to minimize swelling.

Heat should never be applied to an acute injury. Some chronic injuries such as tendinitis, tendinosis, and bursitis may benefit from heating the area prior to activity, either superficially (heat pack, warm whirlpool) or deeply (additional dynamic or cardio warm-up time). Heating tissue increases circulation, muscle excitability, tissue elasticity, cellular metabolism, and nerve conduction. Both chronic and subacute injuries can benefit from cold application after activity (4, 31, 32).

KEY POINT

When soft tissues are injured, proper assessment and initial treatment can reduce the possibility of further trauma and can aid in the healing process. Protection, rest, ice, compression, and elevation (PRICE) are the important steps for immediate care of most musculoskeletal and joint injuries.

Delayed-Onset Muscle Soreness

When starting a new exercise program, some participants may encounter an overload condition called **delayed-onset muscle soreness (DOMS)**. DOMS can occur from an activity that places unaccustomed loads on muscle, resulting in microscopic breakdown of muscle tissue that leads to an inflammatory response over several days. This type of soreness is different from acute soreness, which is pain that develops during or immediately after the activity. Delayed soreness typically begins to develop 12 to 24 hr after the exercise has been performed and may produce the greatest pain between 24 and 72 hr after the exercise. Activities that produce an eccentric force, such as running or walking downhill, weightlifting, and jumping, are often associated with DOMS (6, 10). However, anyone participating in a new activity can experience DOMS.

Although pain is usually the most noticeable symptom of DOMS, people may also experience mild swelling in the affected extremities, stiffness, decreased joint ROM, point tenderness, and muscle weakness. When the signs and symptoms become severe, it may be an indication of exertional rhabdomyolysis (see the next section in this chapter).

One of the best ways to prevent or at least reduce the severity of DOMS is to progress slowly in a new exercise program or activity. The muscles need time to adapt to new stresses, and this should help to minimize the severity of symptoms, although some soreness can be expected. It is also important to allow the muscle time to recover; participating in the same exercises on subsequent days, particularly if exertion is high, is not recommended.

Treatment of DOMS involves decreasing the symptoms. Rest, ice, compression, elevation along with light massage, and NSAID medication may be useful in reducing pain. Return to activity should be gradual to prevent further muscle damage (10, 17, 18).

KEY POINT

Participants starting a new exercise program will often experience DOMS. Muscles should be given an opportunity to adequately recover and adapt to new stresses in order to minimize the pain that accompanies DOMS.

Exertional Rhabdomyolysis

Exertional rhabdomyolysis is a syndrome characterized by skeletal muscle degeneration and muscle enzyme leakage that can occur in normal, healthy people following strenuous exercise. Rhabdomyolysis is the breakdown of muscle tissue that releases a muscle protein called *myoglobin* into the blood, which is then filtered by the kidneys. Myoglobin breaks down into substances that can damage kidney cells, leading to kidney damage. In severe cases, this syndrome can result in renal failure and sudden death (8, 9, 22, 33, 38).

The National Collegiate Athletic Association (NCAA) states, "Novel overexertion is the single most common cause of exertional rhabdomyolysis (ER) and is characterized as too much, too soon, and too fast" (30). This typically involves strength and conditioning programs that increase in intensity and duration too quickly and do not allow for adequate recovery.

The signs and symptoms of exertional rhabdomyolysis may initially resemble DOMS; however, the soreness is more severe, and additional signs and symptoms include the following:

- Dark, red, or cola-colored urine
- Decreased urine output
- Severe muscle stiffness, aching, and swelling
- General weakness
- Abdominal pain
- Nausea or vomiting
- Muscle tenderness
- Muscle weakness

Similar to DOMS, the signs and symptoms of exertional rhabdomyolysis may take several hours to days to develop. Fitness participants with these signs and symptoms should not participate in activity and should see a physician. Medical clearance is recommended before participation resumes.

Risk factors that can increase the likelihood of exertional rhabdomyolysis include the following:

- Being deconditioned
- Having dehydration or heat-related illness
- Having SCT

Research indicates that there may be a relationship between SCT and an increased vulnerability to heat illness and exertional rhabdomyolysis (5, 26). More research is needed in this area to further investigate the possible association.

Prevention of exertional rhabdomyolysis involves gradually increasing the intensity and duration of exercise programs and preventing dehydration. Drinking plenty of fluids after strenuous exercise will help to dilute the urine and enhance the ability of the kidneys to clear large proteins such as myoglobin.

KEY POINT

The single most common cause of exertional rhabdomyolysis is implementing an exercise program that is too much, too soon, too fast. Using progression when introducing any new activity and emphasizing hydration will help prevent exertional rhabdomyolysis. In addition, adequate recovery is essential to protect muscles tissue from excessive breakdown.

Treating Fractures

Fracture occurs when there is a break in the continuity of bone tissue. Acute fracture occurs from a direct force that damages the bone, and stress (chronic) fracture results from repetitive forces that progressively injure the bone. The periosteum is affected initially, followed by damage to the cortical bone. Signs and symptoms of a fracture include pain, point tenderness, swelling, and visual or palpable deformity. There also may be muscle spasms and impairment to nearby blood vessels or nerves. A simple (closed) fracture is one that has no open wound, whereas a compound (open) fracture has one or more bones exposed through the soft tissue and skin around it. An acute fracture should be immobilized by splinting the distal and proximal points to the injured area, and the participant should be referred to a physician. Do not attempt to reduce (push back into place) a fracture. Activate EMS to assist with transport; urgency is a necessity with any skull, spine, compound fracture, or fracture associated with shock, impaired circulation, or nerve damage. A suspected fracture to the skull or spine requires immediate head and neck immobilization until EMS takes over. Table 25.1 gives the possible signs and symptoms and additional procedures to follow when treating a fracture.

KEY POINT

If a fracture is suspected, immobilize the joints above and below the injury, treat for shock, and activate EMS when appropriate. Do not attempt to reduce a fracture.

Treating Wounds and Other Skin Disorders

Wounds are also common injuries associated with activity programs. The fitness professional may need to provide emergency treatment for an open wound to control bleeding and prevent infection. **Universal precautions** are safety measures that prevent exposure to blood and bloodborne pathogens (see the section in this chapter on universal precautions). Once bleeding is controlled, further care can be given to prevent infection. In minor cases, a thorough cleansing and application of a sterile dressing may be all that is needed. Clean with large amounts of soap and water or sterile saline to flush. Use sterile gauze with sterile technique: Begin directly over the wound and sweep, moving away from the injury. Cover with a sterile dressing and apply moderate pressure until bleeding stops. If bleeding continues, apply more gauze on top of the saturated material. When bleeding stops, cover with topical petroleum-based ointment, a sterile nonadherent dressing, and a bandage. Protect open wounds with a sterile dressing; a covered wound heals faster.

If a wound becomes infected, the infection will usually occur several days later and present with an increase in pain, heat, redness, swelling, or dysfunction. Refer immediately to a physician. See table 25.2 for additional care for specific wound types.

A wound involving uncontrolled, severe bleeding is a medical emergency. Excessive blood loss can result in shock and lead to death. Internal bleeding, another serious condition, involves bleeding deep within structures of the body, including the chest, abdominal, or pelvic cavities. The fitness professional should treat for shock and alert EMS immediately. Table 25.3 discusses care of severe bleeding.

KEY POINT

The primary steps of treating an open wound are to control bleeding and prevent infection. Clean the wound and keep it covered until it heals.

Table 25.1 Fractures and Their Treatment

Signs and symptoms	Care
	ACUTE FRACTURE
Loss of function Deformity or bony deviation Swelling Pain Palpable tenderness Referred pain Crepitus False joint Discoloration (usually becomes apparent later)	**Acute closed fracture:** Active EMS if transport is necessary. *Do not* reduce a fracture. Splint the joints above and below the suspected fracture to protect the body part from further injury. Ice can be applied to reduce pain, spasm, and swelling. Treat for shock. (See section on emergency procedures.) Refer to physician. **Acute open fracture:** Activate EMS. Control bleeding and prevent infection by applying a sterile dressing. *Do not* move bones back into place. Follow protocol for closed fracture care.
	CHRONIC STRESS FACTURE
Pain that increases in intensity and duration Swelling Dysfunction Point tenderness	Remove from activity that causes pain. Refer to physician.

Based on Anderson and Parr 2013; Prentice 2007; Prentice 2013.

Table 25.2 Wounds and Their Treatment

Injury	Signs and symptoms	Care
Abrasion—scraping of tissues resulting in removal of outermost skin layers and exposure of numerous capillaries	Superficial, reddish, irregular surface Oozing or weeping from underlying capillaries Dirt, debris, or bacteria may be embedded in tissue	Dirt or debris that is still present after normal cleaning may require gentle scrubbing using sterile technique.
Incision—cutting of skin resulting in an open wound with cleanly cut edges and exposure of underlying tissues	Smooth edges that may bleed freely	Refer to physician if wound needs suturing (e.g., facial cuts, large or deep wounds).
Laceration—tearing of skin resulting in an open wound with jagged edges and exposure of underlying tissues	Jagged edges that may bleed freely	Refer to physician if wound needs suturing.
Puncture—direct penetration of tissues by a pointed object	Small opening that may bleed freely	*Do not* remove object if embedded deeply. Clean wound carefully, moving around embedded object. Apply sterile dressing and protect body part. Activate EMS or refer to physician. Treat for shock.
Blister—friction causing disruption between epidermis and dermis resulting in fluid accumulation between layers of skin	Superficial redness, heat, and pain Pocket of fluid (clear or bloody) under skin Wound may be open or closed	Apply ice. Soft padding, lubricant, or donut pad may decrease pressure. If blister opens, treat as an open wound. Both closed and open blisters have potential for infection (if signs of infection, refer to physician).

Based on Anderson and Parr 2013; Prentice 2007; Prentice 2013.

Table 25.3 Severe Bleeding and Its Treatment

Injury	Signs and symptoms	Care
Excessive bleeding—external-bleeding that results in massive loss of circulating blood volume; often results in shock and can lead to death	External hemorrhage: 1. Arterial Color: bright red Flow: spurts, bleeding usually profuse 2. Venous Color: dark red Flow: steady, oozing	Activate EMS. Elevate affected part above the heart. Put direct pressure over the wound, using a sterile compress if possible. Apply a pressure dressing. Use pressure points. Treat for shock.
Internal bleeding—bleeding within deep structures of the body (chest, abdominal, or pelvic cavity) and bleeding of organs contained within these cavities; may result in shock and can lead to death	Generally, no external signs, except when an individual coughs up blood, finds blood in the urine or feces, or experiences the following: Restlessness Thirst Faintness Anxiety Cold, clammy skin Dizziness Rapid, weak, irregular pulse Significant fall in BP	Activate EMS. Treat for shock. Don't give water or food.

Based on Anderson and Parr 2013; Prentice 2007; Prentice 2013.

Staphylococcus Aureus

Staphylococcus aureus, often referred to as *staph*, is common type of bacteria that lives in our bodies. Plenty of healthy people carry staph without being infected by it. According to the CDC, approximately one-third of the American population is colonized in the nose with *Staphylococcus aureus* and approximately 2% of the population is colonized with methicillin-resistant *Staphylococcus aureus* (MRSA) (15). When MRSA is introduced into the body, often through an open wound, it can cause an infection that has become resistant to the antibiotics commonly used to treat ordinary staph infections.

MRSA is most common among people who have weak immune systems and are in hospitals. However, MRSA is also showing up in healthy people who have not been hospitalized or been to outpatient care facilities. This type of MRSA is classified as community-associated MRSA, or CA-MRSA (community-acquired methicillin-resistant *Staphylococcus aureus*), and this is the form fitness professionals may see in fitness settings. CA-MRSA can be contracted through person-to-person contact, sharing of towels or soaps, and improperly cleaned equipment such as mats, pads, whirlpools, and common surfaces (e.g., weight equipment).

Signs and symptoms of CA-MRSA include skin infections. Patients will present with pimples, pustules, or boils that are often mistaken for spider bites. These irritations are often red, swollen, and painful, and they may produce pus. If left untreated, the bacteria can move from the skin to other tissues, including the bloodstream, heart, lungs, bones, and joints.

Prevention of CA-MRSA is the responsibility of both the fitness professional and the participant. Maintaining good hygiene and avoiding contact with drainage from skin lesions are the best methods for prevention. Fitness personnel and clients should be educated to do the following:

- Cover any suspicious skin lesions until a medical referral can be made.
- Keep hands clean by washing thoroughly with soap and warm water or routinely using an alcohol-based hand sanitizer.
- Remove sweat-soaked athletic wear, especially when worn in common equipment-use areas such as weight rooms or on cardio equipment.

Universal Precautions

When treating skin wounds or when exposed to bodily fluids, the fitness professional needs to follow the Occupational Safety and Health Administration (OSHA) universal precautions for safety of the participant and first aid provider. Wear gloves, and when possible, wash hands or use alcohol-based hand sanitizer before donning the gloves. Use a new set of gloves for each patient and wound site. Rewash hands immediately after removing gloves.

Hand Washing

1. Wash hands with soap and water.
2. Contact with soap at least 15 sec.
3. Cover all surfaces.
4. Dry with a fresh paper towel.
5. Use alcohol-based rub, gel, or foam.
6. Use enough of the product to cover all surfaces.
7. Rub until dry, at least 15 sec.

Glove Removal

1. Grasp outside of glove with opposite gloved hand and peel off.
2. Hold removed glove in gloved hand.
3. Slide fingers of ungloved hand under remaining glove at wrist.
4. Peel glove off over first glove.
5. Discard gloves in a biohazard waste container.

Based on Centers for Disease Control and Prevention, 2014, *How to remove gloves*; United States Department of Labor. Occupational Health and Safety Administration.

- Encourage immediate showering following activity.
- People with open wounds, scrapes, or scratches should avoid pools, whirlpools, and common tubs.
- Avoid sharing towels, razors, and daily athletic gear.
- Wash athletic gear and towels after each use in hot water (140 °F or 60 °C). Designate separate laundry bins for collecting soiled laundry and clean laundry.
- Maintain clean facilities and equipment. Equipment should be routinely sanitized and disinfected with a hospital-grade bactericidal and virucidal cleaner.

Care and treatment of CA-MRSA involves the referral of suspicious lesions to a physician for bacterial cultures in order to establish a diagnosis. If a lesion is determined to be contagious, participants must obtain clearance from their physician before being allowed in common-use areas. Cover skin lesions appropriately before participation (29).

KEY POINT

Follow OHSA guidelines and universal precautions when dealing with open wounds, bodily fluids, and MRSA.

Medical Referral and Exercise Modification

After initial care and treatment of a moderate to severe injury, fitness professionals should refer the client to a medical professional. Conditions that require immediate attention or activating EMS include bone deformity, uncontrolled pain, suspected fracture, severe bleeding, decreased circulation, nerve damage, and any life-threatening emergencies. Possible indications for a nonemergent referral include pain, swelling, and decreased function.

Upon return to exercise after injury, it's helpful to have instructions from a health care provider indicating any exclusions or modifications in activity. Mild injuries may require modifying activity levels until normal function returns. This may be in form of reducing the intensity and duration of an activity or finding an alternative form of exercise. Exercise in a swimming pool is an effective way to decrease forces from body weight. A runner who experiences pain may be able to run without pain in chest-deep water or in deep water with a vest. Examples of strength training modifications include decreasing the number of sets or amount of weight lifted, using machines to assist accessory muscles with the joint stability required during free-weight exercises, and using resistance bands or body-weight exercises. During the recovery phase, the goal is to find activities the participant can perform safely without compromising the healing process. Maintaining communication with the participant and her health care provider is recommended.

Environmental Concerns

Fitness professionals must take into consideration the general health of the population they are working with and the environmental conditions that prevail. The environment can impair performance and contribute to the development of serious medical issues.

Air quality can be a major factor in performance and safety, particularly in urban areas, where pollution from factories and motor vehicles may be more prevalent. Extreme temperatures and lightning can prove deadly in some instances. This section examines these concerns and discusses ways to minimize risk to participants.

Air Quality

Fitness professionals need to consider air quality when training participants both outdoors and indoors. The Air Quality Index (AQI) is a daily air quality measurement of outdoor air pollutants calculated by the Environmental Protection Agency (EPA). See chapter 11 for more information about the AQI and recommendations for participation. Also consider that some indoor facilities may have higher levels of dust, mold, or other allergens. Exercise increases exposure to air pollutants due to participants breathing more deeply and rapidly. They take in more air and have a tendency to mouth breathe, bypassing the nasal filtration system. Pollutants or allergens in the air may adversely affect people with asthma, severe allergies, or other breathing problems.

To minimize the risks:

- Monitor air pollution and allergen levels. Local radio, television, and newspapers often report on daily air quality. Weather apps can provide hour-by-hour updates.
- Exercise should be modified or rescheduled during times of peak pollution or poor air quality. Participants should be advised if there is a high index for certain allergens.
- Avoid high pollution areas such as heavy traffic, industrial, and outdoor smoking areas.
- Exercise indoors on poor air quality days.

Exertional Heat Illnesses

Exertional heat illnesses are a concern for people who participate in intense and long-duration exercise. This section focuses on exertional heat stroke (EHS), heat exhaustion, and exercise-associated muscle cramps (EAMC). Exertional heat illness usually occurs with one or more of the following: elevation in body core temperature, electrolyte imbalance, and dehydration.

KEY POINT

A high pollution index or extreme pollen counts can compromise participants' performance and health. Fitness professionals must be aware of environmental conditions and the sensitivities of the people they are training. Schedule activities for times and places where the participants are unlikely to be affected.

Environmental factors that increase the risk of heat illness include ambient air temperature, relative humidity, air motion, and the amount of radiant heat from the sun. When exercising in high temperatures, participants depend on evaporation of sweat for heat loss. High **relative humidity** inhibits heat loss from the body through evaporation. Intense and long training sessions and the environment can place large heat loads on the body, causing an increase in the core body temperature, or **hyperthermia**. Even the most highly conditioned athlete can experience a heat-related disorder.

Dehydration occurs when more body water is lost via sweat, vomiting, or diarrhea than can be replaced by fluid intake. Participants should weigh themselves before and after activity to monitor fluid loss. A water loss up to 2% of body weight is considered safe. A 3% to 5% loss is cause for concern, and more than a 5% loss is considered serious and activity should be suspended until fluid weight is adequately replaced. The potential for a cascade effect of fluid loss exists; therefore, it is essential to continually replace fluids lost through sweat and urine excretion.

Fluids lost in the sweating process include electrolytes, essential minerals necessary for nerve and muscle function, body-fluid balance, and other critical processes. The balance of electrolytes is constantly shifting due to fluctuations in fluid intake as well as due to exercise and environmental heat conditions. Salt (NaCl) is an important electrolyte in fluid retention, and loss of salt is evident by a white, chalky film on skin and clothing.

In addition to dehydration and environmental conditions, certain predisposing factors can contribute to heat illness:

- Being deconditioned
- Incomplete heat acclimatization
- Sudden increase in physical training
- History of heat illness
- History of SCT
- Illness and medications
- Nutritional supplements
- Poor nutrition
- Obesity
- Sleep deprivation
- Age (children and older populations are more susceptible)

EHS is defined by hyperthermia (core body temperature >40 °C) associated with CNS disturbances and multiple organ system failure (7). It occurs when muscle metabolism creates internal body heat and the thermoregulatory system is overwhelmed. Rectal temperature is the standard used by medical professionals to measure body core temperature and diagnose EHS. This is a life-threatening condition. When a person who has survived EHS is medically cleared to return to activity, exercise should begin in a cool environment and gradually increase in duration, intensity, and heat exposure over a 2 wk period. If any signs and symptoms recur, stop activity and refer to a physician.

Heat exhaustion is the inability to continue exercise associated with any combination of heavy sweating, dehydration, sodium loss, and energy depletion (8). It occurs most frequently in hot, humid conditions and shares many of the signs and symptoms of EHS; therefore, activating EMS is recommended when either condition is suspected. In heat exhaustion, body core temperature can vary from normal to as high as 40 °C (104 °F). Although heat exhaustion does not always involve elevated core temperature, cooling therapy will often improve the medical status (7). In mild cases, participants should not return to activity for a minimum of 24 to 48 hr. When it's safe to resume activity, a gradual increase in intensity and volume is necessary.

EAMC, often called *heat cramps*, are painful, involuntary muscle contractions that occur during or after intense exercise. They are caused by dehydration, electrolyte imbalance, fatigue, or a combination of these factors. Although painful, EAMC often responds positively to conservative treatment and participants can return safely to activity. People who are prone to chronic cramping will benefit from maintaining fluid and salt balance before, during, and after exercise.

KEY POINT

Modify exercise duration and intensity in hot, humid conditions. Encourage hydration and provide water and rest breaks during activity. The fitness professional must be able to recognize the signs of heat illness and take action.

Table 25.4 outlines the stages of heat illness, signs and symptoms, and guidelines for immediate care.

Both the fitness professional and the participant should understand preventive measures to decrease the incidence of heat illness. Do the following to prevent heat injury:

- Develop an EAP with understanding of exertional heat illness prevention, recognition, and treatment.
- Through preparticipation screening, identify participants who have a history of exertional heat illness or SCT.
- Acclimatize by gradually increasing activity levels and heat exposure over 10 to 14 days.
- Educate participants to match fluid intake with sweat and urine losses to maintain adequate hydration.
- Provide adequate fluids (water or sport electrolyte drink) to replace fluids lost during activity sessions.
- Modify activity in high heat and humidity.
- Plan rest breaks, preferably in a cool or shaded environment, to match exercise intensity as well as heat and humidity.
- Measure body weight before and after activity to estimate amount of water loss (replenish by consuming 1-1.25 L [34-42 oz] of fluid per kg of water loss).
- Minimize equipment and clothing if possible.
- Drink sodium-containing fluids to keep urine clear to light yellow.
- Get adequate sleep (at least 6-8 hr).
- Participants should not exercise if they're febrile (temperature >100.3 °F [38.0 °C]), vomiting, or have diarrhea.

Cold-Related Problems

Exercising in cold, wet, windy weather can cause problems if precautions are not taken. Considerable heat loss can occur through convective heat loss from the skin and evaporation of skin moisture. Hypothermia occurs when body heat is lost at a faster rate than it is produced and core body temperature drops below 35 °C (95 °F). Peripheral blood vessels in cold areas constrict, which conserves body heat but increases the risk of frostbite. Exercising in cold, damp weather can compound the problem by increasing the rate of evaporation. A high windchill can result in severe loss of body heat even when the air temperature is above freezing (see chapter 11). Additionally, body temperature drops even more quickly in cold water than in air of the same temperature. Table 25.5 on page 460 describes how to recognize and treat cold-related problems. Cold-related problems are preventable if participants take these precautions:

- Avoid exercising outdoors in extreme cold and wind.
- Modify activity as necessary to prevent overexposure to cold, wet, windy conditions. Consider length of exposure, availability of facilities, and interventions for rewarming if needed. Clothing should provide an internal layer that allows sweat evaporation with minimal absorption, a middle layer that provides insulation, and a removable external layer that is wind and water resistant and allows moisture evaporation (11).
- Cover the face, nose, ears, fingers, and head (a great deal of heat is lost when the head is exposed).
- Warm up before exercise and avoid bouts of inactivity.
- Stay dry.
- Avoid swimming or exercising in cold water, particularly when the surrounding air temperature is low.
- Maintain proper hydration and nutrition. Consume fluids even when not thirsty because the normal thirst mechanism is dampened with cold exposure.

KEY POINT

Cold-related problems may be prevented by avoiding exposure to extreme cold, wearing removable layers, warming up before activity, and constantly remaining active.

Lightning

Lightning is a significant weather hazard that may affect all outdoor fitness and sport activities. Though the probability of being struck by lightning is extremely low, the odds are significantly greater when a storm is in the area and safety guidelines and precautions are not followed. Weather sources and reports should be checked before outdoor activities and when storm conditions exist. Signs of threatening weather include darkening clouds, high winds, thunder, and lightning activity.

The fitness professional should know the location of the closest safe shelter and how long it takes to reach that shelter. A safe shelter is any sturdy building that has metal plumbing, wiring, or both to electrically ground the structure (i.e., not a shed or shack). In the absence of a sturdy building, any vehicle with a hard metal roof (not a convertible car or golf cart) with windows rolled up is considered a safe shelter. If no safe shelter is reachable, look for a dry ditch and instruct clients to crouch with only their feet touching the ground. Minimize body surface area by keeping the feet close together, wrapping the arms around

Table 25.4 Exertional Heat Illnesses and Their Treatment

Exertional heat illness	Signs and symptoms	Care
Exertional heat stroke (EHS)—hyperthermia (elevated core temperature) causing organ system failure; the most serious form of heat-related illness	High core body temperature (>40 °C [104 °F]) CNS system changes: dizziness, drowsiness, irrational behavior, confusion, irritability, emotional instability, hysteria, apathy, aggressiveness, delirium, disorientation, staggering, seizures, loss of consciousness, coma Headache Dehydration Weakness Loss of balance and muscle function Prolonged fatigue Hot and wet or dry skin Tachycardia (100 to 120 bpm) Hypotension Hyperventilation Vomiting Diarrhea	Treat as extreme medical emergency. Activate EMS. Lower core body temperature immediately: Remove clothes and equipment. Immerse body in a pool or tub of cold water. If cold tub not available, place ice or ice towels on head, neck, armpits, and groin. Monitor vital signs. Maintain airway.
Heat exhaustion—inability to continue activity due to heavy sweating, dehydration, sodium loss, and energy depletion	Normal or elevated core body temperature (36-40 °C [97-104 °F]) Dehydration Dizziness Lightheadedness Headache Nausea Diarrhea or urge to defecate Intestinal cramping Decreased urine output Persistent muscle cramps Weakness Profuse sweating Cold, clammy skin Chills Paleness Hyperventilation Thirst	Stop activity. Activate EMS. Move person to a cool or shaded area. Remove equipment and unnecessary clothing. Rapidly cool body by applying ice or ice towels to head, neck, armpits, and groin; use fans and air conditioning if available. Elevate legs. Give cold fluids (if conscious). Monitor vital signs and treat for shock.
Exercise associated muscle cramps (EAMC)—painful, involuntary muscle contractions	Painful muscle cramping often accompanied by thirst, dehydration, and fatigue Subsides within minutes Profuse sweating White residue on clothing (due to sodium depletion)	Remove from activity. Perform mild stretching. Gently massage or put direct pressure on muscle. Ice the muscle. Replace fluids with a sodium-containing drink (sport drink formula). Return to activity when muscle is functional and no other signs or symptoms of heat illness exist.
Heat syncope—fainting or excessive loss of strength due to heat	Headache Nausea Weakness Fatigue Dizziness	Replace lost fluids. Monitor vitals. Cool body and place person in shade. Elevate legs.

Based on Anderson and Parr 2013; Armstrong et al. 2007; Binkley et al. 2002; Casa et al 2000; Casa and Csillan 2009; National Collegiate Athletic Association 2013; Prentice 2007.

Table 25.5 Cold-Related Problems and Their Treatment

Cold-related problems	Signs and symptoms	Care
Superficial frostbite—freezing of skin layers and subcutaneous tissue	Skin: dry, waxy, cold, and firm to the touch; reddening along with white or blue-gray patches Edema Tingling or burning	Remove from cold. Remove jewelry. Slowly rewarm area using water heated to 98-104 °F (37-40 °C). Handle gently and avoid friction or massage. May require medical referral.
Deep frostbite—freezing of deep tissue, including muscle and bone	Skin: hard, cold, waxy, and immobile; white, gray, black, or purple Pain: burning, aching, throbbing, or shooting	Remove from cold exposure. Activate EMS. Protect body part. Remove jewelry from injured body part. Handle gently; avoid friction, rubbing, or massage. Rewarming is best performed in a hospital setting.
Mild hypothermia—body temperature 37-35 °C (98.6-95.0 °F)	Skin: pale Shivering Cold extremities Amnesia, lethargy Impaired motor control Excessive urination Typically conscious	Remove from cold. Rewarm with dry clothing, blankets, heating pad (apply only to trunk, armpit, and groin), and warm drinks. Avoid friction massage. Activate EMS if symptoms don't improve quickly.
Moderate to severe hypothermia—core body temperature 34-32.0 °C (94-90 °F)	Skin: bluish tinge Impaired neuromuscular function Impaired mental function Slurred speech Reduced respiration and pulse Dilated pupils Decreased BP Cessation of shivering Loss of consciousness Muscle rigidity	Treat as a medical emergency. Activate EMS. Remove from cold. Remove wet clothing. Rewarm with dry clothing, blankets, heating pad (apply only to trunk, armpit, and groin). Monitor vital signs. Treat for shock.

Based on Anderson and Parr 2013; Cappaert et al. 2008; National Collegiate Athletic Association 2013.

the knees, and lowering the head. Do not lie flat! Stay away from tall or individual trees, lone objects (e.g., flagpoles), metal objects (fences or bleachers), standing pools of water, and open fields. Avoid being the tallest object in a field.

Fitness professionals should be aware of the proximity of lightning in the area. The flash-to-bang method is used to approximate the distance of a lightning strike. Count the seconds from the flash until the bang (thunder) occurs. Divide this number by 5 to determine how far away (in miles) lightning is occurring. When lightning strikes within 6 mi (9.7 km), or 30 sec from flash to bang, suspend all outdoor activities for 30 min. Table 25.6 explains this 30–30 rule.

Lightning may cause injury to participants and bystanders in five ways:

1. A direct strike to the head
2. Contact with an object that is struck by lightning
3. A side flash where lightning jumps from a struck object to the victim
4. When lightning current that hits the ground radiates outward from the strike point
5. Violent muscular contraction due to lightning current (37)

When caring for the victim of a lightning strike, employ standard emergency care. First, survey the scene for safety and, only if necessary, move the victim to a safer location. Activate the EMS system. Treat the person for shock and perform CPR if indicated.

Table 25.6 The 30–30 Rule

Activity criteria	30–30 rule
Suspension of activities	By the time the flash-to-bang count approaches 30 sec, everyone should already be inside a safe shelter.
Resumption of activities	Wait at least 30 min after the last sound (thunder) or observation of lightning before leaving the safe shelter to resume activities. Each time lightning is observed or thunder is heard, reset the 30 min clock.

Based on Glover 2007; Prentice 2007; Walsh et al. 2000.

KEY POINT

The fitness professional needs to be aware of severe weather conditions. Outdoor activities should stop and participants should take cover if lightning occurs within 6 mi (9.7 km). Do not resume activities for a minimum of 30 min after the last lightning strike.

Medical Conditions

The fitness professional should review each participant's HRA (see chapter 2) to identify medical conditions that may become problematic during activity. This section gives a basic understanding of diabetes, hyperventilation, asthma, concussion, and SCT and how to care for these conditions.

Diabetic Reactions

If managed properly, people with diabetes should be able to exercise without complications. When starting a new exercise program, they should receive medical clearance from their physician, monitor their blood glucose levels more frequently, and gradually progress in the program. Communication between the fitness professional and the participant is vital regarding daily exercise plans. Ideally, 24 to 48 hr notice of the duration and intensity of the exercise session is helpful to ensure proper preparation by the diabetic participant. Exercise has the potential to lower blood glucose levels; therefore, it must be counterbalanced with an increase in food intake or a decrease in insulin dosage. Blood glucose levels should be monitored immediately before and 15 min after activity. Clients should be encouraged to communicate with their physicians regarding their exercise program in order to better manage their diabetes.

The fitness professional should be familiar with the signs and symptoms of diabetic coma and insulin shock (see table 25.7). Diabetic coma occurs when insulin levels drop and the body is unable to metabolize glucose, leading to hyperglycemia. Insulin shock occurs when insulin levels are high and blood glucose is low, leading to hypoglycemia. It is sometimes difficult to differentiate between these two conditions. A person living with diabetes is normally aware of and manages this delicate glucose balance. When the client is in crisis and is conscious but it is unclear whether diabetic coma or insulin shock is present, give the client a sugar substance (orange juice, candy, honey). If the person is in a diabetic coma, there is little chance of seriously worsening the condition by giving sugar. If symptoms do not resolve rapidly, the fitness professional should activate EMS, monitor vital signs, and treat for shock.

KEY POINT

Communication between the fitness professional and the participant living with diabetes regarding daily exercise plans is vital. Exercise has the potential to lower blood glucose levels, and therefore it must be counterbalanced with an increase in food intake or a decrease in insulin dosage.

Respiratory Disorders

Hyperventilation can occur with heavy exhalation or rapid breathing, resulting in breathing out too much carbon dioxide (CO_2) and thereby reducing CO_2 levels in the blood. Low CO_2 levels may cause dizziness, faintness, chest pains, and tingling in the feet and hands. Reassuring the person in a calm manner, encouraging a slower breathing rate, and encouraging the person to talk often improves the situation. If not, helping the person breathe into a paper bag or into hands cupped over the nose and mouth will help restore CO_2 levels.

Asthma is a condition in which the smooth muscles of the bronchial tubes go into spasm. Edema and inflammation of the mucous lining are triggered by exercise, changes

Table 25.7 Diabetic Reactions and Their Treatment

Diabetic reaction	Signs and symptoms	Care
Diabetic coma (hyperglycemia)—loss of consciousness caused by too little insulin; gradual onset	Restlessness and confusion Intense thirst Abdominal cramping and nausea Vomiting Shortness of breath Rapid, weak pulse Sweet, fruity breath Unconsciousness	Activate EMS. If conscious and alert, assist with insulin administration. Treat for shock. Lay person on side to prevent aspiration of vomitus.
Insulin shock (hypoglycemia)—high level of insulin and low glucose levels; rapid onset	Shakiness and anxiety Confusion Pale, cold, clammy skin Profuse sweating Dizziness Rapid HR Intense hunger Nausea Numbness or tingling in face and mouth Headache Aggressive behavior Lack of coordination Seizure Unconsciousness	If conscious, administer sugar (e.g., orange juice, candy). If symptoms do not improve within 15 min, activate EMS. If unconscious, activate EMS. Roll person on side. Place sugar granules or honey under the tongue. Treat for shock.

American Diabetes Association 2014; American Diabetes Association 2015; Anderson and Parr 2013; Casa and Stearns 2014; Jimenex et al. 2007; National Collegiate Athletic Association 2013-2014; Prentice 2007.

in barometric pressure or temperature, viruses, emotional stress, and noxious odors. The affected person may appear anxious, pale, and sweaty; may cough or wheeze; and may seem short of breath. Hyperventilation may occur, resulting in dizziness, and, because of mucous secretions, the person may frequently try to clear his throat.

The fitness professional should be prepared to handle an asthma attack. Generally, people with asthma know how to care for themselves and carry prescription medication to use before exercising or during an attack. People with asthma benefit from staying hydrated and modifying activity in environmental conditions such as high pollen and ozone warnings. If bronchial spasm is excessive and the participant is unable to breathe adequately, activate EMS.

KEY POINT

Respiratory issues can occur in exercise participation. Recognize that absence of normal breathing is a medical emergency.

Seizures

A seizure is caused by an abnormal electrical event in the brain, which can last a few seconds to several minutes. There are many types of seizures, and signs and symptoms are complex and numerous, ranging from a blank stare with unresponsiveness to convulsions with loss of bodily functions. For the management of seizures, see *Care for Seizures*.

Sickle Cell Trait and Exertional Sickling

People with **sickle cell trait (SCT)** have a genetic condition that involves the inheritance of one gene for sickle hemoglobin and one for normal hemoglobin. The prevalence of SCT is approximately 5% to 10% in African Americans and <0.01% in Caucasians. People of Mediterranean descent (e.g., Italy, Spain, France) also have a higher prevalence (5, 6, 26). The U.S. Preventive Services Task Force recommends screening for SCT in newborns (36). However, many people are unaware that they have SCT or are uncomfortable making their status known to others.

Several risk factors have been identified that contribute to the medical problems associated with people with SCT. These risk factors include dehydration, heat, asthma, deconditioning, and high-intensity exercise with little rest and recovery, even in the conditioned athlete. Due to lack of oxygen, exposure to high altitudes from flying, mountain climbing, or visiting a city at higher altitudes puts people with SCT at high risk.

A person with SCT can usually exercise without incidence. However, during intense exertion, exertional

Care for Seizures

Do not place anything in the mouth or attempt to restrain a person having a seizure.

Immediate Care

- Activate EMS.
- Note time of seizure onset.
- Assist individual to supine position.
- Protect head with soft materials or padding.
- Remove nearby objects.
- Remove glasses and loosen clothing.

After Seizure

- Open airway and assess breathing.
- Place individual on side.
- Stay with individual until fully awake.

Critical Care

For seizures lasting 5 min or successive seizures:

- Activate EMS.
- Document length of time and number of seizures.

Based on Anderson and Parr 2013; Prentice 2007; Prentice 2013.

sickling can occur. Some of the normally round-shaped red blood cells form the shape of a sickle and are no longer able to carry oxygen. This sickling leads to the obstruction of small blood vessels in muscle or organs. If intense exercise continues, the condition can escalate.

Prevention is the key to avoiding an exertional sickling emergency. Because the fitness professional may not know which clients have SCT, incorporating sound principles of progression for everyone is the best preventive measure. Gradually increase the intensity of workouts, providing adequate time for rest and recovery. Use submaximal fitness testing early in the training program; more intense testing can be administered after the participant is better conditioned (see chapter 7). Encourage year-round conditioning that includes appropriate cycles of rest and recovery. Keep participants hydrated, especially in high heat and humidity. Encourage them to avoid high levels of caffeine and supplements containing stimulants. Participants with asthma should be instructed to follow their prescribed medical plan. Exercise during illness should be modified or discouraged. No one should exercise with a fever (temperature of 100.3 °F [38.0 °C] or above).

Exertional sickling is a medical emergency, and the fitness professional must act immediately due to the rapid decline of a participant's medical status. Table 25.8 outlines the signs and symptoms, prevention, and care of exertional sickling.

Table 25.8 Exertional Sickling Signs and Symptoms, Prevention, and Care

Signs and symptoms	Prevention	Care
Muscle cramping Muscle weakness Pain Swelling Extreme fatigue Inability to catch breath Elevated core temperature Sudden collapse during activity	Gradually increase exercise intensity. Allow rest and recovery. Modify early exercise testing. Maintain hydration. Avoid caffeine and nutritional stimulants. Modify or stop exercise during illness. No exercise if temperature above 100.3 °F (38.0 °C).	Stop activity immediately. Activate EMS. Monitor vital signs. Support CAB (circulation, airway, breathing) and begin CPR if indicated. Cool the participant if experiencing heat-related illness.

Based on Anzalone 2010; Armstrong 2007; Harrelson, Fincher, and Robinson 1995.

KEY POINT

Reduce the risk of exertional sickling by using exercise programs that include appropriate hydration, rest breaks, and a gradual increase in activity. When exertional sickling is suspected, it is a medical emergency—act immediately.

Traumatic Brain Injury

Traumatic brain injury (TBI) occurs when an external mechanical force causes brain dysfunction. A TBI is caused by a bump, blow, or jolt to the head or a penetrating head injury that disrupts the normal function of the brain. Mild TBI may cause temporary dysfunction of brain cells. More serious TBI can result in bruising, torn tissues, bleeding, and other physical damage to the brain that can result in long-term complications or death (21). TBI can result from severe head injuries such as skull fractures, epidural hematomas, or subdural hematomas.

Severe symptoms of a skull fracture, subdural hematoma, or epidural hematoma include bleeding from a wound, the ears, the nose, or around the eyes; bruising behind the ears (Battle's sign) or around the eyes (raccoon sign); changes in pupils (sizes unequal, not reactive to light); convulsions; drainage of clear or bloody fluid from ears or nose; loss of consciousness; vomiting; slurred speech; and seizures.

Immediate care of severe head injury involves stabilizing the head and neck; checking circulation, airway, and breathing and performing CPR if indicated; controlling bleeding; treating for shock; and activating EMS.

Helmets help prevent or reduce the severity of skull fractures and intracranial hematomas, and experts believe that helmets can also reduce the severity of cerebral concussions. Many sports and fitness activities (American football, ice hockey, lacrosse, softball, baseball, cycling, skateboarding, inline skating, rock climbing, snowboarding, and snow skiing) require or advise the use of helmets (4, 31).

Skull Fracture

The skull provides good protection for the brain; however, a severe impact can fracture the skull. The fracture may be accompanied by concussion or other injury to the brain. Fractures can be simple—a break in the bone without damage to the skin; compound—a splintering of the bone with a break in the skin; or depressed—a crushing of the skull with bone depressed in toward the brain (14). Skull fractures often lead to subdural or epidural hematomas.

Subdural Hematoma

A subdural hematoma is bleeding between the skull and the brain. As blood accumulates, pressure on the brain increases, which may occur suddenly or over several days. The bleeding and increased pressure on the brain from a subdural hematoma can be life threatening.

Subdural hematoma is usually caused by a traumatic head injury, such as from a fall or motor vehicle accident. People with a bleeding disorder and people who take blood thinners are more likely to develop a subdural hematoma even from a relatively minor head injury.

Epidural Hematoma

An epidural hematoma is a type of intracranial hematoma that occurs when a blood clot forms between skull and the dura, the tough covering that surrounds the brain. An epidural hematoma can result from a skull fracture. The jarring of the brain against the sides of the skull can cause shearing (tearing) of the internal lining, tissues, and blood vessels that may result in internal bleeding, bruising, or swelling of the brain (4, 14, 31).

Concussions

The understanding and management of concussions has changed dramatically in recent years. The term *concussion* derives from the Latin term *concutere*, which means to "shake violently." A concussion is a brain injury and is defined as a complex pathophysiological process induced by biomechanical forces (28). It results in a transient disturbance of brain function, encompassing clinical symptoms that may or may not involve loss of consciousness. Concussions have also been referred to as *mild traumatic brain injuries (MTBIs)*; however, it is now widely agreed that concussions are a subset of MTBIs, on the less severe end of the brain injury spectrum, and are generally self-limited in duration and resolution (19, 20, 24, 25, 28).

Concussion may be caused by a blow to head, face, neck, or body that translates to the brain being shaken. It results in the rapid onset of symptoms, which fall into four categories: physical, cognitive, emotional, and sleep. Common symptoms often include headache, dizziness, nausea, mental fog, balance problems, and light and noise sensitivity (for a complete list of symptoms, see table 25.9). Some may appear right away, while others may not be noticed for hours or days after the injury. The damage is functional rather than structural, which is why standard neuroimaging diagnostic studies (e.g., CT scan, X-ray, MRI) often reveal no abnormalities.

KEY POINT

If any signs or symptoms of a concussion are present, the participant must cease all activity until evaluated by a medical professional and should not return to activity until cleared medically.

Table 25.9 Concussion Signs and Symptoms

Physical	Cognitive	Emotional	Sleep
Headache Nausea Vomiting Balance problems Dizziness Visual problems Fatigue Sensitivity to light Sensitivity to noise Numbness, tingling Dazed Stunned	Feels mentally foggy Feels slowed down Difficulty concentrating Difficulty remembering Forgetful of recent information and conversations Confused about recent events Answers questions slowly Repeats questions	Irritable Sad More emotional Nervous	Drowsiness Sleeps more than usual Sleeps less than usual Difficulty falling asleep

Based on Guskiewicz et al. 2004.

If a concussion is suspected, the person should immediately stop participation and see a physician trained in the assessment and management of concussions. Cognitive and physical rest are the main treatments for a concussion. The person must obtain return-to-participation clearance from a physician before returning to fitness activities. If any signs or symptoms recur after returning to activity, stop the activity and refer the participant to her physician.

Around 80% to 90% of concussion cases resolve in 7 to 10 days. In the other 10% to 20% of cases, symptoms can persist for weeks, months, or even years beyond the initial injury (19, 24, 25, 28). The original concussion can turn into persistent concussion symptoms, leading to postconcussion syndrome. This syndrome is simply defined as symptoms and signs of the concussion persisting for weeks to months after the incident.

Basic Life Support and Emergency Procedures

This section addresses the emergency protocols for shock, checking vital signs, CPR, AEDs, and airway obstruction. Fitness professionals are encouraged to be certified in basic life support, minimally in adult CPR with AED. ACSM and other credentialing bodies may require CPR or a more advanced life support certification depending on the fitness professional's certification. Cardiac emergencies require immediate recognition and activation of EMS, early CPR, and rapid defibrillation.

Shock

When attending to injuries or illnesses, the fitness professional must be aware of the possibility of shock. Shock occurs when the heart is unable to circulate adequate oxygen to vital organs. This may result from trauma involving severe pain or blood loss or may be associated with an allergic reaction, heatstroke, severe infection, poisoning, or severe burns. Although shock most often accompanies severe injury, it may also occur with minor injuries. If untreated, this can lead to permanent organ damage or death.

A change in vital signs (pulse, respiratory rate, BP, temperature, pupils, skin color) indicates that a person is going into shock. The signs and symptoms of shock can progress over time. Table 25.10 identifies the signs and symptoms of a person going into shock and the immediate care required.

KEY POINT

The signs and symptoms of shock can develop over time but can also change quickly. It is important to monitor vital signs every 2 to 5 min when shock is likely.

Checking Vital Signs

Monitoring vital signs assists in the recognition and care of the injured patient. Vital signs include pulse, respiratory rate, BP, temperature, and skin color.

- Check HR. Use light finger pressure over an artery to monitor pulse rate. The most common sites for checking HR are the carotid, radial, brachial, and femoral pulses. The average HR for an adult is between 60 and 100 beats · min^{-1}.
- Check breathing. Normal breathing rates vary from 8 to 20 breaths per min. A victim who takes an occasional breath is not receiving adequate ventilation and is in respiratory distress.
- Take BP. Usually BP is taken at the brachial artery with a BP cuff and sphygmomanometer. The following results will help determine the problem:

Table 25.10 Shock Recognition and Treatment

Signs and symptoms	Care
Restless, anxious, fearful, or disorientated Weak, rapid pulse Shallow, irregular breathing Nausea or vomiting Cold, clammy, moist skin Dull, staring eyes with dilated pupils Profuse sweating Dizziness Extreme thirst	Initiate the EAP and call EMS. Check circulation and maintain airway; begin CPR if indicated. Control bleeding, splint fractures, and regulate body temperature. Elevate feet and legs 8-12 in. (20-30 cm) unless suspected lower-extremity, head, or neck injury. Keep the person quiet and still. Even if the person complains of thirst, do not give any liquids by mouth. If the patient vomits, turn her on her side. If a neck injury is suspect, it must be stabilized before rolling the person. Monitor vital signs every 2-5 min until EMS arrives.

Based on Anderson and Parr 2013; Prentice 2007; Prentice 2013.

- Normal BP—<120 mmHg systolic and <80 mmHg diastolic
- Severe hemorrhage, heart attack—marked decrease in BP (20-30 mmHg)
- Damage or rupture of vessels in the arterial circuit—abnormally high BP (>150 SBP and >90 DBP)
- Brain damage—increase in SBP with a stable or falling DBP
- Heart ailment—dec rease in SBP with an increase in DBP

- Body temperature. Normal body temperature is 98.6 °F (37.0 °C). Assess skin quality: Cool, clammy, damp skin suggests shock or heat exhaustion; cool, dry skin indicates exposure to cold air; and hot, dry skin suggests fever or heatstroke.
- Assess color. For light-pigmented people, abnormalities include skin, fingernail beds, lips, sclera of eyes, and mucous membranes that are red or flushed, pale or ashen, or bluish. For dark-pigmented people, it is necessary to assess nail beds and inside the lips, mouth, and tongue. Pink is the normal color for these; a bluish or grayish cast is abnormal.

Cardiopulmonary Resuscitation

Current guidelines in CPR training emphasize circulation, airway, breathing (CAB), stressing the importance of moving the blood in victims of sudden cardiac arrest. Activating EMS and access to an AED are of equal importance. The American Heart Association (AHA) and American Red Cross (ARC) have specific protocols for CPR, depending on certification level. The following list is a basic guide to assist the fitness professional in a sudden cardiac emergency:

1. Check that the scene is safe to assess the participant.
2. Check for responsiveness, pulse, and breathing.
3. Activate EMS and retrieve an AED. Use a bystander if available.
4. If no pulse is detected, begin cycles of 30 chest compressions and 2 breaths. For adults, place the heel of the hand on the middle of the chest (lower half of sternum) and compress the chest 2 to 2.4 in. (5 to 6 cm). Allow the chest to recoil completely. Give 30 compressions at a rate of 100 to 120 per min.
5. If there is a pulse and absent or abnormal breathing, give one breath every 5 to 6 sec. Open the airway using the head tilt–chin lift method. If a head or neck injury is suspected, use jaw-thrust method. Use a barrier or bag mask when available. Give enough breath for the chest to rise, about 1 sec. Recheck the pulse every few minutes.
6. When the AED arrives ensure cell phones are no closer than 6 feet from the victim. Turn AED on and follow audible instructions, placing pads on the right upper chest and left chest below the heart. Continue

KEY POINT

Emergency situations can occur at any time. Cardiac emergencies require immediate recognition and activation of EMS, early CPR, and rapid defibrillation. Fitness professionals need to follow the EAP, including routine practice sessions, and maintain appropriate certification in basic life support to keep up to date with the latest protocols.

CPR while the AED gets set up and analyzes rhythm. If shock is advised, make sure no one is touching the victim. Continue CPR as instructed by the AED until EMS arrives (3).

Airway Obstruction

Airway obstruction can occur when a foreign object or, in case of an unconscious person, the tongue blocks the airway.

CONSCIOUS PERSON

- If breathing is labored and the person is coughing forcefully, stay with him and encourage continued coughing.
- If the person is unsuccessful in expelling the object or has absent or abnormal breathing, activate EMS and begin abdominal thrusts.
  - Stand behind the person, wrap your arms around the midsection, and place your fist with the thumb just above the naval.
  - Thrust in and upward until the object is expelled.

UNCONSCIOUS PERSON

- Treat as a cardiac emergency.
  - Activate EMS.
  - Perform CPR.

LEARNING AIDS

REVIEW QUESTIONS

1. How often should staff be trained in the fitness facility's EAP?
2. How long should ice be applied initially to a suspected sprain?
3. Strength programs that increase in intensity and duration too quickly and do not allow for adequate recovery can result in what serious medical condition?
4. Describe how you would splint a suspected fracture to the fibula.
5. What are three ways to prevent the spread of CA-MRSA in a fitness facility?
6. Describe the appropriate technique for cleaning an open wound.
7. Describe the flash-to-bang and 30–30 rule for assessing lightning.
8. List five vital signs to monitor when an emergency occurs.

CASE STUDIES

1. A participant hurts her ankle performing a plyometric exercise. She falls to the ground, is in moderate pain, and is able to partially bear weight. You suspect she has a sprained ankle. Describe how you would give immediate care.
2. You are conducting a boot camp outdoors that meets 2 times a wk for 8 wk from 5:30 to 6:30 p.m. in Florida beginning June 1. What can you do to prepare for the first class to prevent exertional heat illness in your participants? What recommendations would you give to your participants in an e-mail before the class starts?
3. One of your regular clients comes to you before his weightlifting workout and says that both arms are extremely sore. He challenged his brother to a pull-up contest 2 days ago, and now he has mild swelling in both biceps, stiffness, decreased ROM at the elbow joint, point tenderness in both forearms and upper arms, and difficulty carrying things. What condition do you suspect he has? What treatment would you provide to help him get back to working out?

Answers to Case Studies

1. Do the following:

   - Protection—Splint the ankle above and below the joint.
   - Rest—Discontinue activity.
   - Ice—Apply ice bag for 20 to 30 min.
   - Compression—Apply an elastic bandage, wrapping from the toes up to the lower leg.
   - Elevation—Elevate the ankle above the heart.
   - Refer the participant to a physician.

2. As an instructor, do the following preparation:

   - Screen participants for prior heat illness, SCT, and medications.
   - Provide water and give adequate rest breaks.
   - Monitor the weather and modify activities if heat and humidity are high.
   - Gradually increase the intensity and duration of the activity over a 2 wk period for acclimatization.

   Make the following recommendations to participants:

   - Hydrate before class.
   - Monitor urine color for hydration levels.
   - Get plenty of rest (at least 6-8 hr nightly).
   - Minimize clothing.
   - Weigh in before and after class to monitor fluid loss. Replenish fluids by consuming 1 to 1.25 L [34-42 oz] of fluid per kilogram of body water loss.

3. The client has DOMS (delayed-onset muscle soreness). Give him the following recommendations:

   - No upper-body weight training today. He can work the legs and core.
   - Ice both arms for 20 to 30 min.
   - Provide compression with an elastic wrap on both arms.
   - Lightly massage the muscles.
   - Take an over-the-counter NSAID as directed.
   - Return to activity gradually when soreness has subsided.
   - If signs and symptoms worsen, seek medical advice from a physician.

26

Legal Considerations

JoAnn M. Eickhoff-Shemek

OBJECTIVES

The reader will be able to do the following:

1. Describe why fitness professionals must develop knowledge and skills in the area of legal liability and risk management.
2. Distinguish injuries due to inherent risks, negligence, and product defects.
3. Develop a basic understanding of the law and legal system.
4. Understand the fault basis of tort liability.
5. Define *ordinary negligence* and *gross negligence.*
6. Describe the four elements of negligence that a plaintiff must prove.
7. Explain the primary assumption of risk and waiver defenses.
8. Identify the four elements of a valid contract.
9. Discuss how courts determine duty in negligence cases.
10. Define *risk management* and describe the four steps in the risk management process.
11. Develop risk management strategies to help minimize legal liability in the areas of personnel, preactivity screening, fitness testing and prescription, instruction and supervision, equipment and facilities, and EAPs.
12. Understand the many legal issues that can arise in negligence cases.

As presented in chapter 1, many physiological and psychological health benefits are associated with regular physical activity. Although these benefits outweigh the risks, it is important to understand that risks (e.g., heart attacks, fractured bones, cuts that cause bleeding) do occur, and many people become injured (and sometimes die) each year while participating in physical activity. Unfortunately, in today's litigious society, injured participants do not hesitate to file negligence claims or lawsuits against fitness professionals and their employers. To help minimize injuries and subsequent litigation, it is essential that fitness professionals learn the laws that pertain to the field and how to apply the laws to their daily practices. Studies have shown poor adherence by fitness facilities to laws and safety standards and guidelines published by professional organizations (36). This poor adherence is most likely due to a lack of legal and risk management education among fitness professionals. Therefore, the purpose of this chapter is to help fitness professionals gain knowledge and skills in this area.

This chapter covers various legal concerns to help educate fitness professionals about their legal duties and how they can carry out these duties through the development and implementation of risk management strategies. By no means does this chapter cover all of the legal issues relevant to the fitness field. It would be best for students and professionals to take an entire academic course on legal issues in order to receive a more thorough education on the subject than what this chapter can cover.

Injury Data and Injuries Leading to Litigation

About 11,000 people per day receive treatment in U.S. emergency departments for injuries sustained while participating in sport, recreation, and exercise activities (71). It is unknown how many of these are specifically due to exercise. However, the U.S. Consumer Product Safety Commission's National Electronic Injury Surveillance System (NEISS) does track injuries resulting from exercise and exercise equipment. As table 26.1 shows, the number of these injuries increased more than 30% between 2009 and 2012.

Table 26.1 Exercise and Exercise Equipment Injuries, 2009 to 2012

Year	Number of exercise and exercise equipment injuries*
2009	349,543
2010	382,970
2011	410,024
2012	459,978

*The total number of injuries reflects estimates based on data obtained from U.S. hospital emergency departments through the NEISS. Retrieved December 26, 2014, from www.cpsc.gov/en/Research–Statistics/NEISS-Injury-Data.

Table 26.2 lists selected negligence lawsuits and the type of injury the plaintiff (injured party) suffered. These cases are described later in this chapter. Although most of the injuries listed in table 26.2 would be considered serious, other types of injuries also can result in costly claims and lawsuits. The Association Insurance Group conducted a 12 yr study (1995-2007) of **liability** claims involving both minor and major injuries occurring in fitness facilities, and table 26.3 lists the five most frequent claims and their average cost (36). Member malfunction claims include injuries where participants hurt themselves (e.g., smashing fingers when racking weights, dropping a weight on their foot, straining a muscle). The equipment malfunction claims reflect injuries resulting primarily from poor equipment maintenance (e.g., seats falling off spin bikes, exercise balls that burst, cable failure on machines). The average claim value includes the amount paid to the injured party as well as defense and other costs.

KEY POINT

Several studies have demonstrated that participation in fitness activities and programs can lead to all types of injuries—minor, major, and even death. It also is well established that these injuries can lead to legal claims and lawsuits against fitness professionals and their employers. To help minimize injuries and subsequent litigation, it is essential that fitness professionals learn the laws that pertain to the field and how to apply them to their practices.

Causes of Injuries and Negligence

There are many causes of injuries in fitness facilities and programs. The most common are due to inherent risks, negligence, and product defects. **Inherent risks** are those that happen simply as a result of participation in physical activity—they are no one's fault and are inherent in (or inseparable from) the activity. Almost everyone who has participated in physical activity or sport has experienced an injury due to inherent risks. Injuries caused by **negligence** are due to fault—the fault of a participant (e.g., the

Table 26.2 Types of Injuries Leading to Negligence Lawsuits Against Fitness Professionals and Facilities

Type of injury	Negligence lawsuit
Stroke resulting in death	*Capati v. Crunch Fitness International, Inc.* (15, 16)
Fractured ankle requiring surgical insertion of pins	*Santana v. Women's Workout and Weight Loss Centers, Inc.* (60)
Exertional rhabdomyolysis leading to permanent disabilities	*Proffitt v. Global Fitness Holdings, LLC, et al.* (53, 57) *Mimms v. Ruthless Training Concepts, LLC* (47)
Shattered wrist	*Covenant Health System v. Barnett* (25)
Heart attack	*Rostai v. Neste Enterprises* (58)
Severe head injury resulting in death	*Xu v. Gay* (76)
Fractured ankle and crushed foot	*Thomas v. Sport City, Inc.* (66)
Serious and permanent injuries to mouth and lips	*Alack v. Vic Tanny International of Missouri, Inc.* (4)
Serious neck and back pain	*Goynias v. Spa Health Clubs, Inc.* (39)
Heart attack resulting in death	*DiGiulio v. Gran, Inc.* (29)

Table 26.3 Frequent Injury Claims Occurring in Fitness Facilities

	Number of claims	Average claim value
Member malfunction	388	$8,902
Premises liability (tripping and falling)	350	$18,554
Equipment malfunction	339	$17,063
Slips and falls in wet areas	252	$12,478
Treadmill	233	$8,933

Data from Eickhoff-Shemek, Herbert, and Connaughton 2009.

participant is careless while lifting weights) or of a fitness professional or facility (e.g., the failure to properly instruct and supervise participants, inspect and maintain exercise equipment, and carry out emergency procedures). Injuries also can be caused by **product defects**. Manufacturers can be found liable if an injury was due to a defect in the exercise equipment. This type of liability is called **product liability**.

This chapter focuses on negligence, the major legal concern facing all fitness professionals and facilities. Negligence is failing to do something that a reasonable, prudent professional would do or doing something that a reasonable, prudent professional would not have done under the same or similar circumstances (36). In other words, negligence can be an act of omission (failure to perform) or commission (improper performance). Unfortunately, negligence lawsuits against fitness professionals and facilities continue to increase (1), which reflects negatively upon the profession. However, this problem can be addressed—professionals can learn about their many legal duties toward participants and take steps to adhere to these duties, which will lead to fewer injuries and subsequent negligence claims and lawsuits. To begin this learning process, the next section provides an overview of the law and legal system.

KEY POINT

The most common causes of injuries in fitness programs are inherent risks, negligence, and product defects. Of these, negligence is the major legal concern facing fitness professionals. Negligence is the failure to do something that a reasonable, prudent professional would do or doing something that a reasonable, prudent professional would not have done under the same or similar circumstances.

Law and the Legal System

This section describes primary and secondary sources of law, criminal versus civil law, trial and appellate courts, tort law, and contract law. It also covers certain federal laws applicable to the fitness profession.

Primary and Secondary Sources of Law

In the United States, law is created from the three branches of government at both the federal and state levels: statutory law from the legislative branch, administrative law from the executive branch, and case law from the judiciary branch. **Statutory law** is enacted through the legislative process. Examples of federal statutes are the Americans with Disabilities Act (ADA) and HIPAA. Examples of state statutes include statutes prohibiting the unauthorized practice of medicine or other allied (or licensed) health professions, Good Samaritan statutes, and statutes that require fitness facilities to have an AED. **Administrative law** is formed by numerous administrative agencies that exist at both the federal and state levels. At the federal level, these include the FDA, Internal Revenue Service (IRS), and OSHA. These agencies enact rules and regulations, investigate potential violations, and impose sanctions (e.g., fines) for any violations. **Case law** is derived from written court opinions and is sometimes referred to as *common law*. Courts often rely on the written opinions from previous cases to help form an opinion for a current case in which the facts are similar to those in the previous cases. Terms such as *precedent* or *stare decisis* (to stand by that which is decided) reflect this legal doctrine. Not all litigation results in precedent; most negligence cases are settled out of court and therefore never go to trial.

In addition to these three primary sources of law (statutory, administrative, and case law), there are many secondary sources of law, including books, treatises (e.g., *Restatement of the Law of Torts*), and law review journals. Secondary sources do not reflect the law, but they are helpful for finding primary sources of law or explaining a specific area of law. Both primary and secondary sources of law can be found using electronic legal databases such as LexisNexis Academic and Westlaw Campus Research, often available to students and faculty members through university libraries.

KEY POINT

The law is created from the three branches of government at both the federal and state levels: statutory law from the legislative branch, administrative law from the executive branch, and case law from the judiciary branch. Statutory law is enacted through the legislative process, administrative law is formed by numerous administrative agencies, and case law is derived from written court opinions.

Criminal Law Versus Civil Law

The law also can be categorized into criminal law and civil law. If someone violates a statute, the government can bring criminal charges against that person—the defendant. If the defendant is found guilty, she may have to pay a fine, perform community service, be placed on probation, or go to prison (36). It must be shown that the defendant is guilty beyond a reasonable doubt, meaning she is 100% guilty of the crime. Fitness professionals could face criminal charges for violating state statutes such as assault and battery, theft, and the unauthorized practice of medicine.

Civil law addresses noncriminal matters and deals primarily with civil disputes between individuals, businesses, organizations, and government agencies (36). For example, if a member of a fitness facility is injured while working out in the facility, he could sue the facility for negligence—a civil claim. In this example, the injured member is referred to as the **plaintiff** and the fitness facility is referred to as the **defendant**. The plaintiff in a civil lawsuit has the burden of proof, so he must prove that the defendant was liable for the injury by the preponderance of the evidence, meaning it was more likely than not (51% or greater) that the negligent conduct of the defendant caused the harm to the plaintiff. Note that the term *liable* is used in civil law rather than the term *guilty*, which is used in criminal law. In civil claims such as negligence, the plaintiff seeks monetary damages from the defendant to compensate for the injury (e.g., medical expenses, lost wages).

Trial Courts and Appellate Courts

The U.S. court system is made up of trial and appellate courts at the federal, state, and local levels. Trial courts, the lowest courts, are the first to carry out the legal proceedings. At the end of the trial, the judge or a jury renders a decision in favor of one of the parties. Within a given time frame, the losing party can appeal the trial court's decision to a higher court—an appellate court. Appellate courts are made up of an odd number of judges who review the evidence and proceedings of the trial court. An appellate court has several options when forming its opinion about a case. It can remand it (send it back to trial with instructions), reverse it (disagree with the trial court's decision), affirm it (agree with the trial court's decision), or modify the trial court's decision (36). There are intermediate and supreme (highest) appellate courts at the state and federal levels.

Tort Law and Contract Law

Although there are many types of substantive law, tort law and contract law are most relevant to the fitness field. A tort is "conduct that amounts to a legal wrong that also causes harm on which the courts can impose civil liability" (36, p. 30), and a contract "is an agreement that can be enforceable in court" and is most often "formed when two (or more) parties exchange binding promises" (36, p. 37). The elements of tort law and contract law are described next, along with their applications to the fitness field.

Tort Law

Tort law can be classified into three levels of fault, as shown in figure 26.1: intentional, negligence, and strict liability. Intentional torts involve conduct that requires the intent to cause harm to another. Examples are assault, battery, false imprisonment, defamation of character, and invasion of privacy. Although uncommon in fitness facilities, this type of behavior can occur among fitness staff members and participants. Many times this type of conduct also can be considered a crime (violation of a statute), so the wrongdoer can face both civil claims and criminal charges.

Intentional	Harms such as assault, battery, and invasion of privacy
Negligence	Harms due to ordinary negligence or gross negligence
Strict liability	Product liability and vicarious liability

FIGURE 26.1 Fault basis of tort liability.

Of the three levels of fault, negligence is the most common in the fitness field and can involve both gross negligence (also referred to as *reckless*, *willful*, or *wanton conduct*) and ordinary negligence. An example of gross negligence would be when a piece of exercise equipment is broken and fitness staff do not take any precautions (e.g., posting warning signs) to prevent participants from using it. Gross negligence usually requires prior knowledge of a risk or danger that is clearly foreseeable and then doing little or nothing to minimize that risk. Ordinary negligence is considered careless conduct as defined earlier—the failure to do something (omission) that a reasonable, prudent professional would do or doing something that a reasonable, prudent professional would not have done (commission) given the same or similar circumstances (e.g., the failure to provide proper instruction or maintenance of exercise equipment).

Various forms of strict liability also exist in the fitness field. Two of these are product liability and vicarious liability. Product liability involves a defect in the product (e.g., design defect, manufacturing defect, or marketing defect such as inadequate instructions or warnings). For example, if a plaintiff could show that her injury was due to the manufacturer's defective design of the equipment, then the manufacturer could be held strictly liable for the injury. Product liability is based on public policy (i.e., judicial determination of what is in the best interest of society) rather than fault such as intentional or negligent wrongdoing (36).

Vicarious liability is imposed upon employers even if the employer has not been negligent. Under the legal doctrine of ***respondeat superior***, employers can be held strictly liable for harm to third parties (e.g., fitness participants) caused by negligent acts of their employees while performing their jobs (17). It is common in negligence lawsuits for the plaintiff to name several defendants in the case; for example, it may have been the personal trainer who committed the negligent act, but the plaintiff can name the trainer, his manager, and the owner of the facility as defendants who all could be potentially liable for the plaintiff's injury.

KEY POINT

Tort law involves three levels of fault: intentional, or conduct that requires the intent to cause harm to another; negligence, or careless conduct that causes harm to another (ordinary negligence) and reckless conduct that causes harm to another (gross negligence); and strict liability, such as product liability and vicarious liability. Vicarious liability occurs when employers (e.g., fitness facility managers and owners) are held liable for the negligent acts of their employees through a legal doctrine called *respondeat superior*.

Four Elements to Prove Negligence In a negligence lawsuit, the plaintiff has to prove the following four elements (30):

1. Duty—the defendant owed a duty (or standard of care) to the plaintiff.
2. Breach of duty—the defendant failed to carry out the duty.
3. Causation—the breach of duty was the cause of the harm.
4. Harm and damages—harm occurred to the plaintiff, resulting in damages (losses) to the plaintiff (e.g., medical expenses, lost wages).

Courts (judges) determine the first element of duty—not attorneys, juries, plaintiffs, or defendants. (The approaches that courts use to determine duty are discussed later.) The plaintiff then has to prove that the defendant breached her duty. Therefore, the defendant's conduct becomes a key factor in determining whether or not there was a breach of duty. If the conduct was consistent with the duty owed, even if the plaintiff was seriously hurt or died, it will be difficult for the plaintiff to prevail with his suit. However, if the defendant's conduct was inconsistent with the duty owed, it will be easier for the plaintiff to show that the defendant breached her duty.

To determine if the breach of duty caused the injury, courts often use the "but for" test: "But for the defendant's negligent conduct, would the injury have occurred?" (55). Sometimes injuries are caused by reasons other than the conduct of the defendant, such as inherent causes or the plaintiff's own negligence. There must be a link between the breach of duty and the cause (sometimes referred to as *proximate cause*) of the injury. If the plaintiff can show that the breach of duty caused harm to him (physical or emotional injury or damage to his property), monetary damages can be awarded to compensate for the harm. In ordinary negligence cases, these are called *compensatory damages* and can be both economic, such as medical expenses and lost wages, and noneconomic, such as pain, suffering, and loss of consortium (e.g., loss of companionship of a loved one). In gross negligence cases, plaintiffs usually seek compensatory damages as well as punitive damages (additional damages to punish the defendant for reckless conduct).

Defenses Against Negligence Defendants involved in negligence lawsuits have various defenses they can use to refute (or defend) the negligent claims made against them. The best defense always is to carry out legal duties properly. If the plaintiff cannot prove that the defendant breached a duty, it will be difficult for the plaintiff to win the negligence lawsuit and recover any damages. Two additional defenses, primary assumption of risk and waivers, are discussed next.

Primary assumption of risk is a defense often used by defendants in negligence cases. As discussed, injuries are sometimes due to inherent causes. Primary assumption of risk is a legal theory in which plaintiffs are generally not allowed to seek damages for an injury that was due to inherent risks. However, in order for defendants to successfully use this defense, the following three elements must be met: "(a) The risk must be inherent to the activity, (b) the participant must voluntarily agree to participate, and (c) the participant must know, understand, and appreciate the inherent risk" (36, p. 35).

In determining whether the injury was due to an inherent risk, courts will examine the nature of the activity and the experience of the plaintiff. For example, in *Rutnik v. Colonie Center Court Club, Inc.* (59), a man died from a cardiac arrest while participating in a racquetball tournament. The estate of the decedent sued the club for negligence, claiming they failed to carry out certain duties such as emergency procedures. Using primary assumption of risk, the defendants claimed the decedent assumed the risk of a heart attack and, therefore, they were not liable. The appellate court agreed with the defendants, stating that "relieving an owner . . . of a sporting facility from liability for the inherent risk of engaging in sports is justified when the consenting participant is aware of the risks, has an appreciation of the nature of the risks, and voluntarily assumes the risk" (p. 452). The court also stated that because the decedent was an experienced racquetball player who had played in many previous tournaments, he must have known and appreciated the risk of cardiac arrest while participating in this strenuous sport. The court found no negligence on the part of the club; that is, they carried out emergency procedures properly. In this case, primary assumption of risk protected the defendants from liability.

In another case, *Corrigan v. Musclemakers, Inc.* (23), primary assumption of risk did not protect the defendants from liability. In this case, a personal trainer placed a woman on a treadmill during her first training session, gave her little or no instruction on how to use the treadmill, and then left her unattended. After a short while, she began to drift back on the belt of the treadmill. She tried to walk faster but instead was thrown from the treadmill, which resulted in her fracturing her ankle. Prior to this incident, she had never been in a fitness facility or on a treadmill. She filed a negligence lawsuit against the defendants (the trainer and the facility), claiming the trainer failed to ensure that she understood how to use the treadmill (i.e., failed to provide proper instruction and supervision). The appellate court stated that the "doctrine of primary assumption of risk . . . may be applied in cases where there is an elevated risk of danger typically in sporting and recreational events" (p. 145), but the doctrine was not applicable in this case because fitness activities such as exercising on a treadmill are not the same as sporting activities. In addition, the court ruled that the risks associated with using the treadmill were not known, understood, and appreciated by the plaintiff, a novice exerciser and treadmill user. Therefore, the plaintiff's injury was not due to inherent causes but most likely due to the negligence of the trainer, and thus primary assumption of risk was not an effective defense for negligence.

Strengthening the Primary Assumption of Risk Defense Informing participants of the inherent risks associated with physical activity *may* help to strengthen the primary assumption of risk as a defense. Often, a section that informs a participant of inherent risks (minor, major, and even death) is included in protective legal documents such as waivers, informed consents, express assumptions of risk, and agreements to participate. Examples of these documents and descriptions of the legal protection they provide can be found elsewhere (24, 36, 43). The following text describing inherent risks is taken from an **informed consent** that would be read and signed by a participant prior to fitness testing:

> I understand and have been informed that there exists the possibility of adverse changes during the actual test. I have been informed that these changes could include abnormal blood pressure, fainting, disorders of heart rhythm, stroke, and very rare instances of heart attack

> or even death. Every effort, I have been told, will be made to minimize these occurrences by preliminary examination and by precautions and observations taken during the test. I have also been informed that emergency equipment and personnel are readily available to deal with these unusual situations should they occur. I understand that there is a risk of injury, heart attack, stroke, or even death as a result of my performance of this test, but knowing those risks, it is my desire to proceed to take the test as herein indicated. (43, p. 468)

A **waiver** (or prospective release) is a defense based upon contract law. A waiver, signed by a person before participation, contains an **exculpatory clause** such as the following that was included in the waiver in *Randas v. YMCA of Metropolitan Los Angeles* (54):

> THE UNDERSIGNED HEREBY RELEASES, WAIVES, DISCHARGES AND COVENANTS NOT TO SUE the YMCA, its directors, officers, employees, and agents (hereinafter referred to as "releases") from all liability to the undersigned, his personal representatives, assigns, heirs, and next of kin for any loss or damage, and any claim or demands therefore on account of injury to the person or property or resulting in death of the undersigned, whether *caused by the negligence of the releases* or otherwise while the undersigned is in, upon, or about the premises or any facilities or equipment therein [emphasis added]. (p. 165)

The exculpatory clause in this case was effective because it absolved (protected) the defendant YMCA from its own negligence. Without this waiver, the YMCA may have been found liable for its negligent conduct that caused the injury to the plaintiff. Therefore, when a person signs a waiver, she gives up (waives) her civil right to recover any damages due to the ordinary negligence of the defendant. Waivers do not protect defendants against gross negligence or intentional acts.

For the waiver to be effective and enforceable, it must be written and administered properly. It is also important to realize that the validity and enforceability of a waiver varies significantly from state to state. For example, in some states, the language of the exculpatory clause must be explicit in order for it to be enforceable. In addition, waivers are not enforceable in some states such as Virginia because they are against public policy. Many other factors also need to be considered when preparing an effective waiver; see the book *Waivers and Releases of Liability* for more information (24). Because of the many differences in the requirements for waivers among states, fitness professionals should never adopt a waiver they find in a book or some other source—it must be reviewed and edited by a competent lawyer prior to use.

KEY POINT

Two defenses often used by defendants in negligence cases are primary assumption of risk and waivers. Primary assumption of risk is effective for injuries due to inherent causes if the plaintiff knows, understands, and appreciates the inherent risks and voluntarily assumes those risks. The waiver defense can protect (absolve) defendants of their own negligence if the exculpatory clause within the waiver document is valid and enforceable based on state law. Because waiver law is complex and can vary significantly from state to state, fitness professionals must have a competent lawyer approve any waiver prior to use.

Contract Law

Contracts are commonly used in the fitness field. Examples include waivers, informed consents, employment contracts for employees and independent contractors, membership contracts, and purchase and lease agreements. For a contract to be valid and legally enforceable, it must meet the following four elements (22):

1. *Agreement.* An agreement to form a contract includes an *offer* and an *acceptance*.
2. *Consideration.* Any promises made by the parties to the contract must be supported by legally sufficient and bargained-for consideration.
3. *Contractual capacity.* Both parties entering into the contract must have contractual capacity to do so.
4. *Legality.* The purpose of the contract must be to accomplish some goal that is legal and not against public policy.

An agreement occurs when a fitness facility offers a membership to a person and he accepts. The consideration is the money promised to the fitness facility paid by the member in exchange for programs and services promised by the facility to the member. Contractual capacity means that both parties must be capable and competent to form a contract. For example, minors (children under the age of 18) do not have contractual capacity; only adults can sign contracts such as waivers and informed consents. *Legality* refers to the terms within a contract—they must be legal. For instance, exculpatory clauses in waivers are against public policy in some states and therefore do not meet the legality requirement.

A valid contract meets all four elements. An unenforceable contract is one that violates a statute or law (22). For example, some contracts must be in writing (e.g., contracts involving the sale of goods of $500 or more), and if they are not, they will likely be unenforceable. If one party fails to meets its contractual obligations, it might be considered a breach of contract and the breaching party may be required by a court to pay compensatory damages to the other party.

Federal Laws Applicable to the Fitness Profession

There are several federal laws that fitness professionals should be aware of. However, this section focuses on three major ones: the ADA, OSHA's Bloodborne Pathogens Standard, and the HIPAA Privacy Rule.

The ADA (Americans with Disabilities Act) is a federal statute that was enacted in 1990. The purpose of this law is to prohibit discrimination against people with disabilities. According to the ADA, a person with a disability has a physical or mental impairment that substantially limits one or more major life activities, has a record of such impairment, and is regarded as having such impairment (7). The ADA contains five titles, and two of these, Title I and Title III, pertain to fitness facilities. Title I, Employment, prohibits discrimination in employment procedures for private employers with 15 or more employees (6). These employers must provide reasonable accommodations for disabled employees. A reasonable accommodation is something that will help the employee to perform her job without creating an undue burden (significant difficulty or expense) on the employer.

Title III, Public Accommodations and Services Operated by Private Entities, requires that privately owned or operated places of public accommodation provide access for people with disabilities and make reasonable accommodations with regard to programs and services. There are 12 categories of places of public accommodation according to Title III, including places of exercise or recreation (7). Therefore, fitness facilities not only need to address architectural barriers (e.g., ramps for stairs) but also provide programs and services for people with disabilities. Again, the ADA requires a reasonable accommodation with regard to the provision of programs and services—meaning facilities do not need to purchase expensive, specialized exercise equipment, but they do need to provide appropriate programs and services to people with disabilities. This may require fitness facilities to have staff members who are qualified to conduct health and fitness assessments and design exercise prescriptions for people with disabilities. One credential that fitness professionals should consider in this regard is the Certified Inclusive Fitness Trainer (CIFT) certification established by ACSM and the National Center on Health, Physical Activity and Disability (NCHPAD). See the NCHPAD website (www.nchpad.org) for more information on this certification as well as other helpful information and resources.

OSHA's Bloodborne Pathogens Standard is an administrative law that became effective in March 1992. Exposure to bloodborne pathogens such as the human immunodeficiency virus (HIV) and hepatitis B virus (HBV) can lead to serious illness and death. The major goal of the Bloodborne Pathogens Standard is to reduce or eliminate occupational exposure to these pathogens that can be transmitted via blood or other potentially infectious materials (OPIM). It specifically applies to employers whose employees could come in contact with blood or OPIM while performing their jobs (e.g., fitness staff members who are responsible for carrying out first aid). This law has numerous requirements, including the establishment of a written exposure control plan (ECP) that describes the job classifications where the occupational exposure occurs as well as how and when the provisions within the law will be implemented (12). To assist with the development and implementation of the many provisions within this complex law, fitness professionals can contact their regional OSHA office. A list of these offices is available at www.osha.gov/html/RAmap.html. Each regional office has a Bloodborne Pathogens coordinator.

The HIPAA Privacy Rule, a federal statute, mandates the protection of an individual's private health information. This law became effective on April 14, 2001, and required all covered entities to comply with it by April 14, 2003 (11). Covered entities include those who provide health care services such as health insurance plans and health care providers. Most fitness facilities likely would not be considered a covered entity, but some health promotion and disease prevention programs may be (11). However, it may be wise for fitness facilities to adopt provisions that this law requires with regard to protected health information (PHI)—all individually identifiable health information—because even if this law does not apply, there may be state privacy laws that do apply with regard to PHI. In addition, many professional organizations in the fitness field recommend in their ethical statements that individual health and fitness data be kept confidential. Fitness professionals should consider developing and implementing procedures in their facilities that reflect the following HIPAA-related definitions when handling PHI by paper, electronically, or orally.

- *Privacy* is the right of an individual to enjoy freedom from intrusion or observation, the right to maintain control over certain personal information, and the right to expect health care providers to respect the individual's rights.
- *Confidentiality* is the practice of permitting only certain authorized people to access information, with the understanding that they will disclose it only to other authorized people.

- *Security* refers to the physical, technical, and administrative safeguards used to control access and protect information from accidental or intentional disclosure to unauthorized people and from alteration or destruction to maintain the integrity of the information. (11)

These provisions also apply when fitness professionals want to obtain medical information (e.g., GXT results) from a participant's physician. The participant must first sign a **medical release** granting permission for the physician to release that information. An example of a HIPAA-compliant medical release is available elsewhere (36).

KEY POINT

Federal laws that fitness professionals should be familiar with are the ADA, Bloodborne Pathogens Standard, and HIPAA Privacy Rule. With the assistance of legal counsel, fitness professionals need to develop and implement procedures that reflect the requirements within these laws.

Determining Duty in Negligence Cases

As mentioned, courts (i.e., judges) determine duty in negligence cases. One of the first things courts consider when determining duty is the relationship that is formed between the plaintiff and defendant. Most courts will classify the relationship between fitness professionals and their participants (e.g., members, clients, patients, athletes) as an *inherent relationship*. When an inherent relationship is formed, professionals have a legal duty to provide reasonably safe facilities and programs for their participants. This involves taking precautions (developing and implementing risk management strategies, as discussed later) that will help prevent foreseeable injury risks. Injury risks—minor, major, and even death—are all foreseeable risks that can occur in fitness facilities and programs.

Given the inherent relationship between fitness professionals and their participants, it is likely that courts will hold fitness professionals to what is called the *professional standard of care*. In negligence cases, courts allow expert witnesses to provide testimony to educate the court as to the duty (or standard of care) the fitness professional (defendant) owed to the participant (plaintiff). Expert witnesses provide their opinions regarding the conduct of the fitness professional. If the professional's conduct was consistent with the professional standard of care, then it will be difficult to show a breach of duty (even in cases where a serious injury or death occurred). However, if the professional's conduct was inconsistent with the professional standard of care, then it will be easier to show a breach of duty. Therefore, fitness professionals need to understand not only what the professional standard of care means by definition but also how it is often determined via expert testimony—by situational factors and by adherence to published standards of practice.

Professional Standard of Care

As stated, negligence is the failure to do something that a reasonable, prudent professional would do (omission) or doing something that a reasonable, prudent professional would not have done under the same or similar circumstances (commission). According to the *Restatement of the Law Third. Restatement of the Law Torts: Liability for Physical Harm*, "If an actor has skills or knowledge that exceed those possessed by most others, these skills and knowledge are circumstances to be taken into account in determining whether the actor behaved as a reasonably careful person" (56, p. 18). Because fitness professionals possess special knowledge, skills, and abilities, they are not only required to exercise reasonable care but also a level of care that would be consistent with the knowledge, skills, and abilities expected of fitness professionals.

According to van der Smissen, "If one accepts responsibility for giving leadership to an activity or providing a service, one's performance is measured against the standard of care of a qualified professional **for that situation**" (72, p. 40). The term *qualified professional* in this context means a professional who provides a standard of care that a prudent (competent) professional would provide. In negligence cases, courts will investigate the credentials (e.g., degrees, certifications) and, more importantly, the competence of the professional—that is, what he did (or did not do) given the situation. The phrase "for that situation" means that the professional standard of care is determined using three situational factors: the nature of the activity, the type of participants, and the environmental conditions (72). Each of these is described next. Many of the negligence cases described later in this chapter involve fitness professionals who failed to meet one or more of these three situational factors. To further demonstrate how these situational factors are included in expert testimony, see two articles written by well-known expert witness Dr. Anthony Abbott, who describes cardiac arrest litigations (2) and injury litigations (3) in which he served as an expert witness.

THREE SITUATIONAL FACTORS THAT DETERMINE PROFESSIONAL STANDARD OF CARE

1. **Nature of the activity:** The professional must be aware of the skills and abilities the participant needs to participate safely in the activity (i.e., the fitness professional

must possess adequate knowledge, skills, and abilities to lead safe exercise programs).

Fitness professionals must fully understand and apply numerous safety principles when leading even a basic exercise program. However, professionals who lead complex or advanced exercise programs (e.g., Olympic lifting, high-intensity or extreme conditioning) need to have any additional knowledge and skills necessary to safely teach these programs.

2. **Type of participants:** The professional must be aware of individual factors of the participant (i.e., awareness of medical conditions that impose increased risks and how to minimize those risks).

Fitness professionals who train people with medical conditions need to possess advanced credentials in the exercise sciences, such as academic coursework and certification in clinical exercise (36, 75). For example, when training participants with medical conditions (e.g., pregnancy, diabetes, hypertension, back problems), fitness professionals need to fully understand any risks the conditions might impose and how to minimize those risks. In addition to advanced credentials in clinical exercise, fitness professionals also should refer to the numerous position papers published by professional organizations that address exercise guidelines for all types of medical conditions.

3. **Environmental conditions:** The professional must be aware of any conditions that may increase risks (e.g., heat and humidity, floor surfaces, exercise equipment) and know how to minimize those risks.

Fitness professionals need to have the necessary knowledge, skills, and abilities to safely lead exercise given various environmental conditions. For example, many precautions must be taken to help prevent heat injuries. This would include being familiar with position papers published by professional organizations that describe specific precautions to take in order to minimize the risk of heat injuries. For example, a NATA position statement (10) provides 18 prevention strategies that allied health professionals should understand in order to minimize exertional heat illnesses. The environment also includes properly maintaining floor surfaces and exercise equipment (many injuries in fitness facilities are due to slippery floors and poor equipment maintenance) as well as having policies that require participants to return equipment (exercise balls, dumbbells) to their storage racks to help prevent injuries from tripping and falling.

Adherence to Published Standards of Practice

In recent years, numerous standards of practice (e.g., standards, guidelines, position papers) have been published by both professional organizations (e.g., ACSM, NSCA, YMCA) and independent organizations such as the American Society for Testing and Materials (ASTM) and Consumer Products Safety Commission (CPSC). According to Herbert and Herbert (43), these published standards of practice reflect "benchmark behaviors or actions that are universally exhibited by properly trained and experienced professionals" (pp. 80-81) and should be viewed "as the threshold or minimal acceptable level of service owed to a client, patient, or participant" (pp. 205-206).

Fitness professionals must implement the behaviors and actions described in published standards of practice because of the potential legal impact they can have. Expert witnesses, who educate the court as to the duty the defendant owed to the plaintiff in professional negligence cases, often introduce published standards of practice in their testimony as evidence of the standard of care owed to the plaintiff. Courts often allow these published standards of practice as admissible evidence to help determine duty, as demonstrated in *Elledge v. Richland/Lexington School District Five* (38).

In this case, a 9-yr-old girl was playing on modified monkey bars at school when her foot slipped, resulting in a fall that trapped her right leg between the bars. She suffered a severe spiral fracture in her femur that damaged the growth plate. Prior to this injury, the principal of the school had the monkey bars modified by a playground equipment salesperson who was not trained or licensed as an engineer to modify monkey bars. The child's mother sued the school district, claiming that it was negligent because it deviated from the accepted standard of care (i.e., the modification of the monkey bars did not meet the standards published by ASTM and the guidelines published by CPSC for playground equipment). The trial court excluded the evidence presented by an expert witness that clearly showed that the district did not adhere to industry standards, and it ruled in favor of the school district. Upon appeal, the mother claimed that the trial court erred in excluding the evidence, arguing that such evidence was relevant to establish the appropriate standard of care. The appellate court (an intermediate appellate court) stated the following:

> Safety standards promulgated by government or industry organizations in particular are relevant to the standard of care for negligence. . . . Courts have become increasingly appreciative of the value of national safety codes and other guidelines issued by governmental and voluntary associations to assist in applying the standard of care in negligence cases. . . . A safety code ordinarily represents a consensus of opinion . . . and is not introduced as substantive law but most often as illustrative evidence of safety practices or rules generally prevailing in the industry that provides support for expert testimony concerning the proper standard of care. (38, pp. 477-478)

Given this reasoning, the appellate court reversed the ruling of the trial court. The case was further appealed to the South Carolina Supreme Court, which upheld the intermediate appellate court's ruling.

As previously stated, expert witnesses rely on published standards of practice when providing testimony in negligence cases. For example, two prominent expert witnesses who each have over 30 years of expert witness experience stated: "Not only have we referenced [*ACSM's Health/Fitness Facility Standards and Guidelines*] in our numerous opinions provided in numerous cases, but other prominent standards for fitness facility operation such as those of the NSCA . . . to communicate with courts and juries as to what is appropriate" (74, p. 20-21). Several legal cases described later in this chapter also relied on published standards of practice introduced as evidence by expert witnesses to help establish duty or the standard of care.

The proliferation of standards of practice published by professional and independent organizations in recent years makes it difficult to include all of them in this chapter. Therefore, the section *Strategies to Minimize Legal Liability* only includes selected standards of practice published

Professional Standard of Care and High-Intensity Interval Training (HIIT)

HIIT was rated the number one fitness trend in 2014 and the number two fitness trend in 2015 (69, 70). Although many health and fitness benefits have been associated with high-intensity exercise programs, there are also risks of injuries such as torn ligaments, stress fractures, and exertional rhabdomyolysis (9). Fitness professionals who implement high-intensity programs must understand the increased risks associated with these programs and how to minimize these risks in order to meet the professional standard of care (i.e., nature of the activity). Unfortunately, high-intensity exercise programs (especially those designed with no rest intervals) have led to serious injuries and negligence lawsuits, as demonstrated in legal cases described later in this chapter (*Rostai, Proffitt,* and *Mimms*), because the personal fitness trainers in these cases did not know how to design and deliver a safe and effective program given their client's health and fitness status. Rostai suffered a heart attack and Proffitt and Mimms were both hospitalized for exertional rhabdomyolysis.

Serious injuries such as exertional rhabdomyolysis have also occurred in elite athletes. In 2011, 13 University of Iowa football players were hospitalized with exertional rhabdomyolysis (44). One of these players, William Lowe, who continued to suffer 3 yr after the incident, filed a lawsuit in 2014 against the coaches, trainers, and staff that listed several negligence claims, including that they developed a dangerous and improper training program. Given the increase in exertional rhabdomyolysis cases among collegiate athletes, a consensus statement was published in the *Journal of Athletic Training* (18) that provided 10 recommendations to end morbidity and mortality related to improper conditioning programs. The authors of this consensus statement state that "excesses in strength training and conditioning—workouts that are too novel, too much, too soon, or too intense (or a combination of these)—have a strong connection to exertional rhabdomyolysis" (18, p. 477).

Given the popularity and growth of high-intensity programs, fitness professionals must develop and implement risk management strategies to help minimize the increased risks associated with these programs. These strategies have been discussed in detail elsewhere (37), but one important one is to conduct preactivity screening. People who are sedentary or have certain medical conditions or risk factors should obtain medical clearance before participating in high-intensity exercise. This means that the medical provider does not just clear them for general exercise but specifically for high-intensity exercise (maximal or near-maximal exertion), and this should be clearly indicated on the medical clearance form (e.g., check boxes where the medical provider indicates the level of intensity for which the patient is cleared—low, moderate, vigorous, or high). It is doubtful that any medical provider would clear a sedentary person or one with chronic medical conditions to begin a high-intensity exercise program. If the individual is not medically cleared for high intensity, the fitness professional needs to follow the level of intensity indicated by the medical provider.

Most American adults are sedentary—almost 80% do not meet the U.S. Guidelines for Physical Activity (19) and about half have chronic medical conditions (20). An ACSM position stand (67) states that vigorous exercise increases the risk of a cardiac event (acute MI or sudden death) particularly in habitually sedentary people but also in exercise-conditioned people. Therefore, it is essential to perform preactivity screening and to implement proper progression and design when delivering any exercise program.

by the ACSM (65) and ASTM. According to ACSM (65), *standards* are minimum requirements that fitness facilities must meet and *guidelines* are recommendations to improve the quality of services.

It is often difficult for fitness professionals to know which published standards of practice to follow, especially when inconsistencies exist among them, such as how each defines terms such as *standards* and *guidelines*, and because specific actions provided vary quite a bit among the publications. Therefore, "it is best . . . to adhere to all published standards and guidelines. In the event of inconsistency or conflict . . . follow those that are the most authoritative or safety-oriented in their approach, regardless of how they are defined and/or stated" (36, p. 53).

KEY POINT

Fitness professionals must understand that they will likely be held to the professional standard of care in a negligence case against them. This will involve the court investigating the conduct of the professional, often through the testimony and opinions of expert witnesses. If the conduct is consistent with the standard of care, it will be difficult for the plaintiff (injured participant) to prove that the defendant (fitness professional) breached his duty. However, if the conduct is inconsistent with the standard of care, it will be easier for the plaintiff to prove that the defendant breached his duty, which could lead to the defendant being liable for the plaintiff's injury. Whether or not a fitness professional's conduct met the professional standard of care will most likely be determined by examining three situational factors (nature of the activity, type of participants, and environmental conditions) and adherence to published standards of practice.

Risk Management

Fitness professionals often are employed in management positions within a facility. In these positions, they perform numerous management functions in areas such as human resource management, financial management, facility management, marketing and promotion, strategic planning, customer service, program and service scheduling, and information technology. However, risk management is one of the most important management functions because it focuses on participant safety. Developing and implementing the risk management strategies described in this chapter that help ensure the safety of participants should be the number one priority of all fitness professionals. These risk management strategies also reflect the many legal duties fitness professionals have toward their participants. In addition to minimizing injuries and subsequent litigation, risk management has other benefits such as enhancing operational efficiency and improving the quality of services (36).

Risk management is a broad term that reflects an overall goal of many organizations—to reduce accidental losses to help prevent slowed growth, reduced profits, and general interruption of operations (40). Liability losses (claims and lawsuits due to negligence) are one type of these accidental losses. Because this chapter focuses on legal liability in fitness programs and facilities, *risk management* in this context is defined as "a proactive administrative process that will help minimize liability losses for health/fitness professionals and the organizations they represent" (36, p. 9).

The risk management process involves four steps (36). When assessing legal liability exposures (situations that can lead to injuries or the violation of any laws) in step 1, fitness professionals need to be aware of the many laws and published standards of practice that apply to the field. To assist in this step, as well as steps 2 through 4, a fitness facility should have a risk management advisory committee that is made up of experts (e.g., legal, medical, insurance) who work with the fitness staff members in developing a comprehensive risk management plan for the facility. Because the law is often complex and varies among jurisdictions, it is essential that fitness professionals consult their risk management experts when making the many decisions involved in the four-step risk management process.

Step 2 involves developing three types of risk management strategies that reflect the laws and published standards of practice identified in step 1: *loss-prevention strategies* (i.e., strategies that help prevent injuries from occurring in the first place, such as providing proper instruction and supervision), *loss-reduction strategies* (i.e., strategies that help decrease the severity of an injury once it does occur, such as carrying out proper emergency procedures), and strategies that utilize a *contractual transfer of risks* (e.g., a waiver transfers the liability risks to the participant who signed it, and the liability insurance provider pays for the damages up to the limits of the policy when a defendant is found liable for negligence).

Some fitness facilities have opted for an exposure-avoidance strategy, meaning they don't offer programs (e.g., high intensity) or equipment (e.g., treadmills, free weights) that can pose increased risks of injury (9, 31, 45). Fitness professionals can minimize the increased risks associated with these types of programs and equipment, but a well-informed, concerted effort is needed to do so.

Step 3 involves the implementation of the risk management plan. Once the risk management strategies are developed as written policies and procedures for staff members to follow (step 2), they can be organized into a risk management policy and procedures manual (RMPPM). The policies and procedures should be presented in an organized fashion within the manual, divided into sections such as preactivity screening, equipment inspection and maintenance, EAP, and so on. Another component of step 3 is staff training, which is necessary so that staff members learn how to carry out the policies and procedures. New employees should receive training upon hiring, and there should also be regular in-service trainings throughout the year. An example of an in-service training would be training that includes a review and rehearsal of the EAP. EAP training should occur two to four times a year.

Step 4, evaluation of the risk management plan, includes two types of evaluation—formative and summative. Formative evaluation is ongoing throughout the year. For example, an evaluation as to whether or not the EAP was carried out properly should be conducted after every injury. If the EAP was not carried out properly, staff members may need retraining. Summative evaluation involves a formal, annual review of the entire risk management plan. Laws often change, as do published standards of practice, and therefore the risk management advisory committee and fitness professionals will need to revise and update certain policies and procedures in the RMPPM and then retrain staff members on the changes. For more information on these four important risk management steps, see *Risk Management for Health/Fitness Professionals: Legal Issues and Strategies* (36).

Strategies to Minimize Legal Liability

This part of the chapter includes six sections: (1) personnel, (2) preactivity screening, (3) fitness testing and prescription, (4) instruction and supervision, (5) equipment and facility, and (6) EAPs. Each section provides selected standards of practice published in *ACSM's Health/Fitness Facility Standards and Guidelines* (65), followed by important risk management strategies to help minimize legal liability. By no means do these strategies reflect all of the legal liability exposures that exist.

Personnel

A variety of legal issues can arise with regard to personnel in fitness facilities and programs. This section focuses on hiring qualified, competent employees; incorporating proper procedures in the hiring, training, and supervision of employees; purchasing both general and professional liability insurance; and working with independent contractors.

SELECTED ACSM STANDARDS RELATED TO PERSONNEL

> The health/fitness professionals who have supervisory responsibility and oversight responsibility for the physical activity programs and the staff who administer them shall have an appropriate level of professional education, work experience, and/or certification. Examples of health/fitness professionals who serve in a supervisory role include the fitness director, group exercise director, aquatics director, and program director. (65, p. 32)
>
> The health/fitness and healthcare professionals who serve in counseling, instruction, and physical activity supervision roles for the facility shall have an appropriate level of professional education, work experience, and/or certification. The primary professional staff and independent contractors who serve in these roles are fitness instructors, group exercise instructors, lifestyle counselors, and personal trainers. (65, p. 33)

ACSM (65) provides recommendations regarding the education, certification, and experience needed by professionals serving in supervisory roles as well as instructional roles. For example, those serving in a supervisory role such as fitness director should have a bachelor's degree in fitness, exercise science, or a related field, and fitness instructors, personal trainers, and health and fitness specialists should have certification from a nationally recognized and accredited certifying organization and 3 yr experience.

STRATEGY 1: HIRE QUALIFIED AND COMPETENT EMPLOYEES

Fitness professionals who serve in a supervisory role (e.g., manager, owner, fitness director, group exercise coordinator) need to hire qualified and competent employees. It is important to realize that a qualified professional (one who possesses certain credentials) is not necessarily competent to carry out her legal duties (e.g., knows how to apply safe and effective principles of exercise to meet a participant's specific needs).

Several efforts to address the issue of qualified and competent professionals have been made in the field, including voluntary or self-regulated efforts, such as the accreditation of certifications through independent agencies such as the National Commission for Certifying Agencies (NCCA), and government-regulated efforts, such as legislative bills proposing licensure in various states. However, many unnecessary injuries and subsequent negligence claims and lawsuits continue to occur in the field.

Although many in the field believe that the accreditation of certifications through the NCCA and similar agencies enhances safety and minimizes legal liability, there are no formal education prerequisites for sitting for the accredited exams. Therefore, it is possible that these individuals may be considered qualified by employers because they possess the certification credential, but they may not be competent if they have not received formal educational experiences that included coursework and evaluation of their practical skills (i.e., their ability to apply safe and effective principles of exercise).

In contrast, many of the licensure proposals have required formal education; for instance, the New Jersey proposal to license personal trainers and group exercise leaders requires 200 hr in the classroom and a 50 hr internship or an associate's degree in health and fitness (41). For more on licensure issues, see a three-part article published in *ACSM's Health and Fitness Journal* (33-35). Whether the field remains self-regulated or is regulated by the government in the future, the provision of well-designed formal education programs that prepare both qualified and competent fitness professionals is one of the most important risk management strategies for minimizing injuries and subsequent litigation in the field. Formal education programs to prepare quality personal trainers and group exercise leaders have been described elsewhere (13, 14, 27, 28).

STRATEGY 2: HIRE, TRAIN, AND SUPERVISE EMPLOYEES PROPERLY

Fitness professionals who serve in a supervisory role have a duty to use reasonable care in the hiring, training, and supervising of their employees. To prevent claims of negligent hiring, it is necessary to hire qualified, competent employees, as demonstrated in *Seigneur v. National Fitness Institute, Inc.* (62). In *Seigneur*, the plaintiff, who was injured while using a weight machine during an initial evaluation, claimed that the facility breached its duty to her "by negligently hiring . . . a defendant employee who . . . lacked sufficient training, experience, certification and/or other qualifications and knowledge to properly . . . direct and guide [her] in lifting weights and in the use of the weight equipment" (p. 277).

Fitness facilities also have been sued for negligent hiring because they did not conduct criminal background checks before hiring employees (36, 48). Under the legal principle of *respondeat superior*, employers generally would not be held liable for an employee who conducts a criminal act (e.g., sexual assault) while on the job because the criminal act would not be within the scope of employment. However, employers do have a responsibility to conduct criminal background checks before hiring employees who will be working with vulnerable populations (e.g., children, elderly, people with disabilities), as well as those who work closely with clients, such as massage therapists and personal fitness trainers. In addition, employers have a responsibility to supervise employees serving in these roles. If a fitness supervisor (or any staff member) observes or is made aware of any inappropriate behavior by another staff member or participant, proper steps based on consultation from legal counsel need to be taken in a timely fashion.

The failure to train employees also is a common negligence claim against fitness facilities, as demonstrated by the following claims made in *Chai v. Sports & Fitness Clubs of America, Inc.* (21, p. 55-56):

- Negligently failed to have personnel adequately trained to recognize cardiac arrest and to subsequently start CPR
- Negligently failed to have employees adequately trained in the use and operation of an AED
- Negligently failed to require sufficient training of staff members designated to train the member

These claims demonstrate the importance of staff training as a risk management strategy. Staff members who are well trained are more likely to carry out their legal duties compared with those who receive little or no training.

STRATEGY 3: PURCHASE LIABILITY INSURANCE COVERAGE

If a fitness professional and facility is found liable for negligence, liability insurance will pay for the damages up to the limits of the policy, thus protecting the financial assets of the professional and the facility. Most fitness facilities provide general liability insurance coverage for their employees through a commercial general liability (CGL) policy. This type of liability insurance protects fitness professionals and facilities from ordinary negligence, but not professional negligence. The need for professional liability insurance coverage is demonstrated in *York Insurance Company v. Houston Wellness Center, Inc.* (77).

The plaintiff in *York* claimed that she was injured due to improper instruction given by an employee on how to use an exercise machine. The fitness club contended that their liability insurance provider had a duty to defend and indemnify the club in this negligence case. However, the insurance company claimed they did not have this duty because of a clause in the CGL policy stating that "this insurance does not apply to 'bodily injury' . . . arising out of the . . . failure to render any service, treatment, advice, or instruction relating to the physical fitness . . . or physical training programs" (77, pp. 904-905). A court ruling agreed with the insurance company. The facility had a CGL policy that specifically excluded professional services such as fitness instruction. If they had also purchased professional liability insurance for their staff members, the outcome of this case probably would have been different. Fitness professionals should have both general and professional liability insurance policies and should be sure the policies cover all the programs and services they provide. As a member of a professional organization, a fitness professional can usually purchase professional liability insurance through a low-cost group plan. For example, ACSM has a group plan through the Forrest T. Jones and Company (www.ftj.com/acsm).

STRATEGY 4: HAVE PROCEDURES IN PLACE FOR INDEPENDENT CONTRACTORS

Fitness facilities often hire independent contractors to provide various services. Several legal concerns are involved when hiring independent contractors (36); this discussion will focus on a few of these. First, based on IRS tax law, employers do not have a lot of behavioral control over independent contractors. Therefore, it is essential that they hire only qualified and competent independent contractors. Second, all independent contractors should sign a written contract that specifies the responsibilities of both parties, including a clause stating that the independent contractor must provide proof of having both general and professional liability insurance (the fitness facility's liability insurance does not cover independent contractors—only employees). Third, it is critical that independent contractors do not appear to be employees by their actions or what they wear. For example, they should not wear a shirt with the facility logo on it but perhaps a badge indicating that they are an independent contractor. This is because if they are deemed to be *ostensible agents*, employers could be liable for their negligent acts the same as they would be for employees under the legal principle of *respondeat superior* (36). It is also wise for fitness facilities to inform participants in a membership contract or signage that some services are provided by independent contractors.

KEY POINT

Many injuries (and subsequent litigation) that occur in the field are due to the negligent conduct of staff members. Therefore, it is essential to hire qualified and competent staff members as well as provide them with training and supervision. Additional risk management strategies associated with personnel include conducting criminal background checks before hiring certain staff members, purchasing adequate general and professional liability insurance to cover all programs and services provided by employees, and having several procedures in place when hiring independent contractors.

Preactivity Screening

The failure to conduct a preactivity screening has been a claim in several negligence cases against fitness facilities, especially when there has been a serious injury (e.g., heart attack) or death (36), such as in *Rostai v. Neste Enterprises* (58). During his first personal fitness training session, Rostai, a 46-yr-old, overweight, and inactive male, allegedly suffered a heart attack toward the end of his 60 min session. In his negligence lawsuit against the trainer and the health club, Rostai claimed that the trainer knew he was overweight and was not physically fit but aggressively trained him in his first workout, even though he complained several times during the workout that he needed a break. Rostai claimed that the defendant owed him a duty to investigate his health history, physical condition, and cardiac risk factors. The trainer and the club were not liable in this case because the court ruled that Rostai assumed the risks, even though the trainer was negligent. The court indicated that the trainer and club would only have been liable if the conduct of the trainer was intentional or reckless. Most courts would probably disagree with this ruling because the assumption of risk is usually only effective in protecting defendants against injuries due to inherent causes, not negligence.

SELECTED ACSM STANDARDS RELATED TO PREACTIVITY SCREENING

> Facility operators shall offer a general pre-activity screening tool (e.g., Par-Q) and/or specific pre-activity screening tool (e.g., health risk appraisal [HRA], health history questionnaire [HHQ]) to all new members and prospective users. (65, p. 2)

> All specific pre-activity screening tools (e.g., HRA, HHQ) shall be reviewed and interpreted by qualified staff (e.g., a qualified health/fitness professional or healthcare professional), and the results of the review and interpretation shall be retained on file by the facility for a period of at least one year from the time the tool was reviewed and interpreted. (65, p. 4)

> If a facility operator becomes aware that a member, user, or prospective member has a known cardiovascular, metabolic, or pulmonary disease, or two or more major cardiovascular disease risk factors, or any other self-disclosed medical concern, that individual shall be advised to consult with a qualified healthcare provider before beginning a physical activity program. (65, p. 5)

See chapter 2 for more information on screening and the new Par-Q+, which has replaced the Par-Q.

STRATEGY 1: SELECT PREACTIVITY SCREENING TOOLS FOR SELF-GUIDED AND PROFESSIONALLY GUIDED PROGRAMS

With the assistance of the risk management committee, preactivity procedures need to be established for participants in self-guided and professionally guided programs. According to the eighth edition of *ACSM's Guidelines for Exercise Testing and Prescription* (68), self-guided programs are guided by the participant with little or no input or supervision from a fitness professional, whereas professionally guided programs are guided by a fitness professional with academic training and practical knowledge and skills in assessment, design, and supervision. The ninth edition of the book (52) does not include this same distinction between self-guided and professionally guided screening programs. However, based on a recent national study (26) that focused on preactivity screening procedures, 26% of fitness facilities use self-guided programs, 43% use professionally guided programs, and 31% use both self-guided and professionally guided programs as defined in the eighth edition. Therefore, retaining this distinction between the two types of screening programs makes practical sense.

For self-guided programs, participants would likely complete a tool such as the PAR-Q+, and then on their own they would follow the recommendations of the tool with regard to seeking advice from a doctor (medical provider) or qualified exercise professional prior to participation in physical activity. Some fitness facilities may decide to have participants obtain medical clearance, depending on how they answered certain questions on the PAR-Q+ or other screening tools.

Fitness professionals involved in professionally guided programs may want to consider using the Pre-Activity Screening Questionnaire (PASQ). Developed by faculty members in the exercise science program at the University of South Florida, the PASQ contains screening criteria to classify participants into low-, moderate-, and high-risk categories as established by ACSM (52, 68). Specific screening tools such as an HRA or health history questionnaire (HHQ) may or may not contain these screening criteria. The PASQ has been successfully used at the University of South Florida with both students and employees for several years. This form and related documents (e.g., detailed interpretive guidelines that describe how the PASQ meets the ACSM screening criteria) are available upon request from the author of this chapter (eickhoff@usf.edu).

STRATEGY 2: HAVE ONLY QUALIFIED FITNESS PROFESSIONALS INTERPRET DATA FROM SCREENING TOOLS USED IN PROFESSIONALLY GUIDED PROGRAMS

To comply with the ACSM standards (65), only qualified fitness professionals (e.g., those with academic training) should interpret data from specific screening devices. People who attempt to carry out this interpretation and are not qualified to do so may be practicing outside their scope of practice (discussed later in this chapter). They also would likely not possess the necessary knowledge and skills to meet the professional standard of care needed to conduct the interpretation process, because the professional standard of care is determined from situation-based factors, as described previously.

STRATEGY 3: DEVELOP PROCEDURES FOR MEDICAL CLEARANCE FOR PROFESSIONALLY GUIDED PROGRAMS

When using a screening tool in professionally guided programs to classify participants into low-, moderate-, or high-risk categories, the fitness professional can follow the guidelines in *ACSM's Guidelines for Exercise Testing and Prescription* to determine whether or not medical examination and clinical exercise testing are recommended before initiation of exercise training (see chapter 2). Obviously, only medical providers conduct medical evaluations and prescribe a diagnostic or clinical GXT, whereas fitness professionals obtain medical clearance. (Medical evaluation and medical clearance are distinctly different procedures involved in preactivity screening). For example, once a participant's physician receives the fitness facility's medical clearance form, the physician determines the need for a medical examination and what it would entail, such as a diagnostic or clinical GXT.

KEY POINT

Preactivity screening is essential to help ensure the safety of participants. Risk management strategies include selecting and using appropriate screening tools for both self-guided and professionally guided programs, as well as having only qualified professionals interpret data from specific screening devices and make decisions regarding the need for medical clearance.

Fitness Testing and Prescription

This section focuses on health-related fitness testing and prescription (conducted in fitness facilities) versus clinical exercise testing and prescription (conducted in clinical settings for diagnostic purposes). Fitness testing and prescription procedures require the necessary knowledge and skills in order to carry out these procedures safely. According to *ACSM's Guidelines for Exercise Testing and Prescription* (52, 68), testing procedures include (a) completing preactivity screening procedures as described previously, (b) selecting protocols that safely meet the needs of each individual and proper interpretation of test results, (c) inspecting and calibrating fitness testing equipment, (d) having emergency procedures in place, (e) providing instructions and administering informed consent, and (f) observing participants for any signs and symptoms of overexertion during and after the testing. For fitness prescription, procedures include (a) designing a safe and effective prescription based on the individual's health and fitness needs and (b) prescribing within one's **scope of practice**, or activities a fitness professional engages in when carrying out his practice that are within the boundaries or limitations of his education, training, experience, and certifications (36). (See *Understanding Scope of Practice*.)

SELECTED ACSM STANDARDS RELATED TO FITNESS TESTING AND PRESCRIPTION

In addition to ACSM standards previously listed under personnel, *ACSM's Health/Fitness Facility Standards and Guidelines* (65) offers guidelines that address the additional or higher level of qualifications needed by fitness professionals who provide fitness prescription services for special or clinical populations.

Understanding Scope of Practice

When fitness professionals perform within their scope of practice, they are leading or teaching activities that are within the boundaries or limitations of their education, training, experience, and certifications (36). Scope of practice also can be defined by professional organizations that provide general descriptions (and specific competencies—knowledge and skill) of their various certification levels, but it is most important for fitness professionals to understand how scope of practice is defined legally.

DEFINED BY PROFESSIONAL ORGANIZATIONS

Some certifications offered by ACSM and NSCA are listed here. Both organizations provide descriptions of the job functions associated with each certification level along with the preexam qualifications needed for each (see www.acsm.org and www.nsca.com). Just as there are inconsistencies in standards of practice published by professional organizations, there are also inconsistencies in these descriptions and qualifications.

ACSM

- Certified Personal Trainer (CPT)
- Certified Exercise Physiologist (EP-C)
- Certified Clinical Exercise Physiologist (CEP)

NCSA

- Certified Personal Trainer (CPT)
- Certified Strength and Conditioning Specialist (CSCS)
- Certified Special Population Specialist (CSPS)

DEFINED LEGALLY

Practicing outside one's scope of practice can lead to criminal charges and to negligence claims and lawsuits.

Criminal Charges

If a fitness professional's conduct crosses over the line into a licensed profession, he can face criminal charges for violation of a state statute for practicing medicine or some other licensed profession (e.g., dietetics, physical therapy). No harm is needed to prove the violation; only the conduct.

Negligence Claims and Lawsuits

If a fitness professional's conduct does not meet the professional standard of care as described previously (i.e., does not meet the three situational factors and adhere to practices described in standards of practice published by professional organizations), and the conduct causes harm to a participant, the fitness professional can be found liable for negligence.

STRATEGY 1: DEVELOP SCOPE-OF-PRACTICE GUIDELINES FOR FITNESS PROFESSIONALS WHO CONDUCT FITNESS TESTING AND PRESCRIPTION

The scope-of-practice descriptions that are provided by ACSM and NSCA for their certifications can be useful for fitness supervisors when establishing guidelines for fitness staff. However, the factors involved in how scope of practice is legally defined are the most important to consider when developing these guidelines.

The following cases demonstrate the importance of the fitness professionals having the necessary knowledge and skills to (a) conduct fitness testing, (b) design safe and effective prescriptions based on the participant's needs, and (c) prescribe exercise within their scope of practice. In *Covenant Health System v. Barnett* (25), the plaintiff was performing a 3 min step test as part of a free heart screening held by Covenant for the community when she fell about 2 min into the test, shattering her left wrist. In her negligence lawsuit, Barnett claimed that Covenant failed to have anyone available to observe or supervise the test and stop the test when she became fatigued. The court ruled that Covenant's failure to observe and attend to the plaintiff while performing the test breached the standard of care as established by *ACSM's Guidelines for Exercise Testing and Prescription*.

In *Proffitt v. Global Fitness Holdings, LLC, et al.* (53, 57) and *Mimms v. Ruthless Training Concepts, LLC* (47), both plaintiffs, after their first workout with a personal trainer, were diagnosed with exertional rhabdomyolysis that resulted in permanent injuries and disabilities. Their workouts included numerous bouts of continuous squatting and leg exercises in short periods of time with little or no rest. Both lawsuits included many ordinary and gross negligence claims against the defendants, including failure to assess the health and fitness status of the client, design an exercise program within the client's fitness capacity, respond to the client's complaints of fatigue, and warn of known risks and dangers. The *Proffitt* case was settled for $75,000 awarded to the plaintiff, and in *Mimms*, the plaintiff was awarded $300,000 in damages. An expert witness in Mimms introduced ACSM's position stand *Progression Models in Resistance Training for Healthy Adults* (5) as part of the evidence to show that the plaintiff did not follow these safety recommendations (a breach of duty) with regard to progression and rest periods between sets. It was evident that the personal trainers in these cases and in the *Makris* case, discussed next, were unable to meet the factors as defined by the professional standard of care.

In *Makris v. Scandinavian Health Spa, Inc.* (46), the plaintiff informed her trainer that she felt a sharp pain in her neck that radiated down her arm while using a leg press machine. The trainer told her the pain was due to upper-body weakness and would subside as she got stronger. The trainer had her continue with the exercises despite complaints of intense pain. Later, an MRI revealed she had three herniated cervical disks. She filed a personal injury lawsuit against the defendants (the trainer, Scandinavian Health Spa, and Bally's Total Fitness Corporation) alleging they rendered negligent training, monitoring, instruction, supervision, and advice. It appears that the trainer did not possess the necessary knowledge and skills for training clients. The trainer was not able to distinguish types of pain (i.e., general pain or discomfort associated with training versus pain associated with a possible medical condition). In addition, it appears that the trainer diagnosed the pain—stating it was due to upper-body weakness—and treated the pain by having her continue to perform the exercise to increase her strength. Fitness professionals need to understand that diagnosing and treating medical conditions is outside their scope of practice and they risk violating state statutes such as practicing medicine without a license. An appellate court in this case indicated that the defendant was negligent, and the court remanded (sent back) the case to the trial court for further proceedings.

STRATEGY 2: USE A MEDICAL LIAISON (OR ADVISORY COMMITTEE) AND RESOURCES REGARDING FITNESS TESTING AND PRESCRIPTION PROGRAMS FOR PEOPLE WHO HAVE RISK FACTORS OR MEDICAL CONDITIONS

Because almost all fitness facilities serve people with risk factors or medical conditions, it is important to have a medical liaison or advisory committee that can help establish protocols for fitness professionals to follow when testing and prescribing programs for these participants, as well as the additional or higher qualifications needed for staff members working with these populations. Recommendations by Warburton et al. (75) should be considered. This can help enhance the safety of these participants. In addition, fitness professionals should use published resources such as *ACSM's Exercise Management for Persons With Chronic Diseases and Disabilities* and *Physical Activity and Health Guidelines: Recommendations for Various Ages, Fitness Levels, and Conditions from 57 Authoritative Sources*, both published by Human Kinetics, as well as refer to the many chapters in this text addressing these topics.

STRATEGY 3: DEVELOP SCOPE-OF-PRACTICE GUIDELINES FOR STAFF MEMBERS WHO PROVIDE NUTRITION ADVICE

Fitness professionals often provide nutrition advice, and it is essential that this advice does not cross over into the licensed practice of dietetics (61). To establish scope-of-practice guidelines in this area, it may be wise to use the following, as stated in an Ohio statute, which describes the types of general nonmedical nutrition information that unlicensed nutrition educators can provide (50):

1. Principles of good nutrition and food preparation
2. Foods to include in the normal daily diet

3. Essential nutrients needed by the body
4. Recommended amounts of the essential nutrients
5. Actions of nutrients on the body
6. Effects of deficiencies or excesses of nutrients
7. Food and supplements that are good sources of essential nutrients

Two cases, *Ohio Board of Dietetics v. Brown* (51) and *Capati v. Crunch Fitness International, Inc.* (15, 16), are good examples of individuals practicing outside their scope of practice with regard to nutritional advice. In the first case, the defendant performed nutritional assessments and recommended nutritional supplements to people for the purpose of treating specific complaints and ailments. The court ruled that the defendant was not licensed to practice dietetics in the state of Ohio and was engaged in the practice of dietetics as defined by the Ohio statute. In *Capati*, a personal trainer recommended his client take a variety of over-the-counter nutritional and dietary supplements, including some that contained ephedra. The client also was taking prescribed medications for hypertension, but the trainer did not advise his client that there could be negative health consequences if she took the supplements while on hypertension medication. While exercising at the club, she became ill, lost consciousness, and later died at the hospital from a stroke. This case was settled out of court, with the defendants (trainer and club) liable for $1,750,000 of the total settlement amount of over $4,000,000.

Given recent safety and liability concerns (42, 49), policies regarding supplements, including energy drinks, should be developed and implemented. For example, it may be wise for fitness facilities to refrain from selling supplements and energy drinks and to include a scope-of-practice guideline restricting fitness staff from discussing these topics with participants. A good policy might be providing a list of credible, helpful resources to share with participants to help educate them about the safety issues associated with supplements and energy drinks.

KEY POINT

A variety of risk management strategies can be developed and implemented to help minimize liability associated with fitness testing and prescription. Perhaps the most important strategies involve establishing written scope-of-practice guidelines describing the qualifications that staff members need in order to carry out fitness testing and prescription activities, especially for participants with risk factors and medical conditions. Practicing outside one's scope of practice can lead to civil claims such as negligence and criminal charges such as practicing medicine or dietetics without a license.

Instruction and Supervision

Instruction and supervision involve a variety of legal liability exposures. According to Betty van der Smissen, the "lack of or inadequate supervision is the most common allegation of negligence" (73, p. 163). She also states that there is an inherent duty to supervise, meaning that fitness professionals have a duty to supervise participants who are engaged in activities that are sponsored by them—in other words, virtually all programs and services offered by fitness facilities. She also describes three types of supervision: specific, general, and transitional. *Specific supervision* occurs when a supervisor is directly supervising an individual or small group in an instructional format, such as a personal fitness trainer or group exercise leader. *General supervision* occurs when a supervisor is responsible for overseeing activities going on in a facility, such as a fitness floor supervisor. Finally, *transitional supervision* occurs when a supervisor changes from general to specific supervision while supervising an area, such as a fitness floor supervisor who provides individual instruction to a participant on how to use a piece of exercise equipment and then transitions back to general supervision of the area.

SELECTED ACSM STANDARDS RELATED TO INSTRUCTION AND SUPERVISION

> Once a new member or prospective user has completed a pre-activity screening process, facility operators shall then offer the new member or prospective user a general orientation to the facility. (65, p. 10)

> Facilities shall provide a means by which members and users who are engaged in a physical activity program within the facility can obtain assistance and/or guidance with their physical activity program. (65, p. 11)

> A facility that offers youth services or programs shall provide evidence that it complies with all applicable state and local laws and regulations pertaining to their supervision. (65, p. 40)

STRATEGY 1: PROVIDE A GENERAL ORIENTATION TO THE FITNESS FACILITY AND EQUIPMENT FOR ALL NEW PARTICIPANTS

Providing new participants with an orientation that focuses on fitness safety is an important risk management strategy. For example, the orientation should include information on how to use the exercise equipment and any facilities such as swimming pools and saunas. For instance, regarding exercise equipment, the staff member leading the orientation should give demonstrations on selected pieces of equipment, pointing out posted warning signs and instructional placards as well as explaining the importance of seeking assistance from staff members on the proper use of equipment. As they go through the orientation, participants also should be informed of posted policies and signage, such as facility safety signs (see figure 26.2) and general safety policies, and the importance of following these and other signage (caution, warning, danger). In addition, they should receive information (e.g., handout, booklet [32], or link to a website) that describes principles of safe exercise. It is important to realize that negligence lawsuits have occurred because participants were not taught basic principles of safe exercise, such as proper cool-downs and the concept of blood pooling (2). Lastly, the orientation should promote the facility's programs and services that might best meet the individual's needs and interests.

An excellent case that demonstrates the importance of providing instruction on the proper and safe use of exercise equipment is *Thomas v. Sport City, Inc.* (66). The plaintiff was injured while using a hack squat machine at the defendant's facility. He thought he had properly engaged the hook to secure the weights, but he had not and the rack of weights (180 lbs [81.6 kg]) fell, fracturing his ankle and crushing his foot. Thomas claimed that Sport City failed to instruct and supervise him on the proper use of the hack squat machine, but the court ruled that he did know how to use the machine. He testified that he was an experienced, sophisticated user of the machine and that if he had properly secured the hook, the carriage would not have fallen. Therefore, the failure of the club to instruct and supervise was not the cause of the plaintiff's injury, but his own carelessness (negligence) was. The club was not found negligent in this case. However, the court made the following statement with regard to a fitness professional's duty to instruct: "Members of health clubs are owed a duty of reasonable care to protect them from injury on the premises," and "this duty includes a general responsibility to ensure that their members know how to use gym equipment" (p. 1157), and the failure to instruct or supervise the plaintiff on proper use of the machine would normally be a breach of duty because the machine could easily cause injury.

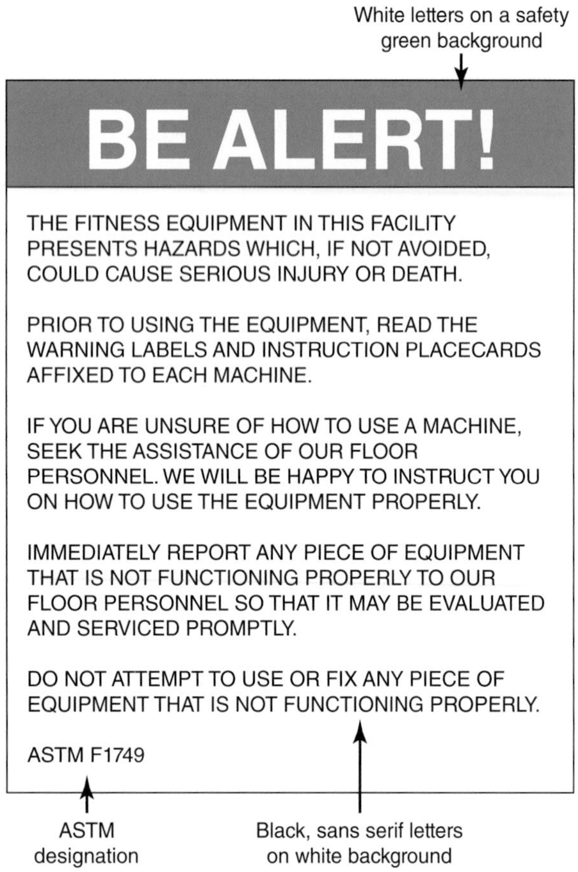

FIGURE 26.2 Facility safety sign to be posted in the equipment room.

Reprinted, with permission, from F1749-09 Standard Specification for Fitness Equipment and Fitness Facility Safety Signage and Labels, copyright ASTM International, 100 Barr Harbor Drive, West Conshohocken, PA 19428.

STRATEGY 2: PROVIDE FITNESS STAFF SUPERVISION DURING ALL OPERATING HOURS

Fitness facilities should have continual staff supervision during all operational hours. A designated manager who has overall responsibility for any situation that might come up, such as a medical emergency, should be on duty at all times. Fitness facilities should have a job description for fitness professionals who serve in this important role as well as train them to handle any number of situations that might arise in a facility. If situations are handled properly and in a timely fashion, there is less potential for liability problems to arise.

STRATEGY 3: CONDUCT JOB PERFORMANCE APPRAISALS OF ALL FITNESS STAFF MEMBERS

In addition to training fitness staff members as discussed earlier, fitness professionals who serve in supervisory roles also should conduct regular job performance appraisals that include direct observation and evaluation of the conduct (actions) of staff members. After a performance appraisal, fitness supervisors should discuss the results of the appraisal with the staff member and design an action plan to address any areas in which the staff member needs improvement, especially those areas that focus on participant safety. More on performance appraisals is available elsewhere (36), as is a sample performance appraisal tool for group exercise leaders. In cases discussed previously (e.g., *Corrigan* and *Rostai*), as well as in the following cases, it is likely that the injuries could have been avoided if the fitness professionals had been trained well and their job performance had been evaluated by a qualified fitness supervisor.

In *Santana v. Women's Workout and Weight Loss Centers, Inc.* (60), the plaintiff was participating in a modified step aerobics class when she fell and fractured her ankle, requiring surgical insertion of pins. She claimed the defendant was negligent because the activity (step aerobics combined with upper-body strengthening exercises using an exercise band) was unreasonably difficult and dangerous. An expert witness testified that the simultaneous activities created a dangerous situation that increased the risks over and above those that were inherent. In other words, the instructor's conduct did not meet the standard of care and was negligent. The defendants claimed that the plaintiff assumed the risks, which should bar her lawsuit against them. The court ruled that "defendants have a duty to use due care not to increase the risks to a participant over and above those inherent in the sport" (p. 26). The *Santana* court also distinguished between sport and exercise when deciding that primary assumption of risk did not protect the defendant from liability. The court stated that sports, by their nature, inherently create extreme risks of injuries due to physical contact between participants and competition aimed at scoring points, racing against time, or accomplishing feats of speed and strength, whereas exercise programs, such as a step aerobics class, are meant to enhance health and fitness and therefore should not create extreme risks of injury. The wavier defense in this case also was ineffective in protecting the defendants from negligence because the exculpatory clause within the waiver was inconspicuous.

In *Stelluti v. Casapenn Enterprises, LLC* (64), the plaintiff suffered serious neck and back injuries in her first stationary cycling class. When she stood, the handlebars on the cycle dislodged and she fell forward while her feet remained strapped to the cycle. The plaintiff claimed that the instructor was negligent because she did not instruct her on safe use of the cycle (i.e., did not inform her to check that the pop pin was fully engaged to make sure the handlebars were secure). An expert witness agreed that the instructor was negligent, stating that "users should be aware of . . . functions and proper operations of the cycle." However, the New Jersey Supreme Court ruled that the waiver protected the defendants from their negligent instruction.

Unfortunately, there are many more negligence cases against fitness instructors like those in *Santana* and *Stelluti* and personal trainers like those in *Corrigan*, *Rostai*, *Proffitt*, *Mimms*, and *Makris* where the failure to provide proper instruction led to the plaintiff's injury. Improper instruction in these cases was most likely due to the instructors and trainers not having adequate formal education and training, as well as the failure of fitness supervisors to observe, evaluate, and correct their job performance. When fitness professionals do not possess the necessary knowledge and skills to deliver safe and effective exercise programs, they subject themselves to negligence claims and lawsuits because their conduct will be judged by factors that make up the professional standard of care that they likely will be unable to meet.

STRATEGY 4: PROVIDE PROPER SUPERVISION OF ALL YOUTH PROGRAMS

All youth programs should be adequately supervised by responsible and well-trained individuals. As mentioned previously, criminal background checks should be performed before hiring employees and volunteers who serve in these roles. Proper supervision also involves preactivity screening procedures as well as having children and their parents or legal guardian sign an *agreement to participate* (24, 36, 43) that not only informs them of the inherent risks associated with the activity or sport but also informs them of the rules and policies they need to follow for safe participation.

KEY POINT

The failure to provide proper instruction and supervision reflects the most common negligence claims made by plaintiffs. To help minimize these types of claims, fitness professionals can (a) provide an orientation for new participants to show them how to use the equipment and facility and inform them of important safety policies, (b) hire qualified and competent fitness staff members and evaluate their job performance (including direct observation and feedback on their teaching behavior) to help ensure they are providing safe and effective programs, and (c) make sure all programs and services are properly supervised at all times.

Equipment and Facility

Fitness professionals have numerous legal duties in this area, but this section focuses on installation and maintenance of exercise equipment, facility access, inspection of premises, and signage. For more information on facilities, fitness professionals should refer to one of the most authoritative and comprehensive resources, *Facility Planning and Design for Health, Physical Activity, Recreation, and Sport* (Sagamore, 2013).

Negligence claims and lawsuits against fitness professionals and facilities are quite common in this area, but sometimes the plaintiff is also negligent (e.g., misuses the equipment, as described in *Thomas v. Sport City, Inc.*), and sometimes the manufacturer may be held strictly liable (i.e., product liability) for a defect in equipment design, manufacturing, or marketing (failure to warn). For example, in the *Thomas* case, the plaintiff claimed that there was a design defect in the hack squat machine, but he was unable to prove that there was a design defect, so the manufacturer was not held liable for his injury.

ACSM (65) has one facility equipment standard related to providing safety equipment in aquatic and pool facilities. It does not include any standards related to exercise equipment, but it does have a few guidelines, including having a preventive maintenance schedule for equipment, a system in place to remove broken or damaged equipment, and a sufficient quantity and quality of equipment. The following standards relate to the fitness facility.

SELECTED ACSM STANDARDS RELATED TO EQUIPMENT AND FACILITY

> Facilities shall have an operational system in place that monitors, either manually or technologically, the presence and identity of all individuals (e.g., members and users) who enter into and participate in the activities, programs, and services of the facility. (65, p. 40)

> Facility operators shall post proper caution, danger, and warning signage in conspicuous locations where facility staff know, or should know, that existing conditions and situations warrant such signage. (65, p. 68)

> All cautionary, danger, and warning signage shall have the required signal icon, signal word, signal color, and layout as specified in ASTM F1749. (65, p. 70)

STRATEGY 1: INSTALL EXERCISE EQUIPMENT PROPERLY

Manufacturers of exercise equipment publish an owner's manual for each piece of equipment. Fitness professionals need to follow the information provided in these manuals, including specifications related to installation, spacing, user safety precautions, warning and caution signage, cleaning, inspections, and maintenance. Other published standards of practice might also apply; for instance, the ASTM standard titled Standard Specification for Motorized Treadmills, F2115, requires 39 in. (99 cm) of space behind treadmills and 19.7 in. (50 cm) on each side of the treadmill.

The importance of treadmill spacing was a key issue in *Xu v. Gay* (76). In this case, Ning Yan died from a severe head injury after falling off a treadmill at a fitness facility. The treadmill only had 2.5 ft (76 cm) clearance behind it. An expert witness for the plaintiff testified that there should be a minimum of 5 ft (152 cm) behind treadmills in order to meet the industry's standard of care for safe distance. He did not indicate which industry standards he was referring to, but he stated they were voluntary. The court stated that the "defendant's ignorance of and failure to implement the standards . . . establish a case of ordinary negligence" (p. 171).

Proper installation also involves bolting certain pieces of equipment to the floor, as demonstrated in *Barnhard v. Cybex International, Inc.* (8, 63). While working with a patient, Barnhard, a physical therapy assistant, stood on the weight-stack side of a Cybex leg extension machine. She placed her hands on top of the machine and pulled on it to stretch her arms and shoulder. While performing the stretch, the machine tipped over, breaking her neck and rendering her a quadriplegic. Barnhard claimed that Cybex was negligent because the machine had design and marketing defects. The court ruled that using the machine for stretching was foreseeable (a common misuse) even though that was not its intended purpose. The court stated that Cybex could have made the machine safer in its design and that it failed to warn of the potential tipping hazard, and thus it was liable for $49.5 million, which was later reduced to $19.5 million in a settlement between Cybex and Barnhard.

STRATEGY 2: MAINTAIN EXERCISE EQUIPMENT PROPERLY

As determined from a 12 yr study of liability claims conducted by the Association Insurance Group, poor maintenance of exercise equipment was one of the most common claims. It is important to maintain exercise equipment based on the specifications provided in the owner's manual. This includes equipment such as exercise balls and resistance tubing. *Alack v. Vic Tanny International of Missouri, Inc.* (4) is an excellent case to demonstrate why this is so important. While the plaintiff was using an upright rowing machine, the handle of the machine disengaged, causing serious and permanent injuries to his mouth and lips. The plaintiff claimed that his injury was due to Vic Tanny's negligence because they did not ensure that the clevis pin was in place. Testimony showed that Vic Tanny did not conduct regular inspections to make sure that the clevis pin was in place, and there was no doubt in the judge's mind that the defendant was negligent. Although the plaintiff had signed a waiver, the court found the waiver to be unenforceable because the exculpatory clause was ambiguous and inconspicuous within the membership agreement. Therefore, Vic Tanny was liable for damages of $17,000 in medical expenses.

STRATEGY 3: HAVE A SYSTEM IN PLACE TO MONITOR FACILITY ACCESS

The main purpose of this strategy is to help ensure that only authorized participants have access to the facility. It also helps to protect participants from anyone entering the facility who might commit crimes such as sexual assault and theft. Many facilities use computerized monitoring systems in which members have an identification card that is scanned upon entry.

KEY POINT

Fitness professionals have many legal duties related to exercise equipment and the fitness facility. These include installing and maintaining exercise equipment according to the manufacturer's specifications in the owner's manual as well as regular inspections of the facility premises (both inside and outside) and all exercise equipment. Given the duty owed to invitees (participants), any dangerous condition found upon inspection must be corrected or a warning must be posted. Fitness professionals also should have a system in place that monitors facility access and includes the posting of signage as required by ASTM.

STRATEGY 4: CONDUCT REGULAR INSPECTIONS OF THE PREMISES

Because participants would be legally classified as invitees, there is a duty to (a) regularly inspect the premises, both inside and outside, including all equipment and facilities, and (b) upon inspection of any reasonable dangerous conditions, warn the invitee of the danger (e.g., post signage) or correct the condition. For example, if inspection of an exercise machine reveals that it is not functioning properly, there is a duty to warn of the danger (e.g., post a sign on the machine), repair the machine, or remove it from use.

The duty to inspect is demonstrated in *Goynias v. Spa Health Clubs, Inc.* (39). The plaintiff in this case was injured from a fall on a wet, slippery floor in the locker area. The court stated: "A property owner is required to exercise reasonable care to provide for the safety of all lawful visitors on his property. . . . [This] includes the duty to exercise ordinary care to keep the premises in a reasonably safe condition and to warn the invitee of hidden perils or unsafe conditions that can be ascertained by reasonable inspection and supervision" (p. 555).

STRATEGY 5: POST SIGNAGE THROUGHOUT THE FACILITY

There are a variety of signage requirements for fitness facilities. To discuss all of these is beyond the scope of this chapter, but two requirements include warning labels that need to be placed on exercise equipment and a facility safety sign that needs to be posted in the exercise equipment area. Requirements for warnings labels and the safety sign are published in ASTM's Standard Specification for Fitness Equipment and Fitness Facility Safety Signage and Labels, F1749. The facility safety sign is shown in figure 26.2. This ASTM publication also provides classifications for danger, warning, and caution to indicate the relative seriousness of a potential hazard.

Emergency Action Plans

All of the risk management strategies presented thus far focus on preventing injuries from occurring in the first place—they are loss-prevention strategies. This section will address loss-reduction strategies—actions that mitigate a medical emergency once it has occurred. Numerous negligence cases have occurred because fitness professionals did not carry out proper emergency procedures. Unfortunately, negligence claims and lawsuits continue to occur in this area, even though published standards of practice requiring facilities to have an EAP have existed for nearly two decades. A variety of factors need to be considered when developing an EAP, as reflected in the following risk management strategies. It is best to designate a professional fitness staff member to serve as the facility's EAP coordinator and to have a medical liaison or adviser who can be directly involved with this effort.

SELECTED ACSM STANDARDS RELATED TO EMERGENCY ACTION PLANS

> Facility operators must have written emergency response policies and procedures, which shall be reviewed regularly and physically rehearsed at least twice annually. These policies shall enable staff to respond to basic first aid situations and emergency events in an appropriate and timely manner. (65, pp. 18)

> In addition to complying with all applicable federal, state, and local requirements relating to automated external defibrillators (AEDs), all facilities (i.e., staffed and unstaffed) shall have as part of their written emergency response policies and procedures a public access defibrillation (PAD) program in accordance with generally accepted practice. (65, p. 21)

> Health/fitness and healthcare professionals engaged in pre-activity screening or prescribing, instructing, monitoring, or supervising of physical activity programs for facility members and users shall have current automated external defibrillation and cardiopulmonary resuscitation (AED and CPR) certification from an organization qualified to provide such certification. A certification should include a practical examination. (65, p. 35)

STRATEGY 1: PREPARE A WRITTEN EMERGENCY ACTION PLAN

Fitness professionals clearly have a legal duty to render aid to a participant who becomes injured while participating in programs and services provided by the fitness facility. Because of this legal duty, every fitness facility should have a written EAP. Some fitness professionals believe that Good Samaritan statutes protect them while on the job, but they do not. These statutes are designed to protect people who voluntarily render aid to someone in need, such as providing first aid to someone while shopping in a store. The written EAP should contain several components, including (a) the job description of the manager on duty who has the overall responsibility for an emergency when it occurs; (b) descriptions of responsibilities of other staff members who are first responders or who should assist in other ways; (c) contingency plans for minor, major, and life-threatening injuries; (d) internal and external (e.g., EMS) communication procedures; and (e) inspection and maintenance procedures for first aid kits and AEDs. Additional components are reflected in the following risk management strategies.

STRATEGY 2: ENSURE THE WRITTEN EMERGENCY ACTION PLAN INCLUDES PROCEDURES FOR HAVING AND USING AN AUTOMATED EXTERNAL DEFIBRILLATOR

In recent years, the failure to have and use an AED has been a common claim in negligence lawsuits filed against fitness facilities when someone has suffered a cardiac arrest while participating in fitness activities. For example, in *DiGiulio v. Gran, Inc.* (29), the plaintiff suddenly fell off a treadmill and collapsed to the floor. An employee began CPR and the assistant manager called 911. The assistant manager knew that the AED was stored in a glass cabinet about 20 yd (18 m) away from the incident but thought the cabinet was locked and did not know where the key was. It turned out that the cabinet was not locked. Paramedics arrived 10 min after the call. They were able to restore DiGiulio's pulse, but he died in the hospital about 6 wk later. A negligence lawsuit claimed the defendant failed to properly train its employees in the use of the AED, properly respond to DiGiulio's cardiac arrest, and notify employees how to access the AED. It also was alleged that the defendant violated a New York statute that requires health clubs to have an AED and an employee trained and certified in its use. The appellate court ruled that although a New York statute requires health clubs to make AEDs available, it does not impose liability on clubs for usage failures.

Fitness professionals need to be aware of AED statutes that have been passed in several states that require fitness facilities to have an AED and to have staff members certified and trained in its use. Provisions within these state statutes vary, and it would be wise to consult with legal counsel on the interpretation of these provisions. It is likely that more states will propose similar legislation.

STRATEGY 3: HAVE QUALIFIED STAFF MEMBERS WHO ARE TRAINED TO CARRY OUT THE EMERGENCY ACTION PLAN

Fitness staff members who have responsibilities to carry out the EAP should maintain current certifications in first aid, CPR, and AED use. It is also a good idea to have a staff member, perhaps the EAP coordinator, be a certified instructor in these areas who can provide recertification classes for staff members. In addition, it is critical that staff members review and rehearse the EAP at least two times a year, as recommended by ACSM (65).

STRATEGY 4: ESTABLISH POSTEMERGENCY PROCEDURES

In addition to completing an incident report form (see figure 26.3) after every medical emergency, the manager on duty should gather and record any evidence, such as photographs of any equipment and conditions involved in the incident and interviews with witnesses who can describe the what, how, why, when, and where of the incident. This evidence may be helpful in defending future negligence lawsuits against staff members and the facility. In addition, after an incident, especially a serious one, a copy of the incident report should be sent to the facility's legal counsel and insurance carrier.

The risk management process in table 26.4 on page 495 depicts seven lines of defense that can help minimize negligence claims and lawsuits for fitness professionals and facilities. The strategies described in this section are reflected in the table along with other legal and risk management principles covered in the chapter (e.g., understanding applicable laws, liability insurance, defenses such as waivers).

KEY POINT

Numerous negligence cases against fitness facilities have occurred for failing to have or properly carry out an EAP. A variety of factors need to be considered when preparing a well-thought-out and effective EAP. To assist with this important risk management strategy, it is recommended that each facility designate a professional staff member as the EAP coordinator and have a medical liaison or adviser who can be directly involved with this effort. Once the EAP is written, staff members should attend in-service trainings that include drills at least two times a year to help ensure the plan will be properly carried out in the event of an emergency.

Record Keeping and Documentation of Evidence

Reference to various documents (e.g., waivers, informed consents) was made throughout this chapter. It is important to store these documents in a secure place because they

HEALTH, FITNESS & RACQUET SPORTS CLUB INCIDENT REPORT
[COMPLETE FOR ALL INCIDENTS AND REPORT IMMEDIATELY – PLEASE PRINT]

Date

Month Day Year	Time of Accident A.M. P.M.	Club Member ☐ Yes ☐ No	Club Name Club Location

Injured Person

FIRST (M.I.) LAST AGE

NUMBER AND STREET

CITY STATE ZIP

BUSINESS PHONE HOME PHONE

HOSPITAL OR FIRST AID SQUAD NOTIFIED
☐ Yes ☐ No

NAME: ____________________

TIME OF INITIAL CALL: ____________________

TIMES OF FOLLOW-UP CALLS: 1. __________
2.__________ 3.__________ 4.__________

TIME OF ARRIVAL: ____________________

TIME OF DEPARTURE: ____________________

TAKEN TO HOSPITAL? ____________________

NAME OF FIRST AID ATTENDANT: ____________________

DESCRIPTION OF ACCIDENT:

CHECK ITEMS THAT APPLY TO INJURED PERSON:

BLEEDING INJURY: ☐ **YES** ☐ **NO** **OTHER VISIBLE INJURY:** ☐ **YES** ☐ **NO**

NO VISIBLE INJURY, BUT COMPLAINT OF PAIN: ☐ **YES** ☐ **NO**

IF EYE INJURY, WEARING EYEGUARDS? ☐ **YES** ☐ **NO**

DESCRIBE EXACT INJURY SUSTAINED:

____
____
____

DESCRIBE FIRST AID ADMINSTERED BY CLUB:

____
____
____

First Witness	**Second Witness**
FIRST (M.I.) LAST	FIRST (M.I.) LAST
NUMBER AND STREET	NUMBER AND STREET
CITY STATE ZIP	CITY STATE ZIP
BUSINESS PHONE HOME PHONE	BUSINESS PHONE HOME PHONE
DESCRIPTION OF ACCIDENT BY WITNESS:	DESCRIPTION OF ACCIDENT BY WITNESS:
SIGNATURE:	SIGNATURE:

FIGURE 26.3 Incident report from Creative Agency Group. *(continued)*

Reprinted, by permission, from Creative Agency Group.

HEALTH, FITNESS & RACQUET SPORTS CLUB INCIDENT REPORT
[continued]

NAME OF CLUB PERSONNEL WHO INSPECTED THE SCENE: | POSITION | DATE OF INSPECTION:

CONDITIONS FOUND: ____________________

ACTION TAKEN, IF PRACTICAL, TO AVOID RECURRENCE: ____________________

Description of Place of Accident

☐ INTERIOR ☐ EXTERIOR ☐ WALKING AREA ☐ PLAYING SURFACE ☐ LOCKER ROOM

☐ PHY. FITNESS ROOM ☐ OTHER: ____________

CONDITIONS: ☐ DRY ☐ WET ☐ SMOOTH ☐ EVEN SURFACE ☐ SLIPPERY

FOREIGN SUBSTANCE? ☐ YES ☐ NO IF 'YES', DESCRIPTION: ____________________

IF INJURY TOOK PLACE OUTSIDE CLUB BUILDING, CHECK APPROPRIATE ITEMS:

WEATHER CONDITION: ☐ DRY ☐ RAIN ☐ SNOW ☐ ICE ☐ DAY ☐ NIGHT LIGHTING CONDITIONS: ____________

IMPORTANT: IF INJURY TOOK PLACE ON A COURT, PROVIDE NAME, ADDRESS AND TELEPHONE NUMBER OF THOSE INDIVIDUALS WHO USED OR RENTED THE COURT DURING THE PRIOR HOUR.

ADDITIONAL COMMENTS

DID POLICE INVESTIGATE? ☐ YES ☐ NO | NAME AND RANK OF OFFICER | DEPARTMENT | PHONE NUMBER

SUBMITTED BY: | SIGNATURE: | TELEPHONE: | DATE / TIME

This information is for reporting purposes only. The information provided is the responsibility of the insured and/or club.

CREATIVE AGENCY GROUP

15 CREATIVE CIRCLE, ROUTE 520, HOLMDEL, NEW JERSEY 07733
800-888-8381 732-946-4000 732-946-2044 FAX

FIGURE 26.3 *(continued)*

Table 26.4 Risk Management Lines of Defense

Line of defense	Strategies and principles
1	Provide a professional environment. Risk managers and liability insurance company executives and underwriters have known for many years that a genuinely friendly, caring, and professional environment will minimize not only the occurrence of incidents, which can lead to claims and suits, but the actual assertion of claims and suits as well!
2	Health/fitness facilities must adhere to the law and should comply with published standards of practice. These standards are the established benchmarks of expected behavior for the profession and will be used to evaluate and judge the care that is provided in the event an incident may occur, which results in claim and suit.
3	Education, training, and certification and/or "national board" testing should serve as the basic starting point for all facility personnel. Only qualified and competent personnel—be they employees or independent contractors—should be permitted to deliver service.
4	Based upon the law and published standards of practice, all health/fitness facilities should adopt written policies and procedures dealing with preactivity health screening, health/fitness assessment and prescription, and instruction and supervision provided to participants as well as a variety of issues related to exercise equipment and the fitness facility.
5	Written and practiced EAPs can help mitigate a medical emergency and minimize any subsequent liability that may occur. Follow-up procedures such as completing an incident report also are important.
6	Protective legal documents (e.g., a waiver, an express assumption of risk) should be read and signed by participants upon joining a facility. These documents can help protect the facility from liability if an injury and subsequent litigation occurs.
7	Both general and professional liability insurance should be considered to protect the financial assets of the facility.

can provide valuable evidence in the event of a claim or lawsuit. For example, if the fitness facility has retained a copy of the waiver signed by a member, it will provide evidence that can help protect the facility if that member ever files a negligence lawsuit against the facility. Other record keeping can help provide evidence that a fitness facility and its staff members properly carried out their legal duties. For example, if a facility keeps records documenting maintenance of exercise equipment, it will be difficult for a plaintiff to prove that the facility failed to carry out this duty. If a plaintiff cannot prove that a defendant breached her duty, it will be difficult for the plaintiff to prevail in a negligence lawsuit. It also is important to have duplicate copies of records (written or electronic) stored at another location in case the original is lost or destroyed. Fitness professionals should seek legal counsel with regard to how long records need to be kept.

Record-Keeping Tips

Keeping records can provide evidence that legal duties were properly carried out. Examples include the following:

- Credentials of staff members (e.g., degrees, current certifications)
- Criminal background checks of personnel
- Staff training meetings (e.g., dates, staff members attending, content covered)
- Preactivity screening forms (e.g., screening device, medical clearance)
- Waivers and informed consents
- Medical release forms
- Written scope-of-practice guidelines for staff members
- Facility orientations for participants (e.g., dates, participants attending, content covered)
- Job performance evaluations of staff members
- Facility and equipment inspections
- Facility and equipment maintenance records
- Written EAP
- Completed incident report forms and related evidence
- Written exposure control plan (OSHA's Bloodborne Pathogens Standard)

LEARNING AIDS

REVIEW QUESTIONS

1. Describe the types of injuries that can occur while participating in physical activity.
2. Describe the three primary sources of law and give an example of each.
3. Define the following legal terms: *stare decisis*, *respondeat superior*, *compensatory damages*, *punitive damages*, and *exculpatory clause*.
4. Define the following risk management terms: *loss-prevention strategies*, *loss-reduction strategies*, *contractual transfer of risks*, *general liability insurance*, and *professional liability insurance*.
5. Describe the type of conduct that would be considered ordinary negligence and gross negligence.
6. Explain why the primary assumption of risk was not an effective defense in the *Corrigan* and *Santana* cases. Also, describe how the courts in these cases distinguished between sport and physical activity with regard to this defense.
7. Describe why fitness professionals should have a competent lawyer review and edit a waiver before having participants signing it.
8. Describe how the professional standard of care can be determined in negligence cases and its application to high-intensity exercise.
9. Explain how a fitness professional could be qualified but not competent. Then describe why it is essential from a legal perspective that fitness professionals be competent.
10. List the names of the negligence cases described in this chapter where the defendant (fitness professional) was likely practicing outside the scope of practice.

CASE STUDIES

Upon joining World's Best Gym (WBG) located in Virginia, Mr. Smith requested an orientation on how to use the gym's exercise equipment. Mr. Smith, a 30-yr-old commercial airline pilot, knew that regular exercise would help him maintain and improve health-related factors that are evaluated annually during his medical flight exam. After he signed a membership contract and a separate document titled Waiver and Release of Liability, he was told that instead of an orientation he should sign up for personal fitness training sessions, which he did. His personal fitness trainer, Bill—an employee of WBG—did not conduct any preactivity screening procedures, nor did he conduct any assessments to determine Mr. Smith's fitness levels. However, Mr. Smith did inform Bill that he had not worked out in years.

Bill did not have any formal education or supervised practical experiences (e.g., an internship) in exercise science prior to becoming a personal fitness trainer at WBG. He possessed a personal trainer certification that was accredited by a nationally recognized accrediting agency, which was the only credential necessary to become a trainer at WBG. Bill's only experience in the field was that he had been a former collegiate football player and thus was familiar with the strength and conditioning program he participated in for many years.

During the first training session, Bill had Mr. Smith perform numerous bouts of strenuous exercises—repeated sets and fast repetitions of squats and other exercises using the quadriceps with little or no rest between sets. As the session continued, Mr. Smith became very fatigued, showing obvious signs and symptoms of overexertion. He requested several breaks during the workout. However, Bill told Mr. Smith that he did not need a break and that he could handle the high-intensity workout because he was young. He said to Mr. Smith, "No pain, no gain," and pushed Mr. Smith to continue performing the strenuous exercises.

After the workout, Mr. Smith went home exhausted, experiencing extreme fatigue. That night and the next day, Mr. Smith was in severe pain and noticed his urine was dark brown. He went to the emergency room and was immediately hospitalized with a diagnosis of severe exertional rhabdomyolysis and a creatine kinase (CK) level that was extremely high. The medical specialists (a nephrologist and a rheumatologist) had never seen such a severe case of exertional rhabdomyolysis in someone like Mr. Smith who had no other underlying medical conditions.

Mr. Smith ended up in the hospital for 8 days, receiving various treatments including kidney dialysis. Although he had several weeks of physical therapy, his injury resulted in a 35% loss of muscle tissue in both quadriceps and permanent disability. It is unlikely that he will be able to ever obtain his medical certificate (clearance) again, which is necessary for him to retain his pilot's license.

Mr. Smith's lawyer has filed a negligence lawsuit against the personal fitness trainer and WBG seeking damages of $1 million to cover medical expenses, future medical expenses, pain and suffering, lost wages, and future lost wages. Note that WBG has a CGL policy but does not have professional liability coverage for any of its employees. Bill also had not purchased any professional liability insurance on his own. The CGL contains an exclusion clause stating it "does not cover any bodily injury that occurred from providing instruction or advice relating to physical fitness or training programs."

1. What negligence claims will Mr. Smith and his lawyer likely file against WBG and the personal fitness trainer?
2. How will the court determine the duties owed to Mr. Smith, the plaintiff in this case?
3. Describe how Bill's conduct would be considered outside his scope of practice.
4. WBG will likely use the waiver and primary assumption of risk as defenses. Will these defenses be effective in protecting WBG? Why or why not?
5. What risk management strategies should WBC have implemented that might have prevented Mr. Smith's injury?
6. Why is it likely that the personal trainer and WBG will be found liable and will have to pay the damages?

Answers to Case Studies

1. WBG failed to do the following:
   - Hire qualified and competent personal fitness trainers.
   - Provide adequate training for their personal fitness trainers.
   - Perform adequate supervision of their personal fitness trainers.

   The personal fitness trainer failed to do the following:
   - Conduct a preactivity screening.
   - Assess fitness levels to evaluate the client's capacity prior to exercise.
   - Design an exercise program within the client's safe capacity.
   - Properly instruct and supervise the client.
   - Recognize signs and symptoms of overexertion.
   - Grant the client's repeated requests for a break throughout the session.
2. The court can determine duty in several ways in this case. For example, the court will likely classify the relationship that was formed between WBG and Mr. Smith as an inherent relationship. In this type of relationship, defendants have a legal duty to provide reasonably safe programs and services, which requires taking steps to prevent foreseeable injury risks. It is likely that an expert witness will testify in this case against the defendants—the personal trainer and WBG. Expert witnesses educate the court as to the standard of care (or duty) that the defendants owed to the plaintiff given the situation. They consider the factors that make up the professional standard of care (nature of the activity, type of participants, and environmental conditions) as well as standards of practice published by professional

organizations when judging the conduct of the defendants. An expert witness in this case will be able to show that Bill (the trainer) did not meet the requirements for (a) nature of the activity (e.g., he did not have the knowledge and skills to design a safe exercise program for Mr. Smith when he did not perform preactivity screening or apply progression, a basic principle of safe exercise) and (b) type of participant (e.g., Bill did not consider the type of client that Mr. Smith was—a novice who was sedentary—when designing and delivering his first exercise session). In addition, an expert witness will be able to show that Bill and WBG breached their duty when they failed to follow standards and guidelines published by professional organizations that, for example, require or recommend preactivity screening.

3. Practicing outside one's scope of practice can occur two ways. If a fitness professional's conduct crosses over the line into a licensed profession, she can face criminal charges for violation of a state statute for practicing medicine or some other licensed profession (e.g., dietetics, physical therapy). No harm is needed to prove the violation; only the conduct.

   If a fitness professional's conduct does not meet the professional standard of care (i.e., does not meet the three situational factors as described in the answer to question 2) or adhere to practices described in standards of practice published by professional organizations, and the conduct caused harm to a participant, the fitness professional can be found liable for negligence.

   The second one is applicable in this case—the personal trainer's conduct was negligent (his breach of several duties, more likely than not, caused the injuries to Mr. Smith) because he did not meet the requirements necessary as defined by the professional standard of care.

4. Neither the waiver nor primary assumption of risk will be effective in protecting the defendants in this case. Though Mr. Smith signed a waiver and release of liability, waivers are against public policy in Virginia for personal injury and, therefore, are unenforceable. It is unlikely that the primary assumption of risk will protect the defendants because this defense is effective for inherent injuries only, not injuries due to negligence. Also, primary assumption of risk requires that the plaintiff knows, understands, and appreciates the inherent risks and voluntarily assumes them. Because Mr. Smith was a novice, it is unlikely that he knew, understood, and appreciated the inherent risks of any exercise program, let alone the increased risks associated with high-intensity exercise.

5. There are several risk management strategies that WBG could have implemented to prevent the injuries and subsequent litigation that occurred in this case. WBG should not assume that a personal trainer who has an accredited certification is both qualified and competent, nor should they assume a former collegiate athlete is qualified and competent to be a personal trainer. WBG should require formal education and training for their trainers—either provided internally or externally by highly qualified and experienced instructors. WBG should have evaluated Bill's knowledge and skills prior to hiring him to help ensure he could meet the requirements that make up the professional standard of care and practices set forth in published standards of practice. Shortly after hiring Bill, WBG should have conducted a performance appraisal to evaluate his on-the-job performance. Bill's improper instruction could have been addressed in this appraisal along with inappropriate statements like "No pain, no gain," which perpetuate a myth of exercise. In addition, WGB should have professional liability insurance to cover their trainers or require that their trainers purchase this coverage on their own.

6. Yes, it is likely both defendants—the personal trainer and WBG (through the legal doctrine *respondeat superior*)—will be liable for negligence (they breached several duties, which likely caused the injuries to the plaintiff). Neither had purchased professional liability insurance coverage to pay out the damages for professional negligence, and the CGL policy contained an exclusion clause stating it "does not cover any bodily injury that occurred from providing instruction or advice relating to physical fitness or training programs." Therefore, both defendants will have to pay out the monetary damages to the plaintiff as awarded by the court (judge) or jury.

APPENDIX A
CALCULATION OF OXYGEN UPTAKE AND CARBON DIOXIDE PRODUCTION

Calculation of Oxygen Consumption ($\dot{V}O_2$)

The air we breathe is composed of 20.93% oxygen (O_2), 0.03% carbon dioxide (CO_2), and the balance, 79.04%, nitrogen (N_2). When we exhale, the fraction of the air represented by O_2 is decreased and the fraction represented by CO_2 is increased. To calculate the volume of O_2 used by the body (VO_2), we simply subtract the number of liters of O_2 exhaled from the number of liters of O_2 inhaled. Equation 1 summarizes these words.

1. Oxygen consumption
= (volume of O_2 inhaled) – (volume of O_2 exhaled).

Now, using VO_2 to mean volume of oxygen used, V_I to mean volume of air inhaled, V_E to mean volume of air exhaled, F_{IO2} to mean fraction of oxygen in inhaled air, and F_{EO2} to mean fraction of oxygen in exhaled air, equation 2 can be written.

2. $VO_2 = (V_I \cdot F_{IO2}) - (V_E \cdot F_{EO2})$.

You know that $F_{IO2} = 0.2093$, and F_{EO2} will be determined on an oxygen analyzer. Consequently, you are left with only two unknowns: the volume of air (liters) inhaled (V_I) and the volume of air (liters) exhaled (V_E). It appears that you must measure both volumes, but fortunately, this is not necessary. It was determined years ago that N_2 is neither used nor produced by the body. Consequently, the number of liters of N_2 inhaled must equal the number of liters of N_2 exhaled. Equation 3 states this equality using the symbols mentioned earlier.

3. $V_I \cdot F_{IN2} = V_E \cdot F_{EN2}$.

This is an important relationship because it permits you to calculate V_E when V_I is known or vice versa. Using equation 3, here are two formulas, one giving V_E when V_I is known and one giving V_I when V_E is known.

$$V_I = \frac{V_E \cdot F_{EN_2}}{F_{IN_2}}, \quad V_E = \frac{V_I \cdot F_{IN_2}}{F_{EN_2}}$$

Now that you know how to do this, you need only one other piece of the puzzle to calculate VO_2. The value for F_{IN2} is constant (0.7904), so we must determine F_{EN2}. When the expired gas sample is analyzed, you will obtain a value for F_{EO2} and F_{ECO2} but not F_{EN2}. However, because all the gas fractions must add up to 1.0000, you can calculate F_{EN2} in the same way we calculated F_{IN2}:

$$1.0000 - 0.0003\ (CO_2) - 0.2093\ (O_2) = 0.7904.$$

QUESTION:

Calculate F_{EN2} when

$$F_{EO2} = 0.1600 \text{ and } F_{ECO2} = 0.0450.$$

ANSWER:

$$F_{EN2} = 1.0000 - 0.1600 - 0.0450 = 0.7950.$$

The following problem shows how these equations are used. Given that V_I equals 100 L, $F_{EO2} = 0.1600$, and $F_{ECO2} = 0.0450$, calculate V_E.

$$V_E \cdot F_{EN_2} = V_I \cdot F_{IN_2}, \text{ so } V_E = \frac{V_I \cdot F_{IN_2}}{F_{EN_2}}$$

$$F_{IN_2} = 0.7904 \text{ and}$$

$$F_{EN_2} = 1.0000 - 0.1600 - 0.0450 = 0.7950$$

$$V_E = 100\ L \cdot \frac{0.7904}{0.7950} = 99.4\ L$$

At this point, the equation for VO_2 can be rewritten using V_I, V_E, F_{IO2}, and F_{EO2}.

$$VO_2 = V_I \cdot F_{IO_2} - V_E \cdot F_{EO_2}$$

Assuming that you measure only V_I, this formula is rewritten:

$$VO_2 = V_I \cdot F_{IO_2} - \frac{V_I \cdot F_{IN_2}}{F_{EN_2}} \cdot F_{EO_2}$$

V_I can be factored out of this equation, so

$$VO_2 = V_I \left[F_{IO_2} - \frac{F_{IN_2}}{F_{EN_2}} \cdot F_{EO_2} \right]$$

We will repeat the last two steps assuming that V_E is the volume that is measured and then factor out V_E.

$$VO_2 = \frac{V_E \cdot F_{EN_2}}{F_{IN_2}} \cdot F_{IO_2} - V_E \cdot F_{EO_2}$$

$$= V_E \left[\frac{F_{EN_2}}{F_{IN_2}} \cdot F_{IO_2} - F_{EO_2} \right]$$

At this point you know how to calculate VO_2. If you ever get stuck, always go back to this formula: $VO_2 = V_I \cdot F_{IO2} - V_E \cdot F_{EO2}$. Simply substitute for V_E or V_I depending on what was measured.

Some comments:

1. You must always match the volume measurement with the F_{EO2} and F_{ECO2} values measured in that expired volume. If you measure V_I for 2 min, you must have a single 2 min bag of expired gas to get F_{EO2} and F_{ECO2} values. If you measure a 30 sec volume, your expired bag must be collected over those 30 sec.
2. VO_2 and VCO_2 are usually expressed in liters per minute: the rate at which O_2 is used or CO_2 is produced per minute. To signify this rate, we write VO_2 (read *vee dot*). You would convert 30 sec or 2 min volumes to 1 min values before calculating $\dot{V}O_2$.

Sample problem:

$\dot{V}_I = 100\ L \cdot min^{-1}$, $F_{EO2} = .1600$, and $F_{ECO2} = .0450$.

Calculate $\dot{V}O_2$.

$$\dot{V}O_2 = V_I \cdot F_{IO_2} - \dot{V}_E \cdot F_{EO_2}, \text{ and}$$

$$\dot{V}_E = \frac{\dot{V}_I \cdot F_{IN_2}}{F_{EN_2}}$$

$$\dot{V}O_2 = \dot{V}_I \cdot F_{IO_2} - \frac{\dot{V}_I \cdot F_{IN_2}}{F_{EN_2}} \cdot F_{EO_2}$$

$$= \dot{V}_I \left[F_{IO_2} - \frac{F_{IN_2}}{F_{EN_2}} \cdot F_{EO_2} \right]$$

$$F_{EN_2} = 1{,}0000 - 0.1600 - 0.0450 = 0.7950$$

$$\dot{V}O_2 = 100\ L \cdot min^{-1} \left[0.2093 - \frac{0.7904}{0.7950} \cdot 0.1600 \right]$$

$$= 5.02\ L \cdot min^{-1}$$

The volume (let's assume that $\dot{V}_E$ was measured) used in the previous equations was measured at room temperature (23 °C) and at the barometric pressure of that moment (740 mmHg). The environmental conditions under which the volume was measured are called *ambient conditions*. If this volume of gas were transported to 10,000 ft (3,050 m) above sea level, where the barometric pressure is lower, the volume would increase because of the reduced pressure. The volume of a gas varies inversely with pressure (at a constant temperature). Another factor influencing the volume of a gas is the temperature. If that volume, measured at 23 °C, were placed in a refrigerator at 0 °C, the volume of gas would decrease. The volume of gas varies directly with the temperature (at constant pressure).

Because the volume ($\dot{V}_E$) is influenced by both pressure and temperature, the value measured as O_2 used ($\dot{V}O_2$) might reflect changes in pressure or temperature rather than a change in workload, training, and so on.

Consequently, it would be convenient to express $\dot{V}_E$ in such a way as to make measurements comparable when they are obtained under different environmental conditions. This is done by standardizing the temperature, barometric pressure, and water vapor pressure at which the volume is expressed. By convention, volumes are expressed at standard temperature and pressure, dry (STPD): 273 K (0 °C), 760 mmHg pressure (sea level), and with no water vapor pressure. When $\dot{V}O_2$ is expressed at STPD, you can calculate the number of molecules of oxygen actually used by the body because at STPD, 1 mole of oxygen equals 22.4 L.

Let's make the correction to STPD one step at a time. Let's assume that a volume ($\dot{V}_E$) was measured at 740 mmHg and 23 °C and equaled 100 L · min⁻¹. This expired volume is always saturated with water vapor.

To correct for temperature, use 273 °K as the standard (0 °C).

$$\text{Volume} \cdot \frac{273\ °K}{273\ °K + °C} = \frac{273\ °K}{273 + 23}$$

$$100\ L \cdot min^{-1} \cdot \frac{273\ °K}{296\ °K} = 92.23\ L \cdot min^{-1}$$

When we correct for pressure, we must remove the effect of water vapor pressure because the gas volume is adjusted on the basis of the standard pressure (760 mmHg), which is a dry pressure.

To correct the volume to the standard 760 mmHg pressure (dry), use this:

$$\text{Volume} \cdot \frac{\text{barometric pressure} - \text{water vapor pressure}}{760\ \text{mmHg (dry)}}$$

Water vapor pressure is dependent on two things: the temperature and the relative humidity. In expired gas, the gas volume is saturated (100% relative humidity). Consequently, you can obtain a value for water vapor pressure directly from the following table.

Temperature (°C)	Saturation water vapor pressure (mmHg)
18	15.5
19	16.5
20	17.5
21	18.7
22	19.8
23	21.1
24	22.4
25	23.8
26	25.2
27	26.7

Going back to our pressure correction:

$$92.23\ L \cdot min^{-1} \cdot \frac{740 - 21.1}{760} = 87.24\ L \cdot min^{-1} (\text{STPD})$$

To combine the temperature and pressure correction:

$$100\ \text{L} \cdot \text{min}^{-1} \cdot \frac{273\ °\text{K}}{273\ °\text{K} + 23} \cdot \frac{740 - 21.1}{760} = 87.24\ \text{L} \cdot \text{min}^{-1}(\text{STPD})$$

A special note must be made here: If you are using an inspired (inhaled) volume ($\dot{V}_I$), you are rarely dealing with a gas saturated with water vapor. Consequently, when you correct for pressure you must find how much water vapor is in the inspired air. You do this by finding the relative humidity of the air. You then multiply this value by the water vapor pressure value for saturated air at whatever the temperature is. To clarify, if your volume in the previous example was $\dot{V}_I$ and had a relative humidity of 50%, the pressure correction would have been as follows:

$$\text{volume} \cdot \frac{740 - (.50 \cdot 21.1\ \text{mmHg})}{760\ \text{mmHg}}$$

This may seem like a minor point, but it is critical to the accurate measurement of $\dot{V}O_2$ that the proper water vapor correction be used. When calculating $\dot{V}O_2$, you usually find the STPD factor first because you will be multiplying this factor by each volume measured.

QUESTION:

Given $\dot{V}_I = 100\ \text{L} \cdot \text{min}^{-1}$, $F_{EO2} = 0.1700$, and $F_{ECO2} = 0.0385$. Temperature = 20 °C, barometric pressure = 740 mmHg, and relative humidity = 30%.

ANSWER:

$$\text{STPD factor} = \frac{740\ \text{mmHg} - (.30)\ 17.5\ \text{mmHg}}{760} \cdot \frac{273\ °\text{K}}{273\ °\text{K} + 20\ °\text{C}} = .900$$

$$100\ \text{L} \cdot \text{min}^{-1} \cdot 0.900 = 90\ \text{L} \cdot \text{min}^{-1}\ \text{STPD}$$

$$\dot{V}O_2 = \dot{V}_{I_{STPD}} \left[F_{IO_2} - \frac{F_{IN_2}}{F_{EN_2}} \cdot F_{EO_2} \right]$$

$$\dot{V}O_2 = 90\ \text{L} \cdot \text{min}^{-1} \left[0.2093 - \frac{0.7904}{0.7915} \cdot 0.1700 \right]$$

$$\dot{V}O_2 = 3.56\ \text{L} \cdot \text{min}^{-1}$$

Carbon Dioxide Production ($\dot{V}CO_2$)

When O_2 is used, CO_2 is produced. The ratio of CO_2 production ($\dot{V}CO_2$) to O_2 consumption ($\dot{V}O_2$) is an important measurement in metabolism. This ratio ($\dot{V}CO_2 \div \dot{V}O_2$) is called the *respiratory exchange ratio* and is abbreviated as *R*.

How do we measure $\dot{V}CO_2$? We start at the same step as for $\dot{V}O_2$:

$$\dot{V}CO_2 = \text{liters of } CO_2 \text{ expired} - \text{liters of } CO_2 \text{ inspired}$$
$$= \dot{V}_E \cdot F_{ECO_2} - \dot{V}_I \cdot F_{ICO_2}$$

The steps to follow are the same as those for measuring $\dot{V}O_2$. Always use an STPD volume in your calculations. The following is the equation to use when $\dot{V}_I$ is measured:

$$\dot{V}CO_2 = \dot{V}_{I_{STPD}} \left[\frac{F_{IN_2}}{F_{EN_2}} \cdot F_{ECO_2} - \dot{V}_I \cdot F_{ICO_2} \right]$$

The following steps summarize the calculations for $\dot{V}CO_2$ and *R* for the previous problem.

$$\dot{V}CO_2 = 90\ \text{L} \cdot \text{min}^{-1} \left[\frac{0.7904}{0.7915} \cdot 0.0385 - 0.0003 \right]$$
$$= 3.43\ \text{L} \cdot \text{min}^{-1}$$
$$R = \dot{V}CO_2 \div \dot{V}O_2 = 3.43\ \text{L} \cdot \text{min}^{-1} \div 3.56\ \text{L} \cdot \text{min}^{-1}$$
$$R = 0.96$$

APPENDIX B
FITNESS ASSESSMENT

This appendix provides a foundation for the areas of fitness assessment covered in part III, allowing you to better explain what fitness test scores mean. In part III, we examined the assessment of cardiorespiratory fitness (CRF), body composition, muscular strength and endurance, and flexibility and low-back function.

The first step in fitness testing is choosing your fitness tests wisely. You must consider the following factors in your selection:

- Reliability: Can I get consistent results with this test?
- Objectivity: Do different test administrators get the same results on this test?
- Validity: Does the test measure the characteristic I'm interested in evaluating?

Although a test can be reliable and objective and still not be valid, tests that are unreliable or lack objectivity cannot be valid. Once the consistency of the test is ensured, there are ways to determine whether the test measures what it is supposed to measure. For example, do experts agree that the test is valid? Does the test compare favorably with an established test (a standard) in the same area?

The fitness tests recommended in this book have been shown to be reliable and objective when carefully administered by trained professionals. There also is evidence that the tests in this book are valid (experts recommend them or the tests compare favorably with valid tests).

Fitness professionals can do several things to maximize accuracy (i.e., minimize error) in testing:

- Properly prepare the person being tested.
- Organize the testing session.
- Attend to details.

Fitness testing has many uses in a fitness setting, from prescribing exercise to refining programs. Fitness professionals must know how to interpret test scores and provide feedback to all program participants.

You can help participants evaluate their fitness test scores by doing the following (2):

- Emphasize health status rather than comparison with others.
- For those needing improvement, emphasize change rather than current status.
- Provide specific recommendations based on the test data and your understanding of the participant.

One common approach to evaluating test scores is to compare the fitness participant with people of the same sex and similar age (i.e., use percentiles). Much of the way the individual compares with others is based on heredity and early experience. There are limits to how much people can change even with great effort. It is unfortunate that many people in fitness programs try to use the performance model of being number one. The emphasis should not be on who can run the fastest or who has the lowest cholesterol but on helping all people understand, achieve, and maintain CRF, healthy body composition, and low-back function.

The current edition of *ACSM's Guidelines for Exercise Testing and Prescription* (1) uses percentiles for evaluation of fitness tests. Much more research is needed before health criteria can be finalized; however, we think that attempting to set health criteria is better, even with its limitations, than relying on percentiles. For example, a person could weigh significantly more now than in 1980 and be at the same percentile because the whole population gained weight. In addition, a person could gain fat and lose muscle with age and stay at the same percentile.

There is general agreement that fitness standards should be based on what is needed for good health. These are called *criterion-referenced standards*, with the fitness score being what is needed for a low risk of health problems (2). Although performance decreases with age, the minimal fitness standards should be the same for adults of all ages. This is similar to a serum cholesterol value $\geq$200 mg $\cdot$ dl^{-1} or SBP $\geq$140 mmHg being the same cutoff values used for risk-factor assessment in adults, independent of age. More research is needed so that we can refine these fitness standards; as we find out more about the relationship between test scores and positive health, some of these standards may need to be modified.

The most important question for a fitness participant is not what her health status is at this moment in life, but what it will be 6 mo, 2 yr, or 20 yr from now. In this way, the person is encouraged to deal with her current status (compared with health standards) so that she can set reasonable, desirable, and achievable goals for the next testing time.

Test results can also help people work toward and eventually achieve specific goals. It may be that the fitness standards are not appropriate or reasonable for an individual.

For example, the standards for running the mile cannot be used for people who swim for their fitness workouts or for people who use wheelchairs. However, individual goals for covering a certain distance in the water or in a wheelchair can be established. Or, the fitness professional may want to set intermediary goals for a person who is very unfit. For example, a person who can only walk a quarter of a mile without stopping would be discouraged by discussing the standards for running 1 mi (1.6 km). The initial goal for that person may be to work up to being able to walk 1 mi without stopping. As indicated in chapter 23, it is important to set goals to help people begin and continue healthy behaviors.

Fitness and lifestyle behaviors (e.g., getting adequate exercise, nutrition, and rest; avoiding substance abuse; coping with stress) and fitness test scores are interrelated. The fitness professional should emphasize fitness behaviors. It is more important for people to begin and continue regular physical activity than to reach a certain level on an exercise test. Likewise, it is more important for people to develop healthy eating habits than to have a certain percentage of body fat. By emphasizing healthy behaviors, fitness professionals can recognize people for their effort, and in the long run, living a consistent, healthy lifestyle is the best way for a client to improve fitness test scores and overall health.

Overemphasizing test scores can discourage some participants. A good example of a program that recognizes the behaviors of regular physical activity and healthy eating is the Presidential Active Lifestyle Award (PALA+) by the President's Council on Fitness, Sports and Nutrition (3). The program recognizes people who do physical activity for a certain number of hours per week and who meet healthy eating goals (e.g., make half your plate fruits and vegetables), thus rewarding behavior rather than a test result.

Many people have one or more disabilities resulting in mild to severe limitations regarding physical activity. It is beyond the scope of this book to recommend specific activities and tests to deal with each possible condition; however, there is clear evidence that regular physical activity provides important health benefits for people with disabilities. The fitness professional can apply the following principles to enhance participation in physical activity for people with disabilities (4):

- Access—Participants with disabilities must have access to equipment and facilities they can use. This includes community (e.g., playgrounds, parks), schools, and fitness facilities.
- Participation—Provide instruction and guidance in the use of exercise equipment and facilities.
- Modifications—Fitness tests and physical activities may have to be modified.
- Adherence—This is enhanced by offering multiple locations and socially engaging activities.
- Regularity—Regular participation is the key to health-related benefits for any population.

The fitness professional should involve experts in adapted physical education, therapeutic recreation, and special education for additional assistance as needed.

Fitness professionals are challenged with determining whether programming is meeting clients' needs, asking themselves, for example, "Is my spin class improving the fitness of my attendees?" Analyzing test scores from various fitness classes can help the fitness professional decide what revisions to make in the overall fitness program. How many people drop out of various classes? What kind of changes in CRF, body fatness, and low-back function are being made? How many injuries relate to the various classes? The answers to such questions help you evaluate, revise, and improve your fitness programs. You might consider your programs to be improving steadily rather than reaching perfection. This improvement can result from program evaluation.

Another use of test scores is to educate the public and to get positive attention for your program. What percentage of the participants stay with the program long enough to make important fitness gains? What is the total amount of fat lost by participants over a year? How many miles have the participants run during the year? Careful testing, record keeping, and analysis can provide helpful information about your program to the public.

GLOSSARY

1-repetition maximum (1RM)—The heaviest weight that can be lifted only once using good form.

A band—Portion of the sarcomere composed of myosin and actin; the length of the A band remains constant during muscle shortening.

abduction—Movement of a bone laterally away from the anatomical position.

abrasion—Scraping of tissues that removes the outermost layers of skin and exposes numerous capillaries.

absolute intensity—Can be expressed in a number of ways: kilocalories of energy produced per min ($kcal \cdot min^{-1}$), milliliters of oxygen consumed per kilogram of body weight per minute ($ml \cdot kg^{-1} \cdot min^{-1}$), or METs, where 1 MET is taken as RMR and is equal to 3.5 $ml \cdot kg^{-1} \cdot min^{-1}$.

acceptable macronutrient distribution range (AMDR)—The percentages of calories from carbohydrate, fat, and protein that are thought to promote good health.

actin—The thin contractile filament of the sarcomere to which myosin binds to release the energy in the activated crossbridges, leading to sarcomere shortening.

adduction—The return to the anatomical position from the abducted position.

adequate intake (AI)—The amount of a nutrient considered adequate although insufficient data exist to establish an RDA.

adipose tissue—Tissue composed of fat cells.

administrative law—A primary source of law (from the executive branch of the government) that is formed by numerous administrative agencies that exist at both the federal and state levels.

aerobic energy—When oxygen is used to help supply energy (ATP) to a person who is working.

agility—Ability to start, stop, and move the body quickly in different directions.

agonist—A muscle that is very effective in causing a certain joint movement; also called the *prime mover*.

air displacement plethysmography—Method of assessing body composition that estimates body density from body volume and body weight.

airway obstruction—Blockage of the airway that can be caused by a foreign object. Swelling is secondary to direct trauma or allergic reaction.

alcohol—Depressant that can affect exercise by impairing motor coordination, balance, and reaction times.

amenorrhea—Absence of menses.

amino acids—Nitrogen-containing building blocks for proteins that can be used for energy.

amortization phase—Time between the eccentric and concentric phases of a muscle action.

amphiarthrodial joint—A joint that allows only slight movement in all directions; also called the *cartilaginous joint*.

anaerobic energy—Energy (ATP) supplied without oxygen. Creatine phosphate and glycolysis supply ATP without using oxygen.

android-type obesity—Obesity in which there is a disproportionate amount of fat in the trunk and abdomen.

aneurysm—A spindle-shaped or saclike bulging of the wall of a blood-filled vein, artery, or ventricle.

angina pectoris—Severe cardiac pain that may radiate to the jaw, arms, or legs. Angina is caused by myocardial ischemia, which can be induced by exercise in susceptible people.

angular momentum—The quantity of rotation. Angular momentum is the product of rotational inertia and angular velocity.

anorexia nervosa—An eating disorder in which a preoccupation with body weight leads to self-starvation.

antagonist—A muscle that causes movement at a joint in a direction opposite to that of the joint's agonist (prime mover).

antiarrhythmics—Drugs that reduce the number of arrhythmias.

anticoagulants—Drugs that delay blood clotting.

antihistamines—Drugs that relieve allergy symptoms, thus making it easier to breathe.

antihypertensives—Drugs that lower BP.

antioxidant vitamins—Substances that attach to free radicals and diminish their effects. Antioxidants are touted as effective in decreasing the risk of CVD and cancer.

aortic valve—Heart valve located between the aorta and the left ventricle.

aponeuroses—Broad, flat, tendinous sheaths attaching muscles to one another.

arterioles—Blood vessels between the artery and the capillary that are involved in the regulation of blood flow and BP.

arteriovenous oxygen difference—Volume of oxygen extraction; calculated by subtracting the oxygen content of mixed venous blood (as it returns to the heart) from the oxygen content of the arterial blood.

arthritis—Inflammation of a joint.

articular capsule—A ligamentous structure that encloses a diarthrodial joint.

articular cartilage—Cartilage covering bone surfaces that articulate (meet or come into contact) with other bone surfaces.

atherosclerosis—A form of arteriosclerosis in which fatty substances are deposited in the inner walls of the arteries.

atrial fibrillation—The atrial rate is 400 to 700 beats $\cdot$ min^{-1}, whereas the ventricular rate is 60 to 160 beats $\cdot$ min^{-1}; P waves cannot be seen on the ECG.

atrial flutter—The atrial rate is 200 to 350 beats $\cdot$ min^{-1}, whereas the ventricular rate is 60 to 160 beats $\cdot$ min^{-1}; ECG shows a sawtooth pattern between QRS complexes.

atrioventricular (AV) node—The origin of the bundle of His in the right atrium of the heart. Normal electrical activity of the heart passes through the AV node before depolarization of the ventricles.

atrophy—A reduction in muscle fiber size.

avascular—Without a blood supply.

balance—Ability to maintain a certain posture or to move without falling.

ballistic movement—A rapid movement with three phases: an initial concentric action by agonist muscles to begin movement, a coasting phase, and a deceleration by the eccentric action of the antagonist muscles.

ballistic resistance training—A type of training in which the athlete accelerates the resistance throughout the entire ROM and eliminates the deceleration phase at the end ROM.

bariatric surgery—A surgical procedure designed to help with weight loss. These surgeries alter the gastrointestinal system to restrict food intake and nutrient uptake.

baroreceptors—Receptors that monitor arterial BP.

behavioral contracts—Written, signed, public agreements to engage in specific goal-directed activities. Contracts include a designated time frame and clear consequences of meeting and not meeting the agreed-upon objectives.

bench stepping—A GXT that can be used for both submaximal and maximal testing to evaluate CRF. The height of the bench and the number of steps per minute determine the intensity of the effort. Bench stepping is also a popular conditioning exercise.

beta-adrenergic blocking medications (beta-blockers)—Drugs that block receptors that respond to catecholamines (epinephrine and norepinephrine); they slow HR.

beta-adrenergic receptors—Receptors in the heart and lungs that respond to catecholamines (epinephrine and norepinephrine).

beta-carotene—A precursor of vitamin A and an important antioxidant.

binge-eating disorder—An eating disorder characterized by consuming large amounts of food in a short time.

bioelectrical impedance analysis (BIA)—Method of body composition assessment based on the electrical conductivity of various tissues in the body.

black-globe temperature (T_g)—A measure of radiant heat energy; a measurement taken in the sunlight to evaluate the potential to gain or lose heat by radiation.

blister—When friction causes disruption between epidermis and dermis, it results in fluid accumulation between the layers of skin.

body composition—Description of the tissues that make up the body; typically refers to the relative percentages of fat and nonfat tissues in the body.

body-fat distribution (fat patterning)—Pattern of fat accumulation that often is inherited.

body mass index (BMI)—Measure of the relationship between height and weight; calculated by dividing weight in kilograms by height in meters squared.

bodybuilding—A competitive sport in which the primary goal is to enhance muscular size, symmetry, and definition.

bone mineral density (BMD)—Amount of bone mineral per unit area. Typically measured with DXA and used for clinical diagnosis of osteoporosis.

bronchodilators—Drugs that dilate the bronchioles, providing relief from an asthma attack.

bulimia nervosa—An eating disorder characterized by consuming large amounts of food followed by food purging.

bundle branch—Bundle of nerve fibers between both ventricles of the heart; conducts impulses.

bundle of His—Conduction pathway that connects the AV node with bundle branches in the ventricles.

bursae—Fibrous sacs lined with synovial membrane that contain a small quantity of synovial fluid. Bursae are found between tendon and bone, between skin and bone, and between muscle and muscle. Their function is to facilitate movement without friction between these surfaces.

calcium channel blockers (CCBs)—Medications that act by blocking the entry of calcium into the cell; used to treat angina, arrhythmias, and hypertension.

caloric equivalent of oxygen—Approximately 5 kcal of energy is produced per liter of oxygen consumed (5 kcal $\cdot$ L^{-1}).

carbohydrate—An essential nutrient composed of carbon, hydrogen, and oxygen that is an energy source for the body.

carbohydrate loading—Increasing carbohydrate intake and decreasing activity in the days preceding competition.

carbon monoxide (CO)—A pollutant derived from the incomplete combustion of fossil fuels; binds to hemoglobin to reduce oxygen transport and thus reduce maximal aerobic power.

cardiac arrest—Failure of the heart to effectively circulate blood because the ventricles cease to contract in a rhythmic fashion.

cardiac output (*Q*)—The volume of blood pumped by the heart per minute; calculated by multiplying HR (beats · min^{-1}) by SV (ml · $beat^{-1}$).

cardiopulmonary resuscitation (CPR)—Established procedures to restore breathing and blood circulation.

cardiorespiratory fitness (CRF)—The ability of the circulatory and respiratory systems to supply oxygen to muscles during dynamic exercise involving a large muscle mass.

case law—A primary source of law (from the judicial branch of government) that is derived from written court opinions at both the federal and state levels.

cholesterol—A fatty substance in which carbon, hydrogen, and oxygen atoms are arranged in rings; may be deposited in the arterial walls, contributing to atherosclerosis.

chronic obstructive pulmonary disease (COPD)—Diseases that obstruct the flow of air in the airways of the lung.

claudication—Interference with the blood supply to the legs, often resulting in limping.

communication—Interaction, often verbal, to share information and emotions.

complex carbohydrate—Polysaccharides formed by combining three or more sugar molecules. Polysaccharides include starches and fiber and are found in high numbers in rice, pasta, and whole-grain breads.

concentric action—Type of muscle contraction in which the muscle shortens. This shortening pulls the points of attachment on each bone closer to each other, causing movement at the joint.

conduction—Heat-exchange mechanism in which heat is lost from warmer to cooler objects in direct contact with each other.

convection—Special case of conduction related to heat loss. Heat is transferred to air or water in direct contact with the skin; warm air or water is less dense and rises, carrying heat away from the body.

coordination—Ability to perform a task that integrates movements of the body and various parts of the body.

core stability—The ability to control the forces across the spine and pelvic girdle while protecting the integrity of the spinal structures, or the ability to achieve and sustain control of the trunk region at rest and during precise movements.

coronary angiography—A diagnostic procedure where a flexible guide wire is inserted into a coronary artery, and a catheter is then passed over it. A radiographic contrast dye is then injected into the artery to reveal any potential blockages.

coronary arteries—Blood vessels that supply the heart muscle.

coronary artery bypass graft (CABG)—Procedure in which arteries or veins are sutured above and below a blocked coronary artery to restore adequate blood flow to that portion of the myocardium.

coronary heart disease (CHD)—Atherosclerosis of the coronary arteries. Also called *coronary artery disease (CAD).*

creeping obesity—Slow accumulation of adipose tissue with aging.

criterion method—Method used as the gold standard, or the method against which other methods are compared.

crossbridge—Part of myosin filament that binds to actin, releasing energy that results in shortening of the sarcomere.

cross-training—An alternative training mode that is outside of the athlete's competition sport.

cycle ergometer—A one-wheeled stationary cycle with adjustable resistance used as a work task for exercise testing or conditioning.

daily caloric need—Number of calories needed to maintain current body weight. This number is composed of RMR, calories for activity, and the thermic effect of food.

daily values (DVs)—Indicate the percentage of daily recommended levels of nutrients that are contained in a food. DVs are based on a calorie intake of 2,000 kcal · day^{-1}.

DASH diet—The DASH (Dietary Approaches to Stop Hypertension) diet was originally designed to help people control their BP. This diet is characterized by sodium restriction; an emphasis on vegetables, fruits, low-fat milk products, whole grains, and lean meats; and elimination or minimization of added sugars and processed meats. Several studies have shown that this dietary approach can be helpful in reducing BP and weight.

decongestants—Drugs that reduce nasal and bronchial congestion and dry out the airways.

deep frostbite—Freezing of deep tissue, including muscle and bone.

defendant—The individual or entity whom the plaintiff (injured party) is suing in a civil law case, such as in a negligence lawsuit, or the individual or entity who is accused of committing a crime (violating a statute) in a criminal law case.

delayed-onset muscle soreness (DOMS)—Soreness experienced when one engages in an activity that places unaccustomed loads on muscle, resulting in microscopic breakdown of muscle tissue that leads to an inflammatory response over several days.

diabetes mellitus—Group of metabolic diseases characterized by high blood glucose concentrations.

diabetic coma—Loss of consciousness caused by too little insulin and extremely high levels of blood glucose.

diaphysis—The shaft of a long bone.

diarthrodial joint—A freely moving joint characterized by its synovial membrane and capsular ligament; also called a *synovial joint*.

diastolic blood pressure (DBP)—The pressure blood exerts on the vessel walls during the resting portion of the cardiac cycle, measured in millimeters of mercury by a sphygmomanometer.

dietary fiber—Substances found in plants that cannot be broken down by the human digestive system.

dietary reference intake (DRI)—Set of values used to evaluate dietary intake.

digitalis—A drug that augments the contraction of the heart muscle and slows the rate of conduction of cardiac impulses through the AV node.

disc—Located between vertebrae; acts as a shock absorber and frequently is involved in low-back pain.

disordered eating—Unhealthy eating pattern that can in some cases be a precursor to eating disorders.

diuretics—Drugs that increase urine production, thereby ridding the body of excess fluid.

dose—The quantity (intensity, frequency, and duration) of exercise needed to bring about a response (e.g., lower resting BP).

double product—See *rate–pressure product*.

dry-bulb temperature (T_{db})—The temperature of the air measured in the shade by an ordinary thermometer.

duration—The length of time for a fitness workout or a bout of physical activity.

dynamic testing—Strength assessment that involves movement of the body (e.g., push-up) or an external load (e.g., bench press).

dyspnea—Difficult or labored breathing beyond what is expected for the intensity of work. The exercise test or activity should be stopped.

dyspnea rating scale—An instrument used to rate the severity of a patient's symptoms of shortness of breath.

eating disorders—Clinical eating patterns that result in severe negative health consequences.

eccentric action—Type of muscle action that occurs when a muscle under tension lengthens. The muscle generates force, but it is inadequate to overcome the force it is working against. Controls speed of movement caused by another force.

ectopic focus—An irritated portion of the myocardium or electrical conducting system; gives rise to extra heartbeats that do not originate from the SA node.

effect—The desired response resulting from exercise training (e.g., lower resting BP).

ejection fraction—The fraction of the EDV ejected per beat (SV divided by EDV).

elasticity—Ability of ligaments and tendons to lengthen passively and return to their resting length.

electrocardiogram (ECG)—Graphic recording of the electrical activity of the heart. The ECG is obtained with the electrocardiograph.

embolism—Sudden obstruction of a blood vessel by a solid body such as a clot carried in the bloodstream.

emergency medical services (EMS)—A system designed to handle medical emergencies; 911 or other community emergency numbers.

emergency action plan (EAP)—A written plan used to facilitate and organize employee actions during workplace emergencies.

empathy—Identification with the thoughts or feelings of another person and the effective communication that the other person's feelings are understood.

end-diastolic volume (EDV)—The volume of blood in the heart just before ventricular contraction; a measure of the stretch of the ventricle.

endothelial cells—Cells that form the interior lining of the blood vessels, heart, and lymphatic vessels.

epimysium—The connective-tissue sheath surrounding a muscle.

epiphyseal plates—The sites of ossification in long bones.

epiphyses—The ends of long bones.

ergogenic aids—Substances taken in hopes of improving athletic performance.

essential amino acids—The eight amino acids that the body cannot synthesize and therefore must be ingested.

essential fat—The minimum amount of body fat needed for good health.

evaporation—Conversion of water from liquid to gas by means of heat, as in evaporation of sweat; results in the loss of 580 kcal for each liter of sweat evaporated.

excess postexercise oxygen consumption (EPOC)—The amount of oxygen used during recovery from work that exceeds the amount needed for rest. Also called *oxygen debt* and *oxygen repayment*.

excessive bleeding—External bleeding that results in massive loss of circulating blood volumes; often results in shock and can lead to death.

exculpatory clause—A clause within a waiver (prospective release) that can absolve (protect) defendants from their ordinary negligence.

exercise—A subset of physical activity that is planned, structured, and repetitive and is meant to improve or maintain physical fitness.

exercise-associated muscle cramps (EAMC)—Painful, involuntary muscle contractions.

exercise-induced asthma—A reactive airway disease in which exercise tends to cause the bronchioles to constrict.

exercise tests—A series of tests that evaluate prospective exercise participants' current level of fitness and commonly include CRF, muscular strength and endurance, body composition, and flexibility.

exertional heat stroke (EHS)—Most severe form of heat-related injury, with body temperature above 41.1 °C (106 °F); treat as medical emergency.

exertional rhabdomyolysis—A syndrome characterized by skeletal muscle degeneration and muscle enzyme leakage that can occur in normal, healthy people following strenuous exercise.

extension—Increasing the angle at a joint, such as straightening the elbow.

external rotation—Movement of a bone around its longitudinal axis away from the midline of the body in the anatomical position.

facet joint—Junction of the superior and inferior articular processes of the vertebrae.

fartlek training—A form of endurance training that combines LSD training with aerobic interval training.

fascicles—Bundles of muscle fibers surrounded by perimysium.

fast glycolytic fiber—See *Type IIx fiber*.

fast oxidative glycolytic fiber—See *Type IIa fiber*.

fat—Non-water-soluble substance composed of hydrogen, oxygen, and carbon that serves a variety of functions in the body, including energy production.

fat mass (FM)—The mass of the fat tissues in the body.

fat-free mass (FFM)—Weight of the nonfat tissues of the body.

fat patterning—See *body-fat distribution*.

female athlete triad—A condition sometimes observed in female athletes that is characterized by disordered eating, amenorrhea, and osteoporosis.

first-degree AV block—The delayed transmission of impulses from atria to ventricles (in excess of 0.20 sec).

flexibility—The ability to move a joint through its full ROM without discomfort or pain.

flexion—Anterior or posterior movement that brings two bones together.

force arm (*FA*)—Perpendicular distance from the axis of rotation to the direction of the application of the force-causing movement.

forced expiratory volume (FEV_1)—The maximal amount of air that can be forcibly exhaled in 1 sec, as measured by spirometry; this variable is used to diagnose COPD. A person who can expel less than 75% of her VC in 1 sec should be referred to a physician.

free radicals—Molecules or fragments of molecules formed during metabolic processes that are highly reactive and can damage cellular components.

frequency—Refers to the number of days per week that physical activity is done.

functional capacity—Maximal oxygen uptake, expressed in milliliters of oxygen per kilogram of body weight per minute, or in METs.

functional curve—Spinal curve (e.g., lordotic curve) that can be removed by assuming different postures.

glucose—A simple sugar that is a vital energy source in the human body.

glycemic index—A rating system used to indicate how rapidly a food causes blood glucose to rise.

glycemic load—A value that reflects the quality and quantity of carbohydrate in a given food.

glycogen—The storage form of carbohydrate in the human body.

glycolysis—The metabolic pathway producing ATP from the anaerobic breakdown of glucose. This short-term source of ATP is important in all-out activities lasting less than 2 min.

goal setting—Goals are desired tasks to accomplish in a specific amount of time; they provide direction and foster persistence in the search for task strategies. Effective goal setting includes establishing objectives that can be measured, concretely defined, and practically achieved.

graded exercise test (GXT)—A multistage test that determines a person's physiological responses to various intensities of exercise and the person's maximal aerobic power.

gynoid-type obesity—Obesity in which there is a disproportionate amount of fat in the hips and thighs.

H zone—The middle area of the sarcomere that contains only myosin.

health—Being alive with no major health problems. Also called *apparently healthy*.

health-related fitness—Refers to muscular strength and endurance, CRF, flexibility, and body composition.

Healthy Mediterranean-Style Eating Pattern—Patterns vary somewhat based on region but generally emphasize grains (particularly whole grains), fruits, vegetables, olive oil, and nuts. More monounsaturated fatty acids than saturated fatty acids are consumed in this pattern.

Healthy U.S.-Style Eating Pattern—A dietary approach based on the previously used USDA Food Patterns and the DASH diet. This approach suggests daily amounts that people should consume from five major food groups (vegetables, fruits, grains, dairy products, and protein) and limited sodium intake.

Healthy Vegetarian-Style Eating Pattern—A balanced dietary approach to consuming a healthy diet without meat.

heart rate (HR)—The number of heartbeats per minute.

heat exhaustion—Inability to continue activity due to heavy sweating, dehydration, sodium loss, and energy depletion.

heat syncope—Fainting or excessive loss of strength due to heat exposure.

hemoglobin A1c—Also called *glycosylated hemoglobin*, hemoglobin A1c is a form of hemoglobin that is typically found in low concentrations but exists in higher concentrations when blood glucose is constantly higher than normal.

high-density lipoprotein cholesterol (HDL-C)—This form of cholesterol protects against the development of CHD by transporting cholesterol to the liver, where it is eliminated. Thus, low levels of HDL-C are related to a high risk of CHD.

high-intensity interval training (HIIT)—A type of training that uses short bursts of maximal (or supramaximal) activity followed by recovery intervals, also known as *anaerobic interval training*.

high-risk situation—An event, thought, or interaction that challenges a person's perceived ability to maintain a desired behavioral change.

hydrostatic weighing—Method of assessing body composition based on Archimedes' principle; also called *underwater weighing*. Hydrostatic weighing is often used as the criterion method for assessing %BF.

hyperglycemia—Blood glucose concentrations above normal (fasting plasma glucose of 110 mg · dl^{-1}).

hypertension—High BP. Normally SBP exceeds 140 mmHg or DBP exceeds 90 mmHg in someone who has hypertension.

hyperthermia—An elevation of the core temperature; if unchecked, it can lead to heat exhaustion or heatstroke and death.

hypertrophy—An enlargement in muscle fiber size.

hyperventilation—A level of ventilation beyond that needed to maintain the arterial carbon dioxide level; can be initiated by a sudden increase in the hydrogen ion concentration attributable to lactic acid production during a progressive exercise test.

hypoglycemia—High insulin levels and low glucose levels.

hypotension—Low BP.

hypothermia—Below-normal body temperature.

hypoxemia—Abnormally low oxygen content in the arterial blood but not total anoxia.

I band—An area of the sarcomere that is bisected by the Z line and is composed of actin; the I band decreases during muscle shortening as the actin slides over the myosin.

impaired fasting glucose—A fasting blood glucose level between 100 and 125 mg · dl^{-1}; commonly considered a precursor to the development of diabetes.

impaired glucose tolerance (IGT)—A condition in which the body does not normally process glucose; often an intermediate step before the development of type 2 diabetes.

incision—Cutting of skin resulting in an open wound with cleanly cut edges and exposure of underlying tissues.

indirect calorimetry—Estimating energy production on the basis of oxygen consumption.

informed consent—A procedure used to obtain a person's voluntary permission to participate in a program. Informed consent requires a description of the procedures to be used as well as the potential benefits and risks and written consent of the participant.

inherent risks—Injury risks that exist during participation in sport or physical activity that are no one's fault; they just happen and are inseparable from the activity.

insulin resistance—A condition in which the body's insulin receptors no longer respond normally to insulin.

insulin shock—A medical condition that results from a high level of insulin and low blood glucose levels.

intensity—Describes the rate of work (e.g., how much energy is being expended per minute) or the degree of effort required to carry out the task (percent of maximal HR).

intercalated discs—Junctions between adjacent cardiac muscle cells that allow electrical impulses to pass from cell to cell into both ventricles (see *bundle of His*).

internal bleeding—Bleeding within deep structures of the body (chest, abdominal, or pelvic cavity) and bleeding of organs contained within these cavities; may result in shock and can lead to death.

internal rotation—Movement of a bone around its longitudinal axis toward the midline of the body in the anatomical position.

interval training—A type of training that alternates periods of exercise with periods of recovery.

intracoronary stent—A device placed within the lumen of the artery to keep the artery open.

iron-deficiency anemia—A condition characterized by a decreased amount of hemoglobin in red blood cells and a resultant decrease in the ability of the blood to transport oxygen.

isokinetic testing—The assessment of maximal muscle tension throughout a range of joint motion at a constant angular velocity (e.g., $60° \cdot sec^{-1}$).

isometric action—A muscle action in which the muscle length is unchanged; the muscle exerts a force that counteracts an opposing force. Isometric action is also called *static action*.

isometric training—Refers to resistance training programs designed to use immovable objects such as a wall or a weight machine loaded with a heavy weight. These programs, also called *static resistance training*, focus on the use of isometric muscle actions.

J point—On an ECG, the point at which the S wave ends and the ST segment begins.

joint cavity—The space between bones enclosed by the synovial membrane and articular cartilage.

kyphotic curve—Describes the condition of kyphosis, a convex curvature of the spine (e.g., the thoracic curve).

laceration—Tearing of skin resulting in an open wound with jagged edges and exposure of underlying tissues.

lactate threshold (LT)—The point during a GXT at which the blood lactate concentration suddenly increases; a good indicator of the highest sustainable work rate. Also called the *anaerobic threshold*.

lean body mass—Term often used synonymously with *fat-free mass*.

liability—Legal responsibility.

ligament—The connective tissue that attaches bone to bone.

lipoproteins—Large molecules responsible for transporting fat in the blood.

local muscular endurance—The ability of a muscle or muscle group to perform repeated contractions against a submaximal resistance.

lordotic curve—Describes the condition of lordosis; a forward, concave curve of the lumbar spine when the spine is viewed from the side.

low-back pain (LBP)—Strong discomfort in the low back, often caused by lack of muscular endurance and flexibility in the midtrunk region or improper posture or lifting.

low-density lipoprotein cholesterol (LDL-C)—The form of cholesterol that is responsible for the buildup of plaque in the inner walls of the arteries (atherosclerosis). Thus, high levels of LDL-C are related to a high risk of CHD.

lumen—The open space inside a structure such as an artery or intestine.

macrocycle—A phase of training that lasts about 1 yr.

malnutrition—A diet in which there is underconsumption, overconsumption, or unbalanced consumption of nutrients that leads to disease or increased susceptibility to disease.

maximal aerobic power or **maximal oxygen uptake ($\dot{V}O_2max$)**—The maximal rate at which oxygen can be used by the body during maximal work; related directly to the maximal capacity of the heart to deliver blood to the muscles. Expressed in $L \cdot min^{-1}$ or $ml \cdot kg^{-1} \cdot min^{-1}$.

maximum voluntary contraction (MVC)—Maximum amount of force that can be elicited during a single repetition.

medical release—A document that is signed by a person that grants permission to release that person's private medical information to a third party. For example, a medical release form can be signed by a client so the personal fitness trainer can obtain medical information from the client's physician such as stress test results, cholesterol, and so on.

menisci—Partial, semilunar-shaped discs between the femur and the tibia at the knee.

mesocycle—A phase of training that lasts for several months.

microcycle—A phase of training that lasts about 1 wk.

minerals—Inorganic atoms or ions that serve a variety of functions in the human body.

mitochondria—Cellular organelles responsible for generating energy (ATP) through aerobic metabolism.

mitral valve—Heart valve located between the left atrium and left ventricle.

Mobitz type I AV block—On an ECG, the PR interval progressively increase s until the P wave is not followed by a QRS complex. The site of the block is within the AV node.

Mobitz type II AV block—On an ECG, a constant PR interval with some but not all P waves followed by QRS. The site of the block is the bundle of His.

moderate intensity—Refers to an absolute intensity of 3 to 5.9 METs and a relative intensity of 40% to 59% $\dot{V}O_2max$.

monounsaturated fatty acids—Fat that has a single double bond between carbon atoms in the fatty acid chain. Examples are olive and canola oil.

motion segment—Fundamental unit of the lumbar spine; made up of two vertebrae and their intervening disc.

motor unit—The functional unit of muscular action that includes a motor nerve and the muscle fibers that its branches innervate.

muscle fiber—Muscle cell. Contains myofibrils that are composed of sarcomeres; uses chemical energy of ATP to generate tension, which, when greater than the resistance, results in movement.

muscle group—A group of specific muscles that are responsible for the same action at the same joint.

muscular endurance—The ability of the muscle to perform repetitive contractions over a prolonged time.

muscular fitness—Describes the integrated status of muscular strength and muscular endurance.

muscular strength—The ability of muscle to generate the maximum amount of force.

myocardial infarction (MI)—Death of a section of heart tissue in which the blood supply has been cut off; commonly called a *heart attack*.

myocardial ischemia—A lack of blood flow to the heart tissue.

myocardium—The middle layer of the heart wall; involuntary, striated muscle innervated by autonomic nerves.

myofibril—Component inside muscle fibers that is composed of a long string of sarcomeres.

myosin—The thick contractile filament in sarcomeres that can bind actin and split ATP to generate crossbridge movement and develop tension.

negative caloric balance—When less energy is consumed than is expended, which decreases body weight.

negative health—Negative health is associated with morbidity (incidence of disease) and premature mortality.

negligence—The failure to do something that a reasonable, prudent professional would do or doing something that a reasonable, prudent professional would not have done under the same or similar circumstances.

nicotine gum—Gum containing nicotine that is used for smoking cessation. Nicotine is absorbed through the oral mucosa, providing sufficient plasma nicotine concentrations to curb the craving to smoke.

nitrates—A class of medications used to treat angina pectoris, or chest pain.

nutrient—A substance that the body requires for the maintenance, growth, and repair of tissues.

nutrient density—The amount of essential nutrients in a food compared with the calories it contains.

obesity—Condition in which a person has an excessive accumulation of fat tissue; also may be classified by the relationship between weight and height.

oligomenorrhea—Irregular menses.

Olympic power lifts—Explosive lifts used to move a barbell from the floor to a position over the head. These include the clean and press (also known as the clean and jerk) and the snatch.

oral antiglycemic agents—Medications used to treat non-insulin-dependent diabetes mellitus; they stimulate the pancreas to secrete more insulin.

ossification—The replacement of cartilage by bone.

Osteoarthritis (OA)—Most common form of arthritis (90%-95% of all cases); affects joints whose articular cartilage is damaged or injured.

osteopenia—When bone has been lost but has not yet reached osteoporotic levels.

osteoporosis—A disease characterized by a decrease in the total amount of bone mineral and a decrease in the strength of the remaining bone.

overload—To place greater than usual demands on some part of the body (e.g., picking up more weight than usual overloads the muscle involved). Chronic overloading leads to increased function.

overspeed training—A type of speed training in which athletes achieve velocities greater than they can attain on their own.

overweight—Condition in which a person is above the recommended weight-to-height range but is below obesity levels.

oxygen consumption ($\dot{V}O_2$)—The rate at which oxygen is used during a specific intensity of an activity; oxygen uptake.

oxygen deficit—The difference between the steady-state oxygen requirement of a physical activity and the measured oxygen uptake during the first minutes of work.

ozone—An active form of oxygen formed in reaction to UV light and as an emission from internal combustion engines; exposure can decrease lung function.

P wave—On an ECG, a small positive deflection preceding a QRS complex, indicating atrial depolarization. The P wave is normally less than 0.12 sec in duration, with an amplitude of 0.25 mV or less.

percent body fat (%BF)—Percentage of the total weight composed of fat tissue; calculated by dividing fat mass by total weight and multiplying by 100.

percentage of HRR (%HRR)—The HR reserve (HRR) is calculated by subtracting resting HR from maximal HR. The %HRR is a percentage of the difference between resting and maximal HR and is calculated by subtracting resting HR from exercise HR, dividing by HRR, and multiplying by 100%.

percentage of maximal HR (%HRmax)—HR expressed as a simple percentage of the maximal HR.

percentage of maximal oxygen uptake (%$\dot{V}O_2$max)—Ratio of submaximal oxygen uptake to maximal oxygen uptake, multiplied by 100%.

percentage of oxygen uptake reserve (%$\dot{V}O_2$R)—$\dot{V}O_2$R is calculated by subtracting 1 MET (3.5 ml · kg^{-1} · min^{-1}) from the subject's $\dot{V}O_2$max. The %$\dot{V}O_2$R is a percentage of the difference between resting $\dot{V}O_2$ and $\dot{V}O_2$max and is calculated by subtracting 1 MET from the measured oxygen uptake, dividing by the subject's $\dot{V}O_2$R, and multiplying by 100%.

percutaneous transluminal coronary angioplasty (PTCA)—A surgical procedure in which a flexible guide wire is inserted into a partially blocked coronary artery, and then a catheter with an inflatable balloon near the tip is passed over the guide wire. The balloon is inflated and then deflated and removed in order to open the coronary artery.

performance—The ability to perform a task or sport at a desired level. Also called *motor fitness* or *skill-related fitness*.

perimysium—The connective tissue surrounding fasciculi within a muscle.

periodization—A process of varying the training stimulus to promote long-term fitness gains and to avoid overtraining.

periosteum—The connective tissue surrounding all bone surfaces except the articulating surfaces.

peripheral artery disease (PAD)—A disease characterized by blockages in the peripheral arteries.

phosphocreatine (PC)—A high-energy phosphate compound that represents the primary immediate anaerobic source of ATP at the onset of exercise. PC is important in all-out activities lasting a few seconds.

phospholipids—Fatty compounds that are essential constituents of cell membranes.

physical activity—Any bodily movement produced by skeletal muscle that results in energy expenditure; associated with occupation, leisure time, household chores, sport, and so on.

physical fitness—A set of health- or skill-related attributes that people have or achieve relating to their ability to perform physical activity.

plaque hemorrhage—Sudden formation of a blood clot that results from the rupture of the fibrous cap covering an atherosclerotic plaque.

plaintiff—The injured party who is seeking damages to recover from a personal injury (or property loss) caused by the conduct of the defendant in a civil law case, such as negligence.

polyunsaturated fatty acid—Fat that has two or more double bonds between carbon atoms in the fatty acid chain. Examples are fish, corn, soybean, and peanut oils.

positive caloric balance—When more calories are consumed than are expended, resulting in weight gain.

positive health—Optimal quality of life, including social, mental, spiritual, and physical fitness components; capacity to enjoy life and withstand challenges, not just the avoidance of disease.

positron emission tomography (PET)—A scanning technique that involves infusing the blood with radionuclides. The photons emitted by destruction of positrons are used to generate color images that correspond to blood flow and uptake of substances in various tissues, such as the heart.

power—Ability to exert muscular strength quickly.

powerlifting—A competitive sport in which athletes attempt to lift maximal amounts of weight in the squat, deadlift, and bench press.

PR interval—The time interval between the beginning of the P wave and the QRS complex. The upper normal limit is 0.2 sec. This segment is normally used as the isoelectric baseline.

PR segment—Forms the isoelectric line, or baseline, from which ST segment deviations are measured.

prediabetes—A condition in which a person has impaired fasting glucose or impaired glucose tolerance. Without treatment, prediabetes typically evolves into type 2 diabetes.

premature atrial contraction—On an ECG, the rhythm is irregular and the R-R interval is short; the origin of the beat is somewhere other than the SA node.

premature junctional contraction (PJC)—On an ECG, the ectopic pacemaker in the AV junctional area causes a QRS complex; frequently seen with inverted P waves.

premature ventricular contraction (PVC)—Wide, bizarrely shaped QRS complex originating from an ectopic focus in the His-Purkinje system. The QRS interval lasts longer than 0.12 sec, and the T wave is usually in the opposite direction.

prevalence—The percentage of a population that has a particular characteristic. For example, obesity prevalence is calculated by dividing the number of people classified as obese by the total number of people.

PRICE principle—The suggested treatment for minor sprains and strains: protection, rest, ice, compression, and elevation.

primary amenorrhea—The absence of menarche (i.e., first menses) in girls aged 16 or older.

primary assumption of risk—A legal theory in which a plaintiff is generally not allowed to seek damages for an injury that was due to inherent risks as long as the plaintiff knew, understood, and appreciated the inherent risks and voluntarily assumed them.

principle of reversibility—A corollary to the principle of overload; loss of a training effect with disuse.

product defects—Various types of defects in exercise equipment (e.g., design, manufacturing, marketing) that can lead to injury.

product liability—A type of liability imposed upon a manufacturer for a defect (design, manufacturing, or marketing) in a product that is considered unreasonably dangerous to the user.

protein—Nutrients composed of amino acids that serve a variety of functions in the human body.

pulmonary function testing—Procedures used to test the capacity of the respiratory system to move air into or out of the lungs.

pulmonary valve—A set of three crescent-shaped flaps at the opening of the pulmonary artery; also called the *semilunar valves*.

pulmonary ventilation—The number of liters of air inhaled or exhaled per minute.

pulse oximeter—Device used to measure the percent saturation of hemoglobin in the arterial blood.

puncture—Direct penetration of tissues by a pointed object.

Purkinje fibers—The fibers found beneath the endocardium of the heart; the impulse-conducting network of the heart.

Q wave—The initial negative deflection of the QRS complex on an ECG.

QRS complex—The largest complex on an ECG, indicating a depolarization of the left ventricle and normally lasting less than 0.1 sec.

QT interval—The time interval from the beginning of the QRS complex to the end of the T wave. The QT interval reflects the electrical systole of the cardiac cycle.

R wave—The positive deflection of the QRS complex in the ECG.

radiation—The process of heat exchange from the surface of one object to another that depends on a temperature gradient but does not require direct contact between objects, for example, heat loss from the sun to the earth.

rate–pressure product—The product of HR and SBP; indicative of the oxygen requirement of the heart during exercise. Training lowers the rate–pressure product at rest and during submaximal work. Also called the *double product*.

rating of perceived exertion (RPE)—Borg's scale used to quantify the subjective feeling of physical effort. The original scale was from 6 to 20; the revised scale is from 0 to 10.

recommended dietary allowance (RDA)—The amount of a nutrient found to be adequate for approximately 97% of the population.

recruitment—Stimulation of additional motor units to increase the strength of a muscle action.

reinforcement—Positive reinforcement involves adding something positive to increase the frequency of the target behavior. Negative reinforcement also increases the frequency of the desired behavior, but it is the removal of something negative, such as losing weight because of a regular walking program. Reinforcement can be administered by oneself (self-reinforcement) or by other people (social reinforcement).

relapse prevention—Way to identify and successfully deal with high-risk situations by educating the client about the relapse process and using a variety of strategies to foster an effective coping response.

relative humidity—A measure of the relative wetness of the air; the ratio of the amount of water vapor in the air to the maximum the air can hold at that temperature times 100%. High relative humidity in a warm environment helps determine the potential for losing heat by evaporation.

relative intensity—Describes the degree of effort required to expend energy and is influenced by the person's maximal aerobic capacity or CRF ($\dot{V}O_2$max). Relative intensity can be expressed as a percentage of $\dot{V}O_2$max or a percentage of maximal HR (HRmax).

relative leanness—The relative amounts of body weight that are fat and nonfat. Also called *body composition*.

repetition—One complete movement of an exercise, which typically consists of a concentric (lifting) and eccentric (lowering) phase.

repetition maximum (RM)—The maximum amount of weight that can be lifted for a predetermined number of repetitions with proper exercise technique. For example, 5RM is the most weight that can be lifted five but not six times.

resistance arm (*RA*)—Perpendicular distance from the axis of rotation to the direction of the application of the force resisting movement.

resistance force (*R*)—The opposing force that is resisting another force.

resistance training—A method of exercise designed to enhance musculoskeletal strength, power, and local muscular endurance. Resistance training encompasses a wide range of training modalities, including weight machines, free weights, medicine balls, elastic cords, and body weight.

respiratory quotient (*RQ*) or **respiratory exchange ratio (*R*)**—The ratio of the volume of carbon dioxide produced to the volume of oxygen used during a given time ($\dot{V}CO_2 \div \dot{V}O_2$).

respondeat superior—A legal doctrine that imposes vicarious liability (a form of strict liability) upon an employer for the negligent acts of its employees while performing their job responsibilities.

resting metabolic rate (RMR)—Number of calories needed to sustain the body under normal resting conditions.

restrictive lung diseases—Diseases that restrict a person's ability to expand the lungs.

rhabdomyolysis—A syndrome characterized by skeletal muscle degeneration and muscle enzyme leakage that can occur in normal, healthy people following strenuous exercise.

rheumatoid arthritis (RA)—Debilitating arthritis of unknown cause that can affect a few joints (pauciarticular) or many joints (polyarticular).

risk factor—A characteristic, sign, symptom, or test score that is associated with increased probability of developing a health problem. For example, people with hypertension have increased risk of developing CHD.

risk management—A proactive administrative process that involves four steps: (1) assessment of legal liability exposures, (2) development of risk management strategies, (3) implementation of the risk management plan, and (4) evaluation of the risk management plan. The major goal of risk management is to minimize injuries and subsequent litigation.

rotational inertia—Reluctance to rotate; proportional to the mass and distribution of the mass around the axis.

R-R interval—The time interval from the peak of the QRS of one cardiac cycle to the peak of the QRS of the next cycle.

S wave—The first negative wave (preceded by Q or R waves) of the QRS complex in the ECG.

sarcomeres—The basic units of muscle contraction. They contain actin and myosin; tension develops as the myosin crossbridges pull the actin toward the center of the sarcomere.

sarcopenia—Loss of muscle mass often associated with aging.

sarcoplasmic reticulum (SR)—The network of membranes that surround the myofibril; stores calcium needed for muscle contraction.

saturation pressure—Water vapor pressure that exists at a particular temperature when the air is saturated with water.

sciatic nerve—Nerve originating in the sacral area; it is involved in low-back problems that can result in loss of feeling and control in the legs.

scoliosis—An abnormal lateral curvature of the spine.

scope of practice—Activities performed by fitness professionals while carrying out their responsibilities that are within the limitations (or boundaries) of their education, training, certifications, and experiences.

secondary amenorrhea—A lack of menses for 3 or more consecutive months occurring in females after menarche.

secondary prevention—Steps taken to prevent the recurrence of a heart attack.

second-degree AV block—On an ECG, some but not all P waves precede the QRS complex and result in ventricular depolarization.

self-determination theory—A theory of human motivation that assumes humans are naturally inclined toward growth and development and have a set of basic psychological needs that are universal.

set—A group of repetitions performed without stopping.

sickle cell trait (SCT)—A genetic condition that involves the inheritance of one gene for sickle hemoglobin and one for normal hemoglobin.

simple sugars—Monosaccharides and disaccharides, such as glucose, fructose, and sucrose. These forms of carbohydrate provide the majority of calories in candy, soft drinks, and fruit drinks.

sinoatrial (SA) node—A mass of tissue in the right atrium of the heart, near the vena cava, that initiates the heartbeat.

sinus arrhythmia—A normal variant in sinus rhythm in which the R-R interval varies by more than 10% per beat.

sinus bradycardia—Normal heart rhythm and sequence, with a slow HR (below 60 beats · min^{-1} at rest). Sinus bradycardia may indicate a high level of fitness or a mental illness such as depression.

sinus rhythm—The normal timing and sequence of the cardiac events, with the sinus node as a pacemaker; resting rate is between 60 and 100 beats · min^{-1}.

sinus tachycardia—The normal heart rhythm and sequence, with a fast HR (above 100 beats · min^{-1} at rest). Sinus tachycardia may indicate illness or stress.

skill-related (performance-related) fitness—Refers to agility, balance, coordination, speed, power, and reaction time that are linked to games, sport, dance, and so on.

sliding-filament theory—The theory that muscular tension is generated when the actin in the sarcomere slides over the myosin because of the action of the myosin crossbridges.

slow oxidative fiber—See *Type I fiber*.

specificity—The principle that states that training effects derived from an exercise program are specific to the exercise done (endurance versus strength training) and the types of muscle fibers involved.

speed—The ability to move the whole body quickly.

speed training—Training program focused on increasing stride frequency to improve sprint performance.

sphygmomanometer—A BP measurement system.

spot reduction—The myth that exercise emphasizing a particular body part will cause that area to lose fat faster than the rest of the body loses it.

sprint-resistance training—A type of training in which the athlete works against a resistance while sprinting.

ST segment—The part of the ECG between the end of the QRS complex and the beginning of the T wave. Depression below (or elevation above) the isoelectric line indicates ischemia.

ST segment depression—When the ST segment of the ECG is depressed below the baseline; may signify myocardial ischemia.

ST segment elevation—When the ST segment of the ECG is elevated above the baseline; may signify the early (acute) stages of an MI.

stability—The ease with which balance is maintained.

stage 1 hypertension—An SBP of 140 to 159 mmHg or a DBP of 90 to 99 mmHg.

stage 2 hypertension—An SBP of 160 to 179 mmHg or DBP of 100 to 109 mmHg; typically controlled through medication.

stage 3 hypertension—A persistent elevation in BP (SBP >180 mmHg or DBP >110 mmHg) with target-organ damage.

standard deviation (SD)—A measure of the deviation from the mean (average) value generalized to the population. One SD above and below the mean includes about 68% of the population, 2 SD includes about 95%, and 3 SD includes about 99% of the population. For example, if the mean $\dot{V}O_2max = 25\ ml \cdot kg^{-1} \cdot min^{-1}$ and SD = $3\ ml \cdot kg^{-1} \cdot min^{-1}$, then you would expect 68% of the population to have $\dot{V}O_2max$ values between 22 (25 – 3) and 28 (25 + 3) $ml \cdot kg^{-1} \cdot min^{-1}$, 95% of the population to be between 19 and 31 $ml \cdot kg^{-1} \cdot min^{-1}$, and almost all of the population to be between 16 and 34 $ml \cdot kg^{-1} \cdot min^{-1}$. The *standard error of estimate (SEE)* is used to indicate the standard deviation of any estimate derived for a prediction formula.

Staphylococcus aureus—Common type of bacteria that lives on the human body and may cause an infection if it enters the skin through a cut or sore.

statutory law—A primary source of law (from the legislative branch of government) that is enacted through the legislative process at both the federal and state levels.

steady-state oxygen requirement—When the oxygen uptake levels off during submaximal work so that the oxygen uptake value represents the steady-state oxygen (ATP) requirement for the activity.

strength—The maximal force a muscle or muscle group can generate at a specified velocity.

strength training—See *resistance training*.

stroke—A vascular accident (embolism, hemorrhage, or thrombosis) in the brain, often resulting in sudden loss of body function.

structural curve—Curve that cannot be removed in normal movement because of chronically shortened musculotendinous units or ligaments.

submaximal—Less than maximal (e.g., an exercise that can be performed with less than maximal effort).

sulfur dioxide (SO_2)—A pollutant that can cause bronchoconstriction in people with asthma.

superficial frostbite—Freezing of skin layers and subcutaneous tissue.

sweating—The process of moisture coming through the pores of the skin from the sweat glands, usually as a result of heat, exertion, or emotion.

synarthrodial joint—Immovable joint.

synovial membrane—The inner lining of the joint capsule; secretes synovial fluid into the joint cavity.

systolic blood pressure (SBP)—The pressure exerted on the vessel walls during ventricular contraction, measured in millimeters of mercury by a sphygmomanometer.

T wave—On an ECG, the wave that follows the QRS complex and represents ventricular repolarization.

tachycardia—HR greater than 100 beats $\cdot\ min^{-1}$ at rest. Tachycardia may be seen in deconditioned people or people who are apprehensive about a situation (e.g., an exercise test).

talocrural joint—Ankle joint.

tapering—The purposeful decrease in training frequency and duration (i.e., total volume) and intensity leading up to a competition to attain peak performance at the time of competition.

target heart rate (THR)—The HR recommended for fitness workouts.

technetium-99m—A radioisotope used in tests of myocardial ejection fraction.

tempo training—An approach to training that uses an intensity at or slightly below that used in the competition.

tendon—A band of tough, inelastic, fibrous connective tissue that attaches muscle to bone.

tetanic contraction—In contrast to a muscle twitch, this is a smooth, sustained muscle contraction associated with a high frequency of stimulation.

thallium-201—A radioactive substance used to diagnose myocardial ischemia.

thermic effect of food—The energy needed to digest, absorb, transport, and store the food that is eaten.

third-degree AV block—On an ECG, the QRS appears independently, the PR interval varies with no regular pattern, and HR is less than 45 beats $\cdot\ min^{-1}$.

threshold—The minimum level needed for a desired effect; often used to refer to the minimum level of exercise intensity needed for improving CRF.

tolerable upper intake level (UL)—The highest intake of a nutrient believed to pose no health risk.

torque (*T*)—The effect produced by a force causing rotation; the product of the force and length of the force arm.

total cholesterol—The sum of all forms of cholesterol in the bloodstream. Because LDL-C is usually the primary factor in the total amount, a high level of total cholesterol is also a risk factor for CHD.

total work—The amount of work accomplished during a workout.

training base—A base level of fitness resulting from an established, routine exercise program.

tranquilizers—Medications that bring tranquility by calming, soothing, quieting, or pacifying. Also known as *anxiolytics*.

trans fat (trans-fatty acid)—Hydrogenated fat created to be solid at room temperature and to be used in cooking. Consuming this type of fat lowers HDL-C and raises LDL-C.

transfer of angular momentum—Angular momentum can be transferred from one body segment to another by stabilizing the initial moving part at a joint.

transtheoretical model—A general model of intentional behavior change in which behavior change is seen as a dynamic process that occurs through a series of interrelated stages. Basic concepts emphasize the person's motivational readiness to change, the cognitive and behavioral strategies for changing behavior, self-efficacy, and the evaluation of the pros and cons of the new behavior.

transverse tubule—Connects the sarcolemma (muscle membrane) to the sarcoplasmic reticulum; action potentials move down the transverse tubule to cause the sarcoplasmic reticulum to release calcium to initiate muscle contraction.

traumatic brain injury (TBI)—Brain dysfunction resulting from an external mechanical force.

treadmill—A machine with a moving belt that can be adjusted for speed and grade, allowing a person to walk or run in place. Treadmills are used extensively for exercise testing and training.

tricuspid valve—A valve located between the right atrium and right ventricle of the heart.

triglycerides—The primary storage form of fat in the human body.

tropomyosin—A protein (part of the thin filament) that regulates muscle contraction; works with troponin.

troponin—A protein (part of the thin filament) that can bind the calcium released from the sarcoplasmic reticulum; works with tropomyosin to allow the myosin crossbridge to interact with actin and initiate crossbridge movement.

two-compartment model—Model that divides the body into fat and fat-free components.

type 1 diabetes—Type of diabetes mellitus in which insulin is not produced. It is caused by damage to the beta cells of the pancreas.

type 2 diabetes—Type of diabetes mellitus in which the insulin receptors lose their sensitivity to insulin.

Type I (slow oxidative) fiber—A muscle fiber that contracts slowly and generates a small amount of tension, with most of the energy coming from aerobic processes; active in light to moderate activities and possesses great endurance.

Type IIa (fast oxidative glycolytic) fiber—A muscle fiber that contracts quickly, can produce energy aerobically, and generates great tension; adds to the tension of Type I fibers tension as exercise intensity increases.

Type IIx (fast glycolytic) fiber—A muscle fiber that contracts quickly and generates great tension; produces energy by anaerobic metabolism and fatigues quickly.

universal precautions—Safety measures taken to prevent exposure to blood or other body fluids.

ventilatory threshold (VT)—The intensity of work at which the rate of ventilation increases sharply during a GXT.

ventricular fibrillation—The heart contracts in an unorganized, quivering manner, with no discernible P waves or QRS complexes on the ECG; requires immediate emergency attention.

ventricular tachycardia—An extremely dangerous condition in which three or more consecutive PVCs occur. Ventricular tachycardia may degenerate into ventricular fibrillation.

vigorous intensity—Refers to an absolute intensity of 6 or more METs and a relative intensity of 60% to 84% $\dot{V}O_2max$.

vital capacity (VC)—The greatest amount of air that can be exhaled after a maximal inspiration. A person whose VC is less than 75% of the value predicted for her age, sex, and height should be referred to a physician for further testing.

vitamins—Organic substances essential to the normal functioning of the human body. They may be subdivided into fat soluble and water soluble.

volume—Refers to the total amount of energy expended or work accomplished in an aerobic activity; equals the product of the absolute intensity, frequency, and time. In resistance training it is the product of the sets, reps, and weight lifted.

waist-to-hip ratio (WHR)—Waist circumference divided by hip circumference; often used as an indicator of android-type obesity.

waiver—A protective legal document, also referred to as a *prospective release*, that contains an exculpatory clause and is signed by a participant before participation in sport or physical activity.

water vapor pressure gradient—The difference between the water vapor pressure in the air and the water vapor pressure of sweat on the body; the greater the gradient (or difference between the two), the easier it is to evaporate sweat and cool the body.

weightlifting—A competitive sport in which athletes attempt to lift maximal amounts of weight in the snatch and the clean and jerk.

wet-bulb globe temperature (WBGT)—Heat stress index that considers dry-bulb, wet-bulb, and black-globe temperatures.

wet-bulb temperature (T_{wb})—Air temperature measured with a thermometer whose bulb is surrounded by a wet wick; an indication of the ability to evaporate moisture from the skin.

windchill index—Indicates the temperature equivalent (under calm air conditions) for any combination of temperature and wind speed.

Z line—Connective-tissue elements that mark the beginning and end of the sarcomere.

REFERENCES

Chapter 1

1. American College of Sports Medicine (ACSM). 1975. *Guidelines for graded exercise testing and exercise prescription.* Philadelphia: Lea & Febiger.
2. American College of Sports Medicine (ACSM). 1978. The recommended quality and quantity of exercise for developing and maintaining fitness in healthy adults. *Medicine and Science in Sports and Exercise* 10:vii-x.
3. American College of Sports Medicine (ACSM). 1990. Position stand: The recommended quantity and quality of exercise for developing and maintaining cardiorespiratory and muscular fitness in healthy adults. *Medicine and Science in Sports and Exercise* 22:265-274.
4. American College of Sports Medicine (ACSM). (in press). *ACSM's guidelines for exercise testing and prescription.* 10th ed. Philadelphia: Lippincott Williams & Wilkins.
5. American Heart Association (AHA). 1972. *Exercise testing and training of apparently healthy individuals: A handbook for physicians.* New York: Author.
6. American Heart Association (AHA). 2014. Women and cardiovascular diseases—statistical fact sheet. www.heart.org/idc/groups/heart-public/@wcm/@sop/@smd/documents/downloadable/ucm_319576.pdf.
7. Artero, E.G., D. Lee, C.J. Lavie, V. España-Romero, X. Sui, T.S. Church, and S.N. Blair. 2012. Effects of muscular strength on cardiovascular risk factors and prognosis. *Journal of Cardiopulmonary Rehabilitation and Prevention* 32:351-358.
8. Bouchard, C., R.J. Shephard, and T. Stephens. 1994. *Physical activity, fitness, and health.* Champaign, IL: Human Kinetics.
9. Bouchard, C., R.J. Shephard, T. Stephens, J.R. Sutton, and B.D. McPherson. 1990. *Exercise, fitness, and health.* Champaign, IL: Human Kinetics.
10. Caspersen, C.J., K.E. Powell, and G.M. Christenson. 1985. Physical activity, exercise, and physical fitness: Definitions and distinctions for health-related research. *Public Health Reports* 100:126-131.
11. Church, T.S., M.J. LaMonte, C.E. Barlow, and S.N. Blair. 2005. Cardiorespiratory fitness and body mass index as predictors of cardiovascular disease mortality among men with diabetes. *Archives of Internal Medicine* 165:2114-2120.
12. Daniels, J.T. 2002. Personal communication.
13. Erlichman, J., A.L. Kerbey, and W.P.T. James. 2002. Physical activity and its impact on health outcomes. Paper 2: Prevention of unhealthy weight gain and obesity by physical activity: An analysis of the evidence. *Obesity Reviews* 3:273-287.
14. Farrell, S.W., L. Braun, C.E. Barlow, Y.J. Cheng, and S.N. Blair. 2002. The relation of body mass index, cardiorespiratory fitness, and all-cause mortality in women. *Obesity Research* 10:417-423.
15. Fletcher, G.F., S.N. Blair, J. Blumenthal, C.J. Caspersen, B. Chaitman, S. Epstein, H. Falls, E.S. Sivarajan Froelicher, V.F. Froelicher, and I.L. Pina. 1992. American Heart Association statement on exercise. *Circulation* 86:340-344.
16. Golding, L.A., C.R. Myers, and W.E. Sinning. 1973. *The Y's Way to Physical Fitness.* Emmaus, PA: Rodale Press.
17. Harris, C.D., K.B. Watson, S.A. Carlson, J.E. Fulton, J.M. Dorn, and L. Elam-Evans. 2013. Adult participation in aerobic and muscle-strengthening physical activities—United States, 2011. *Morbidity and Mortality Weekly Report* 62(17): 326-331.
18. Haskell, W.L. 1985. Physical activity and health: Need to define the required stimulus. *American Journal of Cardiology* 55:4D-9D.
19. Haskell, W.L. 1994. Dose–response issues from a biological perspective. In *Physical activity, fitness and health*, ed. C. Bouchard, R.J. Shephard, and T. Stephens, 1030-1039. Champaign, IL: Human Kinetics.
20. Haskell, W.L., I.M. Lee, R.R. Pate, K.E. Powell, S.N. Blair, B.A. Franklin, C.A. Macera, G.W. Heath, and P.D. Thompson. 2007. Physical activity and public health: Updated recommendation for adults from the American College of Sports Medicine and the American Heart Association. *Medicine and Science in Sports and Exercise* 39:1423-1434.
21. Hoyert, D.L., and J. Xu. 2012. Deaths: Preliminary data for 2011. *National Vital Statistics Reports* 61(6): 1-4.
22. Institute of Medicine (IOM). 2002. *Dietary reference intakes for energy, carbohydrates, fiber, fat, fatty acids, cholesterol, proteins, and amino acids.* Washington, DC: National Academy of Sciences.
23. Jones, W.H.S. 1953. *Regimen (Hippocrates).* Cambridge, MA: Harvard University Press.
24. Lee, C.D., S.N. Blair, and A.S. Jackson. 1999. Cardiorespiratory fitness, body composition, and all-cause and cardiovascular disease mortality in men. *American Journal of Clinical Nutrition* 69:373-380.
25. Maher, C., T. Olds, E. Mire, and P.T. Katzmarzyk. 2014. Reconsidering the sedentary behavior paradigm. *PLOS ONE* 9:e86403.
26. Mokdad, A.H., J.S. Marks, D.F. Stroup, and J.L. Gerberding. 2004. Actual causes of death in the United States, 2000. *Journal of the American Medical Association* 291:1238-1245.
27. Mokdad, A.H., J.S. Marks, D.F. Stroup, and J.L. Gerberding. 2005. Correction: Actual causes of death in the United States, 2000. *Journal of the American Medical Association* 293:293-294.
28. Ogden, C.L., M.D. Carroll, B.K. Kit, and K.M. Flegal. 2014. Prevalence of childhood and adult obesity in the United States, 2011-2011. *Journal of the American Medical Association* 311:806-814.

29. Paffenbarger, R.S.J., A.L. Wing, and R.T. Hyde. 1978. Physical activity as an index of heart attack risk in college alumni. *American Journal of Epidemiology* 108:161-175.
30. Pate, R.R., M. Pratt, S.N. Blair, W.L. Haskell, C.A. Marcera, and C. Bouchard. 1995. Physical activity and public health: A recommendation from the Centers for Disease Control and Prevention and the American College of Sports Medicine. *Journal of the American Medical Association* 273:402-407.
31. Rankinen, T., and C. Bouchard. 2007. Genetic differences in the relationships among physical activity, fitness, and health. In *Physical activity and health*, ed. C. Bouchard, S.N. Blair, and W.L. Haskell. Champaign, IL: Human Kinetics.
32. Ruiz, J.R., X. Sui, F. Lobelo, S. Lee, J.R. Morrow, A.W. Jackson, J.R. Hébert, C.E. Matthews, M. Sjöström, and S.N. Blair. 2009. Muscular strength and adiposity as predictors of adulthood cancer mortality in men. *Cancer Epidemiology Biomarkers Prevention* 18:1468-1476.
33. Saris, W.H.M., S.N. Blair, M.A. Van Baak, S.B. Eaton, P.S. Davies, L. DiPietro, M. Fogelholm, A. Rissanen, D. Schoeller, B. Swinburn, A. Tremblay, K.R. Westerterp, and H. Wyatt. 2003. How much physical activity is enough to prevent unhealthy weight gain? Outcomes of the IASO 1st Stock Conference and consensus statement. *Obesity Reviews* 4:101-114.
34. Sui, X., M.J. LaMonte, J.N. Laditka, J.W. Hardin, N. Chase, S.P. Hooker, and S.N. Blair. 2007. Cardiorespiratory fitness and adiposity as mortality predictors in older adults. *Journal of the American Medical Association* 298:2507-2516.
35. Swain, D.P., and B.A. Franklin. 2006. Comparison of cardioprotective benefits of vigorous versus moderate intensity aerobic exercise. *American Journal of Cardiology* 97:141-147.
36. U.S. Department of Health and Human Services (HHS). 1996. *Physical activity and health: A report of the Surgeon General.* Washington, DC: Author.
37. U.S. Department of Health and Human Services (HHS). 2008. *2008 Physical Activity Guidelines for Americans.* www.health.gov/paguidelines/guidelines/default.aspx.
38. U.S. Department of Health and Human Services (HHS). 2008. *Physical Activity Guidelines Advisory Committee report 2008.* health.gov/paguidelines/report/pdf/committeereport.pdf.
39. U.S. Department of Health and Human Services (HHS). 2014. Heart disease and African Americans. http://minorityhealth.hhs.gov/omh/browse.aspx?lvl=4&lvlid=19.
40. U.S. Department of Health and Human Services (HHS) and U.S. Department of Agriculture (USDA). 2005. *Dietary guidelines for Americans.* Washington, DC: U.S. GPO.
41. U.S. Department of Health, Education, and Welfare. 1979. *Healthy people: The Surgeon General's report on health promotion and disease prevention.* Washington, DC: U.S. GPO.
42. World Health Organization (WHO). 1946. Preamble to the Constitution of the World Health Organization as adopted by the International Health Conference, New York, 19 June-22 July.

Chapter 2

1. American College of Sports Medicine (ACSM). (in press). *ACSM's guidelines for exercise testing and prescription.* 10th ed. Philadelphia: Lippincott Williams & Wilkins.
2. American College of Sports Medicine (ACSM). 2016. *ACSM's resource manual for guidelines for exercise testing and prescription.* 8th ed. Philadelphia: Lippincott Williams & Wilkins.
3. American College of Sports Medicine (ACSM). 2012. *ACSM's health/fitness facility standards and guidelines.* 4th ed. Champaign, IL: Lippincott Williams & Wilkins.
4. American College of Sports Medicine (ACSM). 2012. *ACSM's health-related physical fitness status.* 4th ed. Champaign, IL: Lippincott Williams & Wilkins.
5. American College of Sports Medicine (ACSM) and American Heart Association (AHA). 1998. ACSM/AHA joint position statement: Recommendations for cardiovascular screening, staffing, and emergency policies at health/fitness facilities. *Medicine and Science in Sports and Exercise* 30:1009-1018.
6. American College of Sports Medicine (ACSM) and American Heart Association (AHA). 2007. Exercise and acute cardiovascular events: Placing the risks into perspective. *Medicine and Science in Sports and Exercise* 39:886-897.
7. Canadian Society for Exercise Physiology (CSEP). 2012. Canadian fitness safety standards and recommended guidelines.http://eparmed-x.appspot.com/?locale=en#pub/parmedx.
8. Coutinho, M., H. Gerstein, Y. Wang, and S. Yusuf. 1999. The relationship between glucose and incident cardiovascular events: A metaregression analysis of published data from 20 studies of 95,783 individuals followed for 12.4 years. *Diabetes Care* 22:233-240.
9. Eickhoff-Shemek, J., D.L. Herbert, and D. Connaughton. 2009. Risk management for health/fitness professionals. Philadelphia: Lippincott Williams & Wilkins.
10. Fletcher, G., G. Balady, S. Blair, J. Blumenthal, C. Caspersen, B. Chaitman, S. Epstein, E. Froelicher, V. Froelicher, I. Pina, and M. Pollock. 1996. Statement on exercise: Benefits and recommendations for physical activity programs for all Americans. *Circulation* 94:857-862.
11. Fletcher, G.F., P. Ades, P. Kligfield, R. Arena, et al. 2013. Exercise standards for testing and training: A scientific statement from the American Heart Association. *Circulation* 128:873-934.
12. Ford, E. 2005. Risks for all-cause mortality, cardiovascular disease, and diabetes associated with the metabolic syndrome: A summary of the evidence. *Diabetes Care* 28:1769-1778.
13. Franke, W. 2005. Covering all bases: Working with new clients. *ACSM's Health and Fitness Journal* 9:13-16.
14. Franke, W. 2013. Risk classification: Is it safe for your client to exercise? *ACSM's Health and Fitness Journal* 17:16-22.
15. Gibbons, R., G. Balady, J. Bricker, B. Chaitman, G. Fletcher, V. Froelicher, D. Mark, et al. 2002. ACC/AHA 2002 guideline update to exercise testing: Summary article. A report of the American College of Cardiology/American

Heart Association task force on practice guidelines (committee to update the 1997 exercise testing guidelines). *Journal of the American College of Cardiology* 40:1531-1540.

16. Goff, D., D. Lloyd-Jones, G. Bennett, C. O'Donnell, S. Coady, and J. Robinson. 2014. 2013 ACC/AHA guideline on the assessment of cardiovascular risk. *Journal of the American College of Cardiology* 63:2935-2959.
17. Goodman, J., S. Thomas, and J. Burr. 2011. Evidence-based risk assessment and recommendations for exercise testing and physical activity clearance in apparently healthy individuals. *Applied Physiology, Nutrition, and Metabolism* 36:S14-S32.
18. Grundy, S., R. Pasternak, P. Greenland, S. Smith Jr., and V. Fuster. 1999. Assessment of cardiovascular risk by use of multiple-risk-factor assessment equations: A statement for healthcare professionals from the American Heart Association and the American College of Cardiology. *Circulation* 100:1481-1492.
19. Haskell, W., I.M. Lee, R. Pate, K. Powell, S. Blair, et al. 2007. Physical activity and public health: Updated recommendation for adults from the American College of Sports Medicine and the American Heart Association. *Medicine and Science in Sports and Exercise* 39:1423-1434.
20. Health Insurance Portability and Accountability Act (HIPAA), Subtitle F Section 1171 4(a). August 21, 1996. Public law 104-191, 104th Cong.
21. Li, T., J. Rana, J. Manson, W. Willett, M. Stampfer, G. Colditz, and F.B. Hu. 2006. Obesity as compared with physical activity in predicting risk of coronary heart disease in women. *Circulation* 113:499-506.
22. Lu, Y., K. Hajifathalian, M. Ezzati, M. Woodward, E. Rimm, and G. Danaei. 2014. Metabolic mediators of the effects of body-mass index, overweight, and obesity on coronary heart disease and stroke: A pooled analysis of 97 prospective cohorts with 1.8 million participants. *Lancet* 383:970-983.
23. Magal, M., D. Riebe. (in press). Preparticpation Health Screening Recommendations: What exercise professionals need to know. *ACSM's Health and Fitness Journal.*
24. Riebe, D, B. Franklin, P. Thompson, et al. Updating ACSM's Recommendations for Exercise Preparticipation Health Screening. 2015. *Medicine in Science in Sports and Exercise* 47:2473-79.
25. Stone, N., J. Robinson, A. Lichtenstein, et al. 2013. 2013 ACC/AHA guideline on the treatment of blood cholesterol to reduce atherosclerotic cardiovascular risk in adults. Circulation 2014; 129:S1-S45.
26. Teo, K., S. Ounpuu, S. Hawken, M. Pandey, V. Valentin, D. Hunt, et al. 2006. INTERHEART Study Investigators. Tobacco use and risk of myocardial infarction in 52 countries in the INTERHEART study: A case-control study. *Lancet* 368:647-658.
27. Thompson, P., B. Franklin, and G. Balady. Exercise and acute cardiovascular events placing the risks into perspective: a scientific statement from the American Heart Association Council on Nutrition, Physical Activity, and Metabolism and the Council on Clinical Cardiology. 2007. *Circulation* 115:2358-2368.
28. Warburton, D.E., V.K. Jamnik, S.S. Bredin, and N. Gledhill. 2011. The Physical Activity Readiness Questionnaire for Everyone (PAR-Q+) and electronic Physical Activity Readiness Medical Examination (ePARmed-X+). *Health and Fitness Journal of Canada* 4:3-17.
29. Warburton, D.E., S.S. Bredin, V.K. Jamnik, and N. Gledhill. 2011. Validation of the PAR-Q+ and ePARmed-X+. *Health and Fitness Journal of Canada* 4:38-46.
30. Wilson, P., R. D'Agostino, D. Levy, A. Belanger, H. Silbershatz, and W. Kannel. 1998. Prediction of coronary heart disease using risk factor categories. *Circulation* 97:1837-1847.
31. Yusuf, S., S. Hawken, S. Ounpuu, L. Bautist, M. Franzosi, P. Commerford, and INTERHEART Study Investigators. 2005. Obesity and the risk of myocardial infarction in 27,000 participants from 52 countries: A case-control study. *Lancet* 366:1640-1649.

Chapter 3

1. Burkett, B. 2010. *Sport mechanics for coaches.* 3rd ed. Champaign, IL: Human Kinetics.
2. Floyd, R.T., and C. Thompson. 2014. *Manual of structural kinesiology.* 19th ed. Boston: McGraw-Hill Higher Education.
3. Standring, S., ed. 2008. *Gray's anatomy: The anatomical basis of clinical practice. 40th ed.* New York: Churchill Livingstone.
4. Hall, S. 2014. *Basic biomechanics.* 7th ed. Boston: McGraw-Hill.
5. Hamill, J., K. Knutzen, and T.R. Derrick. 2014. *Biomechanical basis of human movement.* 4th ed. Philadelphia: Lippincott Williams & Wilkins.
6. Hay, J.G., and J.G. Reid. 1988. *Anatomy, mechanics and human motion.* 2nd ed. Englewood Cliffs, NJ: Prentice Hall.
7. Levine, D., J. Richard, and M.W. Whittle. 2012. *Whittle's gait analysis.* 5th ed. New York: Churchill Livingstone.

Chapter 4

1. Åstrand, P.-O. 1952. *Experimental studies of physical working capacity in relation to sex and age.* Copenhagen: Ejnar Munksgaard.
2. Åstrand, P.-O., K. Rodahl, H.A. Dahl, and S.B. Strømme. 2003. *Textbook of work physiology.* 4th ed. Champaign, IL: Human Kinetics.
3. Bassett Jr., D.R. 1994. Skeletal muscle characteristics: Relationships to cardiovascular risk factors. *Medicine and Science in Sports and Exercise* 26:957-966.
4. Bassett, D.R., and E.T. Howley. 1997. Maximal oxygen uptake: Classical versus contemporary viewpoints. *Medicine and Science in Sports and Exercise* 29:591-603.
5. Bassett, D.R., and E.T. Howley. 2000. Limiting factors for maximal oxygen uptake and determinants of endurance performance. *Medicine and Science in Sports and Exercise* 32:70-84.
6. Bouchard, C., R. Lesage, G. Lortie, J. Simoneau, P. Hamel, M. Boulay, L. Perusse, G. Theriault, and C. Leblank. 1986. Aerobic performance in brothers, dizygotic and monozygotic twins. *Medicine and Science in Sports and Exercise* 18:639-646.

7. Brooks, G.A. 1985. Anaerobic threshold: Review of the concept, and directions for future research. *Medicine and Science in Sports and Exercise* 17:22-31.

8. Brooks, G.A., T.D. Fahey, and T.P. White. 2005. *Exercise physiology: Human bioenergetics and its application.* 4th ed. New York: McGraw-Hill.

9. Claytor, R.P. 1985. Selected cardiovascular, sympathoadrenal, and metabolic responses to one-leg exercise training. PhD diss., University of Tennessee at Knoxville.

10. Coggan, A.R., and E.F. Coyle. 1991. Carbohydrate ingestion during prolonged exercise: Effects on metabolism and performance. *Exercise and Sport Sciences Reviews* 19:1-40.

11. Costill, D.L. 1988. Carbohydrates for exercise: Dietary demands of optimal performance. *International Journal of Sports Medicine* 9:1-18.

12. Coyle, E.F. 1988. Detraining and retention of training induced adaptations. In *Resource manual for guidelines for exercise testing and prescription,* ed. S.N. Blair, P. Painter, R.R. Pate, L.K. Smith, and C.B. Taylor, 83-89. Philadelphia: Lea & Febiger.

13. Coyle, E.F., M.K. Hemmert, and A.R. Coggan. 1986. Effects of detraining on cardiovascular responses to exercise: Role of blood volume. *Journal of Applied Physiology* 60:95-99.

14. Coyle, E.F., W.H. Martin III, S.A. Bloomfield, O.H. Lowry, and J.O. Holloszy. 1985. Effects of detraining on responses to submaximal exercise. *Journal of Applied Physiology* 59:853-859.

15. Coyle, E.F., W.H. Martin III, D.R. Sinacore, M.J. Joyner, J.M. Hagberg, and J.O. Holloszy. 1984. Time course of loss of adaptation after stopping prolonged intense endurance training. *Journal of Applied Physiology* 57:1857-1864.

16. Cureton, K.J., P.B. Sparling, B.W. Evans, S.M. Johnson, U.D. Kong, and J.W. Purvis. 1978. Effect of experimental alterations in excess weight on aerobic capacity and distance-running performance. *Medicine and Science in Sports* 10:194-199.

17. Davis, J.H. 1985. Anaerobic threshold: Review of the concept and directions for future research. *Medicine and Science in Sports and Exercise* 17:6-18.

18. Day, J.R., H.B. Rossiter, E.M. Coats, A. Skasick, and B.J. Whipp. 2003. The maximally attainable $\dot{V}O_2$ during exercise in humans: The peak vs. maximal issue. *Journal of Applied Physiology* 95:1901-1907.

19. Ekblom, B., P.-O. Åstrand, B. Saltin, J. Stenberg, and B. Wallstrom. 1968. Effect of training on circulatory response to exercise. *Journal of Applied Physiology* 24:518-528.

20. Faulkner, J.A., D.E. Roberts, R.L. Elk, and J. Conway. 1971. Cardiovascular responses to submaximum and maximum effort cycling and running. *Journal of Applied Physiology* 30:457-461.

21. Fleck, S.J., and L.S. Dean. 1987. Resistance-training experience and the pressor response during resistance exercise. *Journal of Applied Physiology* 63:116-120.

22. Foster, C., E. Kuffel, N. Bradley, R.A. Battista, G. Wright, J.P. Porcari, A. Lucia, and J.J. deKoning. 2007. $\dot{V}O_2$max during successive maximal efforts. *European Journal of Applied Physiology* 102:67-72.

23. Franklin, B.A.1985. Exercise testing, training, and arm ergometry. *Sports Medicine* 2:100-119.

24. Gisolfi, C., and C.B.Wenger. 1984. Temperature regulation during exercise: Old concepts, new ideas. *Exercise and Sport Sciences Reviews* 12:339-372.

25. Gledhill, N., D. Cox, and R. Jamnik. 1994. Endurance athletes' stroke volume does not plateau: Major advantage is diastolic function. *Medicine and Science in Sports and Exercise* 26:1116-1121.

26. Hawkins, M.N., P.B. Raven, P.G. Snell, J. Stray-Gundersen, and B.D. Levine. 2007. Maximal oxygen uptake as a parametric measure of cardiorespiratory capacity. *Medicine and Science in Sports and Exercise* 39:103-107.

27. Hickson, R.C., H.A. Bomze, and J.O. Holloszy. 1977. Linear increase in aerobic power induced by a strenuous program of endurance exercise. *Journal of Applied Physiology: Respiratory, Environmental and Exercise Physiology* 42:372-376.

28. Hickson, R.C., H.A. Bomze, and J.O. Holloszy. 1978. Faster adjustment of O_2 uptake to the energy requirement of exercise in the trained state. *Journal of Applied Physiology: Respiratory, Environmental and Exercise Physiology* 44:877-881.

29. Hickson, R.C., C. Foster, M.L. Pollock, T.M. Galassi, and S. Rich. 1985. Reduced training intensities and loss of aerobic power, endurance, and cardiac growth. *Journal of Applied Physiology* 58:492-499.

30. Hickson, R.C., C. Kanakis Jr., J.R. Davis, A.M. Moore, and S. Rich. 1982. Reduced training duration effects on aerobic power, endurance, and cardiac growth. *Journal of Applied Physiology* 53:225-229.

31. Hickson, R.C., and M.A. Rosenkoetter. 1981. Reduced training frequencies and maintenance of increased aerobic power. *Medicine and Science in Sports and Exercise* 13:13-16.

32. Holloszy, J.O., and E.F. Coyle. 1984. Adaptations of skeletal muscle to endurance exercise and their metabolic consequences. *Journal of Applied Physiology: Respiratory, Environmental and Exercise Physiology* 56:831-838.

33. Howley, E.T. 1980. Effect of altitude on physical performance. In *Encyclopedia of physical education, fitness, and sports: Training, environment, nutrition, and fitness,* ed. G.A. Stull and T.K. Cureton, 177-187. Salt Lake City: Brighton.

34. Howley, E.T., D.R. Bassett Jr., and H.G. Welch. 1995. Criteria for maximal oxygen uptake—Review and commentary. *Medicine and Science in Sports and Exercise* 24:1055-1058.

35. Hultman, E. 1967. Physiological role of muscle glycogen in man, with special reference to exercise. *Circulation Research* 20-21 (Suppl. 1): 99-114.

36. Issekutz, B., N.C. Birkhead, and K. Rodahl. 1962. The use of respiratory quotients in assessment of aerobic power capacity. *Journal of Applied Physiology* 17:47-50.

37. Kasch, F.W., J.L. Boyer, S.P. Van Camp, L.S. Verity, and J.P. Wallace. 1990. The effects of physical activity and inactivity on aerobic power in older men (a longitudinal study). *Physician and Sportsmedicine* 18(4): 73-83.

38. Kasch, F.W., J.P. Wallace, and S.P. Van Camp. 1985. Effects of 18 years of endurance exercise on the physical work capacity of older men. *Journal of Cardiopulmonary Rehabilitation* 5:308-312.
39. Kasch, F.W., J.P. Wallace, S.P. Van Camp, and L.S. Verity. 1988. A longitudinal study of cardiovascular stability in active men aged 45 to 65 yrs. *Physician and Sportsmedicine* 16(1): 117-126.
40. Katch, F.I., and W.D. McArdle. 1977. *Nutrition and weight control.* Boston: Houghton Mifflin.
41. Kenney, W.L., J.H. Wilmore, and D.L. Costill. 2015. *Physiology of sport and exercise.* 5th ed. Champaign, IL: Human Kinetics.
42. Kraemer, W.J., S. Fleck, and M.R. Deschenes. 2016. *Exercise physiology: Integrating theory and application.* 2nd ed. Philadelphia: Wolters Kluwer.
43. Lind, A.R., and G.W. McNicol. 1967. Muscular factors which determine the cardiovascular responses to sustained and rhythmic exercise. *Canadian Medical Association Journal* 96:706-713.
44. MacDougall, J.D., D. Tuxen, D.G. Sale, J.R. Moroz, and J.R. Sutton. 1985. Arterial blood-pressure response to heavy resistance exercise. *Journal of Applied Physiology* 58:785-790.
45. McArdle, W.D., F.I. Katch, and V.L. Katch. 2015. *Exercise physiology, energy, nutrition, and human performance.* 8th ed. Philadelphia: Wolters Kluwer/Lippincott Williams & Wilkins.
46. McArdle, W.D., F.I. Katch, and G.S. Pechar. 1973. Comparison of continuous and discontinuous treadmill and bicycle tests for max $\dot{V}O_2$. *Medicine and Science in Sports* 5 (3): 156-160.
47. McArdle, W.D., and J.R. Magel. 1970. Physical work capacity and maximum oxygen uptake in treadmill and bicycle exercise. *Medicine and Science in Sports* 2 (3): 118-123.
48. Montoye, H.J., T. Ayen, F. Nagle, and E.T. Howley. 1986. The oxygen requirement for horizontal and grade walking on a motor-driven treadmill. *Medicine and Science in Sport s and Exercise* 17:640-645.
49. Nagle, F.J., B. Balke, G. Baptista, J. Alleyia, and E. Howley. 1971. Compatibility of progressive treadmill, bicycle, and step tests based on oxygen-uptake responses. *Medicine and Science in Sports* 3:149-154.
50. Plowman, S.A., and D.L. Smith. 2014. *Exercise physiology for health, fitness and performance.* 4th ed. Philadelphia: Wolters Kluwer/Lippincott Williams & Wilkins.
51. Powers, S.K., S. Dodd, and R.E. Beadle. 1985. Oxygen-uptake kinetics in trained athletes differing in $\dot{V}O_2$max. *European Journal of Applied Physiology* 54:306-308.
52. Powers, S., S. Dodd, R. Deason, R. Byrd, and T. McKnight. 1983. Ventilatory threshold, running economy, and distance-running performance of trained athletes. *Research Quarterly for Exercise and Sport* 54:179-182.
53. Powers, S.K., and E.T. Howley. 2015. *Exercise physiology.* 9th ed. New York: McGraw-Hill.
54. Powers, S., W. Riley, and E. Howley. 1980. A comparison of fat metabolism in trained men and women during prolonged aerobic work. *Research Quarterly for Exercise and Sport* 52:427-431.
55. Raven, P.B., D.H. Wasserman, W.G. Squires Jr., and T.D. Murray. 2013. *Exercise physiology: An integrated approach.* Belmont, CA: Wadsworth Cengage Learning.
56. Raven, P.B., B.L. Drinkwater, R.O. Ruhling, N. Bolduan, S. Taguchi, J. Gliner, and S.M. Horvath. 1974. Effect of carbon monoxide and peroxyacetyl nitrate on man's maximal aerobic capacity. *Journal of Applied Physiology* 36:288-293.
57. Rossiter, H.B., J.M. Kowalchuk, and B.J. Whipp. 2006. A test to establish maximal oxygen uptake despite no plateau in the O_2 uptake response to ramp incremental exercise. *Journal of Applied Physiology* 100:764-770.
58. Rowell, L.B. 1969. Circulation. *Medicine and Science in Sports* 1:15-22.
59. Rowell, L.B. 1986. *Human circulation-regulation during physical stress.* New York: Oxford University Press.
60. Sale, D.G. 1987. Influence of exercise and training on motor unit activation. *Exercise and Sport Sciences Reviews* 15:95-151.
61. Saltin, B. 1969. Physiological effects of physical conditioning. *Medicine and Science in Sports* 1:50-56.
62. Saltin, B., and P.D. Gollnick. 1983. Skeletal muscle adaptability: Significance for metabolism and performance. In *Handbook of physiology,* ed. L.D. Peachey, R.H. Adrian, and S.R. Geiger, 555-631. Baltimore: Williams & Wilkins.
63. Saltin, B., J. Henriksson, E. Nygaard, P. Anderson, and E. Jansson. 1977. Fiber types and metabolic potentials of skeletal muscles in sedentary man and endurance runners. *Annals of the New York Academy of Science* 301:3-29.
64. Saltin, B., and L. Hermansen. 1966. Esophageal, rectal, and muscle temperature during exercise. *Journal of Applied Physiology* 21:1757-1762.
65. Schwade, J., C.G. Blomqvist, and W. Shapiro. 1977. A comparison of the response to arm and leg work in patients with ischemic heart disease. *American Heart Journal* 94:203-208.
66. Sherman, W.M. 1983. Carbohydrates, muscle glycogen, and muscle glycogen supercompensation. In *Ergogenic aids in sports,* ed. M.H. Williams, 3-26. Champaign, IL: Human Kinetics.
67. Taylor, H.L., E.R. Buskirk, and A. Henschel. 1955. Maximal oxygen intake as an objective measure of cardiorespiratory performance. *Journal of Applied Physiology* 8:73-80.
68. Widmaier, E.P., H. Raff, and K.T. Strang. 2014. *Vander's Human physiology.* 13th ed. New York: McGraw-Hill.
69. Zhou, B., R.K. Conlee, R. Jensen, G.W. Fellingham, J.D. George, and A.G. Fisher. 2011. Stroke volume does not plateau during graded exercise in elite male distance runners. *Medicine and Science in Sports and Exercise* 33:1849-1854.

Chapter 5

1. American College of Sports Medicine (ACSM). 2007. Exercise and fluid replacement—position stand. *Medicine and Science in Sports and Exercise* 39(2): 377-390.
2. American College of Sports Medicine (ACSM). 2007. The female athlete triad—position stand. *Medicine and Science in Sports and Exercise* 39(10): 1867-1882.

3. American College of Sports Medicine (ACSM), American Dietetic Association (ADA), and Dietitians of Canada. 2009. Nutrition and athletic performance. *Medicine and Science in Sports and Exercise* 31(3): 709-731.
4. American Dietetic Association (ADA) and Canadian Dietetic Association. 1993. Nutrition for physical fitness and athletic performance for adults. *Journal of the American Dietetic Association* 93:691-696.
5. American Dietetic Association (ADA). 2015. Standards of medical care in diabetes—2015. *Diabetes Care* 38(Suppl. 1): S1-S99.
6. Berning, J.R. 1995. Nutritional concerns of recreational endurance athletes with an emphasis on swimming. In *Nutrition for the recreational athlete,* ed. C.G.R. Jackson, 55-68. Boca Raton, FL: CRC Press.
7. Blume, S.W., and J.R. Curtis. 2011. Medical costs of osteoporosis in the elderly Medicare population. *Osteoporosis International* 22(6): 1835-1844.
8. Driskell, J.A. 2000. *Sports nutrition.* Boca Raton, FL: CRC Press.
9. Durstine, J.L., and W.L. Haskell. 1994. Effects of exercise training on plasma lipids and lipoproteins. *Exercise and Sport Sciences Reviews* 22:477-521.
10. Expert Panel on Detection, Evaluation, and Treatment of High Blood Cholesterol in Adults. 2001. Executive Summary of the Third Report of the National Cholesterol Education Program (NCEP) Expert Panel on detection, evaluation, and treatment of high blood cholesterol in adults (Adult Treatment Panel III). *Journal of the American Medical Association* 285(19): 2486-2497.
11. Food and Nutrition Board, Institute of Medicine. 2000. *Dietary reference intakes: Applications in dietary assessment.* Washington, DC: National Academy Press.
12. Food and Nutrition Board, Institute of Medicine. 2001. *Dietary reference intakes for vitamin A, vitamin K, arsenic, boron, chromium, copper, iodine, iron, manganese, molybdenum, nickel, silicon, vanadium, and zinc.* Washington, DC: National Academy Press.
13. Food and Nutrition Board, Institute of Medicine. 2002/2005. *Dietary reference intakes for energy, carbohydrate, fiber, fat, fatty acids, cholesterol, protein, and amino acids.* Washington, DC: National Academies Press.
14. Food and Nutrition Board, Institute of Medicine. 2005. *Dietary reference intakes for water, potassium, sodium, chloride, and sulfate.* Washington, DC: National Academies Press.
15. Food and Nutrition Board, Institute of Medicine. 2011. *Dietary reference intakes for calcium and vitamin D.* Washington, DC: National Academies Press.
16. Messina, V., V. Melina, and A.R. Mangels. 2003. A new food guide for North American vegetarians. *Canadian Journal of Dietetic Practice and Research* 64:82-86.
17. National Center for Complementary and Alternative Medicine. 2010. Antioxidants and health: An introduction. [Created May 2010; updated Nov 2013; cited June 22, 2015]. https://nccih.nih.gov/health/antioxidants/introduction.htm.
18. National Library of Medicine. 2015. Creatine. [Updated June 9, 2015; cited June 22, 2015]. www.nlm.nih.gov/medlineplus/druginfo/natural/873.html.
19. Peacock, S. 2014. Assessment of nutritional status. In *ACSM's resource manual for guidelines for exercise testing and prescription.* 7th ed. Ed. D.P. Swain, 234-246. Baltimore: Lippincott Williams & Wilkins.
20. Ruud, J.S., and I. Wolinsky. 1995. Nutritional concerns of recreational strength athletes. In *Nutrition for the recreational athlete*, ed. C.G.R. Jackson, 55-68. Boca Raton, FL: CRC Press.
21. Sass, C., J.M. Eickhoff-Shemek, M.M. Manore, and L.J. Kruskall. 2007. Crossing the line: Understanding the scope of practice between registered dietitians and health/fitness professionals. *ACSM's Health and Fitness Journal* 11(3): 12-19.
22. U.S. Department of Health and Human Services (HHS) and U.S. Department of Agriculture (USDA). 2015-2020 *Dietary Guidelines for Americans.* 8th ed. Washington, DC: U.S. Government Printing Office. Available at http://healthgov/dietaryguidelines/2015/guidelines/.
23. U.S. Food and Drug Administration (FDA). 2015. FDA cuts trans fat in processed food. FDA Consumer Health Information. [Updated June 16, 2015; cited June 22, 2015]. www.fda.Gov/ForConsumers/ConsumerUpdates/ucm372915.htm.
24. Westerterp, K.R. 2000. The assessment of energy and nutrient intake in humans. In *Physical activity and obesity,* ed. C. Bouchard, 133-149. Champaign, IL: Human Kinetics.
25. Williams, M.H. 1998. Nutritional ergogenics and sports performance. *PCPFS Physical Activity and Fitness Research Digest* 3(2): 1-14.

Chapter 6

1. Ainsworth B.E., W.L. Haskell, S.D. Herrmann, N. Meckes, D.R. Bassett Jr., C. Tudor-Locke, J.L. Greer, J. Vezina, M.C. Whitt-Glover, and A.S. Leon. 2011. Compendium of Physical Activities: A second update of codes and MET values. *Medicine and Science in Sports and Exercise* 43(8): 1575-1581.
2. American College of Sports Medicine (ACSM). 1980. *Guidelines for graded exercise testing and exercise prescription.* 2nd ed. Philadelphia: Lea & Febiger.
3. American College of Sports Medicine (ACSM). (in press). *ACSM's guidelines for exercise testing and prescription.* 10th ed. Baltimore: Lippincott Williams & Wilkins.
4. Åstrand, P.-O. 1979. *Work tests with the bicycle ergometer.* Verberg, Sweden: Monark-Crescent AB.
5. Åstrand, P.-O., and K. Rodahl. 1986. *Textbook of work physiology.* 3rd ed. New York: McGraw-Hill.
6. Balke, B. 1963. A simple field test for assessment of physical fitness. In *Civil Aeromedical Research Institute report*, 63-66. Oklahoma City: Civil Aeromedical Research Institute.
7. Balke, B., and R.W. Ware. 1959. An experimental study of "physical fitness" of Air Force personnel. *Armed Forces Medical Journal* 10:675-688.
8. Bassett Jr., D.R., M.D. Giese, F.J. Nagle, A. Ward, D.M. Raab, and B. Balke. 1985. Aerobic requirements of overground versus treadmill running. *Medicine and Science in Sports and Exercise* 17:477-481.

9. Bransford, D.R., and E.T. Howley. 1977. The oxygen cost of running in trained and untrained men and women. *Medicine and Science in Sports* 9:41-44.
10. Bubb, W.J., A.D. Martin, and E.T. Howley. 1985. Predicting oxygen uptake during level walking at speeds of 80 to 130 meters per minute. *Journal of Cardiac Rehabilitation* 5(10): 462-465.
11. Dale, D., G.J. Welk, and C.E. Matthews. 2002. Methods of assessing physical activity and challenges for research. In *Physical activity assessments for health-related research*, ed. G.J. Welk, 19-34. Champaign, IL: Human Kinetics.
12. Daniels, J.T. 1985. A physiologist's view of running economy. *Medicine and Science in Sports and Exercise* 17:332-338.
13. Dill, D.B. 1965. Oxygen cost of horizontal and grade walking and running on the treadmill. *Journal of Applied Physiology* 20:19-22.
14. Foster, C., A.S. Jackson, M.L. Pollock, M.M. Taylor, J. Hare, S.M. Sennett, J.L. Rod, M. Sarwar, and D.H. Schmidt. 1984. Generalized equations for predicting functional capacity from treadmill performance. *American Heart Journal* 107:1229-1234.
15. Foster, C., A.J. Crowe, E. Daines, M. Dumit, M.A. Green, S. Lettau, N.N. Thompson, and J. Weymier. 1996. Predicting functional capacity during treadmill testing independent of exercise protocol. *Medicine and Science in Sports and Exercise* 6:752-756.
16. Franklin, B.A. 1985. Exercise testing, training, and arm ergometry. *Sports Medicine* 2:100-119.
17. Haskell, W.L., W. Savin, N. Oldridge, and R. DeBusk. 1982. Factors influencing estimated oxygen uptake during exercise testing soon after myocardial infarction. *American Journal of Cardiology* 50:299-304.
18. Howley, E.T., and M.E. Glover. 1974. The caloric costs of running and walking 1 mile for men and women. *Medicine and Science in Sports* 6:235-237.
19. Knoebel, L.K. 1984. Energy metabolism. In *Physiology*. 5th ed. Ed. E. Selkurt, 635-650. Boston: Little, Brown.
20. Lee, J-M., Y. Kim, and G.J. Welk. 2014. Validity of consumer-based physical activity monitors. *Medicine and Science in Sports and Exercise* 46:1840-1848.
21. Margaria, R., P. Cerretelli, P. Aghemo, and J. Sassi. 1963. Energy cost of running. *Journal of Applied Physiology* 18:367-370.
22. McConnell, T.R., and B.A. Clark. 1987. Prediction of maximal oxygen consumption during handrail-supported treadmill exercise. *Journal of Cardiopulmonary Rehabilitation* 7:324-331.
23. Montoye, H.J., T. Ayen, F. Nagle, and E.T. Howley. 1986. The oxygen requirement for horizontal and grade walking on a motor-driven treadmill. *Medicine and Science in Sports and Exercise* 17:640-645.
24. Nagle, F.J., B. Balke, G. Baptista, J. Alleyia, and E. Howley. 1971. Compatibility of progressive treadmill, bicycle, and step tests based on oxygen-uptake responses. *Medicine and Science in Sport* 3:149-154.
25. Nagle, F.J., B. Balke, and J.P. Naughton. 1965. Gradational step tests for assessing work capacity. *Journal of Applied Physiology* 20:745-748.
26. Sharkey, B.J. 1990. *Physiology of fitness.* 3rd ed. Champaign, IL: Human Kinetics.
27. Storer, T.W., J.A. Davis, and V.J. Caiozzo. 1990. Accurate prediction of $\dot{V}O_2$max in cycle ergometry. *Medicine and Science in Sports and Exercise* 22:704-712.
28. U.S. Department of Health and Human Services (HHS). 2008. *2008 Physical Activity Guidelines for Americans.* www.health.gov/paguidelines/guidelines/default.aspx.

Chapter 7

1. American College of Sports Medicine (ACSM). 2006. *ACSM's guidelines for exercise testing and prescription.* 7th ed. Philadelphia: Lippincott Williams & Wilkins.
2. American College of Sports Medicine (ACSM). 2010. *ACSM's guidelines for exercise testing and prescription.* 8th ed. Philadelphia: Lippincott Williams & Wilkins.
3. American College of Sports Medicine (ACSM). 2016. *ACSM's resource manual for guidelines for exercise testing and prescription.* 8th ed. Baltimore: Lippincott Williams & Wilkins.
4. Åstrand, I. 1960. Aerobic work capacity in men and women with special reference to age. *Acta Physiologica Scandinavica* 49(Suppl. 169): 1-92.
5. Åstrand, P.-O. 1979. *Work tests with the bicycle ergometer.* Varberg, Sweden: Monark-Crescent AB.
6. Åstrand, P.-O. 1984. Principles of ergometry and their implications in sport practice. *International Journal of Sports Medicine* 5:102-105.
7. Åstrand, P.-O., and I. Ryhming. 1954. A nomogram for calculation of aerobic capacity (physical fitness) from pulse rate during submaximal work. *Journal of Applied Physiology* 7:218-221.
8. Åstrand, P.-O., and B. Saltin. 1961. Maximal oxygen uptake and heart rate in various types of muscular activity. *Journal of Applied Physiology* 16:977-981.
9. Bailey, D.A., R.J. Shephard, and R.L. Mirwald. 1976. Validation of a self-administered home test of cardiorespiratory fitness. *Canadian Journal of Applied Sports Sciences* 1:67-78.
10. Balke, B. 1963. A simple field test for assessment of physical fitness. In *Civil Aeromedical Research Institute report,* 63-66. Oklahoma City: Civil Aeromedical Research Institute.
11. Balke, B. 1970. *Advanced exercise procedures for evaluation of the cardiovascular system* (Monograph). Milton, WI: Burdick.
12. Baum, W.A. 1961. *Sphygmomanometers, principles and precepts.* New York: Baum.
13. Blair, S.N., H.W. Kohl III, R.S. Paffenbarger Jr., D.G. Clark, K.H. Cooper, and L.W. Gibbons. 1989. Physical fitness and all-cause mortality. *Journal of the American Medical Association* 262:2395-2401.
14. Borg, G. 1998. *Borg's perceived exertion and pain scales.* Champaign, IL: Human Kinetics.
15. Bransford, D.R., and E.T. Howley. 1977. The oxygen cost of running in trained and untrained men and women. *Medicine and Science in Sports* 9:41-44.

16. Bruce, R.A. 1972. Multistage treadmill test of submaximal and maximal exercise. In *Exercise testing and training of apparently healthy individuals: A handbook for physicians,* ed. American Heart Association, 32-34. New York: American Heart Association.
17. Canadian Society of Exercise Physiology (CSEP). 2013. *Canadian Society for Exercise Physiology—Physical Activity Training for Health.* Ottawa, ON: Author.
18. Chun, D.M., C.B. Corbin, and R.P. Pangrazi. 2000. Validation of criterion-referenced standards for the mile run and progressive aerobic cardiovascular endurance tests. *Research Quarterly for Exercise and Sport* 71:125-134.
19. Cooper, K.H. 1977. *The aerobics way.* New York: Bantam Books.
20. Cooper Institute for Aerobics Research. 1999. *Fitnessgram test administration manual.* Champaign, IL: Human Kinetics.
21. Daniels, J.T. 1985. A physiologist's view of running economy. *Medicine and Science in Sports and Exercise* 17:332-338.
22. Daniels, J., N. Oldridge, F. Nagle, and B. White. 1978. Differences and changes in $\dot{V}O_2$ among young runners 10-18 years of age. *Medicine and Science in Sports* 10:200-203.
23. Ellestad, M. 1994. *Stress testing: Principles and practice.* Philadelphia: Davis.
24. Flouris, A.D., G.S. Metsios, K. Famisis, N. Geladas, and Y. Koutedakis. 2010. Prediction of $\dot{V}O_2$max from a new field test based on portable indirect calorimetry. *Journal of Science and Medicine in Sport* 13:70-73.
25. Frohlich, E.D., C. Grim, D.R. Labarthe, M.H. Maxwell, D. Perloff, and W.H. Weidman. 1988. Recommendations for human blood-pressure determination by sphygmomanometers. *Circulation* 77:501A-514A.
26. George, J.D., W.J. Stone, and L.N. Burkett. 1997. Non-exercise $\dot{V}O_2$max estimation for physically active college students. *Medicine and Science in Sports and Exercise* 29:415-423.
27. Golding, L.A. 2000. *YMCA fitness testing and assessment manual.* 4th ed. Champaign, IL: Human Kinetics.
28. Hagberg, J.M., J.P. Mullin, M.D. Giese, and E. Spitznagel. 1981. Effect of pedaling rate on submaximal exercise responses of competitive cyclists. *Journal of Applied Physiology* 51:447-451.
29. Heil, D.P., P.S. Freedson, L.E. Ahlquist, J. Price, and J.M. Rippe. 1995. Nonexercise regression models to estimate peak oxygen consumption. *Medicine and Science in Sports and Exercise* 27:599-606.
30. Howley, E.T. 1988. The exercise testing laboratory. In *Resource manual for guidelines for exercise testing and prescription,* ed. S.N. Blair, P. Painter, R.R. Pate, L.K. Smith, and C.B. Taylor, 406-413. Philadelphia: Lea & Febiger.
31. Jackson, A.S., S.N. Blair, M.T. Mahar, L.T. Wier, R.M. Ross, and J.E. Stuteville. Prediction of functional aerobic capacity without exercise testing. *Medicine and Science in Sports and Exercise* 22:863-870.
32. Kline, G.M., J.P. Porcari, R. Hintermeister, P.S. Freedson, A. Ward, R.F. McCarron, J. Ross, and J.M. Rippe. 1987. Estimation of $\dot{V}O_2$max from a 1-mile track walk, gender, age, and body weight. *Medicine and Science in Sports and Exercise* 19:253-259.
33. Lamb, K.L., and L. Rogers. 2007. A reappraisal of the reliability of the 20 m multistage shuttle run test. *European Journal of Applied Physiology* 100:287-292.
34. Leger, L.A., and J. Lambert. 1982. A maximal multistage 20 m shuttle run test to predict $\dot{V}O_2$max. *European Journal of Applied Physiology* 49:1-12.
35. Leger, L.A., D. Mercier, C. Gadoury, and J. Lambert. 1982. The multistage 20-meter shuttle run test for aerobic fitness. *Journal of Sport Science* 6:93-101.
36. Maritz, J.S., J.F. Morrison, J. Peter, N.B. Strydom, and C.H. Wyndham. 1961. A practical method of estimating an individual's maximal oxygen uptake. *Ergonomics* 4:97-122.
37. Matthews, C.E., D.P. Heil, P.S. Freedson, and H. Pastides. 1999. Classification of cardiorespiratory fitness without exercise testing. *Medicine and Science in Sports and Exercise* 31:486-493.
38. McArdle, W.D., F.I. Katch, and G.S. Pechar. 1973. Comparison of continuous and discontinuous treadmill and bicycle tests for max $\dot{V}O_2$. *Medicine and Science in Sports* 5(3): 156-160.
39. McNaughton, L., P. Hall, and D. Cooley. 1998. Validation of several methods of estimating maximal oxygen uptake in young men. *Perceptual and Motor Skills* 87:575-584.
40. Montoye, H.J., and T. Ayen. 1986. Body-size adjustment for oxygen requirement in treadmill walking. *Research Quarterly for Exercise and Sport* 57:82-84.
41. Montoye, H.J., T. Ayen, F. Nagle, and E.T. Howley. 1985. The oxygen requirement for horizontal and grade walking on a motor-driven treadmill. *Medicine and Science in Sports and Exercise* 17:640-645.
42. Naughton, J.P., and R. Haider. 1973. Methods of exercise testing. In *Exercise testing and exercise training in coronary heart disease,* ed. J.P. Naughton, H.R. Hellerstein, and L.C. Mohler, 79-91. New York: Academic Press.
43. Oldridge, N.B., W.L. Haskell, and P. Single. 1981. Carotid palpation, coronary heart disease, and exercise rehabilitation. *Medicine and Science in Sports and Exercise* 13:6-8.
44. Pollock, M.L., and J.H. Wilmore. 1990. *Exercise in health and disease.* 2nd ed. Philadelphia: Saunders.
45. President's Council on Physical Fitness and Sports. 2002. *President's Challenge Physical Activity and Fitness Award Program.* Washington, DC: Author.
46. Scott, S.N., D.L. Thompson, and D.P. Coe. 2013. The ability of the PACER to elicit peak exercise response in youth. *Medicine and Science in Sports and Exercise* 45:1139-1143.
47. Shephard, R.J. 1970. Computer programs for solution of the Åstrand nomogram and the calculation of body surface area. *Journal of Sports Medicine and Physical Fitness* 10:206-210.
48. Shephard, R.J. 1980. The current status of the Canadian Home Fitness Test. *British Journal of Sports Medicine* 14:114-125.
49. Shephard, R.J., M. Cox, P. Corley, and R. Smyth. 1979. Some factors affecting accuracy of the Canadian Home Fitness Test scores. *Canadian Journal of Applied Sport Science* 4:205-209.
50. Shephard, R.J., S. Thomas, and I. Weller. 1991. The Canadian Home Fitness Test—1991 update. *Sports Medicine* 11:358-366.

51. Shephard, R.J., D.A. Bailey, and R.L. Mirwald. 1976. Development of the Canadian Home Fitness Test. *Canadian Medical Association Journal* 114:675-679.

52. Strickland, M.K., S.R. Petersen, and M. Bouffard. 2003. Prediction of maximal aerobic power from the 20 m multistage shuttle run test. *Canadian Journal of Applied Physiology* 28:272-282.

53. Weir, L.T., A.S. Jackson, G.W. Ayers, and B. Arenare. 2006. Nonexercise models for estimating $\dot{V}O_2$max with waist girth, percent fat, or BMI. *Medicine and Science in Sports and Exercise* 38:555-561.

54. Weller, I.M.R., S.G. Thomas, M.H. Cox, and P.N. Corey. 1992. A study to validate the Canadian Aerobic Fitness Test. *Canadian Journal of Public Health* 83:120-124.

55. Weller, I.M.R., S. Thomas, N. Gledhill, D. Paterson, and A. Quinney. 1995. A study to validate the modified Canadian Aerobic Fitness Test. *Canadian Journal of Applied Physiology* 20:211-221.

56. Weller, I.M.R., S. Thomas, P.N. Corey, and M.H. Cox. 1993. Prediction of maximal oxygen uptake from a modified Canadian aerobic fitness test. *Canadian Journal of Applied Physiology* 18:175-188.

57. Whaley, M.H., L.A. Kaminsky, G.B. Dwyer, and L.H. Getchell. 1995. Failure of predicted $\dot{V}O_2$peak to discriminate physical fitness in epidemiological studies. *Medicine and Science in Sports and Exercise* 27:85-91.

58. Williford, H.N., M. Scharff-Olson, N. Wang, D.L. Blessing, F.H. Smith, and W.J. Duey. 1996. Cross-validation of nonexercise predictions of $\dot{V}O_2$peak in women. *Medicine and Science in Sports and Exercise* 28:926-930.

Chapter 8

1. American College of Sports Medicine (ACSM). (in press). *ACSM's guidelines for exercise testing and prescription.* 10th ed. Baltimore: Lippincott Williams & Wilkins.

2. Cataldo, D., and V.H. Heyward. 2000. Pinch an inch: A comparison of several high-quality and plastic skinfold calipers. *ACSM's Health and Fitness Journal* 4:12-16.

3. Cornier, M.-A., J.-P. Despres, N. Davis, D.A. Grossniklaus, S. Klein, B. Lamarche, F. Lopez-Jimenez, G. Rao, M.-P. St-Onge, A. Towfighi, and P. Poirier. 2011. Assessing adiposity: A scientific statement from the American Heart Association. *Circulation* 124:1996-2019.

4. Dempster, P., and S. Aitkens. 1995. A new air displacement method for the determination of human body composition. *Medicine and Science in Sports and Exercise* 27:1692-1697.

5. DiPietro, L. 1999. Physical activity in the prevention of obesity: Current evidence and research issues. *Medicine and Science in Sports and Exercise* 31:S542-S546.

6. Fields, D., M. Goran, and M. McCrory. 2002. Body composition assessment via air-displacement plethysmography in adults and children: A review. *American Journal of Clinical Nutrition* 75:453-467.

7. Finkelstein, E.A., J.G. Trogdon, J.W. Cohen, and W. Deitz. 2009. Annual medical spending attributable to obesity: Payer- and service-specific estimates. *Health Affairs* 28(5): w822-w831.

8. Flegal, K.M., B.K. Kit, H. Orpana, and B.I. Graubard. 2013. Association of all-cause mortality with overweight and obesity using standard body mass index categories: A systematic review and meta-analysis. *Journal of the American Medical Association* 309(1): 71-82.

9. Goldman, H.I., and M.R. Becklake. 1959. Respiratory function tests. *American Review of Tuberculosis and Pulmonary Disease* 79:457-467.

10. Heymsfield, S.B., S. Lichtman, R.N. Baumgartner, J. Wang, Y. Kamen, A. Aliprantis, N. Richard, and J. Pierson. 1990. Body composition of humans: Comparison of two improved four-compartment models that differ in expense, technical complexity, and radiation exposure. *American Journal of Clinical Nutrition* 52:52-58.

11. Heyward, V.H., and D.R. Wagner. 2004. *Applied body composition assessment.* 2nd ed. Champaign, IL: Human Kinetics.

12. Jackson, A.S., and M.L. Pollock. 1978. Generalized equations for predicting body density of men. *British Journal of Nutrition* 40:497-504.

13. Jackson, A.S., and M.L. Pollock. 1985. Practical assessment of body composition. *Physician and Sportsmedicine* 13:76-90.

14. Jackson, A.S., M.L. Pollock, and A. Ward. 1980. Generalized equations for predicting body density of women. *Medicine and Science in Sports and Exercise* 12:175-182.

15. Kohrt, W.M. 1995. Body composition by DXA: Tried and true? *Medicine and Science in Sports and Exercise* 27:1349-1353.

16. Lohman, T.G. 1986. Applicability of body composition techniques and constants for children and youth. In *Exercise and Sports Science Reviews*, ed. K.B. Pandolf, 325-357. New York: Macmillan.

17. Lohman, T.G. 1992. *Advances in body composition assessment.* Champaign, IL: Human Kinetics.

18. Lohman, T.G., A.F. Roche, and R. Martorell. 1988. *Anthropometric standardization reference manual.* Champaign, IL: Human Kinetics.

19. McCrory, M.A., T.D. Gomez, E.M. Bernauer, and P.A. Mole. 1995. Evaluation of a new air displacement plethysmograph for measuring human body composition. *Medicine and Science in Sports and Exercise* 27:1686-1691.

20. Ogden, C.L., M.D. Carroll, B.K. Kit, and K.M. Flegal. 2014. Prevalence of childhood and adult obesity in the United States, 2011-2012. *Journal of the American Medical Association* 311(8): 806-814.

21. Ogden, C.L., and K.M. Flegal. 2010. Changes in terminology for childhood overweight and obesity. *National Health Statistics Reports* 25:1-5.

22. Ogden, C.L., R.J. Kuczmarski, K.M. Flegal, Z. Mei, S. Guo, R. Wei, L.M. Gummer-Strawn, L.R. Curtin, A.F. Roche, and C.L. Johnson. 2002. Centers for Disease Control and Prevention 2000 growth charts for the United States: Improvements to the 1977 National Center for Health Statistics version. *Pediatrics* 109:45-60.

23. Ratamess, N. 2014. Body composition status and assessment. In *ACSM's resource manual for guidelines for exercise testing and prescription*. 7th ed. Ed. D.P. Swain, 287-308. Baltimore: Lippincott Williams & Wilkins.

24. Schutte, J.E., E.M. Townsend, J. Hugg, R.F. Shoup, R.M. Malina, and C.G. Blomqvist. 1984. Density of lean body mass is greater in blacks than in whites. *Journal of Applied Physiology: Respiratory, Environmental, and Exercise Physiology* 56:1647-1649.
25. Siri, W.E. 1961. Body composition from fluid spaces and density: Analysis of methods. In *Techniques for measuring body composition*, ed. J. Brozek and A. Henschel, 223-244. Washington, DC: National Academy of Sciences.
26. Weltman, A., S. Levine, R.L. Seip, and Z.V. Tran. 1988. Accurate assessment of body composition in obese females. *American Journal of Clinical Nutrition* 48:1179-1183.
27. Weltman, A., R.L. Seip, and Z.V. Tran. 1987. Practical assessment of body composition in obese males. *Human Biology* 59:523-536.
28. Wilmore, J. 1969. A simplified method for determination of residual volume. *Journal of Applied Physiology* 27:96-100.

Chapter 9

1. Abdul-Hameed, U., P. Rangra, M.Y. Shareef, and M.E. Hussain. 2012. Reliability of 1-repetition maximum estimation for upper and lower body muscular strength measurement in untrained middle-aged type 2 diabetic patients. *Asian Journal of Sports Medicine* 3:267-273.
2. Amarante do Nascimento, M., R. Januário, A. Gerage, J. Mayhew, F. Cheche Pina, and E. Cyrino. 2013. Familiarization and reliability of one-repetition maximum strength testing in older women. *Journal of Strength and Conditioning Research* 27:1636-1642.
3. American Association of Cardiovascular and Pulmonary Rehabilitation (AACVPR). 2006. *AACVPR cardiac rehabilitation resource manual.* Champaign, IL: Human Kinetics.
4. American College of Sports Medicine (ACSM). 2009. Exercise and physical activity for older adults. *Medicine and Science in Sports and Exercise* 41:1510-1530.
5. American College of Sports Medicine (ACSM). 2009. Progression models in resistance training for healthy adults. *Medicine and Science in Sports and Exercise* 41:687-708.
6. American College of Sports Medicine (ACSM). (in press). *ACSM's guidelines for exercise testing and prescription. 10*th ed. Baltimore: Lippincott Williams & Wilkins.
7. Artero, E., V. España-Romero, J. Castro-Piñero, J. Ruiz, D. Jiménez-Pavón, V. Aparicio, M. Gatto-Cardia, P. Baena, G. Vicente-Rodríguez, M.J. Castillo, and F.B. Ortega. 2012. Criterion-related validity of field-based muscular fitness tests in youth. *Journal of Sports Medicine and Physical Fitness* 52:263-272.
8. Barnard, K., K. Adams, A. Swank, E. Mann, and D. Denny. 1999. Injuries and muscle soreness during the one-repetition maximum assessment in a cardiac rehabilitation population. *Journal of Cardiopulmonary Rehabilitation* 19:52-58.
9. Behm, D., and A. Chaouachi. 2011. A review of the acute effects of static and dynamic stretching on performance. *European Journal of Applied Physiology* 111:2633-2651.
10. Bohannon, R.W. 1995. Sit-to-stand test for measuring performance of lower extremity muscles. *Perceptual and Motor Skills* 80:163-166.
11. Borg, G. 1982. Psychophysical bases of perceived exertion. *Medicine and Science in Sports and Exercise* 14:377-381.
12. Brzycki, M. 1993. Strength testing—predicting a one-rep max from reps-to-fatigue. *Journal of Physical Education, Recreation and Dance* 64:88-90.
13. Anton, S.D., D.J. Clark, T.J. Higgins, and M.B. Cooke. 2014. Optimizing the benefits of exercise on physical function in older adults. *Physical Medicine and Rehabilitation* 6:528-543.
14. Canadian Government, Fitness and Amateur Sport. 1986. *Canadian Standardized Test of Fitness operations manual.* 3rd ed. Ottawa: Author.
15. Castro-Piñero, J., F.B. Ortega, E.G. Artero, M.J. Girela-Rejón, J. Mora, M. Sjöström, and J.R. Ruiz. 2010. Assessing muscular strength in youth: Usefulness of standing long jump as a general index of muscular fitness. *Journal of Strength and Conditioning Research* 24:1810-1817.
16. Centers for Disease Control and Prevention (CDC). 2006. Trends in strength training—United States, 1998-2004. *Morbidity and Mortality Weekly Report* 55:769-772.
17. Centers for Disease Control (CDC). 2011. *National Health and Nutrition Examination Survey muscle strength procedures manual.* www.cdc.gov/nchs/data/nhanes/nhanes_11_12/Muscle_Strength_Proc_Manual.pdf.
18. Cogley, R., T. Archambault, J. Fibeger, M. Koverman, J. Youdas, and J. Hollman. 2005, Comparison of muscle activation using various hand positions during the push-up exercise. *Journal of Strength and Conditioning Research* 19:628-633.
19. Cooper Institute. 2010. *Fitnessgram and Activitygram test administration manual.* 4th ed. Champaign, IL: Human Kinetics.
20. Csuka, M., and D.J. McCarty. 1985. Simple method for measurement of lower extremity muscle strength. *Journal of the American Medical Association* 78:77-81.
21. Faigenbaum, A.D., R. Lloyd, and G. Myer. 2013. Youth resistance training: Past practices, new perspectives, and future directions. *Pediatric Exercise Science* 25:591-604.
22. Faigenbaum, A., and J. McFarland. 2014. Criterion repetition maximum testing. *Strength and Conditioning Journal* 36:88-91.
23. Faigenbaum, A., G. Skrinar, W. Cesare, W. Kraemer, and H. Thomas. 1990. Physiologic and symptomatic responses of cardiac patients to resistance exercise. *Archives of Physical Medicine and Rehabilitation* 71:395-398.
24. Faigenbaum, A., J. McFarland, R. Herman, F. Naclerio, N.A. Ratamess, J. Kang, and G. Myer. 2013. Reliability of the one-repetition-maximum power clean test in adolescent athletes. *Journal of Strength and Conditioning Research* 26:432-437.
25. Faigenbaum, A., L. Milliken, and W. Westcott. 2003. Maximal strength testing in healthy children. *Journal of Strength and Conditioning Research* 17:162-166.
26. Featherstone, J.F., R. Holly, and E. Amsterdam. 1993. Physiologic responses to weightlifting in coronary artery disease. *American Journal of Cardiology* 71:287-292.
27. Fleck, S., and W. Kraemer. 2014. *Designing resistance training programs.* 4th ed. Champaign, IL: Human Kinetics.

28. Fleg, J., D. Forman, K. Berra, V. Bittner, J. Blumenthal, M. Chen, S. Cheng, D. Kitzman, M. Maurer, M. Rich, W. Shen, M. Williams, S. Zieman, and American Heart Association Committees on Older Populations and Exercise Cardiac Rehabilitation and Prevention of the Council on Clinical Cardiology, Council on Cardiovascular and Stroke Nursing, and Council on Lifestyle and Cardiometabolic Health. 2013. Secondary prevention of atherosclerotic cardiovascular disease in older adults: A scientific statement from the American Heart Association. *Circulation* 128:2422-2446.

29. Fletcher, G., P.A. Ades, P. Kligfield, R. Arena, G.J. Balady, V.A. Bittner, L.A. Coke, J.L. Fleg, D.E. Forman, T.C. Gerber, M. Gulati, K. Madan, J. Rhodes, P.D. Thompson, M.A. Williams, and American Heart Association Exercise, Cardiac Rehabilitation, and Prevention Committee of the Council on Clinical Cardiology, Council on Nutrition, Physical Activity and Metabolism, Council on Cardiovascular and Stroke Nursing, and Council on Epidemiology and Prevention. 2013. Exercise standards for testing and training: A scientific statement from the American Heart Association. *Circulation* 128:873-934.

30. Garber, C., B. Blissmer, M.R. Deschenes, B.A. Franklin, M.J. Lamonte, I. Lee, D.C. Nieman, D.P. Swain, and American College of Sports Medicine (ACSM). 2011. American College of Sports Medicine position stand. Quantity and quality of exercise for developing and maintaining cardiorespiratory, musculoskeletal, and neuromotor fitness in apparently healthy adults: Guidance for prescribing exercise. *Medicine and Science in Sports and Exercise* 43:1334-1359.

31. Gerodimos, V. 2012. Reliability of handgrip strength test in basketball players. *Journal of Human Kinetics* 31:24-36.

32. Gielen, S., M.H. Laughlin, C. O'Conner, and D.J. Duncker. 2015. Exercise training in patients with heart disease: Review of beneficial effects and clinical recommendations. *Progress in Cardiovascular Diseases* 57:347-355.

33. Golding, L.A., ed. 2000. *YMCA fitness testing and assessment manual.* 4th ed. Champaign, IL: Human Kinetics.

34. Guralnik, J.M., E.M. Simosick, L. Ferrucci, R.J. Glynn, L.F. Berkman, D.G. Blazer, P.A. Scherr, and R.B. Wallace. 1994. A short physical performance battery assessing lower extremity function: Association with self-reported disability and prediction of mortality and nursing home admission. *Journal of Gerontology* 49:M85-M94.

35. Harris, C., K. Watson, S. Carlson, J. Fulton, and J. Dorn. 2013. Adult participation in aerobic and muscle strengthening physical activities—United States. 2011. *Morbidity and Mortality Weekly Reports* 62:326-330.

36. Haslam, K.A., S.N. McCartney, R.S. McKelvie, and J.D. MacDougall. 1988. Direct measurements of arterial blood pressure during formal weightlifting in cardiac patients. *Journal of Cardiopulmonary Rehabilitation* 8:213-225.

37. Hoffman, J. 2006. *Norms for fitness, performance, and health.* Champaign, IL: Human Kinetics.

38. Jones, C.J., R.E. Rikli, and B.C. Beam. 1999. A 30 s chair-stand test as a measure of lower body strength in community residing older adults. *Research Quarterly for Exercise and Sports* 70:113-119.

39. Kim, P., J. Mayhew, and D. Peterson. 2002. A modified YMCA bench press test as a predictor of 1-repetition maximum bench press strength. *Journal of Strength and Conditioning Research* 16:440-445.

40. Kraemer, W., N. Ratamess, A. Fry, and D. French. 2006. Strength training: Development and evaluation of methodology. In *Physiological assessment of human fitness*, ed. P. Maud and C. Foster, 119-150. Champaign, IL: Human Kinetics.

41. Kuo, L. 2013. The influence of chair seat height on the performance of community-dwelling older adults' 30-second chair stand test. *Aging Clinical and Experimental Research* 25:305-309.

42. Labate, V., and M. Guazzi. 2015. Past, present, and future rehabilitation practice patterns for patients with heart failure: The European perspective. *Heart Failure Clinics* 11:105-115.

43. Levinger, I., C. Goodman, D.L. Hare, G. Jerums, D. Toia, and S. Selig. 2009. The reliability of the 1RM strength test for untrained middle-aged individuals. *Journal of Science and Medicine in Sports* 12:310-316.

44. Lloyd, R., A. Faigenbaum, M. Stone, J. Oliver, I. Jeffreys, J.A. Moody, C. Brewer, K. Pierce, T. McCambridge, R. Howard, L. Herrington, B. Hainline, L. Micheli, R. Jaques, W. Kraemer, M. McBride, T. Best, D. Chu, B. Alvar, and G. Myer. 2014. Position statement on youth resistance training: The 2014 International Consensus. *British Journal of Sports Medicine* 48:498-505.

45. Mayhew, J., B. Johnson, M. Lamonte, D. Lauber, and W. Kemmler. 2008. Accuracy of prediction equations for determining one-repetition maximum bench press in women before and after resistance training. *Journal of Strength and Conditioning Research* 22:1570-1577.

46. Mayhew, J., J. Prinster, J. Ware, D. Zimmer, J. Arabas, and M. Bemben. 1995. Muscular endurance repetitions to predict bench press strength in men of different training levels. *Journal of Sports Medicine and Physical Fitness* 35:108-113.

47. McMurdo, M., and L. Rennie. 1993. A controlled trial of exercise by residents of old people's homes. *Age and Aging* 22:11-15.

48. Myer, G., C. Quatman, J. Khoury, E. Wall, and T.E. Hewett. 2009. Youth versus adult "weightlifting" injuries presenting to United States emergency rooms: Accidental versus nonaccidental injury mechanisms. *Journal of Strength and Conditioning Research* 23:2054-2060.

49. National Association for Sport and Physical Education (NASPE). 2011. *Physical education for lifelong fitness.* 3rd ed. Champaign, IL: Human Kinetics.

50. Peolsson, A., Hedlund, R., and B. Oberg. Intra- and intertester reliability and reference values for hand strength. *Journal of Rehabilitation Medicine* 33:36-41.

51. Ratamess, N. 2012. *ACSM's foundations of strength training and conditioning.* Philadelphia: Lippincott Williams & Wilkins.

52. Rikli, R.E., and C.J. Jones. 1999. Development and validation of a functional fitness test for community residing older adults. *Journal of Aging and Physical Activity* 7:129-161.

53. Rikli, R., and C.J. Jones. 2013. Development and validation of criterion-referenced clinically relevant fitness standards for maintaining physical independence in later years. *Gerontologist* 53:255-267.

54. Rikli, R.E., and C.J. Jones. 2013. *Senior fitness test manual. 2nd ed.* Champaign, IL: Human Kinetics.

55. Seo, D., E. Kim, C. Fahs, L. Rossow, K. Young, S.L. Ferguson, R. Thiebaud, V.D. Sherk, J.P. Loenneke, D. Kim, M.K. Lee, K.H. Choi, D.A. Bemben, M.G. Bemben, and W.Y. So. 2012. Reliability of the one-repetition maximum test based on muscle group and gender. *Journal of Sports Science and Medicine* 11:221-225.

56. Simic, L., N. Sarabon, and G. Markovic. 2013. Does pre-exercise static stretching inhibit maximal muscular performance? A meta-analytical review. *Scandinavian Journal of Medicine and Science in Sports* 23:131-148.

57. United States Department of Health and Human Services (HHS). *2008 Physical Activity Guidelines for Americans.* Washington, DC: Author.

58. Westcott, W.L. 2012. Resistance training is medicine: Effects of strength training on health. *Current Sports Medicine Reports* 11:209-216.

59. Westcott, W., and T. Baechle. 2007. *Strength training past 50.* 2nd ed. Champaign, IL: Human Kinetics.

60. Williams, M., W. Haskell, P. Ades, E. Amsterdam, V. Bittner, B. Franklin, M. Gulanick, S. Laing, K. Stewart, American Heart Association Council on Clinical Cardiology, and American Heart Association Council on Nutrition, Physical Activity, and Metabolism. Resistance exercise in individuals with and without cardiovascular disease: 2007 update: A scientific statement from the American Heart Association Council on Clinical Cardiology and Council on Nutrition, Physical Activity, and Metabolism. *Circulation* 116:572-584.

61. Wise, F.M., and J.M. Patrick. 2011. Resistance exercise in cardiac rehabilitation. *Clinical Rehabilitation* 25:1059-1065.

62. Wong, D.P., K.L. Ngo, M.A. Tse, and A.W. Smith. 2013. Using bench press load to predict upper body exercise loads in physically active individuals. *Journal of Sports Science and Medicine* 12:38-43.

63. World Health Organization (WHO). 2010. *Global recommendations on physical activity.* Geneva: Author.

64. Yang, Z., C.A. Scott, C. Mao, J. Tang, and A.J. Farmer. 2014. Resistance exercise versus aerobic exercise for type 2 diabetes: A systematic review and meta-analysis. *Sports Medicine* 44:487-499.

Chapter 10

1. American College of Sports Medicine (ACSM). 2011. *ACSM's complete guide to fitness and health.* Champaign, IL: Human Kinetics.

2. American College of Sports Medicine (ACSM). (in press). *ACSM's guidelines for exercise testing and prescription.* 10th ed. Philadelphia: Lippincott Williams & Wilkins.

3. Aigner, T., J. Rose, J. Martin, and J. Buckwalter. 2004. Aging theories of primary osteoarthritis: From epidemiology to molecular biology. *Rejuvenation Research* 7:134-145.

4. Arthritis Foundation. 2015. Arthritis facts. www.arthritis.org [accessed April 27, 2015].

5. Atamaz, F., B. Ozcaldiran, S. Ozdedeli, K. Capaci, and B. Durmaz. 2011. Interobserver and intraobserver reliability in lower-limb flexibility measurements. *Journal of Sports Medicine and Physical Fitness* 51:689-694.

6. Ayala, F., P.S. de Baranda, M. De Ste Croix, and F. Santonja. 2013. Comparison of active stretching technique in males with normal and limited hamstring flexibility. *Physical Therapy in Sport* 14:98-104.

7. Ayala, F., P. Sainz de Baranda, M. De Ste Croix, F. and F. Santonja. 2012. Reproducibility and criterion-related validity of the sit and reach test and toe touch test for estimating hamstring flexibility in recreationally active young adults. *Physical Therapy in Sport* 13:219-226.

8. Azadinia, F., M. Kamyab, H. Behtash, M.S. Ganjavian, and M.R.M. Javaheri. 2014. The validity and reliability of noninvasive methods for measuring kyphosis. *Journal of Spinal Disorders and Techniques* 27:E212-E218.

9. Baltaci, G., N. Un, V. Tunay, A. Besler, and S. Gerceker. 2003. Comparison of three different sit and reach tests for measurement of hamstring flexibility in female university students. *British Journal of Sports Medicine* 37:59-61.

10. Baykara, R.A., Z. Bozgeyik, O. Akgul, and S. Ozgocmen. 2013. Low back pain in patients with rheumatoid arthritis: Clinical characteristics and impact of low back pain on functional ability and health related quality of life. *Journal of Back and Musculoskeletal Rehabilitation* 26:367-374.

11. Bedekar, N., M. Suryawanshi, S. Rairikar, P. Sancheti, and A. Shyam. 2014. Inter- and intra-rater reliability of mobile device goniometer in measuring lumbar flexion range of motion. *Journal of Back and Musculoskeletal Rehabilitation* 27:161-166.

12. Biering-Sorensen, F. 1984. Physical measurements as risk indicators for low-back trouble over a one-year period. *Spine* 9:106-119.

13. Bohannon, R., R. Gajdosik, and B.F. LeVeau. 1985. Contribution of pelvic and lower limb motion to increases in the angle of passive straight leg raising. *Physical Therapy* 65:474-476.

14. Burton, A.K., K.M. Tillotson, and J.D.G. Troup. 1989. Variation in lumbar sagittal mobility with low-back trouble. *Spine* 14:584-590.

15. Caillet, R. 1988. *Low back pain syndrome.* Philadelphia: Davis.

16. Canadian Society for Exercise Physiology (CSEP). 2013. *CSEP-physical activity training for health.* Ottawa, ON: Author.

17. Centers for Disease Control and Prevention (CDC). 2015. Osteoarthritis. [Accessed Februrary 28, 2015]. http://www.cdc.gov/arthritis/basics/osteoarthritis.htm.

18. Centers for Disease Control and Prevention (CDC). 2015. Osteoporosis. [Accessed Februrary 28, 2015]. http://www.cdc.gov/nchs/fastats/osteoporosis.htm.

19. Centers for Disease Control and Prevention (CDC). 2015. Rheumatoid arthritis. [Accessed February 28, 2015]. http://www.cdc.gov/arthritis/basics/rheumatoid.htm.

20. Cooper Institute for Aerobics Research. 1992. *The prudent Fitnessgram.* Dallas: Author.

21. Corkery, M., H. Briscoe, N. Ciccone, G. Foglia, P. Johnson, S. Kinsman, L. Legere, B. Lum, and P.K. Canavan. 2007. Establishing normal values for lower extremity muscle length in college-age students. *Physical Therapy in Sport* 8:66-74.

22. Deyo, R.A., S.K. Mirza, and B.I. Martin BI. 2006. Back pain prevalence and visit rates: Estimates from U.S. national surveys, 2002. *Spine* 31:2724-2727.

23. Dreischarf, M., L. Albiol, A. Rohlmann, E. Pries, M. Bashkuev, T. Zander, G. Duda, C. Druschel, P. Strube, M. Putzier, and H. Schmidt. 2014. Age-related loss of lumbar spinal lordosis and mobility—a study of 323 asymptomatic volunteers. *PLOS ONE* 9.

24. Ellison, J.B., S.J. Rose, and S.A. Sahrmann. 1990. Patterns of hip rotation range of motion—a comparison between healthy subjects and patients with low-back pain. *Physical Therapy* 70:537-541.

25. Esola, M.A., P.W. McClure, G.K. Fitzgerald, and S. Siegler. 1996. Analysis of lumbar spine and hip motion during forward bending in subjects with and without a history of low back pain. *Spine* 21:71-78.

26. Kendall, F.P., E.K. McCreary, and P.G. Provance. 1993. *Muscles: Testing and function.* Philadelphia: Lippincott Williams & Wilkins.

27. Fairbank, J.C.T., and P.B. Pynsent. 2000. The Oswestry Disability Index. *Spine* 25:2940-2952.

28. Ferber, R., K.D. Kendall, and L. McElroy. 2010. Normative and critical criteria for iliotibial band and iliopsoas muscle flexibility. *Journal of Athletic Training* 45:344-348.

29. Fujiwara, A., K. Tamai, M. Yamato, H.S. An, H. Yoshida, K. Saotome, and A. Kurihashi. 1999. The relationship between facet joint osteoarthritis and disc degeneration of the lumbar spine: An MRI study. *European Spine Journal* 8:396-401.

30. Gellhorn, A.C., J.N. Katz, and P. Suri. 2013. Osteoarthritis of the spine: The facet joints. *Nature Reviews Rheumatology* 9:216-224.

31. Gulick, D. 2009. *Ortho notes: Clinical examination pocket guide.* Philadelphia: F.A. Davis Company.

32. Hamid, M.S.A., M.R.M. Ali, and A. Yusof. 2013. Interrater and intrarater reliability of the active knee extension (AKE) test among healthy adults. *Journal of Physical Therapy Science* 25:957-961.

33. Hasebe, K., K. Sairyo, Y. Hada, A. Dezawa, Y. Okubo, K. Kaneoka, and Y. Nakamura. 2014. Spino-pelvic rhythm with forward trunk bending in normal subjects without low back pain. *European Journal of Orthopaedic Surgery and Traumatology* 24(Suppl. 1): S193-199.

34. Hoy, D., P. Brooks, F. Blyth, and R. Buchbinder. 2010. The epidemiology of low back pain. *Best Practice and Research in Clinical Rheumatology* 24:769-781.

35. Hui, S.S., and P.Y. Yuen. 2000. Validity of the modified back-saver sit-and-reach test: A comparison with other protocols. *Medicine and Science in Sports Exercise* 32:1655-1659.

36. Imrie, D., and L. Barbuto. 1988. *The back power program.* Toronto: Stoddart.

37. Intolo, P., S. Milosavljevic, D.G. Baxter, A.B. Carman, P. Pal, and J. Munn. 2009. The effect of age on lumbar range of motion: A systematic review. *Manual Therapy* 14:596-604.

38. Jones, C.J., and R.E. Rikli. 2002. Measuring functional fitness of older adults. *Journal on Active Aging* March/April: 24-30.

39. Kang, M.-H., D.-H. Jung, D.-H. An, W.-G. Yoo, and J.-S. Oh. 2013. Acute effects of hamstring-stretching exercises on the kinematics of the lumbar spine and hip during stoop lifting. *Journal of Back and Musculoskeletal Rehabilitation* 26:329-336.

40. Keith, N.R., D.O. Clark, T.E. Stump, D.K. Miller, and C.M. Callahan. 2014. Validity and reliability of the Self-Reported Physical Fitness (SRFit) Survey. *Journal of Physical Activity and Health* 11:853-859.

41. Kippers, V., and A.W. Parker. 1987. Toe-touch test: A measure of its validity. *Physical Therapy* 67:1680-1684.

42. Li, W.S., S.B. Wang, Q. Xia, P. Passias, M. Kozanek, K. Wood, and G.A. Li. 2011. Lumbar facet joint motion in patients with degenerative disc disease at affected and adjacent levels: An in vivo biomechanical study. *Spine* 36:E629-E637.

43. Liemohn, W., S.B. Martin, and G.L. Pariser. 1997. The effect of ankle posture on sit-and-reach test performance. *Journal of Strength and Conditioning Research* 11:239-241.

44. Liemohn, W., M. Miller, T. Haydu, S. Ostrowski, S. Miles, and S. Riggs. 2000. An examination of a passive and an active back extension range of motion (ROM) tests. *Medicine and Science in Sports and Exercise* 32:S307.

45. Macrum, E., D. Bell, M. Boling, M. Lewek, and D. Padua. 2011. Effect of limiting ankle-dorsiflexion range of motion on lower extremity kinematics and muscle-activation patterns during a squat. *Journal of Sport Rehabilitation* 21:144-150.

46. Martin, S.B., A. Jackson, J.R. Morrow, and W. Liemohn. 1998. The rationale for the sit-and-reach test revisited. *Measurement in Physical Education and Exercise Science* 2:85-92.

47. Mayer, T.G., A.F. Tencer, S. Kristoferson, and V. Mooney. 1984. Use of noninvasive techniques for quantification of spinal range-of-motion in normal subjects and chronic low-back dysfunction patients. *Spine* 9:588-595.

48. Mayorga-Vega, D., R. Merino-Marban, and J. Viciana. 2014. Criterion-related validity of sit-and-reach tests for estimating hamstring and lumbar extensibility: A meta-analysis. *Journal of Sports Science and Medicine* 13:1-14.

49. McGill, S. 2004. *Ultimate back fitness and performance.* Waterloo, ON: Wabuno.

50. McGill, S.M., V.R. Yingling, and J.P. Peach. 1999. Three-dimensional kinematics and trunk muscle myoelectric activity in the elderly spine—a database compared to young people. *Clinical Biomechanics* 14:389-395.

51. Medeiros, H.B.D., D. de Araujo, and C.G.S. de Araujo. 2013. Age-related mobility loss is joint-specific: An analysis from 6,000 Flexitest results. *Age* 35:2399-2407.

52. Mookerjee, S., and M.J. McMahon. 2014. Electromyographic analysis of muscle activiation during sit-and-reach flexibility tests. *Journal of Strength and Conditioning Research* 28:3496-3501.

53. Nachemson, A. 1975. Towards a better understanding of low back pain: A review of the mechanics of the lumbar spine. *Rheumatology and Rehabilitation* 14:129-143.
54. Nachemson, A.L., and E. Jonsson. 2000. *Neck and back pain: The scientific evidence of causes, diagnosis, and treatment.* Philadelphia: Lippincott Williams & Wilkins.
55. Nadler, S.F., G.A. Malanga, M. DePrince, T.P. Stitik, and J.H. Feinberg. 2000. The relationship between lower extremity injury, low back pain, and hip muscle strength in male and female collegiate athletes. *Clinical Journal of Sport Medicine* 10:89-97.
56. Nadler, S.F., G.A. Malanga, J.H. Feinberg, M. Prybicien, T.P. Stitik, and M. DePrince. 2001. Relationship between hip muscle imbalance and occurrence of low back pain in collegiate athletes: A prospective study. *American Journal of Physical Medicine and Rehabilitation* 80:572-577.
57. Nordin, M.F.V. 2001. *Basic biomechanics of the musculoskeletal system.* Philadelphia: Lippincott Williams & Wilkins.
58. Palmer, K.T., K. Walker-Bone, M.J. Griffin, H. Syddall, B. Pannett, D. Coggon, and C. Cooper. 2001. Prevalence and occupational associations of neck pain in the British population. *Scandinavian Journal of Work Environment and Health* 27:49-56.
59. Rozanska-Kirschke, A., P. Kocur, M. Wilk, and P. Dylewicz. 2006. The Fuller Fitness Test as an index of fitness in the elderly. *Medical Rehabilitation* 10:9-16.
60. Saal, J., and J. Saal. 1991. *Strength training and flexibility.* In *The conservative care of low back pain*, ed. A.H. White and R. Anderson. Baltimore: Williams & Wilkins.
61. Sahrmann, S. 2001. *Diagnosis and treatment of movement impairment syndromes.* Maryland Heights, MD: Mosby.
62. Saur, P.M.M., F.B.M. Ensink, K. Frese, D. Seeger, and J. Hildebrandt. 1996. Lumbar range of motion: Reliability and validity of the inclinometer technique in the clinical measurement of trunk flexibility. *Spine* 21:1332-1338.
63. Tafazzol, A., N. Arjmand, A. Shirazi-Adl, and M. Parnianpour. 2014. Lumbopelvic rhythm during forward and backward sagittal trunk rotations: Combined in vivo measurement with inertial tracking device and biomechanical modeling. *Clinical Biomechanics* 29:7-13.
64. Taylor, J.B., A.P. Goode, S.Z. George, and C.E. Cook. 2014. Incidence and risk factors for first-time incident low back pain: A systematic review and meta-analysis. *Spine Journal* 14:2299-2319.
65. Troke, M., A.P. Moore, F.J. Maillardet, and E. Cheek. 2005. A normative database of lumbar spine ranges of motion. *Manual Therapy* 10:198-206.
66. Walker, B.F. 2000. The prevalence of low back pain: A systematic review of the literature from 1966 to 1998. *Journal of Spinal Disorders* 13:205-217.

Chapter 11

1. American College of Sports Medicine (ACSM). 2007. Exertional heat illness during training and competition. *Medicine and Science in Sports and Exercise* 39:556-572.
2. American College of Sports Medicine (ACSM). 2006. Prevention of cold injuries during exercise. *Medicine and Science in Sports and Exercise* 38:2012-2029.
3. American College of Sports Medicine (ACSM). 2011. The recommended quantity and quality of exercise for developing and maintaining cardiorespiratory, musculoskeletal, and neuromotor fitness in apparently healthy adults: Guidance for prescribing exercise. *Medicine and Science of Sports and Exercise* 43(7): 1334-1359.
4. American College of Sports Medicine (ACSM). (in press). *ACSM's guidelines for exercise testing and prescription. 10th* ed. Philadelphia: Lippincott Williams & Wilkins.
5. Blair, S.N., H.W. Kohl III, R.S. Paffenbarger Jr., D.G. Clark, K.H. Cooper, and L.W. Gibbons. 1989. Physical fitness and all-cause mortality. *Journal of the American Medical Association* 262:2395-2401.
6. Borg, G. 1998. *Borg's perceived exertion and pain scales.* Champaign, IL: Human Kinetics.
7. Burton, A.C., and O.G. Edholm. 1955. *Man in a cold environment.* London: Edward Arnold.
8. Buskirk, E.R., and D.E. Bass. 1974. Climate and exercise. In *Science and medicine of exercise and sport,* ed. W.R. Johnson and E.R. Buskirk, 190-205. New York: Harper & Row.
9. Campbell, M.E., Q. Li, S.E. Gingrich, R.G. Macfarlane, and S. Cheng. 2005. Should people be physically active outdoors on smog alert days? *Canadian Journal of Public Health* 96:24-28.
10. Dehn, M.M., and C.B. Mullins. 1977. Physiologic effects and importance of exercise in patients with coronary artery disease. *Cardiovascular Medicine* 2:365.
11. Dionne, F.T., L. Turcotte, M.-C. Thibault, M.R. Boulay, J.S. Skinner, and C. Bouchard. 1991. Mitochondrial DNA sequence polymorphism, $\dot{V}O_2$max, and response to endurance training. *Medicine and Science in Sports and Exercise* 23:177-185.
12. Dodd, S., S.K. Powers, T. Callender, and E. Brooks. 1984. Blood lactate disappearance at various intensities of recovery exercise. *Journal of Applied Physiology* 57:1462-1465.
13. Dose–response issues concerning physical activity and health: An evidence-based symposium (Suppl.). 2001. *Medicine and Science in Sports and Exercise* 33(6).
14. Drinkwater, B.L., J.E. Denton, I.C. Kupprat, T.S. Talag, and S.M. Horvath. 1976. Aerobic power as a factor in women's response to work within hot environments. *Journal of Applied Physiology* 41:815-821.
15. Folinsbee, L.J. 1990. Discussion: Exercise and the environment. In *Exercise, fitness, and health,* ed. C. Bouchard, R.J. Shephard, T. Stephens, J.R. Sutton, and B.D. McPherson, 179-183. Champaign, IL: Human Kinetics.
16. Frampton, M.W., M.J. Utell, W. Zareba, G. Oberdorster, C. Cox, L.S. Huang, P.E. Morrow, F.E. Lee, D. Chalupa, L.M. Frasier, D.M. Speers, and J. Stewart. 2004. Effects of exposure to ultrafine carbon particles in healthy subjects and subjects with asthma. *Research Report—Health Effects Institute* 126:1-63.
17. Gisolfi, G.V., and J. Cohen. 1979. Relationships among training, heat acclimation, and heat tolerance in men and women: The controversy revisited. *Medicine and Science in Sports and Exercise* 11:56-59.

18. Goodman, L.S., and A. Gilman, eds. 1975. *The pharmacological basis of therapeutics.* New York: Macmillan.
19. Grover, R., J. Reeves, E. Grover, and J. Leathers. 1967. Muscular exercise in young men native to 3,100 m altitude. *Journal of Applied Physiology* 22:555-564.
20. Hanson, P.G., and S.W. Zimmerman. 1979. Exertional heatstroke in novice runners. *Journal of the American Medical Association* 242:154-157.
21. Hardy, J.D., and P. Bard. 1974. Body temperature regulation. In vol. 2 of *Medical physiology.* 13th ed. Ed. V.B. Mountcastle, 1305-1342. St. Louis: Mosby.
22. Haskell, W.L. 1978. Design and implementation of cardiac conditioning programs. In *Rehabilitation of the coronary patient,* ed. N.K. Wenger and H.K. Hellerstein, 203-241. New York: Wiley.
23. Haskell, W.L. 1984. The influence of exercise on the concentrations of triglyceride and cholesterol in human plasma. *Exercise and Sport Sciences Reviews* 12:205-244.
24. Haskell, W.L. 2001. What to look for in assessing responsiveness to exercise in a health context. *Medicine and Science in Sports and Exercise* 33:S454-S458.
25. Haskell, W.L., I.-M. Lee, R.R. Pate, K.E. Powell, S.N. Blair, B.A. Franklin, C.A. Macera, G.W. Heath, P.D. Thompson, and A. Bauman. 2007. Physical activity and public health: Updated recommendations for adults from the American College of Sports Medicine and the American Heart Association. *Medicine and Science in Sports and Exercise* 39:1423-1434.
26. Hayward, M.G., and W.R. Keatinge. 1981. Roles of subcutaneous fat and thermoregulatory reflexes in determining ability to stabilize body temperature in water. *Journal of Physiology* 320:229-251.
27. Hellerstein, H.K., and B.A. Franklin. 1984. Exercise testing and prescription. In *Rehabilitation of the coronary patient.* 2nd ed. Ed. N.K. Wenger and H.K. Hellerstein, 197-284. New York: Wiley.
28. Holmer, I. 1979. Physiology of swimming man. *Exercise and Sport Sciences Reviews* 7:87-123.
29. Horvath, S.M. 1981. Exercise in a cold environment. *Exercise and Sport Sciences Reviews* 9:221-263.
30. Horvath, S.M., P.R. Raven, T.E. Dahms, and D.J. Gray. 1975. Maximal aerobic capacity of different levels of carboxyhemoglobin. *Journal of Applied Physiology* 38:300-303.
31. Howley, E.T. 1980. Effect of altitude on physical performance. In *Encyclopedia of physical education, fitness, and sports: Training, environment, nutrition, and fitness,* ed. G.A. Stull and T.K. Cureton, 177-187. Salt Lake City: Brighton.
32. Howley, E.T. 2001. Type of activity: Resistance, aerobic and leisure versus occupational physical activity. *Medicine and Science in Sports and Exercise* 33:S364-S369.
33. Hughson, R.L., H.J. Green, M.E. Houston, J.A. Thompson, D.R. MacLean, and J.R. Sutton. 1980. Heat injuries in Canadian mass-participation runs. *Canadian Medical Association Journal* 122:1141-1144.
34. Jennings, G.L., G. Deakin, P. Korner, I. Meredith, B. Kingwell, and L. Nelson. 1991. What is the dose–response relationship between exercise training and blood pressure? *Annals of Medicine* 23:313-318.
35. Karvonen, M.J., E. Kentala, and O. Mustala. 1957. The effects of training heart rate: A longitudinal study. *Annales Medicinae Experimentalis et Biologiae Fenniae* 35:307-315.
36. Londeree, B.R., and S.A. Ames. 1976. Trend analysis of the %$\dot{V}O_2$max-HRregression. *Medicine and Science in Sports* 8:122-125.
37. Londeree, B.R., and M.L. Moeschberger. 1982. Effect of age and other factors on maximal heart rate. *Research Quarterly for Exercise and Sport* 53:297-304.
38. McArdle, W.D., J.R. Magel, T.J. Gergley, R.J. Spina, and M.M. Toner. 1984. Thermal adjustment to cold-water exposure in resting men and women. *Journal of Physiology: Respiratory, Environmental and Exercise Physiology* 56:1565-1571.
39. McArdle, W.D., J.R. Magel, R.J. Spina, T.J. Gergley, and M.M. Toner. 1984. Thermal adjustments to cold-water exposure in exercising men and women. *Journal of Applied Physiology* 56:1572-1577.
40. Myers, J., M. Prakash, V. Froelicher, D. Do, S. Partington, and J.E. Atwood. 2002. Exercise capacity and mortality among men referred for exercise testing. *New England Journal of Medicine* 346:793-801.
41. Paffenbarger, R.S., R.T. Hyde, and A.L. Wing. 1986. Physical activity, all-cause mortality, and longevity of college alumni. *New England Journal of Medicine* 314:605-613.
42. Pate, R.R., M. Pratt, S.N. Blair, W.L. Haskell, C.A. Marcera, and C. Bouchard. 1995. Physical activity and public health: A recommendation from the Centers for Disease Control and Prevention and the American College of Sports Medicine. *Journal of the American Medical Association* 273:402-407.
43. Pollock, M.L., L.R. Gettman, C.A. Mileses, M.D. Bah, J.L. Durstine, and R.B. Johnson. 1977. Effects of frequency and duration of training on attrition and incidence of injury. *Medicine and Science in Sports* 9:31-36.
44. Pollock, M.L., and J.H. Wilmore. 1990. *Exercise in health and disease.* 2nd ed. Philadelphia: Saunders.
45. Powers, S.K., and E.T. Howley. 2015. *Exercise physiology. New York: McGraw-Hill.*
46. Pugh, L.G.C. 1964. Deaths from exposure in Four Inns Walking Competition, March 14-15, 1964. *Lancet* 1:1210-1212.
47. Pugh, L.G.C., and O.G. Edholm. 1955. The physiology of Channel swimmers. *Lancet* 2:761-768.
48. Raven, P.B. 1980. Effects of air pollution on physical performance. In vol. 2 of *Encyclopedia of physical education: Physical fitness, training, environment and nutrition related to performance,* ed. G.A. Stull and T.K. Cureton, 201-216. Salt Lake City: Brighton.
49. Raven, P.B., B.L. Drinkwater, R.O. Ruhling, N. Bolduan, S. Taguchi, J. Gliner, and S.M. Horvath. 1974. Effect of carbon monoxide and peroxyacetylnitrate on man's maximal aerobic capacity. *Journal of Applied Physiology* 36:288-293.
50. Roberts, W.O. 2007. Heat and cold: What does the environment do to marathon injury? *Sports Medicine* 37:400-403.

51. Sawka, M.N., R.P. Francesconi, A.J. Young, and K.B. Pandolf. 1984. Influence of hydration level and body fluids on exercise performance in the heat. *Journal of the American Medical Association* 252(9): 1165-1169.
52. Sawka, M.N., A.J. Young, R.P. Francesconi, S.R. Muza, and K.B. Pandolf. 1985. Thermoregulatory and blood responses during exercise at graded hypohydration levels. *Journal of Applied Physiology* 59:1394-1401.
53. Sharman, J.E., J.R. Cockcroft, and J.S. Coombes. 2004. Cardiovascular implications of exposure to traffic air pollution during exercise. *QJM* 97:637-643.
54. Sharkey, B.J. 1990. *Physiology of fitness.* 3rd ed. Champaign, IL: Human Kinetics.
55. Shipe, M. 2009. The effects of a pedometer intervention on the physical activity patterns of cardiac rehabilitation participants. Unpublished PhD dissertation, University of Tennessee.
56. Sutton, J.R. 1990. Exercise and the environment. In *Exercise, fitness, and health,* ed. C. Bouchard, R.J. Shephard, T. Stephens, J.R. Sutton, and B.D. McPherson, 165-178. Champaign, IL: Human Kinetics.
57. Swain, D.P., K.S. Abernathy, C.S. Smith, S.J. Lee, and S.A. Bunn. 1994. Target heart rates for the development of cardiorespiratory fitness. *Medicine and Science in Sports and Exercise* 26:112-116.
58. Swain, D.P., and B.C. Leutholtz. 1997. Heart rate reserve is equivalent to %$\dot{V}O_2$reserve, not to %$\dot{V}O_2$max. *Medicine and Science in Sports and Exercise* 29:410-414.
59. Swain, D.P., B.C. Leutholtz, M.E. King, L.A. Haas, and J.D. Branch. 1998. Relationship between % heart rate reserve and % $\dot{V}O_2$reserve in treadmill exercise. *Medicine and Science in Sports and Exercise* 30:318-321.
60. Swain, D.P., and B.A. Franklin. 2002. $\dot{V}O_2$ reserve and the minimal intensity for improving cardiorespiratory fitness. *Medicine and Science in Sports and Exercise* 34:152-157.
61. Tanaka, H., K.D. Monahan, and D.R. Seals. 2001. Age-predicted maximal heart rate revisited. *Journal of the American College of Cardiology* 37:153-156.
62. U.S. Department of Health and Human Services (HHS). 1996. *Surgeon General's report on physical activity and health.* Washington, DC: Author.
63. U.S. Department of Health and Human Services (HHS). 2010. *Healthy people 2020.* www.healthypeople.gov/2020/topicsobjectives2020/default.aspx.
64. U.S. Department of Health and Human Services (HHS). 2008. *2008 Physical Activity Guidelines for Americans.* www.health.gov/paguidelines/guidelines/default.aspx.
65. U.S. Department of Health and Human Services (HHS). 2008. Physical Activity Guidelines Advisory Committee report 2008. www.health.gov/paguidelines/committeereport.aspx.
66. Zanobetti, A., M.J. Canner, P.H. Stone, J. Schwartz, D. Sher, E. Eagan-Bengston, K.A. Gates, L.H. Hartley, H. Suh, and D.R. Gold. 2004. Ambient pollution and blood pressure in cardiac rehabilitation patients. *Circulation* 110:2184-2189.

Chapter 12

1. American College of Sports Medicine (ACSM). (in press). *ACSM's guidelines for exercise testing and prescription.* 10th ed. Baltimore: Lippincott Williams & Wilkins.
2. American College of Sports Medicine (ACSM). 2009. Appropriate physical activity intervention strategies for weight loss and prevention of weight regain for adults. *Medicine and Science in Sports and Exercise* 41(2): 459-471.
3. American College of Sports Medicine (ACSM). 2007. The female athlete triad. *Medicine and Science in Sports and Exercise* 39(10): 1867-1882.
4. American Psychiatric Association (APA). 1994. *Diagnostic and statistical manual of mental disorders.* Washington, DC: Author.
5. Bassett, D.R., P.L. Schneider, and G.E. Huntington. 2004. Physical activity in an Old Order Amish community. *Medicine and Science in Sports and Exercise* 36:79-85.
6. Beamer, B.A. 2003. Genetic influences on obesity. In *Obesity: Etiology, assessment, treatment and prevention*, ed. R.E. Anderson, 43-56. Champaign, IL: Human Kinetics.
7. Bouchard, C., L. Perusse, C. Leblanc, A. Tremblay, and G. Theriault. 1988. Inheritance of the amount and distribution of human body fat. *International Journal of Obesity* 12:205-215.
8. Cottrell, R.R. 1992. *Weight control.* Guilford, CT: Dushkin.
9. Cunningham, J.J. 1991. Body composition as a determinant of energy expenditure: A synthetic review and a proposed general prediction equation. *American Journal of Clinical Nutrition* 54:963-969.
10. DiPietro, L. 1999. Physical activity in the prevention of obesity: Current evidence and research issues. *Medicine and Science in Sports and Exercise* 31: S542-S546.
11. Flegal, K.M., M.D. Carroll, B.K. Kit, and C.L. Ogden. 2012. Prevalence of obesity and trends in the distribution of body mass index among US adults, 1999-2010. *Journal of the American Medical Association* 307(5): 491-497.
12. Flegal, K.M., M.D. Carroll, C.L. Ogden, and L.R. Curtin. 2010. Prevalence and trends in obesity among U.S. adults, 1999-2008. *Journal of the American Medical Association* 303(3): 235-241.
13. Flegal, K., M. Carroll, C. Ogden, and C. Johnson. 2002. Prevalence and trends in obesity among U.S. adults, 1999-2000. *Journal of the American Medical Association* 288:1723-1727.
14. Food and Nutrition Board, Institute of Medicine. 2002. *Dietary reference intakes for energy, carbohydrate, fiber, fat, fatty acids, cholesterol, protein, and amino acids.* Washington, DC: National Academies Press.
15. Ford, E.S., and W.H. Dietz. 2013. Trends in energy intake among adults in the United States: Findings from NHANES. *American Journal of Clinical Nutrition* 97:848-853.
16. Grundy, S.M., G. Blackburn, M. Higgins, R. Lauer, M.G. Perri, and D. Ryan. 1999. Physical activity in the prevention and treatment of obesity and its comorbidities: Roundtable consensus statement. *Medicine and Science in Sports and Exercise* 31:S502-S508.

17. Hankinson, A.L., M.L. Daviglus, C. Bouchard, M. Carnethon, C.E. Lewis, P.J. Schreiner, K. Liu, and S. Sidney. 2010. Maintaining a high physical activity level over 20 years and weight gain. *Journal of the American Medical Association* 304(23): 2603-2610.
18. Hill, J.O., and E.L. Melanson. 1999. Overview of the determinants of overweight and obesity: Current evidence and research issues. *Medicine and Science in Sports and Exercise* 31:S515-S521.
19. Holden, J.H., L.L. Darga, S.M. Olson, D.C. Stettner, E.A. Ardito, and C.P. Lucas. 1992. Long-term follow-up of patients attending a combination very-low calorie diet and behaviour therapy weight loss programme. *International Journal of Obesity* 16:605-613.
20. Hornbuckle, L.M., D.R. Bassett Jr., and D.L. Thompson. 2005. Pedometer-determined walking and body composition variables in African-American women. *Medicine and Science in Sports and Exercise* 37:1069-1074.
21. Jebb, S.A., and M.S. Moore. 1999. Contribution of a sedentary lifestyle and inactivity to the etiology of overweight and obesity: Current evidence and research issues. *Medicine and Science in Sports and Exercise* 31:S534-S541.
22. Jensen, M.D., D.H. Ryan , C.M. Apovian, J.D. Ard, A.G. Comuzzie, K.A. Donato, F.B. Hu, V.S. Hubbard, J.M. Jakicic, R.F. Kushner, C. Loria, B.E. Millen, C.A. Nonas, F.X. Pi-Sunyer, J. Stevens, V.J. Stevens, T.A. Wadden, B.M. Wolfe, and S.Z. Yanovski. 2013. 2013 AHA/ACC/TOS guideline for the management of overweight and obesity in adults: A report of the American College of Cardiology/American Heart Association Task Force on Practice Guidelines and The Obesity Society. *Circulation* 25(Suppl 2): S102-S138.
23. Johnson, M.D. 1994. Disordered eating. In *Medical and orthopedic issues of active and athletic women*, ed. R. Agostini, 141-151. Philadelphia: Hanley & Belfus.
24. Krumm, E.M., O.L. Dessieux, P. Andrews, and D.L. Thompson. 2006. The relationship between daily steps and body composition in postmenopausal women. *Journal of Women's Health* 15(2): 202-210.
25. Ladabaum, U., A. Mannalithara, P.A. Myer, and G. Singh. 2014. Obesity, abdominal obesity, physical activity, and caloric intake in US adults: 1988 to 2010. *American Journal of Medicine* 127:717-727.
26. Lavery, M.A., and J.W. Loewy. 1993. Identifying predictive variables for long-term weight change after participation in a weight loss program. *Journal of the American Dietetic Association* 93:1017-1024.
27. Lichtman, S.W., K. Pisarska, E.R. Berman, M. Pestone, H. Dowling, E. Offenbacher, H. Weisel, S. Heshka, D.E. Matthews, and S.B. Heymsfield. 1992. Discrepancy between self-reported and actual caloric intake and exercise in obese subjects. *New England Journal of Medicine* 327:1893-1898.
28. Loos, R.J.F. 2009. Recent progress in the genetics of common obesity. *British Journal of Clinical Pharmacology* 68(6): 811-829.
29. Locke, A.E., et al. 2015. Genetic studies of body mass index yield new insights for obesity biology. *Nature* 518:197-206.
30. Loos, R.J.F., and C. Bouchard. 2003. Obesity—is it a genetic disorder? *Journal of Internal Medicine* 254:401-425.
31. Molé, P.A. 1990. Impact of energy intake and exercise on resting metabolic rate. *Sports Medicine* 10:72-87.
32. Montoye, H.J., H.C.G. Kemper, W.H.M. Saris, and R.A. Washburn. 1996. *Measuring physical activity and energy expenditure.* Champaign, IL: Human Kinetics.
33. Must, A., J. Spandano, E.H. Coakley, A.E. Field, G. Colditz, and W.H. Dietz. 1999. The disease burden associated with overweight and obesity. *Journal of the American Medical Association* 282:1523-1529.
34. National Heart, Lung, and Blood Institute. 1998. *Clinical guidelines on the identification, evaluation, and treatment of overweight and obesity in adults* (NIH Publication No. 98-4083). Bethesda, MD: National Institutes of Health—National Heart, Lung, and Blood Institute.
35. Ogden, C.L., M.D. Carroll, B.K. Kit, and K.M. Flegal. 2014. Prevalence of childhood and adult obesity in the United States, 2011-2012. *Journal of the American Medical Association* 311(8): 806-814.
36. Ogden, C.L., C.D. Fryar, M.D. Carroll, and K.M. Flegal. 2004. *Mean body weight, height, and body mass index, United States 1960-2002* (Advance data from vital and health statistics; No. 347). Hyattsville, MD: National Center for Health Statistics.
37. Riera-Crichton, D., and N. Tefft. 2014. Macronutrients and obesity: Revisiting the calories in, calories out framework. *Economics and Human Biology* 14:33-49.
38. Skinner, A.C., and J.A. Skelton. 2014. Prevalence and trends in obesity and severe obesity among children in the United States, 1999-2012. *Journal of the American Medical Association Pediatrics* 168(6): 561-566.
39. Stunkard, A.J., T.I.A. Sørensen, C. Hanis, T.W. Teasdale, R. Charkraborty, W.J. Schull, and F. Schulsinger. 1986. An adoption study of human obesity. *New England Journal of Medicine* 314:193-198.
40. Thompson, D.L., J. Rakow, and S.M. Perdue. 2004. Relationship between accumulated walking and body composition in middle-aged women. *Medicine and Science in Sports and Exercise* 36:911-914.
41. Vimaleswaran, K.S., and R.J.F. Loos. 2010. Progress in the genetics of common obesity and type 2 diabetes. *Expert Reviews in Molecular Medicine* 12:e7. doi:10.1017/S1462399410001389.
42. Volpe, S.L. 2013. Weight management. In *ACSM's resource manual for guidelines for exercise testing and prescription.* 7th ed. Ed. D.P. Swain, 551-564. Baltimore: Lippincott Williams & Wilkins.
43. Wadden, T.A., and A.J. Stunkard. 1993. Psychosocial consequences of obesity and dieting: Research and clinical findings. In *Obesity: Theory and therapy*, ed. A.J. Stunkard and T.A. Wadden, 163-177. New York: Raven Press.
44. Welle, S., G.B. Forbes, M. Statt, R.R. Barnard, and J.M. Amatruda. 1992. Energy expenditure under free-living conditions in normal-weight and overweight women. *American Journal of Clinical Nutrition* 55:14-21.

45. Westerterp, K.R. 2000. The assessment of energy and nutrient intake in humans. In *Physical activity and obesity*, ed. C. Bouchard, 133-149. Champaign, IL: Human Kinetics.
46. Williamson, D.F., J. Madans, R.F. Anda, J.C. Kleinman, H.S. Kahn, and T. Byers. 1993. Recreational physical activity and ten-year weight change in a US national cohort. *International Journal of Obesity* 17:279-286.
47. Wing, R.R., and J.O. Hill. 2001. Successful weight loss maintenance. *Annual Review of Nutrition* 21:323-341.
48. Wright, J.D., J. Kennedy-Stephenson, C.Y. Wang, M.A. McDowell, and C.L. Johnson. 2004. Trends in intake of energy and macronutrients—United States, 1971-2000. *Morbidity and Mortality Weekly Report* 53:80-82.
49. Wright, J.D., and C.-Y. Wang. 2010. Trends in intake of energy and macronutrients in adults from 1999-2000 through 2007-2008. *NCHS Data Brief*, no. 49.

Chapter 13

1. American Association of Cardiovascular and Pulmonary Rehabilitation (AACVPR). 2006. *AACVPR cardiac rehabilitation resource manual.* Champaign, IL: Human Kinetics.
2. American College of Obstetricians and Gynecologists (ACOG). 2002. Exercise during pregnancy and the postpartum period. *International Journal of Gynecology and Obstetrics* 77:79-81.
3. American College of Sports Medicine (ACSM). 2007. *ACSM's health/fitness facility standards and guidelines.* 3rd ed. Champaign, IL: Human Kinetics.
4. American College of Sports Medicine (ACSM). 2009. Exercise and physical activity for older adults. *Medicine and Science in Sports and Exercise* 41:1510-1530.
5. American College of Sports Medicine (ACSM). 2009. Progression models in resistance training for healthy adults. *Medicine and Science in Sports and Exercise* 41:687-708.
6. American College of Sports Medicine (ACSM). (in press). *ACSM's guidelines for exercise testing and prescription.* 10th ed. Philadelphia: Lippincott Williams & Wilkins.
7. Artero, E., D. Lee, C. Lavie, V. España-Romero, X. Sui, T. Church, and S. Blair. 2012. Effects of muscular strength on cardiovascular risk factors and prognosis. *Journal of Cardiopulmonary Rehabilitation and Prevention* 32:351-358.
8. Baechle, T., and W. Westcott. 2010. *Fitness professional's guide to strength training for older adults.* Champaign, IL: Human Kinetics.
9. Barakat, R., A. Lucia, and J. Ruiz. 2009. Resistance exercise training during pregnancy and newborn's birth size: A randomized controlled trial. *International Journal of Obesity* 33:1048-1057.
10. Behm, D., and A. Chaouachi. 2011. A review of the acute effects of static and dynamic stretching on performance. *European Journal of Applied Physiology* 111:2633-2651.
11. Behm, D., A. Faigenbaum, B. Falk, and P. Klentrou. 2008. Canadian Society for Exercise Physiology position paper: Resistance training for children and adolescents. *Applied Physiology Nutrition and Metabolism* 33:547-561.
12. Behm, D., and J. Colado Sanchez. 2013. Instability resistance training across the exercise continuum. *Sports Health* 5:500-503.
13. Behringer, M., A. vom Heede, Z. Yue, and J. Mester. 2010. Effects of resistance training in children and adolescents: A meta-analysis. *Pediatrics* 126:e1199-e1210.
14. Bompa, T., and G. Haff. 2009. *Periodization.* 5th ed. Champaign, IL: Human Kinetics.
15. Brown, L. 2000. *Isokinetics in human performance.* Champaign, IL: Human Kinetics.
16. Campos, G., T. Luecke, H. Wendeln, K. Toma, F. Hagerman, T. Murray, K. Ragg, N. Ratamess, W. Kraemer, and R. Staron. 2002. Muscular adaptations in response to three different resistance training regimens: Specificity of repetition maximum training zones. *European Journal of Applied Physiology* 88:50-60.
17. Chang, Y.K., C.Y. Pan, F.T. Chen, C.L. Tsai, and C.C. Huang. 2012. Effect of resistance-exercise training on cognitive function in healthy older adults: A review. *Journal of Aging and Physical Activity* 20:497-517.
18. Chu, D., and G. Myer. 2013. *Plyometrics.* Champaign, IL: Human Kinetics.
19. Clarkson, P. 2006. Case report of exertional rhabdomyolysis in a 12-year-old boy. *Medicine and Science in Sports and Exercise* 38:197-200.
20. De Onis, M., J. Blössner, and E. Borghi. 2010. Global prevalence and trends of overweight and obesity among preschool children. *American Journal of Clinical Nutrition* 92:1257-1264.
21. De Salles, B.F., R. Simão, F. Miranda, S. Novaes Jda, A. Lemos, and J.M. Willardson. 2009. Rest interval between sets in strength training. *Sports Medicine* 39:765-777.
22. DeLorme, T., and A. Watkins. 1948. Techniques of progressive resistance exercise. *Archives of Physical Medicine and Rehabilitation* 29:263-273.
23. Dempsey, J., C. Butler, and M. Williams. 2005. No need for a pregnant pause: Physical activity may reduce the occurrence of gestational diabetes mellitus and preclampsia. *Exercise and Sport Science Reviews* 33:141-149.
24. DiFiori, J., H. Benjamin, J. Brenner, A. Gregory, N. Jayanthi, G.L. Landry, and A. Luke. 2014. Overuse injuries and burnout in youth sports: A position statement from the American Medical Society for Sports Medicine. *Clinical Journal of Sports Medicine* 24:3-20.
25. Drinkwater, B. 1995. Weight-bearing exercise and bone mass. *Physical Medicine and Rehabilitation Clinics of North America* 6:567-578.
26. Evenson, K.R., R. Barakat, W. Brown, P. Dargent-Molina, M. Haruna, E. Mikkelsen, M. Mottola, K. Owe, E. Rousham, and S. Yeo. 2014. Guidelines for physical activity during pregnancy: Comparisons from around the world. *American Journal of Lifestyle Medicine* 8:102-121.
27. Faigenbaum, A.D., R. Lloyd, and G. Myer. 2013. Youth resistance training: Past practices, new perspectives, and future directions. *Pediatric Exercise Science* 25:591-604.
28. Faigenbaum, A., and G. Myer. 2010. Resistance training among young athletes: Safety, efficacy and injury prevention effects. *British Journal of Sports Medicine* 44:56-63.
29. Faigenbaum, A., W. Kraemer, C. Blimkie, I. Jeffreys, L. Micheli, M. Nitka, and T. Rowland. 2009. Youth resist-

ance training: Updated position statement paper from the National Strength and Conditioning Association. *Journal of Strength and Conditioning Research* 23(Suppl. 5): S60-S79.

30. Faigenbaum, A., and W. Westcott. 2009. *Youth strength training.* Champaign, IL: Human Kinetics.

31. Fiatarone, M.A., E.C. Marks, N.D. Ryan, C.N. Meredith, L.A. Lipsitz, and W. Evans. 1990. High-intensity strength training in nonagenarians: Effects on skeletal muscle. *Journal of the American Medical Association* 263:3029-3034.

32. Fleck, S., and W. Kraemer. 2014. *Designing resistance training programs.* 4th ed. Champaign, IL: Human Kinetics.

33. Fleg, J., D. Forman, K. Berra, V. Bittner, J. Blumenthal, M. Chen, S. Cheng, D. Kitzman, M. Maurer, M. Rich, W. Shen, M. Williams, S. Zieman, and American Heart Association Committees on Older Populations and Exercise Cardiac Rehabilitation and Prevention of the Council on Clinical Cardiology, Council on Cardiovascular and Stroke Nursing, and Council on Lifestyle and Cardiometabolic Health. 2013. Secondary prevention of atherosclerotic cardiovascular disease in older adults: A scientific statement from the American Heart Association. *Circulation* 128:2422-2446.

34. Fletcher, G.F., P.A. Ades, P. Kligfield, R. Arena, G.J. Balady, V.A. Bittner, L.A. Coke, J.L. Fleg, D.E. Forman, T.C. Gerber, M. Gulati, K. Madan, J. Rhodes, P.D. Thompson, M.A. Williams, and American Heart Association Exercise, Cardiac Rehabilitation, and Prevention Committee of the Council on Clinical Cardiology, Council on Nutrition, Physical Activity and Metabolism, Council on Cardiovascular and Stroke Nursing, and Council on Epidemiology and Prevention. 2013. Exercise standards for testing and training: A scientific statement from the American Heart Association. *Circulation* 128:873-934.

35. Fletcher, I., and M. Monte-Colombo. 2010. An investigation into the possible physiological mechanisms associated with changes in performance related to acute response to different preactivity stretch modalities. *Applied Physiology Nutrition and Metabolism* 35:27-34.

36. Fröhlich, M., E. Emrich, and D. Schmidtbleicher. 2010. Outcome effects of single-set versus multiple-set training—an advanced replication study. *Research in Sports Medicine* 18:157-175.

37. Garber, C., B. Blissmer, M.R. Deschenes, B.A. Franklin, M.J. Lamonte, I. Lee, D.C. Nieman, and D.P. Swain. 2011. American College of Sports Medicine position stand. Quantity and quality of exercise for developing and maintaining cardiorespiratory, musculoskeletal, and neuromotor fitness in apparently healthy adults: Guidance for prescribing exercise. *Medicine and Science in Sports and Exercise* 43:1334-1359.

38. Garshasbi, A., and S. Zadeh. 2005. The effect of exercise on the intensity of low back pain in pregnant women. *International Journal of Gynecology and Obstetrics* 88:271-275.

39. Gaston, A., and H. Prapavessis. 2013. Tired, moody and pregnant? Exercise may be the answer. *Psychological Health* 28:1353-1369.

40. Gentil, P., and M. Bottaro. 2010. Influence of supervision ratio on muscle adaptations to resistance training in nontrained subjects. *Journal of Strength and Conditioning Research* 24:639-643.

41. Glass, S., and D. Stanton. 2004. Self-selected resistance training intensity in novice weightlifters. *Journal of Strength and Conditioning Research* 18:324-327.

42. Goldberg, L., and P. Twist. 2007. *Strength ball training.* Champaign, IL: Human Kinetics.

43. Gunter, K., H. Almstedt, and K. Janz. 2012. Physical activity in childhood may be the key to optimizing lifespan skeletal health. *Exercise and Sport Sciences Reviews* 40:13-21.

44. Haff, G., and T. McBride. 2015. *Essentials of strength training and conditioning.* 4th ed. Champaign, IL: Human Kinetics.

45. Harries, S., D. Lubans, and R. Callister. 2014. Systematic review and meta-analysis of linear and undulating periodized resistance training programs on muscular strength. *Journal of Strength and Conditioning Research* (epub ahead of print).

46. Harris, C., M. DeBeliso, K.J. Adams, B. Irmischer, and T. Spitzer Gibson. 2007. Detraining in the older adult: Effects of prior training intensity on strength retention. *Journal of Strength and Conditioning Research* 21:813-818.

47. Harris, C., K. Watson, S. Carlson, J. Fulton, and J. Dorn. 2013. Adult participation in aerobic and muscle strengthening physical activities—United States, 2011. *Morbidity and Mortality Weekly Reports* 62:326-330.

48. Hatfield, D., W.J. Kraemer, B. Spiering, K. Häkkinen, J.S. Volek, T. Shimano, L. Spreuwenberg, R. Silvestre, J. Vingren, M. Fragala, A. Gómez, S. Fleck, R. Newton, and C. Maresh. 2006. The impact of velocity of movement on performance factors in resistance exercise. *Journal of Strength and Conditioning Research* 20:760-766.

49. Hettinger, R., and E. Muller. 1953. Muskelleistung und muskeltraining (Muscle achievement and muscle training). *ArbeitsPhysiologie* 15:111-126.

50. Hibbs, A., K. Thompson, D. French, A. Wrigley, and I. Spears. 2008. Optimizing performance by improving core stability and core strength. *Sports Medicine* 38:995-1008.

51. Hoeger, W., S. Barette, D. Hale, and D. Hopkins. 1987. Relationship between repetitions and selected percentages on the one repetition maximum. *Journal of Applied Sport Science Research* 1:11-13.

52. Karandikar, N., and O. Vargas. 2011. Kinetic chains: A review of the concept and its clinical applications. *Physical Medicine and Rehabilitation* 3:739-745.

53. Keeler, L., L. Finkelstein, W. Miller, and B. Fernhall. 2001. Early phase adaptations to traditional speed vs. super slow resistance training on strength and aerobic capacity in sedentary individuals. *Journal of Strength and Conditioning Research* 15:309-314.

54. Kerr, Z., C. Collins, and R. Comstock. Epidemiology of weight training related injuries presenting to United States emergency room departments, 1990-2007. *American Journal of Sports Medicine* 38:765-771.

55. Kraemer, W., B. Noble, B. Culver, and M. Clark. 1987. Physiologic responses to heavy resistance exercise with very short rest periods. *International Journal of Sports Medicine* 8:247-252.

56. Krieger, J. 2009. Single versus multiple sets of resistance exercise: A meta-regression. *Journal of Strength and Conditioning Research* 23:1890-1901.

57. Liu-Ambrose, T., and M. Donaldson. 2009. Exercise and cognition in older adults: Is there a role for resistance training programmes? *British Journal of Sports Medicine* 43:25-27.

58. Lloyd, R., A. Faigenbaum, M. Stone, J. Oliver, I. Jeffreys, J.A. Moody, C. Brewer, K. Pierce, T. McCambridge, R. Howard, L. Herrington, B. Hainline, L. Micheli, R. Jaques, W. Kraemer, M. McBride, T. Best, D. Chu, B. Alvar, and G. Myer. 2014. Position statement on youth resistance training: The 2014 International Consensus. *British Journal of Sports Medicine* 48:498-505.

59. Loustalot, F., S. Carlson, J. Kruger, D.M. Buchner, and J.E. Fulton. 2013. Muscle-strengthening activities and participation among adults in the United States. *Research Quarterly for Exercise and Sport* 84:30-38.

60. Malina, R. 2006. Weight training in youth—growth, maturation and safety: An evidenced-based review. *Clinical Journal of Sports Medicine* 16:478-487.

61. Mazzetti, S., W. Kraemer, J. Volek, N. Duncan, N. Ratamess, A. Gomez, R. Newton, K. Hakkinen, and S. Fleck. 2000. The influence of direct supervision of resistance training on strength performance. *Medicine and Science in Sports and Exercise* 32:1175-1184.

62. McGuigan, M.R., M. Tatasciore, R.U. Newton, et al. 2009. Eight weeks of resistance training can significantly alter body composition in children who are overweight or obese. *Journal of Strength and Conditioning Research* 23:80-85.

63. Mediate, P., and A. Faigenbaum. 2007. *Medicine ball training for all kids.* Monterey Bay, CA: Healthy Learning.

64. Meeusen, R., M. Duclos, C. Foster, A. Fry, M. Gleeson, D. Nieman, J. Raglin, G. Rietjens, J. Steinacker, A. Urhausen, European College of Sport Science, and American College of Sports Medicine. 2013. Prevention, diagnosis, and treatment of the overtraining syndrome: Joint consensus statement of the European College of Sport Science and the American College of Sports Medicine. *Medicine and Science in Sports and Exercise* 45:186-205.

65. Menezes, A., C. Lavie, R. Milani, D. Forman, M. King, and M. Williams. 2014. Cardiac rehabilitation in the United States. *Progress in Cardiovascular Diseases* 56:522-529.

66. Mudd, L.M., K.M. Owe, M.F. Mottola, and J.M. Pivarnik. 2013. Health benefits of physical activity during pregnancy: An international perspective. *Medicine and Science in Sports and Exercise* 45:268-277.

67. Myer, G., A.D. Faigenbaum, K. Ford, T. Best, M. Bergeron, and T. Hewett. 2011. When to initiate integrative neuromuscular training to reduce sports-related injuries and enhance health in youth? *Current Sports Medicine Reports* 10:155-166.

68. Myer, G., C. Quatman, J. Khoury, E. Wall, and T. Hewett. 2009. Youth vs. adult "weightlifting" injuries presented to United States emergency rooms: Accidental vs. non-accidental injury mechanisms. *Journal of Strength and Conditioning Research* 23:2054-2060.

69. Nelson, M., M. Fiatarone, C. Morganti, I. Trice, R. Greenberg, and W. Evans. 1994. Effects of high intensity strength training on multiple risk factors for osteoporotic fractures. *Journal of the American Medical Association* 272:1909-1914.

70. Ogden, C., M. Carroll, B. Kit, and K. Flegal. 2014. Prevalence of childhood and adult obesity in the United States, 2011-2012. *Journal of the American Medical Association* 311:806-814.

71. Pahor, M., J. Guralnik, W. Ambrosius, S. Blair, D. Bonds, T. Church, M. Espeland, R. Fielding, T. Gill, E. Groessl, A. King, S. Kritchevsky, T. Manini, M. McDermott, M. Miller, A. Newman, W. Rejeski, K. Sink, J. Williamson; LIFE study investigators. 2014. Effect of structured physical activity on prevention of major mobility disability in older adults: The LIFE study randomized clinical trial. *Journal of the American Medical Association* 311:2387-2396.

72. Peterson, M., M. Rhea, and B. Alvar. 2005. Applications of the dose response for muscular strength development: A review of meta-analytic efficacy and reliability for designing training prescription. *Journal of Strength and Conditioning Research* 19:950-958.

73. Petrov Fieril K., A. Glantz, and M. Fagevik Olsen. 2014. The efficacy of moderate-to-vigorous resistance exercise during pregnancy: A randomized controlled trial. *Acta Obstetricia Gynecologica Scandinavica* (epub ahead of print).

74. Petrov Fieril, K., M. Fagevik Olsén, A. Glantz, and M. Larsson. 2014. Experiences of exercise during pregnancy among women who perform regular resistance training: A qualitative study. *Physical Therapy* 94:1135-1143.

75. Pivarnik, J., H. Chambliss, J. Clapp, S. Dugan, M. Hatch, C. Lovelady, M. Mottola, and M. Williams. 2006. Impact of physical activity during pregnancy and postpartum on chronic disease risk. *Medicine and Science in Sports and Exercise* 38:989-1006.

76. Purves-Smith, F., N. Sgarioto, and R. Hepple. 2014. Fiber typing in aging muscle. *Exercise and Sport Science Reviews* 42:45-52.

77. Quatman, C., G. Myer, J. Khoury, E. Wall, and T. Hewett. Sex differences in "weightlifting" injuries presenting to United States emergency rooms. *Journal of Strength and Conditioning Research* 23:2061-2067.

78. Ratamess, N. 2012. *ACSM's foundations of strength training and conditioning.* Philadelphia: Lippincott Williams & Wilkins.

79. Ratamess, N., A. Faigenbaum, J. Hoffman, and J. Kang. 2008. Self-selected resistance training intensity in healthy women: The influence of a personal trainer. *Journal of Strength and Conditioning Research* 22:103-111.

80. Ratamess, N., M. Falvo, G. Mangine, J. Hoffman, A. Faigenbaum, and J. Kang. 2007. The effect of rest interval length on metabolic responses to the bench press exercise. *European Journal of Applied Physiology* 100:1-17.

81. Reid, K., K. Martin, G. Doros, D. Clark, C. Hau, C. Patten, E. Phillips, W. Frontera, and R. Fielding. 2014. Comparative effects of light or heavy resistance power training for improving lower extremity power and physical performance in mobility-limited older adults. *Journals of Gerontology Series A* (epub ahead of print).

82. Rhea, M., B. Alvar, L. Brukett, and S. Ball. 2003. A meta-analysis to determine the dose response for strength development. *Medicine and Science in Sports and Exercise* 35:456-464.

83. Rhea, M., and B. Alderman. 2004. A meta-analysis of periodized versus nonperiodized strength and power training programs. *Research Quarterly for Exercise and Sport* 75:413-422.

84. Robbins, D. 2005. Postactivation potentiation and its practical application. *Journal of Strength and Conditioning Research* 19:453-458.

85. Roberts, C.K., M.M. Lee, M. Katiraie, S.L. Krell, S.S. Angadi, M.K. Chronley, C.S. Oh, V. Ribas, R.A. Harris, A.L. Hevener, and D.M. Croymans. 2014. Strength fitness and body weight status on markers of cardiometabolic health. *Medicine and Science in Sports and Exercise* (epub ahead of print).

86. Rössler, R., L. Donath, E. Verhagen, A. Junge, T. Schweizer, and O. Faude. 2014. Exercise-based injury prevention in child and adolescent sport: A systematic review and meta-analysis. *Sports Medicine* 44:1733-1748.

87. Sáez-Sáez de Villarreal, E., B. Requena, and R.U. Newton. 2010. Does plyometric training improve strength performance? A meta-analysis. *Journal of Science and Medicine in Sport* 13:513-522.

88. Schranz, N., G. Tomkinson, and T. Olds. 2013. What is the effect of resistance training on the strength, body composition and psychosocial status of overweight and obese children and adolescents? A systematic review and meta-analysis. *Sports Medicine* 43:893-907.

89. Schranz, N., G. Tomkinson, N. Parletta, J. Petkov, and T. Olds. 2013. Can resistance training change the strength, body composition and self-concept of overweight and obese adolescent males? A randomised controlled trial. *British Journal of Sports Medicine* 48:1482-1488.

90. Shaibi, G., M. Cruz, G. Ball, M. Weigensberg, G. Salem, N. Crespo, and M. Goran. 2006. Effects of resistance training on insulin sensitivity in overweight Latino adolescent males. *Medicine and Science in Sports and Exercise* 38:1208-1215.

91. Shimano, T., W. Kraemer, B. Sppiering, J. Volek, D. Hatfield, R. Silvestre, J. Vingren, M. Fragala, C. Maresh, S. Fleck, R. Newton, L. Spreuwenberg, and K. Hakkinen. 2008. Relationship between the number of repetitions and selected percentages of one repetition maximum in free weight exercises in trained and untrained men. *Journal of Strength and Conditioning Research* 20:819-823.

92. Sigal, R., A. Alberga, G. Goldfield, D. Prud'homme, S. Hadjiyannakis, R. Gougeon, P. Phillips, H. Tulloch, J. Malcolm, S. Doucette, G. Wells, J. Ma, and G. Kenny. 2014. Effects of aerobic training, resistance training, or both on percentage body fat and cardiometabolic risk markers in obese adolescents: The healthy eating aerobic and resistance training in youth randomized clinical trial. *Journal of the American Medical Association Pediatrics* 168:1006-1014.

93. Silva, N.L., R.B. Oliveira, S.J. Fleck, A.C. Leon, and P. Farinatti. 2014. Influence of strength training variables on strength gains in adults over 55 years old: A meta-analysis of dose–response relationships. *Journal of Science in Medicine and Sport* 17:337-344.

94. Simão, R., B. de Salles, T. Figueiredo, I. Dias, and J. Willardson. 2012. Exercise order in resistance training. *Sports Medicine* 42:251-265.

95. Simic, L., N. Sarabon, and G. Markovic. 2013. Does pre-exercise static stretching inhibit maximal muscular performance? A meta-analytical review. *Scandinavian Journal of Medicine and Science in Sports* 23:131-148.

96. Smith, J., N. Eather, P. Morgan, R. Plotnikoff, A. Faigenbaum, and D. Lubans. 2014. The health benefits of muscular fitness for children and adolescents: A systematic review and meta-analysis. *Sports Medicine* 44:1209-1223.

97. Spaulding, A., and L. Kelly. 2010. *Fitness on the ball.* Champaign, IL: Human Kinetics.

98. Steib, S., D. Schoene, and K. Pfeifer. 2009. Dose–relationship of resistance training in older adults: A meta-analysis. *Medicine and Science in Sports and Exercise* 42:902-914.

99. Stone, M.H., H. O'Bryant, and J. Garhammer. 1981. A hypothetical model for strength training. *Journal of Sports Medicine* 21:342-351.

100. Thiebaud, R., M. Funk, and T. Abe. 2014. Home-based resistance training for older adults: A systematic review. *Geriatrics and Gerontology International* (epub before print).

101. Thompson, W. 2014. *ACSM's resources for the personal trainer.* 4th ed. Philadelphia: Lippincott, Williams & Wilkins.

102. Thompson, W. 2013. Worldwide survey of fitness trends for 2014. *ACSM's Health and Fitness Journal* 17:10-20.

103. United States Department of Health and Human Services (HHS). *2008 Physical Activity Guidelines for Americans.* www.health.gov/paguidelines.

104. Van der Heijden, G., Z. Wang, Z. Chu, G. Toffolo, E. Manesso, P. Sauer, and A. Sunehag. 2010. Strength exercise improves muscle mass and hepatic insulin sensitivity in obese youth. *Medicine and Science in Sports and Exercise* 42:1973-1980.

105. Westcott, W.L. 2012. Resistance training is medicine: Effects of strength training on health. *Current Sports Medicine Reports* 11:209-216.

106. White, E., J. Pivarnik, and K. Pfeiffer. 2014. Resistance training during pregnancy and perinatal outcomes. *Journal of Physical Activity and Health* 11:1141-1148.

107. Wilson, J.M., N. Duncan, P. Marin, L. Brown, J. Loenneke, S. Wilson, E. Jo, R. Lowery, and C. Ugrinowitsch. 2013. Meta-analysis of postactivation potentiation and power: Effects of conditioning activity, volume, gender, rest periods, and training status. *Journal of Strength and Conditioning Research* 27:854-859.

108. Williams, M., W. Haskell, P. Ades, E. Amsterdam, V. Bittner, B. Franklin, M. Gulanick, S. Laing, and K. Stewart. 2007. Resistance exercise in individuals with and without cardiovascular disease: 2007 update. *Circulation* 116:572-584.

109. Williams, M., and K. Stewart. 2009. Impact of strength and resistance training on cardiovascular disease risk factors and outcomes in older adults. *Clinics in Geriatric Medicine* 25:703-714.

110. World Health Organization (WHO). 2010. *Global recommendations on physical activity.* Geneva: Author.

Chapter 14

1. American College of Sports Medicine (ACSM). 2011. *ACSM's complete guide to fitness and health.* Champaign, IL: Human Kinetics.
2. Ahmed, R., S. Shakil-ur-Rehman, and F. Sibtain. 2014. Comparison between specific lumber mobilization and core-stability exercises with core-stability exercises alone in mechanical low back pain. *Pakistan Journal of Medical Sciences* 30:157-160.
3. Akuthota, V., A. Ferreiro, T. Moore, and M. Fredericson. 2008. Core stability exercise principles. *Current Sports Medicine Reports* 7:39-44.
4. Akuthota, V., and S.F. Nadler. 2004. Core strengthening. *Archives of Physical Medicine and Rehabilitation* 85:S86-S92.
5. Axler, C.T., and S.M. McGill. 1997. Low back loads over a variety of abdominal exercises: Searching for the safest abdominal challenge. *Medicine and Science in Sports and Exercise* 29:804-811.
6. Ayala, F., P.S. de Baranda, M. De Ste Croix, and F. Santonja. 2013. Comparison of active stretching technique in males with normal and limited hamstring flexibility. *Physical Therapy in Sport* 14:98-104.
7. Bandy, W.D., J.M. Irion, and M. Briggler. 1998. The effect of static stretch and dynamic range of motion training on the flexibility of the hamstring muscles. *Journal of Orthopaedic & Sports Physical Therapy* 27:295-300.
8. Barker, K.L., D.R. Shamley, and D. Jackson. 2004. Changes in the cross-sectional area of multifidus and psoas in patients with unilateral back pain—the relationship to pain and disability. *Spine* 29:E515-E519.
9. Bergmark, A. 1989. Stability of the lumbar spine: A study in mechanical engineering. *Acta Orthopaedica Scandinavica Supplementum* 230:1-54.
10. Biering-Sorensen, F. 1984. Physical measurements as risk indicators for low-back trouble over a one-year period. *Spine (Phila Pa 1976)* 9:106-119.
11. Bogduk, N. 1998. *Clinical anatomy of the lumbar spine and sacrum.* London: Churchill Livingstone.
12. Borghuis, J., A.L. Hof, and K. Lemmink. 2008. The importance of sensory-motor control in providing core stability implications for measurement and training. *Sports Medicine* 38:893-916.
13. Bressel, E., D.G. Dolny, C. Vandenberg, and J.B. Cronin. 2012. Trunk muscle activity during spine stabilization exercises performed in a pool. *Physical Therapy in Sport* 13:67-72.
14. Chanthapetch, P., R. Kanlayanaphotporn, C. Gaogasigam, and A. Chiradejnant. 2009. Abdominal muscle activity during abdominal hollowing in four starting positions. *Manual Therapy* 14:642-646.
15. Cho, M. 2015. The effects of bridge exercise with the abdominal drawing-in maneuver on an unstable surface on the abdominal muscle thickness of healthy adults. *Journal of Physical Therapy Science* 27:255-257.
16. Cho, M. 2013. The effects of modified wall squat exercises on average adults' deep abdominal muscle thickness and lumbar stability. *Journal of Physical Therapy Science* 25:689-692.
17. Cipriani, D., B. Abel, and D. Pirrwitz. 2003. A comparison of two stretching protocols on hip range of motion: Implications for total daily stretch duration. *Journal of Strength and Conditioning Research* 17: 274-278.
18. Cramer, H., R. Lauche, H. Haller, and G. Dobos. 2013. A systematic review and meta-analysis of yoga for low back pain. *Clinical Journal of Pain* 29:450-460.
19. Critchley, D.J., Z. Pierson, and G. Battersby. 2011. Effect of Pilates mat exercises and conventional exercise programmes on transversus abdominis and obliquus internus abdominis activity: Pilot randomised trial. *Manual Therapy* 16:183-189.
20. De Baranda, P.S., and F. Ayala. 2010. Chronic flexibility improvement after 12 week of stretching program utilizing the ACSM recommendations: Hamstring flexibility. *International Journal of Sports Medicine* 31:389-396.
21. Ellison, J.B., S.J. Rose, and S.A. Sahrmann. 1990. Patterns of hip rotation range of motion: A comparison between healthy subjects and patients with low-back-pain. *Physical Therapy* 70:537-541.
22. Endleman, I., and D.J. Critchley. 2008. Transversus abdominis and obliquus internus activity during Pilates exercises: Measurement with ultrasound scanning. *Archives of Physical Medicine and Rehabilitation* 89:2205-2212.
23. Faries, M.D., and M. Greenwood. 2007. Core training: Stabilizing the confusion. *Strength and Conditioning Journal* 29:10-25.
24. Feland, J.B., J.W. Myrer, S.S. Schulthies, G.W. Fellingham, and G.W. Measom. 2001. The effect of duration of stretching of the hamstring muscle group for increasing range of motion in people aged 65 years or older. *Physical Therapy* 81:1110-1117.
25. Gagnon, L. 2005. Efficacy of Pilates exercises as therapeutic intervention in treating patients with low back pain. PhD diss., University of Tennessee.
26. Garber, C.E., B. Blissmer, M.R. Deschenes, B.A. Franklin, M.J. Lamonte, I.M. Lee, D.C. Nieman, D.P. Swain, and American College of Sports Medicine (ACSM). 2011. American College of Sports Medicine position stand. Quantity and quality of exercise for developing and maintaining cardiorespiratory, musculoskeletal, and neuromotor fitness in apparently healthy adults: Guidance for prescribing exercise. *Medicine and Science in Sports and Exercise* 43:1334-1359.
27. Garcia-Vaquero, M.P., J.M. Moreside, E. Brontons-Gil, N. Peco-Gonzalez, and F.J. Vera-Garcia. 2012. Trunk muscle activation during stabilization exercises with single and double leg support. *Journal of Electromyography and Kinesiology* 22:398-406.
28. Gulick, D. 2009. *Ortho notes: Clinical examination pocket guide.* Philadelphia: F.A. Davis.
29. Hadala, M., and S. Gryckiewicz. 2014. The effectiveness of lumbar extensor training: local stabilization or dynamic

strengthening exercises: A review of literature. *Ortopedia, Traumatologia, Rehabilitacja* 16:561-572.

30. Hajihosseinali, M., N. Arjmand, and A. Shirazi-Adl. 2015. Effect of body weight on spinal loads in various activities: A personalized biomechanical modeling approach. *Journal of Biomechanics* 48:276-282.
31. Hall, A.M., C.G. Maher, P. Lam, M. Ferreira, and J. Latimer. 2011. Tai chi exercise for treatment of pain and disability in people with persistent low back pain: A randomized controlled trial. *Arthritis Care & Research* 63:1576-1583.
32. Hamill, J.K.K. 2003. *Biomechanical basis of human movement.* Philadelphia: Williams & Wilkins.
33. Hasebe, K., K. Sairyo, Y. Hada, A. Dezawa, Y. Okubo, K. Kaneoka, and Y. Nakamura. 2014. Spino-pelvic rhythm with forward trunk bending in normal subjects without low back pain. *European Journal of Orthopaedic Surgery & Traumatology* 24(Suppl. 1): S193-S199.
34. Hides, J., C. Gilmore, W. Stanton, and E. Bohlscheid. 2008. Multifidus size and symmetry among chronic LBP and healthy asymptomatic subjects. *Manual Therapy* 13:43-49.
35. Hides, J., W. Stanton, M.D. Mendis, and M. Sexton. 2011. The relationship of transversus abdominis and lumbar multifidus clinical muscle tests in patients with chronic low back pain. *Manual Therapy* 16:573-577.
36. Hides, J., S. Wilson, W. Stanton, S. McMahon, H. Keto, K. McMahon, M. Bryant, and C. Richardson. 2006. An MRI investigation into the function of the transversus abdominis muscle during "drawing-in" of the abdominal wall. *Spine* 31:E175-E178.
37. Hides, J.A., G.A. Jull, and C.A. Richardson. Long-term effects of specific stabilizing exercises for first-episode low back pain. 2001. *Spine* 26:E243-248.
38. Hides, J.A., C.A. Richardson, and G.A. Jull. 1996. Multifidus muscle recovery is not automatic after resolution of acute, first-episode low back pain. *Spine* 21:2763-2769.
39. Hodges, P.W. 1999. Is there a role for transversus abdominis in lumbo-pelvic stability? *Manual Therapy* 4:74-86.
40. Hodges, P.W., J.E. Butler, D.K. McKenzie, and S.C. Gandevia. 1997. Contraction of the human diaphragm during rapid postural adjustments. *Journal of Physiology* 505(Pt. 2): 539-548.
41. Hodges, P.W., and C.A. Richardson. 1999. Altered trunk muscle recruitment in people with low back pain with upper limb movement at different speeds. *Archives of Physical Medicine and Rehabilitation* 80:1005-1012.
42. Hodges, P.W., and C.A. Richardson. 1997. Contraction of the abdominal muscles associated with movement of the lower limb. *Physical Therapy* 77:132-142; discussion 142-134.
43. Hodges, P.W., and C.A. Richardson. 1997. Feedforward contraction of transversus abdominis is not influenced by the direction of arm movement. *Experimental Brain Research* 114:362-370.
44. Hodges, P.W., and C.A. Richardson. 1996. Inefficient muscular stabilization of the lumbar spine associated with low back pain: A motor control evaluation of transversus abdominis. *Spine* 21:2640-2650.
45. Hoy, D., C. Bain, G. Williams, L. March, P. Brooks, F. Blyth, A. Woolf, T. Vos, and R. Buchbinder. 2012. A systematic review of the global prevalence of low back pain. *Arthritis and Rheumatism* 64:2028-2037.
46. Imai, A., K. Kaneoka, Y. Okubo, I. Shiina, M. Tatsumura, S. Izumi, and H. Shiraki. 2010. Trunk muscle activity during lumbar stabilization exercises on both a stable and unstable surface. *Journal of Orthopaedic & Sports Physical Therapy* 40:369-375.
47. Juker, D., S. McGill, P. Kropf, and T. Steffen. 1998. Quantitative intramuscular myoelectric activity of lumbar portions of psoas and the abdominal wall during a wide variety of tasks. *Medicine and Science in Sports and Exercise* 30:301-310.
48. Kim, B.I., J.H. Jung, J. Shim, H.Y. Kwon, and H. Kim. 2014. An analysis of muscle activities of healthy women during Pilates exercises in a prone position. *Journal of Physical Therapy Science* 26:77-79.
49. Kim, M.J., D.W. Oh, and H.J. Park. 2013. Integrating arm movement into bridge exercise: Effect on EMG activity of selected trunk muscles. *Journal of Electromyography and Kinesiology* 23:1119-1123.
50. Kim, S.J., O.Y. Kwon, C.H. Yi, H.S. Jeon, J.S. Oh, H.S. Cynn, and J.H. Weon. 2011. Comparison of abdominal muscle activity during a single-legged hold in the hook-lying position on the floor and on a round foam roll. *Journal of Athletic Training* 46:403-408.
51. Kim, T.H.M., S. Dogra, B. Al-Sahab, and H. Tamim. 2014. Comparison of functional fitness outcomes in experienced and inexperienced older adults after 16-week tai chi program. *Alternative Therapies in Health and Medicine* 20:20-25.
52. Kolber, M.J., and J. Zepeda. 2004. Addressing hamstring flexibility in athletes with lower back pain: A discussion of commonly prescribed stretching exercises. *Strength and Conditioning Journal* 26:18-23.
53. Kweon, M., S. Hong, G.U. Jang, Y.M. Ko, and J.W. Park. 2013. The neural control of spinal stability muscles during different respiratory patterns. *Journal of Physical Therapy Science* 25:1421-1424.
54. Li, G.C., H. Yuan, and W. Zhang. 2014. Effects of tai chi on health-related quality of life in patients with chronic conditions: A systematic review of randomized controlled trials. *Complementary Therapies in Medicine* 22:743-755.
55. Majewski-Schrage, T., T.A. Evans, and B. Ragan. 2014. Development of a core-stability model: A Delphi approach. *Journal of Sport Rehabilitation* 23:95-106.
56. McGill, S. 2004. Mechanics and pathomechanics of muscles acting on the lumbar spine. In *Kinesiology: The mechanics and pathomechanics of human movement*, ed. C. Otis. Philadelphia: Lippincott Williams & Wilkins.
57. McGill, S. 2004. *Ultimate back fitness and performance.* Waterloo, ON: Wabuno.
58. McGill, S., D. Juker, and P. Kropf. 1996. Quantitative intramuscular myoelectric activity of quadratus lumborum during a wide variety of tasks. *Clinical Biomechanics* 11:170-172.

59. McGill, S.M. 2001. Low back stability: From formal description to issues for performance and rehabilitation. *Exercise and Sport Sciences Reviews* 29:26-31.
60. McGill, S.M., and A. Karpowicz. 2009. Exercises for spine stabilization: Motion/motor patterns, stability progressions, and clinical technique. *Archives of Physical Medicine and Rehabilitation* 90:118-126.
61. Mok, N.W., E.W. Yeung, J.C. Cho, S.C. Hui, K.C. Liu, and C.H. Pang. 2014. Core muscle activity during suspension exercises. *Journal of Science and Medicine in Sport / Sports Medicine Australia*.
62. Natour, J., L.d.A. Cazotti, L.H. Ribeiro, A.S. Baptista, and A. Jones. 2015. Pilates improves pain, function and quality of life in patients with chronic low back pain: A randomized controlled trial. *Clinical Rehabilitation* 29:59-68.
63. Nitz, A.J., and D. Peck. 1986. Comparison of muscle-spindle concentrations in large and small human epaxial muscles acting in parallel combinations. *American Surgeon* 52:273-277.
64. Nordin, M.F.V. 2001. *Basic biomechanics of the musculoskeletal system.* Philadelphia: Lippincott Williams & Wilkins.
65. Okubo, Y., K. Kaneoka, A. Imai, I. Shiina, M. Tatsumura, S. Izumi, and S. Miyakawa. 2010. Electromyographic analysis of transversus abdominis and lumbar multifidus using wire electrodes during lumbar stabilization exercises. *Journal of Orthopaedic & Sports Physical Therapy* 40:743-750.
66. Panjabi, M., K. Abumi, J. Duranceau, and T. Oxland. 1989. Spinal stability and intersegmental muscle forces. A biomechanical model. *Spine (Phila Pa 1976)* 14:194-200.
67. Panjabi, M.M. 2003. Clinical spinal instability and low back pain. *Journal of Electromyography and Kinesiology* 13:371-379.
68. Panjabi, M.M. 1992. The stabilizing system of the spine, part 1: Function, dysfunction, adaptation, and enhancement. *Journal of Spinal Disorders* 5:383-389.
69. Panjabi, M.M. 1992. The stabilizing system of the spine, part 2: Neutral zone and instability hypothesis. *Journal of Spinal Disorders* 5:390-397.
70. Panjabi, M.M., C. Lydon, A. Vasavada, D. Grob, J.J. Crisco, and J. Dvorak. 1994. On the understanding of clinical instability. *Spine* 19:2642-2650.
71. Richardson, C.A., C.J. Snijders, J.A. Hides, L. Damen, M.S. Pas, and J. Storm. 2002. The relation between the transversus abdominis muscles, sacroiliac joint mechanics, and low back pain. *Spine* 27:399-405.
72. Rydeard, R., A. Leger, and D. Smith. 2006. Pilates-based therapeutic exercise: Effect on subjects with nonspecific chronic low back pain and functional disability: A randomized controlled trial. *Journal of Orthopaedic & Sports Physical Therapy* 36:472-484.
73. Sahrmann, S. 2001. *Diagnosis and treatment of movement impairment syndromes.* Maryland Heights, MO: Mosby.
74. Saliba, S.A., T. Croy, R. Guthrie, D. Grooms, A. Weltman, and T.L. Grindstaff. 2010. Differences in transverse abdominis activation with stable and unstable bridging exercises in individuals with low back pain. *North American Journal of Sports Physical Therapy* 5:63-73.
75. Sengupta, D.K., and H.B. Fan. 2014. The basis of mechanical instability in degenerative disc disease: A cadaveric study of abnormal motion versus load distribution. *Spine* 39:1032-1043.
76. Sorosky, S., S. Stilp, and V. Akuthota. 2008. Yoga and Pilates in the management of low back pain. *Current Reviews in Musculoskeletal Medicine* 1:39-47.
77. Stanton, R., P.R. Reaburn, and B. Humphries. 2004. The effect of short-term Swiss ball training on core stability and running economy. *Journal of Strength and Conditioning Research* 18:522-528.
78. Steele, J., S. Bruce-Low, and D. Smith. 2014. A reappraisal of the deconditioning hypothesis in low back pain: Review of evidence from a triumvirate of research methods on specific lumbar extensor deconditioning. *Current Medical Research and Opinion* 30:865-911.
79. Stevens, V.K., P.L. Coorevits, K.G. Bouche, N.N. Mahieu, G.G. Vanderstraeten, and L.A. Danneels. 2007. The influence of specific training on trunk muscle recruitment patterns in healthy subjects during stabilization exercises. *Manual Therapy* 12:271-279.
80. Tidstrand, J., and E. Horneij. 2009. Inter-rater reliability of three standardized functional tests in patients with low back pain. *BMC Musculoskeletal Disorders* 10.
81. Urquhart, D.M., P.W. Hodges, T.J. Allen, and I.H. Story. 2005. Abdominal muscle recruitment during a range of voluntary exercises. *Manual Therapey* 10:144-153.
82. Vera-Garcia, F.J., S.G. Grenier, and S.M. McGill. 2000. Abdominal muscle response during curl-ups on both stable and labile surfaces. *Physical Therapy* 80:564-569.
83. Walker, B.F. 2000. The prevalence of low back pain: A systematic review of the literature from 1966 to 1998. *Journal of Spinal Disorders* 13:205-217.
84. Wilke, H.J., P. Neef, M. Caimi, T. Hoogland, and L.E. Claes. 1999. New in vivo measurements of pressures in the intervertebral disc in daily life. *Spine* 24:755-762.
85. Yue, J.J., J.P. Timm, M.M. Panjabi, and J. Jaramillo-de la Torre. 2007. Clinical application of the Panjabi neutral zone hypothesis: The Stabilimax NZ posterior lumbar dynamic stabilization system. *Neurosurgical Focus* 22:E12.

Chapter 15

1. Aagaard, P., and J.L. Andersen. 2010. Effects of strength training on endurance capacity in top-level endurance athletes. *Scandinavian Journal of Medicine and Science in Sports* 20(Suppl. 2): 39-47.
2. Alcaraz, P.E., J.M. Palao, J.L. Elvira, and N.P. Linthorne. 2008. Effects of three types of resisted sprint training devices on the kinematics of sprinting at maximum velocity. *Journal of Strength and Conditioning Research* 22:890-897.
3. Åstrand, P.-O. 2003. *Textbook of work physiology.* Champaign, IL: Human Kinetics.
4. Bartlett, J.D., G.L. Close, D.P. MacLaren, W. Gregson, B. Drust, and J.P. Morton. 2011. High-intensity interval running is perceived to be more enjoyable than moderate-intensity continuous exercise: Implications for exercise adherence. *Journal of Sports Science* 29:547-553.
5. Bascomb N. 2004. *The perfect mile.* New York: Houghton Mifflin.

6. Billat, L.V. 2001. Interval training for performance: A scientific and empirical practice: Special recommendations for middle- and long-distance running, part I: Aerobic interval training. *Sports Medicine* 31:13-31.
7. Brennan, D.K., and R.P. Wilder. 1996. Cross-training and periodization in running. *Journal of Back and Musculoskeletal Rehabilitation* 6:49-58.
8. Burgomaster, K.A., G.J.F. Heigenhauser, and M.J. Gibala. 2006. Effect of short-term sprint interval training on human skeletal muscle carbohydrate metabolism during exercise and time-trial performance. *Journal of Applied Physiology* 100:2041-2047.
9. Burgomaster, K.A., K.R. Howarth, S.M. Phillips, M. Rakobowchuk, M.J. Macdonald, et al. 2008. Similar metabolic adaptations during exercise after low-volume sprint interval and traditional endurance training in humans. *Journal of Physiology* 586:151-160.
10. Burgomaster, K.A., S.C. Hughes, G.J.F. Heigenhauser, S.N. Bradwell, and M.J. Gibala. 2005. Six sessions of sprint interval training increases muscle oxidative potential and cycle endurance capacity in humans. *Journal of Applied Physiology* 98:1985-1990.
11. Chtara, M., K. Chamari, M. Chaouachi, A. Chaouachi, D. Koubaa, et al. 2005. Effects of intra-session concurrent endurance and strength training sequence on aerobic performance and capacity. *British Journal of Sports Medicine* 39:555-560.
12. Cormie, P., M.R. McGuigan, and R.U. Newton. 2011. Developing maximal neuromuscular power, part 2—training considerations for improving maximal power production. *Sports Medicine* 41:125-146.
13. Costill, D.L. 1986. *Inside running: Basics of sports physiology.* Carmel, IN: Cooper.
14. Daniels, J. 2005. *Daniels' running formula.* Champaign, IL: Human Kinetics.
15. Daniels, J., and N. Scardina. 1984. Interval training and performance. *Sports Medicine* 1:327-334.
16. Delecluse, C. 1997. Influence of strength training on sprint running performance: Current findings and implications for training. *Sports Medicine* 24:147-156.
17. Demarie, S., J.P. Koralsztein, and V. Billat. 2000. Time limit and time at $\dot{V}O_2$max during a continuous and an intermittent run. *Journal of Sports Medicine and Physical Fitness* 40:96-102.
18. Dillman, C.J. 1975. Kinematic analyses of running. *Exercise and Sport Sciences Reviews* 3:193-218.
19. Earle, R.W., and T.R. Baechle. 2008. Resistance training and spotting techniques. In *Essentials of strength training and conditioning*, ed. T.R. Baechle and R.W. Earle. Champaign, IL: Human Kinetics.
20. Ebben, W.P., R.M. Carroll, and C.J. Simenz. 2004. Strength and conditioning practices of National Hockey League strength and conditioning coaches. *Journal of Strength and Conditioning Research* 18:889-897.
21. Ebben, W.P., M.J. Hintz, and C.J. Simenz. 2005. Strength and conditioning practices of Major League Baseball strength and conditioning coaches. *Journal of Strength and Conditioning Research* 19:538-546.
22. Eickhoff-Shemek, J.M., and M.C. Keiper. 2014. High-intensity exercise and legal liability risks. *ACSM's Health and Fitness Journal* 18:30-37.
23. Feito, Y. 2014. Prevalence and incidence rates are not the same: Letter to the editor. *Orthopaedic Journal of Sports Medicine* 2.
24. Fletcher, I.M., and B. Jones. 2004. The effect of different warm-up stretch protocols on 20 meter sprint performance in trained rugby union players. *Journal of Strength and Conditioning Research* 18:885-888.
25. Fyfe, J.J., D.J. Bishop, and N.K. Stepto. 2014. Interference between concurrent resistance and endurance exercise: Molecular bases and the role of individual training variables. *Sports Medicine* 44:743-762.
26. Giordano, B.D., and B.M. Weisenthal. 2014. Prevalence and incidence rates are not the same: Response. *Orthopaedic Journal of Sports Medicine* 2.
27. Hak, P.T., E. Hodzovic, and B. Hickey. (in press). The nature and prevalence of injury during CrossFit training. *Journal of Strength and Conditioning Research.* doi: 10.1519/JSC.0000000000000318.
28. Hakkinen K., P.V. Komi, M. Alen, and H. Kauhanen. 1987. EMG, muscle fibre and force production characteristics during a 1 year training period in elite weight-lifters. *European Journal of Applied Physiology and Occupational Physiology* 56:419-427.
29. Hanc, J. 2007. Your perfect tempo. *Runner's World.* www.runnersworld.com/running-tips/learn-how-to-do-a-perfect-tempo-run [accessed July 2, 2015].
30. Haugen, T., E. Tonnessen, and S. Seiler. 2015. 9.58 and 10.49: Nearing the citius end for 100m? *International Journal of Sports Physiology and Performance* 10:268-272.
31. Hawley, J.A. 2009. Molecular responses to strength and endurance training: Are they incompatible? *Applied Physiology Nutrition, and Metabolism* 34:355-361.
32. Hickson, R.C. 1980. Interference of strength development by simultaneously training for strength and endurance. *European Journal of Applied Physiology and Occupational Physiology* 45:255-263.
33. Hickson, R.C., H.A. Bomze, and J.O. Holloszy. 1977. Linear increase in aerobic power induced by a strenuous program of endurance exercise. *Journal of Applied Physiology: Respiratory, Environmental, and Exercise Physiology* 42:372-376.
34. Hori, N., R.U. Newton, N. Kawamori, M.R. McGuigan, W.A. Andrews, et al. 2008. Comparison of weighted jump squat training with and without eccentric braking. *Journal of Strength and Conditioning Research* 22:54-65.
35. Jaggers, J.R., A.M. Swank, K.L. Frost, and C.D. Lee. 2008. The acute effects of dynamic and ballistic stretching on vertical jump height, force, and power. *Journal of Strength and Conditioning Research* 22:1844-1849.
36. Joyce, D., and D. Lewindon, eds. 2014. *High-performance training for sports.* Champaign, IL: Human Kinetics.
37. Karp, J.R. 2000. Interval training for the fitness professional. *Strength and Conditioning Journal* 22:64-69.

38. Kratky, S., and E. Muller. 2013. Sprint running with a body-weight supporting kite reduces ground contact time in well-trained sprinters. *Journal of Strength and Conditioning Research* 27:1215-1222.
39. Kubukeli, Z.N., T.D. Noakes, and S.C. Dennis. 2002. Training techniques to improve endurance exercise performances. *Sports Medicine* 32:489-509.
40. Laursen, P.B., and D.G. Jenkins. 2002. The scientific basis for high-intensity interval training: Optimising training programmes and maximising performance in highly trained endurance athletes. *Sports Medicine* 32:53-73.
41. Loy, S.F., J.J. Hoffmann, and G.J. Holland GJ. 1995. Benefits and practical use of cross-training in sports. *Sports Medicine* 19:1-8.
42. Lucas, J. 1977. A brief history of modern trends in marathon training. *Annals of the New York Academy of Sciences* 301:858-861.
43. MacDougall, D., and D. Sale. 1981. Continuous vs. interval training: A review for the athlete and the coach. *Canadian Journal of Applied Sport Sciences* 6:93-97.
44. MacDougall, J.D., A.L. Hicks, J.R. MacDonald, R.S. McKelvie, H.J. Green, and K.M. Smith. 1998. Muscle performance and enzymatic adaptations to sprint interval training. *Journal of Applied Physiology* 84:2138-2142.
45. McBride, J.M., T. Triplett-McBride, A. Davie, and R.U. Newton. 2002. The effect of heavy- vs. light-load jump squats on the development of strength, power, and speed. *Journal of Strength and Conditioning Research* 16:75-82.
46. Mero, A., P.V. Komi, and R.J. Gregor. 1992. *Biomechanics of sprint running: A review. Sports Medicine* 13:376-392.
47. Morgan, D.W., F.D. Baldini, P.E. Martin, and W.M. Kohrt. 1989. Ten kilometer performance and predicted velocity at $\dot{V}O_2max$ among well-trained male runners. *Medicine and Science in Sports and Exercise* 21:78-83.
48. Mujika, I., and S. Padilla. 2003. Scientific bases for precompetition tapering strategies. *Medicine and Science in Sports and Exercise* 35:1182-1187.
49. Nader, G.A. 2006. Concurrent strength and endurance training: From molecules to man. *Medicine and Science in Sports and Exercise* 38:1965-1970.
50. Newton, R., W.J. Kraemer, K. Hakkinen, B.J. Humphries, and A.J. Murphy. 1996. Kinematics, kinetics, and muscle activation during explosive upper body movements. *Journal of Applied Biomechanics* 12:31-43.
51. Newton, R.U., and W.J. Kraemer. 1994. Developing explosive power: Implications for a mixed method training strategy. *Strength and Conditioning Journal* 16:20-31.
52. Sandrock, M. 1996. *Running with the legends.* Champaign, IL: Human Kinetics.
53. Scofield, K.L., and S. Hecht. 2012. Bone health in endurance athletes: Runners, cyclists, and swimmers. *Current Sports Medicine Reports* 11:328-334.
54. Sim, A.Y., B.T. Dawson, K.J. Guelfi, K.E. Wallman, and W.B. Young. 2009. Effects of static stretching in warm-up on repeated sprint performance. *Journal of Strength and Conditioning Research* 23:2155-2162.
55. Simenz, C.J., C.A. Dugan, and W.P. Ebben. 2005. Strength and conditioning practices of National Basketball Association strength and conditioning coaches. *Journal of Strength and Conditioning Research* 19:495-504.
56. Smith, M.M., A.J. Sommer, B.E. Starkoff, and S.T. Devor. 2013. CrossFit-based high-intensity power training improves maximal aerobic fitness and body composition. *Journal of Strength and Conditioning Research* 27:3159-3172.
57. Tabata, I., K. Irisawa, M. Kouzaki, K. Nishimura, F. Ogita, and M. Miyachi. 1997. Metabolic profile of high-intensity intermittent exercises. *Medicine and Science in Sports and Exercise* 29:390-395.
58. Tricoli, V., L. Lamas, R. Carnevale, and C. Ugrinowitsch. 2005. Short-term effects on lower-body functional power development: Weightlifting vs. vertical jump training programs. *Journal of Strength and Conditioning Research* 19:433-437.
59. Wang, L., H. Mascher, N. Psilander, E. Blomstrand, and K. Sahlin. 2011. Resistance exercise enhances the molecular signaling of mitochondrial biogenesis induced by endurance exercise in human skeletal muscle. *Journal of Applied Physiology* 111:1335-1344.
60. Weisenthal, B.M., C.A. Beck, M.D. Maloney, K.E. DeHaven, and B.D. Giordano. 2014. Injury rate and patterns among CrossFit athletes. *Orthopaedic Journal of Sports Medicine* 2.
61. Wilson, G., A. Murphy, and A. Walshe. 1997. Performance benefits from weight and plyometric training: Effects of initial strength level. *Coaching and Sport Science Journal* 2:3-8.
62. Yamamoto, L.M., J.F. Klau, D.J. Casa, W.J. Kraemer, L.E. Armstrong, and C.M. Maresh. 2010. The effects of resistance training on road cycling performance among highly trained cyclists: A systematic review. *Journal of Strength and Conditioning Research* 24:560-566.
63. Yamamoto, L.M., R.M. Lopez, J.F. Klau, D.J. Casa, W.J. Kraemer, and C.M. Maresh. 2008. The effects of resistance training on endurance distance running performance among highly trained runners: A systematic review. *Journal of Strength and Conditioning Research* 22:2036-2044.

Chapter 16

1. American College of Sports Medicine (ACSM). (in press). *ACSM's guidelines for exercise testing and prescription.* 10th ed. Philadelphia: Lippincott Williams & Wilkins.
2. American College of Sports Medicine (ACSM). 2006. Prevention of cold injuries during exercise. *Medicine and Science in Sports and Exercise* 38:2012-2029.
3. American College of Sports Medicine (ACSM). 2007. Exertional heat illness during training and competition. *Medicine and Science in Sports and Exercise* 39:556-572.
4. Åstrand, P.-O. 1952. *Experimental studies of physical working capacity in relation to sex and age.* Copenhagen: Ejnar Munksgaard.
5. Bar-Or, O. 1995. Health benefits of physical activity during childhood and adolescence. *PCPFS Research Digest* 2(4).

6. Bar-Or, O., and R.M. Malina. 1995. Activity, fitness, and health of children and adolescents. In *Child health, nutrition, and physical activity,* ed. L.W.Y. Cheung and J.B. Richmond, 79-123. Champaign, IL: Human Kinetics.
7. Blair, S.N., H.W. Kohl III, R.S. Paffenbarger Jr., D.G. Clark, K.H. Cooper, and L.W. Gibbons. 1989. Physical fitness and all-cause mortality. *Journal of the American Medical Association* 262:2395-2401.
8. Bunker, L.K. 1998. Psycho-physiological contributions of physical activity and sports for girls. *PCPFS Research Digest* 3(1).
9. Centers for Disease Control and Prevention (CDC). 1997. Guidelines for school and community programs to promote lifelong physical activity among young people. *Morbidity and Mortality Weekly Report* 44(RR-6): 1-36.
10. Coe, D.P., and M.A. Fiatarone Singh. 2014. Exercise prescription in special populations: Women, pregnancy, children, and older adults. In *ACSM's resource manual for guidelines for exercise testing and prescription*, 7th ed., 565-595. Baltimore: Wolters Kluwer/Lippincott Williams & Wilkins.
11. Corbin, C.B., R.P. Pangrazi, and G.C. LaMasurier. 2004. Physical activity for children: Current patterns and guidelines. *PCPFS Research Digest* 5(2).
12. Cureton, K.J., and G.L. Warren. 1990. Criterion-referenced standards for youth health-related fitness tests: A tutorial. *Research Quarterly for Exercise and Sports* 61:7-19.
13. Fardy, P., and A. Azzollini. 1998. The PATH program. In *Active youth: Ideas for implementing CDC physical activity promotion guidelines,* 81-85. Champaign, IL: Human Kinetics.
14. Hansen, D.M., S.D. Herrmann, K. Lambourne, J. Lee, and J.E. Donnelly. 2014. Linear/nonlinear relations of activity and fitness with children's academic achievement. *Medicine and Science in Sports and Exercise* 46:2279-2285.
15. Hebestreit, H.U., and O. Bar-Or. 2005. Differences between children and adults for exercise testing and exercise prescription. In *Exercise testing and exercise prescription for special cases,* 3rd ed., ed. J.S. Skinner, 68-84. Baltimore: Lippincott Williams & Wilkins.
16. Karila, C., J. de Blic, S. Waernessyckle, M.-R. Benoist, and P. Scheinmann. 2001. Cardiopulmonary testing in children: An individualized protocol for workload increase. *Chest* 120:81-87.
17. Malina, R.M. 2001. Tracking of physical activity across the life span. *PCPFS Research Digest* 3(14).
18. McKenzie, F.D., and J.B. Richmond. 1998. Linking health and learning: An overview of Coordinated School Health programs. In *Health is academic: A guide to coordinated school health programs,* ed. E. Marx, S. Frelick Wooley, and D. Northrop, 1-14. New York: Teachers College Press.
19. Morrow Jr., J.R., and A.W. Jackson. 1999. Physical activity promotion and school physical education. *PCPFS Research Digest* 3(7).
20. National Association for Sport and Physical Education (NASPE). 2009. *Active start: A statement of physical activity guidelines for children birth to age five.* Reston, VA: Author.
21. National Association for Sport and Physical Education (NASPE). 2004. *Physical activity for children: A statement of guidelines for children ages 5-12.* 2nd ed. Reston, VA: Author.
22. National Center for Education in Maternal and Child Health. 2001. *Bright futures in practice: Physical activity.* Arlington, VA: Author.
23. National Federation of State High School Associations (NFHS). 2014. High school participation increases for 25th consecutive year. www.nfhs.org/articles/high-school-participation-increases-for-25th-consecutive-year.
24. National Physical Activity Plan Alliance. 2014. The 2014 United States report card on physical activity for children and youth. www.physicalactivityplan.org/reportcard/NationalReportCard_longform_final%20for%20web.pdf.
25. Ogden, C.L., M.D. Carroll, B.K. Kit, and K.M. Flegal. 2014. Prevalence of childhood and adult obesity in the United States, 2011-2012. *Journal of the American Medical Association* 311:806-814.
26. Park, R.S. 1989. *Measurement of physical fitness: A historical perspective.* Washington, DC: ODPHP National Health Information Center.
27. Plowman, S.A., & M.D. Meredith, eds. (2013). *Fitnessgram/Activitygram reference guide.* 4th ed. Dallas: Cooper Institute.
28. President's Council on Fitness, Sports and Nutrition. 2015. *Presidential Active Lifestyle Award (PALA+).* Washington, DC: Author.
29. Regamey, N., and A. Moeller. 2010. Paediatric exercise testing. *European Respiratory Monograph* 47:291-309.
30. Robinson, S. 1938. Experimental studies of physical fitness in relation to age. *Arbeitsphysiologie* 10:251-323.
31. Rowland, T.W. 1999. Adolescence: A "risk factor" for physical inactivity. *PCPFS Research Digest* 2(4).
32. Rowland, T.W. 1990. *Exercise and children's health.* Champaign, IL: Human Kinetics.
33. Rowland, T.W. 2005. *Children's exercise physiology.* Champaign, IL: Human Kinetics.
34. Sallis, J.F. 1994. Influences on physical activity of children, adolescents, and adults or determinants of active living. *PCPFS Research Digest* 1(7).
35. Sallis, J.F., T.L. McKenzie, J.E. Alcaraz, B. Kolody, N. Faucette, and M. Hovell. 1997. The effects of a 2-year physical education program (SPARK) on physical activity and fitness on elementary school students. *American Journal of Public Health* 87:45-50.
36. Sallis, J.F., T.L. McKenzie, B. Kolody, M. Lewis, S. Marshall, and P. Rosegard. 1999. Effects of health-related physical education on academic achievement: Project SPARK. *Research Quarterly for Exercise and Sport* 70:127-134.
37. Sallis, J.F., K. Patrick, and B.L. Long. 1994. An overview of international consensus conference on physical activity guidelines for adolescents. *Pediatric Exercise Science* 6:299-301.
38. Satcher, D. 1998. Opening remarks. *Childhood obesity: Causes and prevention* (CNPP-6). Washington, DC: USDA Center for Nutrition Policy and Promotion.

39. Seefeldt, V.D., and M.E. Ewing. 1997. Youth sports in America: An overview. *PCPFS Research Digest* 2(11).
40. Strong, W.B., R.M. Malina, C.J.R. Blimkie, S.R. Daniles, R.K. Dishman, B. Gutin, A.C. Hergenroeder, A. Must, P.A. Nixon, J.M. Pivarnik, T. Rowland, S. Trost, and F. Trudeau. 2005. Evidenced-based physical activity for school-age youth. *Journal of Pediatrics* 146:732-737.
41. U.S. Department of Agriculture (USDA). 1999. *Childhood obesity: Causes and prevention. Symposium proceedings* (CNPP-6). Washington, DC: USDA Center for Nutrition Policy and Promotion.
42. U.S. Department of Health and Human Services (HHS). 1996. *Physical activity and health: Report of the Surgeon General.* Atlanta: HHS, CDC, National Center for Chronic Disease Prevention and Health Promotion.
43. U.S. Department of Health and Human Services (HHS). 2010. *Healthy People 2020.* Washington, DC: Author.
44. U.S. Department of Health and Human Services (HHS). 2008. *2008 Physical Activity Guidelines for Americans.* www.health.gov/paguidelines/guidelines/default.aspx.
45. U.S. Department of Health and Human Services (HHS). 2008. *Physical Activity Guidelines Advisory Committee report 2008.* www.health.gov/paguidelines/committee report.aspx.
46. U.S. Department of Health and Human Services (HHS). 2012. *Strategies to increase physical activity among youth: A midcourse report of the Physical Activity Guidelines for Americans Subcommittee of the President's Council on Fitness, Sports & Nutrition.* Washington, DC: Author.
47. Washington, R.L., J.T. Bricker, B.S. Alpert, S.R. Daniels, R.J. Deckelbaum, E.A. Fisher, S.S. Gidding, J. Isabel-Jones, R.-E.W. Kavey, G.R. Marx, W.B. Strong, D.W. Teske, J.H. Wilmore, and M. Winston. 1994. Guidelines for exercise testing in the pediatric age group. *Circulation* 90:2166-2179.
48. Weiss, M.R., and D.M. Wiese-Bjornstal. 2009. Promoting positive youth development through physical activity. *Research Digest* 10:3.
49. Zwiren, L.D. 2001. Exercise testing and prescription considerations throughout childhood. In *ACSM's resource manual for guidelines for exercise testing and prescription,* 4th ed., ed. J.L. Roitman, 520-528. Philadelphia: Lippincott

Chapter 17

1. American College of Sports Medicine (ACSM). 2009. Exercise and physical activity for older adults. *Medicine and Science in Sports and Exercise* 41:1510-1530.
2. American College of Sports Medicine (ACSM). 2011. The recommended quantity and quality of exercise for developing and maintaining cardiorespiratory, musculoskeletal, and neuromotor fitness in apparently healthy adults: Guidance for prescribing exercise. *Medicine and Science in Sports and Exercise* 43(7): 1334-1359.
3. American College of Sports Medicine (ACSM). (in press). *ACSM's guidelines for exercise testing and prescription.* 10th ed. Baltimore: Lippincott Williams & Wilkins.
4. American Council on Exercise. 1998. *Exercise for the older adult.* Champaign, IL: Human Kinetics.
5. Bloomfield, S.A., and S.S. Smith. 2003. Osteoporosis. In *ACSM's exercise management for persons with chronic diseases and disabilities.* 2nd ed. Ed. J.L. Durstine and G.E. Moore, 222-229. Champaign, IL: Human Kinetics.
6. Chodzko-Zajko, W.J. 1998. Physical activity and aging: Implications for health and quality of life in older persons. *PCPFS Research Digest* 3(4).
7. Coe, D.P., and M. Fiatarone Singh. 2014. Exercise prescription in special populations: Women, pregnancy, children, and older adults. In *ACSM's resource manual for guidelines for exercise testing and prescription*, ed. D.P. Swain, 565-595. Baltimore: Wolters Kluwer/Lippincott Williams & Wilkins.
8. Criswell, D.S. 2001. Human development and aging. In *ACSM's health and fitness certification review,* ed. J.L. Roitman and K.W. Bibi, 31-47. Baltimore: Lippincott Williams & Wilkins.
9. Fiatarone, M.A., E.C. Marks, N.D. Ryan, C.N. Meredith, L.A. Lipsitz, and W.J. Evans. 1990. High-intensity strength training in nonagenarians. *Journal of the American Medical Association* 263:3029-3034.
10. Fitzgerald, M.D., H. Tanaka, Z.V. Tran, and D.R. Seals. 1997. Age-related declines in maximal aerobic capacity in regularly exercising vs. sedentary women: A meta-analysis. *Journal of Applied Physiology* 83:160-165.
11. Fitzgerald, P.L. 1985. Exercise for the elderly. *Medical Clinics of North America* 69:189-196.
12. Frontera, W.R., C.N. Meredith, K.P. O'Reilly, and W.J. Evans. 1990. Strength training and determinants of $\dot{V}O_2$max in older men. *Journal of Applied Physiology* 68:329-333.
13. Frontera, W.R., C.N. Meredith, K.P. O'Reilly, H.G. Knuttgen, and W.J. Evans. 1988. Strength conditioning in older men: Skeletal muscle hypertrophy and improved function. *Journal of Applied Physiology* 64:1038-1044.
14. Harris, C.D., K.B. Wayson, S.A. Carlson, J.E. Fulton, J.M. Dorn, and L. Elam-Evans. 2013. Adult participation in aerobic and muscle-strengthening physical activities—United States, 2011. *Morbidity and Mortality Weekly Report* 62:326-330.
15. Holloszy, J.O., and W.M. Kohrt. 1995. Exercise. In *Handbook of physiology, section 11: Aging,* ed. E.J. Masoro, 633-666. New York: Oxford Press.
16. Howley, E.T. 2001. Type of activity: Resistance, aerobic and leisure versus occupational physical activity. *Medicine and Science in Sports and Exercise* 33:S364-S369.
17. Kraemer, W.J., S.J. Fleck, and W.J. Evans. 1996. Strength and power training: Physiological mechanisms of adaptations. *Exercise and Sport Sciences Reviews* 24:363-397.
18. Minor, M.A., and D.R. Kay. 2003. Arthritis. In *ACSM's exercise management for persons with chronic diseases and disabilities,* eds. J.L. Durstine and G.E. Moore, 210-216. Champaign, IL: Human Kinetics.
19. Nybo, L., J.F. Schmidt, S. Fritzdorf, and N.B. Nordsborg. 2014. Physiological characteristics of an aging Olympic athlete. *Medicine and Science in Sports and Exercise* 46:2132-2138.

20. Pate, R.R., M. Pratt, S.N. Blair, W.L. Haskell, C.A. Marcera, and C. Bouchard. 1995. Physical activity and public health: A recommendation from the Centers for Disease Control and Prevention and the American College of Sports Medicine. *Journal of the American Medical Association* 273:402-407.
21. Petit, M.A., J.M. Hughes, and J.M. Warpeha. 2007. Exercise prescription for people with osteoporosis. In *ACSM's resource manual for guidelines for exercise testing and prescription*. 6th ed. Ed. J.K. Ehrman, 635-650. Baltimore: Lippincott Williams & Wilkins.
22. Rikli, R.E., and C.J. Jones. 2001. *Senior fitness test manual*. Champaign, IL: Human Kinetics.
23. Rimmer, J.H. 1994. *Fitness and rehabilitation programs for special populations*. Dubuque, IA: Brown & Benchmark.
24. Rogers, M.A., and W.J. Evans. 1993. Changes in skeletal muscle with aging: Effects of exercise training. *Exercise and Sport Sciences Reviews* 21:65-102.
25. Shephard, R.J. 1997. *Aging, physical activity, and health*. Champaign, IL: Human Kinetics.
26. Skinner, J.S. 2005. Aging for exercise testing and exercise prescription. In *Exercise testing and exercise prescription for special cases*. 3rd ed. Ed. J.S. Skinner, 85-99. Baltimore: Lippincott Williams & Wilkins.
27. Spirduso, W.W., K.L. Francis, and P.G. MacRae. 2005. *Physical dimensions of aging*. 2nd ed. Champaign, IL: Human Kinetics.
28. Spirduso, W.W., and D.L. Cronin. 2001. Exercise dose–response effects on quality of life and independent living in older adults. *Medicine and Science in Sports and Exercise* 33:S598-S608.
29. Trappe, S., E. Hayes, A. Galpin, L. Kaminsky, B. Jemiolo, W. Fink, T. Trappe, A. Jansson, T. Gustafsson, and P. Tesch. 2013. New records in aerobic power among octogenarian lifelong endurance athletes. *Journal of Applied Physiology* 114:3-10.
30. U.S. Department of Health and Human Services (HHS). 2008. *2008 Physical Activity Guidelines for Americans*. www.health.gov/paguidelines/guidelines/default.aspx.
31. U.S. Department of Health and Human Services (HHS). 2008. Physical Activity Guidelines Advisory Committee report 2008. http://health.gov/paguidelines/report/pdf/committeereport.pdf.
32. U.S. Department of Health and Human Services (HHS). 2013. *A profile of older Americans: 2013*. Washington, DC: Author.
33. World Health Organization (WHO). 1997. *A summary of the physiological benefits of physical activity for older persons*. Geneva: Author.
34. Wroblewski, A.P., F. Amati, M.A. Smiley, B. Goodpaster, and V. Wright. 2011. Chronic exercise preserves lean muscle mass in masters athletes. *Physician and Sportsmedicine* 39:172-178.

Chapter 18

1. American College of Sports Medicine (ACSM). 1995. Position stand: Osteoporosis and exercise. *Medicine and Science in Sports and Exercise* 27:i-vii.
2. American College of Sports Medicine (ACSM). 2007. Position stand: The female athlete triad. *Medicine and Science in Sports and Exercise* 39:1867-1882.
3. American College of Sports Medicine (ACSM). 2004. Physical activity and bone health. *Medicine and Science in Sports and Exercise* 36:1985-1996.
4. American College of Sports Medicine (ACSM). (in press). *ACSM's guidelines for exercise testing and prescription*. 10th ed. Baltimore: Lippincott Williams & Wilkins.
5. American College of Obstetricians and Gynecologists (ACOG). 2015. Exercise during pregnancy and the postpartum period. Committee Opinion No. 650. *Obstetrics and Gynecology* 126:e135-142.
6. Artal, R., C. Sherman, and N.A. DiNubile. 1999. Exercise during pregnancy. *Physician and Sportsmedicine* 27:51-60+.
7. Blume, S.W., and J.R. Curtis. 2011. Medical costs of osteoporosis in the elderly Medicare population. *Osteoporosis International* 22(6): 1835-1844.
8. Bonci, C.M., L.J. Bonci, L.R. Granger, C.L. Johnson, R.M. Malina, L.W. Milne, R.R. Ryan, and E.W. Vanderbunt. 2008. National Athletic Trainers' Association position statement: Preventing, detecting, and managing disordered eating in athletes. *Journal of Athletic Training* 43:80-108.
9. Coe, D.P., and M.A. Fiatarone-Singh. 2014. Exercise prescription in special populations: Women, pregnancy, children and older adults. In *ACSM's resource manual for guidelines for exercise testing and prescription*. 7th ed. Ed. D.P. Swain, 565-595. Baltimore: Lippincott Williams & Wilkins.
10. Drinkwater, B.L., K. Nilson, C.H. Chesnut, W.J. Bremner, S. Schainholtz, and M.B. Southworth. 1984. Bone mineral content of amenorrheic and eumenorrheic athletes. *New England Journal of Medicine* 311:277-281.
11. Heffernan, A.E. 2000. Exercise and pregnancy in primary care. *Nurse Practitioner* 25:42, 49, 53-56, 59-60.
12. Hobart, J.A., and D.R. Smucker. 2000. The female athlete triad. *American Family Physician* 61:3357-3364, 3367.
13. Johnson, M.D. 1994. Disordered eating. In *Medical and orthopedic issues of active and athletic women*, ed. R. Agostini, 141-151. Philadelphia: Hanley & Belfus.
14. Khan, K., H. McKay, P. Kannus, D. Bailey, J. Wark, and K. Bennell. 2001. *Physical activity and bone health*. Champaign, IL: Human Kinetics.
15. Melzer, K., Y. Schutz, M. Boulvain, and B. Kayser. 2010. Physical activity and pregnancy: Cardiovascular adaptations, recommendations and pregnancy outcomes. *Sports Medicine* 40:493-507.
16. Metcalfe, L., T. Lohman, S. Going, L. Houtkooper, D. Ferriera, H. Flint-Wagner, T. Guido, J. Martin, J. Wright, and E. Cussler. 2001. Postmenopausal women and exercise for prevention of osteoporosis: The Bone, Estrogen, Strength Training (BEST) study. *ACSM's Health and Fitness Journal* 5:6-14.
17. National Institutes of Health (NIH). 2000. Osteoporosis prevention, diagnosis, and therapy. NIH Consensus Development Conference. Bethesda, MD: Author.

18. Petit, M.A., J.M. Hughes, and L. Scibora. 2014. Exercise prescription for people with osteoporosis. In *ACSM's resource manual for guidelines for exercise testing and prescription*. 7th ed. Ed. D.P. Swain, 699-712. Baltimore: Lippincott Williams & Wilkins.
19. Smith, S.S., C.H.E. Wang, and S.A. Bloomfield. 2009. Osteoporosis. In *ACSM's exercise management for persons with chronic diseases and disabilities*. 3rd ed. Ed. J.L. Durstine, G.E. Moore, P.L. Painter, and S.O. Roberts, 270-279. Champaign, IL: Human Kinetics.
20. Smolak, L., S.K. Murnen, and A.E. Ruble. 2000. Female athletes and eating problems: A meta-analysis. *International Journal of Eating Disorders* 27:371-380.
21. Streuling, I., A. Beyerlein, E. Rosenfeld, H. Hofmann, T. Schulz, and R. von Kries. 2011. Physical activity and gestational weight gain: A meta-analysis of intervention trials. *British Journal of Obstetrics and Gynaecology* 118:278-284.
22. Tobias, D.K., C. Zhang, R.M. van Dam, K. Bowers, and F.B. Hu. 2011. Physical activity before and during pregnancy and risk of gestational diabetes mellitus. *Diabetes Care* 34:223-229.
23. U.S. Department of Health and Human Services (HHS). 2008. *2008 Physical Activity Guidelines for Americans.* www.health.gov/paguidelines/guidelines/default.aspx.
24. Wang, T.W., and B.S. Apgar. 1998. Exercise during pregnancy. *American Family Physician* 57:1846-1852, 1857.
25. Wright, N.C., A.C. Looker, K.G. Saag, J.R. Curtis, E.S. Delzell, S. Randall, and B Dawson-Hughes. 2014. The recent prevalence of osteoporosis and low bone mass in the United States based on bone mineral density at the femoral neck or lumbar spine. *Journal of Bone and Mineral Research* 29(11): 2520-2526.

Chapter 19

1. Ades, P.A., P.G. Gunter, W.L. Meyer, T.C. Gibson, J. Maddalena, and T. Orfeo. 1990. Cardiac and skeletal muscle adaptations to training in systemic hypertension and effect of beta blockade (metoprolol or propranolol). *American Journal of Cardiology* 166(5): 591-596.
2. American Association for Cardiovascular and Pulmonary Rehabilitation (AACVPR). 2013. *Guidelines for cardiac rehabilitation and secondary prevention programs.* 5th ed. Champaign, IL: Human Kinetics.
3. American College of Sports Medicine (ACSM). 2004. Position stand: Exercise and hypertension. *Medicine and Science in Sports and Exercise* 36(3): 533-553.
4. American College of Sports Medicine (ACSM). (in press). *ACSM's guidelines for exercise testing and prescription. 10th* ed. Baltimore: Lippincott Williams & Wilkins.
5. American Heart Association (AHA). 2015. *Heart and stroke statistics—2015 update.* Dallas: Author.
6. American Hospital Formulary Service. 2015. *Drug information 2015.* Bethesda, MD: American Society of Hospital Pharmacists.
7. Brubaker, P.H. 2008. Contemporary approaches to cardiovascular disease diagnosis. In *Pollock's textbook of cardiovascular disease and rehabilitation*, 83-94. Champaign, IL: Human Kinetics.
8. Brubaker, P.H., L.A. Kaminsky, and M.H. Whaley. 2002. *Coronary artery disease: Essentials of prevention and rehabilitation programs.* Champaign, IL: Human Kinetics.
9. Clausen, J.P. 1977. Circulatory adjustments to dynamic exercise and physical training in normal subjects and in patients with coronary artery disease. In *Exercise and the heart,* ed. E.H. Sonnenblick and M. Lesch, 39-75. New York: Grune & Stratton.
10. Dubin, D. 2000. *Rapid interpretation of EKGs.* 6th ed. Tampa: Cover.
11. Enos, W., R. Holmes, and J. Beyer. 1953. Coronary disease among United States soldiers killed in action in Korea. *Journal of the American Medical Association* 152:1090-1093.
12. Franklin, B.A. 2009. Myocardial infarction. In *ACSM's exercise management for persons with chronic diseases and disabilities. 3rd ed.* Ed. J.L. Durstine and G.E. Moore, 49-57. Champaign, IL: Human Kinetics.
13. Franklin, B.A. 2009. Revascularization: CABGS and PTCA or PCI. In *ACSM's exercise management for persons with chronic diseases and disabilities. 3rd ed. Ed.* J.L. Durstine, G.E. Moore, P.L. Painter, and S.O. Roberts, 58-65. Champaign, IL: Human Kinetics.
14. Franklin, B.A., J.E. Trivax, and T.E. Vanhecke. 2008. Coronary artery disease, myocardial infarction, and angina pectoris. In *Pollock's textbook of cardiovascular disease and rehabilitation*, 271-284. Champaign, IL: Human Kinetics.
15. Grines, C.L. 1996. Aggressive intervention for myocardial infarction: Angioplasty, stents, and intra-aortic balloon pumping. *American Journal of Cardiology* 78:29-34.
16. Hagberg, J.M. 1990. Exercise, fitness, and hypertension. In *Physical activity, fitness, and health,* ed. C. Bouchard, R.J. Shephard, and T. Stephens, 993-1005. Champaign, IL: Human Kinetics.
17. Hargens, T. 2014. Pathophysiology and treatment of cardiovascular disease. In *ACSM's resource manual for guidelines for exercise testing and prescription.* 7th ed. Ed. J.K. Ehrman, 110-119. Baltimore: Lippincott Williams & Wilkins.
18. Hillegass, E.A., and W.C. Temes. 2001. Therapeutic interventions in cardiac rehabilitation and prevention. In *Essentials of cardiopulmonary physical therapy.* 2nd ed. Ed. E.A. Hillegass and H.S. Sadowsky, 676-726. Philadelphia: Saunders.
19. Hossack, K.F., R.A. Bruce, and L.J. Clark. 1980. Influence of propranolol on exercise prescription of training heart rates. *Cardiology* 65:47-58.
20. Kaplan, N.M. 1994. *Clinical hypertension.* 6th ed. Baltimore: Williams & Wilkins.
21. Kinderman, W. 1987. Calcium antagonists and exercise performance. *Sports Medicine* 4(3): 177-193.
22. Koester Qualters, W. 2014. Diagnostic procedures for cardiovascular disease. In *ACSM's resource manual for guidelines for exercise testing and prescription.* 7th ed. Ed. J.K. Ehrman, 382-396. Baltimore: Lippincott Williams & Wilkins.
23. Libby, P. 2002. Atherosclerosis: The new view. *Scientific American* 286(5): 46-55.

24. MacGowan, G.A., D. O'Callaghan, and J.H. Horgan. 1992. The effects of verapamil on training in patients with ischemic heart disease. *Chest* 101(2): 411-415.

25. Ornish, D., L.W. Scherwitz, and J.H. Billings. 1998. Intensive lifestyle changes for reversal of coronary heart disease. *Journal of the American Medical Association* 280:2001-2007.

26. Pavia, L., G. Orlando, J. Myers, M. Maestri, and C. Rusconi. 1995. The effect of beta-blockade therapy on the response to exercise training in postmyocardial infarction patients. *Clinical Cardiology* 18(12): 716-720.

27. Pollock, M.L., and J.H. Wilmore. 1990. *Exercise in health and disease.* 2nd ed. Philadelphia: Saunders.

28. Savage, P.D., and S.J. Keteyian. 2014. Exercise prescription for patients with cardiovascular disease. In *ACSM's resource manual for guidelines for exercise testing and prescription.* 7th ed. Ed. D.P. Swain, 619-634. Baltimore: Lippincott Williams & Wilkins.

29. Tesch, P.A. 1985. Exercise performance and beta-blockade. *Sports Medicine* 2(6): 389-412.

30. Thompson, P.D. 1988. The benefits and risks of exercise training in patients with chronic coronary artery disease. *Journal of the American Medical Association* 259:1537-1540.

31. Wenger, N.K., and J.W. Hurst. 1984. Coronary bypass surgery as a rehabilitative procedure. In *Rehabilitation of the coronary patient,* ed. N.K. Wenger and H.K. Hellerstein, 115-132. New York: Wiley.

Chapter 20

1. American College of Sports Medicine (ACSM). (in press). *ACSM's guidelines for exercise testing and prescription.* 10th ed. Baltimore: Lippincott Williams & Wilkins.

2. American College of Sports Medicine (ACSM). 2009. Appropriate physical activity intervention strategies for weight loss and prevention of weight regain for adults. *Medicine and Science in Sports and Exercise* 41(2): 459-471.

3. Allison, D.B., K.R. Fontaine, J.E. Manson, J. Stevens, and T.B. VanItallie. 1999. Annual deaths attributable to obesity in the United States. *Journal of the American Medical Association* 282:1530-1538.

4. Ball, K., D. Crawford, and N. Owen. 2000. Too fat to exercise? Obesity as a barrier to physical activity. *Australian and New Zealand Journal of Public Health* 24:331-333.

5. Beamer, B.A. 2003. Genetic influences on obesity. In *Obesity: Etiology, assessment, treatment and prevention*, ed. R.E. Anderson, 43-56. Champaign, IL: Human Kinetics.

6. Bouchard, C., L. Perusse, C. Leblanc, A. Tremblay, and G. Theriault. 1988. Inheritance of the amount and distribution of human body fat. *International Journal of Obesity* 12:205-215.

7. DiPietro, L. 1999. Physical activity in the prevention of obesity: Current evidence and research issues. *Medicine and Science in Sports and Exercise* 31:S542-S546.

8. Expert Panel on the Identification, Evaluation and Treatment of Overweight and Obesity in Adults. 1998. Executive summary of the clinical guidelines on the identification, evaluation, and treatment of overweight and obesity in adults. *Archives of Internal Medicine* 158:1855-1867.

9. Faith, M.S., P.E. Matz, and D.B. Allison. 2003. Psychosocial correlates and consequences of obesity. In *Obesity: Etiology, assessment, treatment, and prevention*, ed. R.E. Andersen, 17-31. Champaign, IL: Human Kinetics.

10. Finkelstein, E.A., J.G. Trogdon, J.W. Cohen, and W. Deitz. 2009. Annual medical spending attributable to obesity: Payer- and service-specific estimates. *Health Affairs* 28(5): w822-w831.

11. Flegal, K.M., B.I. Graubard, D.F. Williamson, and M.H. Gail. 2005. Excess deaths associated with underweight, overweight, and obesity. *Journal of the American Medical Association* 293:1861-1867.

12. Flegal, K.M., B.I. Graubard, D.F. Williamson, and M.H. Gail. 2007. Cause-specific excess deaths associated with underweight, overweight, and obesity. *Journal of the American Medical Association* 298:2028-2037.

13. Flegal, K.M., B.K. Kit, H. Orpana, and B.I. Graubard. 2013. Association of all-cause mortality with overweight and obesity using standard body mass index categories: A systematic review and meta-analysis. *Journal of the American Medical Association* 309(1): 71-82.

14. Food and Nutrition Board, Institute of Medicine. 2002. *Dietary reference intakes for energy, carbohydrate, fiber, fat, fatty acids, cholesterol, protein, and amino acids.* Washington, DC: National Academies Press.

15. Ford, E.S., L.M. Maynard, and C. Li. 2014. Trends in mean waist circumference and abdominal obesity among U.S. adults, 1999-2012. *Journal of the American Medical Association* 312(11): 1151-1153.

16. Gortmaker, S., A. Must, A. Sobel, K. Peterson, G.A. Colditz, and W.H. Dietz. 1996. Television viewing as a cause of increasing obesity among children in the United States. *Archives of Pediatric Adolescent Medicine* 150:356-362.

17. Grundy, S.M., G. Blackburn, M. Higgins, R. Lauer, M.G. Perri, and D. Ryan. 1999. Physical activity in the prevention and treatment of obesity and its comorbidities: Roundtable consensus statement. *Medicine and Science in Sports and Exercise* 31:S502-S508.

18. Jakicic, J.M. 2003. Exercise in the treatment of obesity. *Endocrinology and Metabolism Clinics of North America* 32:967-980.

19. Jakicic, J.M. 2003. Exercise strategies for the obese patient. *Primary Care* 30:393-403.

20. Jebb, S.A., and M.S. Moore. 1999. Contribution of a sedentary lifestyle and inactivity to the etiology of overweight and obesity: Current evidence and research issues. *Medicine and Science in Sports and Exercise* 31:S534-S541.

21. Locke, A.E., et al. 2015. Genetic studies of body mass index yield new insights for obesity biology. *Nature* 518:197-206.

22. National Heart, Lung, and Blood Institute. 1998. *Clinical guidelines on the identification, evaluation, and treatment of overweight and obesity in adults.* NIH Publication No. 98-4083. Bethesda, MD: National Institutes of Health—National Heart, Lung, and Blood Institute.

23. National Institute of Diabetes and Digestive and Kidney Diseases. 2009. *Bariatric surgery for severe obesity.* NIH Publication No. 08-4006 (update June 2011).

24. Ng, M., et al. 2013. Global, regional, and national prevalence of overweight and obesity in children and adults 1980-2013: A systematic analysis for the Global Burden of Disease Study 2013. *Lancet* 384:766-781.
25. Ogden, C.L., M.D. Carroll, B.K. Kit, and K.M. Flegal. 2014. Prevalence of childhood and adult obesity in the United States, 2011-2012. *Journal of the American Medical Association* 311(8): 806-814.
26. Ratamess, N. Body composition status and assessment. 2014. In *ACSM's resource manual for guidelines for exercise testing and prescription*. 7th ed. Ed. D.P. Swain, 287-308. Baltimore: Lippincott Williams & Wilkins.
27. Robinson, T.N. 1998. Does television cause childhood obesity? *Journal of the American Medical Association* 279:959-960.
28. Saris, W.H.M., S.N. Blair, M.A. van Baak, S.B. Eaton, P.S.W. Davies, L. Di Pietro, M. Fogelholm, A. Rissanen, D. Schoeller, B. Swinburn, A. Tremblay, K.R. Westerterp, and H. Wyatt. 2003. How much physical activity is enough to prevent unhealthy weight gain? Outcome of the IASO 1st Stock Conference and consensus statement. *Obesity Reviews* 4:101-114.
29. Sarma, S., G.S. Zaric, M.K. Campbell, and J. Gilliland. 2014. The effects of physical activity on adult obesity: Evidence from the Canadian NPHS panel. *Economics and Human Biology* 14:1-21.
30. Shungin, D., et al. 2015. New genetic loci link adipose and insulin biology to body fat distribution. *Nature* 518:187-196.
31. Skinner, A.C., and J.A. Skelton. 2014. Prevalence and trends in obesity and severe obesity among children in the United States, 1999-2012. *Journal of the American Medical Association Pediatrics* 168(6): 561-566.
32. Snow, V., P. Barry, N. Fitterman, A. Qaseem, and K. Weiss. 2005. Pharmacologic and surgical management of obesity in primary care: A clinical practice guideline for the American College of Physicians. *Annals of Internal Medicine* 142:525-531.
33. Stubbs, C.O., and A.J. Lee. 2004. The obesity epidemic: Both energy intake and physical activity contribute. *Medical Journal of Australia* 181:489-491.
34. Tsai, A.G., D.F. Williamson, and H.A. Glick. 2011. Direct cost of overweight and obesity in the USA: A quantitative systematic review. *Obesity Reviews* 12:50-61.
35. U.S. Department of Health and Human Services (HHS). 2001. *The Surgeon General's call to action to prevent and decrease overweight and obesity.* Rockville, MD: U.S. GPO.
36. U.S. Department of Health and Human Services (HHS). 2008. *2008 Physical Activity Guidelines for Americans.* www.health.gov/paguidelines/guidelines/default.aspx.
37. U.S. Department of Health and Human Services (HHS). 2010. *The Surgeon General's vision for a healthy and fit nation.* Rockville, MD: U.S. GPO.
38. Wallace, J.P., and S. Ray. 2009. Obesity. In *ACSM's exercise management for persons with chronic diseases and disabilities.* 3rd ed. Ed. J.L. Durstine, G.E. Moore, P.L. Painter, and S.O. Roberts, 192-200. Champaign, IL: Human Kinetics.
39. Welk, G.J., and Blair, S.N. 2000. Physical activity protects against the health risks of obesity. *PCPFS Research Digest* 3:1-7.
40. Wing, R.R. 1999. Physical activity in the treatment of adulthood overweight and obesity: Current evidence and research issues. *Medicine and Science in Sports and Exercise* 31:S547-S552.
41. Wing, R.R., and Hill, J.O. 2001. Successful weight loss maintenance. *Annual Review of Nutrition* 21:323-341.
42. Wing, R.R., and S. Phelan. 2005. Long-term weight loss maintenance. *American Journal of Clinical Nutrition* 82(Suppl.): 222S-225S.
43. Withrow, D., and D.A. Alter. 2010. The economic burden of obesity worldwide: A systematic review of the direct costs of obesity. *Obesity Reviews.* doi: 10.1111/j.1467-789X.2009.00712.x.

Chapter 21

1. American College of Sports Medicine (ACSM). (in press). *ACSM's guidelines for exercise testing and prescription.* 10th ed. Baltimore: Lippincott Williams & Wilkins.
2. American College of Sports Medicine (ACSM) and American Diabetes Association (ADA). 2010. Joint position statement: Exercise and type 2 diabetes. *Medicine and Science in Sports and Exercise* 42:2282-2303.
3. American Diabetes Association (ADA). 2013. Economic costs of diabetes in the U.S. in 2012. *Diabetes Care* 36(4): 1033-1046.
4. American Diabetes Association (ADA). 2015. Foundations of care: Education, nutrition, physical activity, smoking cessation, psychosocial care, and immunization. *Diabetes Care* 38(Suppl. 1): S20-S30.
5. American Diabetes Association (ADA). 2015. Classification and diagnosis of diabetes mellitus. *Diabetes Care* 38(Suppl. 1): S8-S16.
6. Barnes, D.E. 2004. *Action plan for diabetes: Your guide to controlling blood sugar.* Champaign, IL: Human Kinetics.
7. Bassuk, S.S., and J.E. Manson. 2005. Epidemiological evidence for the role of physical activity in reducing risk of type 2 diabetes and cardiovascular disease. *Journal of Applied Physiology* 99:1193-1204.
8. Centers for Disease Control and Prevention (CDC). 2014. National diabetes statistics report: Estimates of diabetes and its burden in the United States, 2014. Atlanta: U.S. Department of Health and Human Services.
9. Colberg, S.R. 2014. Exercise prescription in patients with diabetes. In *ACSM's resource manual for guidelines for exercise testing and prescription*. 7th ed. Ed. D.P. Swain, 661-681. Baltimore: Lippincott Williams & Wilkins.
10. Eriksson, J.G. 1999. Exercise and the treatment of type 2 diabetes mellitus: An update. *Sports Medicine* 27:381-391.
11. Grundy, S.M., J.L. Cleeman, S.R. Daniels, K.A. Donato, R.H. Eckel, B.A. Franklin, D.J. Gordon, R.M. Krauss, P.J. Savage, S.C. Smith, J.A. Spertus, and F. Costa. 2005. Diagnosis and management of the metabolic syndrome: An American Heart Association/National Heart, Lung, and Blood Institute scientific statement (executive summary). *Circulation* 112:285-290.

12. Hornsby, W.G., and A.L. Albright. 2009. Diabetes. In *ACSM's exercise management for persons with chronic diseases and disabilities*. 3rd ed. Ed. J.L. Durstine, G.E. Moore, P.L. Painter, and S.O. Roberts, 182-191. Champaign, IL: Human Kinetics.
13. Kriska, A. 2000. Physical activity and the prevention of type 2 diabetes mellitus: How much for how long? *Sports Medicine* 29:147-151.
14. Roitman, J.L., and N. Moodie. 2014. Diagnostic procedures in patients with metabolic disease. In *ACSM's resource manual for guidelines for exercise testing and prescription*. 7th ed. Ed. D.P. Swain, 413-423. Baltimore: Lippincott Williams & Wilkins.
15. U.S. Department of Health and Human Services (HHS). 2000. *Healthy People 2010: Understanding and improving health.* Washington, DC: U.S. GPO.
16. Zhao, G., E.S. Ford, C. Li, and A.H. Mokdad. 2008. Compliance with physical activity recommendations in U.S. adults with diabetes. *Diabetic Medicine* 25:221-227.

Chapter 22

1. American Association of Cardiovascular and Pulmonary Rehabilitation (AACVPR). 2011. *Guidelines for pulmonary rehabilitation programs.* 4th ed. Champaign, IL: Human Kinetics.
2. American College of Sports Medicine (ACSM). (in press). *ACSM's guidelines for exercise testing and prescription.* 10th ed. Baltimore: Lippincott Williams & Wilkins.
3. American Lung Association. 2008. *Lung disease data: 2008.* New York: Author.
4. American Lung Association. 2012. *Trends in asthma morbidity and mortality.* New York: Author.
5. American Lung Association. 2013. *Trends in COPD (chronic bronchitis and emphysema): Morbidity and mortality.* New York: Author.
6. Barr, R.N. 2001. Pulmonary rehabilitation. In *Essentials of cardiopulmonary physical therapy.* 2nd ed. Ed. E.A. Hillegass and H.S. Sadowsky, 727-751. Philadelphia: Saunders.
7. Berman, L.B., and J.R. Sutton. 1986. Exercise and the pulmonary patient. *Journal of Cardiopulmonary Rehabilitation* 6:52-61.
8. Borg, G.A. 1998. *Borg's perceived exertion and pain scales.* Champaign, IL: Human Kinetics.
9. Brubaker, P.H., L.A. Kaminsky, and M.H. Whaley. 2002. *Coronary artery disease: Essentials of prevention and rehabilitation programs.* Champaign, IL: Human Kinetics.
10. Cahalin, L.P., and H.S. Sadowsky. 2001. Pulmonary medications. In *Essentials of cardiopulmonary physical therapy.* 2nd ed. Ed. E.A. Hillegass and H.S. Sadowsky, 587-607. Philadelphia: Saunders.
11. Clough, P. 2001. Restrictive lung dysfunction. In *Essentials of cardiopulmonary physical therapy.* 2nd ed. Ed. E.A. Hillegass and H.S. Sadowsky, 183-255. Philadelphia: Saunders.
12. Cooper, C.B. 1995. Determining the role of exercise in patients with chronic pulmonary disease. *Medicine and Science in Sports and Exercise* 27:147-157.
13. Cooper, C.B. 2009. Chronic obstructive pulmonary disease. In *ACSM's exercise management for persons with chronic diseases and disabilities*, ed. J.L. Durstine, G. Moore, P. Painter, and S. Roberts, 129-135. Champaign, IL: Human Kinetics.
14. Cooper, C.B., and T.W. Storer. 2010. Exercise prescription in patients with pulmonary disease. In *ACSM's resource manual for guidelines for exercise testing and prescription.* 4th ed. Ed. J.K. Ehrman, 575-599. Baltimore: Lippincott Williams & Wilkins.
15. Davidson, A.C., R. Leach, R.J.D. George, and D.M. Geddes. 1988. Supplemental oxygen and exercise ability in chronic obstructive airways disease. *Thorax* 43:965-971.
16. Davis, P.B. 1991. Cystic fibrosis: A major cause of obstructive airway disease in the young. In *Chronic obstructive pulmonary disease,* ed. N.S. Cheniack, 297-307. Philadelphia: Saunders.
17. Environmental Protection Agency (EPA). 2010. Chronic obstructive pulmonary disease prevalence and mortality. https://cfpub.epa.gov/roe/indicator.cfm?i=76 [accessed March 10, 2016].
18. Garritan, S.L. 1994. Chronic obstructive pulmonary disease. In *Essentials of cardiopulmonary physical therapy,* ed. E.A. Hillegass and H.S. Sadowsky, 257-284. Philadelphia: Saunders.
19. Guyton, A.C., and J.E. Hall. 2010. *Textbook of medical physiology.* 12th ed. Philadelphia: Saunders.
20. Lacroix, V.J. 1999. Exercise-induced asthma. *Physician and Sportsmedicine* 27:75-92.
21. Mahler, D.A., and M.B. Horowitz. 1994. Perception of breathlessness during exercise in patients with respiratory disease. *Medicine and Science in Sports and Exercise* 26:1078-1081.
22. Rundell, K.W., and D.M. Jenkinson. 2002. Exercise-induced bronchospasm in the elite athlete. *Sports Medicine* 32:583-600.

Chapter 23

1. Biddle, S., and C.R. Nigg. 2000. Theories of exercise behavior. *International Journal of Sport Psychology* 31:290-304.
2. Buckworth, J., R.K. Dishman, P. O'Connor, and P. Tomporowski. 2013. *Exercise psychology.* 2nd ed. Champaign, IL: Human Kinetics.
3. Deci, E., and N.D. Ryan. 2008. Self-determination theory: A macrotheory of human motivation, development and health. *Canadian Psychology* 49(3): 182-185. doi: 10.1037/a0012801.
4. Dishman, R.K., and J. Buckworth. 1996. Adherence to physical activity. In *Physical activity and mental health,* ed. W.P. Morgan, 63-80. Washington, DC: Taylor & Francis.
5. Hagger, M.S., N.L.D. Chatzisarantis, and S.J.H. Biddle. 2002. A meta-analytic review of the theories of reasoned action and planned behavior in physical activity: Predictive validity and the contribution of additional variables. *Journal of Sport and Exercise Psychology* 24:3-32.
6. Keller, C., B. Ainsworth, K. Records, M. Todd, M. Belyea, S. Vega-López, et al. 2014. A comparison of a social support physical activity intervention in weight management among post-partum Latinas. *Biomedical Central Public Health* 14(1): 1-15.

7. King, A.C., J.E. Martin, and C. Castro. 2006. Behavioral strategies to enhance physical activity participation. In *ACSM's resource manual for guidelines for exercise testing and prescription,* ed. L.A. Kaminsky and K.A. Bonzheim, 572-580. Philadelphia: Lippincott Williams & Wilkins.
8. King, A.C., D. Stokols, E. Talen, G.S. Brassington, and R. Killingsworth. 2002. Theoretical approaches to the promotion of physical activity: Forging a transdisciplinary paradigm. *American Journal of Preventive Medicine* 23:15-25.
9. Knapp, D.N. 1988. Behavioral management techniques and exercise promotion. In *Exercise adherence,* ed. R.K. Dishman, 203-236. Champaign, IL: Human Kinetics.
10. Kyllo, L.B., and D.M. Landers. 1995. Goal setting in sport and exercise: A research synthesis to resolve the controversy. *Journal of Sport and Exercise Psychology* 17:117-137.
11. Marcus, B., and L. Forsyth. 2009. *Motivating people to be physically active.* 2nd ed. Champaign, IL: Human Kinetics.
12. Marcus, B.H., P.M. Dubbert, L.H. Forsyth, T.L. McKenzie, E.J. Stone, A.L. Dunn, and S.N. Blair. 2000. Physical activity behavior change: Issues in adoption and maintenance. *Health Psychology* 19:32-41.
13. Markland, D., and L. Hardy. 1993. The exercise motivation inventory: Preliminary development and validity of a measure of individuals' reasons for participation in regular physical exercise. *Personality and Individual Differences* 15:289-296.
14. Marlatt, G.A., and J.R. Gordon. 1985. *Relapse prevention: Maintenance strategies in the treatment of addictive behaviors.* New York: Guilford Press.
15. McCormack, G.R, and A. Shiell. 2011. In search of causality: A systematic review of the relationship between the built environment and physical activity among adults. *International Journal of Behavioral Nutrition and Physical Activity* 8:125.
16. Nigg, C., ed. 2014. *ACSM's behavioral aspects of physical activity and exercise.* Philadelphia: Lippincott Williams & Wilkins.
17. Prochaska, J.O., and B.H. Marcus. 1994. The transtheoretical model: Applications to exercise. In *Advances in exercise adherence,* ed. R.K. Dishman, 161-180. Champaign, IL: Human Kinetics.
18. Prochaska, J.O., and W.F. Velicer. 1997. The transtheoretical model of behavior change. *American Journal of Health Promotion* 12:38-48.
19. Rollnick, S., W.R. Miller, and C.C. Butler. 2007. *Motivational interviewing in health care: Helping patients change behavior.* New York: Guilford Press.
20. Ryan, R., C. Frederick, D. Lepes, N. Rubio, and K. Sheldon 1997. Intrinsic motivation and exercise adherence. *International Journal of Sport Psychology* 28:335-354.
21. Sonstroem, R.J. 1988. Psychological models. In *Exercise adherence: Its impact on public health,* ed. R.K. Dishman, 125-153. Champaign, IL: Human Kinetics.
22. Stetson, B.A., A.O. Beacham, S.J. Frommelt, K.N. Boutelle, J.D. Cole, C.H. Ziegler, et al. 2005. Exercise slips in high-risk situations and activity patterns in long-term exercisers: An application of the relapse prevention model. *Annals of Behavioral Medicine* 30(1): 25-35.
23. Teixeira, P.J., E.V. Carraca, D. Markland, M.N. Silva, and R.M. Ryan. 2012. Exercise, physical activity, and self-determination theory: A systematic review. *International Journal of Behavioral Nutrition and Physical Activity* 9:78.
24. Trost, S.G., N. Owen, A. Bauman, J.F. Sallis, and W.J. Brown. 2002. Correlates of adults' participation in physical activity: Review and update. *Medicine and Science in Sports and Exercise* 34:1996-2001.
25. Wallace, J.P., J.S. Raglin, and C.A. Jastremski. 1995. Twelve month adherence of adults who joined a fitness program with a spouse vs. without a spouse. *Journal of Sports Medicine and Physical Fitness* 35:206-213.
26. Whiteley, J.A., B.A. Lewis, M.A. Napolitano, and B.H. Marcus. 2009. Health behavior counseling. In *ACSM's resource manual for guidelines for exercise testing and prescription*, ed. J.K. Ehrman, 723-733. Baltimore: Williams & Wilkins.
27. Wilson, K., and D. Brookfield. 2009. Effect of goal setting on motivation and adherence in a six-week exercise program. *International Journal of Sport and Exercise Psychology* 7:89-100.

Chapter 24

1. American College of Sports Medicine (ACSM). (in press). *Guidelines for exercise testing and prescription. 10th* ed. Baltimore: Lippincott Williams & Wilkins.
2. American College of Sports Medicine (ACSM) and American Heart Association (AHA). 2002. Joint position statement: Automated external defibrillators in health/fitness facilities. *Medicine and Science in Sports and Exercise* 34(3): 561-564.
3. American Hospital Formulary Service. 2015. *Drug information 2015.* Bethesda, MD: American Society of Hospital Pharmacists.
4. Berne, R.M., and M.N. Levy. 2001. *Cardiovascular physiology.* 8th ed. St. Louis: Mosby.
5. Chang, K., and K.F. Hossack. 1982. Effect of diltiazem on heart rate responses and respiratory variables during exercise: Implications for exercise prescription and cardiac rehabilitation. *Journal of Cardiac Rehabilitation* 2:326-332.
6. Conover, M.B. 1996. *Understanding electrocardiography.* 7th ed. St. Louis: Mosby.
7. Donnelly, J.E. 1990. *Living anatomy.* 2nd ed. Champaign, IL: Human Kinetics.
8. Dubin, D. 2000. *Rapid interpretation of EKGs.* 6th ed. Tampa: Cover.
9. Ellestad, M.H. 2003 *Stress testing: Principles and practice. 5th ed.* New York: Oxford University Press.
10. Hurst, J.W. 1994. *Diagnostic atlas of the heart.* Philadelphia: Lippincott-Raven.
11. Kannel, W.B., and R.D. Abbot. 1984. Incidence and prognosis of unrecognized myocardial infarction. *New England Journal of Medicine* 311:1144-1147.
12. Kelbaek, H., T. Gjorup, S. Floistrup, O. Hartling, N. Christensen, and J. Godtfredsen. 1985. Acute effects of alcohol on left ventricular function in healthy subjects at rest and during upright exercise. *American Journal of Cardiology* 55:164-167.

13. Stein, E. 2000. *Rapid analysis of electrocardiograms: A self-study program.* 3rd ed. Philadelphia: Lea & Febiger.
14. Williams, M.H. 1991. Alcohol, marijuana and beta blockers. In *Perspectives in exercise science and sports medicine: Vol. 4. Ergogenics: Enhancement of performance in exercise and sport,* ed. D.R. Lamb and M.H. Williams, 331-372. Dubuque, IA: Brown & Benchmark.

Chapter 25

1. American Diabetes Association (ADA). 2014. Hypoglycemia. www.diabetes.org/living-with-diabetes/treatment-and-care/blood-glucose-control/hyperglycemia.html.
2. American Diabetes Association (ADA). 2015. Preventing and treating severe hypoglycemia. www.diabetes.org/living-with-diabetes/treatment-and-care/blood-glucose-control/hypoglycemia-low-blood.html.
3. American Heart Association (AHA). 2015. Highlights of the 2015 American Heart Association Guidelines Update for CPR and ECC. http://eccguidelines.heart.org/wp-content/uploads/2015/10/2015-AHA-Guidelines-Highlights-English.pdf.
4. Anderson, M. K., and G.P. Parr. 2013. *Foundations of athletic training: Prevention, assessment, and management.* 5th ed. Philadelphia: Lippincott Williams & Wilkins.
5. Anzalone, M.L., V.S. Green, M. Buja, R.I. Harrykissoon, and E.R. Eichner. 2010. Sickle cell trait and fatal rhabdomyolysis in football training: A case study. *Medicine and Science in Sports and Exercise* 42(1): 3-7.
6. Armstrong, A.B. 1984. Mechanisms of exercise-induced delayed onset muscular soreness: A brief review. *Medicine and Science in Sports and Exercise* 16(6): 529-538.
7. Armstrong, L.E., D.J. Casa, M. Millard-Stafford, D.S. Moran, S.W. Pyne, and W.O. Roberts. 2007. ACSM's position stand: Exertional heat illness during training and competition. *Medicine and Science in Sports and Exercise* 39(3): 556-572.
8. Binkley, H.M., J. Beckett, D.J. Casa, D.M. Kleiner, and P.E. Plummer. 2002. National Athletic Trainers' Association position statement: Exertional heat illnesses. *Journal of Athletic Training* 37(3): 329-343.
9. Bosh, X., P. Esteban, and J. Grau. 2009. Rhabdomyolysis and acute kidney injury. *New England Journal of Medicine* 361:62-72.
10. Byrnes, W.C., P.M. Clarkson, J.S. White, S.S. Hsieh, P.N. Frykman, and R. J. Maughan. 1985. Delayed onset muscle soreness following repeated bouts of downhill running. *Journal of Applied Physiology* 59(3): 710-715.
11. Cappaert, T.A., J.A. Stone, J.W. Castellani, B.A. Krause, D. Smith, and B.A. Stephens. 2008. National Athletic Trainers' Association position statement: Environmental cold injuries. *Journal of Athletic Training* 43(6): 640-658.
12. Casa, D.J., L.E. Armstrong, S.K. Hillman, S.J. Montain, R.V. Reiff, B.S.E Rich, W.O. Roberts, and J.A. Stone. 2000. National Athletic Trainers' Association position statement: Fluid replacement for athletes. *Journal of Athletic Training* 35(2): 212-224.
13. Casa, D.J., and D. Csillan. 2009. Preseason heat-acclimatization guidelines for secondary school athletics. *Journal of Athletic Training* 44(3): 332-333.
14. Casa, D.J., and R.L. Stearns. 2014. *Emergency management for sport and physical activity.* Burlington, MA: Jones & Barlett.
15. Centers for Disease Control and Prevention (CDC). 2014. General Information About MRSA in Healthcare Settings. http://www.cdc.gov/mrsa/healthcare/index.html
16. Centers for Disease Control and Prevention (CDC). How to remove Gloves. http://www.cdc.gov/vhf/ebola/pdf/poster-how-to-remove-gloves.pdf.
17. Cheung, K., P.A. Hume, and L. Maxwell. 2003. Delayed-onset muscle soreness: Treatment strategies and performance factors. *Sports Medicine* 33(2): 145-164.
18. Connolly, D.A., S.E. Sayers, and M.P. Mchugh. 2003. Treatment and prevention of delayed onset muscle soreness. *Journal of Strength and Conditioning Research* 17(1): 197-208.
19. Covassin, T., and R.J. Elbin. 2010. The cognitive effects and decrements following concussion. *Journal of Sports Medicine* 1:55-61.
20. Eckner, J.T., and J.S. Kutcher. 2010. Concussion symptom scales and sideline assessment tools: A critical literature update. *Current Sports Medicine Reports ACSM* 9(1): 8-15.
21. Faul M., L. Xu, M.M. Wald, and V.G. Coronado. 2010. *Traumatic brain injury in the United States: Emergency department visits, hospitalizations and deaths 2002–2006.* Atlanta: Centers for Disease Control and Prevention, National Center for Injury Prevention and Control.
22. Gardner, J.W., and J.A. Kark. 1994. Fatal rhabdomyolysis presenting as mild heat illness in military training. *Military Medicine* 159:160-163.
23. Glover, J. 2007. *Sports medicine essentials: Core concepts in athletic training and fitness instruction.* 2nd ed. Clifton Park, NY: Thompson Delmar Learning.
24. Guskiewicz, K.M., S.L. Bruce, R.C. Cantu, M.S. Ferrara, J.P. Kelly, M. McCrea, M. Putukian, and T.C. Valovich McLeod. 2004. National Athletic Trainers' Association position statement: Management of sport-related concussion. *Journal of Athletic Training* 39(3): 280-297.
25. Harmon, K.G., et al. 2013. American Medical Society for Sports Medicine position statement: Concussion in sport. *Clinical Journal of Sports Medicine* 23:1-18.
26. Harrelson, G.L., A.L. Fincher, and J.B. Robinson. 1995. Acute exertional rhabdomyolysis and its relationship to sickle cell trait. *Journal of Athletic Training* 30(4): 309-312.
27. Jimenez, C.C, M.H. Corcoran, J.T. Crawley, W.G. Hornsby, K.S. Peer, R.D. Philbin, and M.C. Riddell. 2007. National Athletic Trainers' Association position statement: Management of the athlete with type 1 diabetes mellitus. *Journal of Athletic Training* 42(4): 536-545.
28. McCrory, P., et al. 2013. Consensus statement on concussion in sport: The 4th International Conference on Concussion in Sport, Zurich, November 2012. *British Journal of Sports Medicine* 47:250-258.
29. National Athletic Trainers' Association (NATA). 2005. Official statement from the National Athletic Trainers' Association on community-acquired MRSA infections (CA-MRSA). www.nata.org/sites/default/files/MRSA.pdf.

30. National Collegiate Athletic Association (NCAA). *2013-2014 NCAA sports medicine handbook.* 24th ed. Ed. D. Klossner. Indianapolis: Author.
31. Prentice, W.E. 2007. *Essentials of athletic injury management.* 7th ed. New York: McGraw-Hill.
32. Prentice, W. 2013. *Principles of athletic training: A competency-based approach.* 15th ed. New York: McGraw-Hill Higher Education.
33. Sayers, S.P., P.M. Clarkson, P.A. Pierre, and G. Kamen. 1999. Adverse events associated with eccentric exercise protocols: Six case studies. *Medicine and Science in Sports and Exercise* 31(12): 1697.
34. Tharrett, S.J., and J.A. Peterson, eds. 2012. *ACSM's health/fitness facility standards and guidelines.* 4th ed. Champaign, IL: Human Kinetics.
35. United States Department of Labor. Occupational Health and Safety Administration universal precautions. www.osha.gov/SLTC/etools/hospital/hazards/univprec/univ.html.
36. U.S. Preventive Services Task Force (USPSTF). 2016. Sickle cell disease (hemoglobinopathies) in newborns: Screening. www.uspreventiveservicestaskforce.org/uspstf07/sicklecell/sicklers.htm.
37. Walsh, K.M., B. Bennett, M.A. Cooper, R.L. Holle, R. Kithil, and R.E. Lopez. 2000. National Athletic Trainers' Association position statement: Lightning safety for athletics and recreation. *Journal of Athletic Training* 35(4): 471-477.
38. Ward, M.M. 1988. Factors predictive of acute renal failure in rhabdomyolysis. *Archives of Internal Medicine* 148(7): 1553-1557.

Chapter 26

1. Abbott, A.A. 2009. Fitness professionals: Certified, qualified, and justified. *Exercise Standards and Malpractice Reporter* 23(2): 17, 20-22.
2. Abbott A.A. 2013. Cardiac arrest litigations. *ACSM's Health & Fitness Journal* 17(1): 31-34.
3. Abbott A.A. 2013. Injury litigations. *ACSM's Health & Fitness Journal* 17(3): 28-32.
4. *Alack v. Vic Tanny International of Missouri, Inc.* 923 S.W.2d 330 (Mo., 1996).
5. American College of Sports Medicine (ACSM). 2009. Position stand. Progression models in resistance training for healthy adults. *Medicine and Science in Sports and Exercise* 41(3): 687-708.
6. Americans with Disabilities Act (ADA). 2004. 42 U.S.C. 12181(7) (L) and 12182.
7. Americans with Disabilities Act Title III Regulations: Part 36 nondiscrimination on the basis of disability by public accommodation and commercial facilities. 2010. www.ada.gov/regs2010/titleIII_2010/titleIII_2010_regulations.htm#a102 [accessed January 16, 2015].
8. *Barnhard v. Cybex International, Inc.,* 933 N.Y.S.2d 794 (N.Y. App. Div. LEXIS 8278, 2011).
9. Bergeron M.F., B.C. Nindl, P.A. Deuster, et al. 2011. Consortium for health and military performance and American College of Sports Medicine consensus paper on extreme conditioning programs in military personnel. *Current Sports Medicine Reports* 10(6): 383-389.
10. Binkley, H.M., J. Beckett, D.J. Casa, D.M. Kleiner, and P.E. Plummer. 2002. National Athletic Trainers' Association position statement: Exertional heat illnesses. *Journal of Athletic Training* 37(3): 329-343.
11. Blair, S.A. 2003. Implementing HIPAA. *ACSM's Health & Fitness Journal* 7(5): 25-27.
12. *Bloodborne pathogens.* 2009. 29 C.F.R. § 1910.1030. New York: Thomson Reuters.
13. Brathwaite, A., D. Davidson, and J.M. Eickhoff-Shemek. 2006. Recruiting, training, and retaining qualified group exercise leaders: Part I. *ACSM's Health & Fitness Journal* 10(2): 14-18.
14. Brathwaite, A., and J.M. Eickhoff-Shemek. 2007. Preparing quality personal trainers: A successful pilot program. *Exercise Standards and Malpractice Reporter* 21(2): 25-31.
15. *Capati v. Crunch Fitness International, Inc., et al.* Analyzed in: Herbert, D.L. 1999. $320 million lawsuit filed against health club. *Exercise Standards and Malpractice Reporter* 13(3): 33, 36.
16. *Capati v. Crunch Fitness International, Inc., et al.* Analyzed in: Herbert, D.L. 2006. Wrongful death case of Anne Marie Capati settled for in excess of $4 million. *Exercise Standards and Malpractice Reporter* 20(3): 36.
17. Carper, D.L., N.J. Mietus, and B.W. West. 2000. *Understanding the law.* 3rd ed. Cincinnati: West Legal Studies in Business/Thomson.
18. Casa D.J., S.A. Anderson, L. Baker, et al. 2012. The inter-association task force for preventing sudden death in collegiate conditioning sessions: Best practices recommendations. *Journal of Athletic Training* 47(4): 477-480.
19. Centers for Disease Control and Prevention (CDC). 2014. *State indicator report on physical activity, 2014.* Atlanta: U.S. Department of Health and Human Services. www.cdc.gov/physicalactivity/downloads/pa_state_indicator_report_2014.pdf [accessed January 5, 2015].
20. Centers for Disease Control and Prevention (CDC). 2014. *Chronic diseases: The leading causes of death and disability in the United States.* Atlanta: U.S. Department of Health and Human Services. www.cdc.gov/chronicdisease/overview/index.htm [accessed January 5, 2015].
21. *Chai v. Sports & Fitness Clubs of America, Inc.* Analyzed in: Failure to defibrillate results in new litigation. 1999. *Exercise Standards and Malpractice Reporter* 13(4): 55-56.
22. Clarkson, K.W., R.L. Miller, G.A. Jentz, and F.B. Cross. 2001. *West's business law.* 8th ed. St. Paul: West.
23. *Corrigan v. Musclemakers, Inc.,* 258 A.D.2d 861 (N.Y. App. Div., 1999).
24. Cotten, D.J., and M.B. Cotten. 2016. *Waivers and releases of liability.* 9th ed. Statesboro, GA: Sport Risk Consulting.
25. *Covenant Health System v. Barnett,* 342 S.W.3d 226 (Tex. App. LEXIS 3665, 2011).
26. Craig, A.C. (2014). A national investigation of pre-activity health screening procedures in fitness facilities: Perspectives from American College of Sports Medicine certified health fitness specialists (3667189). PhD diss., University of South Florida.

27. Craig, A., and J.M. Eickhoff-Shemek. 2009. Educating and training the personal fitness trainer: A pedagogical approach. *ACSM's Health & Fitness Journal* 13(2): 8-15.
28. Davidson, D., A. Brathwaite, and J.M. Eickhoff-Shemek. 2006. Recruiting, training, and retaining qualified group exercise leaders: Part II. *ACSM's Health & Fitness Journal* 10(3): 22-26.
29. *DiGiulio v. Gran, Inc.*, 903 N.Y.S.2d 359 (N.Y. App. Div. LEXIS 4620, 2010).
30. Dobbs, D.B. 2000. *The law of torts.* St. Paul: West.
31. Eickhoff-Shemek, J. 2010. Treadmill injuries: An analysis of case law. *ACSM's Health & Fitness Journal* 14(1): 39-41.
32. Eickhoff-Shemek, J., and K. Berg. (2012). *Physical fitness: Guidelines for safe and effective exercise.* www.fitnesslawacademy.com.
33. Eickhoff-Shemek, J.M., and D.L. Herbert. 2007. Is licensure in your future? Issues to consider—part 1. *ACSM's Health & Fitness Journal* 11(5): 35-37.
34. Eickhoff-Shemek, J.M., and D.L Herbert. 2008. Is licensure in your future? Issues to consider—part 2. *ACSM's Health & Fitness Journal* 12(1): 36-38.
35. Eickhoff-Shemek, J.M., and D.L. Herbert. 2008. Is licensure in your future? Issues to consider—part 3. *ACSM's Health & Fitness Journal* 12(3): 36-38.
36. Eickhoff-Shemek, J.M., D.L. Herbert, and D.P. Connaughton. 2009. *Risk management for health/fitness professionals: Legal issues and strategies.* Baltimore: Lippincott Williams & Wilkins.
37. Eickhoff-Shemek, J., and M. Keiper, M. 2014. High-intensity exercise and the legal liability risks. *ACSM's Health & Fitness Journal* 18(5): 30-37.
38. *Elledge v. Richland/Lexington School District Five*, LEXIS 108 (S.C. Ct. App. 2000).
39. *Goynias v. Spa Health Clubs, Inc.*, 148 N.C.App. 554 (N.C. Ct. App., 2002).
40. Head, G.L., and S. Horn. 1997. *Essentials of risk management: Vol. I.* 3rd ed. Malvern, PA: Insurance Institute of America.
41. Herbert, D.L. 2010. New Jersey reintroduces personal trainer legislation. *Exercise Standards and Malpractice Reporter* 24(3): 37-41.
42. Herbert, D.L. 2014. Stroke during personal training session leads to suit. *Exercise, Sports and Sports Medicine Standards and Malpractice Reporter* 3(3): 43-44.
43. Herbert, D.L., and W.G. Herbert. 2002. *Legal aspects of preventive, rehabilitative and recreational exercise programs.* 4th ed. Canton, OH: PRC.
44. Jordin, E. 2014. Former Hawkeye sues over 2011 football training hospitalization: 13 players hospitalized after intense workout. *Gazette*, March 11. http://thegazette.com/2014/03/11/former-hawkeye-sues-state-over-2011-rhabdo-incident. [accessed June 27, 2014].
45. Kerr Z.Y., C.L. Collins, and R.D. 2010. Epidemiology of weight-training-related injuries presenting to the United States emergency departments, 1990 to 2007. *American Journal of Sports Medicine* 38(4): 765-771.
46. *Makris v. Scandinavian Health Spa, Inc.*, Ohio App. LEXIS 4416 (Ct. of Appeals, 7th Dist., 1999).
47. *Mimms v. Ruthless Training Concepts, LLC*, (Case No. 78584, Cir. Ct. of Prince William County, VA, 2008).
48. Moorman, A.M., and J.M. Eickhoff-Shemek. 2007. Risk management strategies for avoiding and responding to sexual assault complaints. *ACSM's Health & Fitness Journal* 11(3): 35-37.
49. New lawsuit against energy drink manufacturer 2013. *Exercise, Sports and Sports Medicine Standards and Malpractice Reporter* 2(1): 13-15.
50. Ohio Board of Dietetics. 2009. *Bulletin #8, general non-medical nutrition information.* www.dietetics.ohio.gov/bulletins/bulletin8.pdf [accessed January 16, 2015].
51. *Ohio Board of Dietetics v. Brown*, 83 Ohio App. 3rd 242 (Ohio App. LEXIS 88, 1993).
52. Pescatello L.S., ed. 2013. *ACSM's guidelines for exercise testing and prescription.* 9th ed. Philadelphia: Lippincott Williams & Wilkins.
53. *Proffitt v. Global Fitness Holdings, LLC, et al.* In: Herbert D.L. 2013. New lawsuit against personal trainer and facility in Kentucky—rhabdomyolysis alleged. *Exercise, Sports and Sports Medicine Standards and Malpractice Reporter* 2(1): 1, 3-10.
54. *Randas v. YMCA of Metropolitan Los Angeles*, 17 Cal. App. 4th 158 (Cal. App. 2 Dist., 1993).
55. *Restatement of the law third. Restatement of the law torts.* 2006. Philadelphia: American Law Institute.
56. *Restatement of the law third. Restatement of the law torts: Liability for physical harm.* 2005. Proposed final draft No. 1, § 12. Knowledge and skills. Philadelphia: American Law Institute.
57. Rhabdomyolysis lawsuit in Kentucky settled. 2013. *Exercise, Sports and Sports Medicine Standards and Malpractice Reporter* 2(4): 58.
58. *Rostai v. Neste Enterprises*, 41 Cal. Reptr. 3rd 411 (Cal. Ct. App., 4th Dist. 2006).
59. *Rutnik v. Colonie Center Court Club, Inc.*, 672 N.Y.S 2d 451 (1998 N.Y. App. Div. LEXIS 4845).
60. *Santana v. Women's Workout and Weight Loss Centers, Inc.* (2001 Cal. App. LEXIS 1186).
61. Sass, C., J.M. Eickhoff-Shemek, M.M. Manore, and L.J. Kruskall. 2007. Crossing the line: Understanding the scope of practice between registered dietitians and health/fitness professionals. *ACSM's Health & Fitness Journal* 11(3): 12-19.
62. *Seigneur v. National Fitness Institute, Inc.*, 132 Md. App. 271 (Md. Ct. Spec. App., 2000).
63. Stebbins, T. 2012. Cybex reaches $19.5m settlement in product liability case. Lawsuit Reform Alliance of New York, February 17. [accessed January 16, 2015]. http://www.nylawsuitreform.org/2012/02/cybex-reaches-19-5m-settlement-in-product-liability-case-tort-reform-lrany
64. *Stelluti v. Casapenn Enterprises, LLC*, 203 N.J. 286 (N.J. LEXIS 750, 2010).

65. Tharrett, S.J. and J.A. Peterson, eds. 2012. *ACSM's health/fitness facility standards and guidelines.* 4th ed. Champaign, IL: Human Kinetics.

66. *Thomas v. Sport City, Inc.* 738 So. 2d 1153 (La. Ct. App. 2 Cir., 1999).

67. Thompson P.D., B.A. Franklin, and G.J. Balady, et al. 2007. Exercise and acute cardiovascular events: Placing the risks into perspective. *Medicine and Science in Sports and Exercise* 39(5): 886-897.

68. Thompson, W.R., ed. 2010. *ACSM's guidelines for exercise testing and prescription.* 8th ed. Philadelphia: Lippincott Williams & Wilkins.

69. Thompson, W.R. 2013. Now trending: Worldwide survey of fitness trends for 2014. *ACSM's Health & Fitness Journal* 17(6): 10-20.

70. Thompson, W. R. (2013). Worldwide survey of fitness trends for 2015: What's driving the market. *ACSM's Health & Fitness Journal* 18(6): 8-17.

71. U.S. Department of Health and Human Services (HHS). 2009. *CDC injury research agenda 2009-2018.* Atlanta: U.S. Department of Health and Human Services, Centers for Disease Control and Prevention, National Center for Injury Prevention and Control. www.cdc.gov/injury/ResearchAgenda/pdf/CDC_Injury_Research_Agenda-a.pdf [accessed January 16, 2015].

72. Van der Smissen, B. 2007. Elements of negligence. In *Law for recreation and sport managers*, 4th ed. Ed. D.J. Cotton and J.T. Wolohan. Dubuque, IA: Kendall/Hunt.

73. Van der Smissen, B. 1990. *Legal liability and risk management for public and private entities: Vol. 2.* Cincinnati: Anderson.

74. Voris, H.C., and M. Rabinoff. 2011. When is a standard of care not a standard of care? *Exercise Standards and Malpractice Reporter* 25(2): 20-21.

75. Warburton, D.E.R., S.S.D. Bredin, and S.A. Charlesworth, et al. 2011. Evidence-based risk recommendations for best practices in the training of qualified exercise professional working with clinical populations. *Applied Physiology Nutrition and Metab*olism 36:S232-S265.

76. *Xu v. Gay*, 668 N.W.2d 166 (Mich. App., 2003).

77. *York Insurance Company v. Houston Wellness Center, Inc.*, 261 Ga. App. 854 (Ga. Ct. App., 2003).

Appendix B

1. American College of Sports Medicine (ACSM). (in press). *ACSM's guidelines for exercise testing and prescription.* 10th ed. Philadelphia: Lippincott Williams & Wilkins.

2. Plowman, S.A., and M.D. Meredith, eds. 2013. *Fitnessgram/Activitygram reference guide.* 4th ed. Dallas: Cooper Institute.

3. President's Council on Fitness, Sports and Nutrition. 2015. Presidential Active Lifestyle Award. www.presidentschallenge.org/challenge/active/index.shtml.

4. Rimmer, J.H. 2014. A focus and pathway to inclusive physical activity for people with disabilities. *Elevate Health* 4(15).

INDEX

Page numbers ending in an *f* or a *t* indicate a figure or table, respectively.

Q

R

ABOUT THE EDITORS

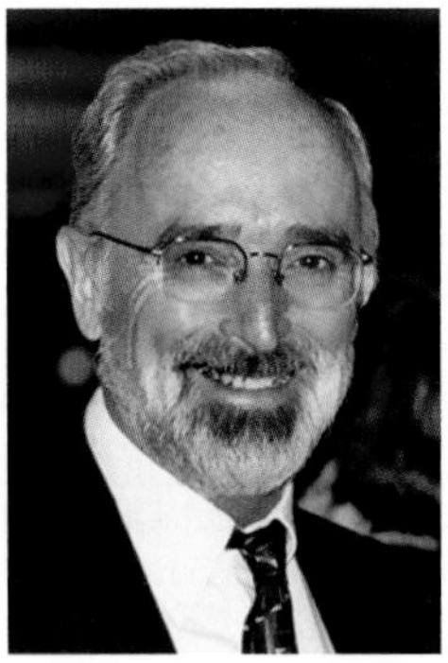

© Edward Howley

Edward T. Howley, PhD, FACSM, FNAK, earned his bachelor's degree from Manhattan College and his master's and doctorate degrees from the University of Wisconsin at Madison. He then completed a one-year postdoctoral appointment at Penn State University and was hired in 1970 as a faculty member at the University of Tennessee at Knoxville. Howley taught a variety of courses, including an undergraduate course in fitness testing and prescription and undergraduate and graduate courses in exercise physiology. He retired in 2007 and holds the rank of professor emeritus.

In addition to the previous editions of this book, Dr. Howley has authored three books, four book chapters, and more than 60 research articles dealing with exercise physiology, fitness testing, and prescription. He is a fellow in the National Academy of Kinesiology and served as chair of the Science Board of the President's Council on Physical Fitness and Sports in 2006-2007. In 2007-08 he served on the Physical Activity Guidelines Advisory Committee that evaluated the science related to physical activity and health and generated a report for use by the U.S. Department of Health and Human Services to write the *2008 Physical Activity Guidelines for Americans*.

Most of Dr. Howley's volunteer efforts have been with the American College of Sports Medicine (ACSM). He was involved in the development of certification programs and served as president in 2002-03. He served as editor in chief of *ACSM's Health & Fitness Journal* for seven years and as chair of the program planning committee for the annual ACSM Health and Fitness Summit meeting. In 2007, Howley was recognized for his professional contributions with the ACSM Citation Award. In his leisure time, he likes to golf, ride his bike, travel, and play with his grandchildren.

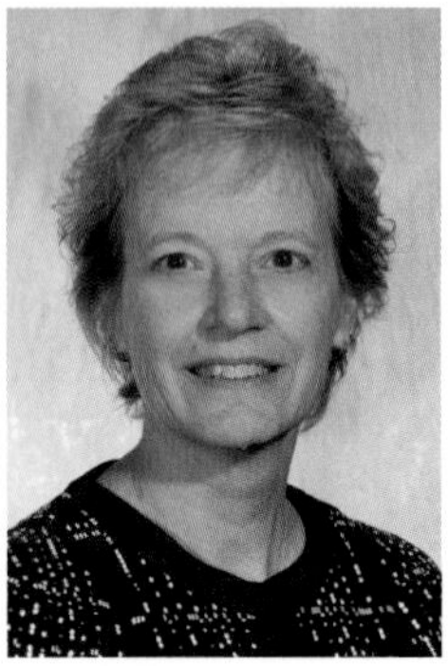

Photo courtesy of University of Tennessee photography services.

Dixie L. Thompson, PhD, FACSM, FNAK, is vice provost and dean of the graduate school at the University of Tennessee at Knoxville and is a professor in the department of kinesiology, recreation, and sports studies. She graduated from the 2008 class of the Higher Education Resource Services (HERS) Bryn Mawr Summer Institute, held at Bryn Mawr College. The Summer Institute is a professional development program dedicated to the advancement of female leaders in administration of higher education. She also participated in the 2009-2010 Academic Leadership Development Program sponsored by the Southeastern Conference Academic Consortium.

Dr. Thompson focuses her research on the health benefits of exercise for women and techniques used for body composition assessment. She is the author of over 70 peer-reviewed publications and numerous articles for fitness professionals and general audiences. She is a former associate editor in chief for *ACSM's Health & Fitness Journal* and former editor in chief for *ACSM's Fit Society Page Newsletter.*

Dr. Thompson is a fellow of the American College of Sports Medicine (ACSM) and a member of the ACSM Board of Trustees. She is a fellow of the National Academy of Kinesiology. She is a past president of the Southeast Chapter of ACSM and former chair of the Physical Fitness Council for the American Alliance for Health, Physical Education, Recreation and Dance.

Dr. Thompson received her BA in physical education and MA in exercise physiology from the University of North Carolina at Chapel Hill. She earned her PhD from the University of Virginia.

ABOUT THE CONTRIBUTORS

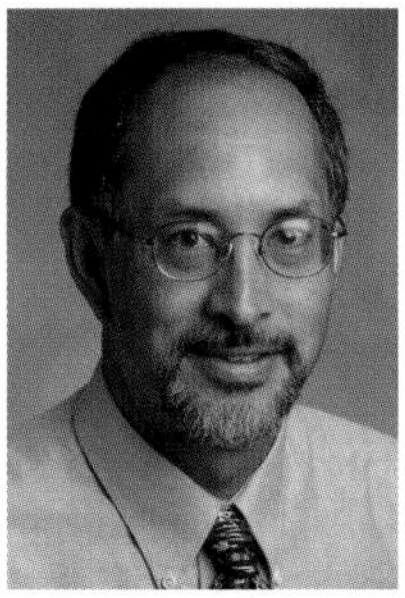

Photo courtesy of the University of Tennessee.

David R. Bassett Jr., PhD, is a professor in the department of kinesiology, recreation, and sport studies at the University of Tennessee in Knoxville. He is a fellow of the American College of Sports Medicine and the National Academy of Kinesiology. He is also a frequent reviewer for several scientific journals. Dr. Bassett teaches courses in exercise physiology, clinical exercise physiology, and physiology of athletes. His primary research focus is on objective methods of measuring physical activity, including pedometers, accelerometers, and heart rate monitors. He also studies the role of the built environment as a determinant of physical activity and health at the community level. In his spare time he enjoys hiking, bicycling, and swimming.

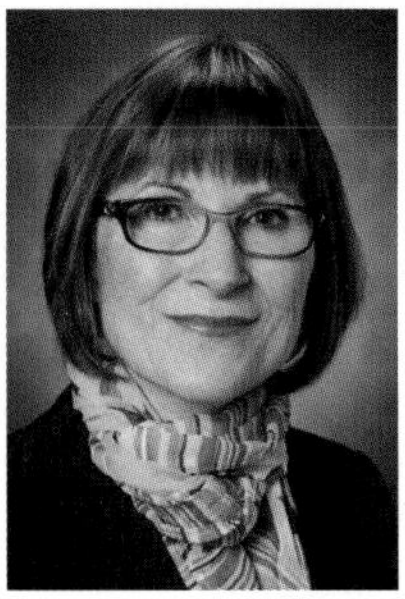

Photo courtesy of the College of Education, University of Georgia.

Janet Buckworth, PhD, FACSM, is a professor and head of the department of kinesiology at the University of Georgia. Her academic and professional background includes master's degrees in clinical social work and health education and a PhD in exercise psychology as well as work experiences in medical and college settings. Her research areas are exercise adherence and the psychobiology of exercise, mental health, and obesity. Dr. Buckworth teaches a graduate course on weight management coaching that is part of the graduate certificate in obesity and weight management. She also has expertise in theory-based interventions to increase exercise adoption and adherence with an emphasis on motivation and related psychosocial constructs. Dr. Buckworth has been invited as the keynote presenter for several conferences on exercise psychology and is the coauthor of *Exercise Psychology*, which is in its second edition. She is also a fellow of the American College of Sports Medicine and has served on the Behavioral Strategies Special Interest Group since 2002.

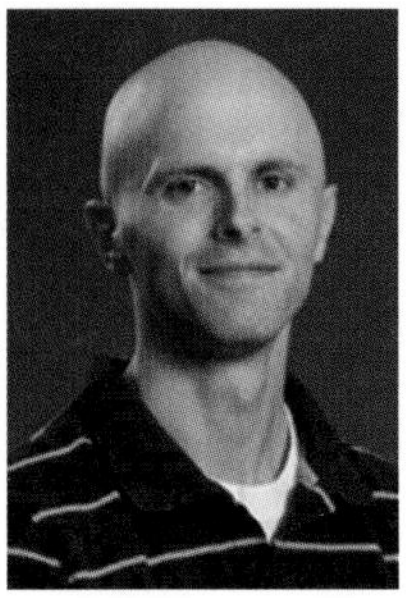

Photo courtesy of Boise State University.

Scott A. Conger, PhD, is an assistant professor in the department of kinesiology at Boise State University. Prior to his current position, he held research appointments at the University of Pittsburgh, University of Arkansas, and University of Michigan medical schools. He is a certified clinical exercise physiologist and a certified exercise physiologist through the American College of Sports Medicine. Dr. Conger teaches undergraduate and graduate courses in exercise physiology, sport nutrition, and exercise testing and prescription.

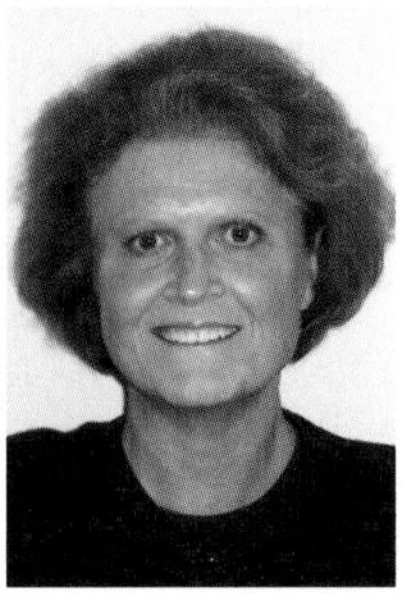

© JoAnn Eickhoff-Shemek

JoAnn M. Eickhoff-Shemek, PhD, FACSM, is a professor in the exercise science program at the University of South Florida (USF) in Tampa. Her teaching and research focus on legal liability and risk management issues in the health and fitness field. She is the lead author of a comprehensive textbook titled *Risk Management for Health/Fitness Professionals: Legal Issues and Strategies* and a coauthor of *The Australian Fitness Industry Risk Management Manual*. Dr. Eickhoff-Shemek also is the president of the Fitness Law Academy, a company devoted to advancing the fitness profession by providing educational programs to enhance fitness safety and minimize legal liability. Dr. Eickhoff-Shemek was an associate editor and the legal columnist for *ACSM's Health & Fitness Journal* from 2001 to 2010. She has been a fellow of the ACSM since 1997 and received her PhD from the University of Nebraska at Lincoln in 1995.

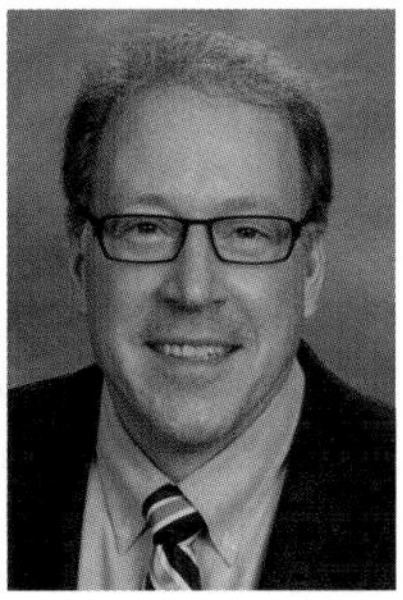

© Avery Faigenbaum

Avery Faigenbaum, EdD, FACSM, FNSCA, is a full professor in the department of health and exercise science at the College of New Jersey. His research interests focus on pediatric exercise science, resistance exercise, and preventive medicine. As an active researcher and practitioner, he has coauthored more than 200 peer-reviewed publications, 40 book chapters, and 9 books, including *Youth Strength Training* and the *ACE Youth Fitness Manual*. He has been an invited speaker at more than 300 regional, national, and international conferences. Dr. Faigenbaum is a fellow of the American College of Sports Medicine and the National Strength and Conditioning Association.

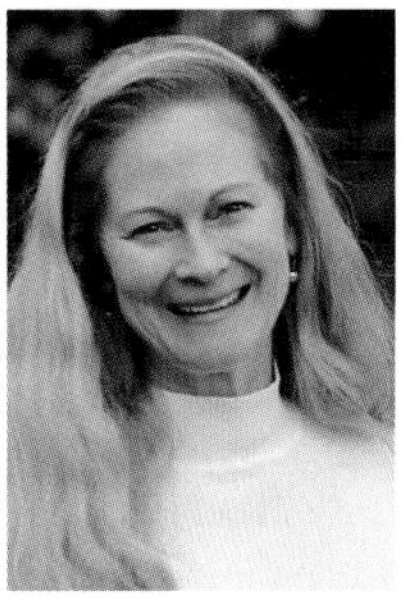

Photo courtesy of Chelsey Williams.

Laura Horvath Gagnon, PT, DPT, PhD, OCS, IMT, received her BFA in dance from Florida State University. She danced professionally with the Martha Graham Dance Company and was a member of the faculty at the Martha Graham School before pursuing a career in physical therapy. She received her MS in physical therapy from Columbia

University College of Physicians and Surgeons, her PhD in biomechanics and sports medicine from the University of Tennessee at Knoxville, and her doctorate in physical therapy from the University of Tennessee at Chattanooga. Dr. Gagnon is a board-certified orthopedic specialist and is certified in integrative manual therapy. She has served as adjunct faculty at the University of Tennessee in both the dance and exercise science programs. Dr. Gagnon's research has included pelvic girdle alignment, core stability, and Pilates. She is currently researching the application of integrative manual therapy and its influence on the central and autonomic nervous systems at the University of Tennessee Hospital. She was a contributing author to the book *Exercise Prescription and the Back* (McGraw-Hill Medical, 2000). Dr. Gagnon currently operates her own physical therapy practice, A Moving Experience. She and her husband live in Maryville, Tennessee, with her twins. In her spare time she enjoys choreographing and dancing in church and competing in triathlons.

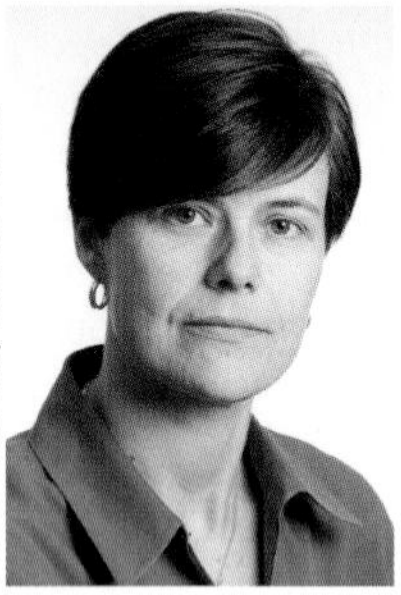

Photo courtesy of Jeff Fusco.

Clare E. Milner, PhD, FACSM, is an associate professor in the department of physical therapy and rehabilitation sciences at Drexel University in Philadelphia. Her research interests are in the biomechanics of lower-extremity injury, injury prevention, and rehabilitation. She focuses on overuse injuries in runners, knee injuries in recreationally active women, and activities of daily living in older adults and people with obesity. Dr. Milner teaches graduate classes in biomechanics and research methods. She is a fellow of the American College of Sports Medicine.

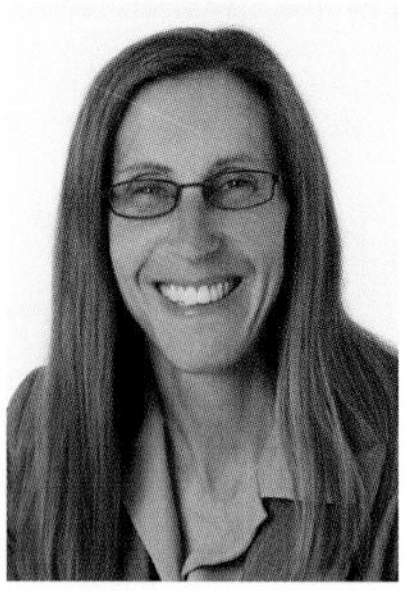

Jenny Moshak, MS, ATC, CSCS, is currently providing rehabilitation and strength and conditioning services to the UMMC Basketball Club, a women's professional team in Yekaterinburg, Russia. She retired from the University of Tennessee in August 2013 after a 24-year career heading up the sports medicine department for women's athletics, primarily working with Lady Volunteers basketball. Her vision led to the creation of Team ENHANCE, a unique program that creates a healthy culture for the Lady Vol student-athletes so they can achieve personal bests in their sports and in their lives. Under her leadership, the program was established to assist student-athletes in the nutritional, mental, and emotional aspects of performance with the guidance of UT professional staff and a comprehensive group of medical experts from the private sector. Ms. Moshak's book, *Ice 'n' Go: Score in Sports and Life,* was released in May 2013. The book presents a model for healthy living that focuses on physical, mental, and emotional development, which tells her story of achieving her "national championship" as she discovered the thrills of the journey. She is an avid cyclist

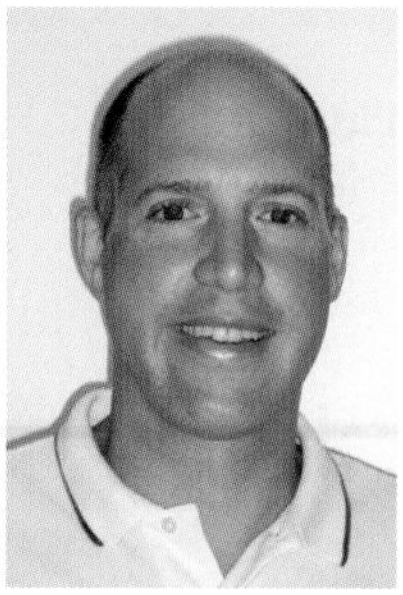

Photo courtesy of Stephanie M. Shipe.

Michael Shipe, PhD, RCEP, is an associate professor and the chair of the department of kinesiology at Charleston Southern University in South Carolina. He teaches courses in exercise physiology, clinical exercise physiology, physical activity epidemiology, and movement analysis. He attained his registered clinical exercise physiologist certification in 1999. Dr. Shipe was the fitness director for the Blount Memorial Wellness Center from 1997 to 2001. He was director of the medical fitness and cardiac rehabilitation programs at Blount Memorial Hospital from 2002 to 2004 and the chair of the department of exercise science at Carson Newman University from 2005 to 2012.